Handbuch
der allgemeinen Pathologie

Herausgegeben von

H.-W. Altmann · F. Büchner · H. Cottier · E. Grundmann

G. Holle · E. Letterer · W. Masshoff · H. Meessen

F. Roulet · G. Seifert · G. Siebert

Sechster Band, Achter Teil

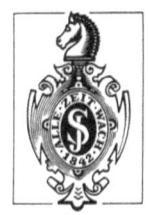

Springer-Verlag Berlin Heidelberg New York 1977

Transplantation

By

K.T. Brunner · C.E. Calkins · J.-C. Cerottini · C.C. Congdon · E.L. Cooper
H. Cottier · D.A.L. Davies · F. Eitel · J. Hagmann · E.S. Henderson
M. Hess · M.W. Hess · E.N. Hinzpeter · H.P. Hobik · T. Hraba · M. Jäger
P.H.K. Jap · M. Jeannet · C.R. Jerusalem · G.R.F. Krueger · H.U. Keller
Z.J. Lucas · G.O.H. Naumann · R. Pichlmayr · L. Schweiberer
M. Segall · R. Storb · O. Stutman · C.J. Wirth · K. Wonigeit

Edited by

Johann Wilhelm Masshoff

With 233 Figures

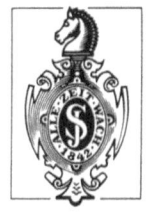

Springer-Verlag Berlin Heidelberg New York 1977

ISBN-13: 978-3-642-66394-9   e-ISBN-13: 978-3-642-66392-5

DOI: 10.1007/978-3-642-66392-5

Library of Congress Catalog Card Number 56-2297

Preface

Organ transplantation has almost disappeared from headlines in the daily press, possibly because it failed to fulfill exaggerated expectations. Transplantation pathology has become more and more important, not only with relation to therapeutic transplantations but even more in its fundamental theories. There is some analogy here to the development in space science where spectacular achievements were followed by sobering frustrations and where, for the time being, the effect on technology is more fruitful than the outcome of the original far-reaching projects. That transplant rejection was defined, in most of its stages, as an immunologic process, has given many new impulses to immunology in general. Transplantation assays have become a pet experiment in immunobiology and an abundant source of general information and knowledge.

The implications of such a development could not be predicted when the present volume was outlined and planned. In accordance with the concept of WILLI MASSHOFF, general transplantion pathology was given a central position as a fundamental science, while the chapters on the transplantation of various tissues are of a more paradigmatic character. It was MASSHOFF who invited competent authors and who managed to balance their articles, despite some overlapping, so as to draw a comprehensive picture of contemporary transplantation pathology. WILLI MASSHOFF died while he was editing the first manuscripts. As co-editors we have undertaken to complete the publication that we began together.

Some delays were unavoidable. The progress of evolution, especially in immunology, is so rapid that some of the articles written nearly 2 years ago no longer correspond to the present status of knowledge. Our readers will notice this by comparing the dates of bibliographic references. The decision of the authors who approved of publication in spite of the delay is very much appreciated because a new editing and updating of these chapters would in turn have outdated the more recent ones. The chapter on "Cell Systems Participating in Graft Rejections" by HAGMANN was added to update the volume in this important aspect of cellular immunology.

The first chapters deal with the genetic background of transplant reactions, their clinical significance, and the mixed leucocyte culture test (MLC). In its phylogenetic and ontogenetic aspects, transplant theory adheres to the field of general biology; the discussion of humoral and cell-mediated mechanisms and of tolerance phenomena relates it to general immunology. Subsequent chapters report on the transplantation of cells—mostly from bone marrow—and of skin, connective tissue, cornea and bone. An overview is given in the central comprehensive chapter by CH.R. JERUSALEM and P.H.K. JAP. Therapeutic possibilities and their implications for general pathology are discussed in chapters on radiation-induced tolerance, and the application of antisera and various medications. The volume ends with a presentation of the graft-versus-host reaction as an inverted transplant rejection.

The editors have often questioned the utility of this kind of review volume in a large handbook. The rapid progress of science will outstrip, as a rule, their work in editing and preparing contributions. Whoever wants to keep abreast of recent developments will find the latest publications in scientific periodicals. The fundamental facts of contemporary knowledge, however, can only be gathered from comprehensive presentations where the widespread results are collected, compared and evaluated. Here we see the role of our volume and the reason for its publication.

WILLI MASSHOFF began his editing under these aspects, and we have endeavoured to complete his work. Having been in close contact with him over many years we felt sufficiently informed about his plans, and we hoped to fulfill them to the best of our ability. WILLI MASSHOFF had to die without having seen the final shape of this volume which we dedicate to his memory as a token of friendship and reverence.

HANS COTTIER
EKKEHARD GRUNDMANN

Vorwort

Die Organtransplantation ist aus den Überschriften der Tagespresse verschwunden. Mag sein, daß sie manche übersteigerte Erwartung nicht erfüllt hat. Die Transplantations-Pathologie ist um so wichtiger geworden. Das gilt sowohl für die Transplantation als klinische Therapie als auch in noch stärkerem Maße für ihre theoretischen Grundlagen. Eine gängige Parallele bietet sich an: Die Weltraumforschung brachte neben spektakulären Höhepunkten auch Ernüchterung; der Gewinn an Technologie ist vorerst größer als der der primär projektierten Ziele. Die Erkenntnis, daß die Abstoßung eines Transplantates in nahezu allen Phasen ein immunologischer Vorgang ist, brachte der Immunologie eine Fülle von Impulsen. Die Transplantation wurde ein bevorzugtes Experiment der Immunbiologie, und viel allgemeingültiges Wissen wurde so gewonnen.

Als der jetzt vorliegende Band geplant wurde, war diese Entwicklung noch nicht in dieser Konsequenz vorauszusehen. Es ist das Verdienst von WILLI MASSHOFF, den Band schließlich so gegliedert zu haben, daß die allgemeine Transplantations-Pathologie als Grundlagenwissenschaft in den Mittelpunkt kam, während die speziellen Gewebskapitel mehr paradigmatische Stellung erhielten. MASSHOFF gelang es, kompetente Autoren zu gewinnen und die Beiträge im Ansatz so aufeinander abzustimmen, daß sie trotz mancher Überschneidungen ein geschlossenes Bild der Transplantations-Pathologie liefern. Während der Bearbeitung der eingehenden Manuskripte verstarb WILLI MASSHOFF. Die unterzeichnenden Mitherausgeber haben es übernommen, gemeinsam das begonnene Werk zu Ende zu führen.

Dabei waren Verzögerungen nicht zu vermeiden. Die Erkenntnisse gerade in der Immunologie schritten in raschem Tempo weiter, und es ist mancher Beitrag — vor fast zwei Jahren abgeschlossen — schon nicht mehr auf dem aktuellen Stand. Der Leser kann das leicht an den Jahreszahlen der Literaturzitate erkennen. Wir sind den Autoren dieser Beiträge besonders dankbar, daß sie trotzdem ihre Zustimmung zur Veröffentlichung gegeben haben: eine nochmalige Überarbeitung dieser Artikel hätte wiederum die anderen veralten lassen. Durch Einfügung des Beitrages von HAGMANN et al. über „Cell Systems Participating in Graft Rejection" wurde wenigstens dieser für die zelluläre Immunologie wichtige Aspekt aktualisiert.

Der Band beginnt mit Artikeln über die genetischen Grundlagen der Trans-

plantatreaktion, deren klinische Bedeutung und die Testmöglichkeiten mit der
mixed leukocyte culture (MLC). Die phylogenetischen und ontogenetischen
Aspekte stellen die Transplantatlehre in den Bereich der Allgemeinen Biologie;
die Erörterungen der humoralen und zellvermittelten Mechanismen sowie der
Toleranzphänomene geben allgemein-immunologische Beziehungen. Es folgen
Abhandlungen über die Transplantation von Zellen — im wesentlichen des
Knochenmarkes, der Haut, des Bindegewebes, der Cornea, des Knochens; als
zentraler Beitrag bringt der Artikel von Ch.R. Jerusalem und P.H.K. Jap das
Résumé der vorangegangenen Beispiele. Den therapeutischen Möglichkeiten und
ihren Folgen für die Allgemeine Pathologie widmen sich die Artikel über die
strahlen-induzierte Toleranz, die Anwendung von Antiseren und von verschiedenen Medikationen. Eine Darstellung der Graft-versus-Host-Reaktion als einer
umgekehrten Transplantat-Abstoßung schließt diesen Band.

Die Herausgeber haben oft über den Sinn solcher zusammenfassenden Hand-
buchbände diskutiert. Das wissenschaftliche Erkenntnistempo überholt in der
Regel die redaktionelle Bearbeitung. Wer das Allerneueste wissen will, findet
es in den wissenschaftlichen Zeitschriften. Die Grundlage des heutigen Wissens-
standes kann er aber nur aus zusammenfassenden Darstellungen erfahren, die
das weit verbreitete Wissensgut sammeln, ordnen und werten. Hier liegt nach
unserer Ansicht die Daseinsberechtigung auch dieses Bandes.

Unter dieser Vorstellung hatte Willi Masshoff die Redaktion übernommen.
Wir, die Unterzeichnenden, haben versucht, seine Arbeit abzuschließen. Wir
standen über viele Jahre in engem Kontakt mit ihm, glauben, seine Pläne zu
kennen, und hoffen, sie wenigstens nach unserem Vermögen verwirklicht zu
haben. Es ist Willi Masshoff nicht vergönnt gewesen, den fertigen Band vor
sich zu haben. Wir widmen ihn in Freundschaft und Verehrung seinem Gedächt-
nis.

Hans Cottier
Ekkehard Grundmann

List of Contributors

BRUNNER, K.T., Dr., Schweizerisches Institut für Experimentelle Krebsforschung, Ch. des Boveresses, CH-1066 Épalinges s/Lausanne (Switzerland)

CALKINS, C.E., Dr., Memorial Sloan-Kettering Cancer Center, Cellular Immunbiology Section, 1275 York Avenue, New York, N.Y. 10021 (USA)

CEROTTINI, J.-C., Dr., Ludwig Institute for Cancer Research, Ch. des Boveresses, CH-1066 Épalinges s/Lausanne (Switzerland)

CONGDON, C.C., Dr., The University of Tennessee, Memorial Research Center, 1924 Alcoa Highway, Knoxville, Tenn. 37920 (USA)

COOPER, E.L., Prof. Dr., University of California, Department of Anatomy, School of Medicine, The Center for the Health Sciences, Los Angeles, Calif. 90024 (USA)

COTTIER, H., Prof. Dr., Pathologisches Institut der Universität, Freiburgstraße 30, CH-3010 Bern (Switzerland)

DAVIES, D.A.L., Prof. Dr., G.D. Searle & Co. Ltd., Research Division, P.O. Box 53, Lane End Road, High Wycombe, Bucks. HP12 4HL (England)

EITEL, F., Dr., Chirurgische Universitätsklinik, Abt. Unfallchirurgie, 6650 Homburg/Saar (Fed. Rep. of Germany)

HAGMANN, J., Dr., Pathologisches Institut der Universität, Freiburgstraße 30, CH-3010 Bern (Switzerland)

HENDERSON, E.S., Dr., Chief of Medicine A, Roswell Park Memorial Institute, Department of Health, State of New York, 666 Elm Street, Buffalo, N.Y. 14263 (USA)

HESS, M., Dr., G.D. Searle & Co. Ltd., Research Division, P.O. Box 53, Lane End Road, High Wycombe, Bucks. HP12 4HL (England)

HESS, M.W., Prof. Dr., Pathologisches Institut der Universität, Freiburgstraße 30, CH-3010 Bern (Switzerland)

HINZPETER, E.N., Dr., Allgemeines Krankenhaus Heidelberg, Augen-Abteilung, Tangstedter Landstr. 400, 2000 Hamburg 62 (Fed. Rep. of Germany)

HOBIK, H.P., PD Dr., Pathologisches Institut der Universität, Westring 17, 4400 Münster/Westf. (Fed. Rep. of Germany)

HRABA, T., Dr., Institute of Experimental Biology and Genetics, Czechoslovak Academy of Sciences, Budějovická 1083, 142 20 Prague 4 (ČSSR)

JÄGER, M., Prof. Dr., Orthopädische Klinik, Harlachinger Straße 51, 8000 München 90 (Fed. Rep. of Germany)

JAP, P.H.K., Dr., Katholieke Universiteit, Faculteit der Geneeskunde, Laboratorium voor Cytologie en Histologie, Geert Grooteplein Noord 21, Nijmegen (Holland)

JEANNET, M., Dr., Hôpital Cantonal, Unité d'Immunologie de Transplantation, 64, av. de la Roseraie, CH-1211 Genève 4 (Switzerland)

JERUSALEM, C.R., Prof. Dr., Katholieke Universiteit, Faculteit der Geneeskunde, Laboratorium voor Cytologie en Histologie, Geert Grooteplein Noord 21, Nijmegen (Holland)

KRUEGER, G.R.F., Prof. Dr., Pathologisches Institut der Universität, Immunpathologische Laboratorien, Joseph-Stelzmann-Str. 9, 5000 Köln 41 (Fed. Rep. of Germany)

Keller, H.U., PD Dr., Pathologisches Institut der Universität, Freiburgstraße 30, CH-3010 Bern (Switzerland)

Lucas, Z.J., Prof. Dr., Stanford University Medical Center, Department of Surgery, Stanford, Calif. 94305 (USA)

Naumann, G.O.H., Prof. Dr., Universitäts-Augenklinik, Abteilung und Lehrstuhl II, Schleichstraße 12, 7400 Tübingen (Fed. Rep. of Germany)

Pichlmayr, R., Prof. Dr., Medizinische Hochschule, Klinik für Abdominal- und Transplantationschirurgie, Department Chirurgie, Karl-Wiechert-Allee 9, 3000 Hannover-Kleefeld (Fed. Rep. of Germany)

Schweiberer, L., Prof. Dr., Chirurgische Universitätsklinik, Abteilung für Unfallchirurgie, 6650 Homburg/Saar (Fed. Rep. of Germany)

Segall, M., Dr., Institut für Genetik der Universität, Weyertal 121, 5000 Köln 41 (West-Germany)

Storb, R., Prof. Dr., University of Washington, Department of Medicine, Division of Oncology, Seattle, Washington 98122 (USA)

Stutman, O., Dr., Memorial Sloan-Kettering Cancer Center, Cellular Immunbiology Section, 1275 York Avenue, New York, N.Y. 10021 (USA)

Wirth, C.J., Dr., Orthopädische Klinik, Harlachinger Straße 51, 8000 München 90 (Fed. Rep. of Germany)

Wonigeit, K., Dr., Medizinische Hochschule, Klinik für Abdominal- und Transplantationschirurgie, Department Chirurgie, Karl-Wiechert-Allee 9, 3000 Hannover-Kleefeld (Fed. Rep. of Germany)

Contents

General Pathology of the Transplantation Reaction in Experimental and Clinical Organ Grafts. CHRISTOPH R. JERUSALEM and PAUL H.K. JAP. With 61 Figures

Medications and Their Toxicity. EDWARD S. HENDERSON and GERHARD R.F. KRUEGER.
With 23 Figures and 2 Tables 745

Graft-Versus-Host-Reactions. H.P. HOBIK. With 26 Figures 793

The Main Histocompatibility System in Man

M. Jeannet

With 2 Tables

A. Introduction

It is now well established that the intensity of graft rejection is conditioned by the degree of antigenic difference between the donor and the recipient. The phenomenon of rejection is the result of an immune response of the host, directed against transplantation or histocompatibility antigens present on the donor cells. Histocompatibility testing represents the identification by serological techniques or other methods of the transplantation antigens. Many studies conducted in inbred mice have led to the recognition of at least 30 histocompatibility systems. One of them, the H-2 system, is considered to be the major histocompatibility system, because incompatibility with respect to H-2 antigens will result in rapid rejection of grafts. Transplants performed between strains of mice differing only in antigens belonging to the minor system will survive for a longer time. Now similar major systems have been identified in other animals: the AgB system in the rat, the B system in the chicken, the DL-A system in the dog, the H-I system in the rabbit, the ChL-A system in the chimpanzee. So far, two major antigenic systems have been observed to be histocompatibility barriers in man: the ABO system and the HL-A system. In this review, we will discuss the HL-A system only and concentrate on the serology, the genetics, and the clinical applications, especially for transplantation, of this recently discovered immunogenetic system.

B. Historical Background

In the early days of leukocyte immunology, before the discovery of human leukocyte groups in 1954, the main stream of research in this field dealt with the possible role of leukocyte antibodies in cases of neutropenia (DAUSSET, 1953; MIESCHER, 1953). But despite intensive research, no important progress has been made in the understanding of the mechanisms of leukocyte autoimmune disorders. However, the detection of leukocyte agglutinins in the serum of poly-transfused patients (DAUSSET and NENNA, 1952) led to the discovery of the

existence of leukocyte groups in man (DAUSSET, 1954; MIESCHER and FAUCON-
NET, 1954). The first leukocyte antigen (Mac) was described by DAUSSET (1958)
and, in the same period, the presence of leukocyte antibodies in the serum
of multiparous women was recognized for the first time (PAYNE and ROLFS,
1958; VAN ROOD et al., 1958). With the help of ingenious computer techniques,
VAN ROOD and VAN LEEUWEN (1963) used antibodies from this source to define
the first diallelic system with antigens 4a and 4b and, later, an other system
with the antigens 6a, 6b, and 6c (VAN ROOD and VAN LEEUWEN, 1965). The
same statistical approach, which was made necessary by the multispecific nature
of the antisera available at the time, was used by PAYNE et al. (1964) to define
the HL-A system, including the antigens now called HL-A 1, HL-A 2, and
HL-A 3 (BODMER et al., 1966). At the 1st Histocompatibility Workshop, which
was organized in 1964 at Duke University, new techniques, specifically complement fixation (SHULMAN et al., 1962; SHULMAN et al., 1964) and cytotoxicity
(WALFORD et al., 1964; TERASAKI and McCLELLAND, 1964) were compared with
leukoagglutination, which had been widely used up to that time. The first
attempts to correlate leukocyte antigen compatibility and skin graft (VAN ROOD
et al., 1962; COLOMBANI et al., 1963) or kidney graft (TERASAKI et al., 1965)
also date from this time. Soon thereafter, at the 2nd Histocompatibility Workshop, organized in Leiden in 1965, it became clear that many of the antigens
described independently by different investigators using different techniques
were, in fact, closely related. DAUSSET et al. (1965) suggested that all these
antigens were components of a single complex immunogenetic system. The
view was confirmed in 1967 at the 3rd workshop organized in Torino, when
the segregation of these antigens was analyzed in a number of families (CEPPELLI-
NI et al., 1967). The single system hypothesis was further confirmed by BACH
and AMOS (1967) based on evidence from the mixed lymphocyte culture technique. Shortly thereafter, by common agreement, this system was named the
human leukocyte locus A, or HL-A system (WHO, 1968).

Following the conference, a number of new antigens were described, and
the notion that they were governed by two separate but closely linked subloci
began to emerge (KISSMEYER-NIELSEN et al., 1968; SINGAL et al., 1968). However,
the fact that all the workers in the field used different nomenclatures led to
great confusion. This problem was solved by a WHO committee and the first
seven HL-A antigens were defined (WHO, 1968). After the 4th workshop organized in Los Angeles in 1970, four additional HL-A specificities received official
recognition, and a dozen others have been identified by more than one group
of investigators (TERASAKI, 1970). During the 5th workshop, organized in Evian,
more than 50 different populations were studied, and significant differences
in distribution of HL-A antigens between the various populations were found
(DAUSSET and COLOMBANI, 1973). Moreover, it appeared that some antigens
previously thought to be homogeneous could be subdivided into two or more
specificities and that some recently identified antigens did not belong to the
two known series, but to a third segregant series, also called AJ. The complexity
of the HL-A chromosomal region now often called the MHC (major histocompatibility complex) has been further increased by the recognition of an additional
closely linked locus on the HL-A chromosome. The corresponding genes cannot

be serologically defined (SD) and have been named LD (lymphocyte defined) (BACH, 1973), because they are defined by the outcome of the mixed leukocyte culture test (see chapter on Testing Methods). In the following sections an attempt will be made to summarize the present knowledge of the HL-A system and its medical and biological relevance.

C. Methodology and Serological Considerations

Three different techniques have been widely used for the identification of leukocyte antigens: *leukoagglutination*, which has been almost completely abandoned now, *lymphocytoxicity*, which is used most commonly, and *platelet complement fixation*, which deserves to be more largely employed. Reproducibility has always been a problem and continues to be a major challenge of HL-A typing. Leukoagglutination seems to be the worst technique and platelet complement fixation the best in this regard. Many efforts have been made to standardize the methods, especially the lymphocyte cytotoxicity technique, which was chosen as the common technique for all laboratories participating at the 4th and 5th histocompatibility workshops. The results of these international cooperative studies have shown that, even in the hands of the most experienced investigators, the same technique used with the same antisera may yield divergent results from one laboratory to another.

I. Leukoagglutination

This is the oldest method used in the field of leukocyte immunology (DAUSSET and NENNA, 1952; MIESCHER, 1953; DAUSSET, 1954). The first leukocyte antigens described were all defined by leukoagglutinating sera (DAUSSET, 1958; VAN ROOD and VAN LEEUWEN, 1963; PAYNE et al., 1964). Three slightly different leukoagglutination techniques have been described: the *so-called defibrination* (DAUSSET and NENNA, 1952), *EDTA* (VAN ROOD and VAN LEEUWEN, 1965), and *polybrene* (LALEZARI, 1962) *methods*. A micromethod has also been more recently described (PAYNE et al., 1967). The defibrination technique is the most sensitive of all leukocyte typing techniques in current use and, therefore, may still be useful for the screening of antibodies, particularly in patients waiting for a kidney transplant. However, it is characterized by poor reproducibility and is not suitable for typing purposes. EDTA agglutination is less sensitive and somewhat more reproducible. Apparently, there are some antigens which are detected only by leukoagglutination, such as 5a and 5b (VAN ROOD and EERNISSE, 1969) and the granulocyte antigens. But since these antigens probably do not belong to the HL-A system, this does not justify the mandatory use of leukoagglutination for routine typing. An extensive discussion on the respective advantages and disadvantages of the different leukoagglutination techniques may be found in the excellent review by WALFORD (1969).

II. Lymphocyte Cytotoxicity

This reaction, first used in humans by WALFORD et al. (1964, 1965), TERASAKI and McCLELLAND (1964), ENGELFRIET and BRITTEN (1965), and AMOS (1965), is currently the most widely used technique for leukocyte typing. Micromethods, all derived from the ingenious technique of TERASAKI and McCLELLAND (1964), are now used exclusively because of the very short supply of valuable reagents. Reproducibility of the technique is generally in the 95% range or better, but sensitivity may vary considerably depending on whether a two-stage (MITTAL et al., 1968) or a one-stage (KISSMEYER-NIELSEN and KJERBYE, 1967) modification is used. The smaller amount of complement added and the shorter period of incubation account for the decreased sensitivity of the one-stage method (KISSMEYER-NIELSEN et al., 1970). This loss of sensitivity is not necessarily a disadvantage in typing leukocytes; as a result more sera may behave as monospecific, and weak contaminating antibodies will not be detected. The way the lymphocyte suspension is prepared does not seem to influence the sensitivity of the test (JEANNET et al., 1970a). The Ficoll-Isopaque method, devised by BOYUM (1968) and the most simple and reliable method proposed so far, is now in general use in all tissue typing laboratories. More elaborate cytotoxicity techniques such as fluorochromasia (BODMER et al., 1967), ^{51}Cr release (ROGENTINE, 1967), lymphocyte-dependent antibody assay (HERSEY et al., 1973), antiglobulin test (JOHNSON et al., 1972), and also immunofluorescent (BERNOCO et al., 1973; VAN LEEUWEN et al., 1973) techniques have been designed mostly for research purposes. These techniques are less suitable for routine typing, but some are very sensitive and they have obvious advantages for quantitative work.

III. Platelet Complement Fixation

This method, described by SCHULMAN et al. (1962) and modified later by VAN DER WEERDT (1965), COLOMBANI et al. (1967), and SVEJGAARD and KISSMEYER-NIELSEN (1968a), is now available as a micro-method (D'AMARO et al., 1970; GABB and BODMER, 1970; SMITH and WALFORD, 1970). This technique is the least sensitive, but probably the most quantitative and reproducible of all procedures used for HL-A typing. In addition, storage of antigen is possible for many months at 4° C. It seems that almost all the HL-A specificities presently defined can be detected by this method.

IV. Serum Sources

Antisera which react with human leukocyte antigens may be found in polytransfused patients, during or after pregnancy, after organ transplantation, or induced by immunization of human volunteers and animals. Lymphocytotoxins were also occasionally found in sera of males without transfusion or organ transplantation (PERKINS et al., 1974) and in patients with various diseases (WATERS et al., 1971a; COLLINS et al., 1973).

1. Polytransfused Patients

It is now well documented that leukocyte antibodies are very often formed after multiple transfusions (DAUSSET, 1954). The incidence of antibodies found ranges from 8–90% depending on the method of detection and the number of previous transfusion (DAUSSET, 1962; ENGELFRIET, 1966; PERKINS *et al.*, 1974). The sera obtained from polytransfused patients are usually multispecific, because the antibodies are induced by immunization with leukocytes from several individuals. However, these sera may provide very valuable monospecific reagents when they are used in the complement fixation technique with platelets.

2. Pregnancy

These antibodies are formed by fetomaternal immunization which occurs when leukocytes from the fetus cross the placental barrier (PAYNE and ROLFS, 1958; VAN ROOD *et al.* 1958). They tend to be less multispecific than the antibodies which are formed following transfusions, since they are induced by a restricted number of leukocyte antigens, specifically those the fetus inherits from the father. Their incidence is relative to the number of pregnancies and the technique used for detection. Usually the percentage of positive sera found in multiparous women varies between 15% and 25% (ENGELFRIET, 1966; GERT-JENSEN, 1966).

3. Immunization of Human Volunteers

This method is being used more and more for production of specific leukocyte antisera. Its main advantage is that donors and recipients can be screened by lymphocyte typing so that the pairs selected are incompatible for only one HL-A antigen (THORSBY and KISSMEYER-NIELSEN, 1969). Immunization experiments are also very valuable in producing sera directed against new antigens. Specific immunization can be done by transfusing normal blood (CEPPELLINI *et al.*, 1964), by skin grafting (WALFORD *et al.*, 1962), or by multiple intradermal injections of leukocytes (SHANBROM *et al.*, 1968). Seven or eight weekly intradermal injections of approximately 1.5×10^8 leukocytes each time (SHANBROM *et al.*, 1968) or three injections of $30–40 \times 10^6$ mononuclear cells at monthly intervals (THORSBY and KISSMEYER-NIELSEN, 1970) are usually sufficient to obtain excellent cytotoxic antibodies. It is important to stop immunization as soon as antibodies are detected in order to get monospecific sera. Prolonged immunization may induce cross-reacting antibodies and thus "broaden" the specificity. As shown by THORSBY and KISSMEYER-NIELSEN (1970), this may be avoided by immunization within donor-recipient pairs where the recipient possesses another antigen belonging to the same group of "cross-reacting antigens" as the incompatible antigen of the donor, although LEGRAND *et al.* (1973) showed that it is not always true.

4. After Organ Transplantation

The sera of patients who have rejected a renal allograft often contain leukocyte antibodies. These antibodies have been found in 90% of the patients whose transplanted kidney was removed due to rejection, whereas the incidence was much lower in the group of patients with functioning grafts (Morris *et al.*, 1968). In our own experience, too, humoral antibodies specific for histocompatibility antigens can be detected with very sensitive methods in the majority of renal allograft recipients with bad clinical courses (Jeannet *et al.*, 1970b). However, as almost all patients receive blood transfusions, the specificity of the antibodies does not always show a close correlation with the HL-A incompatibility between donor and recipient. Some sera from this source can be used effectively as leukocyte typing reagents. This problem will be discussed further in a later chapter.

5. "Natural" Lymphocytotoxins

Numerous studies have documented the occurrence of lymphocytotoxic antibodies in the sera of patients with various diseases such as autoimmune disorders, including systemic lupus erythematosus, scleroderma, and rheumatoid arthritis, in viral diseases including infectious mononucleosis, rubella, and measles (Terasaki *et al.*, 1970), and in various bacterial and parasitic infections (Williams *et al.*, 1971; Mayer *et al.*, 1973). These antibodies have been usually of low titer, more reactive at 15° C than at room temperature or 37° C, and have often shown no serologic correlation to the HL-A system. Using the patients' own cells, an autoimmune activity could often be demonstrated. It has been suggested that these cold lymphocytotoxins might be biologically active at body temperature and responsible for the acute lymphopenia associated with immune deficiency sometimes observed during various viral or mycoplasma infections (Huang *et al.*, 1973). Interestingly, specific anti-HL-A antibodies have been occasionally found in sera from patients with infections or multiple myeloma, without previous stimulation by pregnancy or transfusions (Waters *et al.*, 1971a; Collins *et al.*, 1973; Falk *et al.*, 1973).

6. Immunization of Animals

As heteroantisera can be used to demonstrate individual antigenic differences in human erythrocytes (e.g., antigens M, N, etc.) and serum proteins, likewise, antisera-detecting isoantigens on human leukocytes can be prepared by immunizing animals with human material. For instance, Balner *et al.* (1967) have produced good typing sera in the chimpanzee. Attempts by Albert *et al.* (1969) and Einstein *et al.* (1971) to produce anti-HL-A sera by immunizing rabbits have been successful only in certain instances; it seems that good reagents can be obtained only by the immunization of rabbits with purified human lymphoid membrane components bearing HL-A antigens (Einstein *et al.*, 1971) or with soluble HL-A antigens from human serum (Billing and Terasaki, 1974).

D. Genetics of the HL-A System

As mentioned before, the serologically detectable antigens of the HL-A system are now thought to be controlled by three adjacent series of genes, located on the autosomal chromosome C6 (CEPPELLINI and VAN ROOD, 1974; RYDER et al., 1974; THORSBY, 1974; LAMM et al., 1974) (Fig. 1). Other genes have been recently located on the same chromosome: blood groups P (HRONKOVA-ZOULKO-VA et al., 1968) and Chido (MIDDLETON et al., 1974), enzyme markers such as phosphoglucomutase 3 (PMG_3) (LAMM et al., 1971), cytoplasmic malic enzyme (ME_1) (VAN SOMEREN et al., 1974), tetrameric indophenol oxidase (IPO-B) (VAN SOMEREN et al., 1974), and proteins of the properdin system (glycin-rich B-glyco-protein, GBG) (ALLEN, 1974) and the complement system (C2) (FU et al., 1974).

Each of the three HL-A loci code for a number of mutually exclusive allelic antigens. Every individual will have only two alleles, one paternally and one maternally derived at each locus. The antigens belonging to the three segregant series are listed in Table 1 with their phenotypic frequencies in a Caucasian (Swiss) population. Now there are 11 antigens officially accepted by the WHO Nomenclature Committee: HL-A 1, 2, 3, 9, 10, and 11 of the first locus and HL-A 5, 7, 8, 12, and 13 of the second locus (WHO, 1972). The antigens mentioned by the letter W have been recognized by several investigators at the 4th and 5th histocompatibility workshops but have not yet received a WHO designation (WHO, 1972). In addition, several antigens can be recognized only in individual laboratories and are designated by a local terminology (e.g., Sabell, TY, etc.).

Table 1. HL-A antigens and their approximate phenotype frequencies in a caucasian (Swiss) population

1st (LA) locus	%	2nd (four) locus	%	3rd (AJ) locus[a]	%
HL-A 1	27.6	HL-A 5	16.6	T1 (W20, AJ)	9.4
HL-A 2	50.6	HL-A 7	21.6	T2 (170)	7.2
HL-A 3	25.0	HL-A 8	17.2	T3 (UPS)	21.6
HL-A 9	22.4	HL-A 12	25.6	T4 ("W5"!, 315)	20.1
– W23		HL-A 13	5.6	T5 (TW)	13.7
– W24					
		W 5	23.5		
HL-A 10	9.4	W10	8.2		
– W25		W14	7.6		
– W26					
HL-A 11	10.6	W15	11.8		
W28	9.6	W16	7.4		
W29	7.4	W17	8.0		
W30	5.8	W18	10.4		
W31	2.4	W21	4.2		
W32	8.2	W22	3.8		
W19.6	3.9	W27	7.2		
		SABELL	1.2		
		TY	2.4		

[a] According to CEPPELLINI and VAN ROOD (1974).

Family studies have shown that the genes coding for the HL-A antigens at each locus behave as mutually exclusive alleles. Each parent always transmits only one antigen from each series to any given child. Family studies have also shown that the three antigens governed by one parental chromosome (or haplotype) are almost always transmitted together (or "en bloc") to the children, indicating that the three loci are located very closely to each other or, in other words, they are closely linked. In fact, very few recombinations (crossing-over) between the first and the second loci have been described (BODMER et al., 1970), while separation of the second and third loci by crossing-over has not yet been observed. The individuality of these three HL-A loci has been recently confirmed by "capping" experiments demonstrating that the antigens belonging to different loci are carried at the cell surface by different polypeptides (BERNOCO et al.,1973; SOLLHEIM et al., 1973).

An example of the inheritance of the four parental haplotypes in five children is shown in Table 2. Since the father's and mother's haplotypes are all different, there will be four and only four possible combinations of antigens in the children. However, if one of the parents in a family possesses two identical haplotypes (homozygosity at the three loci), there will be only two phenotypes in the children. In both families, all the children will have only one HL-A haplotype in common with each parent. This fact is important when one considers a parent as a possible transplant donor for a child. In most families, parents and children will not be genotypically identical for HL-A antigens and the success of the graft may be compromised in this situation. On the other hand, two siblings have usually one chance out of four to be HL-A identical (one chance out of two in the rare case of a homozygote parent). HL-A identity is rarely encountered between parents and children; it occurs when the same haplotype is possessed by the father and the mother. In this situation, one child out of two will be identical with the father or the mother, and one out of four will inherit the same haplotype from both parents.

In many populations, it has been observed that certain combinations of antigens from different loci (for instance, HL-A 1, 8 or HL-A 2, 12 or W10, T3 or W5, T4, etc.) occur more frequently than expected by chance, on the

Table 2. Family P.U. illustrating the inheritance of HL-A Haplotypes

	First series			Second series				Third series			HL-A haplo-types	HL-A genotypes
	HL-A1	HL-A2	W32	HL-A12	W15	W17	W27	T1	T4	T5		
Father	+	−	+	−	+	−	+	+	+	−	a/b	1, W15,T4/W32, W27, T1
Mother	+	+	−	+	−	+	−	−	−	+	c/d	1, W17,−/2, 12, T5
Sib 1	+	−	+	−	−	+	+	+	−	−	b/c	W32, W27, T1/1, W17,−
Sib 2	+	−	−	−	+	+	−	−	+	−	a/c	1, W15, T4/1, W17,−
Sib 3	+	−	−	−	+	+	−	−	+	−	a/c	1, W15, T4/1, W17,−
Sib 4	+	−	+	−	−	+	+	+	−	−	b/c	W32, W27, T1/1, W17.−

basis of the frequencies of the individual genes. These associations reflect a linkage disequilibrium, an interesting characteristic of the HL-A system which is probably due to some selective pressure favoring certain associations (CEPPELLINI, 1971).

E. Heterogeneity and Cross-Reactivity of HL-A Antigens

Several previously defined antigens have subsequently been found to be heterogeneous and appear to include different antigenic determinants (JEANNET and VASSALLI, 1971). This apparent heterogeneity of some antigens is obvious when one uses a battery of sera supposedly directed against the same factor. Some sera appear "shorter" than others and seem to detect only a part of the corresponding antigen ("subtypic" or "private" antigen). Other sera are "broader" (although apparently monospecific as judged by absorption experiments) and are probably directed against a "supertypic" or "public" determinant shared by molecules carrying different private specificities. Recent studies (BERNOCO et al., 1973; SOLLHEIM et al., 1973; RICHIARDI et al., 1973) have confirmed that private and public HL-A specificities are determined by separate determinants on the cell membrane, but may represent different parts of the same molecule. The heterogeneity of HL-A antigens may also be explained by the presence of "cross-reacting" antigens. Some private antigens may be very similar, so that some antibodies formed against one of them also react with the others. Those cross-reacting antibodies will demonstrate a broader reactivity than antibodies formed against one private determinant; absorption of the cross-reacting antibody with cells possessing only one of the private determinants will remove all reactivity against cells carrying the other cross-reacting determinants. A number of cross-reacting groups of antigens have been described (SVEJGAARD and KISSMEYER-NIELSEN, 1968b; COLOMBANI et al., 1970): They include HL-A 2 and W28; HL-A 3 and HL-A 11; HL-A 1 and HL-A 3; HL-A 10 and W19; HL-A 5 and W5; HL-A 7 and W22, etc. Interestingly enough, cross-reactive antigens always belong either to the first or to the second segregant series, showing that there is probably a certain structural similarity between antigens of the same series. In fact, the majority of the antigens of the 2nd series can be grouped according to their reactivity with sera showing either 4a (W4) of 4b (W6) specificity (CEPPELLINI and VAN ROOD, 1974). The latter represent typical examples of supertypic or public specificities (CEPPELLINI and VAN ROOD, 1974).

The existence of cross-reacting antigens may imply that HL-A antigens show a decreased immunogenecity in certain cases: if, for instance, the donor and the recipient of a kidney graft differ only by two HL-A antigens belonging to the same group of cross-reactive antigens (i.e., HL-A 5 and W5), one might expect a weaker immunologic rejection than if they differed by two non-cross-reacting antigens (i.e., HL-A 5 and HL-A 8). This assumption still needs to be proved. The fact that pregnant women frequently produce HL-A antibodies against cross-reacting antigens of their husbands speaks against the existence of such a phenomenon. The heterogeneity and cross-reactivity of HL-A antigens greatly complicates their precise definition and an unknown number of HL-A alleles remains to be identified; thus, the already considerable polymorphism of this system is likely to increase even more in the future.

F. HL-A, Mixed Lymphocyte Culture (MLC) Cell-Mediated Lympholysis (CML) and Cellular Immunity

Among the different nonserologic tests used for assessment of histocompatibility in clinical transplantation, the mixed lymphocyte culture (MLC) test has been the best studied (BAIN and LOWENSTEIN, 1964; BACH and HIRSCHORN, 1964; BACH and AMOS, 1967; JEANNET et al., 1969; JEANNET, 1970; BACH et al., 1970; YUNIS and AMOS, 1971). In fact, it has been shown that the MLC test is a model of the recognition phase of the homograft reaction (BACH, 1973, EIJSVOO-GEL, 1974). As extensively discussed in another chapter of this book, this test measures the reciprocal stimulation of two populations of allogeneic lymphocytes differing at the major histocompatibility locus. In the great majority of cases, lymphocytes of siblings with the same HL-A genotype fail to stimulate each other. However, a few exceptions have been observed, leading to the assumption that the MLC activation is controlled by a genetic locus closely linked, but not identical, with the HL-A locus, the so-called MLC or LD locus (YUNIS and AMOS, 1971). This possibility is also supported by the observation that the majority of unrelated individuals who have identical phenotypes do stimulate each other, although the degree of stimulation seems lower than that elicited in mixture of cells from randomly selected, unrelated individuals (FREIESLEBEN-SØRENSEN and STAUB-NIELSEN, 1970). The MLC test is now extensively used to define the alleles of the MLC or LD locus (MLC typing), but it has recently been shown that a serologic definition of the LD antigens might become possible in the near future (VAN ROOD et al., 1975a).

Many observations indicate that the MLC test can also be used to demonstrate the existence in the plasma from uremic patients, polytransfused individuals, and also pregnant women, of a special class of IgG antibodies, the so-called blocking or enhancing antibodies (KASAKURA and LOWENSTEIN, 1967; LEVEN-THAL et al., 1970; CEPPELLINI, 1971; BUCKLEY et al., 1972; THORSBY, 1974). Similar "blocking" immunoglobulins have also been eluted from human placentas and are assumed to represent maternal blocking antibodies protecting the placenta from maternal cell-mediated immunity directed to fetal antigens (FAULK et al., 1974). "Blocking" or "enhancing" factors (thought to play a role in the acceptance of human kidney grafts) have also been found in the plasma of kidney transplant patients (HATTLER et al., 1971) and in eluates from grafted kidneys (JEANNET and LAMBERT, 1974). The exact specificity of the "blocking" factor activity has not been established yet, but it seems independent from HL-A specificity and may be directed against antigens of the MLC locus. In fact, MLC inhibition might be a very sensitive tool for detecting anti-LD antibodies either alone or complexed with antigen.

The great importance of the MLC reaction stems not only from its close correlation with the main transplantation antigens and its ability to measure the overall amount of tissue antigenic disparity between two individuals; the MLC test is also of fundamental interest in transplantation immunology because it probably represents an in vitro approximation of cell-mediated immunity. It has been shown in experiments using thymectomized animals that reactivity in the MLC may not be a property of all lymphocytes but a function of the thymus-derived cells only (WILSON et al., 1967; KISKEN and SWENSON, 1969). The MLC can also distinguish between immunologic tolerance, a central failure of immune reactivity, and enhancement, a peripheral inhibition. Cells from animals rendered tolerant by the injection of lymphoid cells neonatally are specifically unreactive against the donor-strain cells in the MLC (SCHWARZ, 1968). In contrast, cells from animals which have accepted kidney transplant following the administration of donor bone-marrow cells or isoantisera directed against the graft or both, do react fully in the MLC against lymphoid cells derived from the kidney donors (GORDON, 1972). In the course of a study of the MLC test in kidney transplant patients, we observed in three patients who were HL-A incompatible with their donors a specific inhibition of the reactivity of their lymphocytes versus donor lymphocytes treated with mitomycin. In contrast, the patients' lymphocytes were quite normally stimulated by phytohemagglutinin and by unrelated lymphocytes (JEANNET, 1970). These findings have been confirmed by BACH et al. (1972). Whether the low level of stimulation by the donor cells observed in these subjects after transplantation represents a state of specific tolerance toward the donor or an example of the production of blocking antibodies cannot be decided, because further investigation of the recipients' sera was not performed at the time.

As also discussed in detail elsewhere in this volume, it is now known that human lymphocytes stimulated in MLC display cytotoxicity toward target lymphocytes carrying the same histocompatibility antigens as the stimulating cells in the MLC. This model of the "effector phase" of the homograft reaction is called cell-mediated lympholysis (CML). It appears, from experiments in families with crossing-over within the HL-A region conducted by EIJSVOOGEL (1974), that MLC incompatibility between the stimulator and responder cell is a prerequisite for subsequent cytotoxicity by the responder cell. But the specificity of the cytotoxic or "effector" phase seemed to be directed towards the HL-A antigens (or antigens determined by very closely linked loci) of the target cells. However, SCHAPIRA and JEANNET (1974) found a significant proportion of positive CML between HL-A identical unrelated individuals, and there is also evidence from recent experiments by MAWAS et al. (1974) that the CML specificity might be different from the HL-A antigens. Although more studies are necessary to elucidate completely its genetic aspects, the MLC-CML system appears promising for a better in vitro evaluation of human histocompatibility in vivo.

G. HL-A System and Clinical Transplantation

I. Skin Graft Survival

The influence of the HL-A system on the results of clinical transplantation is currently a subject of much debate and controversy. The relevance of HL-A antigens in transplantation was first established by experimental skin transplants between ABO-matched individuals. Exchange of first-set skin grafts between related individuals showed a mean survival time of about 20–30 days among HL-A identical siblings as compared to about 11–15 days for siblings differing by one or two haplotypes (CEPPELLINI et al., 1969; AMOS et al., 1969; DAUSSET et al., 1970). These results clearly demonstrate the influence of the chromosomal region which codes for the HL-A antigens in graft survival. However, these findings do not tell which locus of the HL-A chromosome is really important for human histocompatibility, since these siblings are identical for the three series of HL-A (SD) antigens, the MLC (LD) antigens, and also for the products of the Ir locus. In unrelated, nonimmunized donor-recipient combinations, skin grafts are rejected rapidly (9–13 days), and in early studies no significant correlation between number of HL-A antigenic differences and survival time has been found (CEPPELLINI et al., 1969; WALFORD et al., 1969). However, preimmunization against a specific transplantation antigen was shown to shorten the survival of subsequent skin grafts carrying that antigen (VAN ROOD et al., 1965). More recently, KOCH et al. (1973) compared skin graft rejection times between HL-A identical unrelated subjects known to be stimulatory or nonstimulatory in mixed lymphocyte culture with rejection of skin from stimulatory HL-A nonidentical unrelated individuals. The grafts from HL-A and MLC nonidentical donors were rejected in 10 days, those from the HL-A identical and MLC stimulating in 12 days, and those from HL-A and MLC identical donors in 15 days. SASPORTES et al. (1973) and WARD et al. (1973), in experiments conducted in HL-A different, but MLC nonstimulating, parent-child and sib-sib combinations, observed a prolongation of skin graft survival to 17 days. This critical experiment has however not been performed yet in unrelated individuals. Thus, MLC nonresponsiveness appears to correlate better with first-set rejection than HL-A identity; but there is a clear difference between HL-A/MLC identical related and unrelated combinations which remains to be explained.

II. Kidney Transplantation

A correlation between the compatibility of the HL-A antigens of donor and recipient and the clinical results of human kidney transplantation had been found by several investigators, even before adequate knowledge of the HL-A antigens was available (TERASAKI et al.,1965; VREDEVOE et al., 1965; PATEL et al., 1968; BATCHELOR and JOYSEY, 1969; MORRIS and TING, 1970). In all studies, a better correlation has been found with related than with unrelated (cadaveric) donors. Results from the 11th report of the human renal transplant registry

(1973) show a 1-year kidney survival in 1972 of 74% of first grafts from sibling donors, 76% when the donor is a parent, and 45% in cadaver transplantation. These differences in graft survival between related and unrelated donors can at least partially be explained by the influence of the HL-A system. A statistically significant correlation between HL-A typing and the clinical outcome of kidney transplantation in related donors has been documented in practically all studies published so far. The influence of the HL-A system is especially evident when the graft donor is an HL-A identical sibling. Hors *et al.* (1971), among others, have shown that in such a group the graft survival is close to 100% after 1 or 2 years. According to the same authors, when the donor is an HL-A haplo-identical sibling of a parent, the probability of 2 years' survival is 84% for the more compatible as compared to 64% for the more incompatible transplants; this difference was, however, not statistically significant. In another report, Opelz *et al.* (1974) have also found that 215 transplants from HL-A identical siblings had an excellent 1-year survival (90%), compared to 343 transplants from HL-A nonidentical sibling donors (70%). Of 126 sibling transplants which were clearly one-haplotype different 67% had a 1-year graft survival compared to 59% in 30 HL-A two-haplotype different sibling transplants. HL-A matching also seemed to influence survival rates in parent-to-child transplants: small differences could be shown between grafts in pairs with no, one, or two incompatible HL-A antigens detected (81%, 72%, and 69%, respectively). These differences, however, were again statistically not significant. Kissmeyer-Nielsen *et al.* (1971a), on the other hand, found a very convincing correlation between HL-A matching and graft survival even in the parental group, using only the cases where it was possible to account for all four HL-A antigens in the donor. Interestingly, it was found repeatedly in all series that an unusually high percentage of mismatched parent-child transplants have good clinical courses.

A major controversy surrounds recipients of unrelated (cadaver) allografts. In early studies, many investigators found a significant correlation between HL-A typing and graft survival or function, despite the fact that at the time, the number of HL-A antigens determined was low (Patel *et al.*, 1968; Batchelor and Joysey, 1969; Morris and Ting, 1970). However, in a study including more than 600 cases, Terasaki *et al.* (1971) found no significant correlation between clinical rank and matching. This study, which led to considerable confusion, has been subsequently criticized, mainly because the important material analyzed was very heterogeneous and included many cases tested several years before, at a time when HL-A typing was still rather inaccurate. In a recent study including more than 2,000 cadaver kidneys transplanted since 1969 in the USA, Opelz *et al.* (1974) mention that HL-A matching seemed of some influence, although not statistically significant. In patients who had no preformed anti-HL-A antibodies, grafts with identical HL-A antigens had the highest survival at one year (68%), while 156 grafts with three or four incompatible antigens had a survival of 51%. Transplants in patients with preformed antibodies had a significantly lower mean 1-year (41%) survival than those in recipients without lymphocytotoxins (56%). Moreover, the lowest 1-year survival (29%) was found in 67 recipients sensitized against more than 50% of the donor panel. This last finding has been confirmed in the recent analysis of a series of more than 400 cadaver kidneys transplanted in Switzerland since 1969 (JEANNET, 1975) and will be discussed more extensively in another section of this chapter. No significant correlation was found in the latter study between HL-A matching and graft survival in nonsensitized patients. On the other hand, several recently published studies have shown a marked influence of HL-A antigen matching on long-term graft survival of cadaver kidney transplants (VAN HOOFF et al., 1972, 1974; DAUSSET et al., 1974a; Scandiatransplant Report, 1975). A joint analysis of 918 cases performed by France-Transplant and the London Transplant Group showed a 70% 2-year survival of grafts identical for four antigens, as compared to 34% for these with one or zero identities (DAUSSET et al., 1974a). The effect of HL-A antigen matching was greatest in recipients who had a previously failed graft, but no influence of anti-HL-A presensitization was demonstrable. Another extensive European study showed, on the contrary, a striking difference between grafting of presensitized patients, as compared with nonsensitized patients (VAN HOFF et al., 1972). A highly significant correlation between matching and graft survival was found only in patients with antibodies and especially in those mismatched for the antigens of the 2nd locus. In addition, ten grafts compatible for the three most common haplotypes (HL-A 1, 8, HL-A 3, 7, and HL-A 2, 12) had a significantly better prognosis (70% after 18 months) than forty grafts mismatched for these haplotypes (41% after 18 months) (VAN HOFF et al., 1974). These findings were not confirmed in another recent European series including 523 kidney transplants (Scandiatransplant Report, 1975). Although a weak but significant correlation was found between graft survival and the HL-A match, it was not possible to show any effect of matching for the antigens of the 2nd locus nor for the haplotypes HL-A 1, 8, HL-A 3, 7, or HL-A 2, 12. In addition, compatible as well as incompatible grafts did only slightly worse in patients with antibodies as compared with patients without antibodies. The disagreement among the various statistics is troublesome and has led to a great deal of confusion. Several explanations have been proposed for the conflicting results, such as differences between centers in the management of patients, genetic differences between populations in Europe and in the United States, differences in the sensitivity of the antibodies screening and cross-match tests, possible differences in the immunogenicity of HL-A antigens, particularly in the case of a donor and a recipient incompatible for cross-reacting antigens, etc. However, as emphasized by OPELZ et al. (1974), despite these discrepancies, one fact emerges clearly from the statistics: that kidney transplants can frequently survive for years in spite of well-documented mismatches for HL-A antigens. In our view, at least two not-mutually exclusive hypotheses can be put forward to explain this observation: (1) MLC or Ir gene products, rather than HL-A antigens, as such, are the relevant histocompatibility antigens in human organ transplantation. In fact, recent studies by COCHRUM et al. (1973) have confirmed, in unrelated kidney-donor pairs, earlier observations (JEANNET et al., 1969; JEANNET, 1970; BACH et al., 1970) showing that kidney graft prognosis in parent-child and sibling combinations correlated better with MLC reactivity than with HL-A differences. (2) Individual variability in the immune response on the part of the host, perhaps genetically controlled, plays a major role besides differences in histocompatibility antigens in the rejection of allografts in the human. The first hypothesis is fully discussed elsewhere in this book, so that only the second will be considered briefly in the following section.

III. Variability in the Host Immune Response

In animals, genetic control of specific immune response has been demonstrated for a wide variety of antigens. This genetic control has been shown to be dependent on autosomal dominant genes closely linked to the major histocompatibility locus of the species (McDevitt et al., 1971; McDevitt and Landy, 1972; Katz and Benacerraf, 1975). These histocompatibility-linked, specific, immune response (Ir) genes control the ability to respond to a number of antigens, including transplantation antigens. They are expressed by immunocompetent cells, and responsiveness can be transferred to irradiated nonresponders with thymus-dependent lymphocytes (T cells). High responder strains exhibit both an IgM and IgG antibody response and delayed hypersensitivity after antigenic challenge, while a low responding strain exhibits only an IgM response. Recent observations have demonstrated the critical role of histocompatibility gene products in governing the cell-cell interactions concerned with development and regulation of immune responses (Katz and Benacerraf, 1975). In addition, the development of genetic recombinant mice differing at precise loci in the H-2 chromosome has led to the identification of new antigens which are probably the products of the Ir genes (David et al., 1973).

Nothing is known at the present time about the possible existence of such genes in man, but it can be predicted that the HL-A genotype of an individual will also influence his capacity for specific immune response against certain antigens, for instance, foreign histocompatibility antigens. Kissmeyer-Nielsen et al. (1971) and Mickey et al. (1971) found a high incidence of the phenotype HL-A 1, 8 in kidney graft recipients with rejection. This was reported as the first possible indication that in the human, genetic control of the immune response is linked to the HL-A system. However, these observations have not been confirmed in later studies. Many instances of nonresponse to certain antigens are known in man; e.g., 40% of Rh-negative individuals will not produce anti-Rh antibodies even when repeatedly immunized with Rh-positive blood (Mollison et al., 1970). Among Rh-negative multiparous women whose husbands were ABO-compatible and Rh-positive, there was no significant difference between women with and without anti-D antibody, in the frequency of any of the HL-A antigens tested (van Rood et al., 1975b). Nor was a significant difference observed in volunteers submitted to a planned schedule of anti-D immunization (Dausset and Hors, 1975). In a recent study of dizygotic twin pairs, however, evidence was shown of a possible linkage between HL-A loci and loci involved in the immune response against measles (Haverkorn et al., 1975).

The possible association between certain diseases and the HL-A system will be discussed in a later section. These observations may be relevant for the prognosis of kidney grafts. It is not impossible that the apparent absence of immune response of certain recipients to a strongly incompatible kidney graft may be explained by the existence of a genetic control of the response linked to the HL-A system.

The different classes of antibodies produced after HL-A immunization represent an additional source of variability in the immune response of the host. Whereas many patients produce complement-dependent antibodies after blood transfusions, others may produce "blocking or enhancing" antibodies. Perhaps the strongest evidence of the importance of the HL-A system in transplantation depends on the observation that patients with preformed cytotoxic HL-A antibodies, capable of reacting with donor tissues, will reject their transplant in an hyperacute manner. This hyperacute rejection, first described by KISSMEYER-NIELSEN et al. (1966), is characterized by extensive microthrombosis of glomerular capillaries with subsequent renal cortical necrosis; in most cases so far described, complement-dependent (KISSMEYER-NIELSEN et al., 1966; MORRIS et al., 1968; PATEL and TERASAKI, 1969; JEANNET et al., 1970b; TERASAKI et al., 1971) or lymphocyte-dependent (JEANNET et al., 1975; TING and TERASAKI, 1975) HL-A antibodies active against donor lymphocytes have been detected in the recipient serum prior to transplantation. The way these antibodies act to bring about destruction of transplanted kidneys is unclear, but the speed of the reaction and the distribution of the antigens supposedly involved suggest that antibodies react with isoantigens on the outer cell membrane of the vascular endothelium. As mentioned in a previous section, the source of sensitization may be through blood transfusion, previous pregnancies, exposure to certain cross-reacting bacterial or viral antigens, or a previous kidney allograft. In most centers, the number of blood transfusions is kept to a minimum and leukocyte-poor blood is used when red cells are absolutely needed. If feasible, the use of HL-A-compatible blood may be an even better alternative, because in our experience, "leukocyte free" blood may still sensitize the recipients in certain cases. Sensitization by a previous allograft can, of course, be avoided only by a very careful selection of the donor. The more compatible the donor, the less likely the recipient to produce multispecific antibodies after graft rejection and the less difficult it will be to find a second compatible kidney. The frequency of sensitization by previous allograft is difficult to establish, because nearly all patients receive blood transfusions during the surgical procedure. As mentioned before, recipients with preformed cytotoxic antibodies of broad spectrum, even though not reactive with donors' antigens, have significantly fewer successful grafts than those without detectable antibodies (CLARK et al., 1974; JEANNET, 1975).

On the other hand, it has been reported that recipients of cadaver kidneys who had not developed cytotoxic antibodies during hemodialysis treatment of more than 1 year before transplantation subsequently had a much higher graft survival rate than recipients who remained negative for cytotoxins for periods less than a year (OPELZ et al., 1972). This higher survival rate was attributed to unresponsiveness of the patients, both to HL-A-incompatible blood transfusions for long periods during hemodialysis and to HL-A-incompatible kidney transplants. Four possible mechanisms were suggested to explain this unresponsiveness, namely production of enhancing antibodies by transfusions, acquired immunologic tolerance induced by the injection of blood, cross-reactions with autologous HL-A antigens resulting in no response, and finally the existence of a genetically determined trait in certain patients (OPELZ *et al.*, 1972). One of the conclusions drawn from these observations was that blood transfusion in patients waiting for a kidney transplant were not necessarily harmful but perhaps beneficial to subsequent transplants. When patients were studied according to the number of transfusions they had received at the time they were found negative for cytotoxins, it was found that recipients who had received more than 10 transfusions had a graft survival of 80% at 1 year compared to 40% in recipients with no transfusions and 48% in recipients with 1–10 transfusions (OPELZ *et al.*, 1973). The most plausible explanation was, therefore, that nonresponsiveness was actively induced by blood transfusions, which lead to "blocking or enhancing" antibodies. Evidence was in fact presented that MLC "blocking" antibodies appear in the plasma of hemodialysis patients as a consequence of blood transfusions and that these factors seem to have a beneficial effect on human renal allografts (SENGAR *et al.*, 1973). It should not be concluded, however, that all patients waiting for a kidney transplant must be largely transfused to find out whether they are responders or nonresponders. In our experience, nonresponders appear to represent only a small proportion of patients·waiting for a kidney transplant. An in vitro technique is urgently needed to identify these low failure risk patients, without the hazard of inducing broad spectrum lymphocytotoxins by unnecessary blood transfusions. The division between responders and nonresponders in clinical transplantation represents an appealing concept because it would satisfactorily explain why so many HL-A incompatible kidney transplants survive so well for longer periods of time.

IV. Donor Selection
for Kidney Transplantation

The existence of a correlation between HL-A compatibility and the clinical results of human kidney transplantation is now sufficiently established to justify the use of strict criteria for the selection of donors. For ethical reasons this is especially important when living donors are concerned. In our opinion, only ABO compatible HL-A genotypically identical donors from the same family should be used, unless the patient is in desperate condition, no cadaver kidney is available, and dialysis cannot be continued further. Especially in presensitized patients, the use of an HL-A incompatible living donor should be avoided. For cadaver donors, the polymorphism of the HL-A system sometimes makes it difficult to find closely matched recipients. The probability of finding an unrelated donor and recipient with identical HL-A phenotypes is less than 1 in 1,000 for most individuals and still less for rare phenotypes.

The creation of large pools of several hundred recipients within organ exchange programs (KISSMEYER-NIELSEN *et al.*, 1971; VAN ROOD *et al.*, 1971; JEANNET *et al.*, 1971; DAUSSET and HORS, 1972; OPELZ and TERASAKI, 1974) has proved an efficient means of providing HL-A compatible cadaver kidneys for most recipients. In such exchange programs, it is difficult to establish strict criteria for HL-A compatibility. As a rule, the determination of an acceptable level of incompatibility must be left to the patients' doctors, who will take into consideration many factors such as degree of urgency, level of presensitization, transportation facilities, etc., before accepting a cadaver kidney offered by another center. Collaboration on a wide scale between regional or national organizations is especially necessary for heavily sensitized patients that require HL-A identical donors in order to have a reasonable chance of prolonged survival. For the "difficult" cases it is, in our opinion, indispensable to establish very carefully the specificity of the antibodies formed before transplantation in order to select a donor who does not possess the corresponding or cross-reacting antigen. The use of a highly sensitive cross-match test is mandatory and one must be careful to test not only the most recent but also the strongest and broadest, reactive serum of the recipient, because the level of circulating antibody may have fallen below detectable levels at the time of transplantation. Moreover, the selection of a donor identical for all HL-A antigens will decrease still further the chances of an accelerated rejection reaction in these heavily presensitized patients. It is well known that even sensitive cross-match tests may sometimes be falsely negative, due to the so-called CYNAP phenomenon (cytotoxicity negative, but absorption positive). A more extensive discussion of the problem linked with the selection of donors and recipients for cadaveric kidney transplantation will be found in a recent paper by van Rood (1974).

V. Bone Marrow Transplantation

Transplantation of bone marrow involves not only an immunologic response of the host lymphoid cells against the graft, but also a reaction of immunologically competent cells of the donor against the incompatible HL-A antigens of the recipient. The graft-versus-host reaction (GVHR), also called secondary disease, results in a syndrome characterized by dermatitis, diarrhea, liver symptoms, infections, lymphatic aplasia, thrombocytopenia, and hemolytic anemia. Early clinical attempts to transplant patients with aplastic anemias, acute leukemias, and congenital immunologic deficiencies were generally unsuccessful. Although a "take" of the bone marrow graft was often observed in the immunosuppressed recipients, the transplant was eventually rejected, and the original disease recurred or severe GVHR caused the death of the patient. Recently, a number of advances have led to a revival of interest in bone marrow transplantation; the most important progress has been better selection of donors due to the improved understanding of the HL-A system. However, the use of better immunosuppressive treatment and especially the introduction of anti-lymphocyte globulin has led to impressive clinical successes.

Successful bone marrow transplants using ABO, HL-A, and MLC identical siblings as donors have been reported in children with lymphopenic immunologic deficiencies (de Koning et al., 1969; Levey et al., 1971; Meuwissen et al., 1971; Buckley, 1971; van Bekkum, 1974). With HL-A and MLC identical donors, the majority of grafts resulted in a successful take and more than half of the children are alive more than 6 months after transplantation (with a functional graft) (DOOREN et al., 1974). In contrast, only one recipient survived more than 6 months after receiving a graft from an HL-A and MLC incompatible donor (BUCKLEY et al., 1971). Although the GVHR may occasionally be severe (RUBIN-STEIN et al., 1971), the patients grafted with HL-A and MLC identical donors have usually survived, whereas if the graft is HL-A and MLC incompatible, the GVHR has resulted in the rapid death of the patient, except when measures like cell separation techniques or administration of allogeneic sera have been undertaken. So far, no patients have been permanently reconstituted immunolog-ically with incompatible bone marrow, showing clearly the importance of the HL-A chromosomal region in this type of transplantation. Matching for the MLC locus might be more important than matching for HL-A antigens, as demonstrated in a child with combined immunodeficiency by a successful bone marrow transplantation from an uncle who carried, as a result of a crossing over, the same LD determinants but different HL-A antigens as the recipient (DUPONT et al., 1973).

In the past, many attempts have been made to treat severe bone marrow aplasia by transplantation of normal bone marrow. These trials have been sucessful only when the donor was an identical twin, and yet because of the absence of "markers" on the donor cells, it was impossible to prove a "take." Recently, the use of HL-A identical donors combined with the use of cyclophos-phamide as an immunosuppressive agent in the recipient has led to prolonged successes in about half of the cases (THOMAS et al., 1972; FEFER et al., 1974). For patients with no HL-A identical donors, a promising approach appears to be the use of ALG for immunosuppression. Using this procedure, MATHE et al. (1969) have obtained prolonged successes, without GVHR, in about 50% of their cases. We have also obtained remissions of aplastic anemias using ALG alone to prepare the recipient before bone marrow grafting (JEANNET et al., 1974). The remarkable advantage of this form of therapy is the complete absence of signs of GVHR despite the use of incompatible HL-A donors. Howev-er, in several cases, there was no evidence of a "take," but recovery may occur even if the graft is rejected. The results of bone marrow transplantation in patients with acute leukemia are also encouraging. About 25% of the leukemic patients have survived for more than 3 months with a functioning graft when an HL-A and MLC identical donor was available (FEFER et al., 1974). The recent observation that leukemia had recurred in the donor cells, however, casts some doubt on the future of bone marrow transplantation in leukemic patients (FIALKOW et al., 1971). The greatest problem, however, is the GVHR which occurs in almost 70% of patients with substained grafts, despite HL-A and MLC identity. One of the most urgent problems is the identification of non-HL-A antigens that are probably responsible for this high frequency of GVHR (JEANNET et al., 1973). The feasibility of using as donors HL-A and MCL identical unrelated individuals, when HL-A identical siblings are not available, is currently evaluated. As suggested by VAN ROOD (1974), when MLC typing becomes available as a routine procedure, large groups of potential bone marrow donors should be typed under the auspices of an international organization (Europdonor).

H. HL-A System and Human Diseases

I. HL-A and Hematologic Malignant Diseases

It has been suggested that the considerable degree of polymorphism of the HL-A system may be an immunologic surveillance mechanism directed against oncogenic viral infections and somatic mutations. In mice, susceptibility to leukemogenic virus (Lilly et al., 1964; Dausset, 1971) and specific immune responses (McDevitt et al., 1971; McDevitt and Landy, 1972) are linked to the major histocompatibility locus. It has been shown that mice homozygotes for the allele H-2^k are highly susceptible to Gross leukemia virus, whereas mice with the H-2^b allele are resistant. The influence of the H-2 system has also been demonstrated for susceptibility to the Tennant virus and the Friend virus. It seems that genes other than H-2 might determine the success or failure of the virus to infect the host's cells, whereas H-2 genes influence whether or not the infection, once established, will lead to the appearance of leukemia and to death (Tennant, 1970). The resistance to leukemogenesis seems to be the result of an immunologic response of the host to the tumor-specific transplantation antigens induced by the virus in the tumor cells. The antigenic change induced by the virus is apparently histocompatible in strains sharing certain H-2 alleles. It was tempting to speculate that in man, too, susceptibility to leukemia was also linked to the major histocompatibility system, the HL-A system. The discovery that the immune response is genetically determined, as discussed before, and that the responsible genes are linked with the genes governing the cell surface histocompatibility antigens, also stimulated many investigators to look for a similar relationship in man.

A number of early studies in man showed no differences in the frequencies of the HL-A antigens of leukemic patients compared to those of normal individuals (Peacocke et al., 1966; Kourilsky et al., 1968; van Rood et al., 1968; Schlesinger and Amos, 1968). More recently, Thorsby and Lie (1971) and Walford et al. (1971) studied a small number of children with acute leukemia and their families in order to determine the HL-A genotypes of the patients. In both studies, an increase of the haplotype HL-A 2, 12 was found in children with acute leukemia. However, a number of studies found a normal distribution of HL-A antigens or haplotypes in acute lymphoblastic leukemia (Lawler et al., 1971; Batchelor et al., 1971; Jeannet and Magnin, 1971; Dick et al., 1972; Davey et al., 1973), while an excess of HL-A 2 (Rogentine et al., 1973) and also of HL-A 9 (Klouda et al., 1974), observed by others, has been attributed to a longer survival of patients possessing these particular HL-A antigens. Conflicting results have also been reported in similar studies of acute myeloblastic leukemias, chronic myelocytic and lymphocytic leukemias, and malignant lymphomas (Walford et al., 1971; Jeannet and Magnin, 1971; Morris, 1974; Dausset et al., 1974b; Svejgaard et al., 1975). The frequencies of a number of HL-A antigens were found to be slightly altered, but these antigens were different in each study and usually the variations were only of borderline significance.

Conflicting results have also been reported in patients with Hodgkin's disease. Whereas AMIEL (1967) found a higher incidence of the broad antigen 4c, ZERVAS et al. (1970) and THORSBY et al. (1971) observed an increased frequency of HL-A 5. However, FORBES and MORRIS (1970) and also VAN ROOD and VAN LEEUWEN (1971) found that, of the specificities HL-A 5 and W5 (now known to be included in the broad antigen 4c), only W5 had an increased frequency among patients with Hodgkin's disease. In our own study (JEANNET and MAGNIN, 1971), the frequency of HL-A 5 was found to be rather low and that of W5 only slightly increased. The frequency of W15, a specificity belonging to the second segregant series, cross-reacting with HL-A 5 and W5, was increased. KISSMEYER-NIELSEN et al. (1971b) found an increase of HL-A 1 and HL-A 8 and also of the antigen CM* (W18) also cross-reacting with HL-A 5 and W5, and BERTRAMS et al. (1972) observed an excess of their antigen 4c^r, which seems to be identical with CM* (W18). By contrast, COUKELL et al. (1971), using the serum Rafter (which originally defined the antigen 4c), were unable to confirm its excess of reactivity in 44 patients with Hodgkin's disease. As mentioned by DAUSSET (1971), it is interesting to notice that almost all the increased frequencies reported concerned the same cross-reacting group HL-A 5, W 5, W 15, and W 18 (probably including also CM* and 4c^r). A recent survey of 17 different studies involving about 1,500 patients with Hodgkin's disease has shown a highly significant deviation of antigens HL-A 1, 5, 8, and W18 (SVEJGAARD et al., 1975).

Serologic problems, however, cannot be the sole explanation for the divergent results obtained so far in the study of the distribution of HL-A antigens in hematopoietic malignancies. Other factors must be considered. Perhaps the most important is the small number of patients tested in most studies. As mentioned above, the statistical significance of most variations reported is low. When a great number of correlations is done, it is expected that a small proportion of them will be significant by chance alone. Another factor which could explain these conflicting results is the possible heterogeneity of malignant diseases. As demonstrated for Burkitt's tumor, geographical factors may play a role in the susceptibility to an oncogenic virus and therefore different associations may be found in different regions. For instance, in some studies reported, as noted by DAUSSET (1971), a very low incidence of certain HL-A antigens has been observed: thus no HL-A 1 antigen was detectable in the Los Angeles patients with acute myeloblastic leukemia (WALFORD et al., 1971), whereas in Geneva we did not find a single patient with HL-A 11 (JEANNET and MAGNIN, 1971).

It is known that H-2 antigens may be lost or inactivated on some tumor cells in mice (HELLSTRÖM and MÖLLER, 1965). In man, very few instances of antigen loss on lymphocytes of patients with leukemia or lymphoma have been reported (NELKEN, 1963; SEIGLER and METZGAR, 1971; BERTRAMS et al., 1971). In the studies mentioned above, it is somewhat surprising that no deletions of HL-A antigens were reported, despite the fact that often the HL-A genotype of the patient could be compared to the genotype of the parents. In our own experience, too, although many patients with hematologic malignancies were retyped at different stages of the disease, no differences in the HL-A antigens were observed during relapses or remissions.

It is also remarkable that until now there has been no evidence of the existence of additional specific HL-A tumor antigens on leukemic cells. Such a possibility has been suggested by the exceptional stimulatory capacity of certain lymphoma cell lines in culture (HARDY et al., 1969) and by the demonstration that leukemic cells are mitogenic to autologous lymphocytes in some cases of leukemia in remission (FRIDMAN and KOURILSKY, 1969).

II. HL-A and Cancer (other than Lymphomas)

Almost 600 patients with carcinoma of the breast and 350 with malignant melanoma have been studied by many different groups (DAUSSET et al., 1974b), but in the combined analysis of these data, no particular association was found to be significant. In a smaller number of patients with multiple myeloma, an increased incidence of W18 was observed (BERTRAMS et al., 1972), whereas in retinoblastoma the frequency of W5 was increased and that of HL-A 12 decreased (BERTRAMS et al., 1973). Only weak deviations were found in nasopharyngeal carcinoma in Chinese (SIMONS et al., 1974), Burkitt's disease (BODMER et al., 1975), and in cancer of the bladder, prostate, lung, colon, cervix, rectum, stomach, endometrium, and ovary (TAGASUKI et al., 1973). The role of histocompatibility in choriocarcinoma, which can be considered as a malignant fetal allograft, has been investigated by several groups of workers, but so far the influence of the HL-A system in this peculiar tumor has not been clearly demonstrated.

In contrast, the influence of the ABO groups on the risk for a woman to develop choriocarcinoma has been recently confirmed (BAGSHAWE et al., 1971). The concept has been put forward that choriocarcinoma can occur only if the tumor is antigenically compatible with the maternal host. That this is not, in fact, always the case has been clearly shown (LAWLER, 1971; MOGENSEN and KISSMEYER-NIELSEN, 1971; KLOUDA et al., 1972). The presence of antibodies against the incompatible HL-A antigens of the child does not seem to have any prognostic value either. More data will be necessary before the role of the HL-A system in trophoblastic neoplasia can be clearly assessed.

III. HL-A and Immunopathic Diseases

Systemic lupus erythematosus (SLE) is known, like the other autoimmune diseases, to be characterized by a genetic predisposition. A possible correlation between the HL-A system and susceptibility to this disease has been studied by several investigators. Both WATERS et al. (1971b) and GRUMET et al. (1971) found an excess of W15, whereas only the latter group found an increase of HL-A 8. This antigen was found in excess in several other studies (DAUSSET et al., 1974b; MORRIS, 1974), while no significant deviation was observed in a recent study (KISSMEYER-NIELSEN et al., 1975). An increase in the frequency of HL-A 8 has been found in other autoimmune diseases, such as active chronic hepatitis (MACKAY and MORRIS, 1972; BERTRAMS et al., 1974; FREUDENBERG et al., 1973), Graves' disease (GRUMET et al., 1973), Addison's disease (PLATZ et al., 1974), myasthenia gravis (BEHAN et al., 1973; SÄFWENBERG et al., 1973; FELTKAMP et al., 1974; FRITZE et al., 1974), and in patients showing IgG or complement coating on their red cells (DA COSTA et al., 1974). Often this increase in HL-A 8 was accompanied by a significant increase in HL-A 1. HL-A 8 was also found associated with adult coeliac disease, which probably represents a hypersensitivity to gluten (ALBERT et al., 1973; LUDWIG et al., 1973; MCNEISH et al., 1973; STOKES et al., 1973), in dermatitis herpetiformis, another probable immunopathic disorder (KATZ et al., 1972; WHITE et al., 1973), and in juvenile diabetes mellitus, also an endocrine autoimmune condition (SINGAL and BLAJCH-MAN, 1973; NERUP et al., 1974). In allergic diseases, no significant deviation has been observed, although HL-A 8 is perhaps increased in endogen asthma (THORSBY and LIE, 1971). LEVINE et al. (1972) and BLUMENTHAL et al. (1974) reported that, in families, ragweed hypersensitivity segregated with HL-A but with a different haplotype in each family. They suggested that an immune response (Ir) locus linked to HL-A is involved in the pathogenesis of ragweed hay fever and asthma by affecting the level of the production of reagin (IgE) as well as IgG antibodies to ragweed. MARSH et al. (1973), on the other hand, found that sensitivity to ragweed was associated with the HL-A 7 cross-reacting group in unrelated patients. In atopic dermatitis, no significant deviation was found (KRAIN and TERASAKI, 1973).

IV. HL-A and Infectious Diseases

Few significant associations have been found so far in infectious diseases. However, only a few studies have been performed and it is likely that interesting associations will be found, since it is not impossible that the great epidemics in the past have influenced by natural selection the distribution of HL-A antigens observed today in world populations. It is known, for instance, that susceptibility to leprosy is determined by the immunologic reactivity of the host towards *Mycobacterium leprae*. Recently, an excess of W21 has been observed among patients with leprosy, suggesting that individuals possessing that antigen may be more susceptible to the disease (THORSBY et al., 1973). Other investigators have reported an association between W17 and infection due to *Haemophilus influenzae* (ROBBINS et al., 1973) and between HL-A 3 and HL-A 7 and paralytic poliomyelitis (PIETSCH and MORRIS, 1974), but the latter observation was not confirmed in another study (DAUSSET and HORS, 1975). In tuberculosis, no particular deviation was observed (ROSENTHAL et al., 1973).

It has been shown that group A streptococci are able to induce transplantation immunity in animals (RAPAPORT and CHASE, 1964). Moreover, group A streptococci membrane antigens and mice histocompatibility H-2 antigens appear to have a very similar structure. Recently, cross-reactions have been described between streptococcal M1 protein and human transplantation antigens (HIRATA and TERASAKI, 1970). It was therefore tempting to speculate that susceptibility to certain diseases associated with streptococcal infection, such as glomerulonephritis, might be linked with a particular HL-A genotype. In fact, HL-A 2 was found in excess in one series of patients with glomerulonephritis (MICKEY *et al.*, 1970), but this finding has not been confirmed (McDEVITT and LANDY, 1972). Associations between possible viral diseases and the HL-A system have also been investigated; for example, in infectious mononucleosis, MORRIS and FORBES (1971) found an excess of W5, as in Hodgkin's disease. This finding is especially interesting, since an increase in titer of antibodies against the Epstein-Barr virus has been reported in both diseases. Recently, we found in healthy carriers of hepatitis B viral antigen a significant excess of the specificity Sabell, a new antigen of the 2nd locus (JEANNET and FARQUET, 1974). Again, one could explain these findings by a possible cross-reactivity of a causative virus with the antigen Sabell or a genetically controlled defect in the immune response of these patients toward the virus which could be linked with HL-A. A third hypothesis, the so-called receptor hypothesis, according to which HL-A antigens would be the receptors of the viruses, appears less likely (DAUSSET and HORS, 1975).

Interesting associations have been reported in multiple sclerosis, a neurologic disorder in which both autoimmune and viral etiologies have been suggested. HL-A 3, HL-A 7, and W18 were found significantly increased in several studies (BERTRAMS and KUWERT, 1972; NAITO *et al.*, 1972; DAUSSET and HORS, 1975). In addition, JERSILD *et al.* (1973) found an even greater excess of the recently identified LD antigen 7a, which is known to be in strong linkage disequilibrium with the HL-A 7 and HL-A 3. This was the first indication that there may be in some diseases stronger associations with certain MLC determinants than with serologically detectable HL-A antigens.

V. HL-A and Rheumatoid Diseases

The most impressive association between HL-A and disease is certainly that of ankylosing spondylitis and W27. BREWERTON *et al.* (1973a) and SCHLOSSTEIN *et al.* (1973) reported that W27 was present in about 90% of the patients, whereas its frequency in the normal population is about 8%. Many rheumatologists already use W27 in the diagnosis of ankylosing spondylitis, since in other arthropathies, such as rheumatoid arthritis, the frequency of W27 seems to be normal. The same W27 antigen has been found strikingly increased in Reiter's syndrome (BREWERTON *et al.*, 1973b) and acute anterior uveitis (BREWERTON *et al.*, 1973c), two disorders having many similarities with ankylosing spondylitis. W27 and Da 31 were also found in excess in patients suffering from psoriatic arthritis associated with sacroileitis (DAUSSET and HORS, 1975). Although in rheumatoid arthritis no strong deviations have been reported (RYDER *et al.*, 1974), in the juvenile form the frequency of W27 seems to be also increased (RACHELEFSKY *et al.*, 1974).

VI. HL-A System and Various other Diseases

In several studies involving more than 800 patients with psoriasis, a dermatologic disease with a strong genetic influence, HL-A 13 and W17 were found to be increased (WHITE et al., 1972; RUSSELL et al., 1972; RYDER et al., 1974). In Behçet's disease and in Hurler's disease an important excess of HL-A 5 has been found, and the same antigen also appeared associated with polycystic disease (DAUSSET and HORS, 1975). Negative or equivocal results have been published for many other diseases, such as sarcoidosis, rheumatic fever, regional enteritis, ulcerative colitis, gout, and cystic fibrosis (RYDER et al., 1974; DAUSSET et al., 1974 b).

I. HL-A System and Blood Transfusion

Because leukocytes and platelets possess HL-A antigens on their membrane, blood transfusions will lead to immunization of the recipient against certain HL-A antigens. It has been estimated that about 50% of individuals who have received 25 or more transfusions develop antileukocyte antibodies. These antibodies may react with HL-A antigens present in the donor blood and result in febrile transfusion reactions. On rare occasions, febrile reactions are caused by leukocyte antibodies in the donor active against antigens of the recipient. Typical reactions are characterized by the abrupt onset of chills, fever, tachycardia, and dyspnea. The acute symptoms last only a few hours and most of these reactions run a mild course. A few more serious cases with pulmonary infiltrates have been described (WARD, 1970). These reactions can be prevented by transfusion of "leukocyte poor" blood. Prevention of anti-HL-A immunization is particularly important in patients in chronic dialysis waiting for a kidney transplant or in patients with aplastic anemia or leukemia who will receive a large number of transfusions over many months or years. In these patients, the transfusion of platelets and leukocytes is very often necessary in order to reduce the risk of thrombocytopenic hemorrhage and infection. If the patient has been immunized against HL-A by numerous transfusions, the platelets and leukocytes infused will be destroyed very rapidly and become ineffective. It has been shown that the transfusion of platelets of an HL-A identical donor selected from the family of the patient will allow a normal lifespan of the platelets even in the face of a strong anti-HL-A immunization (YANKEE et al., 1969; VAN ROOD et al., 1969; VAN ROOD, 1974). Patients refractory to platelets from unrelated donors could be kept alive for prolonged periods with HL-A identical platelets from siblings, but HL-A identical unrelated donors can also be used (YANKEE et al., 1973). Similarly, it has been shown for leukocyte transfusions that the presence of preformed leukocyte alloantibodies directed against donor cells, predisposed to transfusion reactions and failure of the transfused cells to survive and circulate in the recipient (GRAW et al., 1970; GOLDSTEIN et al., 1971; GRAW et al., 1972). Selection of HL-A compatible donors, either related or unrelated, for leukocyte transfusion, although still difficult, is certainly feasible. In order to facilitate the procurement of blood with infrequent HL-A types, it has recently been proposed to constitute national or international pools of blood donors typed for HL-A (JEANNET, 1974; VAN ROOD, 1974). The exclusive use of unrelated donor blood over blood from family members would have in addition the advantage of not jeopardizing the chances of a subsequent marrow transplant, as suggested recently by STORB *et al.* (1974).

J. HL-A System and Disputed Paternity Cases

The extreme polymorphism of the HL-A system and the fact that there are no HL-A alleles which are very common suggest that it will be a potentially much more informative tool in paternity testing than most other systems. MAYR (1971) has recently calculated that the total chances of exclusions of paternity by the HL-A system alone is about 76%. Using erythrocyte serum and erythrocyte enzymatic groups together with the HL-A system brings the overall chances of exclusion to 98.3%. Before using the HL-A system in paternity studies, one must of course be sure that a sufficient number of families have been studied to ascertain the mode of inheritance of these antigens. According to MAYR's (1971) recent review of the literature, for most of the HL-A antigens more than 200 "critical cases" have now been observed. In addition, under the condition that at least two and, if possible, highly specific sera are used for each HL-A specificity, the microlymphocytotoxicity technique now used by the overwhelming majority of investigators is both accurate and highly reproducible. Therefore, assuming that the dominant inheritance of the HL-A antigens is now well established and that their serologic determination is sufficiently safe in experienced hands, HL-A antigens are now systematically determined in disputed paternity cases, in addition to the usual erythrocyte, serum proteins, and enzyme groups (JEANNET *et al.*, 1972; SPEISER, P., 1975). As in the other systems, two different situations can be found in which a falsely accused father can be excluded. In the first one, the most frequent, the child possesses one or two HL-A antigens not possessed by his mother or the presumptive father. In the second one, which is much rarer, the four HL-A antigens of the child are all possessed either by the mother or by the presumptive father, but the child has neither of the two alleles of the same locus possessed by the presumptive father. The exclusion in this case is also clear-cut, because one of the two alleles of the first locus of the child must come from his father. However, it must be used only when the four HL-A antigens of the child and the father can be detected. In conclusion, the HL-A system certainly represents the most potent system now available for paternity testing, provided that the investigator is experienced and uses well standardized and "potent" reagents. Its generalized application in the field of disputed paternity appears quite promising.

K. Conclusions

The biological function of the HL-A system is still largely unknown. It is likely that its high degree of polymorphism has an advantage for the survival of the species. HL-A antigens could be considered as markers to distinguish self from nonself and would thus play a role of immune surveillance; the deletion or alteration by viruses of these histocompatibility antigens occurring in cell variants would distinguish them from normal cells and lead to their elimination by an immune response. Many experimentally produced tumors possess tumor-specific antigens against which an immune response can be elicited. As was discussed above, similar mechanisms may play a role in human malignant diseases, and the ability of the organism to develop the response may depend on the HL-A genotype. Recently, DOHERTY and ZINKERNAGEL (1975) have suggested that the correlation between HL-A and susceptibility to a particular infectious disease or oncogenic process may reflect absence of an immunogenic modification in HL-A antigens, rather than operation of controlling immune response (Ir) genes. They presented experimental evidence that immune T cells in three of the most prevalent, naturally occurring virus diseases of mice are apparently sensitized to altered-self histocompatibility antigens. Some pathogens or oncogenic processes may not cause an immunogenic modification of self associated with a particular HL-A antigen. This would explain why the major histocompatibility system in animals and in men shows such an extreme genetic polymorphism. Multiple polymorphism tends to minimize the risk of general unresponsiveness throughout the population and reflects evolutionary pressure exerted by this immunologic surveillance mechanism. JERNE (1971) has suggested that the function of histocompatibility antigens may be the generation of self-tolerance and antibody diversity. The latter, according to this hypothesis, would be the result of proliferation during early ontogeny of those cells which produce antibodies against histocompatibility antigens of the individual himself. During proliferation, somatic mutation would occur and new clones of cells would appear, producing antibody molecules with specificities different from the individual's own histocompatibility antigens. Cells which do not mutate will persist only if they do not produce antibodies against the organism's own antigens. As assumed by Burnet's clonal selection theory, this will produce self-tolerance. This theory explains the finding that immune response to certain antigens is linked to the main histocompatibility system and also the intensity of the immune response against foreign histocompatibility antigens. Although very stimulating, these hypotheses are still unproven and extensive studies will be necessary to elucidate the exact biological significance of the HL-A system.

References

ALBERT, E., HARM, K., WANK, R., STEINBAUER-ROSENTHAL, I., SCHOLZ, S.: Segregation analysis of HL-A antigens and haplotypes in 50 families of patients with coeliac disease. Transplant. Proc. **5**, 1785 (1973)

ALBERT, E., KANO, K., ABEYOUNIS, C.J., MILGROM, F.: Detection of human lymphocyte isoantigens by rabbit homotransplantation sera. Transplantation **8**, 466 (1969)

ALLEN, F.H.: Linkage of HL-A and GBG. Vox Sang. **27**, 382 (1974)

AMIEL, J.: Study of the leucocyte phenotypes in Hodgkin's disease. In: Histocompatibility Testing. Copenhagen: Munksgaard, 1967, p. 79

AMOS, D.B.: Some results on the cytotoxicity test. In: Histocompatibility Testing. Copenhagen: Munksgaard, 1965, p. 151

AMOS, D.B., SEIGLER, H.F., SOUTHWORTH, J.G., WARD, F.E.: Skin graft rejection between subjects genotyped for HL-A. Transplant. Proc. **1**, 342 (1969)

BACH, F.H., AMOS, D.B.: Hu-1: Major histocompatibility locus in man. Science **156**, 1506 (1967)

BACH, F.H.: The major histocompatibility complex in transplantation immunology. Transplant. Proc. **5**, 23 (1973)

BACH, F.H., HIRSCHHORN, K.: Lymphocyte interaction: a potential histocompatibility test in vitro. Science **143**, 813 (1964)

BACH, J.F., DEBRAY-SACHS, M., CROSNIER, J., KREIS, H., DORMONT, J.: Correlation between mixed lymphocyte culture performed before transplantation and kidney function. Clin. Exper. Immunol. **6**, 821 (1970)

BACH, M.L., ENGSTROM, M.A., BACH, F.H., ETHEREDGE, E.E., NAJARIAN, J.S.: Specific tolerance in human kidney allograft recipients. Cell Immuno. **3**, 161 (1972)

BAGSHAWE, K.D., RAWLINS, G., PIKE, M.C., LAWLER, S.D.: The ABO blood groups in trophoblastic neoplasia. Lancet **1**, 553 (1971)

BAIN, B., LOWENSTEIN, L.: Genetic studies on the mixed lymphocyte reaction. Science **145**, 1315 (1964)

BALNER, H., VAN LEEUWEN, A., DERSJANT, H., VAN ROOD, J.J.: Defined leucocyte antigens of chimpanzees: use of chimpanzee isoantisera for leucocyte typing in man. Transplantation **5**, 624 (1967)

BATCHELOR, J.R., JOYSEY, V.: Influence of HL-A incompatibility on cadaveric renal transplantation. Lancet **1**, 790 (1969)

BATCHELOR, J.R., EDWARDS, J.H., STUART, J.: Histocompatibility and acute lymphoblastic leukemia. Lancet **1**, 699 (1971)

BERNOCO, D., CULLEN, S., SCUDELLER, G., TRINCHIERI, B., CEPPELLINI, R.: HL-A molecules at the cell surface. In: Histocompatibility Testing 1972. Copenhagen: Munksgaard, 1973, p. 527

BEHAN, P.O., SIMPSON, J.A., DICK, H.: Immune response genes in myasthenia gravis. Lancet **2**, 1033 (1973)

BERTRAMS, J., KUWERT, E., BOHME, V., REIS, H.E., GALLMEIER, W.M., WETTER, O., SCHMIDT, C.G.: HL-A antigens in Hodgkin's disease and multiple myeloma. Increased frequency of W18 in both diseases. Tissue Antigens **2**, 41 (1972)

BERTRAMS, J., KUWERT, E., GALLMEIER, W.M., REIS, H.E., SCHMIDT, C.G.: Transient lymphocyte HL-A antigen loss in a case of irradiated M Hodgkin. Tissue Antigens **1**, 105 (1971)

BERTRAMS, J., KUWERT, E.: HL-A frequencies in multiple sclerosis. Europ. Neurol. **7**, 74 (1972)

BERTRAMS, J., REIS, H.E., KUWERT, E., SELMAIR, H.: Hepatitis associated antigen (HAA), HL-A antigens and auto-lymphocytotoxins (CoCoCy) in chronic agressive and persistent hepatitis. Z. Immun.-Forsch. **146**, 300 (1974)

BERTRAMS, J., SCHILDBERG, P., HOPPING, W., BOHME, V., ALBERT, E.: HL-A antigens in retinoblastoma. Tissue Antigens **3**, 78 (1973)

BILLING, R.J., TERASAKI, P.I.: Rabbit antisera to HL-A 9 isolated from normal serum. Transplantation **17**, 231 (1974)

BLUMENTHAL, M.N., NOREEN, H., AMOS, D.B., MENDELL, N.R., YUNIS, E.: Genetic mapping of Ir gene in man: linkage with second locus of HL-A. Science **184**, 1301 (1974)

BODMER, J.G., BODMER, W.F., PICKBOURNE, P., DEGOS, L., DAUSSET, J., DICK, H.M.: Combined analysis of three studies of patients with Burkitt's lymphoma. Tissue Antigens **5**, 63 (1975)

BODMER, W.F., BODMER, J., ADLER, S., PAYNE, R., BIALEK, J.: Genetics of 4 and LA human leucocyte groups. Ann. N.Y. Acad. Sci. **129**, 673 (1966)

BODMER, W.F., TRIPP, M., BODMER, J.: Application of a fluorochromatic cytotoxicity assay to human leucocyte typing. In: Histocompatibility Testing. Copenhagen: Munksgaard, 1967, p. 341

BODMER, W.F., BODMER, J.G., TRIPP, M.: Recombination between the LA and 4 loci of the HL-A system. In: Histocompatibility Testing. Copenhagen: Munksgaard, 1970, p. 187

BOYUM, A.: Separation of leucocytes from blood and bone marrow. Scand. J. Clin. Lab. Invest. **21**, suppl. 97 (1968)

BREWERTON, D.A., CAFFREY, M., HART, F.D., JAMES, D.C.D., NICHOLLS, A., STURROCK, R.D.: Ankylosing spondylitis and HL-A 27. Lancet **I**, 904 (1973a)

BREWERTON, D.A., CAFFREY, M., NICHOLLS, A., WALTERS, D., DATES, J.K., JAMES, D.C.: Reiter's disease and HL-A 27. Lancet **II**, 996 (1973b)

BREWERTON, D.A., CAFFREY, M., NICHOLLS, A., WALTERS, D., JAMES, D.C.O.: Acute anterior uveitis and HL-A 27. Lancet **II**, 994 (1973c)

BUCKLEY, R.H.: Reconstitution: grafting of bone-marrow and thymus. In: Progress in Immunology. New York: Academic Press, 1971, p. 1061

BUCKLEY, R.H., AMOS, O.B., KREMER, W.P., STICKEL, D.L.: Incompatible bone-marrow transplantation in lymphopenic immunologic deficiency. New Engl. J. Med. **285**, 1035 (1971)

BUCKLEY, R.H., SCHIFF, R.I., AMOS, B.: Blocking of autologous and homologous leucocyte responses by human alloimmune plasmas: A possible in vitro correlate of enhancement. J. Immunol. **108**, 34 (1972)

CEPPELLINI, R.: Old and new facts and speculations about transplantation antigens of man. In: Progress in Immunology. New York: Academic Press, 1971

CEPPELLINI, R., CELADA, F., MATTIUZ, P.L., ZENALDA, A.: Study of the possible correlation between blood antigens and histocompatibility in man. I. Production of leukoagglutinins by repeated transfusions from one donor. Ann. N.Y. Acad. Sci. **120**, 335 (1964)

CEPPELLINI, R., CURTONI, E.S., MATTIUZ, P.L., MIGGIANO, V., SCUDELLER, G., SERRA, A.: Genetics of leucocyte antigens. A family study of segregation and linkage. In: Histocompatibility Testing. Copenhagen: Munksgaard, 1967, p. 169

CEPPELLINI, R., MATTIUZ, P.L., SCUDELLER, G., VISETTI, M.: Experimental allotransplantation in man. I. The role of the HL-A system in different genetic combinations. Transplant. Proc. **1**, 385 (1969)

CEPPELLINI, R., VAN ROOD, J.J.: The HL-A system. I. Genetics and biology. Sem. Hematol. **11**, 233 (1974)

CLARK, E.A., TERASAKI, P.I., OPELZ, G., MICKEY, M.R.: Cadaver-kidney transplant failures at one month. New Engl. J. Med. **291**, 1099 (1974)

COCHRUM, K., PERKINS, H., PAYNE, R., KOUNTZ, S., BELZER, F.: The correlation of MLC with graft survival. Transplant. Proc. **5**, 391 (1973)

COLLINS, Z.V., ARNOLD, P.F., PEETOM, F., SMITH, G., WALFORD, R.L.: A naturally occuring mono-specific anti-HL-A 8 isoantibody. Tissue Antigens **3**, 350 (1973)

COLOMBANI, J., COLOMBANI, M., BENAJAM, A., DAUSSET, J.: Leucocyte and platelet antigens defined by platelet complement fixation test. (Antigens 1, 5, 11 and 16). In: Histocompatibility Testing. Copenhagen: Munksgaard, 1967, p. 413

COLOMBANI, J., COLOMBANI, M., DAUSSET, J.: Cross-reactions in the HL-A system with special reference to DA 6 cross-reacting group. In: Histocompatibility Testing. Copenhagen: Munksgaard, 1970, p. 79

COLOMBANI, J., DAUSSET, J., PREAUX, J.: Homogreffe de peau chez l'homme en relation avec les isoantigènes leucocytaires. Nouv. Rev. Fr. Hémat. **3**, 499 (1963)

COUKELL, A., BODMER, J.G., BODMER, W.F.: HL-A types of 44 Hodgkin's patients. Transplant. Proc. **3**, 1291 (1971)

DA COSTA, J.A.G., WHITE, A.G., PARKER, A.C., GRIGOR, G.B.: Increased incidence of HL-A 1 and 8 in patients showing IgG or complement coating on their red cells. J. Clin. Path. **27**, 353 (1974)

D'AMARO, J., VAN LEEUWEN, A., SVEJGAARD, A., VAN ROOD, J.J.: The microcomplement fixation test. II. Serologic and comparative studies. In: Histocompatibility Testing. Copenhagen: Munksgaard, 1970, p. 539

DAUSSET, J.: Immuno-hématologie des plaquettes et des leucocytes. Presse Méd. **61**, 1533 (1953)

DAUSSET, J.: Leuco-agglutinins. IV. Leuco-agglutinins and blood transfusion. Vox Sang. **6**, 190 (1954)

DAUSSET, J.: Iso-leuco-anticorps. Acta Haemat. **20**, 156 (1958)

DAUSSET, J.: The leucoagglutinins. Transfusion **2**, 209 (1962)

DAUSSET, J.: Correlation between histocompatibility antigens and susceptibility to illness. In: Progress in Clinical Immunology. New York: Grune and Stratton, 1971, p. 183

DAUSSET, J., COLOMBANI, J. (ed.). Histocompatibility Testing 1972. Copenhagen: Munksgaard, 1973

DAUSSET, J., DEGOS, L., HORS, J.: The association of the HL-A antigens with diseases. Clin. Immunol. Immunopath. 3, 127 (1974b)

DAUSSET, J., HORS, J.: L'association France-Transplant. II. Les transplantations de reins effectuées entre donneurs et receveurs groupés dans le système HL-A. Nouv. Presse Méd. 1, 1273 (1972)

DAUSSET, J., HORS, J.: Some contributions of the HL-A complex to the genetics of human diseases. Transplant. Rev. 22, 44 (1975)

DAUSSET, J., HORS, J., FESTENSTEIN, H., OLIVER, R.T.D., PARIS, A.M.I., SACHS, J.A.: Serologically defined HL-A antigens and long-term survival of cadaver kidney transplants. New Engl. J. Med. 290, 979 (1974a)

DAUSSET, J., IVANYI, P., IVANYI, D.: Tissue alloantigens in human. Identification of a complex system (Hu-1). In: Histocompatibility Testing. Copenhagen: Munksgaard, 1965, p. 51

DAUSSET, J., NENNA, A.: Présence d'une leucoagglutinine dans le sérum d'un cas d'agranulocytose chronique. C.R. Soc. Biol. 140, 1534 (1952)

DAUSSET, J., RAPAPORT, F.T., LEGRAND, L., COLOMBANI, J., MARCELLI-BARGE, A.: Skin allograft survival in 238 human subjects. Role of specific relationships at the four gene sites of the first and the second HL-A loci. In: Histocompatibility Testing. Copenhagen: Munksgaard, 1970

DAVEY, F.R., HENRY, J.B., GOTTLIEB, A.J.: HL-A antigens in lymphatic leukemia. Lancet II, 802 (1973)

DAVID, C.S., SHREFFLER, D.C., FRELINGER, J.A.: New lymphocyte antigens controlled by the region of the mouse H-2 complex. Proc. Nat. Acad. Sci. 70, 2509 (1973)

DE KONING, J., DOOREN, L.J., VAN BEKKUM, D.W., VAN ROOD, J.J., DICKE, K.A., RADL, J.: Transplantation of bone marrow cells and fetal thymus in an infant with lymphopenic immunological deficiency. Lancet I, 1223 (1969)

DICK, F.R., FORTUNY, I., THEOLOGIDES, A., GREALLY, J., WOOD, N., YUNIS, E.J.: HL-A and lymphoid tumors. Cancer Res. 32, 2608 (1972)

DOHERTY, P.C., ZINKERNAGEL, R.M.: A biological role for the major histocompatibility antigens. Lancet I, 1406 (1975)

DOOREN, L.J., KAMPHUIS, R.P., DE KONING, J., VOSSEN, J.M.: Bone marrow transplantation in children. Sem. Hematol. II, 369 (1974)

DUPONT, B., ANDERSEN, V., ERNST, P., FABER, V., GOOD, R.A., HANSEN, G.S., HENRIKSEN, K., JENSEN, K., JUHL, F., KILLMANN, S.A., KOCH, C., MULLER-BERAT, N., PARK, B.H., SVEJGAARD, A., THOMSEN, M., WILK, A.: Immunological reconstitution in severe combined immunodeficiency with HL-A incompatible bone marrow graft: donor selection by mixed lymphocyte culture. Transplant. Proc. 5, 905 (1973)

EIJSVOOGEL, V.P.: The cellular recognition in vitro of antigens related to human histocompatibility. Sem. Hematol. II, 305 (1974)

EINSTEIN, A.B., MANN, D.L., GORDON, H.G., TRAPANI, R.J., FAHEY, J.L.: Heterologous antisera against specific HL-A antigens. Transplantation 12, 299 (1971)

ENGELFRIET, C.P.: Cytotoxic isoantibodies against leucocytes. Thesis, Amsterdam, 1966

ENGELFRIET, C.P., BRITTEN, A.: The cytotoxic test for leucocyte antibodies. Vox Sang. 10, 660 (1965)

FALK, J.A., SARGENT, A.V., BROWN, M.R., FALK, R.E.: Monospecific HL-A 2 cytotoxic activity in a M-protein. In: Internat. Symp. on Standardization of HL-A Reagents. Basel: S. Karger, 1973, p. 294

FAULK, W.P., JEANNET, M., CREIGHTON, W.D., CARBONARA, A.: Immunological studies on the human placenta. Characterization of immunoglobulins on trophoblastic basement membranes. J. Clin. Invest. 54, 1011 (1974)

FEFER, E.D., THOMAS, C.D., BUCKNER, C.D., STORB, R., NEIMAN, P., GLUCKSBERG, H., CLIFT, R.A., LERNER, K.G.: Marrow transplants in aplastic anemia and leukemia. Sem. Hematol. II, 353 (1974)

FELTKAMP, T.E.W., BERG-LOONEN, P.M. VAN DER, NIJENHUIS, L.E., ENGELFRIET, C.P., ROSSUM, A.L. VAN, LOGHEM, J.J. VAN, OOSTERHUIS, H.J.G.H.: Myasthenia gravis, auto-antibodies and HL-A antigens. Brit. Med. J. I, 131 (1974)

FIALKOW, J., THOMAS, E.D., BRYANT, J.I., NEIMANN, P.E.: Leukemic transformation of engrafted human marrow cells in vivo. Lancet I, 251 (1971)

FORBES, J.F., MORRIS, P.J.: Leucocyte antigens in Hodgkin's disease. Lancet II, 849 (1970)

FREIESLEBEN-SØRENSEN, S., STAUB-NIELSEN, L.: The genetic basis for reactivity in human mixed lymphocyte culture. II. Studies of unrelated subjects identical at the HL-A subloci "LA and Four". Acta Path. Microbiol. Scand. 78b, 719 (1970)

FREUDENBERG, J., ERDMAN, K., MEYER ZUM BUSCHENFELDE, K., FORSTER, H., BERGER, J.: HL-A in liver diseases. Klin. Wschr. 51, 1075 (1973)

FRIDMAN, W.H., KOURILSKY, F.M.: Stimulation of lymphocytes by autologous leukemic cells in acute leukemia. Nature (Lond.) 224, 277 (1969)

FRITZE, D., HERMANN, C., NAEIM, F., SMITH, G.S., WALFORD, R.L.: HL-A antigens in myasthenia gravis. Lancet I, 240 (1974)

FU, S.M., HUNKEL, H.P., BRUSMAN, F.H., ALLEN, J.R., FOTINO, F.: Evidence for linkage between HL-A histocompatibility genes and those involved in the synthesis of the second component of complement. J. Exp. Med. 140, 1108 (1974)

GABB, B.W., BOOMER, W.F.: A microcomplement-fixation test for platelets antibodies. In: Histocompatibility Testing. Copenhagen: Munksgaard, 1970, p. 543

GERT-JENSEN, K.: Leucocyte antibodies and pregnancy. A survey. Thesis. Copenhagen: Munksgaard, 1966

GOLDSTEIN, I. M., EYRE, H. J., TERASAKI, P. I., HENDERSON, E. S., GRAW, R. G.: Leucocyte transfusions: role of leucocyte alloantibodies in determining transfusion response. Transfusion II, 19 (1971)

GORDON, J.: The mixed leucocyte culture reaction. Med. Clin. N. Amer. 56, 337 (1972)

GRAW, R.G., GOLDSTEIN, I.M., EYRE, H.J., TERASAKI, P.I.: Histocompatibility testing for leucocyte transfusion. Lancet II, 77 (1970)

GRAW, R.G., HERZIG, G., PERRY, S., HENDERSON, E.S.: Normal granulocyte transfusion therapy. New Engl. J. Med. 287, 367 (1972)

GRUMET, E.C., COUKELL, A., BODMER, J.G., BODMER, W.F., McDEVITT, H.O.: Increased incidence of two leucocyte antigen specificities in systemic lupus erythematosus. New Engl. J. Med. 285, 193 (1971)

GRUMET, C., KONISHI, J., PAYNE, R.D., KRIS, J.P.: Association of Grave's disease with HL-A 8. Clin. Res. 21, 493 (1973)

HARDY, D.A., LING, N.R., KNIGHT, S.C.: Exceptional lymphocyte stimulating capacity of cells from lymphoid cell lines. Nature (Lond.) 223, 511 (1969)

HATTLER, B.G., KARESH, C., MILLER, J.: Inhibition of the mixed lymphocyte culture response by antibody following successful human renal transplantation. Tissue Antigens 1, 270 (1971)

HAVERKORN, M.J., HOFMAN, B., MASUREL, N., VAN ROOD, J.J.: HL-A linked genetic control of immune response in man. Transplant. Rev. 22, 120 (1975)

HELLSTRÖM, K.E., MÖLLER, G.: Immunological and immunogenetic aspects of tumor transplantation. Prog. Allergy 9, 158 (1965)

HERSEY, P., CULLEN, P., MacLENNAN, I.C.M.: Lymphocyte-dependent cytotoxic antibody activity against human transplantation antigens. Transplantation 16, 9 (1973)

HIRATA, A.A., TERASAKI, P.I.: Cross-reactions between streptococcal M proteins and human transplantation antigens. Science 168, 1095 (1970)

HORS, J., FEINGOLD, N., FRADELIZI, D., DAUSSET, J.: Critical evaluation of histocompatibility in 179 renal transplants. Lancet I, 609 (1971)

HRONKOVA-ZOULKOVA, J., IVASKOVA, E., KLOUDA, P., IVANYI, P.: A possible correlation between antigens of the HL-A system and P system. Folia Biol. 14, 402 (1968)

HUANG, S.W., LATTOS, D.B., NELSON, D.B., REEB, K., HONG, R.: Antibody-associated lymphotoxin in acute infection. J. Clin. Invest. 52, 1033 (1973)

JEANNET, M.: Histocompatibility testing using leucocyte typing and mixed lymphocyte culture in kidney transplants. Helv. med. Acta 35, 168 (1970)

JEANNET, M.: Selection of compatible platelet donors by lymphocyte HL-A matching. In: Strahlen, Blutgerinnung und Hämostase. Stuttgart: F.K. Schattauer Verlag, 1974, p. 147

JEANNET, M.: Unpublished observations, 1975

JEANNET, M., DE WECK, A., FREI, P.C., GROB, P., HORISBERGER, B., THIEL, G.: A collaborative program for tissue typing between six Swiss hospitals. In: Histocompatibility Testing. Copenhagen: Munksgaard, 1970a, p. 435

JEANNET, M., DE WECK, A., GROB, P., HORISBERGER, B., LARGIADER, F., THIEL, G.: HL-A typing and cadaver kidney transplants. Transplant. Proc. 3, 1015 (1971)

JEANNET, M., FARQUET, J.J.: HL-A antigens in asymptomatic chronic HBAg carriers. Lancet II, 1383 (1974)

JEANNET, M., HÄSSIG, A., BERNHEIM, J.: Use of the HL-A antigen system in disputed paternity cases. Vox Sang. 23, 197 (1972)

JEANNET, M., LAMBERT, P.H.: Propriétés immunologiques des anticorps élués à partir du rein transplanté. In: Cours International de Transplantation. Villeurbane: Simep, 1974, p. 171

JEANNET, M., MAGNIN, C.: HL-A antigens in haematological malignant-diseases. Europ. J. Clin. Invest. 2, 39 (1971)

JEANNET, M., PINN, V.W., FLAX, M.H., WINN, H.J., RUSSELL, P.S.: Humoral antibodies in renal allotransplantation in man. New Engl. J. Med. 282, 111 (1970b)

JEANNET, M., RUBINSTEIN, A., PELET, B.: Studies on non-HL-A cytotoxic and blocking factor in a patient with immunological deficiency successfully reconstituted by bone-marrow transplantation. Tissue Antigens 3, 411 (1973)

JEANNET, M., RUBINSTEIN, A., PELET, B., KUMMER, H.: Prolonged remission of severe aplastic anemia after ALG pretreatment and HL-A semi-incompatible bone-marrow cell transfusion. Transplant. Proc. 6, 359 (1974)

JEANNET, M., VASSALLI, P.: Studies on new HL-A antigens of the first segregant series. Vox Sang. 20, 317 (1971)

JEANNET, M., VASSALLI, P., BOTELLA, F.: Lymphocyte-dependent cytotoxic antibody (LDA) in kidney transplantation. Transplant. Proc. 7, 631 (1975)

JEANNET, M., WONHAM, V.A., WINN, H.J., RUSSEL, P.S.: Donor selection for kidney transplantation based on lymphocyte pheno- and genotyping and mixed lymphocyte cultures. Transplant. Proc. 1, 382 (1969)

JERNE, N.K.: The somatic generation of immune recognition. Europ. J. Immunol. 1, 71 (1971)

JERSILD, C., FOG, T., HANSEN, G.S., THOMSEN, M., SVEJGAARD, A., DUPONT, B.: Histocompatibility determinants in multiple sclerosis with special reference to clinical course. Lancet II, 1221 (1973)

JOHNSON, A.H., ROSSEN, R.D., BUTLER, W.T.: Detection of alloantibodies using a sensitive antiglobulin microcytotoxicity test: identification of low levels of preformed antibodies in accelerated allograft rejection. Tissue Antigens 2, 215 (1972)

KASAKURA, S., LOWENSTEIN, L.: The effect of uraemic blood on mixed leucocyte reactions and on cultures of leucocytes with phytohaemagglutinin. Transplantation 5, 283 (1967)

KATZ, D.H., BENACERRAF, B.: The function and interrelationships of T-cell receptors, Ir genes and other histocompatibility gene. Transplant. Rev. 22, 175 (1975)

KATZ, S.I., FALCHUK, E.M., DAHL, M.V., ROGENTINE, G.N., STROBER, W.: HL-A 8: a genetic link between dermatitis herpetiformis and glutensensitive enteropathy. J. Clin. Invest. 51, 2977 (1972)

KISKEN, W.A., SWENSON, N.A.: Unresponsiveness of mixed leucocyte cultures from thymectomized adults dogs. Nature 224, 76 (1969)

KISSMEYER-NIELSEN, F., OLSEN, S., POSBORG-PETERSEN, V., FJELDBORG, O.: Hyperacute rejection of kidney allografts, associated with pre-existing humoral antibodies against donor-cells. Lancet II, 662 (1966)

KISSMEYER-NIELSEN, F. et al.: Scandiatransplant. Preliminary report of a kidney exchange program. Transplant. Proc. 2, 1019 (1971a)

KISSMEYER-NIELSEN, F., BJORN-JENSEN, K., FERRARA, G.B., KJERBYE, K.E., SVEJGAARD, A.: HL-A phenotypes in Hodgkin's disease. Preliminary report. Transplant. Proc. 3, 1287 (1971b)

KISSMEYER-NIELSEN, F., KJERBYE, K.E.: Lymphocytotoxic microtechnique. Purification of lymphocytes by flotation. In: Histocompatibility Testing. Copenhagen: Munksgaard, 1967, p. 381

KISSMEYER-NIELSEN, F., KJERBYE, K.E., ANDERSEN, E., KALBERG, P.: HL-A antigens in systemic lupus erythematosus. Transplant. Rev. 22, 164 (1975)

KISSMEYER-NIELSEN, F., STAUB-NIELSEN, L., LINDHOLM, A., SNADBERG, L., SVEJGAARD, A., THORSBY, E.: The HL-A system in relation to human transplantations. In: Histocompatibility Testing. Copenhagen: Munksgaard, 1970, p. 105

KISSMEYER-NIELSEN, F., SVEJGAARD, A., HAUGE, M.: Genetics of the human HL-A transplantation system. Nature 219, 116 (1968)

KLOUDA, P.T., LAWLER, S.D., BAGSHAWE, K.D.: HL-A matings in trophoblastic neoplasia. Tissue Antigens 2, 280 (1972)

KLOUDA, P.T., LAWLER, S.D., TILL, M.M., HARDISTY, R.M.: Acute lymphoblastic leukemia and HL-A: a prospective study. Tissue Antigens **4**, 262 (1974)

KOCH, C.T., VAN HOOFF, J.P., VAN LEEUWEN, A., VAN DER TWEEL, J.G., FREDERIKS, E., VAN DER STEEN, G.J., SCHIPPERS, H.M.A., VAN ROOD, J.J.: The relative importance of matching for the MLC versus the HL-A loci in organ transplantation. In: Histocompatibility Testing, 1972. Copenhagen: Munksgaard, 1973, p. 521

KRAIN, L.S., TERASAKI, P.I.: HL-A types in atopic dermatitis. Lancet I, 1059 (1973)

KOURILSKY, F.M., DAUSSET, J., FEINGOLD, N., DUPUY, J.M., BERNARD, J.: Etude de la répartition des antigènes leucocytaires chez des malades atteints de leucémie aiguë en rémission. In: Advance in Transplantation. Copenhagen: Munksgaard, 1968, p. 515

LALEZARI, P.: A new technique for separation of human leucocytes. Blood **19**, 109 (1962)

LAMM, L.U., FRIEDRICH, U., PETERSEN, G.B., JÖRGENSEN, J., NIELSEN, J., THERKELSEN, A.J., KISS-MEYER-NIELSEN, F.: Assignment of the major histocompatibility complex to chromosome No. 6 in a family with a pericentric inversion. Hum. Hered. **24**, 273 (1974)

LAMM, L.U., SVEJGAARD, A., KISSMEYER-NIELSEN, F.: PGM₃: HL-A is another linkage in man. Nature New Biol. **231**, 109 (1971)

LAWLER, S.D.: Histocompatibility and trophoblastic neoplasia. Transplant. Proc. **3**, 1265 (1971)

LAWLER, S.D., KLOUDA, P.T., HARDISTY, R.M., TILL, M.M.: Histocompatibility and acute lymphoblastic leukemia. Lancet I, 699 (1971)

LEGRAND, L., DAUSSET, J.: Serological evidence of the existence of several antigenic determinants (or factors) on the HL-A gene products. In: Histocompatibility Testing 1972. Copenhagen: Munksgaard, 1973, p. 441

LEVENTHAL, B.G., BUELL, D.N., YANKEE, R., ROGENTINE, G.N., TERASAKI, P.I.: The mixed leucocyte response: effect of maternal plasma. In: Proc. 5th Leucocyte Culture Conference. New York: Academic Press, 1970, p. 473

LEVEY, R.H., KLEMPERER, M.R., GELFAND, E.W., SANDERSON, A.R., BATCHELOR, J.R., BERKEL, A.I., ROSEN, F.S.: Bone marrow transplantation in severe combined immuno-deficiency syndrome. Lancet II, 571 (1971)

LEVINE, B.B., STEMBER, R.H., FOTINO, M.: Ragweed hay fever: genetic control and linkage to HL-A haplotypes. Science **178**, 1201 (1972)

LILLY, F., BOYSE, E.A., OLD, L.J.: Genetic basis of susceptibility to viral leukaemogenesis. Lancet II, 1207 (1964)

LUDWIG, H., POLYMENIDIS, Z., GRANDITSCH, G., WICK, G.: Association of HL-A 1 and HL-A 8 with childrood coeliac disease. Z. Immun. Forsch. **146**, 158 (1973)

MACKAY, I.R., MORRIS, P.J.: Association of autoimmune active chronic hepatitis with HL-A 1, 8. Lancet II, 793 (1972)

MARSH, D.G., BIAS, W.B., HSU, S.H., GOODFRIEND, L.: Association of the HL-A 7 cross-reacting group with a specific reaginic antibody response in allergic man. Science **179**, 691 (1973)

MATHE, G., AMIEL, J.L., SCHWARZENBERG, L., CHOAY, J., TROLARD, P., SCHNEIDER, M., HAYAT, M., SCHLUMBERGER, J.R., JASMIN, C.: Bone marrow transplantation in man. Transplant. Proc. I, 16 (1969)

MAWAS, C., CHRISTEN, Y., LEGRAND, L., SASPORTES, M., DAUSSET, J.: Cellular and humoral response against determinants other than the classical HL-A specifities. Transplantation **18**, 256 (1974)

MAYER, S., FALKENRODT, A., TONGIO, M.M.: Cold lymphocytotoxins in infections and parasitic infestations. Tissue Antigens **3**, 431 (1973)

MAYR, W.: Die Genetik des HL-A Systems. Populations- und Familienuntersuchungen, unter besonderer Berücksichtigung der Paternitätsserologie. Humangenetik **12**, 195 (1971)

McDEVITT, H.O., BECHTOL, K.B., GRUMET, F.C., MITCHELL, G.F., WEGMANN, T.G.: Genetic control of the immune response to branched synthetic polypeptide antigens in inbred mice. In: Progress in Immunology. New York: Academic Press, 1971, p. 495

McDEVITT, H.O., LANDY, M. (ed.): Genetic Control of Immune Responsiveness: Relationship to Disease Susceptibility. New York: Academic Press, 1972

McNEISH, A.S., NELSON, R., MACKINTOSH, P.: HL-A 1 and 8 in childhood coeliac disease. Lancet I, 668 (1973)

MEUWISSEN, H.J., RODNEY, G., McARTHUR, J., PABST, H., GATTI, R., CHILGREN, R., HONG, H., FROMMEL, D., COIFMAN, R., GOOD, R.A.: Bone marrow transplantation. Therapeutic usefulness and complications. Amer. J. Med. **51**, 513 (1971)

MICKEY, M.R., KREISLER, M., ALBERT, E.D., TANAKA, N., TERASAKI, P.I.: Analysis of HL-A incompatibility in human renal transplants. Tissue Antigens 1, 57 (1971)

MICKEY, M.R., KREISLER, M., TERASAKI, P.I.: Leucocyte antigens and disease. II. Alterations in frequencies of haplotypes associated with chronic glomerulonephritis. In: Histocompatibility Testing. Copenhagen: Munksgaard, 1970, p. 237

MIDDLETON, J., CROOKSTON, M.C., FALK, J.A., ROBSON, E.B., COOK, P.J.L., BATCHELOR, J.R., BODMER, J., FERRARA, G.B., FESTENSTEIN, H., HARRIS, R., KISSMEYER-NIELSEN, F., LAWLER, S.D., SACHS, J.A., WOLF, E.: Linkage of Chido and HL-A. Tissue Antigens 4, 366 (1974)

MIESCHER, P.: Leucopénie chronique par auto-anticorps. Helv. med. Acta 20, 420 (1953)

MIESCHER, P., FAUCONNET, M.: Mise en évidence de différents groupes leucocytaires chez l'homme. Schweiz. Med. Wschr. 89, 597 (1954)

MITTAL, K.K., MICKEY, M.R., SINGAL, D.P., TERASAKI, P.I.: Serotyping for homotransplantation. XVIII. Refinement of microdroplets lymphocyte cytotoxicity test. Transplantation 6, 913 (1968)

MOGENSEN, B., KISSMEYER-NIELSEN, F.: Current data on HL-A and ABO typing in gestational choriocarcinoma and invasive mole. Transplant Proc. 3, 1267 (1971)

MOLLISON, P.L., FRAME, M., ROSS, M.E.: Differences between Rh (s) negative subjects in response to Rh (D) negative subjects in response to Rh (D) antigen. Brit. J. Haemat. 19, 257 (1970)

MORRIS, P.J.: Histocompatibility systems, immune response and disease in man. In: Contemporary Topics in Immunobiology. New York: Plenum Publishing, 1974, Vol. 3

MORRIS, P.J., FORBES, J.F.: HL-A in follicular lymphoma, reticulum cell sarcoma, lymphosarcoma and infectious mononucleosis. Transplant. Proc. 3, 1315 (1971)

MORRIS, P.J., TING, A.: Leukocyte antigens in renal transplantations. 9. Matching for the HL-A system and the early course of cadaveric renal grafts. Med. J. Austr. 14, 517 (1970)

MORRIS, P.J., WILLIAMS, G.M., HUME, D.M., MICKEY, M.R., TERASAKI, P.I.: Serotyping for homotransplantation. XII. Occurence of cytotoxic antibodies following kidney transplantation in man. Transplantation 6, 392 (1968)

NAITO, S., NAMEROW, N., MICKEY, M.R., TERASAKI, P.I.: Multiple sclerosis: Association with HL-A 3. Tissue Antigens 2, 1 (1972)

NELKEN, D.: Loss of leukocyte individual specific antigen in a case of acute leukemia. Vox Sang. 8, 638 (1963)

NERUP, J., LYNGSØE, J., ORTED-ANDERSEN, O., CHRISTY, M., KROMANN, H., PLATZ, P., POULSEN, J.E., RYDER, L.P., STAUB-NIELSEN, L., SVEJGAARD, A., THOMSEN, M.: HL-A antigens in diabetes mellitus. Lancet II, 864 (1974)

OPELZ, G., MICKEY, M.R., TERASAKI, P.I.: Identification of unresponsive kidney transplant recipients. Lancet I, 868 (1972)

OPELZ, G., MICKEY, M.R., TERASAKI, P.I.: HL-A and kidney transplants: reexamination. Transplantation 17, 371 (1974)

OPELZ, G., SENGAR, D.P.S., MICKEY, M.R., TERASAKI, P.I.: Effect of blood transfusions on subsequent kidney transplants. Transplant. Proc. 5, 523 (1973)

OPELZ, G., TERASAKI, P.I.: National utilization of cadaver kidneys for transplantation. J. A. M. A. 228, 1260 (1974)

PATEL, R., MICKEY, M.R., TERASAKI, P.I.: Serotyping for homotransplantation. XVI. Analysis of kidney transplants from unrelated donors. New Engl. J. Med. 297, 501 (1968)

PATEL, R., TERASAKI, P.I.: Significance of the positive cross-match test in kidney transplantation. New Engl. J. Med. 280, 735 (1969)

PAYNE, R., PERKINS, H.A., NAJARIAN, J.S.: Compatibility for seven leucocyte antigens in renal homografts: Utilization of a micro-agglutination test with few sera. In: Histocompatibility Testing. Copenhagen: Munksgaard, 1967, p. 237

PAYNE, R., ROLFS, M.R.: Foetomaternal leucocyte incompatibility. J. Clin. Invest. 37, 1756 (1958)

PAYNE, R., TRIPP, M., WEIGLE, J., BODMER, W., BODMER, J.: A new leucocyte isoantigen system in man. Cold Spring Harbor Symp. Quant. Biol. 29, 285 (1964)

PEACOCKE, I., AMOS, B., LASZLO, I.: The detection of isoantigens on leukemic cells using the cytotoxicity test. Blood 28, 665 (1966)

PERKINS, H.A., HOWELL, E., GANTAN, Z., MIMS, M.C., DICKERSON, T., SENECAL, I.: Variation in cytotoxic antibody response to transfusion in prospective allograft recipients. Transplantation 17, 216 (1974)

PIETSCH, M.C., MORRIS, P.J.: An association of HL-A 3 and HL-A 7 with paralytic poliomyelitis. Tissue Antigens **4**, 50 (1974)

PLATZ, P., RYDER, L., STAUB-NIELSEN, L., SVEJGAARD, A., THOMSEN, M., NERUP, J., CHRISTY, M.: HL-A and idiopathic Addison's disease. Lancet **II**, 289 (1974)

RACHELEFSKY, G.S., TERASAKI, P.I., KATZ, R., STIEHM, E.R.: Increased prevalence of W27 in juvenile rheumatoid arthritis. New Engl. J. Med. **290**, 892 (1974)

RAPAPORT, F.T., CHASE, R.M.: Homograft sensitivity induction by Group A streptococci. Science **165**, 407 (1964)

RICHIARDI, P., CARBONARA, A.D., MATTIUZ, P.L., CEPPELLINI, R.: Inhibition of cytotoxic anti-HL-A sera by their $F(a^b)_2$. In: Histocompatibility Testing. Copenhagen: Munksgaard, 1973, p. 455

ROBBINS, J.B., SCHNEERSON, R., ARGAMAN, M., HANDZEL, T.: Hemophilus influenza type B disease and immunity in humans. Ann. Intern. Med. **78**, 259 (1973)

ROGENTINE, G.N.: Detection of isoantigens on human lymphocytes and tissue culture cells by ^{51}Cr cytotoxicity technique. In: Histocompatibility Testing 1967. Copenhagen: Munksgaard, 1967, p. 371

ROGENTINE, G.N., TRAPANI, R.J., YANKEE, R.A., HENDERSON, E.S.: HL-A antigens and acute lymphatic leukemia: the nature of the HL-A 2 association. Tissue Antigens **3**, 470 (1973)

ROSENTHAL, I., SCHOLZ, S., KLIMEK, R., ALBERT, E.D., BLAHA, H.: HL-A antigens and haplotypes in patients with tuberculosis. Z. Immun-Forsch. **144**, 424 (1973)

RUBINSTEIN, A., SPECK, B., JEANNET, M.: Successful bone-marrow transplantation in a lymphopenic immunologic deficiency syndrom. New Engl. J. Med. **285**, 1399 (1971)

RUSSELL, T.J., SCHULTES, L.M., KUBAN, D.J.: Histocompatibility (HL-A) antigens associated with psoriasis. New Engl. J. Med. **287**, 738 (1972)

RYDER, L.P., STAUB-NIELSEN, L., SVEJGAARD, A.: Associations between HL-A histocompatibility antigens and non-malignant diseases. Humangenetik **25**, 251 (1974)

SÄFWENBERG, J., LINDBLOM, J.B., OSTERMAN, P.D.: HL-A frequencies in patients with myasthenia gravis. Tissue Antigens **3**, 465 (1973)

SASPORTES, M., LEBRUN, A., RAPAPORT, F.T., DAUSSET, J.: Skin allografts survival in relation to HL-A incompatibilities and response in MLC. Transplant. Proc. **5**, 353 (1973)

SCANDIATRANSPLANT REPORT. HL-A matching and kidney-graft survival. Lancet **I**, 240 (1975)

SCHAPIRA, M., JEANNET, M.: Cell-mediated lympholysis in HL-A identical unrelated individuals. Tissue Antigens **4**, 178 (1974)

SCHLESINGER, M., AMOS, B.: Antigenic alterations of host tissues during tumor growth. In: Human Transplantation. New York: Grune and Stratton, 1968, p. 601

SCHLOSSTEIN, L., TERASAKI, P.I., BLUESTONE, R., PEARSON, C.M.: High association of an HL-A antigen, W27, with ankylosing spondylitis. New Engl. J. Med. **288**, 704 (1973)

SCHULMAN, N.R., MARDER, V.J., ALEDORT, L.M., HILLER, M.C.: Complement-fixing isoantibodies against antigens common to platelets and leucocytes. Trans. Ass. Amer. Phys. **75**, 89 (1962)

SCHULMAN, N.R., MARDER, V.J., HILLER, M.C., COLLIER, E.M.: Platelet and leucocyte isoantigens and their antibodies: serologic, physiologic and clinical studies.. Progr. Hemat. **4**, 222 (1964)

SCHWARZ, M.R.: The mixed lymphocyte reaction: an in vitro test for tolerance. J. Exp. Med. **127**, 879 (1968)

SEIGLER, H.F., METZGAR, R.S.: HL-A in malignant lines. J. Nat. Cancer Inst. **46**, 577 (1971)

SENGAR, D.P.S., OPELZ, G., TERASAKI, P.I.: Outcome of kidney transplants and suppression of mixed leucocyte culture by plasma. Transplant. Proc. **5**, 641 (1973)

SHANBROM, E., FEINGOLD, E., SHEPERD, L., WALFORD, R.L.: Antisera for tissue typing: the production of cytotoxic and agglutinating antibodies following intradermal leucocyte injection in man. Blood **32**, 402 (1968)

SIMONS, M.J., WEE, G.B., DAY, N.E., MORRIS, P.J., SHANMUGARATNAM, K., DE THE, G.B.: Immunogenetics aspects of nasopharyngeal carcinoma. 1. Differences in HL-A antigen profiles between patients and comparison groups. Internat. J. Cancer **13**, 122 (1974).

SINGAL, D.P., BLAJCHMAN, M.A.: Histocompatibility (HL-A) antigens, lymphocytotoxic antibosies and tissue antibodies in patients with diabetes mellitus. Diabetes **22**, 429 (1973)

SINGAL, D.P., MICKEY, M.R., MITTAL, K.K., TERASAKI, P.I.: Serotyping for homotransplantation. XVII. Preliminary studies of HL-A sub-units and alleles. Transplantation **6**, 904 (1968)

SMITH, G.S., WALFORD, R.L.: A micro-complement fixation method for determining isoantigens of human platelets. In: Histocompatibility Testing. Copenhagen: Munksgaard, 1970, p. 549

SOLLHEIM, B.G., BRATLIE, A., SANDBERG, L., STAUB-NIELSEN, L., THORSBY, E.: Further evidence of a third HL-A locus. Tissue Antigens **3**, 439 (1973)

SPEISER, P.: Das HL-A System im Paternitatsprozeß mit Berücksichtigung des Beweiswertes. In: 5. Tagung der Gesellschaft für forensische Blutgruppenkunde. In press (1975)

STOKES, P.L., ASQUITH, P., HOLMES, G.K.T., MACKINTOSH, P., COOKE, W.T.: Inheritance and influence of histocompatibility (HL-A) antigens in adult coeliac disease. Gut **14**, 627 (1973)

STORB, R., THOMAS, E.D., BUCKNER, C.D., JOHNSON, F.L., FEFER, A., GLUCKSBERG, H., GIBLETT, E.R., LERNER, K.G., NEIMANN, P.: Allogenic marrow grafting for treatment of aplastic anaemia. Blood **43**, 157 (1974)

SVEJGAARD, A., KISSMEYER-NIELSEN, F.: Complement-fixing platelet iso-antibodies. I. A quantitative technique for their detection. Vox Sang. **14**, 106 (1968a)

SVEJGAARD, A., KISSMEYER-NIELSEN, F.: Cross-reacting iso-antibodies. Nature (Lond.) **219**, 868 (1968b)

SVEJGAARD, A., PLATZ, P., RYDER, L.P., STAUB-NIELSEN, L., THOMSEN, M.: HL-A and disease associations. A survey. Transpl. Rev. **22**, 3 (1975)

TAGASUKI, M., TERASAKI, P.I., HENDERSON, B., MICKEY, M.R., MENCK, H., THOMPSON, R.W.: HL-A antigens in solid tumors. Cancer Res. **33**, 648 (1973)

TENNANT, J.R.: Immunogenetic approach to neoplasia. Transplant. Proc. **2**, 104 (1970)

TERASAKI, P.I. (ed.): Histocompatibility Testing. Copenhagen: Munksgaard, 1970

TERASAKI, P.I., MARCHIORO, T.L., STARZL, T.E.: Serotyping of human lymphocyte antigens: preliminary trials on long-term kidney graft survivors. Histocompatibility testing. Nat. Acad. Sci. Washington Publ. **1229**, 83 (1965)

TERASAKI, P.I., MCCLELLAND, J.D.: Microdroplet assay of human serum cytotoxins. Nature (Lond.) **204**, 998 (1964)

TERASAKI, P.I., MICKEY, M.R., KREISLER, M.: Presensitization and kidney transplant failures. Posgrad. Med. J. **47**, 89 (1971)

TERASAKI, P.I., MOTTIRONI, V.D., BARNETT, E.V.: Cytotoxins in disease. Autotoxins in lupus. New Engl. J. Med. **283**, 724 (1970)

THE 11 TH. REPORT OF THE HUMAN RENAL TRANSPLANT REGISTRY. J.A.M.A. **226**, 1197 (1973)

THOMAS, E.D., BUCKNER, C.O., STORB, R., NEIMAN, P.E., FEFER, A., CLIFT, R.A., SLICHTER, S.J., FUNK, D.D., BRYANT, J., LERNER, K.E.: Aplastic anaemia treated by marrow transplantation. Lancet II, 284 (1972)

THORSBY, E.: The human major histocompatibility system. Transplant. Rev. **18**, 51 (1974)

THORSBY, E., FALK, J., ENGESETH, A., OSOBA, O.: HL-A antigens in Hodgkin's disease. Transplant. Proc. **3**, 1279 (1971)

THORSBY, E., GODAL, T., MYRVANG, B.: HL-A antigens and susceptibility to diseases. II. Leprosy. Tissue Antigens **3**, 373 (1973)

THORSBY, E., KISSMEYER-NIELSEN, F.: HL-A antigens and genes. III. Production of HL-A typing antisera of desired specificity. Vox Sang. **17**, 102 (1969)

THORSBY, E., KISSMEYER-NIELSEN, F.: New alleles of the HL-A system. Identification by planned immunization. Vox Sang. **18**, 134 (1970)

THORSBY, E., LIE, S.D.: Relationship between the HL-A system and susceptibility to diseases. Transplant. Proc. **3**, 1305 (1971)

TING, A., TERASAKI, P.I.: Lymphocyte dependent antibody cross-matching for transplant patients. Lancet I, 304 (1975)

VAN BEKKUM, D.W.: The double barrier in bone-marrow transplantation. Sem. Hematol II, 325 (1974)

VAN DER WEERDT, CH.: Platelets antigens and iso-immunization. Thesis. Amsterdam: Drukkerij, 1965

VAN HOOFF, J.P., HENDRIKS, G.F.J., SCHIPPERS, H.M.A., VAN ROOD, J.J.: Influence of possible HL-A haploidentity on renal-graft survival in Eurotransplant. Lancet I, 1130 (1974)

VAN HOOFF, J.P., SCHIPPERS, H.M.A., VAN DER STEEN, G.J., VAN ROOD, J.J.: Efficacy of HL-A matching in Eurotransplant. Lancet II, 1385 (1972)

VAN LEEUWEN, A., SCHUIT, H.R.E., VAN ROOD, J.J.: Typing for MLC. II. The selection of non-stimulator cells by MLC inhibition tests using SD identical stimulator cells (MISIS) and fluorescent antibody studies. Transplant. Proc. **5**, 1539 (1973)

VAN ROOD, J.J.: The HL-A system. II. Clinical relevance. Sem. Hematol. II, 253 (1974)

VAN ROOD, J.J., EERNISSE, J.G., VAN LEEUWEN, A.: Leucocyte antibodies in sera from pregnant women. Nature (Lond.) **181**, 1735 (1958)

VAN ROOD, J.J., EERNISSE, J.G.: The detection of transplantation antigens in leucocytes. In: Progress in Surgery. Basel/New York: Karger, 1969, Vol. 7, p. 217

VAN ROOD, J.J., FREUDENBERG, J., VAN LEEUWEN, A., SCHIPPERS, A., ZWEERUS, R., TERPSTRA, J.L.: Eurotransplant. Transplant. Proc. **3**, 933 (1971)

VAN ROOD, J.J., VAN HOOFF, J.P., KEUNING, J.J.: Disease predisposition, immune responsiveness and the fine structure of the HL-A supergene. Transplant. Rev. **22**, 75 (1975 b)

VAN ROOD, J.J., VAN LEEUWEN, A., BOSCH, L.J.: Leucocyte antigens and transplantation immunity. In: Proc. 8th Congr. Europ. Soc. Haemat., Vienna, 1961. Basel/New York: Karger, 1962, p. 199

VAN ROOD, J.J., VAN LEEUWEN, A.: Leukocyte grouping. A method and its application. J. Clin. Invest. **62**, 1382 (1963)

VAN ROOD, J.J., VAN LEEUWEN, A., SCHIPPERS, A.M.J., VOOYS, W.H., FREDERIKS, E., BALNER, H., EERNISSE, J.G.: Leucocyte groups, the normal lymphocyte transfer test and homograft sensitivity. In: Histocompatibility Testing 1965. Copenhagen: Munksgaard, 1965, p. 37

VAN ROOD, J.J., VAN LEEUWEN, A.: Defined leukocytic antigenic groups in man. In: Histocompatibility Testing. Washington: Nat. Acad. Sci. Publ., 1965, p. 21

VAN ROOD, J.J., VAN LEEUWEN, A., SCHIPPERS, A., BALNER, H.: Human histocompatibility antigens in normal and neoplastic tissues. Cancer Res. **28**, 1415 (1968)

VAN ROOD, J.J., VAN LEEUWEN, A., RUBINSTEIN, P.: Isoantigens of leucocytes and platelets. In: Textbook of Immunopathology. New York: Grune and Stratton, 1969, p.469

VAN ROOD, J.J., VAN LEEUWEN, A.: HL-A and the group Five system in Hodgkin's disease. Transplant. Proc. **3**, 1283 (1971)

VAN ROOD, J.J., VAN LEEUWEN, A., KEUNING, J.J., BLUSSE VAN OUD ABLAS, A.: The serological recognition of the human MLC determinants using a modified cytotoxicity technique. Tissue Antigens **5**, 73 (1975 a)

VAN SOMEREN, H., WESTERVELD, A., HAGEMEISTER, A., MEES, J.R., MEERA KHAN, P., ZAALBERG, O.B.: Human antigen and enzyme markers in man-Chinese hamster somatic cell hybrids: evidence for a synteny between the HL-A, PGM_3, ME and IPO-B loci. Proc. Nat. Acad. Sci. **71**, 962 (1974)

VREDEVOE, D.L., TERASAKI, P.I., MICKEY, M.R., GLASSOCK, R., MERRIL, J.P., MURRAY, J.E.: Serotyping of human lymphocyte antigens. III. Long term kidney homograft survivors. In: Histocompatibility Testing. Copenhagen: Munksgaard, 1965, p. 25

WALFORD, R.L.: The isoantigenic system of human leucocytes. medical and biological significance. Series Haemat. **2**, 1 (1969)

WALFORD, R.L., COLOMBANI, J., DAUSSET, J.: Retrospective leucocyte typing of unrelated human donor-recipient pairs in relation to skin allograft survival times. Transplantation **7**, 188 (1969)

WALFORD, R.L., CARTER, P.K., ANDERSON, R.E.: Leucocyte antibodies following skin homografting in man. Transplant. Bull. **29**, 16 (1962)

WALFORD, R.L., GALLAGHER, R., SJAARDA, J.R.: Serologic typing of human lymphocytes with immune serum obtained after homografting. Science **144**, 868 (1964)

WALFORD, R.L., GALLAGHER, R., TROUP, F.M.: Human lymphocyte typing with isologous antisera. Technical consideration and a preliminary study of the cytotoxic reaction system. Transplantation **3**, 387 (1965)

WALFORD, R.L., ZELLER, E., COMBS, L., KONRAD, P.: HL-A specificities in acute and chronic lymphatic leukemia. Transplant. Proc. **3**, 1297 (1971)

WARD, F.E., SEIGLER, F.H.: Mixed lymphocyte reactions and skin graft survival in an HL-A recombinant family. Transplant. Proc. **5**, 359 (1973)

WARD, H.N.: Pulmonary infiltrates associated with leucoagglutinin transfusion reactions. Ann. Intern. Med. **73**, 689 (1970)

WATERS, H., KONRAD, P., WALFORD, R.L.: The distribution of HL-A histocompatibility factors and genes in patients with systemic lupus erythematosus. Tissue Antigens **1**, 68 (1971 b)

WATERS, H., SMITH, G.S., FISHKIN, B., TANAKA, K.R., WALFORD, R.L.: Lymphocyte isoantibodies in autoallergic and dysgammaglobulinemic states. Transplant. Proc. **3**, 145 (1971 a)

WHITE, A.G., BARNETSON, R.ST.C., DA COSTA, J.A.G., MCLELLAND, D.B.L.: The incidence of HL-A antigens in dermatitis herpetiformis. Brit. J. Dermat. **89**, 133 (1973)

WHITE, S.H., NEWCOMER, V.D., MICKEY, M.R., TERASAKI, P.I.: Disturbance of HL-A antigen frequency in psoriasis. New Engl. J. Med. **287**, 740 (1972)

WHO, 1968: Nomenclature for factors of the HL-A system. Bull-WHO **39**, 483 (1968)

WHO: Nomenclature for factors of the HL-A system. Bull-WHO **47**, 659 (1972)

WILLIAMS, R.C., EMMONS, J.D., YUNIS, E.J.: Studies of human sera with cytotoxic activity. J. Clin. Invest. **50**, 1514 (1971)

WILSON, D.B., SILVERS, W.K., NOWELL, P.C.: Quantitative studies on the mixed lymphocyte interaction in rats. II. Relationship of the proliferative response to the immunologic status of the donors. J. Exp. Med. **126**, 655 (1967)

YANKEE, R.A., GRAFF, K.S., DOWLING, R., HENDERSON, E.S.: Selection of unrelated compatible platelet donors by lymphocyte HL-A matching. New Engl. J. Med. **288**, 760 (1973)

YANKEE, R.A., GRUMET, F.C., ROGENTINE, G.N.: Platelet transfusion therapy. The selection of compatible platelet donors for refractory patients by lymphocyte HL-A typing. New Engl. J. Med. **281**, 1208 (1969)

YUNIS, E.J., AMOS, D.B.: HL-A, mixed leucocyte reaction (MLR) and hypersensitivity delayed reactions (HDR). Three closely linked genetic systems relevant to transplantation. Proc. Nat. Acad. Sci. U.S. **68**, 3031 (1971)

ZERVAS, J.D., DELAMORE, J.M., ISRAEL, M.C.G.: Leucocyte phenotypes in Hodgkin's disease. Lancet **II**, 634 (1970)

Gene Products of the Major Histocompatibility Complex: Biology and Chemistry

D. A. L. DAVIES and M. HESS

With 19 Figures and 8 Tables

1. Introduction

Of the several approaches which led to the elucidation of transplantation immunogenetics a key study was that of mouse blood groups by GORER (1942, 1953) along lines already established in human erythrocyte serology (RACE and SANGER, 1962). Recent studies of human ABO blood groups in transplantation show that incompatibility constitutes a significant barrier to acceptance of skin grafts in man and ABO matching is preferable, and is normal practice in human kidney transplantation. Mice do not now appear to have a closely similar homologue of human ABO polymorphism but are, in general terms, "B-like". The early mouse hemagglutination studies showed that red cells had at least 3 different alloantigens (then called isoantigens) and one of these (the second) proved, in the light of further work, to be of special importance in the context of transplantation. It was subsequently called H-2 (=histocompatibility-2) (SNELL, 1953; AMOS et al., 1955). Mice are now known to have at least 30 other histocompatibility "H" loci (KLEIN, 1973a) (referred to as "non-H-2") and as this includes at least one on the X (ROSENAU and HORWITZ, 1968) and one on the Y (KOO et al., 1973) chromosome it seems likely that all the twenty chromosomes have one or more H loci. There is every reason to believe that a similar situation exists in man. In this chapter, however, we will be concerned primarily with the human analog of mouse H-2 which is called HLA. Much evidence exists for non-HLA loci in man but they have not been studied extensively. Reasons for supposing that human HLA is not only analogous to, but is actually a genetic homologue of mouse H-2 will be given shortly. Presupposing this to be the case a few general ideas about the importance of mouse H-2 will not be out of place at this point. Rodents played a special role in the development of this subject because, while suitable for genetic studies, they are also large enough as subjects for experimental transplantation. Our review of HLA will therefore be liberally supplemented by data from mice, and to some extent rats and guinea pigs. The serology of mouse H-2 histocompatibility antigens developed rapidly because these antigens are expressed on red cells and could be detected by hemagglutination. The development can also be attributed to the existence of inbred, homozygous strains of mice. Later, great value acrued from the use of congenic lines of mice where two strains result from a particular mating pattern such that they differ by one small segment of chromosome; it can be arranged that the segment carries the genes required for study. H-2 proved to be more than just a gene, but actually a chromosomal segment, in linkage group IX, more recently identified as chromosome 17. Thus each mouse strain was distinguished by a set of multiple antigenic specificities, shared to differing degrees by other inbred strains. The direction in which mouse work developed led to some divergence from the human studies, which began with the discovery of leukocyte alloantigens (DAUSSET et al., 1960; VAN ROOD et al., 1961) and where the methods available were necessarily quite different. It was some time before H-2 and HLA took up parallel lines of development. Especially mouse work revealed many specificities because of the relative ease of the mouse serology based on hemagglutination, but few "individuals" were available, if we liken an inbred line to an individual in this context. In man, many individuals were available but the serology was more difficult because HLA antigens are not expressed by human red cells; for this reason there was little development until leukocyte cytotoxicity serology was perfected.

The complexity of the H-2 and HLA genetic regions is much greater than that of non-H-2 (H-1, H-3…H-30) and non-HLA histocompatibility loci and the former play a special role in transplantation immunity which is, even now, not wholly elucidated. For these and other reasons to become apparent, we refer to mouse H-2, human HLA, and the genetic homologue of other species as the major histocompatibility complex or MHC. The MHC is highly polymorphic and its gene products are widely expressed on many types of tissue cells. They are located particularly on the external cell membranes and the alloantigenicity expressed as a result of MHC differences between individuals leads to rapid graft rejection which can be, to some extent, accelerated by preimmunization, ("second set response", BILLINGHAM et al., 1956). The weaker non-MHC loci usually lead to a slower rejection, which can, however, be much more substantially accelerated by preimmunization (high "factor of immunization", SIMONSEN, 1962).

Before committing ourselves to a description of the MHC, it is necessary to point out briefly, because of its practical importance in human transplants, that ABO "blood groups" constitute a human "non-HLA" histocompatibility system, as already mentioned, of special importance in skin grafts. Its role in transplants which are surgically vascularized is not so clear and it is possible that the necessity for skin to vascularize itself may render ABO of special importance in that context. ABO specificity is expressed widely among mucopolysaccharides through the nature of the polysaccharide chain end group sugars (galactosamine, galactose, and fucose respectively, in the broadest terms) and occurs on red cells as mucopolysaccharide and also glycolipid (WATKINS, 1970). Leukocytes also express ABO specificity on their surface (DAUSSET, 1954).

2. The MHC in Man and Animals

2.1. Similarities

2.1.1. General Similarities

In all species of mammals studied, strong incompatibility, as seen by the rapid rejection of grafted tissue, is usually attributed to incompatibility at a particular locus which always proves to be highly polymorphic and referable to an MHC. There are two main kinds of exceptions to this general rule. (1) ABO rejection of human skin in fully HLA matched siblings, and mouse skingraft rejection, due to multiple non-MHC incompatibility. (2) there are certain privileged sites (e.g. hamster cheek pouch) and tissues (e.g. cornea) where rejection does not occur in spite of MHC incompatibility. The MHC in mouse and man can be subdivided into several regions and for two of these the gene products are readily detected serologically, i.e. K and D in the mouse (DÉMANT, 1973), and A and B in man (KISSMEYER-NIELSEN and THORBY, 1970). There may, in each species, be a third region with somewhat similar characters, i.e. where the gene products induce a cytotoxic humoral alloantibody, (originally detected by a serum A/J in man and a serum "H-2.7" in the mouse). These regions were called "subloci" or "segregant series". The extent of the H-2 and HLA regions are somewhat similar in the sense that the crossover rate between the presently known outer limits is about 0.5% in both species. The mouse MHC is linked to "T" locus, which is a region responsible for the regulation of development of the animal on its long axis and some of whose alleles lead to various developmental defects from death of embryos at some early stage to spina bifida or incompletely developed tail, etc. (GLUECHSOHN-WAELSH and ERICKSON, 1970). In man also, spina bifida is linked with HLA (AMOS et al., 1975). This suggests that a chromosomal region considerably greater in extent than the MHC has been preserved with no major alterations over a very long evolutionary period. The preservation of T-locus is easy to visualize; the fundamental importance of MHC is not fully clarified but a study of its "I" region (see below) shows some basic connection with control of the immune response. Thus we would only have to invoke a role for immunity in homoeostasis to provide a functional link between the MHC and the T-locus. Animals other than mice show features always agreeing with what we know of MHC characteristics, and never disagreeing with them. The genetic homology has not been formally proven but broad similarities exist over all of the following MHC characters:

1. Strong transplantation immunity
2. Multiple serologic characters
3. Similar tissue distribution of gene products
4. Similar location in and on cells (including sperms)
5. Chemical structures of gene products
6. Association with immune responsiveness (Ir) genes
7. Control of mixed lymphocyte reaction (MLR)

   8. Association with diseases
   9. Size of locus
   10. Division of the chromosome segment into regions with similar properties

These are all subjects enlarged upon below.

2.1.2. Serologic Similarities

Antigens which are assembled by enzymes, and are not themselves direct gene products, may have specific determinant structures which are e.g. sugars substituted onto carrier molecules by glycosyl transferases. Considering the small number of different kinds of sugars entering into the structure of the mammalian body, it is not surprising that there should be serologic cross reactions between human and bacterial products if it is due to e.g. galactose, when similarly linked on a bacterial endotoxin and blood group "B" substance. By contrast it is indeed surprising to find cross reactions between distantly related species if the epitope is an amino acid in a protein, unless the substances are products of genes subject to evolutionary conservation. No immunologic feature of the MHC has been attributed to its carbohydrate moiety but only to its protein structure, nevertheless serologic cross reactivity between H-2 and HLA is on record from many studies. Very suggestive direct interactions have long been known and recently indirect studies show H-2, HLA relationships e.g. by immunization of some other animal with partly purified antigen (DAVID et al., 1973a), which showed an involvement of allospecific sites, or by reactivity of human lymphocytes with mouse antisera when allospecific sites were not so clearly implicated (PELLEGRINO et al., 1974). The clearest case is that of congenically derived mouse H-2 alloantiserum reacting with a restricted number of a panel of human lymphocytes, where cross reactivity was attributed to something close to HLA-B7 and HLA-B27 (IVAŠKOVÁ and IVANYÍ, 1974).

2.2. Differences

The most obvious difference between H-2 and HLA, and one which delayed clarification of homology, was the expression of H-2 antigens on mouse red cells. This led to different methodology in mouse and human studies although H-2 hemagglutination in the mouse is now essentially obsolete as a typing method. Expression of "H" specificities on rodent red cells is not complete, as some specificities cannot be detected, at least by direct hemagglutination (DÉMANT et al., 1971). On the other hand some HLA specificities are expressed by human reticulocytes (HARRIS and ZERVAS, 1969; SILVESTRE et al., 1970); thus it is felt that the difference is almost a matter of degree, trivial and not basic. The MHC includes, in those species adequately studied, an immune responsiveness (Ir) region where genes exist, responsible for high (good) or low (poor) responsiveness to a variety of antigens (see 3.3 and 3.4). The ability to react exists in low responders. It is the degree to which such a recognition

event can be amplified into a useful degree of response that is controlled by
Ir genes. In the mouse the "*I*" region lies between the two regions (*K* and
D), whose gene products are responsible for eliciting, by appropriate alloimmunization, humoral antibody, as used for mouse tissue typing. In man the evidence
presently favors an "*I*" region outside the *B* region but still very closely linked
to it. *B* and *A* region gene products elicit the humoral response which provides
HLA tissue typing sera in man. A difference in the sequential arrangement of
regions in the MHC is not difficult to accommodate into genetic events considering
the period which has elapsed since mouse and man had a common ancestor (about
10^8 years); it does suggest, however, that the region is not subject to sequential
reading of genes in transcription.

3. Biology of Human MHC Products

3.1. HLA Antigens

It is usually more difficult to study a human product than its animal homologue
and in the transplantation field, animals have made a particularly handsome
contribution to our knowledge (see Section 4.1). Information about in vivo
effects is very sparse where soluble products are concerned but "cellular antigen"
has been studied as discussed below. The in vitro studies have agreed throughout
with the animal data, which gives us more confidence in their interpretation.
These data are dealt with extensively elsewhere in this volume, but a few aspects
are mentioned below.

3.1.1. In Vitro Studies

In the early days of transplantation immunobiology consideration was given
to the possibility that there were distinguishable H (histocompatibility) and
T (transplantation) antigens. By the early 1960s it had been generally accepted
that in vitro methods of assessing antigen by its binding with alloantibody
were a measure of the antigen which sensitized for graft rejection. This assumption led us all astray and now we known that the HLA antigen measured
by its ability, when solubilized and purified, to bind HLA cytotoxic "tissue
typing" alloantibody is indeed the foreignness itself, but is not the substance
("Ia" antigen) whose difference from a graft recipient permits the recognition
of nonself.

HLA alloantisera are either 'H' sera or H+I sera. They are probably rather
rarely I antisera, because we do not know a source of human material that
is I positive and H negative. I antisera may arise by cross immunization between
HLA identical unrelated individuals who would be expected to have I-region
differences. Anti-"LADS"[1] (=anti-I?) antibody blocks the stimulator cell (CEP-
PELLINI, 1973), as can be seen if the HLA antibody is removed by absorption
with H-positive, I-negative material (e.g. platelets, fibroblasts, liver cells) (VAN

[1] *Lymphocyte activating determinant*

Rood, personal communication). Ia antibodies are only very weakly cytotoxic and not easy to use in cytotoxic inhibition tests (unpublished observations). Other kinds of tests are applicable, e.g. LDA (Zighelboim *et al.*, 1974) or MISIS (van Leeuwen *et al.*, 1973).

The number of HLA molecules on a peripheral lymphocyte is approximately 30,000 (Sanderson and Welsh, 1974a). This provides enough material of each of the four specificities in a doubly heterozygous individual to allow antibody mediated cell surface redistribution ("capping") (Kourilsky *et al.*, 1972 and see also 5.2.1.). Antigen distribution data are less extensive than for animals but otherwise correspond as e.g. for trophoblast (Loke *et al.*, 1971), and seminal plasma (Singal and Berry, 1972). Existence of HLA antigens on man-mouse hybrid cells has been studied (Kano *et al.*, 1972) and HLA changes have been documented for neoplastic cells (Seigler *et al.*, 1971).

In relation to what follows it is important to allude to studies of cell mediated lympholysis carried out by Eijsvoogel *et al.* (1973a, b). These experiments show that activation to make killer cells is due to incompatibility at the "MLC locus" (I-region?) although for actual destruction of target cells by such killer cells, incompatibility at the HLA locus itself was necessary (see Section 4.1.2.).

The in vitro complexes of soluble antigen with HLA alloantibody are themselves soluble, probably because particular HLA specific sites are only represented once on the molecule, thus not permitting cross linking (Sanderson and Welsh, 1974b). This is important in the context of kidney damage which might otherwise ensue. Circulating 'H' antibody is found e.g. in rats bearing enhanced kidney allografts (Burgos *et al.*, 1974), where we take it that no cellular response arises because of anti-Ia suppression of sensitization.

3.1.2. In Vivo Studies

3.1.2.1. Induction of Humoral Antibody

Because different HLA specificities can, to some extent, be separated from each other by fractionation of soluble antigens, then it should be possible to use these for purposeful immunization to prepare tissue typing antisera of a desired restricted specificity. The precedent exists in animals (Davies, 1969; Staines *et al.*, 1973). Papain-solubilized HLA antigen from various tissue cultured lymphoid cell lines were used to immunize rabbits, and the antisera, after suitable absorptions, were reactive with some HLA alloantigenic specificities (Einstein *et al.*, 1971). Reagents, possibly more closely akin to alloantisera, have been prepared from nonhuman primates (Metzgar and Miller, 1972; Sanderson and Welsh, 1973). Purposeful immunization of human volunteers is not on record with purified antigens but carefully selected donor lymphocytes have been used to elicit sera with particularly desired alloantibodies (Carvalho *et al.*, 1973). A line of work not adequately interpreted is that of heterophile antibodies arising concomitantly with transplantation immunity (Kano *et al.*, 1975).

3.1.2.2. *Other in Vivo Data*

Clearly no experiments have been intentionally carried out to study hastened organ graft rejection in man, but much has been written on the circumstances attending situations where hastened rejection was, unfortunately, the outcome. Earlier studies have associated presensitization of transplant recipients through blood transfusions with poor prognosis for kidney grafts. More recently the situation appears by no means so simple. In one study subliminal amounts of preformed HLA antibody (measured by a sensitive inhibition of binding of radioiodine labeled IgG fraction of anti-HLA sera), and also higher levels of preformed antibody led to rapid destruction of renal transplants (LUCAS *et al.*, 1970). More recent studies in an extensive series of first cadaver renal transplants showed a poor outcome for low levels of preformed antibody, and improved prospects for those with intermediate levels (MYBURGH *et al.*, 1974). As we now believe that HLA antibodies are damaging to grafts by direct toxicity, we can interpret the results to mean that only when anti-Ia antibodies have been adequately elicited does the effect of active enhancement outweight the disadvantage of HLA antibody also present in the patients. Active enhancement has had a degree of success with canine renal allografts, using solubilized antigen as immunogen (HOLL-ALLEN *et al.*, 1970). In man, passive enhancement was tried using father anti-mother antiserum; toxicity was reduced by making Fab fragments of antibody from the Ig fraction (BATCHELOR *et al.*, 1970). The outcome of such trails has not been encouraging and might be due to the use of the wrong specificity, i.e. HLA rather than Ia.

That graft survival is not necessarily shortened, but may indeed be prolonged by preimmunization in man is supported by in vivo data collected by VAN ROOD (1973) and VAN ROOD *et al.*, 1975b. This leads to the conclusion that the in vivo events are as defined in the in vitro studies of cell mediated lympholysis described by EIJSVOOGEL *et al.* (1973a, b) and already referred to.

3.2. β2-Microglobulin (β2m)

Although not a gene product of the MHC, β2m will be discussed here for two reasons. (1) In man, mouse, and guinea pig the molecule has been found to be associated with H-antigens (see 5.5); (2) because of the role attributed to β2m-antibodies in cellular immunity and in the membrane redistribution

3.2.1.

While HL-A antigens are governed by a complex genetic region on the 6th chromosome, β2m is controlled by a gene on the 15th chromosome (GOODFEL-LOW *et al.*, 1975). As for H- and L-chains in immunoglobulins however, (which are also governed by different genes on separate chromosomes) this does not preclude the contribution of two separate entities to form one functional molecule (HLA (H-2)+β2m).

3.2.2. Tissue Distribution of β2m

Originally isolated by BERGGÅRD and BEARN (1968) from the urine of patients with tubular malfunction (e.g. chronic cadmium poisoning, Wilson's disease), β2m was later found in biological fluids (human serum, cerebrospinal fluid, saliva, and colostrum) (EVRIN et al., 1971), and on the surface of nucleated cells (BERNIER and FANGER, 1972; EVRIN and PERTOFT, 1973; EVRIN and NILSSON, 1974; POULIK, 1973; POULIK and BLOOM, 1973). Secreted by lymphoid cells in culture (in marked contrast to HLA antigens), β2m has also been isolated from spent culture media (POULIK and BLOOM, 1973; NAKAMURO et al., 1973). The rate of secretion for permanent human cell lines varies between 38 and

Table 1. Production of β2-microglobulin in cultures of freshly explanted cells (taken from NILSSON et al., 1974)

Designation of cells	Origin of cells	Type of cell	β_2-μ-production/65 h (ng/ml)
U-605	Non malignant tonsil	Tonsil cells	64
U-605 P	Non malignant tonsil, PHA stimulated	PHA stimulated tonsil cells	120
U-864	Non malignant thymus	Thymus cells	24
U-874	Non malignant lymph node	Lymph node cells	19
U-850	Burkitt's lymphoma	Lymphoma cells	10
U-615	Burkitt's lymphoma	Lymphoma cells	34
U-624	Burkitt's lymphoma	Lymphoma cells	61
U-626	Burkitt's lymphoma	Lymphoma cells	37
U-811	Histiocytic lymphoma	Lymphoma cells	61
U-878	Histiocytic lymphoma	Lymphoma cells	26
U-882	Histiocytic lymphoma	Lymphoma cells	15
U-857	Hand-Schüller-Christian's disease	Lymphoma cells	29
U-875	Lymphocytic lymphoma, poorly differentiated	Lymphoma cells	21
U-698	Lymphocytic lymphoma, poorly differentiated	Lymphoma cells	25
U-701	Lymphocytic lymphoma, poorly differentiated	Lymphoma cells	50
U-704	Lymphocytic lymphoma, poorly differentiated	Lymphoma cells	42
U-719	Lymphocytic lymphoma, poorly differentiated	Lymphoma cells	67
U-838	Hodgkin's disease, mixed type	Lymphoma cells + normal lymph node cells	273
U-839	Hodgkin's disease, mixed type	Lymphoma cells + normal lymph node cells	136
U-858	Hodgkin's disease, mixed type	Lymphoma cells + normal lymph node cells	230
U-863	Hodgkin's disease, mixed type	Lymphoma cells + normal lymph node cells	150

Table 2. Production of β2-microglobulin by human malignant and nonmalignant cell lines of mesenchymal or epithelial origin

Designation of cell line	Origin of cell line	Type of cell	β_2-μ-production/65 h (ng/ml)[a]
2 T*	Osteosarcoma	Sarcoma cell	103
393 T*	Osteosarcoma	Sarcoma cell	957
16 Hel	Embryonic lung	Fibroblastoid cell	255
377 Hel	Embryonic lung	Fibroblastoid cell	270
460 Hel	Embryonic lung	Fibroblastoid cell	284
141 S	Adult skin	Fibroblastoid cell	250
87 MG*	Glioma	Glioma cell	700
118 MG*	Glioma	Glioma cell	392
138 MG*	Glioma	Glioma cell	65
178 MG*	Glioma	Glioma cell	225
251 MG*	Glioma	Glioma cell	195
706 MG*	Glioma	Glioma cell	190
622 CG	Normal brain tissue	Glia cell	237
787 CG	Normal brain tissue	Glia cell	244
316 Nj	Kidney (embryonic)	Epithelial cell	53
143 Ne	Nephroblastoma	Nephroblastoma cell?	699
KB*	Carcinoma (oral)	Carcinoma cell	1190
HeLa*	Carcinoma (cervix)	Carcinoma cell	1190
T 24*	Carcinoma (urinary bladder)	Carcinoma cell	2150
RT 4*	Carcinoma (urinary bladder)	Carcinoma cell	2850

[a] The concentration is given for an initial number of 5×10^5 cells/ml; * denotes permanent lines. (Modified after NILSSON et al., 1974.)

$550 \, \text{ng}/5 \times 10^5$ cells/65 h; lymphoblastoid cell lines show a higher secretion rate than e.g. myeloma cell lines (NILSSON et al., 1974; HÜTTEROTH et al., 1973). Compared with short term culture biopsy cells and various malignant cells (Table 1), it would appear that Epstein-Barr virus infected cells (i.e. lymphoblastoid cell lines) are characterized by a higher rate of β2m secretion. A comparison between malignant and nonmalignant cell lines of mesenchymal or epithelial origin is given in Table 2. β2m has been shown to bear structural similarities to the constant region domains of IgG₁ heavy chains; however, no correlation between Ig synthesis and β2m secretion was found. The amount of β2m present on the cell surface was not correlated with the secretion rate and no correlation was detected between β2m secretion and cell proliferation (NILSSON et al., 1974).

3.2.3.

As mentioned above, indirect evidence, using β2m antibodies, points towards these antibodies having (1) a mitogenic effect (SOLHEIM and THORSBY, 1974), and (2) being able to inhibit lymphocyte activation in MLR (SOLHEIM and THORSBY, 1974; LINDBLOM et al., 1974; BACH et al., 1973), possibly by affecting the responding cells.

3.2.3.1.

The mitogenic effect of anti-β2m antibodies is presumed to result from stimulation of B-lymphocytes (SOLHEIM and THORSBY, 1974).

3.2.3.2.

Inhibition of the mixed lymphocyte reaction (MLR) is attributed to reactions with the subset of thymus derived (T-) cells involved in antigenic recognition (Responder T-cell) (SOLHEIM and THORSBY, 1974; LINDBLOM et al., 1974), whereas the effector T-cells in cell mediated lympholysis (CML) are not inhibited by anti-β2m (LIGHTBODY et al., 1974).

3.2.4.

Antigen redistribution on the cell surface ("capping") can be induced by antibodies (TAYLOR et al., 1971). This also renders the cells resistant to C'-dependent lysis when they are rechallenged with excess antibody (BERNOCO et al., 1972). The topography of HLA antigens on the cell surface has been investigated (BERNOCO et al., 1972; MAYR et al., 1973; NEAUPORT-SAUTES et al., 1972) in elegant studies using either fluorescein − or rhodamine − isothiocyanate conjugates of the appropriate antibodies (see 5.2.1.) Using this technique the relationship of β2m, Ig, and HLA molecules has been studied in various laboratories (POULIK et al., 1973; NEAUPORT-SAUTES et al., 1974; BISMUTH et al., 1974; SOLHEIM and THORSBY, 1974). HLA antigens were shown to "cocap" with β2m when the antiserum used in the first instance was anti-β2m, whereas, although some β2m aggregated in the HLA "cap", HLA antisera failed to induce the redistribution of all the β2m molecules present on the cell surface (Fig. 1). This shows that only part of the β2m molecules present on the cell surface are associated with HLA antigens.

The significance of this association in particular and of β2m in general remains an intriguing problem.

3.3. Ir-region in Man

Human studies of genetically controlled MHC associated immune responsiveness was prompted by the discovery in guinea pigs and mice that the ability to mount a specific immune response is under genetic control (BENACERRAF and McDEVITT, 1972); that this regulation of the immune response was linked to the major histocompatibility complex (McDEVITT et al., 1972) and that these immune response (Ir) genes map between the K- and D-regions of the MHC (see 4.1). As certain diseases (see 3.4 and Chapter 1) can be associated with a definite HLA specificity, then, because of the genetic association of immune response genes with the mouse MHC, one should also be able to define Ir-genes in man. The assumption, of course, is that susceptibility to a certain disease

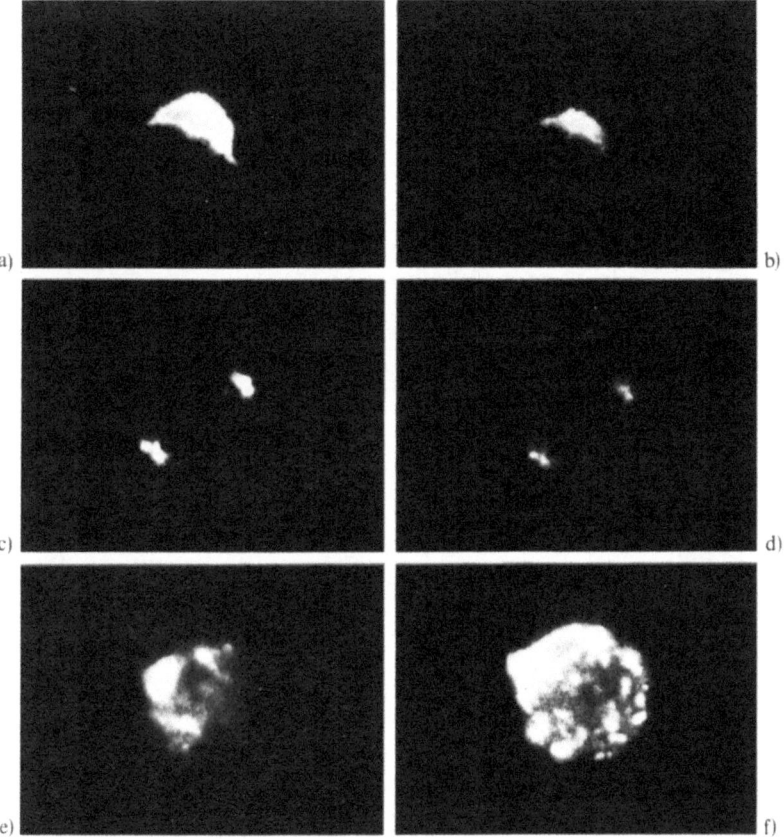

Fig. 1. Redistribution of β2-microglobulin and HLA antigens as shown by immunofluorescence. (a, b) Lymphocyte labeled with rabbit anti β2-m serum and FITC-conjugated goat anti-rabbit IgG, incubated at 37° C, and finally stained at 0° C with the TRITC-conjugated anti-β2-m. (a) Clusters of fluorescein anti-β2-m; (b) No rhodamine labeling (anti-β2-m) is seen outside green caps. (c, d) Lymphocyte labeled with rabbit anti-β2-m antiserum and FITC-conjugated goat anti-rabbit Ig, incubated at 37° C, and finally stained at 0° C, with the R anti-HLA conjugate. (c) Cap of fluorescein (anti-β2-m); (d) No rhodamine labeling (anti-HLA) found outside cap. (e, f) Lymphocyte labeled with anti-HLA serum and FITC-conjugated goat antihuman γ-chain, incubated at 37° C, and finally stained at 0° C with anti-β2-m antiserum and TRITC-conjugated goat anti-rabbit Ig. (e) Cap of fluorescein (anti-HLA); (f) Rhodamine labeling (anti-β2-m) is seen outside anti-HLA cap. (Taken from NEAUPORT-SAUTES et al., 1974.) FITC = fluorescein isothiocyanate (green); R = rhodamine (red); TRITC, tetramethyl-rhodamine-isothiocyanate

is associated with low immunologic responsiveness towards the etiologic agents responsible for the disease. In this respect, the level of IgE reaginic antibodies in human sera, the degree of ragweed skin sensitivity and the association with a given HLA haplotype have led to the demonstration and mapping of an "Ir E" locus in man (LEVINE et al., 1972; BLUMENTHAL et al., 1974; MARSH et al., 1974). An association between HLA-B7 (and its cross reacting group) and IgE and IgG antibody production to a low molecular weight ragweed pollen allergen (Ra5) has been demonstrated recently (MARSH et al., 1973).

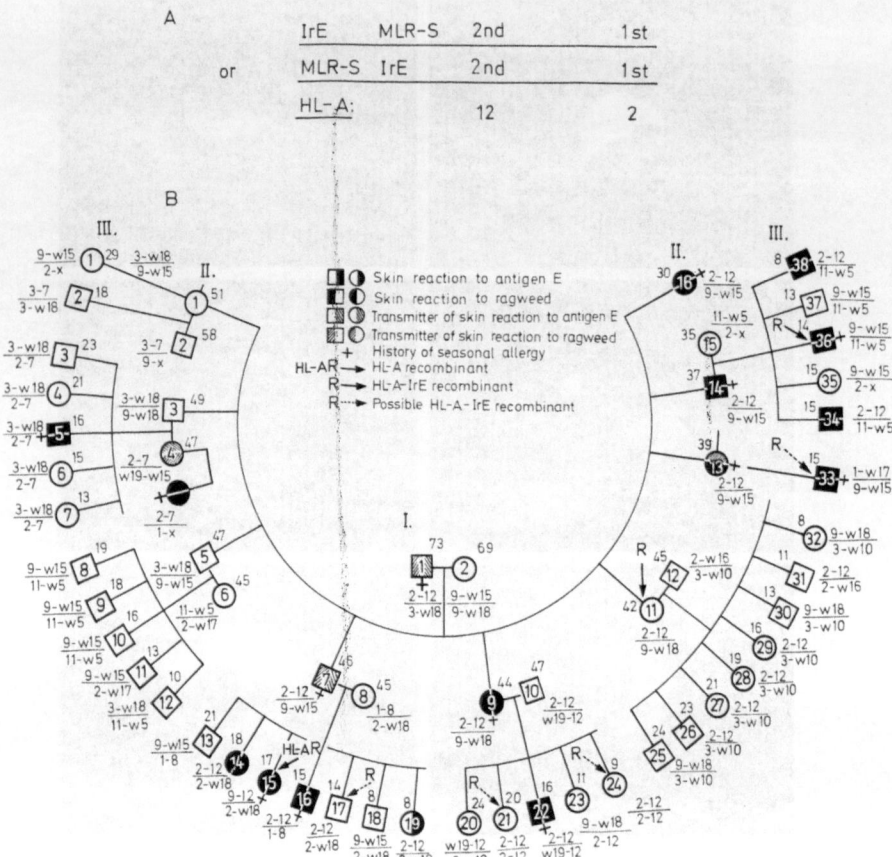

Fig. 2. Linkage of HLA haplotype and Ir E. (*A*) Tentative mapping of IrE locus. (*B*) Linkage in family B. Subjects are indicated by numbers (squares and circles), whereas superscripts give age of subjects. The HLA haplotype is given for each individual (2–12)/(2–12) (taken from BLUMEN-THAL *et al.*, 1974)

A further association (antigen E, ragweed skin sensitivity and HLA-A2; HLA-B12) led to a tentative mapping of the *Ir-E* locus in man on the left of the *B* locus (BLUMENTHAL *et al.*, 1974), i.e. between the centromere and the *B* locus. This is in contrast to the mouse MHC, where the *Ir* region maps between the *K* and *D* regions of the H-2 complex. (Fig. 2 and 4.1.1.).

3.4. Association of HLA with Disease (see also Chapter 1)

Studies in this sphere followed guidelines which also emerged from experiments in mice, where there were clear associations of some diseases with certain H-2 haplotypes, for example some inbred lines have particular susceptibilities to oncogenic viruses (MUHLBOCK and DUX, 1974). The association is not always simple; thus there are examples where an H-2 linked gene and some other autosomal gene in a different linkage group contribute to viral oncogenic susceptibility (LILLY, 1968). Study of H-2 congenic lines clarified some examples.

In any event, the HLA association with disease is a rapidly expanding field (DAUSSET et al., 1975). Associations extend from some which are very strong in the sense that an HLA haplotype may be almost diagnostic of the disease, or that virtually all sufferers from the disease show a particular HLA specificity (e.g., ankylosing spondylitis with HLA-B27, CAFFREY and JAMES, 1973). On the other hand there are situations were there is disagreement even on the statistical significance. The latter can have at least two obvious causes. (1) The disease has not been adequately defined; thus association with leukemia may not be obvious but association with a particular category of leukemia is clear. (2) Common HLA haplotypes in one ethnic group may be rare in or even missing from another. This is on record from one of the histocompatibility workshops (DAUSSET and COLOMBANI, 1973). For example in Bantu-speaking negroids in Zambia there is no HLA-A11, HLA-BW22 and HLA-B27 and while some "Caucasian type" specificities are much reduced (HLA-A1, A2, A3, B8), others are increased (BW7, AW19.3); there are also new antigens not recorded in Caucasians (Mo. MWA, A10, A3), (FESTENSTEIN et al., 1973a). East Bengalis living in London had no AW19.1, AW19.3, B14 and B18 (FESTENSTEIN, 1973b). Thus disease association with HLA type will be more complex than it might have been at first sight. We mean that, for example, the rather strong association of BW17 with psoriasis (SCHUNTER and SCHIEFERSTEIN, 1974), would not be found in an ethnic group lacking BW17, although the disease is found world-wide; in such a situation, psoriasis might be associated with some other genetic marker, if such exists, in some ethnic groups. This is a widespread phenomenon and reminds us of mouse demes which, even living in the same haystack, may be characterized by different (unique) "private" H-2 (K-D) antigenic specificities (KLEIN, 1971; 1973b).

There are two main possibilities to explain these phenomena at the immunologic level, (1) failure to respond to, or (2) high response with respect to some particular antigen, be it an etiologic agent, or a purely autoimmune situation.

For those who do not believe in a purely autoimmune situation (re-emergence of forbidden clone) then an altered "self" antigen due to viral or other presence intracellularly, but giving no overt disease, (or even giving overt disease), could be the antigen focused upon. In either case there are also two models still to choose from at the genetic level. (1) If the MHC is regarded as a continuum or spectrum of specificities, some having prominent epitopes leading to humoral immunity (mouse K and D, human B and A) others having poorly defined epitopes or differing little from self, and hence leading to cellular immunity (humoral and cellular have been visualized as opposite ends of a mutually exclusive spectrum (PARISH, 1973)), e.g. "I" region specificities, – then functionally all these genes could have much in common. The immune responsiveness related to MHC-disease associations could then actually "belong" to particular gene products (B27 to ankylosing spondylitis) or be merely associated (BW17 with psoriasis) because the appropriate true marker has not been recognized in the latter (has yet no alloantibody). (2) We could visualize the model where "H" and "I" gene products are functionally different; in that event MHC associated diseases will have weak or strong association merely through the closeness of genetic linkage between the HLA serologic marker and the "I" region gene which is responsible for the effect.

While many publications focus on each of the diseases so far studied, most authors agree to a strong association of some HLA antigen(s) with the following neoplastic conditions: acute lymphoblastic leukemia; chronic lymphocytic leukemia; Hodgkin's disease; multiple myeloma; retinoblastoma.

There are many statistically valid associations which are less strong. Among non-neoplastic conditions there are many strong associations e.g. as follows: celiac disease; myasthenia gravis; dermatitis herpetiformis; active chronic hepatitis; ankylosing spondylitis; Reiter's disease; as well as multiple sclerosis with DW2.

There are also some surprising discrepancies in this literature which we refer to through the review of DAUSSET et al. (1975).

4. Additional Information from Animal Studies

The mouse model has been and still is proving to be of paramount importance regarding genetics and biology of the MHC. As a point of fact, due to the establishment of strains differing at the H-2 complex only (congenic lines) and to recombination studies performed with these (inbred) animals the H-2 complex represents the best investigated stretch of any mammalian chromosome.

4.1. Genetics of the H-2 Complex

(For more extensive information on this topic we would like to refer to review articles by SNELL and STIMPFLING (1966); KLEIN and SHREFFLER (1971); SNELL et al. (1973); DEMANT (1973); KLEIN (1974), and SHREFFLER and DAVID (1975); the latter reference contains the most comprehensive information available so far on Ia-antigens.)

Like HLA, the *H-2* complex contains two segregant series, K and D, which code for the classical H-2 antigens. The *H-2* complex is located on the 17th chromosome. Increasingly complex *H-2* maps emerged from the genetic localization of a mouse serum protein (Ss) in the *H-2* complex (PASSMORE and SHREFFLER, 1970); the mapping of genes which regulate the immune response to different antigens at the *K-end* of the mouse MHC (McDEVITT et al., 1972); the findings that the resistance to RNA tumor viruses is *H-2* linked (LILLY, 1966) and the identification of a new type of antigen associated with the *I* region of the MHC (Ia antigens) (DAVID et al., 1973b). These discoveries were illuminated by extensive recombination studies carried out mainly in the laboratories of George D. Snell, Jackson Laboratories, Bar Harbor, Maine, and Donald C. Shreffler, University of Michigan, Ann Arbor, and led to the definition of four main regions and their subregions. These have been shown to control

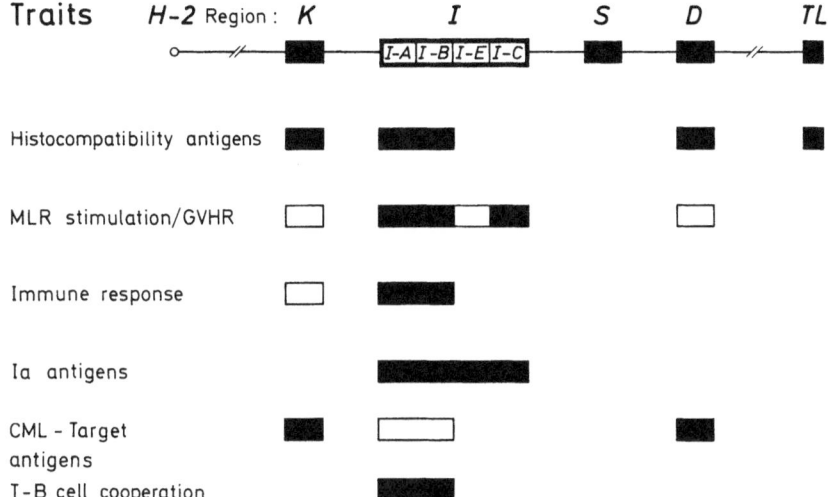

Fig. 3. The genetic map of the H-2 complex. Traits and functions associated with different regions and subregions. The S-region controls level of an α_2-serum protein as well as C' levels in different strains. Open squares indicate preliminary evidence. (Modified after SHREFFLER and DAVID, 1975.)
TL-region controls alloantigens found in some thymus leukemias (BOYSE *et al.*, 1968)

serologically detectable antigens (H-2 and Ia) as well as different traits and functions related to and of importance for basic immunologic phenomena. These are shown in Fig. 3. Thus, the classical H-2 genes seem to control cell surface components serving as targets in transplant rejection and cell mediated lysis, whereas I-region genes code for membrane structures responsible for sensitization, antigen recognition, and cellular interaction (see below).

The fine structure of the K- and D- (or B and A) regions has not yet been elucidated. Only biochemical data, not yet available, will reveal whether K- and D- (or B and A) are single loci and thus controlling a system of multiple alleles or whether K- and D- (or B and A) are complex multigenic regions composed of duplicated genes. The latter possibility could account for the unprecedented genetic polymorphism of the $H-2$ (HLA) system. As cautiously pointed out by SHREFFLER and KLEIN (1970) the 0.5 map units of the $H-2$ complex would encompass some 500–600 genes, each of which could code for proteins with an average molecular weight of about 35,000, assuming that the DNA is all functional. Similar figures were deduced for the HLA region by BODMER (1972). Studies carried out in wild mouse populations further emphasized the extent of the H-2 polymorphism, since, in a relatively small sample of wild mice from a restricted area, at least 30 different H-2 chromosomes were identified compared to the 11 chromosomes which had been defined in inbred animals (KLEIN, 1974). This resembles, of course, the "outbred" situation encountered in man. One of the major recent achievements in the H-2 field is the production (genetic engineering) by SHREFFLER and DAVID of I-congenic mice, i.e. animals which are identical for the K- and/or D-regions but differ at either the whole I-region or for one or more of its subregions. These animals are invaluable for studies concerning the functional dichotomy (first described in man) (Yunis and Amos, 1971; Eijsvoogel *et al.*, 1973a; Schendel and Bach, 1974), according to which in in vivo as well as in vitro systems, membrane structures controlled by *I*-region genes have a predominant role in sensitization, whereas gene products of the *K*- and *D*-regions are the primary targets in cell destruction (see 4.1.2. and 4.2.).

4.1.1. H-2 Genetics

4.1.1.1. Alloantigens Controlled by the K- and D-regions

As pointed out by Snell *et al.* (1973) and Klein and Shreffler (1971), classic H-2 antigens are controlled by two chromosomal regions (*K*- and *D*-) separated by about 0.5cM. In a homozygous haplotype (e.g. *H-2^d* or *H-2^k*) each region i.e. *K*- or *D*-, codes for an antigenic determinant *specific* for this inbred strain and therefore called "private" (Fig. 4). The private K^d determinant, for instance, is H-2.31, whereas the private D^d specificity is H-2.4; i.e. D4 *and* K31 occur only in H-2^d mice; whereas D4 *or* K31 will characterize a recombinant animal. Thus K23/D4 is a recombinant haplotype between an *H-2K^k* and *H-2D^d* mouse (see Fig. 4). This particular recombinant is called *H-2^a*. An F$_1$ hybrid, e.g. (*H-2^d* × *H-2^k*) on the other hand, will have the following haplotype: K^{k}23;D^{k}32/ K^{d}31; D^{d}4.

Furthermore, each of the four private specificities will be expressed on the cell surface, i.e. H-2 antigens are inherited in a *codominant* fashion (Cullen *et al.*, 1972). The private specificities are most probably true alleles. Less clear, in genetic and structural terms, is the picture regarding the "public" specificities, i.e. those antigenic determinants which *do not* characterize a particular haplotype, since they are shared by different inbred strains (not shown in Figure 4 below). To complicate the picture, some public determinants are not even specific for the *K*- or *D*-region, since e.g. 1,3 and 28 can be present in *both* regions of the H-2 complex. This led Shreffler *et al.* (1971) to propose a duplication

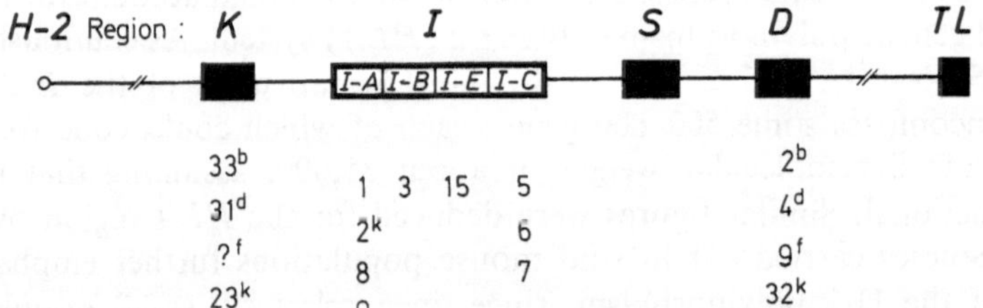

Fig. 4. Simplified chart of the H-2 complex. The K- and D-region antigens shown represent "private" specificities of a given hyplotype (*b, d, f*, etc.). Arrows indicate I-region alloantigens not yet mapped conclusively: Ia4, for instance, could map in *I-A, I-B* or *I-E*. The haplotype superscript (Ia4^s) indicates antigens *so far* restricted to this particular haplotype

model, assuming that these *serologic* data also reflect *structural* phenomena. It is worth mentioning that the wild mice analyzed so far by KLEIN (1972, 1974) share, as one might expect, some public determinants (or "supertypic" specificities as they have been called by CEPPELLINI (1973) in the HLA system); each deme however, possesses a new private antigen.

A functional dichotomy is emerging from data indicating that in in vitro systems effector cells will only recognize private differences (FORMAN and MÖLLER, 1974; BRONDZ et al., 1975), whereas in in vivo systems graft rejection has also been demonstrated across public H-2 barriers (KLEIN and MURPHY, 1973) (see 4.2).

4.1.1.2. Antigens Controlled by the I-Region

(It should be pointed out that *I*-region *associated* antigens (Ia) have not been shown to be identical with receptors involved in antigen recognition and/or regulation of the immune response.)

The Ia antigen system is also characterized by a marked genetic polymorphism as shown in Figure 4 above. The generation of new recombinants established the existence of four *I*-subregions (*I-A, I-B, I-E, I-C*) coding for different specificities. Ir-genes have, so far, been allotted only to *I-A* and *I-B* subregions. *I-C*, on the other hand, seems to code for Ia-antigens predominantly present on thymus derived (T-) cells, whereas the other specificities are mainly B-cell antigens (LONAI and McDEVITT, 1974a; SHREFFLER and DAVID, 1975; FRELINGER et al., 1974). Thus in contrast to H-2 antigens, Ia-antigens are not detectable on all cells. For instance, recent data (not yet confirmed) would suggest that different T-cell populations can be classified according to the presence or absence of Ia-antigens on the cell surface (LONAI, personal communication). Preliminary data about the tissue distribution of these antigens (DAVID et al., 1973; HAUPT-FELD, HAUPTFELD and KLEIN, 1974) suggest a possible role for Ia-antigens in cell differentiation from their presence on all cells of the cleavage stage embryo (McDEVITT et al., 1974).

A possible role for Ia-antigens in cell proliferation will be described below (see 4.1.2. and 4.2.).

4.1.2. In Vitro Studies

The events taking place when two cell types, which belong to different H-2 haplotypes, are cultured together (mixed lymphocyte reaction or MLR) are considered the in vitro correlates of the mechanisms leading to sensitization for allograft rejection.

4.1.2.1.

The MLR is controlled by the major histocompatibility complex (DUTTON, 1966). As early as 1968 however, AMOS and BACH (1968) suggested that, in man, in addition to H-loci, other genetic differences were responsible for a proliferative response in MLR. Later, reports by RYCHLIKOVA et al. (1971), showed that the transformation of allogeneic mouse lymphocytes could easily be induced in vitro in K-end incompatible combinations, whereas D-end differences had little or no effect in MLR. These results were later confirmed, and the strong activation observed in K-end incompatible animals was shown to be associated not with K-region itself, but with I-region differences since recombinants differing at the K- (or D-) region only were weakly stimulatory (or not at all) (WIDMER et al., 1973[2]). On similar lines are results showing that a graft versus host (g.v.h.) reaction (see 4.1.3.) can occur in strain combinations which are identical for the SD determinants and will therefore accept each others skin grafts permanently (LIVNAT et al., 1973). With regard to the genetic control of allograft rejection this situation already suggested that its in vitro correlates — (the MLR corresponding to the sensitization or recognition phase, whereas the cell mediated lympholysis (CML[3]) resembles the rejection phase) — seemed to involve different genetic loci and therefore possibly separate membrane structures. This was born out by the fact that SD-differences, although known to lead to graft rejection (see 4.1.3.), were apparently not necessary to elicit cell proliferation or transformation (WIDMER et al., 1973).

This functional dichotomy was first demonstrated in man in elegant studies by EIJSVOOGEL et al. (1973a). These data provided suggestive evidence for a distinct genetic control of lymphocyte activating and CML target antigens. Since then this has been clearly demonstrated in the mouse.

4.1.2.2. Genetic Control of MLR and CML

a) MEO et al. (1975) have shown that anti-Ia sera added to mixed lymphocyte cultures will block the stimulating cell, and thus prevent responder cell proliferation. Similar observations have been reported from several laboratories (Table 3). MEO et al. (1975) however, devised an experiment, outlined below, which strongly suggests that Ia-antigens or closely related products are involved in MLR stimulation: in a MLR, cells of genotype A will respond to cells of genotype B (stimulating cell) when A and B differ only for Ia-antigens and are identical at the K- and D-regions of the MHC. An anti-B (Ia) serum will, as mentioned above, inhibit the stimulation (whereas an anti-A (Ia) serum will *not* block proliferation). These results were further substantiated when the same responder (A) was used in a MLR involving (AxB)F$_1$ cells as stimulator. Anti-B (Ia) still inhibited stimulation, whereas anti-A (Ia) had no effect (the same applied to reciprocal cells and antisera). Furthermore, antisera directed against the K- or D-region products failed to inhibit stimulation (or proliferation). In turn, these experiments also imply that Ia-antigens must be present on T-cells since purified T-cells will also stimulate in MLR (FRELINGER et al., 1974; LONAI and MCDEVITT, 1974a; DAVIES and HESS, 1974; HESS and DAVIES, 1975).

b) In a three cell experiment (Table 4), based on EIJSVOOGEL's data mentioned above, SCHENDEL and BACH (1974) provided direct evidence for the separate

---

[2] At that time these I region antigenic differences were not detectable serologically and were therefore termed LD (=lymphocyte-defined) antigens in contrast to the serologically detectable (SD) H-2 K+D antigens, (BACH et al., 1972).

[3] See CEROTTINI and BRUNNER (1974).

Table 3. Roles and functions attributed to Ia-antigens or antisera

MLC-CML:	Stimulation by Ia antigens; H-2 antigens as target for effector T-cells	SCHENDEL and BACH, 1974
	Ia antibodies inhibit stimulation	MEO et al., 1975; FATHMAN and SACHS, pers. commun.
	All Ia-regions involved in stimulation	LONAI and McDEVITT, pers. commun. FISH et al., pers. commun.
	Inhibition even in the absence of complete blocking by Ia antibodies	MEO et al., 1975
Immune response:	1° Inhibited by Ia-antibodies	FRELINGER et al., 1975
	2° Inhibited by (K + I)-region antibodies	PIERCE et al., 1974
	Inhibited by Ia antibodies	FRELINGER et al., 1975
Generation of Killer T-cells:	Ia differences essential in 1° response	WAGNER, pers. commun.
	Killer T-cells devoid of detectable Ia Ag.	LONAI, pers. commun.
Soluble mediators:	Antigen specific factor blocked by (K + I) as	TAUSSIG and MUNRO, 1974
	Controlled by I-A or I-B subregion	MUNRO et al., 1974
	Nonspecific factor removed by Ia antisera	ARMERDING et al., 1974
T-B cell cooperation:	(K + I)-region identity necessary	KATZ et al., 1973
	Controlled by I-A or I-B subregion	KATZ et al., 1975
Ir-gene Effect:	In vitro response in high responders Inhibited by H-2 antisera	LONAI and McDEVITT, 1974b
Enhancement:	Ia antibodies enhance hemizygous heart grafts	DAVIES and ALKINS, 1974
	Ia antibodies enhance incompatible skin grafts	STAINES et al., 1974
No role in:	Antigen binding to T- or B-cells	HAMMERLING and McDEVITT, 1974a, b
	Blocking responder cell	see "MLC-CML"
	CML-target	NABHOLZ et al., 1974

MLC = Mixed lymphocyte culture.
CML = Cell mediated lysis.
1° and 2° immune response refers to inhibition of IgM or IgG production by plaque-forming cells.

genetic control of MLR and CML, since only the combination involving *I*-plus *D*-region differences were effective in generating killer T-cell activity. These data confirm the observations reported above (RYCHLIKOVA *et al.*, 1971) in as much as LD *plus* SD differences i.e. "K-end" in this particular case, were necessary to obtain CML. An *I*-region difference alone resulted in marked proliferation, whereas neither MLR nor CML was achieved when the only

Table 4. Genetic control of cell mediated lympholysis

Responder	Stimulator			Difference	MLC	CML
	q	k	d	I-region	+ + +	−
q q d	q	q	q	D-region	−	±
	q	k	d	I + D-region	+ + +	+ + +
	q	q	q			

The three letters in the first 2 columns stand for K-, I-, and D-regions of the MHC, in that order. The allogeneic differences existing between responder and stimulator are emphasized and listed along corresponding lines. (Modified after SCHENDEL and BACH, 1974.)

difference was in the *H-2D* region. Furthermore, these results clearly demonstrate that (1) a stimulation is possible in H-2 D + K identical cells; (2) the target in CML can be identical to the responder cell with regard to the *I*-region without affecting the outcome, and (3) LD and SD determinants can be present on different cells and still provide effective generation of killer T-cells.

c) NABHOLZ *et al.* (1974), also showed that specific killer activity was directed against *K* or *D*-region antigens, whereas no significant killing was observed in cell combinations involving strains differing at the *I*-region only. Effector cell activity could not be blocked by anti H-2 sera directed against H-2 determinants of the killer cell (showing that H-2 itself is not the recognizing molecule in CML), whereas specific inhibition of killer cell activity was observed when *K*-(or *D*-) end antigens of the target cell were blocked by the appropriate anti-H-2 reagents (showing that H-2 or closely related structures on the cell surface are the CML target). Killer cells directed against H-2K-or D- determinants were removed by macrophages carrying these determinants (BRONDZ *et al.*, 1975), showing that specific effector cell receptors react with H-2 or closely related antigens on the surface of the target cells. No dissociation between H-2 determinants and CML-specificities has been observed so far. The question still remains, however, as to whether CML and H-2 determinants represent identical structures or different antigenic determinants on the same H-2 molecule, or even different molecules.

4.1.2.3.

New light has been shed on this aspect of the problem by reports from two laboratories which would indicate that killer T-cells generated in MLR will selectively react with the private specificity of the target cell (FORMAN and MÖLLER, 1974; BRONDZ *et al.*, 1975). As a point of fact T-cells will not even recognize public H-2 specificities, since macrophages sharing these specificities (but not the private antigen) with the original stimulating cell will not remove the specific killer cell (BRONDZ *et al.*, 1975). This point is of some importance because some public and private specificities reside on the same molecules (see 5.4.4.). The problem of molecular representation, therefore, does not concern the whole H-2 molecule, but an antigenic determinant closely associated or identical with the immunodominant private specificity.

4.1.3. In Vivo Studies

In vivo data from animal experiments necessarily form part of other sections of this chapter. Here we collect some data we cannot afford to overlook and which are not easily obtained from studies in man. While very many papers in the literature describe experiments using organs, tissues, or whole cell suspensions, and refer to these as "antigen", we would discourage this misusage because such material is truly a *source* of antigen and usually a source of many different antigens. We use "antigen" to mean some material, less than whole cell membranes and preferably at least to some extent purified. The former, in any case, constitutes the bulk of general transplantation biology, a subject which is at once vast, dealt with in many reviews of its different aspects (LENGEROVA, 1969; BILLINGHAM and SILVERS, 1971), and still unrewarding in its practical outcome from the clinical point of view. The early and inappropriate use of the prefixes homo- and hetero- (e.g. homograft) was put in order by GORER (1960) and SNELL (1964), providing the terms auto- (e.g. autograft), allo- (e.g. allogeneic), syn- (e.g. syngeneic), xeno- (=hetero-, e.g. xenogeneic) and the derived terminology.

In their simplest form the rules of transplantation are illustrated by considering inbred animals of one genotype, P1 (first parental line) and of another genotype P2 (second parental line) and their first generation (F1) hybrids. Transplants behave thus:

1. P1 to P2,   rejected, incompatible.
2. P2 to P1   rejected, incompatible.
3. P1 (or P2) to F1,   accepted, no foreignness.
4. F1 to P1 (or P2)   rejected by foreignness of antigens
                       inherited from the other parent (see also Fig. 5).

These are the gross expectations for a tissue transplant in respect to the host versus graft component.

Situation 3 shows that if the graft is one composed of immunologically competent cells (I.C.C.), then these cells react against the foreignness of the host (derived from the other parent) to highlight the graft-versus-host (g.v.h.) reaction (SIMONSEN, 1962). This constitutes the basic problem in bone marrow transfusion. A g.v.h. component inevitably forms part of situations 1, 2 and 4 due to "passenger" leukocytes in tissue transplants but is most frequently obscured.

G.v.h. reactions between mice related allogeneically is lethal in newborn recipients, which are immunologically incompetent. There is rarely a lethal outcome in the parent to F1 model, which we must presume is due to some reverse immunologic reaction on the part of the animal to the supposedly "compatible" graft. This may be accounted for by the only foreignness one can visualize as present on P1-I.C.C. and absent from F1-I.C.C., that is the molecule by means of which P1 recognizes P2; whatever that molecule is, it is clearly absent from the F1 hybrid. This may be the idiotype of the alloantibody which P1 is able to make against P2, and hence the aliotype or anti-receptor site (Anti-RS). Such antisera as can be raised in F1 hybrid mice by immunization

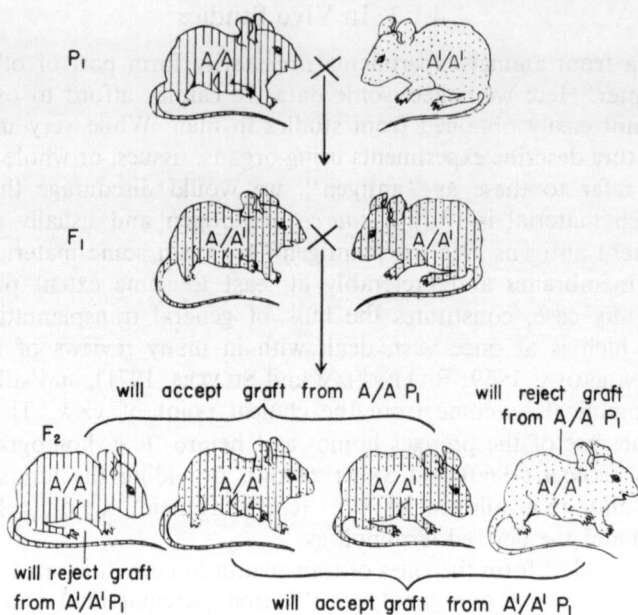

will accept graft from A/A P_1 will reject graft
                                          from A/A P_1

will reject graft
from A^1/A^1 P_1 will accept graft from A^1/A^1 P_1

Fig. 5. Transplantation rules. If parental strain (P_1) animals differ at only a single histocompatibility locus, one being of genotype A/A and the other of genotype A'/A', then four possible genetic combinations, two of which produce similar offspring, can occur in animals of the second generation (F_2). Thus, three out of four animals of F_2 generation will posses at least one specific histocompatibility gene from one of the P_1 grandparents and, consequently, will tolerate a skin graft taken from any member of inbred strain to which that grandparent happens to belong. One of four members of F_2 population will reject grafts from this strain since it has not received a histocompatibility allele from it. The same situation holds true for grafts taken from the other P_1 strain. Regardless of number of genes by which any P_1 pair differs, all first-generation (F_1) offsprings will accept a graft donated by member of either P_1 inbred strain (taken from Billingham and Silvers, 1971)

with parental strain cells do have the ability to delay the rejection of skin grafts between the parental lines (P2 to P1) although the specificity of the reaction is not clarified (Davies, 1971). The subject has been reviewed by Ramseier and Lindenmann (1972).

The distribution of H-2 antigens will be briefly mentioned and it should be noted that data from absorption methods should be assessed with care because they predate the discovery of anti-I region antibodies, which are present in many (most?) typing sera. H-2 antigens appear at different times in tissues in the embryo (Möller, G., 1963; Möller, E., 1965). They are present on most, perhaps all, adult cells, most on lymphocytes, possibly least in muscle; they are present on sperm but haploid expression is not likely although the situation is confused by H-2 antigen in seminal plasma (Vojtíšková et al., 1969). Expression on the cell surface of leukocytes changes in the course of the cell cycle (Cikes, 1970) and regenerates in much less than the division time, viz. about 6 h, if it is removed enzymically from the cell surface without otherwise damaging the cells (SCHWARTZ and NATHENSON, 1971 b). H-2 and HLA antigens coexist on man-mouse hybrid cells.

It is clear that the biological consequence of H-2 expression cannot easily be predicted. While inability to induce transplantation immunity (to hasten graft rejection) using rodent red cells is clear, this can now be attributed to lack of Ia antigen (DAVIES and ALKINS, 1974). No such simple explanation provides for the long-term phenomenon that liver extracts do not sensitize in the same way as those from spleen cells. Liver, however, is an effective source of H-2 antigen for serum-antibody clearance (MANDEL et al., 1965; NI-MELSTEIN et al., 1973). It does not absorb out Ia antibodies (DAVIES, 1975), which could account for the non-sensitizing capacity of liver (CALNE, 1973) but the ability of liver to abrogate the sensitizing capacity of spleen derived antigen could be enzymic destruction of I antigen. Presence of H-2 antigen in brain cannot be demonstrated serologically, which led to early suggestions of its absence from that tissue; the antigen was demonstrated by the capacity of brain to sensitize for hastened rejection of skin grafts between appropriate H-2 congenic strains of mice (BARNES, 1964). Neoplastic cells generally possess 'H' antigens and obey transplantation rules; there are many exceptions to these generalizations which cannot be dealt with here. Intracellular distribution has been extensively studied and the rather simple outcome is that 'H' antigens are surface expressed, but there may be more material in a membrane than can readily be measured as exposed on the surface. There is no 'H' antigen on internal membranes, except the nuclear membrane (ALBERT and DAVIES, 1973) and little (or none) can be detected in cytoplasm.

While liver, perhaps because of its paucity of Ia antigen (lymphocyte activating property) may be regarded as a privileged tissue there are certain classical privileged sites and situations, e.g. the cheek pouch of the hamster, from which transplants are not rejected. The cornea, not being vascularized, usually accepts corneal allografts, but there is a significant level of immunologic rejection nevertheless. The fetus, viewed as a privileged allograft, has been the subject of many reviews (EDWARDS et al., 1975).

Histocompatibility (H) alloantibody will not, at least when acting alone, lead to rejection of an allograft; on the contrary such an outcome is confined to elicitation of a cellular immunity. There are situations where antibody will cause graft destruction but these are exceptional and generally concern xenografts, e.g. rat skin on immunosuppressed mice (WINN et al., 1973). Hence we may anticipate that isolated and purified H antigens may have different properties when given parenterally in vivo and depending on the conditions of the experiment. Firstly, H antigen injected into mice will hasten the rejection of skin grafts (GRAFF and NATHENSON, 1971), if injection schedules favor a cellular response. Secondly, H antigen injected into mice will prolong graft survival (a) if it is used in conjunction with some other immunosuppressive treatment such as irradiation (ROSENBERG et al., 1971) or drugs (HALLE-PANNEN-KO et al., 1971 a), or (b) if it is injected long enough before grafting (about 2 weeks) and in such a way as to encourage a *humoral* response (e.g. BRENT and PINTO, 1974) and using some accessory agent in the case of skin grafts. We can allocate this to active enhancement (see 4.3.1.2.).

It is possible that the category (a) above is true tolerance but one which, for some reason, cannot be achieved with antigen alone. Many experiments have aimed at tolerance induction directly by treatment with soluble H antigen, e.g.: groups of mice were maintained at in vivo molarities of 10^{-8} to 10^{-14} with respect to H antigen by daily injections of antigen for up to 3 months without affecting rejection time of allografts (unpublished observations). By contrast, such treatment, or even quite short courses of soluble antigen injections will suppress the *humoral* alloantibody response to H-2 antigens. This may be "true" tolerance, but if so, it is 'B' cell tolerance and not 'T' cell tolerance. Whatever its basis, it has no clinical usefulness at the present time (see also LAW *et al.*, 1974).

H-2 antigen pretreatment is claimed to prevent g.v.h. reactivity (HALLE-PAN-NENKO *et al.*, 1971 b). Antigen-antibody complexes will suppress graft rejection when tested in a rat kidney allograft model (STUART *et al.*, 1970). In general, i.e. with no special interfering factors, H-2 antigens are immunogenic in allogeneically related individuals to give circulating alloantibody. More purified soluble preparations are less immunogenic than whole cells. We should now be cautious to recall that most 'H' antigen preparations which were used in the past can now be seen to be mixtures of H and Ia-antigen and that many experimental results will have been confused by this fact. The immunogenicity of H + I soluble antigens might, in retrospect, be an anti-Ia response (e.g. NATHENSON and DAV-IES, 1966), especially where solubilization was carried out by some method other than papain treatment (e.g. autolysis or KCl). The physical separation of H from I antigens is referred to in section 5.6.

4.2. *I*-region Traits and Functions

Although the implications of the data given above will be discussed in Section 6, we feel that a few remarks about *I*-region associated functions are justified here.

Table 3 is a summary of the different roles attributed to Ia-antigens or their antibodies and it would seem at first glance, that virtually the whole field of cellular and humoral immunity is governed by this region of the *H-2* complex. This is particularly relevant (1) to responder cell stimulation in the mixed lymphocyte reaction (MLR), (2) to cell cooperation and mediation of cooperation by soluble factors, (3) to the (genetic) control of the immune response and (4) to enhancement of allografts (see 4.3.).

4.2.1.

It is now generally accepted that cell cooperation (involving T-cells, B-cells, and macrophages) is a prerequisite to antibody formation (MILLER and MITCH-ELL, 1969; MITCHISON *et al.*, 1970; RAFF, 1973; FELDMAN *et al.*, 1975). Early reports, confirmed by various different methods, suggest the involvement, in cell cooperation, of soluble mediators released by T-cells and, moreover, able to replace T-cells under appropriate conditions (KATZ and BENACERRAF, 1972; SCHIMPL and WECKER, 1972; TAUSSIG, 1974; DUTTON, 1974). Some of these factors are claimed to be antigen specific (TAUSSIG and MUNRO, 1974; MUNRO *et al.*, 1974; FELDMAN *et al.*, 1973; TAUSSIG *et al.*, 1974) while others are not (ARMERDING and KATZ, 1974). The importance which attaches to *H-2* gene products is best documented by the fact that physiologic T-B cell cooperation (KATZ *et al.*, 1973; KATZ *et al.*, 1975), as well as the action of the factors mentioned previously, can be specifically inhibited by anti Ia sera directed against *I-A* or *I-B* gene products (ARMERDING *et al.*, 1974; MUNRO *et al.*, 1974; FELDMAN personal communication) implying that both phenomena are *H-2* associated, i.e. controlled or generated by cell surface components coded for by *I*-genes of the MHC.

It would be very surprising, in the light of the homology of H-systems among different species, if dissimilar genetic functions would apply to man.

4.2.2.

The *I-A* and *I-B* subregions are, in fact, the subregions in which the *Ir*-genes so far identified have been mapped (MCDEVITT *et al.*, 1972; SHREFFLER and DAVID, 1975). This genetic association does not imply that the gene products involved are necessarily identical. This restriction applies also to the phenomena briefly discussed above. Antibodies, however, directed against such products might be "masked" by Ia-antibodies in anti-Ia-sera in the same way as Ia-antibodies were shown to be masked by H-2 antibodies in anti-"H-2" reagents (DAVID and SHREFFLER, 1974; DAVIES and HESS, 1974; HESS and DAVIES, 1975; STAINES *et al.*, 1974; ARCHER *et al.*, 1974). It is therefore not surprising—and raises some expectations regarding the characterization of these Ir-gene receptors—that different laboratories were able to show (Table 3) that H-2 antisera do indeed inhibit the in vitro response against a synthetic antigen (or red blood cells) in animals which otherwise mount a normal humoral response against this particular antigen (high responders) (PIERCE *et al.*, 1974; LONAI and MCDEVITT, 1974b; MCDEVITT *et al.*, 1974; FRELINGER *et al.*, 1975). The situation is complicated by preliminary results indicating that antigen binding to *presensitized* T- or B-cells is not inhibited by anti-Ia-sera (HÄMMERLING and MCDEVITT, 1974a), whereas antisera against K- or D-region antibodies will block antigen binding (HÄMMERLING and MCDEVITT, 1974b). These data make it rather difficult to envisage a simple mechanism for the mode of action of *Ir*-gene (*I-A* or *I-B*) products present (on T-cells) as receptors which control the immune response to synthetic antigens (MCDEVITT *et al.*, 1974). A more complex situation with regard to the regulatory function of *Ir*-genes is evidenced by two observations: (1) that I-region genes might influence or be influenced by other *Ir*-genes not closely linked to *H-2* (ZALESKY and KLEIN, 1974; ZALESKY personal communication), and (2) that a "lesion of cooperation" rather than direct genetic control could be the defect in genetic nonresponders (FELDMAN *et al.*, 1975). (For a discussion of the hapten-carrier function not mentioned in this paragraph see MITCHISON *et al.* (1970) and BENACERRAF and MCDEVITT (1972)).

4.3. Donor Specific Prolongation of Transplant Survival

4.3.1.

The primary expectation from animal studies in the field of transplantation biochemistry and immunogenetics was to provide a practical means for suppressing the immune response to the chosen donor, leaving a patient's immune capacity otherwise unimpaired. Only in this way can we visualize overcoming the disadvantages of the treatment now in use (synthetic immunosuppressive drugs and antithymocyte globulin) which, useful though they may be, leave patients with greatly reduced protection against infection because of the nonspecific mode of their action. Whereas an enormous new subject of transplantation biology has grown up in the last two decades, this expectation has perhaps only just been realized.

4.3.1.1. Passive Enhancement

Immunologic enhancement got its name from the ability of an alloantiserum, raised in an animal of one inbred strain (A) against one of another (B), to allow a strain B tumor to grow in and kill a mouse of strain A (FLEXNER and JOBLING, 1907; KALISS, 1958). Normally a strain A mouse would reject a strain B tumor in the same way as it would reject any other allograft (Fig. 6).

The full power of this method might have been appreciated sooner, but for its limited efficacy in prolonging mouse skin grafts. The skin is, of all tissues, "difficult" to maintain as a transplant, perhaps affected by more H loci and by its content of immunologically competent cells as evidenced by the local immunity which can be mounted by skin tissue.

It was not until inbred rats became available, and methods for rat kidney grafting, that the great potential of enhancement became clear for specific kidney transplant prolongation (ENOMOTO and LUCAS, 1973); there was minimal effect on skin, even in the same recipients from the same donor (MULLEN et al., 1973). It is true that hemizygous transplants (example F1 to parent) are normally used to obtain good results, but this in any case corresponds to a 2/4 mismatch in human terms. In spite of all this, the theories proposed to account for enhancement extend from peripheral to afferent to central to efferent, and none, nor is any combination fully in accord with the available data (FRENCH and BATCHELOR, 1972; CRUSE et al., 1974). This problem now seems to have been resolved by questioning the validity of the rules, in particular the specificity of the enhancing serum. It was assumed that ordinary "cytotoxic" Ag-B (rat, corresponding to H-2 and HLA) typing serum antibody was responsible for enhancement. This was, indeed, the only antibody then known to be present. The following experiment showed the defect in this assumption and provides an explanation that is as practically useful as it is conceptionally satisfactory.

Alloantisera elicited by conventional spleen cell injections between two inbred strains of rat, Wag and Agus, which differ at their MHC, administered in 6×1 ml amounts over the first 9 days were able to enhance, for the lifetime of the animals, auxiliary heart transplants sewn in abdominally, aorta to aorta

ACTIVE   ENHANCEMENT

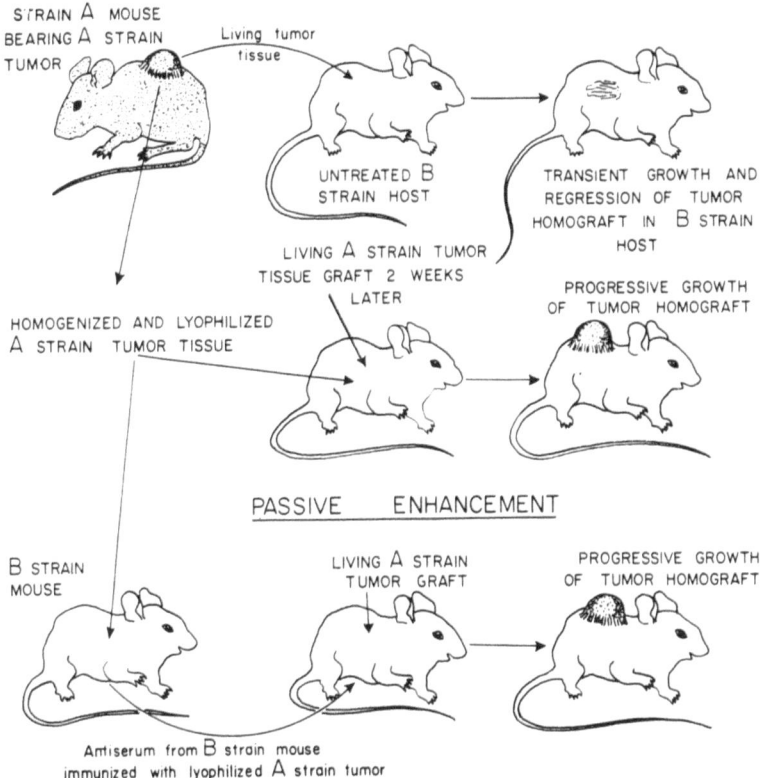

STRAIN A MOUSE
BEARING A STRAIN
TUMOR

Living tumor
tissue

UNTREATED B
STRAIN HOST

TRANSIENT GROWTH AND
REGRESSION OF TUMOR
HOMOGRAFT IN B STRAIN
HOST

LIVING A STRAIN TUMOR
TISSUE GRAFT 2 WEEKS
LATER

PROGRESSIVE GROWTH
OF TUMOR HOMOGRAFT

HOMOGENIZED AND LYOPHILIZED
A STRAIN TUMOR TISSUE

PASSIVE   ENHANCEMENT

B STRAIN
MOUSE

LIVING A STRAIN
TUMOR GRAFT

PROGRESSIVE GROWTH
OF TUMOR HOMOGRAFT

Antiserum from B strain mouse
immunized with lyophilized A strain tumor

Fig. 6. Passive and active enhancement. In active enhancement, a tumor of *A* strain origin is removed, homogenized, and freeze-dried. The material is reconstituted in distilled water and inoculated into a *B* strain host. If untreated, the host would normally reject a challenge graft of *A* strain tumor tissue. However, as a result of pretreatment, *B* strain mouse sustains growth of tumor homograft inoculated two weeks later. In passive enhancement, lyophilized strain *A* tumor tissue is first inoculated into *B* strain host. This animal is bled two weeks later and its antiserum injected into a second strain *B* host, which will now accept an allograft from the *A* strain tumor (taken from BILLINGHAM and SILVERS, 1971)

and pulmonary artery to posterior vena-cava (DAVIES and ALKINS, 1974). The transplants were (Wag×Agus)F_1 to Agus recipients, using anti-Wag serum. When the cytotoxic alloantibodies (Ag-B=H-1) were completely removed from these sera by repeated absorption with Wag red cells or platelets, the enhancing capacity was not diminished. This kind of absorbing material was chosen for its expression of the serologic determinants of the MHC and for its lack of expression of "I" associated traits, as shown, for example, by failure to participate in mixed lymphocyte reactions (MLR). Whereas all enhancing activity could be removed by absorption with *donor* strain lymphocytes, it was not impared by similar absorption with *recipient* lymphocytes (DAVIES, 1975). These experiments could not show if the absorbed sera were more effective than the unabsorbed, but to the extent that they influenced much more "difficult" skin grafts, only with absorbed serum was there measurable prolongation.

Mouse studies using MHC congenic strains and employing skin grafts amply confirmed this phenomenon (STAINES et al., 1974), and in both rat and mouse systems the absorbed sera had all the in vitro properties of I region antisera, which could be substantiated by appropriate genetic studies in mice (STAINES et al., 1976) (see 4.1.1.) and where only partial coverage of the Ia specificities was sufficient to give substantial enhancement (STAINES et al., 1975).

For these reasons we believe that mouse H-2, K/D (serologic determinant = "SD", BACH et al., 1972) directed antibody has no role in immunologic enhancement of normal tissue allografts. On the contrary, we attribute the effect wholly to antibodies against I region gene products. We consider the same to be true in the rat and hence in man where cytotoxic = HLA = tissue typing alloantisera are not merely irrelevant but actually damaging to the graft. The Ia antibody by attaching to I sites (= lymphocyte activating determinants = "LADS", FESTENSTEIN, 1973) of resident and passenger I positive cells of the transplant are thus rendered incapable of exciting host cells to recognize their (HLA) foreignness, as seen by the way in which these sera interfere with MLR reactions (MEO et al., 1975). Human sera prepared by absorption as described in rodents (using for example platelets) have the same in vitro properties, including, as for mouse enhancing sera, that of inhibiting the stimulating cell in MLR (VAN ROOD et al., 1975a).

Human sera have yet to be tested for enhancement in this kind of situation, but if they did not we would be unable to explain the fall in kidney transplant survival rate since blood transfusions came to be discouraged, or their white cells removed, to avoid "presensitization" as seen by cytotoxic HLA antibody (MURRAY et al., 1974). In addition the human heart transplant success rate of about 40% (at one year) does not extend to patients previously transfused for open heart surgery, who enjoy the enhanced success rate of 10/11 (CAVES et al., 1973). Thus the defect in the original thinking turned on the nature of the antibody concerned which clearly is that related to the I region of the MHC.

The prospects in this area are now very promising for the reason that enhancement with pooled "unrelated" serum has been achieved in a baboon kidney transplant model (MYBURGH and SMIT, 1972; SMIT and MYBURGH, 1974); this agrees with the mouse experiment on partial coverage of I differences already referred to (STAINES et al., 1975). Damage to transplants by cytotoxic antibody is well documented both experimentally and clinically (JEANNET et al., 1970), but this is now presumed to be attributable to HLA, (not anti-I antibodies), which the rat experiments show to be dispensable. Damage by HLA antibody is likely to be related to the degree of HLA antigen expression by grafted cells (high for lymphocytes, endothelium etc., low for muscle). The sensitizing action of a tissue in the way it induces "transplantation immunity" is related to its I content (high in skin, low in liver). Unfortunately it is difficult to induce "I" antibodies without also raising "H" antibodies (offspring of first cousin marriages might help) (VAN DEN TWEEL et al., 1973) and generally absorption is necessary because H + ve, I-ve material does exist, while H-ve, I + ve material is not known.

There are data to show a synergistic effect between enhancing serum and antilymphocyte serum (ALS), (RUSSELL, 1971; BATCHELOR *et al.*, 1972), which can, in the light of the above reasoning, be interpreted in that the enhancing serum is directed against the stimulating cell derived from the transplant, while the ALS is directed at the host cell which is responsible for receiving the stimulating message to perform the recognition event. Synergism of enhancing serum with drugs is also to be expected. On the other hand ALS would not act synergistically with the immunosuppressive drugs, because they impinge on the same target cells of the host.

4.3.1.2. Active Enhancement

This has been widely studied in animals both in the early mouse tumor enhancement work, (KANDUTSCH and REINERT-WENCK, 1957) (see also Fig. 6) and more recently in the context of tissue transplants, sometimes under the guise of "tolerance". Treatment of animals with "antigen", whether partly purified or given as whole cells is frequently very effective in leading to specific prolongation of grafts if administered about 2 weeks preoperatively. This has been found in many systems, e.g. rat auxiliary heart grafts (MACDONALD *et al.*, 1972) and also with mouse skin grafts if "helped" with ALS (KILSHAW *et al.*, 1974) (skin being too "difficult" to actively enhance directly in some cases). We take it that the two weeks delay is for I antibody to be elicited and that this accounts for the relative ineffectiveness of antigen injected at or just before grafting time. It may be noted that effective ALS is induced with thymocytes, which are H +, and I poor (DAVIES and HESS, 1974) so that anti-I antibodies actively acquired might not be neutralized thereby. This risk exists for anti-spleen ALS which is consistently ineffective.

Clinically, active enhancement has clearly played a hitherto unrecognized role in skin (VAN ROOD *et al.*, 1973), kidney and heart transplantation, but in the face of unwelcomed HLA preimmunization. Indeed purposeful active enhancement of human skin was tried some years ago and with measurable success (RAPAPORT *et al.*, 1968).

4.3.2. Tolerance

The high/low tolerance model using soluble proteins and finding conditions where they minimise a humoral response (MCDEVITT, 1974) has not extended to any degree of control, on the part of the manipulator, over the cellular immunity which is presumed to be largely responsible for rejection of transplants. Purified H-2 antigens have been used over a wide range of concentrations and durations but have failed to promote the prolongation of skin grafts, although they are capable of suppressing the humoral immune response against H-2 (K/D) antigens (LAW *et al.*, 1972). When tolerance is induced by injection of leukocytes very shortly after birth in the mouse, it is clear that the tolerant features of the adult mouse are due to its residual chimeric state (Brent *et al.*, 1972).

The relationship between a particular small subpopulation of lymphocytes and a particular antigenic recognition capability is clearly established (Humphrey and Keller, 1970). If true tolerance is the elimination of the appropriate clone, then such tolerance has probably never been achieved for transplants, experimentally or clinically.

While enhancement provides a block in the ability to recognize a foreignness the facility still exists to make that recognition when enhancing antibody decays. Drugged antibodies exist to specifically attack chosen target cells (Davies and O'Neill, 1974); perhaps similarly drugged antigens could specifically eliminate the relevant lymphocyte clone to achieve real tolerance.

5. Chemistry of Human and Mouse MHC Gene Products

5.1. Homology

HLA gene products in man and their homologue from H-2 in the mouse are cell surface antigens which form an integral part of cell membranes, especially those of lymphoid cells. As outlined above (4.1.) these antigens are under the genetic control of the major histocompatibility complex (MHC) which governs such basic immunologic phenomena as T-cell proliferation, regulation of the immune response (=antigen recognition), T-B cell cooperation, and allograft rejection. The latter phenomenon is directly related to the products of the three main regions of the MHC in man (*A*, *B* and *C*) and the *K* and *D* regions in the mouse. ('HLA' and 'H-2'-antigens (=H-antigens) refer exclusively to those products which are identical with so-called SD (serologically defined) antigens; since some I-region products have also been defined serologically, these antigens will be termed Ia-antigens.)

5.2. Membranes and Models

Singer and Nicholson (1972) have proposed a model according to which biological membranes have a fluid structure under physiologic conditions. A mosaic of proteins is embedded in a discontinuous lipid bilayer, in which nonpolar fatty acid chains are sequestered in the interior of the membrane (Fig. 7). This implies that a membrane is a dynamic, viscous 'solution' (at 37° C) of proteins and lipids. Protein molecules with nonpolar groups are buried in the hydrophobic part of the fluid bilayer, whereas ionic, polar groups, protrude into the aqueous phase. Two fundamental implications can be derived for (1) the antibody induced redistribution of cell surface antigens (capping) and (2) the solubilization of membrane bound proteins (see 5.3.2.).

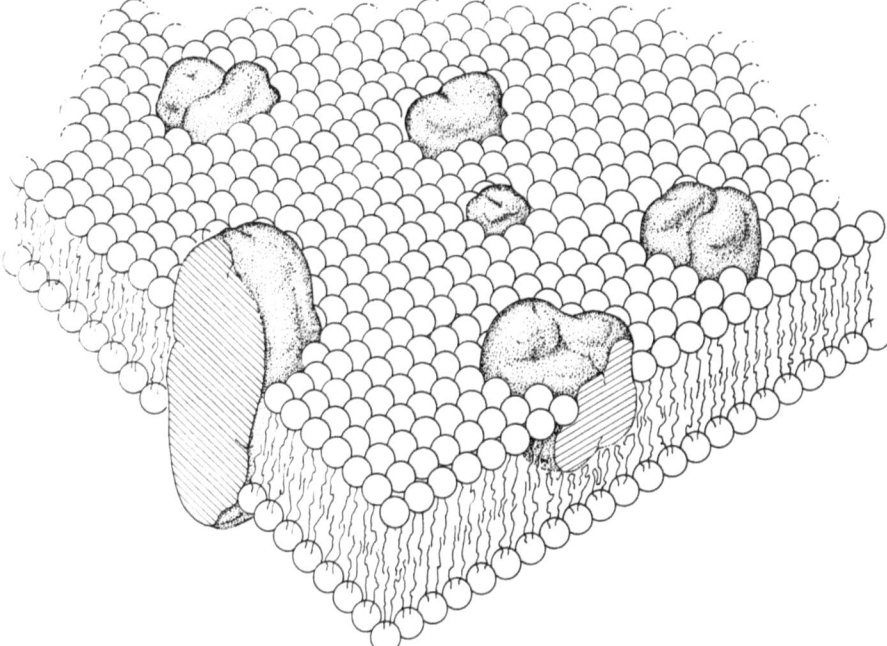

Fig. 7. The fluid mosaic model of membranes. Schematic three dimensional and cross sectional view. In a discontinuous phospholipid bilayer (circles=ionic and polar groups; lines= fatty acid chains) integral proteins (solid bodies) will be partially embedded (lypophilic part) or protruding into the aqueous environment (taken from SINGER and NICHOLSON, 1972)

5.2.1.

The molecular independence of ántigenic determinants controlled by different regions of the MHC has been demonstrated by KOURILSKY and colleagues by an elegant method which takes advantage of the membrane properties described above (NEAUPORT-SAUTES *et al.*, 1973a, b). The principle of this method is shown in Figure 8. It is evident that antigenic determinants migrating indepen-

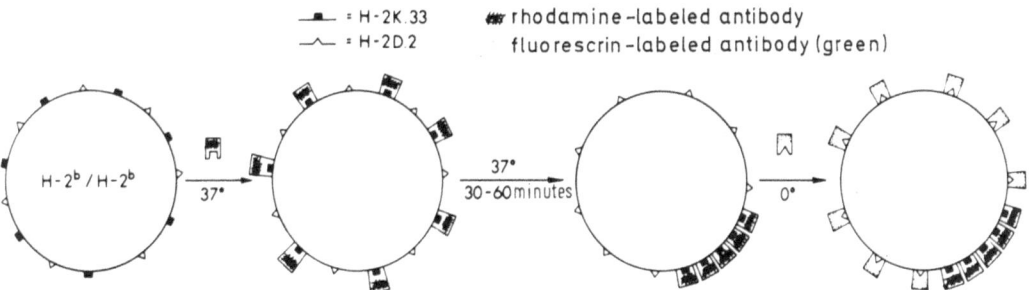

Fig. 8. Antibody induced redistribution of cell surface antigens. Incubation of rhodamine labeled antialloantibody (K33) at 0° C followed by 37° C incubation will result in "cap" formation. Second incubation at 0° C with fluorescein labeled antibody directed against H-2.2D reagent shows diffuse staining of whole cell surface, showing that K and D determinants are independent molecules on cell surface (taken from NEAUPORT-SAUTES *et al.*, 1973b)

dently on the lymphoid surface are located on different molecules. Thus it has been shown that H-2 molecules controlled by the *H-2D* and *H-2K* regions as well as HLA antigens controlled by the *A* and *B* loci migrate independently (NEAUPORT-SAUTES *et al.*, 1973a, b; NEAUPORT-SAUTES *et al.*, 1972; BERNOCO *et al.*, 1972). A similar approach has been used to demonstrate that some public (e.g. H-2.28D^d) and private (e.g. H-2.4D^d) specificities are controlled by different genes (DÉMANT *et al.*, 1975) and that Ia-antigens are on molecules distinct from H-2K or D region antigens (UNANUE *et al.*, 1974).

5.3. Methods

5.3.1. Membrane Preparation and Fractionation

A crude membrane suspension can be obtained after hypotonic cell lysis and disruption by shearing forces according to the flow chart in Figure 9. The

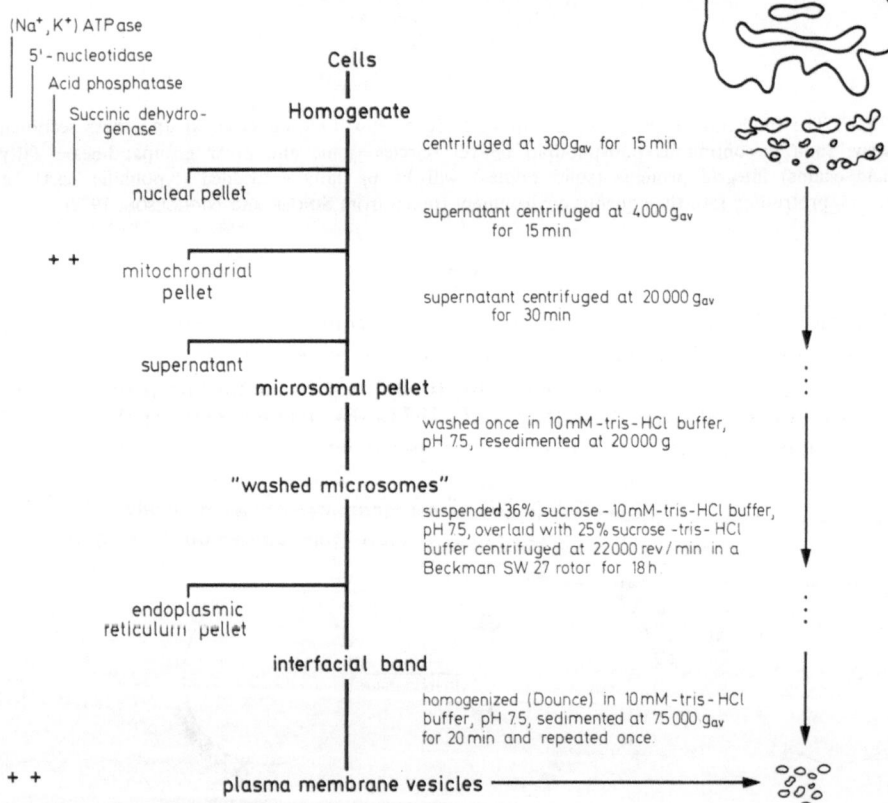

Fig. 9. Plasma membrane preparation: subcellular fractions and enzyme markers. The flow scheme details a procedure used, with minor modifications, in many laboratories. Enzyme markers should be taken as guideline, since no enzyme is strictly speaking specific for the respective fraction (taken from CRUMPTON and SNARY, 1974; WALLACH and LIN, 1973)

Table 5. Composition of lymphocyte plasma membrane fractions

	Human BRI 8 cells	Mouse Leukemia cells
Protein (% dry weight)	42	n.d.
Lipid (% dry weight)	51	n.d.
Cholesterol	260	147
Phospholipid	510	316
Neutral sugar	117	778
Sialic acid	14	10
RNA	17	1.5
DNA	0	n.d.
5'-Nucleotidase	5.6	1.6
(Na^+, K^+) ATPase	8.7	12.7
Succinic dehydrogenase	0	0.27
Acid phosphatase	0	0.61
Lactic dehydrogenase	0	n.d.
Glucose 6-phosphatase	0.18	0.81

Chemical compositions are expressed, except where otherwise stated, as µg/mg protein and enzymic activities as µmole of product liberated per h per mg protein. A value of 0 indicates that no material or activity was detected under the assay conditions used; n.d. = not determined. (Modified after CRUMPTON and SNARY, 1974.)

actual membrane fractionation is achieved by differential centrifugation and centrifugation on sucrose density gradients. As shown in Figure 9 the different subcellular fractions obtained can be monitored with appropriate marker enzymes (CRUMPTON and SNARY, 1974). The composition and properties of human lymphoid cells and mouse leukemia cell plasma membranes is given in Table 5. It is worth mentioning that about 0.1% of the membrane protein fraction represents the average amount of histocompatibility antigen present on the cell surface (see also 5.3.3.).

5.3.2. Solubilization

The solubilization of proteins embedded in a phospholipid bilayer requires either detergents (or organic solvents) to solubilize the whole protein; or enzymic degradation which will attack the protuding protein molecules that are in contact with the aqueous environment. (A protein present in the liquid supernatant after centrifugation at 120,000 xg for 120' is regarded as operationally "soluble".)

5.3.2.1.

Nonionic *detergents*, e.g. Triton X-114, NP.40 (Triton X-100) Brij 99 (KAN-DUTSCH and STIMPFLING, 1963; HILGERT et al., 1969; SCHWARTZ and NATHENSON, 1971a; SPRINGER et al., 1974), (i.e. detergents which can be removed from a protein by ion exchange chromatography in 8M urea or 6M guanidine−HCl) are now in use in many laboratories. The advantages obtained by solubilizing the whole protein in this way must be weighed against certain difficulties such as the formation of high molecular weight detergent micelles, and the necessity to use high concentrations of urea to remove the detergent, resulting in a complete loss of biological activity. Used in conjunction with either cell surface iodination (^{125}I) or incorporation, during in vitro culture, of ^{3}H or ^{14}C amino acid precursors the method can, however, be extremely useful (see 5.3.5.).

5.3.2.2.

Among the *enzymes* used for the solubilization of H-antigens papain has become the method of choice (DAVIES *et al.*, 1968; SHIMADA and NATHENSON, 1969; HESS and DAVIES, 1974) and is usually used at pH 8.0, for 60′ at 37° C at enzyme/substrate ratios varying from 1:100 to 1:20.

5.3.2.3.

Among other extraction methods are autolyis (NATHENSON and DAVIES, 1966), sonication (REISFELD and KAHAN, 1970), and solubilization by chaotropic agents (i.e. agents which will disturb the ordered water structure and thus affect the physicochemical properties of the membrane in water (HANSTEIN *et al.*, 1971)), like 3M KCl (REISFELD and KAHAN, 1970).

   H-antigens solubilized by the techniques mentioned above retain their serologic and biological activities; i.e. they will induce accelerated graft rejection, elicit the formation of alloantibodies and according to early reports induce blast transformation in mixed lymphocyte cultures (MLC) (REISFELD and KAHAN, 1970). Most important for following purification is their retention of ability to inhibit the cytotoxic potential of specific alloantisera.

5.3.3. Detection of H-Antigens

The alloantibody and complement (C′) dependent cytotoxicity test using $Na_2{}^{51}CrO_4$ labeled target cells was first described by WIGZELL (1965) and SANDERSON (1965) and was developed from the dye exclusion methods which are still widely used in tissue typing and are also useful to detect a reactive subpopulation in a target cell suspension. More recently an antibody binding assay (SCHWARTZ and NATHENSON, 1971a), and a radioimmunoassay (TANIGAKI *et al.*, 1973a) have also been introduced.

5.3.3.1. The cytotoxicity Test and its Inhibition

Viable target cells, which have incorporated ^{51}Cr, will retain this as a convenient label which can be released by, and used as an indicator of, cell damage. The amount of ^{51}Cr released by alloantibodies in the presence of C′ is therefore a direct measure of the cytotoxic activity of these antibodies. The rationale is given in Figure 10A. The titer of an antiserum (e.g. anti H-2.4 raised by cross immunizing animals differing only for the H-2 complex = H-2 congenic

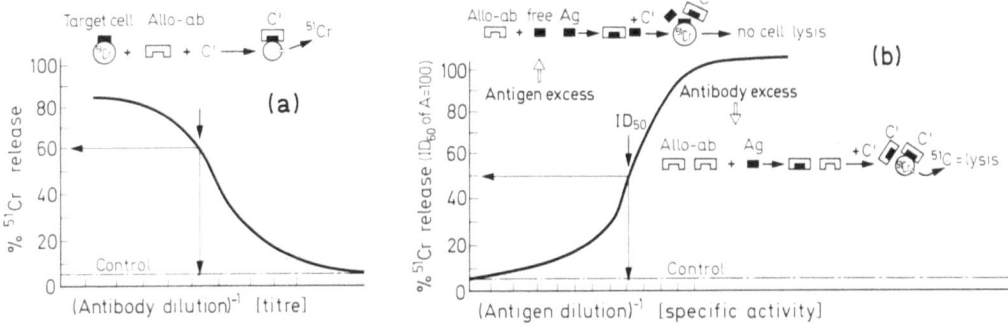

Fig. 10. Complement dependent cytotoxicity assay. (*a*) Titer of an antiserum established by reacting serial dilutions of this antiserum with appropriate target cells in presence of C'. (*b*) Reactivity of this antiserum inhibited by presence of excess antigen; i.e. no cell lysis (=inhibition of ^{51}Cr release) will occur under such circumstances. Serial dilution of antigen used to measure specific inhibitory activity of soluble or particulate antigens. Controls must be included to eliminate nonspecific inhibition (=anticomplementarity)

animals) is given by adding e.g. 10^4 cells and guinea pig serum as C' source to serial dilutions of antiserum. The C' is used at a dilution which is not directly toxic for the target cell but still fulfils its functions in antibody-mediated lysis. The antiserum is now used (Fig. 10 B) at a final concentration (f.c.) corresponding to a ^{51}Cr-release of 60% (in A). The release is calculated according to:

$$\frac{R - C}{cells} \times 100 \ \text{ in which}$$

R = ^{51}Cr release in cpm.
C = Control, i.e. release in the presence of (diluted) C' only.
Cells = cpm given by 10^4 ^{51}Cr labeled cells.

The inhibition of solubilized (or even particulate) material is now tested on serial dilutions of this antigen (B.). The ID_{50}, i.e. the reciprocal of antigen dilution at a point corresponding to 50% ^{51}Cr-release, is a measure of the specific activity of the antigen. This activity is expressed as ID_{50} units/mg antigen and serves to monitor the purification of any cell surface expressed antigens (such as H-substances, see 5.3.4.) for which antisera are available.

5.3.3.2.

The antibody binding assay is used extensively for the *isolation* of radiolabeled alloantigens. The method, shown in Figure 11, is based on an indirect "sandwich" technique. The present limitations lay in the minute amounts of antigenic material thus recovered.

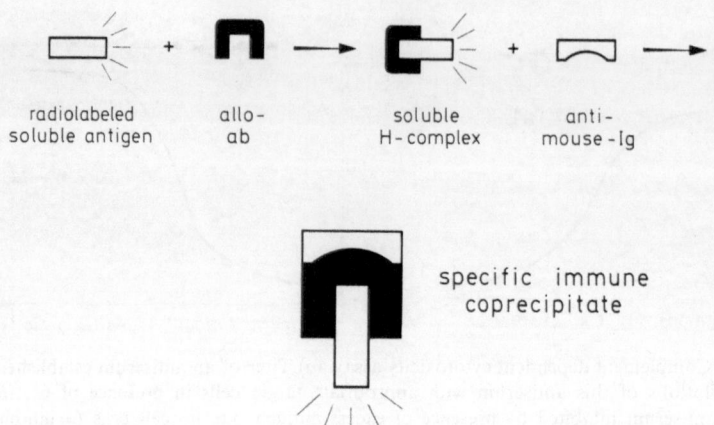

Fig. 11. Indirect immune coprecipitation technique. Immune complexes of H-alloantigen and anti-body do not form precipitates. Such a complex is brought down in the following way: (Mouse alloantiserum + antigen) + (rabbit anti-mouse-Ig). To eliminate rabbit antiserum this complex is precipitated with goat anti-rabbit Ig. The precipitate, once dissolved by boiling in 0.2% SDS or 8M Urea, is now used for further characterization of the alloantigen (Sieve chromatography, electro-phoresis, peptide maps, etc.)

5.3.4. Purification

The numerous trails followed by many investigators attempting to obtain chem-ically pure H-substances from various sources reflect inherent problems en-countered with membrane proteins characterized by an unprecedented genetic (and structural?) polymorphism.

A detailed analysis of the purification methods employed using lymphoid tissue as original source is far beyond the scope of this chapter but the outline shown in Figure 12 will suffice to provide a general view of the diversity of the techniques employed. A fair idea about the problems being faced can be seen from the total amounts of H-antigen present on the normal lymphoid cell surface (ca. 10^{-16}g/cell/haplotype) (SANDERSON and WELSH, 1974a; HESS and DAVIES, 1974). This corresponds to about 0.1–0.01% of the total membrane protein. Hence at least a 1000-fold purification has to be achieved in order to obtain pure H-antigen.

Purification up to 700–800 fold has been reported for H-2D antigens (SHIMA-DA and NATHENSON, 1969; HESS and DAVIES, 1974; HESS and SMITH, 1974) thought to be about 70% pure. SPRINGER et al. (1974) obtained a 220-fold purification of HLA-A2 material estimated to be about 50% homogeneous on SDS-gel electrophoresis. Electrophoretic homogeneity was also achieved for HLA-A1 and A2 after a 240–530 fold purification (MIYAKAWA et al., 1973). In recent attempts to isolate HLA antigens from normal human serum a 120 fold increase in specific activity was obtained after a purification sequence involving QAE-ion-exchange chromatography, affinity chromatography (Con A-Sepharose), and PAGE (BILLING and TERASAKI, 1974). Whether this implies

Soluble H-antigens

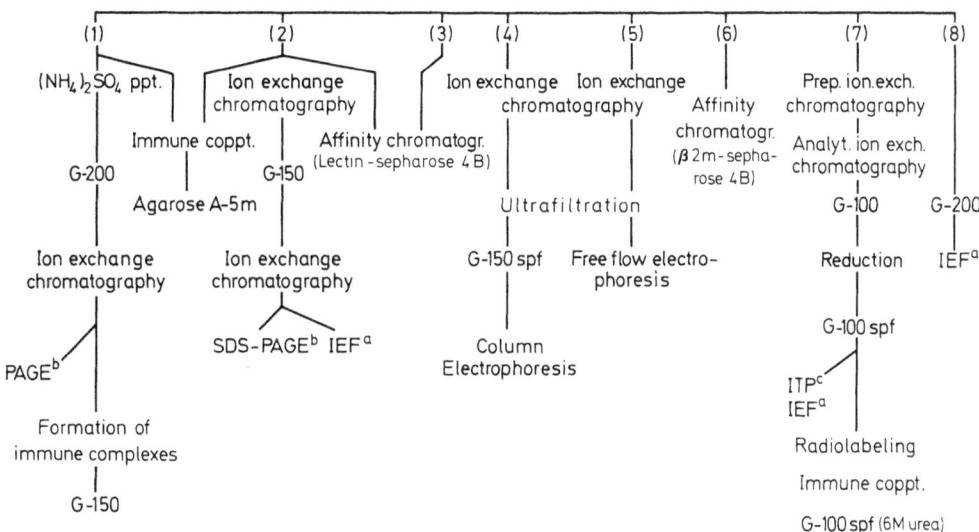

Fig. 12. Purification of soluble H-antigens. A Comparison

[1] SHIMADA and NATHENSON, 1969; SCHWARTZ and NATHENSON, 1971a.
[2] SPRINGER et al., 1974; CRESSWELL et al., 1974a.
[3] SNARY et al., 1974.
[4] TANIGAKI and PRESSMAN, 1974.
[5] KOUBEK et al., 1973.
[6] CRESSWELL and DAWSON, 1975; OH et al., 1975.
[7] HESS and DAVIES, 1974; HESS and SMITH, 1974.
[8] BERNIER et al., 1974.

[a] *IEF* = isoelectric focusing.
[b] *PAGE* = polyacrylamide gel electrophoresis.
[c] *ITP* = isotachophoresis.

that normal serum might be a better source for H-antigens than lymphoid tissues remains to be seen, particularly in the light of the different figures and claims obtained, as outlined above, by various laboratories. Cultured lymphoblastoid cells may, however, in some instances, contain up to 10–25 times as much HLA protein as peripheral white blood cells or spleen lymphocytes (STROMINGER et al., 1974), a fact which may greatly facilitate HLA antigen purification.

5.3.5.

Among the special techniques which will prove to be important for the eventual determination of the primary structure of H-antigens are (1) the incorporation of amino acid precursors, and (2) the radiolabeling (e.g. by acetylation or amidination) of highly purified H-antigens.

5.3.5.1.

The incorporation of ^{3}H or ^{14}C labeled amino acid precursors is the method of choice when permanent lymphoid cell lines or tumour cells growing in culture are available (Nathenson and Cullen, 1974; Strominger et al., 1974). A judicious choice of amino acids (e.g. Arginine or Lysine to determine differences in tryptic peptides (see 5.4.4.), enables valid interpretations to be made, provided the radiolabeled H-antigens isolated consist, after additional purification, of single polypeptide chains.

5.3.5.2.

Less versatile but still very useful, is the introduction of chemical groups such as 4-hydroxy-3,5diiodo-phenylacetyl azide, which will react with accessible amino groups by peptide bond formation according to the following reaction (Brownstone et al., 1966):

$$OH\langle\bigcirc\rangle^{^{125}I}_{_{125}I}CH_2CON_3 + H_2N\text{—Protein} \longrightarrow OH\langle\bigcirc\rangle^{^{125}I}_{_{125}I}CH_2\overset{O}{\overset{\|}{C}}\text{—}\underset{H}{N}\text{—Protein} + \text{azide}.$$

It is evident that the introduction of ^{125}I in positions 3 and 5 provides a powerful tool which can be used for the general characterization of the antigen, as well as in two dimensional peptide mapping and in ion exchange peptide chromatography.

5.4. Biochemistry of HLA/H-2 Antigens

We summarize below the most recent data (1975). For additional information we would like to refer to recent comprehensive reviews (Nathenson, 170; Mann and Fahey, 1971; Reisfeld and Kahan, 1970). In order to emphasize the chemical homology existing between histocompatibility antigens of man and mouse the results obtained for both species will be treated in parallel.

H-antigens are glycoproteins composed of about 10–20% carbohydrate and 80–90% protein, the polypeptide chains bearing the alloantigenic determinant. Pronase digestion results in extensive degradation of the protein backbone to yield glycopeptides of molecular weight (M_r) 4–5000 containing about:

HL-A	H-2
4–6% neutral sugars[a]	3–4% neutral sugars[b]
3–5% N-Acetyl-Glucosamine	2–3% N Acetyl glucosamine
–N-Acetyl Galactosamine	1% N-Acetyl galactosamine
1% sialic acid	1% sialic acid
[a] Nathenson and Cullen (1974) Nathenson and Muramatsu (1971)	[b] Sanderson et al., 1971.

The carbohydrate moiety does not seem to contribute to the alloantigenic activity since enzymatic removal of the carbohydrate does not impair the reactivity of the remaining intact protein with (H-2) alloantisera (Nathenson and Muramatsu, 1971).

5.4.2.

Early reports by PRESSMAN and coworkers, later confirmed by the group of STROMINGER, as well as observations from other laboratories (MIYAKAWA et al., 1973; CRESSWELL et al., 1973; PETERSON et al., 1974; SILVER and HOOD, 1974; RASK et al., 1974a, b; HESS, 1975a) indicate that the HLA/H-2 molecule in its monomeric form is composed of two polypeptide chains with M_r (after detergent solubilization) of about 44,000 and 12,000 respectively. Recent data (see Fig. 13) even suggest an Immunoglobulin-like structure, with HLA and H-2 molecules composed in situ of two disulfide linked heavy chains and two non covalently linked light chains (STROMINGER et al., 1974; SCHWARTZ et al., 1973).

The homology can be further extended in as much as, like in Ig molecules, papain cleavage will release an antigenic molecule containing both a 34,000 (heavy) and the 12,000 (light) chain but devoid of disulphide bonds, since, as shown in Figure 14 no changes in the M_r were apparent when SDS polyacrylamide gels were run in the *presence* or *absence* of 2-mercaptoethanol; this reagent will reduce covalent disulphide bridges (as seen in Fig. 13). As will be discussed later the small M_r component has been shown to correspond to β2-microglobulin.

5.4.3.

In addition to M_r differences reported for D and K end antigens of the mouse (SCHWARTZ et al., 1973), and for A and B antigens in man (SNARY et al., 1974), differences in the overall charge and isoelectric points have also been demonstrated (SHIMADA and NATHENSON, 1969; HESS and DAVIES, 1974; HESS and SMITH, 1974; KOUBEK et al., 1973) (Fig. 15).

5.4.4.

The advent of automated sequencing (EDMAN and BEGG, 1967), new types of amino acid analyzers as well as new developments confidently to be anticipated (MCKEAN et al., 1974) should help in the determination of partial amino acid sequences obtained from minute amounts of purified material. The judicious incorporation of radiolabeled amino acids (see 5.3.5.1.) followed, after indirect immune coprecipitation, by automated sequencing and scintillation counting will help to establish a (partial) determination of the primary structure of H-antigens. Using this approach SILVER and HOOD have assigned leucyl and tyrosyl residues to positions 5 and 7 respectively in H-2.4 antigens (personal communication). NATHENSON's group as well as HESS (1975b) were able to obtain structural information by using more conventional techniques (see Fig. 16). Figure 16b depicts two dimensional peptide maps obtained with radiolabeled H-2 substances recovered as "heavy" and "light" chains after fractionation on SDS-chromatography. According to NATHENSON and CULLEN (1974), only 2–3 out of the 12 peptides resolved on ion exchange chromatography showed identical elution behavior when products of the H-2D and H-2K end were compared after

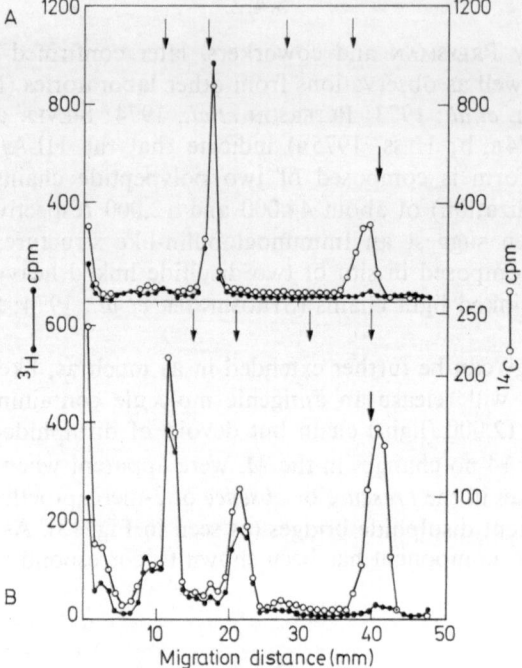

Fig. 13. Dimeric and monomeric forms of H-antigens. (*A, B*) Radioactive immune complexes of
^{3}H glucosamine and ^{14}C amino acid labeled HLA antigens. SDS gel electrophoresis (*A*) in presence
of 2-mercaptoethanol (monomer and ^{14}C labeled β2-microglobulin); (*B*) without 2-mercaptoethanol
(dimer, monomer, and β2-m) (taken from Cresswell and Dawson, 1975). (*C, D*) Radioactive
immune complexes of H-2.4D and H-2.31K alloantigens. SDS electrophoresis without (*C*) and
with 2-mercaptoethanol (*D*). Marker molecules are ^{14}C-labeled IgG (150,000, 75,000 and 25,000)
in (*C*) and H and L chains in (*D*). Only the dimeric (*C*) and monomeric (*C* and *D*) forms
are visible (taken from Schwartz et al., 1973)

incorporation of ^{14}C-Arginine (H-2.31 K^d) and ^{3}H-Arginine (H-2.4D^d) and trypic
cleavage of immune coprecipitated H-2 material. On the other hand comparing,
in the same haplotype, products of the D-end only, i.e. the private specificity 4D
with the public determinant 28D, the peptide maps indicated that not all the
public specificities were located on the polypeptide chains bearing the private
determinant (Hess, 1975b). Both results are suggestive evidence that the genetic
polymorphism apparent in the H-system is reflected at the structural level.

5.4.5.

5.4.5.1. General Implications

A comparison of the different molecular weights obtained for detergent and
papain solubilized H-antigens, confirmed by various laboratories (Schwartz
et al., 1973; Springer *et al.*, 1974) indicates that a portion of the H-molecule

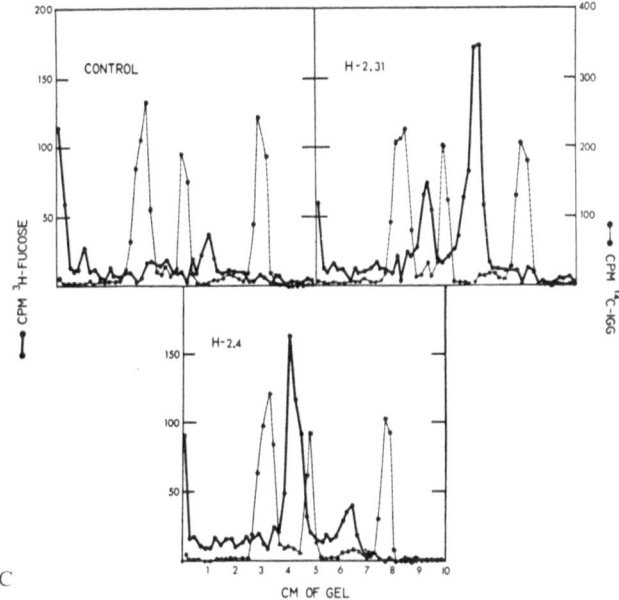

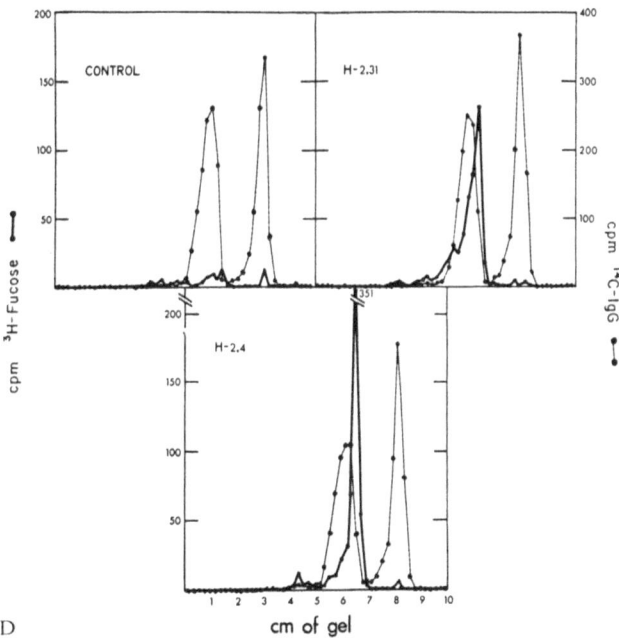

Fig. 13 C and D

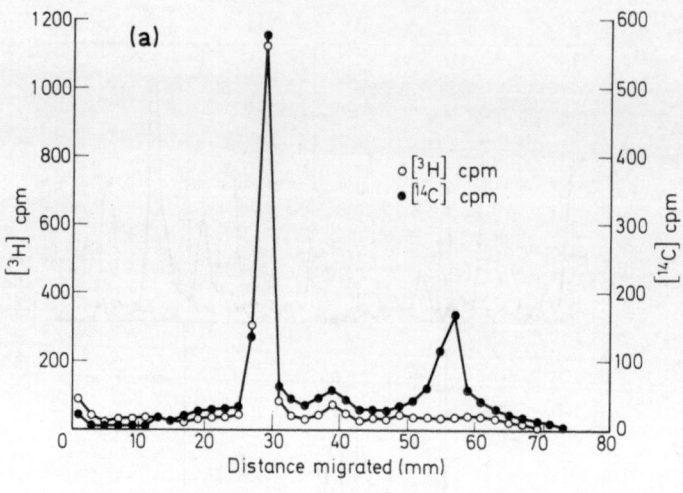

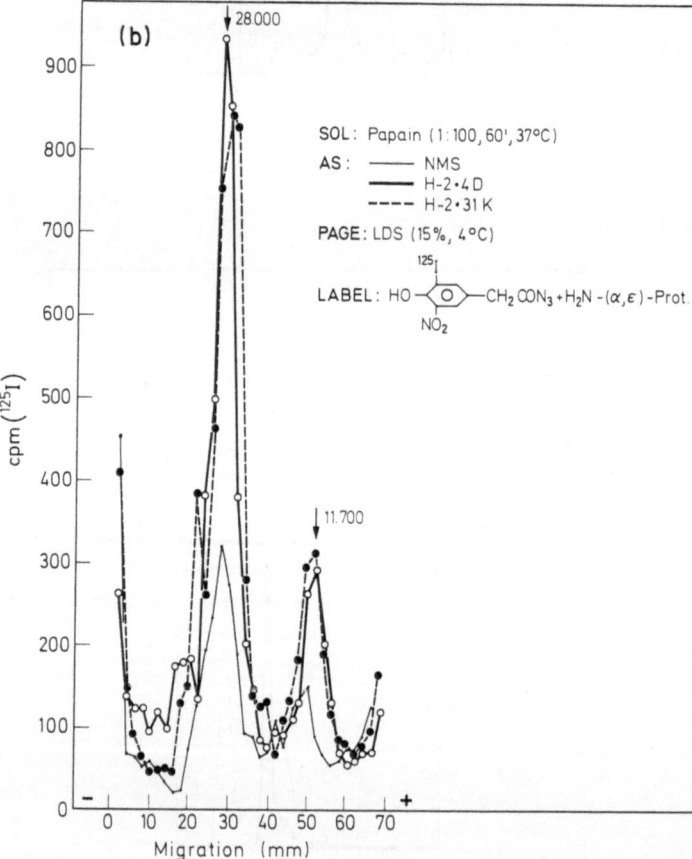

Fig. 14. "Heavy" and "light" chains of papain-solubilized H-antigens. (a) HLA complexes chromatographed on polyacrylamide gel electrophoresis (PAGE) in SDS. The "light" chain fails to incorporate ^{3}H-glucosamine (o——o); ●——● = ^{14}C amino acid label (taken from CRESSWELL et al., 1973). (b) H-products of the K and D region, radiolabeled (4-hydroxy-3-nitro-5-^{125}iodo-phenylacetylazide) after extensive purification and complexed with antisera monospecific for the private determinants K31 (●) and D4 (o). ·——· = normal mouse serum control (HESS, 1975a)

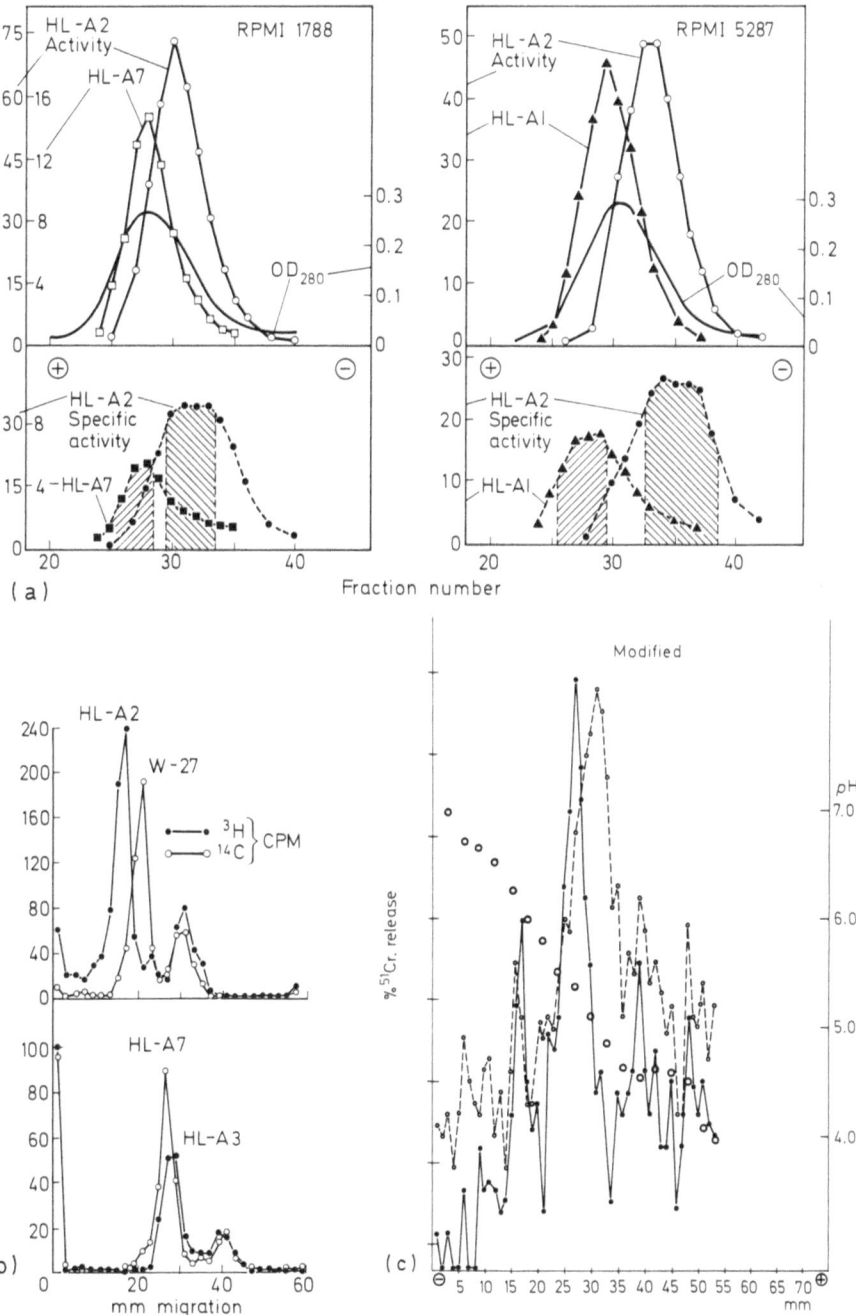

Fig. 15. Charge heterogeneity of papain solubilized H-antigens. (*a*) Electrophoretic pattern of soluble HLA antigens of different origin. Compared to HLA-A2, HLA-A1 and HLA-B7 have a higher electrophoretic mobility (taken from Miyakawa *et al.*, 1971). (*b*) Gel electrophoresis of immune complexes in 6M urea shows similar results with regard to HLA-A2, since B27 as well as HLA-A3 and HLA-B7 migrate faster. The cellular antigens, obtained from different sources, were labeled by in vitro incorporation with ^{3}H- (●) or ^{14}C-amino acids (○) (taken from Cresswell *et al.*, 1974a). (*c*) On isotachophoresis H-2.4 (●——●) displays a maximum at pH (5.4) distinct from H-2.31K (○---○) with an apparent pI of 5.0 (modified after Hess and Smith, 1974)

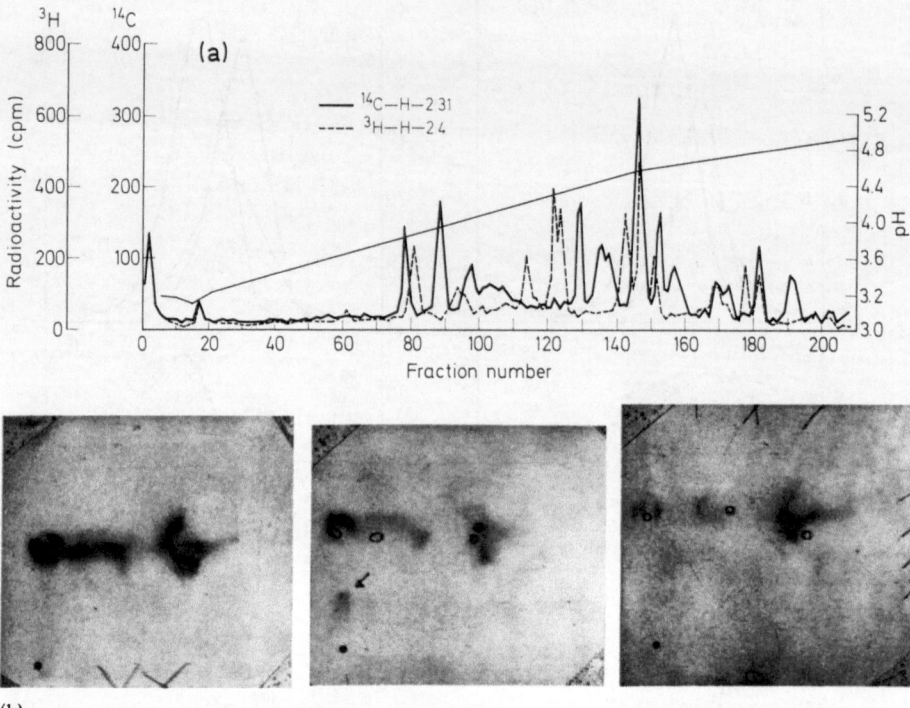

(b)

Fig. 16. Chromatography of radiolabeled peptides. (a) Tryptic peptides from ^{14}C-Arginine labeled H-2.31K and ^{3}H-Arginine labeled H-2.4D preparations, showing substantial differences in elution behavior after cation exchange fractionation (taken from Nathenson and Cullen, 1974). (b) Peptide maps of "heavy" and "light" chains of H-2D^d antigens. N^{125}IP labeled antigens, present as a mixture of K- plus D-region specificities even after extensive purification, were fractionated by indirect immune coprecipitation and subjected, after denaturation, to (i) trypsin and (ii) elastase digestion. Three two dimensional maps (fingerprints) obtained by autoradiography after thin layer chromatography in two different solvent systems are shown. The H-2.4 map is taken as 'master'. Peptides present in H-2.4 but absent from H-2.28, and the light chain are encircled. Arrows indicate peptides not detectable in H-2.4 coprecipitates of N^{125}IP labeled papain products (taken from Hess, 1975b)

corresponding to M_r of about 10,000 is either buried in the membrane bilayer or not susceptible to papain cleavage. As mentioned earlier (5.2.1.), however, this does not imply a rigid static structure for these antigens since these molecules can be induced to redistribute on the cell surface.

The antibody induced redistribution (capping) (Neauport-Sautes et al., 1973a, b) as well as sequential immune coprecipitation techniques (Cullen et al., 1972; Thieme et al., 1974), provided additional information about the genetic-structural relationship of H-antigens.

5.4.5.2.

Molecules which move independently in the membrane will also represent different structures. This was shown by Kourilsky and colleagues for antigens of the K (2nd) and D (1st) region of the mouse (man) MHC (NEAUPORT-SAUTES *et al.*, 1973a, b).

5.4.5.3.

Since these molecules are inherited in a codominant manner (i.e. expressed independently in the F_1 generation) one should expect the four "SD" antigens present in an F_1 genotype (i.e. K+D from ♂ plus K+D from ♀) also to be present on four separate molecules. This is indeed the case (CULLEN *et al.*, 1972; THIEME *et al.*, 1974).

5.4.5.4.

Only partially resolved, however, is the relationship between private and public specificities at the structural level. Will the complete set of public determinants (see 4.1.1.1.) be represented on the same polypeptide chain, also carrying the private specificity (PANCAKE and NATHENSON, 1973; CEPPELLINI, 1973; RICHIARDI *et al.*, 1972), or will the results obtained for H-2.28 (HESS, 1975b) be extended to other public specificities (see 5.4.4.)?

5.4.5.5.

In addition to having important biological implications (FORMAN and MÖLLER, 1974; BRONDZ *et al.*, 1975) (see 4.1.2.), this is also of significance for interpretation of the evolution of H-antigens, and the gene duplication (SHREFFLER *et al.*, 1971; MURPHY and SHREFFLER, 1975) which led to the formation of two (or three) H-regions in the mouse and in man.

5.4.5.6.

With regard to the MHC gene product structure a comparison with immunoglobulins has been made by various authors (AMOS *et al.*, 1972; NATHENSON and CULLEN, 1974; STROMINGER *et al.*, 1974). For reasons partly outlined above (5.4.2.) these comparisons center on the genetic polymorphism of H-antigens and the existence of v- (variable) and c- (constant) regions in Ig molecules. Particularly attractive in this context is a notion put forward by STROMINGER *et al.* (1974) according to which the covalent association of the c- and v-parts in immunoglobulins "was a late evolutionary event, necessitated by the step in which these substances became secretory proteins and thus circulated in an aqueous environment rather than being localized in the membrane." There is a point, however, which we would like to make: in immunoglobulins of any species the *immunodominant* feature is the allotypic marker, due to amino acid exchange(s) in the *constant* region of the molecule, rather than the idiotypic distinction resulting from amino acid differences in the *v-regions*. This is despite the fact that these v-regions are identical for about 40 out of about 100 amino acids present. This is to say that the "strong" private, mutually exclusive, H-specificity *is* likely to represent a difference in a relatively "constant" part, whereas the "weak", public specificities, which are shared by more than one haplotype (duplicated in both D and K regions) are more likely to correspond to the subgroup phenomenon observed among Ig v-regions.

5.5. β2-Microglobulin [4]

The low molecular weight component described in 5.4.2. (β2m-H) has been shown by different investigators, using biochemical and immunologic approaches, to be β2-microglobulin (β2m) (TANIGAKI et al., 1973b; SOLHEIM, 1974; RASK et al., 1974b; STROMINGER et al., 1974). The complete amino acid sequence of this molecule (β2m) has been determined and shown to be homologous to constant domains of human IgG (CUNNINGHAM et al., 1973; CUNNINGHAM and BERGGARD, 1974), and to be associated on the cell surface and after solubilization with H-antigens in man and mouse (NAKAMURO et al., 1973; CRESSWELL et al., 1974b; PETERSON et al., 1974; LINDBLOM et al., 1974; NEAUPORT-SAUTES et al., 1974; POULIK et al., 1973; SOLHEIM and THORSBY, 1974).

5.5.1.

Unlike the H-substances, β2m, in addition to being present on the cell surface and in normal serum, is also found in urine and spent culture medium (BERGGARD and BEARN, 1968; POULIK and BLOOM, 1973; MIYAKAWA et al., 1973).

5.5.2.

In the species studied so far, man, mouse, guinea pig, rabbit and dog, and independent of source and haplotype, β2m-H is a protein with a molecular weight of ca. 12,000 (BERGGARD and BEARN, 1968; NATORI et al., 1974; FINKELMAN et al., 1975; BERGGARD, 1974; SMITHIES and POULIK, 1972).

5.5.3.

At pH 9.5 β2m-H migrates with an R_f value of 0.47; upon isoelectric focusing β2m-H displays a pI of 5.0 (TANIGAKI et al., 1973b) or 6.4 (PARHAM et al., 1974) in man, and 7.5 in mice (TANIGAKI, pers. comm.).

5.5.4.

The amino acid composition of β2m-H and β2m is virtually identical (SMITHIES and POULIK, 1972; TANIGAKI et al., 1973b; CUNNINGHAM and BERGGARD, 1974). Moreover, TANIGAKI et al. (1973b) reported that the first 24 N-terminal residues of β2m-H were identical when compared with the complete amino acid sequence of the β2m given in Figure 17.

---

[4] β2-microglobulin, as described in 3.2 will be referred to as β2m, the component present in H-antigens as β2m-H.

```
1                        10                              20
Ile-Gln-Arg-Thr-Pro-Lys-Ile-Gln-Val-Tyr-Ser-Arg-His-Pro-Ala-Glu-Asn-Gly-Lys-Ser-

21                       30                              40
Asn-Phe-Leu-Asn-[Cys]-Tyr-Val-Ser-Gly-Phe-His-Pro-Ser-Asp-Ile-Glu-Val-Asp-Leu-Leu-

41                       50                              60
Lys-Asp-Gly-Glu-Arg-Ile-Glu-Lys-Val-Glu-His-Ser-Asp-Leu-Ser-Phe-Ser-Lys-Asp-Trp-

61                       70                              80
Ser-Phe-Tyr-Leu-Leu-Tyr-Ser-Tyr-Thr-Glu-Phe-Thr-Pro-Thr-Glu-Lys-Asp-Glu-Tyr-Ala-

81                       90                             100
[Cys]-Arg-Val-Asn-His-Val-Thr-Leu-Ser-Gln-Pro-Lys-Ile-Val-Lys-Trp-Asp-Arg-Asp-Met
```

Fig. 17. The amino acid sequence of β2-microglobulin (taken from CUNNINGHAM *et al.*, 1973)

5.5.5.

A comparison of the partial sequences obtained in different species displays an extensive homology (CUNNINGHAM and BERGGÅRD, 1974) (see Fig. 18). This would suggest that β2m has been highly conserved in evolution (for the evolutionary implications with regard to immunoglobulins see CUNNINGHAM and BERGGÅRD (1974)).

```
           1         5           10          15          20          25
HUMAN    ILE GLN ARG THR PRO LYS ILE GLN VAL TYR SER ARG HIS PRO ALA GLU ASN GLY LYS SER ASN PHE LEU ASN CYS

RABBIT   [VAL] GLN ARG [ALA] PRO [ASN][VAL] GLN VAL TYR SER ARG HIS PRO ALA GLU ASN GLY LYS [ASP] ASN PHE LEU ASN CYS

DOG      [VAL] GLN [HIS][PRO] PRO LYS ILE GLN VAL TYR SER ARG HIS PRO ALA GLX ASX GLY LYS [PRO] ASX PHE LEU ASX CYS

          26         30          35
         TYR VAL SER GLY PHE HIS PRO SER ASP ILE
         TYR VAL SER GLY PHE HIS PRO SER ASP ILE
         TYR VAL SER GLY PHE HIS PRO  ?  [GLX] ILE
```

Fig. 18. Comparison of partial amino acid sequences of β2-microglobulin. Differences from human amino acid sequence are emphasized (taken from CUNNINGHAM and BERGGÅRD, 1974)

5.5.6.

β2m-H is not, strictly speaking, a gene product of the MHC (see also 3.2.). β2m-H has been treated briefly in this chapter because of its association with H-antigens in all the species so far investigated. The biological significance of this association is not clarified and the physical association by noncovalent bonds might still be fortuitous. In this respect we would particularly draw attention to the fact that antibody induced "capping" of HLA antigens fails to provoke the redistribution of all detectable β2m molecules on the cell surface (NEAUPORT-SAUTES *et al.*, 1974), and that NILSSON *et al.* (1974) have calculated a ratio of β2m to HLA of 6:1 on the cell surface.

5.6. Immune Response Region Associated Antigens (Ia)

We justify a brief description of mouse Ia antigens here because of a fundamental role assigned to these molecules in cellular immunology (see 4.2.), and the paucity of data available so far for the human homologues.

5.6.1.

With the exception of the results from our own laboratory (DAVIES and HESS, 1974; HESS and DAVIES, 1975), most of the information concerning Ia-antigens has been obtained after incorporation of radioactive markers (sugars or amino acids) (CULLEN et al., 1974), or cell surface labeling (VITETTA et al., 1974; FINKEL-MAN et al., 1975). According to CULLEN et al. (1975), these antigens will incorporate mannose and are therefore glycoproteins. In agreement with these data is the fact that Ia antigens will bind to lectin columns from which they can be eluted with excess α-methyl-mannoside. As for H-antigens, however, the carbohydrate moiety is not the alloimmunogenic determinant.

5.6.2.

Upon electrophoresis (CULLEN et al., 1974; VITETTA et al., 1974), Ia antigens display a greater heterogeneity of molecular weights which vary between 35,000 and 25,000. On gel chromatography papain solubilized Ia- (like H-) antigens, elute in a position corresponding to M_r of about 35,000 whereas on LDS chromatography the M_r of Ia. 11 antigen varies between 26,000 and 28,000 as compared to 35,000 after lysine, arginine, or histidine incorporation (Fig. 19A), (DAVIES and HESS, 1974; HESS and DAVIES, 1975; HESS, 1975a).

5.6.3.

In overall charge and pI, however, Ia antigens differ markedly from H-antigens (DAVIES and HESS, 1974; HESS and DAVIES, 1975) as can be seen from Figure 19B.

5.6.4.

Basic structural differences between Ia and H-2 antigens can be inferred, in addition to the different molecular weights mentioned above, from the following observations: (1) acid incubation (0.01 M HCl, 30′) or exposure to 56° C (30′) leaves Ia-substances intact (both treatments would destroy H-antigens). Most striking is the difference in the susceptibility to papain (see Table 6), which,

Fig. 19. Some physicochemical properties of H-2 and Ia-antigens. (A) LDS gel electrophoresis ▷ (15%) of specific immune coprecipitates of detergent (BRIJ 98) solubilized Ia antigens after incorporation of arginine (o—o), lysine (●---●), and histidine (●—●); and after ^{125}I labeling of partially purified papain-solubilized material (o---o). (B, a) Polyacrylamide gel electrophoresis and (B, b) isotachophoresis of H-2 and Ia-antigens. The maxima of antigenic activity are drawn (for Ia.6,11) and indicated for H-2 (K31 and D4). Higher electrophoretic mobility (a) and lower apparent pI (b) characterize Ia antigens as compared to H-2. The molecular weights of the papain-solubilized products are very similar (ca. 26,000). pH: o---o (taken from HESS, 1975a; DAVIES and HESS, 1974)

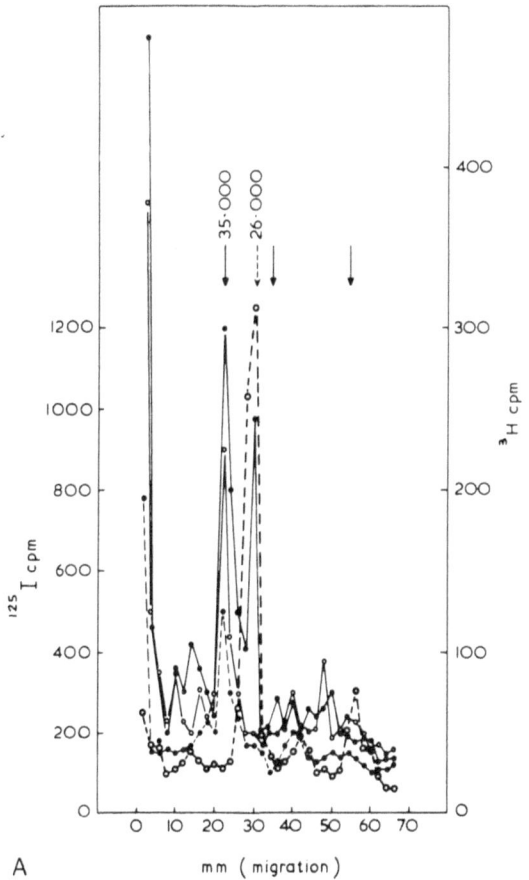

A

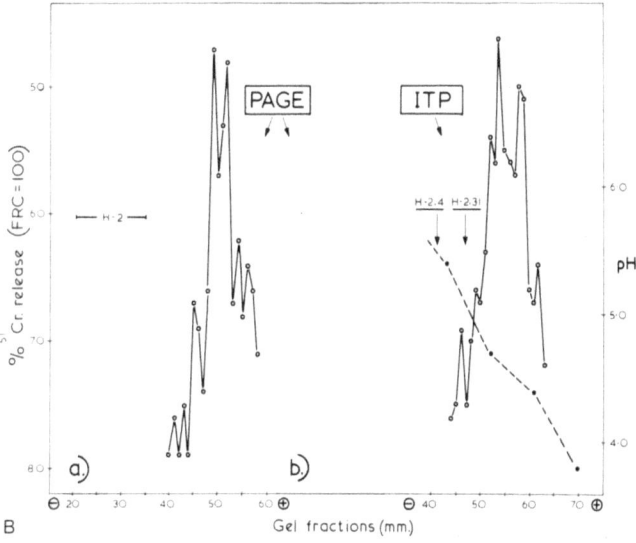

B

Fig. 19 A and B

Table 6. H-2 and Ia antigens: Susceptibility to papain

Fraction	Controlled papain digestion						Autolysis		
	Inhibition of cytotoxic activity determined for								
	H-2.31			Ia.6, 11, 16					
	U/mg	Total activ.	Yield %	U/mg	Total activ.	Yield %	U/mg	Total activ.	Yield %
Crude membrane suspension									
a) before hydrolysis	284	2.2×10^6	100	130	3.3×10^5	100	130	3.3×10^5	100
b) after hydrolysis	309	1.8×10^6	*86*	15	2.4×10^4	*7.4*	65	1.5×10^5	45
Soluble fraction	203	2.3×10^5	*11*	10	1.0×10^4	*3.1*	20	1.2×10^4	3.8
Membrane pellet	348	1.3×10^6	*63*	4	4.7×10^3	*0.15*	140	1.4×10^5	43

The very low yields obtained in the soluble fraction after papain hydrolysis of membrane suspension and the absence of Ia-activity in the residual membrane pellet are the main features characterizing Ia antigen solubilization by enzymic digestion (taken from Hess and Davies, 1975).

Table 7. Factors associated with the mouse MHC

	Character studied	B10.A	B10
1	H-2 haplotype	a	b
2	Serum substance (β-lipoprotein)	Ss-high Slp	Ss-high Slp
3	Hemolytic complement level (C'-H50)	C'-high (35, 60)	C'-low (20, 06)
4	Immune response to synthetic polypeptides (Ir-1)		
	(T, G)-A-L	low	high
	(H, G)-A-L	high	low
	(Phe, G)-A-L	high	low
5	Ir-1 region T cell specific antigen	Ir-1.1 +	Ir-1.1 −
6	H-2 MLC stimulating genes	a	b
7	Non-H-2 MLC capacitating gene	high	low
8	Immune response to various antigens (Ir)[a]		
	Thyroglobulin	medium	low
	Trinitrophenyl conjugate-MSA	low	high
	Random linear copolymer-GAT$_{10}$	high	low
9	Immune responsiveness to IgA allotypes (Ir-IgA)	high	low
10	Immune responsiveness to IgG allotypes (Ir-IgG)	low	high

Two congenic lines showing major differences were chosen. One (H-2^b) is from an original haplotype, the other (H-2^a) is a k × d recombinant (not F_1).
[a] The magnitude of response to a number of further antigens is associated with H-2 but was not tested on B10.A and B10 congenic strains.

Table 7 (continued)

	Character studied[c]	B10.A	B10
11	Viral leukemogenesis; Gross leukemia incidence per cent[b]	93	27
12	Viral leukemogenesis; Tennant-leukemia incidence per cent	73	37
13	Immune response to sex-linked histocompatibility antigens (H-Y)	medium	high
14	Θ-1 antigen manifestation on lymph node cells (anti-Θ-1 cytotoxic score)	high	low
15	PFC number per spleen[c]	high	low
16	cAMP level in liver cells (moles/ng)	3.8	2.6
17	Blood testosterone level (ng/ml)	2.81	2.10
18	Testosterone binding globulin level (ng/ml)	6.70	5.65
19	Vesicular gland weight (mg) (mg/g body weight)	228.9 0.87	320.7 1.08
20	Testes weight (mg) (mg/g body weight)	174.0 0.60	157.6 0.53
21	Thymus weight (mg) (mg/g body weight)	49.0 1.74	38.7 1.29
22	Lymph node weight (mg) (mg/g body weight)	35.8 1.28	25.3 0.88
23	Mandible skeletal characters (13 measurements of the mandible bone)	B10.A differ from B10	
24	Absorbing capacity of lymph node cells for anti-H-2.5	high	low
25	Developmental expression of H-2 antigens (first to third day)[c]	late	early
26	Hybrid-histocompatibility (Hh), (H-2.D end)	Hh	Hh
27	Thymus leukemia[d]	TL+	TL−

[b] (C3H × C57BL)F$_2$ H-2^k/H-2^k are high and H-2^b/H-2^b are low and included in this table because these were the first data on H-2 associated characters.

[c] The difference was found between A (H-2^a/H-2^a) and A.BY (H-2^b/H-2^b) mice.

[d] TL is located about 1% of recombination to the right of the H-2.D gene (taken from IVANYI and FOREIJT, 1974).

under similar conditions, will barely affect H-2K antigen activity; Ia activity, however, is almost completely abolished (HESS and DAVIES, 1975). Preliminary results indicate that Ia antigens of different genetic subregions are, as one would expect, on separate molecules (e.g. Ia. 3 or 9 and Ia. 7, which map in *I-B*, *I-A* and *I-C* respectively); on the other hand, two antigens of the *I-A*^{d} subregion (8 and 11) appear to be antigenic sites present on the same molecule (CULLEN *et al.*; 1975).

5.6.5.

The great importance which attaches to Ia-antigens lies in the fact that they represent the first gene products isolated from the immune response (*Ir*) region of the mouse. The implication for Ia and H-2 antigen functions have been discussed in paragraph 4.2.

Table 8. Experimental models in preclinical transplantation. (*A*) mouse, (*B*) rat,

A				B		
infor- mation about MHC **H-2**	SD LD IR	excellent detailed information excellent detailed information excellent detailed information	"mapping" very advanced	infor- mation about MHC **H-1** or **Ag-B**	SD LD IR	existance of major system demonstrated but detailed information lacking (no evidence for 2-locus model) HC-linked major locus demonstrated; location within MHC unknown HC-linked genes demonstrated; location within MHC unknown
ad- vantages	excellent information about MHC; economy, rapid reproduction; inbred strains (internationally standardized); genetic manipulation possible (recombinants, congenic strains etc.)			ad- vantages	adequate size for microsurgery; economy, rapid reproduction; inbred strains (internationally standardized); genetic manipulation possible (recombinants, congenic strains etc.)	
disad- vantages	small size; little information about *outbred* populations; some immunologic peculiarities: relatively weak GvH across strong H-2 barriers, induction of tolerance/ enhancement relatively "easy"; large phylogenetic distance to man			disad- vantages	poor knowledge of SD antigens; number of H-1 "alleles" very limited; little information about *outbred* populations; many immunologic peculiarities such as weak GvH after bone marrow transplantation; induction of tolerance/enhancement often "too easy"; large phylogenetic distance to man	

6. Concluding Remarks

As the outcome of biological studies certain approaches that appear to be interesting to investigate in donor specific immunosuppression (D.S.I.) are these:

(i) Prevent recognition of H antigen by blocking sensitization with antibody against Ia antigen. This is "enhancement" in the strict sense and may be achieved actively or passively. At the moment, passive enhancement is the method of choice because active induction of anti-Ia produces also anti-H.

(ii) Eliminate Ia antigen from the graft and thus prevent sensitization. This is clearly impossible for Ia positive tissue such as skin, but Ia positive leukocytes could be minimized by thorough perfusion of prospective transplants of some organs.

(C) dog, (D) rhesus monkey (Taken from BALNER, 1974)

C		D	

information about MHC **DL-A**	SD 2 linked loci
	    ± 15 specificities
	    fairly well defined
	LD one major locus with several
	    identified determinants;
	    location within MHC known
	    evidence for minor LD loci;
	IR indications for HC-linked
	    IR genes (unpublished)
		information about MHC **RhL-A**	SD 2 linked loci
			    20 specificities well defined
			LD one major locus with several
			    identified determinants;
			    location within complex known;
			    evidence for minor LD loci
			IR HC-linked Ir loci demonstrated,
			    location probably near major
			    LD locus

advantages	MHC rather well defined (very similar to HL-A); international agreement about typing reagents; usually *outbred* populations; size, temperament and availability of animals o.k.; relatively rapid reproduction (large litters)	advantages	MHC well defined (very similar to HL-A); international agreement about typing reagents; usually *outbred* populations; size of animals o.k.; phylogenetic closeness to man; immunological reaction patterns similar to those of man: ("difficult" matching, severity of GvH etc.)
disadvantages	rather expensive; danger of "inbreeding" in some colonies; some immunologic peculiarities: matching on basis of SD antigens "too easy", GvH after bone marrow transplantation mild; phylogenetic distance to man unknown	disadvantages	expensive; maintenance and handling difficult; slow reproduction; acquisition from the wild increasingly difficult

(iii) Block the (H) foreignness by anti-H antibody. This does not seem to work effectively.

(iv) Eliminate the (H) foreignness; there does not seem to be any way to achieve this beyond a degree of matching for donors and recipients.

(v) Eliminate the recognizing clone ("true tolerance"?). At the moment this can only be done nonspecifically e.g. with drugs or ALG.

It is now clear that active enhancement has been playing a part in kidney transplant success for patients who were blood transfused.

We can now propose the double hierarchy as follows:

H+++ (e.g. endothelium) to H+ve (e.g. muscle).

I +++ (e.g. skin) to I−ve (e.g. liver).

Thus in sensitized patients endothelium suffers badly because it is a "good" target; muscle fares least badly because it is a "poor" target. Skin is a powerful sensitizer, liver is a poor sensitizer. The interaction of these two parameters explains many of the unaccountable results of earlier experiments.

Quite apart from all this, non HLA antigens reject skin grafts exchanged between HLA identical siblings in 20–30 days and such incompatibility may not be subject to control by D.S.I. as referred to above. Fortunately it can be controlled by minimal immunosuppression at least for some kinds of transplants.

We see the device of an H-2 pattern subject to scanning by the Ia system for detection of foreignness (e.g. of viral infected or neoplastic cells) as that which causes the immunologic problems of allotransplantation. A deeper role may reside in homeostasis, to account for the variety of physiologic effects attributable to the MHC, as listed on Table 7 (taken from IVANYI and FOREIJT, 1974).

Practical clinical needs will be apparent from all chapters of this volume. Beyond that the animal species most suited to different experimental requirements have been selected by BALNER (1974) from whose paper Table 8 has been prepared. Why, in this context, study biochemistry of cell surface molecules controlled by different regions of the major histocompatibility complex? For practical purposes the points mentioned above provide a direct, and in the not too distant future, possibly the only successful approach. The solution, however, presupposes a satisfactory resolution of the genetic problem posed by the extensive polymorphism encountered in in vivo and in vitro alloimmune reactions. This outcome will only be achieved by an insight into the structure of molecules responsible for functions like e.g. antigen recognition, control of the immune response, cell-cell interations, and cellular differentiation—i.e. functions involving cell surface determinants governed by closely related genes of the MHC.

References

ALBERT, W.H.W., DAVIES, D.A.L.: H-2 antigens on nuclear membranes. Immunology **24**, 841–850 (1973)

AMOS, D.B., BACH, F.H.: Phenotypic expression of the major histocompatibility locus in man (HL-A): leucocyte antigens and mixed leucocyte culture reactivity. J. Exp. Med. **128**, 623–634 (1968)

AMOS, B., CORLEY, R., KOSTYN, D., DELMAS-MARSALET, Y., WOODBURY, N.: The serologic structure of HL-A as indicated by cross-reactivities. In: Histocompatibility Testing. Copenhagen: Munksgaard, 1972, p. 359–366

AMOS, D.B., GORER, P.A., MIKULSKA, Z.B.: Analysis of an antigenic system (the *H-2* system) in the mouse. Proc. Roy. Soc. B. **144**, 369–380 (1955)

AMOS, D.B., RUDERMAN, R., MENDELL, N., JOHNSON, A.H.: Linkage between HL-A and spinal development. Proc. 5th Internat. Congress Transplantation Soc., Jerusalem, 1975

AMOS, D.B., RUDERMAN, R., MENDELL, N., JOHNSON, A.H.: Linkage between HL-A and spinal development. Transpl. Proc. **7** Supp. 1, 93–99 (1975)

ARCHER, J.R., SMITH, D.A., DAVIES, D.A.L., STAINES, N.A.: A skin graft enhancing antiserum which recognizes two new B-cell alloantigens determined by the Major Histocompatibility Locus of the mouse. J. Immunogenetics **1**, 377–384 (1974)

ARMERDING, D., KATZ, D.H.: Activation of T and B lymphocytes in vitro. II. Biological and biochemical properties of an allogeneic effect factor (AEF) active in triggering specific B-lymphocytes. J. Exp. Med. **140**, 19–37 (1974)

ARMERDING, D., SACHS, D.H., KATZ, D.H.: Activation of T and B lymphocytes in vitro. III. Presence of Ia determinants on allogeneic effect factor. J. Exp. Med. **140**, 1717–1722 (1974)

BACH, F.H., WIDMER, M.B., BACH, M.L., KLEIN, J.: Serologically defined and lymphocyte-defined components of the major histocompatibility complex in the mouse. J. Exp. Med. **136**, 1430–1444 (1972)

BACH, M.L., HUANG, S.W., HONG, R., POULIK, M.D.: β2-microglobulin.: Association with lymphocyte receptors. Science (Wash.) **182**, 1350–1352 (1973)

BALNER, H.: Choice of animal species for modern transplantation research. Transpl. Proc. **6**, 19–25 (1974)

BARNES, A.D.: A quantitative comparison study of immunizing ability of different tissues. Ann. N.Y. Acad. Sci. **120**, 237–250 (1964)

BATCHELOR, J.R., ELLIS, F., FRENCH, M.E., BEWICK, M., CAMERON, J.S., OGG, C.S.: Immunological enhancement of human kidney graft. Lancet **2**, 1007–1010 (1970)

BATCHELOR, J.R., FABRE, J., MORRIS, P.J.: Passive enhancement of kidney allografts: Potentiation with antithymocyte serum. Transplantation **13**, 610–613 (1972)

BENACERRAF, B., McDEVITT, H.O.: Histocompatibility linked Immune Response genes. Science (Wash.) **175**, 273–279 (1972)

BERGGÅRD, I.: Isolation and characteristics of a rabbit β2-microglobulin: comparison with human β2-microglobulin. Biochem. Biophys. Res. Comm. **57**, 1159–1165 (1974)

BERGGÅRD, I., BEARN, A.G.: Isolation and properties of a low molecular weight β2globulin occuring in human biological fluids. J. Biol. Chem. **243**, 4095–4103 (1968)

BERNIER, G.M., FANGER, M.W.: Synthesis of β2-microglobulin by stimulated lymphocytes. J. Immunol. **109**, 407–409 (1972)

BERNIER, I., DAUTIGNY, A., COLOMBANI, J., JOLLÈS, P.: Detergent solubilized HL-A antigens from human platelets: A comparative study of various purification techniques. Biochem. Biophys. Acta. **356**, 82–90 (1974)

BERNOCO, D., CULLEN, S., SCUDELLER, S., TRINCHIERI, G., CEPPELLINI, R.: HL-A molecules at the cell surface. In: Histocompatibility Testing. Copenhagen: Munksgaard, 1972, 527–537

BILLING, R.J., TERASAKI, P.I.: Purification of HL-A antigens from normal serum. J. Immunol. **112**, 1124–1130 (1974)

BILLINGHAM, R.E., BRENT, L., MEDAWAR, P.B.: The antigenic stimulus in transplantation immunity. Nature (Lond.) **197**, 514–519 (1956)

BILLINGHAM, R., SILVERS, W.: The immunobiology of transplantation. New Jersey: Prentice Hall, 1971

BISMUTH, A., NEAUPORT-SAUTES, C., KOURILSKY, F.M., MANUEL, U., GREENLAND, T., SILVESTRE, D.: Distribution and mobility of β2-microglobulin on the human lymphocyte membrane: Immunofluorescence and Immunoferritin studies. J. Immunol. **112**, 2036–2046 (1974)

BLUMENTHAL, M.W., AMOS, D.B., NOREEN, H., MENDELL, N.R., YUNIS, E.J.: Genetic mapping of *Ir*-locus in Man: Linkage to Second Locus of HL-A. Science (Wash.) **184**, 1301–1303 (1974)

BODMER, W.F.: Evolutionary significance of the HL-A system. Nature (Lond.), **237**, 139–145 (1972)

BOYSE, E.A., OLD, L.J., STOCKERT, E., SHIGENO, N.: Genetic origin of tumour antigens. Cancer Res. **28**, 1280–1287 (1968)

Brent, L., Brooks, C., Lubling, N., Thomas, A.V.: Attempts to demonstrate an in vivo role for serum blocking factors in tolerant mice. Transplantation 14, 382–387 (1972)

Brent, L., Pinto, M.: Induction of specific unresponsiveness by donor antigen and non-specific immunosuppression. In: Immunological Aspects of Transplantation Surgery. Lancaster: M.T.P. 1974, 317–337

Brondz, B.D., Egorov, I.K., Dreizlikh, G.I.: Private specificities of H-2K and H-2D loci as possible selective targets for effector lymphocytes in cell mediated immunity. J. Exp. Med. 141, 11–26 (1975)

Brownstone, A., Mitchison, N.A., Pitt-Rivers, R.: Chemical and serological studies with an Iodine-containing synthetic immunological determinant 4-hydroxy-3-iodo-5-nitrophenylacetic acid (NIP) and related compounds. Immunology 10, 465–479 (1966)

Burgos, H., French, M.E., Batchelor, J.R.: Humoral and cell mediated immunity in rats with enhanced kidney allografts. Transplantation 18, 328–335 (1974)

Caffrey, M.F.P., James, D.C.O.: Human lymphocyte antigen association in ankylosing spondylitis. Nature (Lond.) 242, 121 (1973)

Calne, R.Y.: Allografting in the pig. In: Immunological Aspects of Transplantation Surgery. Lancester: M.T.P. 1973, 296–316

Carvalho, A.S., Summerell, J.M., Wentzel, J., Harris, R.: The production of HL-A antisera by planned immunization. Internat. Symp. Standardization of HL-A reagents. Symp. Series Immunobiol. Standard. 18, 11–19. Basel: Karger 1973

Caves, P.K., Stinson, E.B., Griepp, R.B., Rider, A.K., Dong, E., Shumway, N.E.: Results of 54 cardiac transplants. Surgery 74, 307–314 (1973)

Ceppellini, R.: Old and new facts and speculations about transplantation antigens of man. In: Progress in Immunology. New York: Academic Press, 1973, Vol. I, 973–1025

Cerottini, J.C., Brunner, K.T.: Cell-mediated Cytotoxicity, allograft rejection and tumour immunity. Adv. Immunol. 18, 67–132 (1974)

Cikes, M.: Relationship between growth rate, cell volume, cell cycle kinetics, and antigenic properties of cultured murine lymphoma cells. J. Nat. Cancer Inst. 40, 979–988 (1970)

Cresswell, P., Dawson, J.R.: Dimeric and monomeric forms of HL-A antigens solubilized by detergent. J. Immunol. 114, 523–525 (1975)

Cresswell, P., Robb, R.J., Turner, M.J., Strominger, J.L.: Papain solubilised HL-A antigens. Chromatographic and electrophoretic studies of the two sub-units from different specificities. J. Biol. Chem. 249, 2828–2832 (1974a)

Cresswell, P., Springer, T., Strominger, J. L., Turner, M. J., Grey, H. M., Kubo, R. T.: Immunological identity of the small sub-unit of HL-A antigens and β2-microglobulin and its turnover on the cell membrane. Proc. Nat. Acad. Sci. U.S.A. 71, 2123–2127 (1974b)

Cresswell, P., Turner, M.J., Strominger, J.L.: Papain solubilized HL-A antigens from cultured human lymphocytes contain two peptide fragments. Proc. Nat. Acad. Sci. U.S.A. 70, 1603–1607 (1973)

Crumpton, M.J., Snary, D.: Preparation and properties of lymphocyte plasma membranes. In: Current Topics in Molecular Immunology 3, 27–56 (1974)

Cruse, J.M., Lewis, G.K., Whitten, H.D., Watson, E.S., Fields, J.F., Adams, S.T., Harvey, G.F., Paslay, J.W., Porter, M.: Mechanisms of Immunological Enhancement. Progr. Exp. Tumor Res. 19, 110–156 (1974)

Cullen, S.E., David, C.S., Shreffler, D.C., Nathenson, S.G·: Membrane molecules determined by the H-2 associated Immune Response region: Isolation and some properties. Proc. Nat. Acad. Sci. U.S.A. 71, 648–652 (1974)

Cullen, S.E., Freed, J.H., Atkinson, P.H., Nathenson, S.G.: Evidence that protein determines Ia antigenic specificity. Transplant. Proc. 7, 237–239 (1975)

Cullen, S.E., Schwartz, B.D., Nathenson, S.G., Cherry, M.: The molecular basis of codominant expression of the Histocompatibility-2 genetic region. Proc. Nat. Acad. Sci. U.S.A. 69, 1394–1397 (1972)

Cunningham, B., Berggård, I.: Structure, evolution and significance of β2-microglobulin. Transpl. Rev. 21, 3–14 (1974)

Cunningham, B., Wang, J.L., Berggård, I., Peterson, P.A.: The complete amino acid sequence of β2-microglobulin. Biochemistry 12, 4811–4822 (1973)

DAUSSET, J.: Présence des antigènes A et B dans les leucocytes décélée par des épauves d'agglutina-tion. Comptes Rendus Soc. Biol. **148**, 1607-1608 (1954)

DAUSSET, J., COLOMBANI, J.: Histocompatibility Testing 1972. Copenhagen: Munksgaard 1973

DAUSSET, J., COLIN, M., COLOMBANI, J.: Immune platelet isoantibodies. Vox. Sang. **5**, 4–31 (1960)

DAUSSET, J., DEGOS, L., HORS, J.: The Association of HL-A antigens with diseases. Clin. Immunol. and Immunopath., **3**, 127–149 (1974) and Transplant. Revs. **22** (1975)

DAVID, C.S., SHREFFLER, D.C.: Lymphocyte antigens controlled by the *Ir* region of the mouse *H-2* complex. Detection of new specificities with anti-H-2 reagents. Transplantation **17**, 462–469 (1974)

DAVID, C.S., KLEIN, J., SHREFFLER, D.C.: Serologic Homology between H-2 and HL-A system. Transplant. Proc. **5**, 461–466 (1973 a)

DAVID, C.S., SHREFFLER, D.C., FRELINGER, J.: New lymphocyte antigen system (Lna) controlled by the *Ir* region of the mouse *H-2* complex. Proc. Nat. Acad. Sci. U.S.A. **70**, 2509–2514 (1973 b)

DAVIES, D.A.L.: The molecular individuality of different mouse H-2 histocompatibility specificities determined by single genotypes. Transplantation **8**, 51–70 (1969)

DAVIES, D.A.L.: Transplantation antigens and tolerance. In: Immunological Tolerance to Tissue Antigens. Oswestry: Orthopaedic Hospital, 1971, 89–100

DAVIES, D.A.L.: The mechanism of transplant enhancement. Transpl. Proc. **7**, 443–447 (1975)

DAVIES, D.A.L., ALKINS, B.J.: What abrogates heart transplant rejection in immunological enhance-ment? Nature (Lond.) **247**, 294–297 (1974)

DAVIES, D.A.L., HESS, M.: New alloantigen genetically linked to the Major Histocompatibility Locus of the mouse. Nature **250**, 228–230 (1974)

DAVIES, D.A.L., MANSTONE, A.J., VIZA, D.C., COLOMBANI, J., DAUSSET, J.: Human transplantation antigens: The *HL-A* system and its homology with the mouse *H-2* system. Transplantation **6**, 571–586 (1968)

DAVIES, D.A.L., O'NEILL, G.J.: Methods of Cancer Immuno-chemotherapy (DRAB and DRAC) using antisera against tumour specific cell membrane antigens. Proc. XI Internat. Cancer Con-gress, Florence, 1974

DAVIES, D.A.L., O'NEILL, G.J.: Methods of Cancer Immuno-chemotherapy (DRAB and DRAC) using antisera against tumour specific cell membrane antigens. Printed in Excerpta Medica International Congress Series No. 349 Vol. 1 Cell biology and humour immunology. 218–221. Proceedings of the XI International Cancer Congress, Florence, 1974. Excerpta Medica Amster-dam

DÉMANT, P.: *H-2* gene complex and its role in alloimmune reactions. Transpl. Rev. **15**, 162–200 (1973)

DÉMANT, P., CHERRY, M., SNELL, G.D.: Hemagglutination and cytotoxic studies of H-2. Transplanta-tion **11**, 238–241 (1971)

DÉMANT, P., SNELL, G.D., HESS, M., LEMONNIER, F., NEAUPORT-SAUTES, C., KOURILSKY, F.: Separate and polymorphic loci controlling two types of polypeptide chains bearing the H-2 private and public specificities. J. Immunogenetics **2**, 263–271 (1975)

DUTTON, R.W.: Spleen cell proliferation in response to homologous antigens studied in congenic resistant strains of mice. J. Exp. Med. **123**, 665–672 (1966)

DUTTON, R.W.: T-cell factors in the regulation of the B-cell response. In: The Immune system: Genes, Receptors, Signals. New York: Academic Press, 1974, 485–496

EDMAN, P., BEGG, G.: A protein sequenator. Eur. J. Biochem. **1**, 80–91 (1967)

EDWARDS, R.G., HOWE, C.W.S., JOHNSON, M.H.: Immunology of Trophoblast. Cambridge: Univer-sity Press, 1975

EIJSVOOGEL, V.P., DUBOIS, M.J.G.J., MELIEF, C.J.M., DEGROOT-KOOY, M.L., KONING, C., VAN ROOD, J.J., VAN LEEUWEN, A., DUTOIT, E., SCHELLEKENS, P.TH.: Position of a locus determining mixed lymphocyte reaction (MLR), distinct from the known HL-A loci, and its relation to cell-mediated lympholysis. In: Histocompatibility Testing. Copenhagen: Munksgaard, 1973 a, 501–508

EIJSVOOGEL, V.P., DUBOIS, R., MELIEF, C.J.M., ZEYLEMAKER, W.P., ROOS-KONING, L., DEGROOT KOOY, L.: Lymphocyte activation and destruction in vitro in relation to MLC and HL-A. Transplant. Proc. **5**, 1301–1307 (1973 b)

EINSTEIN, A.B., MANN, D.L., GORDON, H.G., TRAPANI, R.J., FAHEY, J.L.: Heterologous antisera against specific HL-A antigens. Transplantation **12**, 299–304 (1971)

ENOMOTO, K., LUCAS, Z.J.: Immunological enhancement of renal allografts in the rat. Transplantation 15, 8–16 (1973)

EVRIN, P.E., NILSSON, K.: β2-microglobulin production in vitro by human hematopoietic, mesenchymal and epithelial cells. J. Immunol. 112, 137–144 (1974)

EVRIN, P.E., PERTOFT, H.: β2-microglobulin in human blood cells. J. Immunol. 111, 1147–1154 (1973)

EVRIN, P.E., PETERSON, P.A., WIDE, L., BERGGÅRD, I.: Radioimmunassay of β2-microglobulin in human biological fluids. Scand. J. Clin. Lab. Invest. 28, 439–443 (1971)

FELDMAN, M., BASTEN, A., BOYLSTON, A., ERB, P., GORCZYNSKI, R., GREAVES, M., HOGG, N., KILBURN, D., KONTIAINEN, S., PARKER, D., PEPYS, M., SCHRADER, J.: Interaction between T and B lymphocytes and accessory cells in antibody production. Progr. Immunol. 2, 65–75 (1975)

FELDMAN, M., CONE, R.E., MARCHALONIS, J.J.: Cell interactions in the immune responses in vitro. Cell Immunol. 9, 1–11 (1973)

FESTENSTEIN, H.: Immunogenetic and biological aspects of in vitro lymphocyte allotransformation (MLR) in the mouse. Transplant Rev. 15, 62–88 (1973)

FESTENSTEIN, H., ADAMS, E., BROWN, J., BURKE, J., LINCOLN, P., OLIVER, R.T.D., RONDIAK, G., SACHS, J.A., WELCH, S.G., WOLF, E.: The Distribution of HL-A antigens and other polymorphism in Bantu-speaking negroids living in Zambia. In: Histocompatibility Testing 1972. Copenhagen: Munksgaard, 1973 a, 397–407

FESTENSTEIN, H., ADAMS, E., BURKE, J., OLIVER, R.T.D., SACHS, J.A., WOLF, E.: The distribution of HL-A antigens in expatriates from East Bengal living in London. In: Histocompatibility Testing 1972. Copenhagen: Munksgaard, 1973 b, 175–178

FINKELMAN, F.D., SVEHACH, E.M., VITETTA, E.S., GREEN, I., PAUL, W.E.: Guinea pig Immune Response-related Histocompatibility antigens. J. Exp. Med. 141, 27–41 (1975)

FLEXNER, S., JOBLING, J.W.: On the promoting influence of heated tumor emulsions on tumour growth. Proc. Soc. Exp. Biol. and Med. 4, 156–157 (1907)

FORMAN, J., MÖLLER, G.: Generation of cytotoxic lymphocytes in mixed lymphocyte reactions. II. Importance of Private and Public H-2 alloantigens on the expression of cytotoxicity. Immunogenetics 3, 211–225 (1974)

FRELINGER, J.A., NIEDERHUBER, J.E., DAVID, C.S., SHREFFLER, D.C.: Evidence for the expression of Ia (H-2-associated) antigens on thymus-derived lymphocytes. J. Exp. Med. 140, 1273–1284 (1974)

FRELINGER, J.A., NIEDERHUBER, J.E., SHREFFLER, D.C.: Inhibition of immune responses in vitro by specific anti-Ia sera. Science (Wash.) 188, 268–270 (1975)

FRENCH, M.E., BATCHELOR, J.R.: Enhancement of renal allografts in rats and man. Transplant. Rev. 13, 115–141 (1972)

GLUECKSOHN-WAELSCH, S., ERICKSON, R.P.: The T-Locus of the mouse: Implications for mechanisms of development. Current Topics in Developmental Biol. 5, 281–316 (1970)

GOODFELLOW, P.N., JONES, E.A., VAN HEYNINGEN, V., SOLOMON, E., BORROW, M., MIGGIANO, V., BODMER, W.F.: The β2-microglobulin gene is on chromosome 15 and not in the HL-A region. Nature 254, 267–269 (1975)

GORER, P.A.: The role of antibodies in immunity to transplanted leukaemia in mice. J. Path. Bact. 54, 51–65 (1942)

GORER, P.A.: The genetic and antigenic basis of tumour transplantation. J. Path. Bact. 44, 691–697 (1953)

GORER, P.A.: Transplantese. Ann. N.Y. Acad. Sci. 87, 604–607 (1960)

GRAFF, R.J., NATHENSON, S.G.: Immunogenic properties of papain solubilized alloantigen. Transplant. Proc. 3, 249–252 (1971)

HALLE-PANNENKO, O., MARTYRE, M.C., JOLLÈS, P.: Conditioning of allogeneic mice with crude and purified H-2 extracts, alone and combined with cyclophosphamide for skin graft prolongation. Transplant. Proc. 3, 257–259 (1971 a)

HALLE-PANNENKO, O., MARTYRE, M.C., MATHÉ, G.: Prevention of graft-versus-host reaction by donor pretreatment with soluble H-2 antigens. Transplantation 11, 414–416 (1971 b)

HÄMMERLING, G.J., MCDEVITT, H.O.: Comparative analysis of antigen-binding T cells in genetic high and low responder mice. J. Exp. Med. 140, 1180–1188 (1974 a)

HÄMMERLING, G.J., MCDEVITT, H.O.: Antigen binding T and B lymphocytes. J. Immunol. 112, 1734–1740 (1974 b)

HANSTEIN, W.G., DAVIES, K.A., HAFETI, Y.: Water structure and the chaotropic properties of haloacetates. Arch. Biophys. Biochem. **147**, 534–544 (1971)

HARRIS, R., ZERVAS, Z.D.: Reticulocyte HL-A antigens. Nature (Lond.) **221**, 1062 (1969)

HAUPTFELD, V., HAUPTFELD, M., KLEIN, J.: Tissue distribution of I-region associated antigens in the mouse. J. Immunol. **113**, 181–188 (1974)

HESS, M., DAVIES, D.A.L.: Basic structure of mouse histocompatibility antigens. Eur. J. Biochem. **41**, 1–13 (1974)

HESS, M.: I-A^d alloantigens of the murine *Histocompatibility-2* complex. Folia Biol. (Prague) **21**, 428–430 (1975a)

HESS, M., DAVIES, D.A.L.: Membrane alloantigens controlled by the *I*-region of the *H-2* complex. Biochemical characterization using absorbed H-2 antisera. Transpl. Proc. **7**, 209–212 (1975)

HESS, M.: Private and public specificities of the Major murine Histocompatibility Complex (*H-2*): Molecular representation of H-2D^d antigens. Folia Biol. (Prague) **21**, 420–423 (1975b)

HESS, M., SMITH, W.: Comparative studies of mouse (H-2) and Human (HL-A) Histocompatibility antigens. Eur. J. Biochem. **43**, 471–477 (1974)

HILGERT, I., KANDUTSCH, A.A., CHERRY, M., SNELL, G.D.: Fractionation of murine H-2 antigens with the use of detergents. Transplantation **8**, 451–461 (1969)

HOLL-ALLEN, R.T.J., SCHARLI, A.P., MAGGS, P.R., BUSCH, G.J., SIMONIAN, S.J., WILSON, R.E.: Active enhancement of canine renal allografts using solubilized lymphocyte antigen. Transplantation **10**, 472–483 (1970)

HUMPHREY, J., KELLER, H.V.: Some evidence for specific interaction between immunologically competent cells and antigen. In: Developmental Aspects of Antibody Formation and Structure. Praha: Academia, 1970, 485–502

HÜTTENROTH, T.H., CLEEVE, H., LITWIN, S.D., POULIK, M.D.: The relationship between β2-microglobulin and immunoglobulin in cultured human lymphoid cell lines. J. Exp. Med. **137**, 838–840 (1973)

IVANYI, P., FOREIJT, J.: Genetic factors closely associated with the major histocompatibility system: Structural and/or regulatory genes. In: Present Problems in Haematology. Amsterdam-Prague: Excerpta Media-Czechoslovak Medical Press, 1974, 143–152

IVAŠKOVÁ, E., IVÁNYI, P.: Cytotoxic effect of anti-H-2 sera on human lymphocytes: Association with HL-A7 and W27. Folia Biol. **20**, 283–285 (1974)

JEANNET, M., PINN, V.W., FLAX, M.H., WINN, H.J., RUSSEL, P.S.: Humoral antibodies in renal allotransplantation in man. New England J. Med. **282**, 111–117 (1970)

KALISS, N.: Immunological enhancement of tumour homografts in mice: a review. Cancer Res. **18**, 992–1003 (1958)

KANDUTSCH, A.A., REINERT-WENCK, V.: Studies on a substance that promotes tumor homograft survival (the "enhancing substance"). Its distribution and some properties. J. Exp. Med. **105**, 125–139 (1957)

KANDUTSCH, A.A., STIMPFLING, J.H.: Partial purification of isoantigens from a mouse sarcoma. Transplantation **1**, 201–216 (1963)

KANO, K., KNOWLES, B.B., KOPROWSKI, H., MILGROM, F.: HL-A antigens on man-mouse hybrid cells. Eur. J. Immunol. **2**, 198–202 (1972)

KANO, K., LOZA, U., GERBASI, J.R., MILGROM, F.: Studies on heterophile antibodies in transplantation sera. Transplantation **19**, 20–26 (1975)

KATZ, D.H., BENACERRAF, B.: The regulatory influence of activated T cells on B cell responses to antigen. Adv. Immunol. **15**, 1–25 (1972)

KATZ, D.H., GRAVES, M., DORF, M.E., DIMUZIO, H., BENACERRAF, B.: Cell interactions between histoincompatible T and B lymphocytes. VII. Co-operative responses between lymphocytes are controlled by genes in the *I* region of the *H-2* complex. J. Exp. Med. **141**, 263–268 (1975)

KATZ, D.H., HAMAOKA, T., DORF, M.E., BENACERRAF, B.: Cell interactions between histoincompatible T and B lymphocytes. The H-2 gene complex determines successful physiologic lymphocyte interactions. Proc. Nat. Acad. Sci. U.S.A. **70**, 2624–2628 (1973)

KILSHAW, P.J., BRENT, L., THOMAS, A.V.: Specific unresponsiveness to skin allografts in mice. Transplantation **17**, 57–69 (1974)

KISSMEYER-NIELSEN, F., THORSBY, E.: Human transplantation antigens. Transplant. Rev. **4** (1970)

KLEIN, J.: Private and public antigens of the mouse H-2 system. Nature (Lond.) **229**, 635–637 (1971)

KLEIN, J.: Histocompatibility-2 system in wild mice. I. Identification of five new *H-2* chromosomes. Transplantation 13, 291–299 (1972)

KLEIN, J.: List of congenic lines of mice. Transplantation 15, 137–153 (1973a)

KLEIN, J.: The H-2 system: past and present. Transpl. Proc. 5, 11–21 (1973b)

KLEIN, J.: Genetic polymorphism of the histocompatibility loci of the mouse. Ann. Rev. Genetics 8, 63–79 (1974)

KLEIN, J., MURPHY, D.B.: The role of 'private' and 'public' antigens in skingraft rejection. Transpl. Proc. 5, 261–265 (1973)

KLEIN, J., SHREFFLER, D.C.: The H-2 model for the major histocompatibility systems. Transpl. Rev. 6, 3–29 (1971)

KOO, G.C., STACKPOLE, C.W., BOYSE, E.A., HÄMMERLING, U., LARDIS, M.P.: Topographic location of H-Y antigen on mouse spermatozoa by immunoelectronmicroscopy. Proc. Nat. Acad. Sci. U.S.A. 70, 1502–1505 (1973)

KOUBEK, K., HILGERT, I., KRIŠTOFOVÁ, H.: Chemical Nature of mouse histocompatibility antigens (II). Folia Biol. (Prague) 19, 397–401 (1973)

KOURILSKY, F.M., SILVESTRE, D., NEAUPORT-SAUTES, C., LOOSFELT, Y., DAUSSET, J.: Antibody induced redistribution of HL-A antigens at the cell surface. Eur. J. Immunol. 2, 249–257 (1972)

LAW, L.W., APPELLA, E., STROBER, S., WRIGHT, P.W., FISCHETTI, T.: Induction of immunological tolerance to soluble histocompatibility-2 antigens of mice. Proc. Nat. Acad. Sci. U.S.A. 69, 1858–1862 (1972)

LAW, L.W., APPELLA, E., STROBER, S., WRIGHT, S., WRIGHT, P.W., FISCHETTI, Y.: Soluble transplantation antigens, further studies of their tolerogenic properties. Transplantation 18, 487–495 (1974)

LENGEROVÁ, A.: Immunogenetics of Tissue Transplantation. Amsterdam-London: North Holland Publishing Company, 1969

LEVINE, B.B., STEMBER, R.H., FOTINO, M.: Ragweed hay fever: genetic control and linkage to HL-A haplotypes. Science 178, 1201–1203 (1972)

LIGHTBODY, J.J., URBANI, L., POULIK, M.D.: Effect of β2-microglobulin antibody on effector function of T-cell mediated cytotoxicity. Nature (Lond.) 250, 227–228 (1974)

LILLY, F.: The inheritance of susceptibility to the Gross leukaemia virus in mice. Genetics 53, 529–539 (1966)

LILLY, F.: The effect of histocompatibility-2 type on response to the Friend leukaemia virus in mice. J. Exp. Med. 127, 465–473 (1968)

LINDBLOM, J.B., ÖSTBERG, L., PETERSON, P.A.: β2-microglobulin on the cell surface. Relationship to HL-A antigens and the mixed leucocyte culture reaction. Tissue Antigens 4, 186–196 (1974)

LIVNAT, S., KLEIN, J., BACH, F.H.: Graft versus host reaction in strains of mice identical for H-2K and H-2D antigens. Nature New Biol. 243, 42–44 (1973)

LOKE, Y.W., JOYSEY, V.C., BORLAND, R.: HL-A antigens on human trophoblast cells. Nature (Lond.) 232, 403–404 (1971)

LONAI, P., McDEVITT, H.O.: *I*-region genes are expressed on T and B lymphocytes. J. Exp. Med. 140, 1317–1323 (1974a)

LONAI, P., McDEVITT, H.O.: Genetic control of the immune response. In vitro stimulation of lymphocytes by (T, G)-A–L, (H,G)-A–L and (Phe, G)-A–L. J. Exp. Med. 140, 977–994 (1974b)

LUCAS, Z.J., COPLON, N., KEMPSON, R., COHN, R.: Early renal transplant failure associated with subliminal sensitization. Transplantation 10, 522–529 (1970)

MANDEL, M.A., MONACO, A.P., RUSSEL, P.S.: Destruction of splenic transplantation antigens by a factor present in liver. J. Immunol. 95, 673–679 (1965)

MANN, D.L., FAHEY, J.L.: Histocompatibility antigens. Annu. Rev. Microbiol. 25, 679–710 (1971)

MAYR, W.R., BERNOCO, D., DE MARCHI, M., CEPPELLINI, R.: Genetic analysis and biological properties of products of the third SD (AJ) locus of the HL-A region. Transpl. Proc. 5, 1581–1593 (1973)

MacDONALD, A.S., DAVIES, D.A.L., CALNE, R.Y.: Factors governing antigen and antibody enhancement of the rat heart allografts. Transplantation Abstracts of the Fourth International Congress of the Transplantation Society. New York: Grune and Stratton, 1972, p. 180

MARSH, D.G., BIAS, W.B., HSU, S.H., GOODFRIEND, L.: Association of the HL-A. 7 cross reacting group with a specific antibody response in allergic man. Science (Wash.) 179, 691–693 (1973)

MARSH, D.G., BIAS, W.B., ISHIZAKA, K.: Genetic control of basal serum immunoglobulin E level and its effect on specific reagenic sensitivity. Proc. Nat. Acad. Sci. U.S.A. **71**, 3588–3592 (1974)

McDEVITT, H.: Mechanisms of B cell tolerance. In: Immunological Tolerance: Mechanisms and Potential Therapeutic Applications. New York: Academic Press, 1974, p. 247

McDEVITT, H.O., BECHTOL, K.B., HÄMMERLING, G.J., LONAI, P., DELOVITCH, T.L.: *Ir* genes and antigen recognition. In: The immune system: Genes, Receptors, Signals. New York: Academic Press, 1974, pp.597–632

McDEVITT, H.O., DEAK, B.D., SHREFFLER, D.C., KLEIN, J., STIMPFLING, J.H., SNELL, G.D.: Genetic control of the immune response. Mapping of the *Ir-1* locus. J. Exp. Med. **135**, 1259–1278 (1972)

McKEAN, D.J., PETERS, E.H., WALKBY, J.I., SMITHIES, O.: Amino acid sequence determination with radioactive proteins. Biochemistry **13**, 3048–3051 (1974)

MEO, T., DAVID, C.S., RIJNBECK, A.M., NABHOLZ, M., MIGGIANO, V.C., SHREFFLER, D.C.: Inhibition of mouse MLR by anti Ia-sera. Transpl. Proc. **7**, 127–130 (1975)

METZGAR, R.S., MILLER, J.L.: Production of HL-A specific antibodies in monkeys by immunization with soluble HL-A antigens. Transplantation **13**, 407–471 (1972)

MILLER, J.F.A.P., MITCHELL, G.F.: Thymus and antigen reactive cells. Transplant. Rev. **1**, 3–42 (1969)

MITCHISON, N.A., RAJEWSKY, K., TAYLOR, R.B.: Co-operation of antigenic determinants in the induction of antibodies. In: Developmental Aspects of Antibody Formation and Structure. New York: Academic Press, 1970, pp. 547–564

MIYAKAWA, Y., TANIGAKI, N., KREITER, V.P., MOORE, G.E., PRESSMAN, D.: Characterization of soluble substances in the plasma carrying HL-A alloantigen activity and HL-A common antigenic activity. Transplantation **15**, 312–319 (1973)

MIYAKAWA, Y., TANIGAKI, N., YAGI, Y., PRESSMAN, D.: An efficient method for isolation of HL-A antigens from hematopoietic cell lines. J. Immunol. **107**, 394–401 (1971)

MÖLLER, E.: Quantitative studies on the differentiation of isoantigens in newborn mice. Transplantation **1**, 165–173 (1965)

MÖLLER, G.: Phenotypic expression of isoantigens of the H-2 system in embryonic and newborn mice. J. Immunol. **90**, 271–279 (1963)

MUHLBOCK, O., DUX, A.: Histocompatibility Genes (the H-2 Complex) and susceptibility to mammary tumour virus in mice. J. Nat. Cancer Inst. **53**, 993–996 (1974)

MULLEN, Y., TAKASUGI, M., HILDEMANN, W.H.: The Immunological status of rats with long surviving (enhanced) kidney allografts. Transplantation **15**, 238–246 (1973)

MUNRO, A.J., TAUSSIG, M.J., CAMPBELL, R., WILLIAMS, H., LAWSON, Y.: Antigen specific T-cell factor in cell cooperation: Physical properties and mapping in the left-hand (K) half of *H-2*. J. Exp. Med. **140**, 1579–1587 (1974)

MURPHY, D.B., SHREFFLER, D.C.: Cross reactivity between H-2K and H-2D products. J. Exp. Med. **141**, 374–391 (1975)

MURRAY, S., DEWAR, P.J., ULDALL, P.R., WILKINSON, R., KERR, D.N.S., TAYLOR, R.M.R., SWINNEY, J.: Some important factors in cadaver-donor kidney transplantation. Tissue Antigens **4**, 548–557 (1974)

MYBURGH, J.A., MAIER, J., SMIT, J.A., SHAPIRO, M., MEYERS, A.M., RABKIN, R., VAN BLERK, P.J.P., JERSKY, J.: Presensitization and clinical kidney transplantation. Transplantation **18**, 206–212 (1974)

MYBURGH, J.A., SMIT, J.A.: Passive and active enhancement in baboon liver allografting. Transplantation **14**, 227–235 (1972)

NABHOLZ, M., VIVES, J., YOUNG, H.M., MEO, T., MIGGIANO, V., RIJNBEEK, A., SHREFFLER, D.C.: Cell mediated lysis in vitro: Genetic control of killer cell production and target specificities in the mouse. Eur. J. Immunol. **4**, 378–387 (1974)

NAKAMURO, K., TANIGAKI, N., PRESSMAN, D.: Multiple common properties of human β2-microglobulin and the common portion fragment derived from HL-A antigen molecules. Proc. Nat. Acad. Sci. U.S.A. **70**, 2863–2865 (1973)

NATHENSON, S.G.: Biochemical properties of histocompatibility antigens. Annu. Rev. Genetics **4**, 69–90 (1970)

NATHENSON, S.G., CULLEN, S.: Biochemical properties and immunochemical genetic-relationships of mouse H-2 alloantigens. Biochem. Biophys. Acta **344**, 1 25 (1974)

NATHENSON, S.G., DAVIES, D.A.L.: Solubilization and partial purification of mouse histocompatibility antigens from a membranous lipoprotein fraction. Proc. Nat. Acad. Sci. **56**, 476–483 (1966)

NATHENSON, S.G., MURAMATSU, T.: Properties of the carbohydrate portion of mouse H-2 alloantigen glycoproteins. In: Glycoproteins of Blood Cells and Plasma. Philadelphia: Lippincott, Co., 1971, pp. 245–262

NATORI, T., KATAGIRI, M., TANIGAKI, N., PRESSMAN, D.: The 11,000-dalton component of mouse H-2. Isolation and identification. Transplantation **18**, 550–555 (1974)

NEAUPORT-SAUTES, C., BISMUTH, A., KOURILSKY, F.M., MANUEL, Y.: Relationship between HL-A antigens and β2-microglobulin as studied by immunofluorescence on the lymphocyte membrane. J. Exp. Med. **139**, 957–968 (1974)

NEAUPORT-SAUTES, C., LILLY, F., SILVESTRE, D., KOURILSKY, F.M.: Independence of *H-2K* and *H-2D* antigenic determinants on the surface of mouse lymphocytes. J. Exp. Med. **137**, 511–526 (1973a)

NEAUPORT-SAUTES, C., SILVESTRE, D., KOURILSKY, F.M., DAUSSET, J.: Independence of HL-A antigens from the first and second locus at the cell surface. In: Histocompatibility Testing. Copenhagen: Munksgaard, 1972, 539–544

NEAUPORT-SAUTES, C., SILVESTRE, D., LILLY, F., KOURILSKY, F.M.: Molecular Independence of H-2K and H-2D antigens on the cell surface. Transpl. Proc. **5**, 443–446 (1973b)

NILSSON, K., EVRIN, P.E., WELSH, K.I.: Production of β2-microglobulin by normal and malignant human cell lines and peripheral lymphocytes. Transpl. Rev. **21**, 53–84 (1974)

NIMELSTEIN, S.H., HOTTI, A.R., HOLMAN, H.R.: Transformation of a histocompatibility immunogen into a tolerogen. J. Exp. Med. **138**, 723–733 (1973)

OH, S.K., PELLEGRINO, M.A., FERRONE, S., SEVIER, E.D., REISFELD, R.A.: Soluble HL-A antigens in serum. I. Isolation and purification.

PANCAKE, S.J., NATHENSON, S.G.: Selective loss of H-2 antigenic reactivity after chemical modification. J. Immunol. **111**, 1086–1092 (1973)

PARHAM, P., HUMPHREYS, R.E., TURNER, J., STROMINGER, J.L.: Heterogeneity of HL-A antigen preparations is due to variable sialic acid content. Proc. Nat. Acad. Sci. U.S.A. **71**, 3998–4001 (1974)

PARISH, C.R.: Immune response to chemically modified flagellin. IV. Further studies on the relationship between humoral and cell-mediated immunity. Cellular Immunol. **6**, 66–79 (1973)

PASSMORE, H.C., SHREFFLER, D.C.: A sex-limited serum protein variant in the mouse: Inheritance and association with the H-2 region. Biochem. Genet. **4**, 351–365 (1970)

PELLEGRINO, M.A., FERRONNE, S., MITTAL, K.K., GÖTZE, D., TERASAKI, P.I., REISFELD, R.A.: Cross-reactivity between human and murine lymphocyte antigens. Immunogenetics **1**, 158–173 (1974)

PETERSON, P.A., RASK, L., LINDBLOM, J.B.: Highly purified papain solubilized HT-A antigens contain β2-microglobulin. Proc. Nat. Acad. Sci. U.S.A. **71**, 35–39 (1974)

PIERCE, C.W., KAPP, J.A., SOLLIDAY, S.M., DORF, M.E., BENACERRAF, B.: Immune responses in vitro. XI. Suppression of primary IgM and IgG plaque forming cell responses in vitro by alloantisera against leucocyte alloantigens. J. Exp. Med. **140**, 921–938 (1974)

POULIK, M.D.: Presence of β2-microglobulin on B- and T-cells and lymphocytotoxicity of anti β2-microglobulin sera. Immunol. Commun. **2**, 403–414 (1973)

POULIK, M.D., BERNOCO, M., BERNOCO, D., CEPPELLINI, R.: Aggregation of HL-A antigens at the lymphocyte surface induced by antiserum to β2-microglobulin. Science (Wash.) **182**, 1352–1355 (1973)

POULIK, M.D., BLOOM, A.D.: β2-microglobulin production and secretion by lymphocytes in culture. J. Immunol. **110**, 1430–1433 (1973)

RACE, R.R., SANGER, R.: Blood Groups in Man, 4th ed. Oxford: Blackwell 1962

RAFF, M.C.: T and B lymphocytes and immune responses. Nature **242**, 19–23 (1973)

RAMSEIER, H., LINDENMANN, J.: Aliotypic antibodies. Transplant. Rev. **10**, 57–96 (1972)

RAPAPORT, F.T., DAUSSET, J., LAWRENCE, H.W., CONVERSE, J.M.: Enhancement of skin allograft survival in man. Surgery **64**, 25–30 (1968)

RASK, L., LINDBLOM, J.B., PETERSON, P.A.: Subunit structure of H-2 alloantigens. Nature **249**, 833–834 (1974a)

RASK, L., ÖSTBERG, L., LINDBLOM, B., FERNSTEDT, U., PETERSON, P.A.: The subunit structure of transplantation antigens. Transpl. Rev. **21**, 85–105 (1974b)

REISFELD, R.R., KAHAN, B.D.: Transplantation antigens. Adv. Immunology **12**, 117–200 (1970)

RICHIARDI, P., CARBONARA, H.O., MATTIUZ, P.L., CEPPELLINI, R.: Inhibition of cytotoxic anti HL-A sera by their F(ab')₂. In Histocompatibility Testing. Copenhagen: Munksgaard, 1972, p. 455–464

ROSENAU, W., HORWITZ, C.: Graft rejection in paternal to F_1 hybrid and reciprocal hybrid grafts indicating a histocompatibility gene on the mouse X chromosome. Lab. Invest. **18**, 298–303 (1968)

ROSENBERG, E.B., MANN, D.L., HILL, J.J., FAHEY, J.L.: Prolonged skin allograft survival in mice pretreated with soluble transplantation antigens. Transplantation **12**, 402–405 (1971)

RUSSELL, P.S.: Immunological enhancement. Transplant. Proc. **3**, 960–966 (1971)

RYCHLIKOVA, M., DÉMANT, P., IVANYI, P.: Histocompatibility gene organisation and mixed lymphocyte reaction. Nature New Biol. **320**, 271–272 (1971)

SANDERSON, A.R.: Quantitative titration, kinetic behaviour and inhibition of cytotoxic mouse isoantisera. Immunology **9**, 287–300 (1965)

SANDERSON, A.R., CRESWELL, P., WELSH, K.I.: Involvement of Carbohydrate in the immunochemical determinant area of HL-A substances. Nature **230**, 11–12 (1971)

SANDERSON, A.R., WELSH, K.I.: HL-A reagents from primates. Transplantation **16**, 304–312 (1973)

SANDERSON, A.R., WELSH, K.I.: Site density of antigens of the two HL-A segregant series on peripheral human lymphocytes. Transplantation **17**, 281–289 (1974a)

SANDERSON, A.R., WELSH, K.I.: Properties of histocompatibility (HL-A) determinants. Transplantation **18**, 197–205 (1974b)

SCHENDEL, D.J., BACH, F.H.: Genetic control of cell-mediated lympholysis in the mouse. J. Exp. Med. **140**, 1534–1546 (1974)

SCHIMPL, A., WECKER, B.: Replacement of T-cell function by a T-cell product. Nature New Biol. **237**, 15–17 (1972)

SCHUNTER, F., SCHIEFERSTEIN, G.: HL-A Antigene bei psoriasis vulgaris. Der Hautarzt **25**, 82–83 (1974)

SCHWARTZ, B.D., KATO, K., CULLEN, S.E., NATHENSON, S.G.: H-2 Histocompatibility alloantigens. Some biochemical properties of the molecules solubilized by NP-40 detergent. Biochemistry **12**, 2157–2164 (1973)

SCHWARTZ, B.D., NATHENSON, S.G.: Isolation of H-2 alloantigens solubilized by the detergent NP-40. J. Immunol. **107**, 1363–1367 (1971a)

SCHWARTZ, B.D., NATHENSON, S.G.: Regeneration of transplantation antigens on mouse cells. Transplant. Proc. **3**, 180–182 (1971b)

SEIGLER, H.F., KREMER, W.B., METZGAR, R.S., WARD, F.E., HAUNG, A.T., AMOS, D.B.: HL-A antigenic loss in malignant transformation. J. Nat. Cancer Inst. **46**, 577–584 (1971)

SHIMADA, A., NATHENSON, S.G.: Murine histocompatibility-2 (H-2) alloantigens. Purification and some chemical properties of soluble products from H-2ᵇ and H-2ᵈ genotypes released by papain digestion of membrane fractions. Biochemistry **8**, 4048–4062 (1969)

SHREFFLER, D.C., DAVID, C.S.: The *H-2* major histocompatibility complex and the *I* immune response region: Genetic variation, function and organization. Adv. Immunol. **20**, 125–195 (1975)

SHREFFLER, D.C., DAVID, C.S., PASSMORE, H.C., KLEIN, J.: Genetic organization and evolution of the mouse *H-2* region: A duplication model. Transpl. Proc. **3**, 176–179 (1971)

SHREFFLER, D.C., KLEIN, J.: Genetic organization and gene action of mouse *H-2* region. Transpl. Proc. **2**, 5–14 (1970)

SILVER, J., HOOD, L.: Detergent solubilized H-2 alloantigen is associated with a small molecular weight peptide. Nature **249**, 764–765 (1974)

SILVESTRE, D., KOURILSKY, F.M., NICCOLAI, M.G., LEVY, J.P.: Presence of HL-A antigens on human reticulocytes as demonstrated by electron microscopy. Nature (Lond.) **228**, 67–68 (1970)

SIMONSEN, M.: The Factor of immunization: clonal selection theory investigated by spleen assays of graft versus host reaction. In: Transplantation. London: Ciba Foundation Symposium, Churchill, 1962, p. 185–215

SINGAL, D.P., BERRY, R.: Soluble HL-A antigens, localization in the human seminal plasma fraction. Transplantation **13**, 441–442 (1972)

SINGER, S.J., NICHOLSON, G.L.: The fluid mosaic model of the structures of cell membranes. Science (Wash.) **175**, 720–731 (1972)

Smit, J.A., Myburgh, J.A.: Enhancement of baboon liver allografts with noncytotoxic preparations of alloimmune IgG. Transplantation 18, 63–70 (1974)

Smithies, O., Poulik, M.D.: Dog homologue of human β2-microglobulin. Proc. Nat. Acad. Sci. U.S.A. 69, 2914–2917 (1972)

Snary, D., Goodfellow, P., Hayman, M. J., Bodmer, W.F., Crumpton, M. J.: Subcellular separation and molecular nature of human histocompatibility antigens (HL-A). Nature 247, 457–461 (1974)

Snell, G.D.: The genetics of transplantation. J. Nat. Cancer Inst. 14, 691–700 (1953)

Snell, G.D.: The terminology of tissue transplantation. Transplantation 2, 655–657 (1964)

Snell, G.D., Cherry, M., Demant, P.: H-2: Its structure and similarity to HL-A. Transpl. Rev. 15, 3–25 (1973)

Snell, G.D., Stimpfling, J.H.: Genetics of tissue transplantation. In: Biology of the Laboratory Mouse. New York: McGraw-Hill, 1966, p. 457–491

Solheim, B.G.: Association between the β2m/HL-A molecule and membrane structures responsible for lymphocyte activation. Transpl. Rev. 21, 35–52 (1974)

Solheim, B.G., Thorsby, E.: β2-microglobulin. Part of the HL-A molecule in the cell membrane. Tissue Antigens 4, 83–94 (1974)

Springer, T.A., Strominger, J.L., Mann, D.: Partial purification of detergent soluble HL-A antigen and its cleavage by papain. Proc. Nat. Acad. Sci. U.S.A. 71, 1539–1543 (1974)

Staines, N.A., Ashton, J., Cuthbertson, J., Davies, D.A.L.: The detection of Ia antibodies in polyspecific H-2 alloantisera absorbed with erythrocytes. Tissue Antigens, 7, 1–14 (1976)

Staines, N.A., Guy, K., Davies, D.A.L.: Passive enhancement of mouse skin allografts. Specificity of the antiserum for major histocompatibility antigens. Transplantation 18, 192–195 (1974)

Staines, N.A., Guy, K., Davies, D.A.L.: The dominant role of Ia antibodies in the passive enhancement of H-2 incompatible skin grafts. Europ. J. Immunol., 5, 782–789 (1975)

Staines, N.A., O'Neill, G.J., Guy, K., Davies, D.A.L.: Xenoantisera against lymphoid cells, specificity and use in monitoring purification of mouse and human histocompatibility antigens. Tissue Antigens 3, 1–21 (1973)

Strominger, J.L., Cresswell, P., Grey, H., Humphreys, R.H., Mann, D., McCune, J., Parham, P., Robb, R., Sanderson, A.R., Springer, T.A., Perhorst, C., Turner, M.J.: The immunoglobulin-like structure of human histocompatibility antigens. Transplantation Rev. 21, 126–143 (1974)

Stuart, F.P., Fitch, F.W., Rowley, D.A.: Specific suppression of renal allograft rejection by treatment with antigen and antibody. Transplant. Proc. 2, 483–488 (1970)

Tanigaki, N., Miyakawa, U., Yagi, Y., Kreiter, V.P., Pressman, D.: Radioiodinated soluble HL-A antigens: HL-A alloantigenic characterization and use in radioimmunoassay. J. Immunol. Methods 3, 109–126 (1973a)

Tanigaki, N., Nakamuro, K., Appella, E., Poulik, M.D., Pressman, D.: Identity of the human HL-A common fragment and human β2-microglobulin. Biochem. Biophys. Res. Commun. 55, 1234–1239 (1973b)

Tanigaki, N., Pressman, D.: The basic structure and the antigenic characteristics of HL-A antigens. Transpl. Rev. 21, 15–34 (1974)

Taussig, M.J.: T-cell factor which can replace T-cells in vivo. Nature 248, 234–236 (1974)

Taussig, M.J., Mozes, E., Isac, R.: Antigen specific thymus cell factor in the genetic control of the immune response to poly (Tyrosyl, Glutamyl)-Poly-D, L-Alanyl-Poly-lysyl. J. Exp. Med. 140, 301–312 (1974)

Taussig, M.J., Munro, A.J.: Removal of specific cooperative T-cell factor by anti-H-2 but not by anti-Ig sera. Nature 251, 63–64 (1974)

Taylor, R.B., Duffus, W.P.H., Raff, M.C., De Petris, S.: Redistribution and pinocytosis of lymphocyte surface immunoglobulin molecules induced by anti-immunoglobulin antibody. Nature New Biol. 233, 225–229 (1971)

Thieme, T.R., Raley, R.A., Fahey, J.L.: Demonstration of molecular individuality of HL-A antigens. J. Immunol. 113, 323–328 (1974)

Unanue, E.B., Dorf, M.E., David, C.S., Benacerraf, B.: The presence of I-region-associated antigens on B-cells in molecules distinct from immunoglobulin and H-2K and H-2D. Proc. Nat. Acad. Sci. U.S.A. 71, 5014–5016 (1974)

van den Tweel, J.G., van Oud Alblas, A.B., Keuning, J.J., Goulmy, E., Termijtelen, A., Bach, M.L., van Rood, J.J.: Typing for MLC (LD): I. Lymphocytes from cousin-marriage offspring as typing cells. Trans. Proc. 5, 1535–1538 (1973)

VAN LEEUWEN, A., SCHUIT, H.R.E., VAN ROOD, J.J.: Typing for MLC (LD): II. The selection of nonstimulator cells by MLC inhibition tests using SD-identical stimulator cells (MISIS) and fluorescence antibody studies. Transplant. Proc. **5**, 1539–1542 (1973)

VAN ROOD, J.J.: LD-SD interaction in vivo and the allograft reaction. Transplant. Proc. **5**, 1747–1750 (1973)

VAN ROOD, J.J., KOCH, C.T., VAN HOOFF, J.P., VAN LEEUWEN, A., VAN DEN TWEEL, J.G., FREDERIKS, E., SCHIPPERS, H.M.A., HENDRIKS, G., VAN DER STEEN, G.J.: Graft survival in unrelated donor-recipient pairs matches for MLC and HL-A. Transplant. Proc. **5**, 409–414 (1973)

VAN ROOD, T.J., VAN LEEUWEN, A., BOSCH, L.J.: Leucocyte antigens and transplantation immunity. Proc. 8th Congr. Europ. Soc. Haematol (Vienna). Basel: Karger, 1961, p. 109–199

VAN ROOD, J.J., VAN LEEUWEN, A., KEUNING, J.J., TERMIJTELEN, A.: Serotyping for MLC III. Family and population studies with an MLC inhibiting serum Pl. Transpl. Proc., **7**, Suppl. 1, 31–34 (1975a)

VAN ROOD, J.J., VAN OUD ALBLAS, A.B., KEUNING, J.J., FREDERIKS, E., TERMIJTELEN, A., VAN HOOFF, J.P., PENA, A.S., VAN LEEUWEN, A.: Histocompatibility genes and transplantation antigens. In: Proc. 5th Internat. Congr. Transplantation, Jerusalem. (1975b)

VAN ROOD, J.J., VAN OUD ALBLAS, A.B., KEUNING, J.J., FREDERIKS, E., TERMIJTELEN, A., VAN HOOFF, J.P., PENA, A.S., VAN LEEUWEN, A.: Histocompatibility genes and transplantation antigens. Transpl. Proc. **7** Supp. 1, 25–30 (1975)

VITETTA, E.S., KLEIN, J., UHR, J.W.: Isolation and partial characterization of Ia antigens from murine lymphoid cells. Immunogenetics **1**, 82–90 (1974)

VOJTÍŠKOVÁ, M., POLÁČKOVÁ, M., POKORNÁ, Z.: Histocompatibility antigens on mouse spermatozoa. Folia Biol. **15**, 322–332 (1969)

WALLACH, D.F.H., LIN, P.S.: A critical evaluation of plasma membrane fractionation. Biochem. Biophys. Acta **300**, 211–254 (1973)

WATKINS, W.M.: Biosynthesis of blood group substances. In: Blood and Tissue antigens. New York: Academic Press, 1970, p. 441–459

WIDMER, M.B., OMEIDI-ZORINI, C., BACH, M.L., BACH, F.H., KLEIN, J.: Importance of different regions of *H-2* for MLC stimulation. Tissue Antigens **3**, 309–315 (1973)

WIGZELL, H.: Quantitative titrations of mouse H-2 antibodies using ^{51}Cr labelled target cells. Transplantation **33**, 423–431 (1965)

WINN, H.J., BALDAMUS, C.A., JOOSTE, S.V., RUSSELL, P.S.: Acute destruction by humoral antibody of rat skin grafted to mice. J. Exp. Med. **137**, 593–610 (1973)

YUNIS, E.J., AMOS, B.D.: Three closely linked genetic systems relevant to transplantation. Proc. Nat. Acad. Sci. (Wash.) **68**, 3031–3035 (1971)

ZALESKY, M.B., KLEIN, J.: Immune response of mice to Thy-1.1 antigen: Genetic control by alleles at the *Ir-5* locus loosely linked to the *H-2* complex. J. Immunol. **113**, 1170–1177 (1974)

ZIGHELBOIM, J., THIEME, T., GALE, R.P., OSSORIO, R.C., FAHEY, J.L.: A sensitive method for detecting antibodies in human sera used for tissue typing. Transplantation **18**, 180–185 (1974)

Lymphocyte – Defined Components of the Major Histocompatibility Complex *

Miriam Segall

With 7 Figures and 10 Tables

A. Introduction. General Principles of MLC

The mixed leukocyte culture (MLC) test has come into increasing use in the last few years, both in experimental studies and as a clinical test in matching potential donors and recipients for transplantation. It is considered a model of the "recognition phase" of the homograft reaction, representing the initial recognition by, and subsequent proliferation of, lymphocytes responding to histocompatibility differences. In this "classical" MLC no attempt is made to identify individual factors responsible for histoincompatibility; rather, the total disparity between two individuals is measured. The way in which this measurement is made, the genetic control of reactivity, and the experimental evidence for the relationship of MLC reactivity to other forms of histocompatibility testing and to the actual fate of transplanted cells or organs, will be discussed in the sections which follow.

The MLC reaction was originally described by Bain et al. (1964) and Hirsch-horn et al. (1964) as a proliferative response induced in human leukocytes in culture by allogeneic leukocytes. Proliferation was measured either by determination of the uptake of radioactive thymidine, a DNA precursor, or by estimation of the percentage of dividing or transformed (blast) cells in the mixed cultures of allogeneic leukocytes. The transformed cells were of lymphoblastoid type, morphologically similar to those seen in cultures stimulated with nonspecific mitogens such as phytohemagglutinin (PHA) or with antigens to which the cell donor was sensitized, and it was thought that these cells were small lymphocytes which were stimulated to division in response to foreign histocompatibility antigens.

That the proliferative response in MLC was an immunologic reaction was not immediately clear. Early in the study of MLC responses it was learned that cells of identical twins were mutually non-stimulatory in mixed culture, that a certain percentage of siblings were mutually non-stimulatory, and that cells of two unrelated individuals were stimulatory if culture conditions were

* Supported by training grant NIGMS 00398.
This is paper no. 1835 from the Laboratory of Genetics; and paper no. 28 from the Immunobiology Research Center. The University of Wisconsin, Madison Wisconsin.

adequate. Work by Wilson *et al.* (1967) established the immunologic nature of the MLC response by showing that this response was specifically abolished in tolerant animals which did not reject skin grafts. Tolerant rats were non-responsive to stimulating cells of the strain to which the animal was tolerant, and normally responsive to cells of third-party strains. The effects of preimmunization, especially in humans, on MLC responses are not well defined.

B. Technical and Statistical Aspects of Human MLC

I. Macro- and Micro-Methods

The early techniques established for MLC required rather large numbers of cells; it was therefore difficult to do MLC tests in certain clinical situations, especially with leukopenic patients or young children. The development of "micro-" methods, utilizing much smaller numbers of cells, has made it possible to perform such tests. Several methods are now in use which require $0.5-2 \times 10^5$ responding cells and $0.5-4 \times 10^5$ stimulating cells per replicate culture; three or four replicates of each combination are generally made. Such "micro-" cultures can be incubated in small tubes or in small-volume wells in tissue-culture plates.

The MLC response as originally studied was a "two-way" response, i.e., in a mixed culture of cells from individuals A and B, there would be a proliferative response of A lymphocytes to B histocompatibility antigens, and a proliferative response of B lymphocytes to A histocompatibility antigens. A "one-way" response can be obtained by treating the cells which are to provide the stimulus with mitomycin-C, or x-irradiating them, to prevent division. The incorporation of labeled thymidine in a culture AB_m or AB_x would thus measure only the division of A cells stimulated by histocompatibility antigens on B cells, since the treated B cells would be unable to divide. However, the stimulating cells may not behave simply as passive carriers of antigens. The treated cells are not immediately killed and may survive for two or three days, perhaps even longer. It is known that mitomycin-treated cells can liberate blastogenic and other factors into the medium, so they may be able to influence the response of the untreated cells in some non-specific way. Several reports in the literature indicate that killed cells or cell extracts are non-stimulatory; it is not clear whether the killing or extracting procedure destroys some structure essential for stimulating ability, or whether some function of a live cell is required. In the absence of any definitive work, the assumption that labeled thymidine incorporation in a culture AB_m represents a reaction of responsive A cells to passive B cells is suspect, although it is clear that the cells incorporating thymidine are A cells.

The general procedure in setting up mixed cultures is as follows: Blood is drawn in anticoagulants. Leukocytes are isolated either by allowing the blood to settle or by centrifuging the whole blood and removing the buffy coat. The cells are then purified to remove most of the polymorphonuclear leukocytes and red cells, leaving lymphocytes, monocytes, and any remaining platelets. The whole blood may be diluted and purified without prior isolation of leukocytes if defibrinated blood is used. Purified cells are washed, treated with mitomycin-C or X-ray where required, and resuspended in culture medium. Appropriate dilutions of responding and stimulating cells are then distributed into culture tubes or plates. After a period of incubation a radioactive compound, usually tritiated (H^3-) or C^{14}-thymidine, is added to the culture, and after a further period of incubation with a labeled compound the cultures are harvested and prepared for scintillation counting.

Mononuclear cells are separated from granulocytes since the granulocyte contamination in the final cultures affects the MLC response which is obtained. Either X-ray or mitomycin-C treatment may be used for inactivation; we have found no difference between the two methods, and the choice will generally be dictated by convenience and/or availability of equipment.

Recently several laboratories, including our own, have begun to use cryopreserved cells for MLC. In such procedures, mononuclear cells are purified in the same way as for MLC, then frozen at $-1°C/min$ in a controlled-rate freezing apparatus and stored in liquid nitrogen. With some experience good yields of cells with very high viability can be obtained on thawing, and we find that these cells can be used in MLC and behave in the same way, as either stimulators or responders, as fresh cells from the same individual. The usefulness of such a method, both for cooperation between laboratories and for experiments where fresh cells of a particular individual may not be available (e.g., post-transplant testing of cadaver kidney recipients), is obvious.

II. Determination of Non-Stimulation

1. Controls

In attempting to determine stimulation or non-stimulation in MLC, it is essential that certain controls be included in the experiment. These will be discussed using letters of the alphabet (A, B, C etc.) to indicate the different cells involved in an experiment, and the subscript "m" to indicate mitomycin treatment (or X-ray if this is used). The letter X indicates cells of a normal unrelated donor which must be included in any experiment involving tests for non-stimulation, as discussed below.

If the mixture AB_m shows no stimulation, one must be able to demonstrate in the same experiment a mixture AX_m in which there is stimulation (indicating that the A cells are capable of response) and a mixture XB_m in which there is stimulation (indicating that the B_m cells are capable of stimulation). Should either of these control combinations be negative, the experiment is considered a technical failure. A control mixture A_mB_m is also useful to demonstrate the efficacy of the inactivation procedure.

In determining stimulation or non-stimulation, the control AA_m should be used in preference to the control A cells alone, and this control should be done using A_m cells at every concentration at which B_m is used. I.e., for the experimental mixture A cells $1 \times 10^5 + B_m$ 2×10^5, the proper control is A $1 \times 10^5 + A_m$ 2×10^5. At high concentrations of stimulating cells, a culture AA_m will incorporate appreciable amounts of tritiated thymidine, and this phenomenon must be controlled for. A typical protocol for a clinical MLC is shown in Table 1.

Table 1. General Clinical Protocol. A = potential recipient, B = potential donor, X = normal unrelated

Responder	Cells/Well	Stimulator	Cells/Well
A	1×10^5	B_m	1×10^5
A	1×10^5	B_m	2×10^5
A	1×10^5	X_m	1×10^5
A	1×10^5	X_m	2×10^5
A	1×10^5	A_m	1×10^5
A	1×10^5	A_m	2×10^5
X	1×10^5	B_m	1×10^5
X	1×10^5	B_m	2×10^5
X	1×10^5	X_m	1×10^5
X	1×10^5	X_m	2×10^5

Given that, where a combination AB_m is being tested, it has been shown that the A cells can respond and the B_m cells can stimulate, other technical or quasitechnical problems may arise in attempting to determine stimulation or non-stimulation. One deceptive situation is the case where the mixture AB_m is negative and the incorporation in the mixture AX_m is very low. Such a negative result may represent simply a very low response of A cells, in effect a failure due to lack of sensitivity of the method, and a conclusion of non-stimulation between A and B is not warranted in these circumstances. Another false interpretation of non-stimulation due to insensitivity of the method may occur in the situation where AB_m at one concentration of B_m cells is negative, but AB_m at a higher concentration of B_m (if it has been done) will be positive. With the micro-method, in our hands, this has been exceedingly infrequent, but clinical experiments in our laboratory are still routinely run at two concentrations of stimulating cells.

2. Statistical Analysis

The most difficult interpretive problems are raised in those cases where incorporation in the mixture AB_m is above that in the AA_m control, but the significance of the differences is not immediately clear. A number of methods of statistical analysis are available in such situations; all have their drawbacks. (For a brief definition of terms used in the following discussion, the reader is referred to Appendix I.)

a) Stimulation Index. The stimulation index, expressed as the ratio of counts per minute in the experimental mixture divided by counts per minute in the control, has been used by a number of groups; a stimulation index above a certain level is designated a positive test, and below that level, a negative test. An examination of the statistics of the MLC test will reveal the difficulties of using this criterion.

Control values in the MLC are generally quite low and have a high standard deviation (in our micromethod, frequently 25–30% of the mean or greater, as compared to 5–15% of the mean in experimental combinations). If in replicate cultures of a control AA_m we obtain, for example, 304, 196, 406 and 252 cpm, this set of replicates has a mean of 290 cpm and a standard deviation of 89 cpm, or almost 31%. The 95% confidence limits of this mean of 290 cpm are 110 and 470 cpm. If the 95% confidence limits are considered, it will be seen that a mixture AB_m with a mean of 580 counts, which at first glance has a stimulation index of 2.0 (usually considered positive), may actually have a stimulation index anywhere between 1.2 and 4.4, without even considering the 95% confidence limits which may be placed on the figure of 580 cpm. Stimulation indices are entirely valid, of course, in considering a series of stimulators tested against one responder (AB_m, AC_m, AD_m, etc.). They can also be useful in pooling data from large numbers of experiments provided the statistical limitations are kept in mind; but for the evaluation of stimulation or non-stimulation in doubtful cases they are less than ideal and may be very misleading.

b) T-test and Mann-Whitney U-test. Statistical methods for determining the significance of differences in the mean of two populations may be applied to the two sets of replicates, AA_m and AB_m. One of the most familiar is the Student's t-test, which we have frequently used in evaluating stimulation. The t-test is a parametric test and therefore makes several requirements of the data. One is that both samples be drawn from a population normally distributed with respect to the parameter in question (which may not be true for AA_m); another is that the variances of the two populations be equal (a situation which we have approximated by using the $\log_{10}$ cpm values rather than the actual cpm as the raw data for the t-test). Another test, with similar purpose but less restrictive, is the Mann-Whitney U-test (also known as the Wilcoxon rank test), which evaluates whether the means of two populations are significantly different by examining the degree of overlap between the two populations when the members of both populations (in this case, the cpm in the two sets of replicates) are ranked in order from lowest to highest. The Mann-Whitney test has the advantage that it makes no requirements of the data with respect to normality, variances, etc.

c) Wilcoxon signed rank test. Both the t-test and the Mann-Whitney U-test have the disadvantage that relative degree of stimulation, simply considered as whether the combination AB_m incorporates *significantly* more cpm than the combination AC_m, is not completely reproducible. That is, in one experiment AB_m might have been significantly higher than AC_m at the 5% significance level by t-test; in a repeat experiment the two combinations might not be significantly different. This suggests a third possibility for evaluating stimulation in doubtful cases, namely considering whether (in several experiments) the experimental mean is usually higher than the control although it may not be significantly higher. The Wilcoxon signed rank test may be useful for this purpose to give a level of statistical significance for the observed data.

In discussing this problem the assumption is frequently, although tacitly, made that the difference between non-stimulation and low stimulation has some biological significance. That this assumption is valid is not at all clear. The distinction may be entirely artificial, a result of the sensitivity of the method and the type of control employed, or it may be "real" in some biological sense but of no particular significance in evaluating histocompatibility differences; i.e. a low stimulator may be as good an organ donor for a particular recipient as a non-stimulator. This question is discussed further below (Sections F, H).

3. Quantitation of MLC Results

The question of low versus non-stimulation also brings up another problem in the evaluation of MLC data, that of quantitating the results. It is generally assumed that a low-stimulating combination is more histocompatible than a high-stimulating one. Given this assumption, which will be considered in detail later, two questions remain: how great a degree of incompatibility is indicated by a given degree of stimulation, and how does one define a given degree of stimulation. We will take the second question first, and postpone the first question to the discussion of the correlation of MLC with graft results.

Evidence that the MLC can be a quantitative as well as a qualitative test comes from family studies in which siblings who differ by one HL-A haplotype (e.g., an a/c sibling responding to an a/d sibling) generally stimulate less than siblings who differ by two alleles (e.g., an a/c sibling responding to a b/d sibling). The difference between one- and two-allele-different stimulators is usually approximately two-fold. However, in certain families we have seen that one particular allele may give relatively low stimulation, e.g. a/c responding to a/d is always lower than the reciprocal combination, and b/c responding to b/d is always lower than the reciprocal combination; the test is sensitive enough to detect such differences.

a) Counts per minute. The simplest method for quantitating degree of stimulation would appear to be by the number of counts per minute incorporated in the allogenic mixture AB_m. However, this number is probably not in itself a reliably quantitative index.

First, there can be considerable variation in the total cpm incorporated in a given mixture if the same A and B cells are set up in mixed culture on different days. Some of this variation may be technical; some may be a reflection of real biological differences in stimulatory or responsive capability of the same individual's cells on different days. Regardless of its source, this variability is an important consideration in quantitation of MLC responses.

Second, it is clear that different responders are different in the maximum response they will give. In experiments where a responder was tested against 15 or 20 stimulators, the average stimulation (average of the cpm incorporated

Table 2. Illustration of Range of MLC stimulation

	Responder			
	A	B	C	D
Average of stimulation with stimulators G_m-Z_m	12,000[a]	20,000	27,000	18,000
Lowest combination	AX_m 5,000	BH_m 7,000	CZ_m 5,000	DR_m 6,500
Highest combination	AQ_m 25,000	BK_m 55,000	CG_m 63,000	DL_m 45,000

[a] Average of counts per minute of tritiated thymidine incorporated in replicate cultures.

in the 15 or 20 mixtures of allogeneic stimulators with that responder) of different responders with the same set of stimulators was different. Hence, as shown in Table 2, 5,000 cpm in the mixture AX_m, where the mean stimulation with responder A was 12,000 cpm and the highest individual stimulation was 25,000 cpm, may have an entirely different significance (in terms of degree of histoincompatibility) from 5,000 cpm in the mixture CZ_m, where the mean stimulation with responder C was 27,000 cpm and the highest individual stimulation was 63,000 cpm.

Several different approaches have been used to control for the day-to-day variability of cpm in a given mixture.

b) Stimulation index. Some investigators have used the stimulation index, discussed previously, to indicate degree of stimulation. The difficulties inherent in the use of a low-value, high-variability number as the foundation for a quantitative measurement have been discussed in connection with the determination of non-stimulation. The use of the stimulation index as a measure of degree of stimulation contains the further assumption that the control (AA_m) value is a quantitative measurement of the "degree of responsiveness" of a particular responder. For example, if the control AA_m incorporates 200 cpm, the control BB_m 1,000 cpm, and the incorporation in the mixtures AC_m and BC_m is 10,000 and 50,000 cpm respectively, according to the stimulation index both AC_m and BC_m have values of 50, and C_m stimulates both A and B to the same extent (see Table 3). While it is entirely possible that there is a tendency

Table 3. Illustration of Stimulation Indices

Stimu-lator	Responder					
	A		B		C	
	cpm[a]	S.I.[b]	cpm	S.I.	cpm	S.I.
A_m	200	—	25,000	25	5,000	10
B_m	4,000	20	1,000	—	20,000	40
C_m	10,000	50	50,000	50	500	—

[a] Average of counts per minute of tritiated thymidine incorporated in replicate cultures.
[b] S.I.=cpm in experimental cultures/cpm in control (autologous) cultures.

for individuals who are high responders to have high levels of spontaneous cell division, this is probably not sufficiently reliable for quantitation.

Moreover, experiments in our laboratory indicate that the spontaneously dividing cells in the AA_m control are not directly related to the stimulated dividing cells in the AB_m culture. Treatment of cells with 5-bromo-deoxyuridine (BUdR) followed by exposure to light inactivates the dividing cells, as determined by subsequent failure of treated AB_m mixtures to incorporate tritiated thymidine. A responding cells were treated with BUdR and light and subsequently cultured with either A_m or B_m stimulating cells. The BUdR pre-treatment reduced the cpm incorporated in the AA_m mixtures, but did not reduce the cpm incorporated in the AB_m mixtures.

This is not to argue that the stimulation index is useless. It can be used (we among others have used it), for example, to pool data from a large number of repeat experiments. However, in the individual instance, it should be used and regarded with full consideration of the technical and statistical difficulties involved.

c) Standard stimulating cells or reagents. The next approach is to use some other stimulator as a standard. In a clinical experiment (see Table 1) cells of one or two random unrelateds are routinely included, along with cells of the potential donor, as stimulators of the cells of the potential recipient, as controls for the response of the recipient, as previously discussed. However, in view of the wide variability in stimulation of a given responder by a series of stimulating cells, it may be difficult to compare response to a potential donor with response to one or two randomly chosen unrelateds in any quantitatively meaningful way (but see Section H).

We have tried, on the basis of the experiments with 15–20 stimulators discussed above, to use a panel of 20 randomly chosen cells as representatives of the "general population", and to express the stimulation in a mixture AB_m in terms of its relative position in the range of stimulation $AX_{1m} \ldots AX_{20m}$. This approach is obviously not suited to the routine clinical situation, even had it proved entirely satisfactory for certain experimental purposes (which it did not). The use of pools of stimulating cells seemed more practical. If, instead of using stimulating cells from one donor, one uses a pool of cells from different donors (but maintaining the final concentration of stimulating cells constant), with increasing pool size one should eventually reach a point where all responding cells capable of being stimulated would be stimulated, and a plateau of labeled thymidine uptake should be reached, with larger pool sizes not stimulating a greater uptake. This expectation has been verified in several experiments. We have also found that once this plateau is reached (usually with pools of 20–30 cells), different non-overlapping pools of this size all give approximately the same amount of stimulation (in terms of cpm incorporated) with a given responder in a given experiment, even though the pools are composed of different cells.

In a number of large experiments we found that the mean stimulation of a given responder by three pools of 20 stimulating cells (pool mean) correlated very highly with the mean stimulation of the responder by a group of 12–15 individual stimulating cells (Segall *et al.*, to be published). This suggested that the pools were indeed able to correct for both the technical and biological components of the day-to-day variability of cpm. In these experiments both the control (AA_m) and stimulation with concanavalin A (another non-specific mitogen, similar to PHA) showed a much poorer correlation with the experimental mean than did the pool mean.

Another approach to the use of pools as standard stimulators has been reported, using pools of three cells which among them covered a spectrum of cross-reacting HL-A SD specificities (OSOBA and FALK, 1974).

The demonstration of some sort of standard stimulating agent is obviously extremely important for any precise quantitation of MLC results, and it is hoped that a satisfactory and generally acceptable standard will be forthcoming.

d) Technical and Statistical Aspects of Quantitation. In considering quantitative measurements in MLC, certain technical and statistical imperatives must be kept in mind. The first is the kinetics of response in mixed leukocyte cultures. Different mixtures may reach their peak incorporation of label on different days, even in a system where medium is replaced to replenish nutrients and the buffering is designed to prevent pH changes resulting from rapid cell division. In cases where exhaustion of nutrients or pH changes may play a role, the kinetics may also be affected by these essentially extraneous factors. For this reason the choice of a day of assay is important, especially where quantitative considerations are involved. An experiment looking for MLC-identical siblings in a family requires much less attention to details of kinetics than an experiment designed to detect small differences in degree of stimulation between unrelateds.

In our micromethod, we have generally used a 5- or 6-day assay, considering the day of setting up the cultures as day 0, labeling in the afternoon or evening of day 4 and harvesting the cultures on the morning of day 5, or labeling in the afternoon or evening of day 5 and harvesting on the morning of day 6. In numerous time-course experiments we have not seen mixtures which peak on day 4 or are on a plateau when harvested at day 4 and day 5, and we thus feel confident that an experiment harvested on the morning of day 5 is still in the exponential growth stage. We have observed combinations which are on a plateau when harvested at day 5 and day 6, or where the rate of increase in thymidine incorporation has slowed substantially between day 5 and day 6; for this reason, in quantitative experiments, cultures are harvested on the morning of day 5. By day 7, in these small-volume cultures without replenishment of medium, there are frequently marked pH changes and a decrease in thymidine incorporation from that found on day 5 or 6.

Another technical consideration is the dose-response curve. In theory, in a culture system where all nutritional and other requirements are met, the incorporation of tritiated thymidine should depend only on the amount of stimulus provided (number of stimulating cells) and the amount of response available (number of responding cells). Thus the response should increase in a linear fashion if responding cell number is held constant and stimulating cell number increased. Such linearity is important if one wishes to state that stimulation in the technique employed is directly related to degree of histoincompatibility between stimulator and responder, and not influenced in some undefined fashion by technical factors in the culture system. Obviously it is important

Table 4. Example of MLC Data

Combi-nation	Mean	S.D.	%S.D.	Log Mean	Log S.D.	%Log S.D.	cpm in individual cultures			
AA$_m$	1,241	1,005	81.0	3.0001	0.3162	10.5	2,706	534	640	1,082
AB$_m$	25,155	1,478	5.9	4.4001	0.0249	0.6	24,577	24,561	27,349	24,131
AC$_m$	18,366	1,554	8.5	4.2628	0.0371	0.9	16,514	19,930	19,325	17,696
CA$_m$	8,119	1,087	13.4	3.9065	0.0590	1.5	7,605	9,261	8,747	6,861
CB$_m$	11,297	1,089	9.6	4.0514	0.0422	1.0	11,382	11,241	9,950	12,614
CC$_m$	473	123	26.0	2.6630	0.1157	4.3	553	599	395	343
CD$_m$	12,755	448	3.5	4.1055	0.0151	0.4	13,374	12,785	12,372	12,489
DA$_m$	17,845	1,091	6.1	4.2509	0.0259	0.6	17,347	19,459	17,071	17,503
DB$_m$	14,657	3,070	20.9	4.1581	0.0987	2.4	17,627	15,934	14,629	10,436
DC$_m$	19,745	2,368	12.0	4.2931	0.0517	1.2	17,499	18,111	20,793	22,576
DD$_m$	724	500	69.0	2.7701	0.3407	12.3	688	592	1,407	210

Mean = arithmetic mean of cpm incorporated in replicate cultures; S.D. = standard deviation; %S.D. = coefficient of correlation (S.D./mean); log mean = geometric mean (mean of the logs) of cpm incorporated in replicate cultures.

to work at cell concentrations where such linearity can be demonstrated, and not to use concentrations so high that inhibition results.

Statistically, an important parameter of a test which one wishes to quantitate is the degree of discrimination between different combinations which is possible. A convenient indicator is the variability in replicate cultures of a single stimula-tor-responder combination. A coefficient of variation (standard deviation divided by the mean) of 0.10 or less will give excellent discrimination between combinations; 0.15 is still very good. Large coefficients of variation imply wide 95% confidence limits for the average cpm of a given mixture and make it unlikely that differences will be statistically distinguishable. In Table 4 are given some MLC data from a single experiment, and the statistical parameters calculated from that data.

C. Mouse MLC Techniques

The laboratory mouse offers a number of advantages in the study of histocom-patibility and these advantages have been evident in work concerning MLC. Mice are readily available as highly inbred strains, strains in which all individuals are virtually identical and which therefore provide a large uniform population for experimental studies. Not only are inbred strains available, but some of these strains have been developed so as to be identical except for their major histocompatibility (H-2) regions (congenic resistant strains); e.g. the strains C57BL/10, B10.D2, B10.BR, B10.A, etc. carry different H-2 alleles but are otherwise genetically identical. Studies over the last thirty years have produced a large body of information concerning the genetics of H-2 (and other histocompatibility loci) in the mouse; the serologically defined H-2 specificities have been extensively studied. This accumulation of information makes the mouse an extremely useful object for study of problems in histocompatibility.

In the past few years, a number of relatively simple culture systems for cells of the mouse spleen and other lymphoid organs have been developed. The method in use in our laboratory for mixed cultures of mouse spleen or lymph node cells is rather similar to the one used for human peripheral blood cells. In general, the results of mouse MLC discussed in the following sections hold true for various methods and have been verified in several laboratories. Required controls and statistical procedures are the same as those previously discussed for human cultures.

D. Genetics of MLC in Humans

I. Basic Principles

In order to discuss the genetics of MLC it is of course necessary to have an understanding of certain basic principles of genetics and of some genetic terminology. Many genetic terms have entered the general vocabulary, although not necessarily with the same meanings as those given to them by geneticists; therefore, to make sure that author and readers are speaking the same language, definitions of some terms used in this discussion are given in Appendix II. A brief explanation of some principles of inheritance is given below.

In the somatic cells each human being carries 23 pairs of chromosomes (total 46), both members of a pair, except for the pair of sex chromosomes, being morphologically alike and having the same loci but not necessarily the same alleles at each locus. Two loci may be either on different chromosomes or on the same one.

The first possibility, that of two loci on different chromosomes, is shown in Figure 1 where parent 1 carries the alleles 1a and 1b at locus 1 on a certain chromosome. On another chromosome he (or she) carries the alleles 2a and 2b at locus 2. For simplicity, Parent 2 carries the allele 1a at locus 1 on both chromosomes of one pair, and the allele 2a at locus 2 on both chromosomes of the other pair. During meiosis or gamete formation, the pairs of chromosomes are separated so that a given gamete receives only one chromosome of each pair, a process known as segregation. However, as can be seen from Figure 1, the chromosomes of each pair are randomly assorted into the gametes; a gamete which receives the chromosome carrying 1a has an equal probability of receiving the chromosome carrying 2a or the one carrying 2b. Since Parent 2 is homozygous at both loci, the gametes contributed by Parent 2 can be of only one type. Considering the offspring, it is clear that although the parent carrying allele 1b also had allele 2b, the offspring carrying allele 1b (Types III and

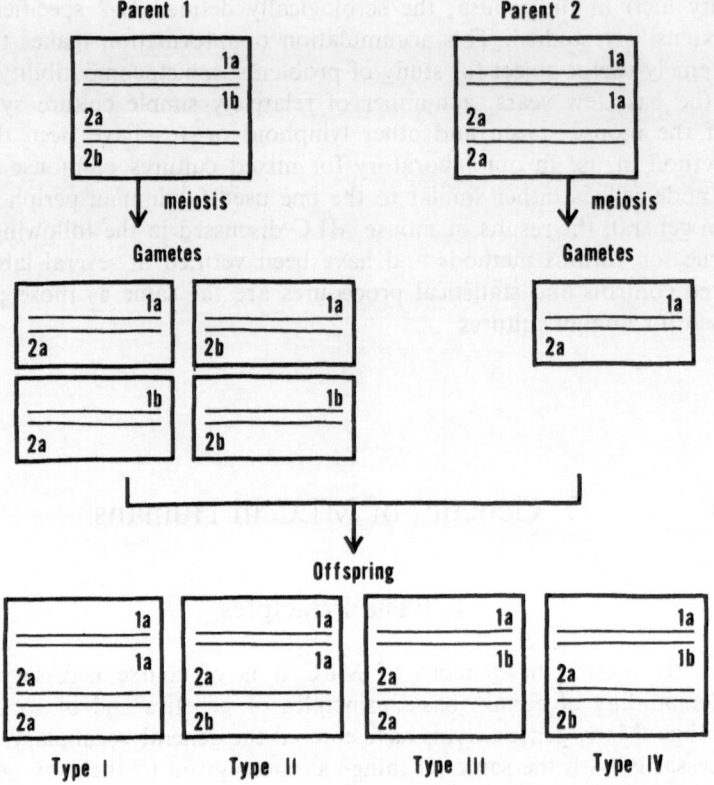

Fig. 1. Independent assortment of alleles of loci on different chromosomes. See text for details

IV) are equally likely to have or not to have the allele 2b. We say that alleles at these two loci, 1 and 2, show independent assortment; in the individual case one cannot predict, knowing which alleles the child has at locus 1, which alleles he has at locus 2.

It will be seen from Figure 1 that the physical unit of assortment is the chromosome; it is the whole chromosome which goes to a particular gamete. Hence it is not surprising that the assortment of alleles of loci on the same chromosome is somewhat different from that of alleles of loci on different chromosomes. The situation is shown diagrammatically in Figure 2. The loci 5 and 6 are on the same chromosome; locus 2 is on a different chromosome. Alleles at locus 2 assort independently of those at loci 5 and 6. However, the alleles which are on the same chromosome at loci 5 and 6 tend to remain together; i.e., the proportion of offspring receiving 5a and 6a or 5b and 6b (non-recombinant chromosomes) will be greater than the proportion of offspring receiving 5a and 6b or 5b and 6a (recombinant chromosomes). This phenomenon is called linkage between the two loci. Recombinant chromosomes are generated by crossover events; during meiosis, before their separation, the two chromosomes of a pair become tightly apposed and crossing over, or exchange

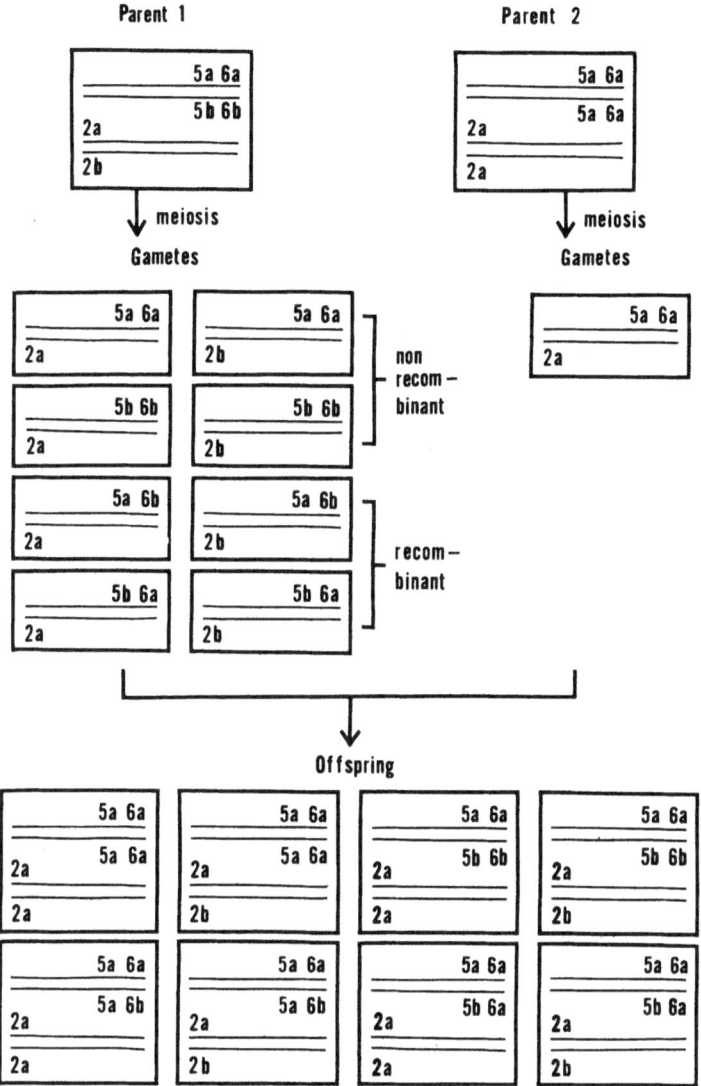

Fig. 2. Assortment of alleles of different loci on the same chromosome. Two alleles on the same chromosome (e.g. 5a and 6a) will be inherited together unless separated by crossing-over. See text for details

of genetic material, may occur between them. If a crossover occurs between loci 5 and 6 in Parent 1, for example, recombinant chromosomes carrying 5a–6b and 5b–6a will be generated. The probability of a crossover occurring between two loci is a function of the distance between them on the chromosome; hence the frequency of recombinants gives an index of how far apart the loci are. Loci which are very close together show very low recombination frequencies and are said to be closely linked genetically.

II. Correlation of MLC Non-Stimulation in Siblings with Inheritance of the Same HL-A Haplotype

Early in the course of MLC studies, it was observed that some siblings in the normal families studied did not stimulate each other. The non-stimulation was clear-cut when compared with the stimulation obtained in other sibling combinations (see Table 5), and was reciprocal; that is, in a one-way mixed culture, if the combination AB_m showed no stimulation, there was no stimulation in the combination BA_m, and the two-way culture (AB, with neither cell treated to prevent division) also showed no stimulation. When these families were HL-A typed, it was found that siblings who were non-stimulatory were those that had inherited the same HL-A haplotypes (Fig. 3 and Table 6). This correlation has generally been found to hold in the many hundreds of families which have been HL-A typed and tested in MLC.

Table 5. Data of a Family MLC Test[a]

	A_m	B_m	C_m	D_m	E_m	X_m
A	578	2,055	25,028	6,094	3,420	19,592
B	30,807	500	32,087	398	501	20,258
C	26,623	23,101	502	28,720	27,419	15,876
D	28,309	500	66,082	334	848	27,446
E	28,513	301	32,335	224	252	28,668
X	63,544	59,639	42,711	57,514	42,271	1,174

[a] cpm incorporated in quadruplicate cultures. A is the mother; B, D, and E are HL-A SD identical siblings; X is a normal unrelated.

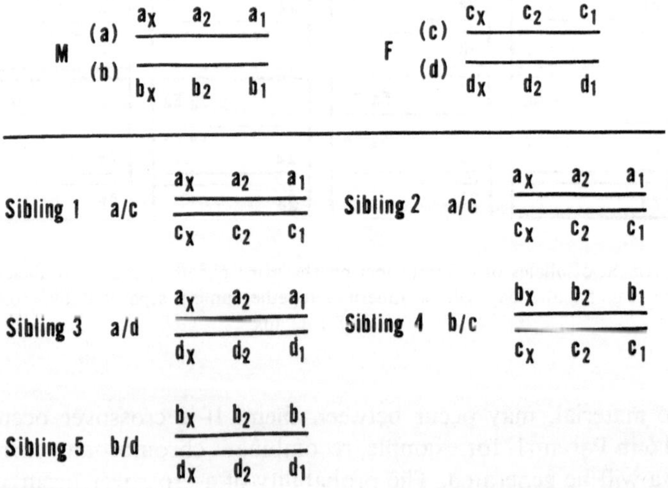

Fig. 3. Inheritance of HL-A haplotypes in a family. The mother's haplotypes are designated a and b, with the serologically defined specificities a_1 and b_1 of LA (first segregant series) and a_2 and b_2 of Four (second segregant series); the father's haplotypes are designated c and d. a_x, b_x, etc. are alleles at a hypothetical LD locus (see text for details). MLC stimulation is shown in Table 6

Table 6. Pattern of MLC Stimulation in a Family[a]

Sibling Combination	Serological Haplotypes	MLC Stimulation (one-way test in both directions)
1+2	a/c+a/c	−
1+3	a/c+a/d	+
1+4	a/c+b/c	+
1+5	a/c+b/d	+
2+3	a/c+a/d	+
2+4	a/c+b/c	+
2+5	a/c+b/d	+
3+4	a/d+b/c	+
3+5	a/d+b/d	+
4+5	b/c+b/d	+

[a] MLC stimulation in the family shown in Figure 3.

These findings suggest that MLC reactivity, if it does not directly involve the HL-A antigens defined by typing, is controlled by something very closely linked genetically to HL-A. "Very closely linked" means that in the chromosome the loci determining MLC reactivity are very near the loci determining the LA and Four antigens, so that these loci are usually not separated when the chromosomes are distributed into the gametes. Thus, a child who inherits a certain HL-A haplotype inherits a particular MLC allele or alleles associated in his family with that HL-A haplotype.

III. Exceptional Cases of Stimulation and Non-Stimulation

The first suggestion that MLC reactivity might indeed by separable from LA and Four antigens came in the studies by Amos and Bach (1968) and by Bach et al. (1969) in which the general correlation of HL-A typing identity and MLC non-stimulation was demonstrated. In one of the families tested in each of these studies, one pair of siblings showed anomalous behavior: they were HL-A typing-identical but were mutually stimulatory in MLC. The finding of these particular sib pairs (and others which were seen later) indeed raised the possibility that siblings might inherit the same LA and Four determinants but different determinants for MLC reactivity. However, other explanations of the phenomenon were also possible.

A clear demonstration of the separation of serologically detected HL-A antigens and MLC reactivity came in a study by Yunis et al., discussed in Yunis and Amos (1971). These investigators studied a family in which one pair of HL-A typing-identical siblings was mutually stimulatory, and found the pattern of response shown in Table 7. Sibling 1, although his haplotype by HL-A typing is a/c, behaves in MLC like the siblings of type a/d, stimulating and responding to another sibling of type a/c and neither stimulating nor responding to siblings of type a/d. The doubly anomalous situation (mutual stimu-

Table 7. Pattern of MLC Stimulation in a Family with Mutually Stimulatory SD-identical Sibs[a]

Sibling Combination	Serological Haplotypes	MLC Stimulation (one-way cultures in both directions)
1+2	a/c+a/c	+
1+3	a/c+a/d	−
1+4	a/c+b/c	+
1+5	a/c+b/d	+
2+3	a/c+a/d	+
2+4	a/c+b/c	+
2+5	a/c+b/d	+

[a] MLC stimulation in the family shown in Figure 4.

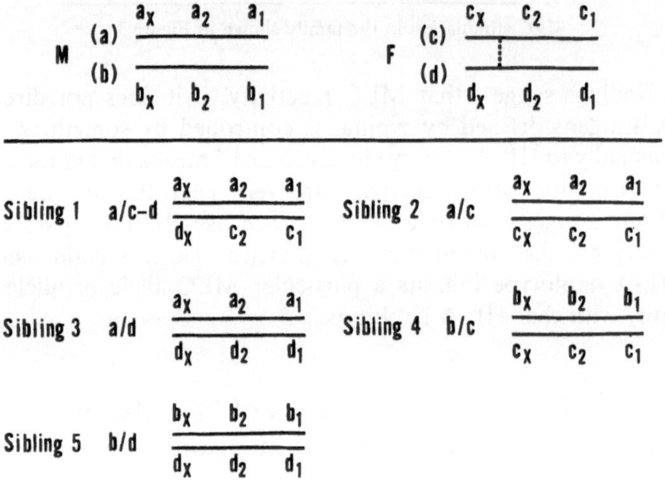

Fig. 4. Inheritance of HL-A haplotypes in a family. Symbols as in Figure 3. The MLC data (Table 7) is accounted for by the following hypothesis: As indicated a crossover has occurred between the father's chromosomes, producing a recombinant chromosome carrying c_1, c_2, and d_x which was inherited by Sibling 1. Siblings 1 and 2 thus differ at the hypothetical LD locus and are MLC stimulatory. See text for details

lation between a pair of typing-identical sibs, and mutual non-stimulation between one member of the pair and a typing-non-identical sib) clearly suggested that MLC reactivity was functionally independent of, although genetically linked to, the LA and Four antigens.

This conclusion is drawn as follows: Individuals who inherit the same HL-A haplotypes (determined by typing) are generally non-stimulatory. The exceptional cases show that these individuals are non-stimulatory not because they are identical for LA and Four, but because they are identical for some other locus (or loci) which is usually inherited along with LA and Four, i.e., is closely linked genetically. In the exceptional cases, this "other" locus or loci has become separated from LA and Four, presumably by some event of genetic recombination in the precursor cells of sperm or egg (Fig. 4). Recombination rather than mutation is inferred because of the mutual non-stimulation between the exceptional sib and a sib differing by one haplotype.

This situation results in some terminological confusion: siblings who are "HL-A identical" by serological criteria are nevertheless stimulatory in MLC. A similar situation is seen in the mouse, as will be discussed later. We have therefore distinguished between serologically defined (SD) antigens such as those of the LA and Four loci, and lymphocyte-defined (LD) differences which can cause strong MLC stimulation but do not seem to provoke formation of cytotoxic or agglutinating antibodies. The genetic basis for this distinction can be seen more clearly in the mouse studies discussed later.

IV. Association of Stimulation with Four-Locus Region

Other information on the genetics of the region which includes the HL-A SD and LD loci has come from studies of families in which a crossover has occurred between the LA and Four loci. Such families are recognized by a situation where, with the parental haplotypes defined, one sibling carries, for example, the LA antigen of the mother's a haplotype and the Four antigen of the mother's b haplotype (Fig. 5). (The haplotype inherited from the other parent will usually be non-recombinant, since such crossovers are relatively rare.) Such a sibling is recombinant for one of his two HL-A haplotypes, and provides a situation in which differences of one LA allele, one Four allele, etc., can be studied, provided that siblings of the other haplotypes are available. A number of studies have established that strong stimulation is usually associated with differences at the Four locus; siblings differing by one LA specificity show no or weak stimulation (Table 8). Coupled with the finding of mutually stimulatory SD-identical sibs discussed above, these data suggest that the locus or loci controlling reactivity in MLC lies near the Four locus, on the side away from LA rather than between LA and Four. Different results of genetic mapping are found in the mouse, as will be discussed later.

V. Minor Loci

Data collected in families also suggest that there is little or no effect on MLC stimulation of loci not in the HL-A region. Many "minor" histocompatibility loci, unlinked to H-2, have been identified in the mouse, and presumably such loci exist also in man. However, these loci do not appear to play a role in stimulation in human MLC. If the number of minor loci in man is at all comparable to the number in the mouse (more than 15) siblings inheriting the same HL-A haplotypes should nevertheless differ for some minor loci, yet there is no stimulation in such HL-A identical sibling pairs, with the exceptions discussed above. The argument may be advanced that differences at the minor loci may not stimulate in MLC without a difference for the HL-A region. Experiments with identical twins and MLC-non-stimulatory, SD-identical siblings have suggested that non-HL-A-linked differences do not have a detectable

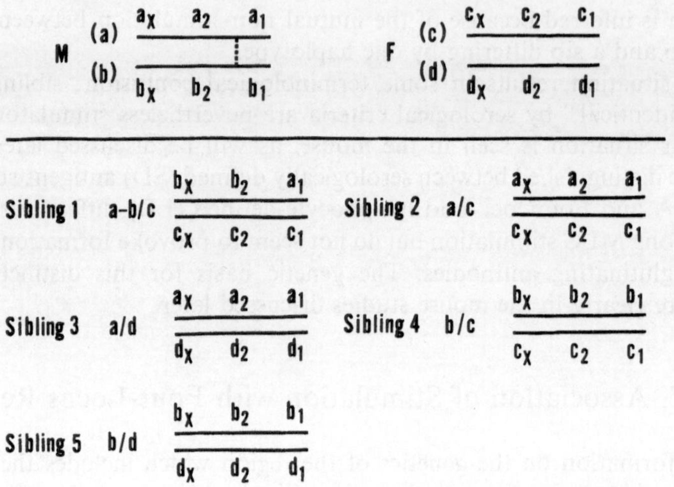

M (a) a_x a_2 a_1
M (b) b_x b_2 b_1
F (c) c_x c_2 c_1
F (d) d_x d_2 d_1

Sibling 1 a–b/c b_x b_2 a_1 / c_x c_2 c_1

Sibling 2 a/c a_x a_2 a_1 / c_x c_2 c_1

Sibling 3 a/d a_x a_2 a_1 / d_x d_2 d_1

Sibling 4 b/c b_x b_2 b_1 / c_x c_2 c_1

Sibling 5 b/d b_x b_2 b_1 / d_x d_2 d_1

Fig. 5. Inheritance of HL-A haplotypes in a family. Symbols as in Figure 3. A crossover has occurred at the indicated point between the mother's chromosomes, producing a recombinant chromosome carrying a_1, b_2, and b_x which was inherited by Sibling 1. MLC combinations and results are indicated in Table 8

Table 8. Pattern of MLC stimulation in a Family with a Sibling Recombinant between LA and Four[a]

Sibling combination		Specificities Recognized[b]	MLC Stimulation
Responder	Stimulator		
1	2	a_2, a_x	+
2	1	b_2, b_x	+
1	4	b_1	−, ±
4	1	a_1	−, ±
All other combinations			+

[a] In various combinations among the siblings of the family shown in Figure 5. Sibling 1 is recombinant.

[b] In the column headed "Specificities Recognized" are listed those specificities of the stimulating cell which are not present on the responding cell. See Figure 5 for details.

influence. In view of evidence in the mouse that non-H-2-linked loci stimulate, the disparity between human and mouse may be attributable to differences in sensitivity of the methods or to failure to study the right individuals.

VI. MLC and HL-A Typing in Unrelateds

For these interested in the selection of donor-recipient pairs for transplantation, one question posed by these results is: Do HL-A SD identical unrelated individuals behave like HL-A SD identical siblings? The answer is clearly that they do not.

That this result is in accord with genetic understanding can be seen by making the distinction between phenotypically and genotypically identical individuals. Siblings in a family who are identical for serologically defined antigens and non-stimulatory in MLC are genotypically identical for HL-A; not only are they the same so far as we can determine from serological testing, but we are justified in assuming that they have actually inherited the same SD and LD alleles. Unrelated individuals who are identical for HL-A SD antigens are phenotypically identical: they are the same so far as we can determine by serological testing, but we cannot make the assumption that the alleles they carry are the same. If two such unrelated "HL-A identical" individuals are mutually stimulatory in MLC, two types of differences (or a combination of the two) can be involved: either the SD alleles of the individuals are different, although in ways that we do not detect by serological testing, or the SD alleles are the same but alleles at other (LD) loci are not.

The data we have indicate that most unrelated individuals who are HL-A SD identical are mutually stimulatory in MLC. This result is not surprising in view of the evidence previously cited that the SD antigens themselves do not determine MLC reactivity; however, two aspects of these results may be of great practical and theoretical importance.

The first point is that some pairs of unrelated HL-A SD identical individuals are mutually non-stimulatory. This point assumes considerable significance in view of the fact that the overwhelming majority of randomly chosen unrelated pairs that have been studied are mutually stimulatory, although there are a few instances of non-stimulation between unrelated SD-non-identicals. If HL-A SD antigens are not themselves determining reactivity, then why should selection for identity of SD antigens help to select for MLC-identical pairs? The answer to this question rests on population genetics.

Human population may be considered, with certain limitations, as random-breeding populations with respect to HL-A SD antigens. That is, within a population, the choice of mates is random with respect to SD antigens; the fact that an individual has a certain HL-A SD phenotype does not influence his or her choice of, or chances of selection as, a mate. (Between different populations, e.g., between different races or different religious groups, breeding barriers may exist, and this is why the human race should be considered genetically as a series of populations, each random-breeding within itself but having incomplete exchange of genetic material with other populations.) Within such a random-breeding population, over a long period of time, alleles become distributed randomly throughout the population; i.e., the possession of one allele is independent of the possession of any other allele at the same or another locus. This is easily seen in the case of alleles at a single locus, which segregate from each other at gamete formation. It is also clear for alleles of loci which are on different chromosomes (as diagrammed in Figure 1) and hence not genetically linked to one another. Obviously, in such situations, if the mating of the offspring of all parents is random with respect to the trait in question, alleles will gradually be distributed throughout the population.

It was stated earlier that independent assortment means that the alleles carried by an individual at locus 2 cannot be inferred from a knowledge of his genotype for locus 1. However, on a population level one can predict the relative frequencies of individuals having given alleles at any one locus or at a number of different loci. If a population has been random-breeding for long enough so that alleles are randomly distributed through it, it is said to be in Hardy-Weinberg equilibrium with respect to the locus or loci in question. In equilibrium alleles at a given locus will be distributed according to a formula known as the Hardy-Weinberg law, and the distribution of genotypes (and hence of phenotypes) can be calculated knowing only the relative frequencies of the alleles at that locus. The formula applies regardless of how many alleles there are.

The situation of linked genes, such as the SD and LD loci of HL-A, is essentially similar. As will be seen from Figure 2, alleles of closely linked loci will be separated at a certain rate by crossing-over; that is, a certain proportion of the offspring in each generation will be recombinant between the loci in question, the proportion depending on the distance between the loci. After a number of generations, in each of which recombinations will occur, the alleles will be distributed randomly with respect to one another throughout the population, although the linkage will be evident if inheritance is studied in families.

This Hardy-Weinberg equilibrium can, however, be upset if for some reason the expected independent assortment or the expected frequency of recombinants does not occur. If, for example, certain combinations of alleles have an advantage in natural selection, or if other combinations are selected against, there will no longer be a random distribution of alleles; favorable combinations will be more frequent, or unfavorable combinations less frequent, than predicted by the Hardy-Weinberg formula. In the case of alleles at linked loci, this situation is known as linkage disequilibrium and can be demonstrated in large population studies by calculating the actual and expected frequencies of the various combinations of alleles. If the actual frequency of a particular combination of alleles is significantly higher than expected from the frequencies of the individual alleles in the combination, these alleles are said to exhibit linkage disequilibrium. Linkage disequilibrium has been demonstrated between some specificities of LA and Four, such as HL-A 1 and 8, or HL-A 3 and 7, in Caucasian populations; these haplotypes occur more frequently than expected on the basis of a random distribution of alleles, although other haplotypes occur with no more than the expected frequency. This situation may of course be mimicked in a population where the alleles have not yet come to equilibrium, as in the case of several small populations with different gene frequencies which have recently been mixed.

Applying this picture of linkage disequilibrium to the case of the unrelated HL-A SD identical, MLC-non-stimulating individuals, we may think of MLC reactivity (LD locus or loci) as being genetically separate from LA and Four but closely linked to them. For some reason certain LD alleles tend to remain linked with certain LA and Four alleles, i.e., there is a linkage disequilibrium between SD and LD in these cases. Such a disequilibrium could account for the selection of non-stimulating pairs by identity for SD antigens, since individuals identical for LA and Four would have a much higher probability of being identical for the linked LD alleles than would random unrelateds. Such a linkage has been demonstrated for certain alleles identified by LD typing (see Section F).

The second point which has emerged from MLC studies of HL-A SD identical unrelateds is that such individuals stimulate each other less, on the average, than randomly chosen pairs. Despite the difficulties in quantitation of MLC discussed earlier, this distinction has been made with great statistical significance in studies employing different experimental designs (SORENSON and STAUB-NIELSEN, 1970; SEGALL et al., 1973). This situation raises questions which cannot be answered with any assurance in our present state of knowledge, although hypotheses can be suggested.

One possibility is that stimulation between unrelateds is actually due to SD differences; stimulation between SD-identical unrelateds would therefore be due to small differences between their SD antigens which are not detected with present serological methods. The non-stimulatory pairs would represent cases of complete SD antigen identity. This seems unlikely in view of the data on anomalous stimulation and non-stimulation in sibling pairs discussed above. Another possibility emerges from consideration of linkage disequilibrium. It would be assumed that a given HL-A haplotype would include alleles of the LD locus or loci. Due to linkage disequilibrium, individuals with the same SD antigens would also carry the same or similar LD alleles. Stimulation among the SD-identical unrelateds would then be the result of small differences in LD alleles; such small differences would arise either from mutational changes, at a single locus or at several loci, or from rare crossing-over events within a complex composed of several loci.

More refined analyses of MLC in unrelated individuals with different degrees of SD disparity have recently been made. MEMPEL et al. (1973) have presented data on MLC in a large number of unrelated combinations, using the stimulation index (AB_m/AA_m) as a measure of degree of stimulation; these authors find that the mean stimulation index of the groups increases in the order SD-identical <1 SD-1 difference <2 SD-1 differences <1 SD-2 difference <2 SD-2 differences <differences for all four SD specificities. We have analyzed in detail several sets of SD-identical unrelateds (SEGALL and BACH, 1974). It is clear from our results that apparent SD identity is not always correlated with low stimulation in MLC. Further, in the combinations where low stimulation was seen between SD-identical unrelateds, individuals differing by SD-1 specificities only were also low stimulators.

Our data and those of MEMPEL et al. are both consistent with the hypothesis, previously discussed, that a region important in MLC activation is associated with the Four locus. Our data also suggest, however, that the situation may be more complex than a simple linkage disequilibrium between Four and LD. Combinations having the Four (SD-2) antigens HL-A8 and HL-A7, or HL-A8 and HL-A W15, in common are significantly low stimulators of one another, while combinations having the SD-2 antigens HL-A7 and HL-A W15 in common are not. This result suggests the possibility that the low stimulation is due, not simply to linkage disequilibrium for LD alleles associated with HL-A7, HL-A8 and HL-A W15, but to some more complicated phenomenon having to do with HL-A8 and/or its associated LD alleles. There may be some form of interaction, at either the genotypic or phenotypic level, between the LD alleles of the two haplotypes or between the LD and SD alleles. If such interactions do occur, they will be difficult to study experimentally; however, they may be of great importance in assessing compatibility for transplantation (see also Section F II).

E. Genetics of MLC in the Mouse

The existence of LD specificities in the mouse has been demonstrated in essentially the same way as in humans: by showing that cells of animals from two different congenic resistant strains, identical for the SD specificities of H-2, are nevertheless in certain strain combinations stimulatory in MLC. The availability of congenic resistant strains of mice, and the possibility of making planned matings, has however permitted more precise mapping of the LD locus or loci.

A map of the mouse major histocompatibility complex is shown in Figure 6. At the ends of the region are the SD loci, called H-2K and H-2D. The region between them is divided by the Ss marker, determining an antigenic variant of a serum protein but apparently unrelated to lymphocyte surface antigen determinants. A "strong" LD locus or loci, controlling strong proliferative responses in MLC, can be mapped on the H-2K side of Ss, but within the region bounded by H-2K and H-2D (unlike the situation in man). A "weak" locus lies on the H-2D side of Ss. A number of other marker genes have now been identified in the major histocompatibility complex: a series of Ir genes, controlling the immune response to certain antigens, and a series of loci controlling the Ia antigens, surface antigens of mouse lymphocytes. The relationships, genetic and functional, of LD to these other markers are as yet unknown.

In addition to the LD loci mapped within the H-2 region, a non-H-2-linked locus, the M locus, in the mouse can also cause strong proliferative responses in MLC (FESTENSTEIN and DEMANT, 1973). So far no human parallel to the M locus is known.

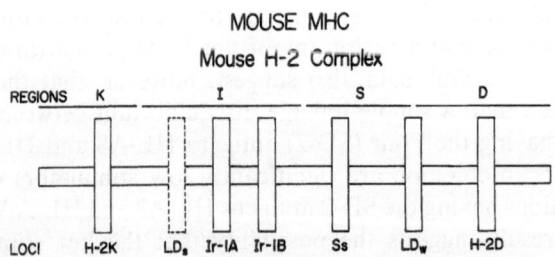

Fig. 6. The major histocompatibility complex of the mouse. A strong LD locus (LD$_s$) lies somewhere in the I region between H-2K and Ss. A weak LD locus (LD$_w$) lies between Ss and H-2D. See text for details

Recent results have suggested that "weak" LD loci may be present in the H-2K and H-2D regions, although it is not clear whether these are the same as or different from the loci determining the serologically defined antigens. This may also prove to be the case in man.

F. MLC Typing

I. Principle of Typing – Use of Homozygous Cells

As stated in the Introduction, the "classical" MLC provides a measure of the total histoincompatibility (of this type) between two individuals without defining any individual factors responsible for the stimulation. One of the most exciting recent developments in this field has been the establishment of a method of identifying individual stimulating factors, known as "MLC Typing".

The principle of MLC typing is elegantly simple. In order to define the individual factors one must have some kind of "reagent", such as antisera in SD typing, which can be used to define the presence or absence of a given factor on an individual's cells by positive or negative reactions with those cells. The identity of cells of two individuals for LD specificities is established by non-stimulation in MLC. Cells of most individuals cannot be used as "reagents" because they are heterozygous, carrying two different HL-A haplotypes, and thus do not define one individual factor. HL-A homozygous cells, however, can be used as reagents or "typing cells", as shown in Table 9.

HL-A homozygotes should be found among offspring of first-cousin marriages, as shown in Figure 7. In each generation there is a certain probability that a particular haplotype (haplotype a, in this example) from one of the common ancestors will be inherited by both of the relevant children, resulting eventually in a certain proportion of HL-A homozygous (a/a, in this example) children. The two HL-A haplotypes of the apparent homozygote, barring crossing-over, should be identical by descent. This being the case, the MLC pattern shown in Table 9 should be obtained. Any heterozygote carrying the haplotype of the homozygote should not be stimulated by homozygous cells, since the homozygote has no major histocompatibility antigens foreign to the heterozygote, but the homozygote should be stimulated by the heterozygote. Thus, non-stimulation of cells of any individual by a given homozygous cell indicates that individual has the LD specificity defined by the homozygote.

Individuals homozygous for LD specificites should also be found among offspring of parents who share one haplotype as defined by SD specificites; a certain percentage of these, depending on the haplotype, will also share linked LD specificities. However, the probability of an LD-homozygote from such matings is lower than that of an LD-homozygote from a first cousin marriage, and in screening for homozygotes it is easier to start by screening offspring of first-cousin marriages.

Table 9. Possible MLC results and interpretations in a Family with an SD-homozygous Sib

Combination		MLC stimulation if	
Stimulator	Responder	$a_m = a_p$	$a_m \neq a_p$
Sib 2 (a_p/f) or mother (a_m/f)	Sib 1 (a_m/a_p)	+	+
Sib 3 (a_m/g) or father (a_p/g)	Sib 1 (a_m/a_p)	+	+
Sib 1 (a_m/a_p)	Sib 2 (a_p/f) or mother (a_m/f)	−	+
Sib 1 (a_m/a_p)	Sib 3 (a_m/g) or father (a_p/g)	−	+
mother (a_m/f)	Sib 2 (a_p/f)	−	+
Sib 2 (a_p/f)	mother (a_m/f)	−	+
father (a_p/g)	Sib 3 (a_m/g)	−	+
Sib 3 (a_m/g)	father (a_p/g)	−	+

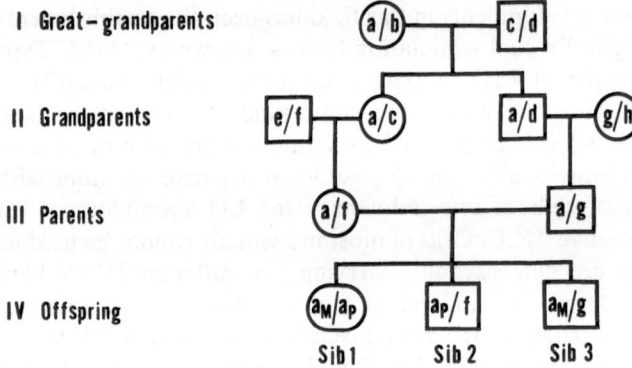

Fig. 7. Pattern of inheritance in a family with an HL-A homozygous sibling. Both of the parents (Generation III), who are first cousins, have inherited the a haplotype from the common great-grandmother. In their offspring (Generation IV), A_m and a_p designate the maternal and paternal a haplotypes, which are identical by descent. Identity of a_m and a_p can be established by MLC testing (see Table 9). o = female, □ = male

The procedure followed in such a screening is to type a number of first-cousin couples for SD specificities, select those with a common haplotype, and test the children of these selected couples for SD and LD-homozygotes by the procedure given in Table 9. LD-homozygous cells can then be tested among themselves and those which are mutually non-stimulatory can be considered to define an LD specificity, in the same way that a group of antisera with highly correlated reaction patterns define an SD specificity. These LD homozygotes can then be used as stimulators against unrelated responders, non-stimulation again indicating that the responder being tested carries the same specificity as the homozygous "typing cell". Such screening programs, and the construction of panels of unrelated "MLC-typed" individuals, are already well under way in several laboratories.

II. Problems in Defining a "Typing" Response

Some difficulties in the definition of non-stimulation have already been discussed. An additional problem in MLC typing is that there is frequently some response by the heterozygous responder to the homozygous stimulator, and this so-called "paradoxical stimulation" may clearly represent a real stimulation by the homozygous cell. This occurs in families where there is no stimulation between the parents and their SD-identical children (see Table 9), indicating that the shared haplotype is indeed LD- as well as SD-identical. This phenomenon may be considered to represent an instance of interactive effects (see Section D II): the behavior of a particular haplotype appears to be influenced by the haplotype which accompanies it, and may vary in a predictable way depending on the second haplotype.

This "paradoxical stimulation" must be taken into account for MLC typing; that is, a "negative" reaction indicating the presence of the allele on the cell being tested (a "typing" response) must be defined to include reactions which one would usually classify as "positive". One must therefore set a level of stimulation and consider all values below that level as negative; which returns us to the problem of quantitation discussed in Section B. 3. The relative response (JORGENSEN et al., 1973) of the cell being tested, i.e. its response to the typing cell compared to its response to several random unrelated stimulating cells, is frequently being used to analyze typing results. For recent results in this area, the reader should consult the proceedings of the MLC section of the VIth Histocompatibility Workshop (Histocompatibility Testing 1975).

Eventually, it is hoped that MLC typing will be clinically applicable, especially in the area of cadaver kidney transplantation. The MLC is not now prospectively applicable to cadaver kidney transplantation because four or five days of incubation are required, although strenuous efforts are being made to develop a "rapid" MLC. However, the possibility has been raised that LD specificities may be serologically detectable by tests other than standard cytotoxicity or agglutination assays, for example by fluorescent antibody staining (VAN LEEUWEN et al., 1973). Should this prove to be the case, it could provide a rapid and reliable method of matching for histocompatibility antigens which appear to be important in the success or failure of kidney grafts.

It is apparent from early results that some LD specificities defined by MLC typing are in strong linkage disequilibrium with particular SD alleles. This supports the theoretical conclusions given earlier (Section D. VI). Also, some specificities may be in linkage disequilibrium with more than one SD specificity. Such information may be useful in many ways in increasing the number of successful cadaver kidney transplants, as discussed below (Section H). MLC typing may also be extremely useful in selecting unrelated (and possibly non-SD-identical) donors for patients in need of a bone marrow transplant (see below, Section H).

G. The Cell-Mediated Lympholysis (CML) Reaction

I. CML in Humans

In addition to the proliferative "recognition" response in MLC, it is now known that another event or series of events occurs in a mixed culture. This latter leads to the generation of "killer" lymphocytes, cells which will recognize and destroy target lymphocytes carrying the same histocompatibility antigens as the stimulating cells in the original mixed culture. The genetics of this reaction of cell-mediated lympholysis, and its relationship to the proliferative MLC response, will be discussed in this section.

The CML is generally assayed by the release of radioactive chromium (Cr^{51}) from the cytoplasm of labeled target cells. Mixed cultures are set up as usual (generally in large volumes to allow the recovery of enough responder cells after the incubation to perform the CML test), and cultured for 5 or 6 days. Target cells are cultured with phytohemagglutinin (PHA) so that the peak of PHA reactivity (3 days) coincides with the day of setting up the CML. The PHA-stimulated blast cells are used rather than normal cells because they appear to be better targets, in the sense of showing a higher percentage of Cr^{51} release under a given set of conditions than do normal cells. The cells recovered from the mixed culture ("effector" or "killer" cells) are incubated with the labeled target cells, in a ratio of 50–100 effectors: 1 target, for 3–6 hours, and the amount of Cr^{51} released into the supernatant by lysis of the target cells is then determined.

As is amply demonstrated in family studies in man, CML reactivity is not directed against the LD antigens which appear to be the most important stimulus in MLC. For example, EIJSVOOGEL et al. (1973a) have studied families with a recombinant sibling and their results illustrate certain general rules (Table 10). In families with a pair of SD-identical siblings who were mutually stimulatory in MLC, neither member of this pair when acting as responder produced effector cells against the other member of the pair (combinations 1 and 2, Table 10). In other combinations it was demonstrated that cells of either of these sibs, as responders to another cell, could function as CML effectors (combinations 9 and 10), and as targets could be killed by other cells (combinations 7a and 8b). However, a non-identical sibling, stimulated by either of these two SD-identical sibs, produced effector cells against both of them (7a, 7b; 8a, 8b). Indeed, sibling #3, although non-responsive in MLC and CML to sibling #1 (combination 4), when stimulated by sibling #2 produced effector cells cytotoxic for cells of both sibling #1 and sibling #2.

These results indicate that SD antigens serve at least as an important target in CML. That LD antigens do not serve as targets, at least not to an extent which is detectable in this system, is indicated by combinations 1 and 2, and 5a and 5b. In combinations 1 and 2, the SD-identical sibs recognize LD differences between them but do not generate effector cells directed against these

Table 10. MLC and CML in a Family with an LD-Recombinant Sibling[a]

MLC Combination		Serological Haplotypes	MLC Stimulation	Target Cell	CML Cytotoxicity
(1)	$1+2_m$	a/c+a/c	+	2	−
(2)	$2+1_m$	a/c+a/c	+	1	−
(3)	$1+3_m$	a/c+a/d	−	3	−
(4)	$3+1_m$	a/d+a/c	−	1	−
(5a)	$2+3_m$	a/c+a/d	+	3	+
(5b)				1	−
(6a)	$3+2_m$	a/d+a/c	+	2	+
(6b)				1	+
(7a)	$5+1_m$	b/d+a/c	+	1	+
(7b)				2	+
(8a)	$5+2_m$	b/d+a/c	+	1	+
(8b)				2	+
(9)	$1+5_m$	a/c+b/d	+	5	+
(10)	$2+5_m$	a/c+b/d	+	5	+

[a] MLC and CML results in the family shown in Figure 4.

differences. In combination 5a, sibling ∄2 gives both a proliferative and a cytotoxic response to cells of sibling ∄3. Yet the cytotoxic cells are directed only against the SD antigens of sibling ∄3, since there is no CML activity against cells of sibling ∄1 (combination 5b) although these are LD-identical with the stimulating cell.

There appears to be a correlation between the specificities defined by anti-HL-A antisera and by CML, although on the basis of available evidence they may not be entirely the same. Both LA and Four locus specificites may act as targets for effector cells if the appropriate MLC mixtures are used to generate such cells.

The precursors of the effector cells can be removed from the responder population by incubation on a monolayer of adherent leukocytes from the donor of the stimulating cells, although MLC proliferation does not seem to be affected by this preadsorption (BACH et al., 1973). It is not clear whether the cells that are removed are non-proliferating cytotoxic precursors or proliferating cytotoxic precursors which amount to only a small proportion of the proliferating cells.

II. CML in Mouse

The general principles outlined above (CML directed against SD antigens and not against LD antigens) also appear to be true for CML in the mouse, although several exceptions have been noted here. Some MLC-stimulatory, SD-identical combinations do not appear to generate cytotoxic cells in MLC. However, the MLC combination between the strain C57BL/6 and the Bailey mutant of that strain produces strong cytotoxicity in both directions (as well as MLC proliferation) although no cytotoxic or agglutinating antibody has been produced in extensive cross-immunization. Similarly, the mutant of Egorov produces both MLC reactivity and skin graft rejection with the parental strain, although this mutation apparently affects the parental H-2D specificity.

III. Relation of CML and MLC

In the human experiments discussed above it appeared that there was no generation of CML effector cells in the absence of an MLC response. However, several authors have observed that mixed cultures of mouse cells apparently differing only by serologically defined H-2K or H-2D specificities will generate effector cells, although less efficiently than in cases where an LD difference is also present (e.g. Schendel and Bach, 1974). Eijsvoogel et al. (1973b) and Schendel and Bach (1974) have also shown that heat-treatment of stimulating cells (45° C for one hour) destroys their MLC-stimulating ability but does not destroy SD antigens, as judged by absorption of antisera, or the ability to provoke the formation of cytotoxic cells in mixed culture if an LD stimulus is provided. Heat-treatment of the stimulating cell, in an SD-different combination where CML effector cells can be generated by mitomycin-treated stimulators, abrogates the CML response (Schendel and Bach, 1974). This suggests that there is a heat-labile LD stimulus coded for in the H-2D and H-2K regions, although it is not clear whether this is a different molecule from the one carrying the SD antigens. From this result it would appear that some MLC response is necessary for the generation of CML effector cells, although this is not yet certain, and it is possible that yet another response is involved.

H. Correlations of MLC with Grafting

From the clinician's point of view, the most important question about LD is whether it plays any significant role in transplant success or failure and whether, as a corollary, matching for LD can be helpful in selecting donors and recipients for organ transplantation.

It is clear from all studies in this area that kidney transplants between HL-A identical siblings have an extremely high success rate, much higher than that of any other category of transplant. This may be due to SD identity, LD identity, or both (or neither). Several reports suggest that LD identity does play a role in the success of kidney grafts.

In two early studies Jeannet (1970) and Hamburger et al. (1971) suggested that the MLC might serve as a matching test for potential donors and recipients. (In both of these studies, a relatively insensitive MLC technique and/or the current state of SD typing may have made interpretation more difficult.) Jeannet found, in a series of living-related-donor transplants, that a mismatch by MLC in the presence of apparent SD compatibility appeared to predict a relatively poor clinical course, as did a mismatch by both typing and MLC, although the number of cases was small. There was a suggestion in the data that SD-mismatched, MLC-matched transplants did relatively well. HAMBURGER *et al.*, in a sample containing both related and unrelated donor-recipient pairs, found that non-SD-identicals with a "negative" MLC test had significantly better graft survival at two years post-transplant than those with positive MLCs. In both of these studies a two-way MLC was used.

COCHRUN *et al.* (1973) have studied recipients of kidneys from living related donors and recipients of cadaver kidney. In both samples these authors found that graft survival at more than four months or more than two years was considerably higher in the group of recipients where MLC stimulation was low (stimulation index <8) than in the group where stimulation was high (index >8). This difference in survival was seen even within groups where donor and recipient were mismatched for the same number of SD antigens. In this study a two-way MLC was used.

THOMPSON *et al.* (1973) have reported several SD-"compatible" transplants where the donor was homozygous and the recipient heterozygous for a given SD haplotype ("compatible" meaning that the donor had no SD antigens not possessed by the recipient). Those compatible transplants with a high stimulation index in one-way MLC were rejected within a short period of time; those with a low stimulation index are still surviving.

On the basis of available information concerning linkage disequilibrium between SD and LD determinants (see sections D. VI and F. II), VAN HOOFF *et al.* (1974) have analyzed a large series of cadaver kidney transplants and found that two-year graft survival was much higher in a group matched for antigens of a haplotype with a strong linkage disequilibrium (HL-A 1 and 8, 3 and 7, or 2 and 12) than in a group mismatched for these antigens. THOMPSON *et al.* (1974) have studied a group of cadaver kidney recipients matched for one SD haplotype (the haplotypes were determined by family typing of donor and recipient) and found that these grafts had a higher survival rate than those which were not matched for a haplotype, also suggesting a possible effect of LD-SD linkage. MLC's were not performed in these studies, but the assumption from other data is that, had they been done, many of them would have been negative or low.

We have studied a group of recipients of kidneys from living related donors (SEGALL *et al.*, 1975), using one-way MLC and defining level of stimulation by means of an incompatibility index (comparing stimulation of recipient by donor to stimulation of recipient by random unrelateds; see section B. 3). There were no significant differences in graft survival between high and low stimulating pairs. However, when the incompatibility index was low, the clinical course (judged by number and severity of rejection episodes and general level of renal function) was significantly better than when the incompatibility index was high. In fact, recipients of grafts with low incompatibility index had as good a clinical course as recipients of SD- and LD-identical grafts, indicating that the difference between low- and non-stimulation may not be of great importance in this type of transplant. When results of those grafts where the donor and recipient had a clearly demonstrable one-haplotype, two-antigen mismatch were analyzed, the pairs with low incompatibility index again had a significantly better clinical course.

It will be noted that some of these studies utilized a two-way and some a one-way MLC. Since both tests appear to correlate with clinical results it may be assumed that regardless of the differences between them, both tests are assessing some factor(s) important in the success or failure of kidney transplants.

The results cited here suggest that, in the non-immunized recipient of a kidney transplant, the most critical single histocompatibility factor is matching for LD specificities. The success of SD matching, where it appears to be successful, in such recipients may actually be the result of concurrent matching for LD due to linkage disequilibrium. In preimmunized recipients the story may be completely different (VAN ROOD et al., 1973).

That SD and LD identity are not the whole story in clinical transplantation is, however, demonstrated by the fact that some grafts between SD- and LD-identical sibling donors and recipients are rejected in spite of immunosuppressive treatment. The question is raised even more strikingly in the case of bone marrow transplants, where a substantial percentage of transplants between SD- and LD-identical siblings lead to an acute graft-versus-host (GvH) reaction (STORB et al., 1974). The determinants against which this reaction is directed are unknown, but many laboratories are currently involved in trying to identify them. Following the studies of MAWAS et al. (1973), much attention has been centered on the possibility that these determinants are CML target specificities not coded for by the HL-A region. However, the importance of LD in GvH reactions is indicated by successful transplants between MLC-negative, SD-non-identical bone-marrow donors and recipients (DUPONT et al., 1973; GATTI et al., 1971).

I. Conclusion

The lymphocyte-defined (LD) specificities are histocompatibility determinants which provoke a strong proliferative response in the mixed leukocyte culture test. In this chapter the techniques for study of these specificities, their mode of inheritance, and some information concerning their clinical significance have been presented. I especially hope that this material will be useful to those using, or intending to use, the mixed lymphocyte culture test in transplantation or in other clinical situations.

Appendix I. Statistical Definitions

Confidence limits: Upon obtaining from a population experimental data with, for example, a certain mean and standard deviation, we can state the probability that on repeated sampling from this population we will obtain means within certain limits of the first mean obtained. The usual limits are 95% or 99% confidence limits. The 95% confidence limits used in this discussion represent the mean ± 1.96 standard deviations from the mean. In the example given in the discussion of stimulation index, 4 AA_m replicates with mean 290 and standard deviation 89, if we continue to draw sets of 4 from a population of replicate cultures AA_m, the means of 95% of these sets will lie within 464 and 116 cpm. The 95% confidence limits thus give an estimate of the reliability of a given experimental mean as an estimator of the true population mean.

Standard deviation and standard error: Both are measurements of the variability or "spread" of replicates around the mean in an experimental population, and are calculated, according to formulae (which may be found in any statistics book), from the deviation of each replicate from the mean. Large standard deviations or standard errors mean a wide variability in replicates. The difference between the two is that the standard deviation is a statistic of the sample studied and the standard error is a statistic of the population sampled; $S.E. = S.D.$ divided by the square root of the number of observations in the sample. Hence the standard error is smaller than the standard deviation and this should be kept in mind when looking at data.

These definitions are intended to be adequate for an understanding of the statistical discussion in the text. For more detail or a consideration of any of the statistical tests mentioned, the reader should consult a book on statistics.

Appendix II. Definition of Genetic Terms

Chromosome: A piece of genetic material (nucleic acids and associated proteins), containing a number of genes, physically connected, and presumed to be in a beads-on-a-string, longitudinal arrangement.

Region: A segment of chromosome, usually thought of as a unit because it contains a number of genes whose products appear to be related to the same function, although apparently unrelated genes may also be present. For example, the chromosomal segment containing LA, Four, and an unknown number and distribution of LD loci can be considered the HL-A region.

Gene: A unit of genetic function. This word has several meanings in genetics; for example, one may speak of a gene for eye color or a gene for blue eyes. To avoid this confusion I have used the terms locus and allele, respectively.

Locus: A point or section of the chromosome which is inherited as a unit, and has a given product (message). For example, one may speak of a locus determining eye color or one determining hair color.

Allele: A particular form of the locus, producing a particular phenotype. For example, one may speak of an allele for blue or brown eyes at a locus determining eye color.

Homozygous: Having the same allele at a given locus on both chromosomes of a pair.

Heterozygous: Having different alleles at a given locus on the two chromosomes.

Genotype: The actual alleles carried by an individual.

Phenotype: The manifestation of alleles at some physical level. In the case of dominant and recessive alleles, as discussed below, genotype cannot always be inferred from phenotype.

Dominant: An allele which is expressed in the same way in both the homozygous and heterozygous condition. I.e., if the phenotype 1a/1b is the same as the phenotype 1a/1a, 1a is dominant to 1b, and 1b is recessive to 1a.

Codominant: Alleles both of which are expressed in the heterozygote as in the homozygote. Transplantation antigens are usually codominant; for example, in an individual who carries alleles for HL-A1 and HL-A2 at the first segregant series, each allele is apparently expressed as if the other were not present, and the expression of HL-A1, for example, is not affected by the presence of any other first-series allele in the genotype. The simple term "dominant" is not used because there is no recessive allele.

Recessive: See Dominant.

These definitions are intended to be adequate for an understanding of the discussion in the text. For more detail, the reader should consult a book on genetics. The terms independent assortment, segregation, linkage and linkage disequilibrium are defined in the text.

Addendum

Since this section was written, a great deal of progress in several areas has been made.

Homozygous-cell typing for products of the strong LD locus (now called HLA-D) is being caried out in a number of laboratories. Through collaborative efforts several HLA-D specificities are now internationally recognized and readily identifiable. The possibility of using re-stimulation of previously specifically stimulated responder cells to type for LD is also being explored.

VAN LEEUWEN *et al.* (Transplantation Proc. 5:1539, 1973) suggested that it might be possible to identify LD alleles by serological means (see Section F II). The antigens identified by these and other workers are present on B (bone marrow derived) lymphocytes, which act as stimulating cells in MLC, but so far have not been detected on T (thymus-derived) lymphocytes which act as responding cells. They are therefore analogous to the Ia antigens of mouse B lymphocytes, which are genetically controlled by the H-2 region. The presence of particular human B-cell antigens on cells of a given individual appears to be closely correlated with the possession by that individual of particular HLA-D specificities as defined by homozygous cell typing; for example most individuals having specificity HLA-Dw1 will also have one particular B cell antigen. However, these are only strong statistical correlations and do not prove that the B cell antigens are identical with HLA-D specificities.

Papers concerning these topics will be published in a proposed supplement to the Journal of Experimental Medicine in late 1976, and in the reports of the Seventh Histocompatibility Workshop to be held in 1977.

References

Every effort has been made not to provide a comprehensive bibliography. The papers listed are references to work of current interest and very few "historical" papers have been included. The reader is especially referred to the following reviews:

BACH, F.H., VAN ROOD, J.J.: The major histocompatibility complex: genetics and biology. New England J. Med., in press (1975)

SORENSEN, S.F.: The mixed lymphocyte culture interaction. Techniques and immunogenetics. Acta Path. Microbiol. Scand. Sect. B, suppl. 230 (1972)

THORSBY, E.: The human major histocompatibility system. Transplant. Rev. **18**, 51 (1974)

Also to be consulted are the Proceedings of the Congresses of the Transplantation Society (in Trans-plantation Proceedings) and the MLC section of the Proceedings of the Sixth Histocompatibility Workshop.

AMOS, D.B., BACH, F.H.: Phenotypic expressions of the major histocompatibility locus in man (HL-A): leukocyte antigens and mixed leukocyte culture reactivity. J. Exp. Med. **128**, 623 (1968)

BACH, F.H., ALBERTINI, R.J., AMOS, D.B., CEPPELLINI, R., MATTIUZ, P.L., MIGGIANO, V.C.: Mixed leucocyte culture studies in families with known HL-A genotypes. Transplant. Proc. **1**, 339 (1969)

BACH, F.H., SEGALL, M., ZIER, K.S., SONDEL, P.M., ALTER, B.J., BACH, M.L.: Cell mediated immunity: separation of cells involved in recognition and destruction phases. Science **180**, 403 (1973)

BAIN, B., VAS, M.R., LOWENSTEIN, L.: The development of large immature mononuclear cells in mixed leucocyte cultures. Blood **23**, 108 (1964)

COCHRUN, K.C., PERKINS, H.A., PAYNE, R.O., KOUNTZ, S.L., BELZER, F.O.: The correlation of MLC with graft survival. Transplant. Proc. **5**, 391 (1973)

DUPONT, B., ANDERSON, V., ERNST, P., FABER, V., GOOD, R.A., HANSEN, G.S., HENRIKSEN, K., JENSEN, K., JUHL, F., KILLMANN, S.Aa., KOCH, C., MULLER-BERAT, N., PARK, B.H., SVEJGAARD, A., THOMSEN, M., WIIK, A.: Immunologic reconstruction in severe combined immunodeficiency with HL-A-incompatible bone-marrow graft: donor selection by mixed lymphocyte culture. Transplant. Proc. **5**, 905 (1973)

EIJSVOOGEL, V.P., DUBOIS, M., MELIEF, C.J.M., ZEYLEMAKER, W.R., RAAT-KONING, L., DE GROOT-KOOY, L.: Lymphocyte activation and destruction in vitro: relation to MLC and HL-A. Transplant. Proc. **5**, 415 (1973a)

EIJSVOOGEL, V., DUBOIS, M., MEINESZ, A., BIERHORST-EIJSLANDER, A., ZEYLEMAKER, W., SCHELLE-KENS, P.: The specificity and activation mechanism of cell-mediated lympholysis (CML) in man. Transplant. Proc. **5**, 1675 (1973b)

FESTENSTEIN, H., DEMANT, P.: Workshop summary on genetic determinants of cell-mediated immune reactions in the mouse. Transplant. Proc. **5**, 1321 (1973)

GATTI, R.A., MEUWISSEN H.J., TERASAKI, P.I., GOOD, R.A.: Recombination within the HL-A locus. Tissue Antigens **1**, 239 (1971)

HAMBURGER, J., CROSNIER, J., DESCAMPS, B., ROWINSKA, D.: Value of present methods used for selection of organ donors. Transplant. Proc. **3**, 260 (1971)

HIRSCHHORN, K., BACH, F.H., RAPAPORT, F.T., CONVERSE, J.M., LAWRENCE, H.S.: The relationship of in vitro lymphocyte compatibility to homograft sensitivity in man. Ann. N.Y. Acad. Sci. **120**, 303 (1964)

VAN HOOFF, J.P., HENDRIKS, G.F.J., SCHIPPERS, H.M.A., VAN ROOD, J.J.: Influence of possible HL-A haploidentity on renal-graft survival in Eurotransplant. Lancet **1**, 1130 (1974)

JEANNET, M.: Histocompatibility typing using leukocyte typing and MLC in kidney transplants. Helv. Med. Acta **35**, 168 (1970)

JORGENSEN, F., LAMM, L.U., KISSMEYER-NIELSEN, F.: Mixed lymphocyte cultures with inbred individuals: an approach to MLC typing. Tissue Antigens **3**, 323 (1973)

VAN LEEUWEN, A., SCHUIT, H.R.E., VAN ROOD, J.J.: Typing for MLC (LD) II. The selection of non-stimulator cells by MLC inhibition tests using SD-identical stimulator cells (MISIS) and fluorescent antibody studies. Transplant. Proc. **5**, 1539 (1973)

MAWAS, C., SASPORTES, M., CHRISTEN, Y., BERNARD, A., DAUSSET, J., ALTER, B.J., BACH, M.L.: Cell-mediated lympholysis (CML) in the absence of LD2 mixed lymphocyte reaction and CML in the presence of SD1-SD2 identity in two HL-A-genotyped families. Transplant. Proc. **5**, 1683 (1973)

MEMPEL, W., GROSSE-WILDE, H., ALBERT, E., THIERFELDER, S.: Atypical MLC reactions in HL-A typed related and unrelated pairs. Transplant. Proc. **5**, 401 (1973)

OSOBA, D., FALK, J.: The mixed leukocyte reaction in man: effect of pools of stimulating cells selected on the basis of cross-reacting HL-A specificities. Cellular Immunol. **10**, 117 (1974)

VAN ROOD, J.J., KOCH, C.T., VAN HOOFF, J.P., VAN LEEUWEN, A., VAN DEN TWEEL, J.G., FREDERIKS, E., SCHIPPERS, H.M.A., HENDRIKS, G., VAN DER STEEN, G.J.: Graft survival in unrelated donor-recipient pairs matched for MLC and HL-A. Transplant. Proc. **5**, 409 (1973)

SCHENDEL, D.J., BACH, F.H.: Genetic control of cell-mediated lympholysis in the mouse. J. Exp. Med. **140**, 1534 (1974)

SEGALL, M., OMODEI-ZORINI, C., BACH, F.H., JORGENSEN, F., KISSMEYER-NIELSEN, F.: HL-A antigens and mixed leukocyte culture (MLC) reactivity. Transplant. Proc. **5**, 383 (1973)

SEGALL, M., BACH, F.H.: Possible relationships among HL-A histocompatibility components. Transplant. Proc. **5**, 1595 (1974)

SEGALL, M., BACH, F.H., BACH, M.L., HUSSEY, J.L., UEHLING, D.T.: Correlation of MLC stimulation and clinical course in kidney transplants. Transplant. Proc., in press (1975)

SORENSEN, S.F., STAUB-NIELSEN, L.: Studies of unrelated subjects identical at the HL-A subloci "LA" and "Four". Acta Path. Microbiol. Scand. **B78**, 719 (1970)

STORB, R., THOMAS, E.D., BUCKNER, C.D., CLIFT, R.A., FEFER, A., GLUCKSBERG, H., NEIMAN, P.E.: Transplantation of bone marrow in refractory marrow failure and neoplastic diseases. Amer. J. Clin. Path. **62**, 212 (1974)

THOMPSON, J.S., FLINK, R.J., CALDWELL, J.L., SEVERSON, C.D., BONNEY, W.W.: Relationship of mixed lymphocyte culture response, HL-A histocompatibility antigens, and renal transplantation. Transplant. Proc. **5**, 1763 (1973)

THOMPSON, J.S., BONNEY, W.W., LAWTON, R.L., FLINK, R.J., CORRY, R.J.: Effect of HL-A haplotype matching on renal transplantation. Transplantation **17**, 438 (1974)

WILSON, D.B., SILVERS, W.K., NOWELL, P.C.: Quantitative studies on the mixed lymphocyte interaction in rats. II. Relationships of the proliferative response to the immunological status of the donors. J. Exp. Med. **126**, 655 (1967)

YUNIS, E., AMOS, D.B.: Three closely linked genetic systems relevant to transplantation. Proc. Nat. Acad. Sci. USA **68**, 3031 (1971)

Phylogenetic Aspects of Transplantation *

Edwin L. Cooper

With 4 Figures

A. Introduction

Central to the phylogenesis of transplantation immunity is the ability to distinguish between self and not-self (BURNET, 1974). How the recognition response is mediated and the degree of its complexity depend upon an animal's taxonomic position. Transplantation immunity is detected by transplanting cells, tissues, or entire organs. Acceptance of a graft confirms the presence of self antigens and, conversely, rejection suggests the presence of foreign, not-self antigens. It was recognized earlier as LOEB (1945) noted: "Strange or foreign individuality differentials (non-self provoke incompatibility, but self tissue (nonforeign) individuality differentials lead to no incompatible reactions."

Fishes, amphibians and reptiles, and coelomate invertebrates are unique (see HILDEMANN, 1972; DU PASQUIER, 1973; COOPER, 1974). Both the temperature and the length of experimentation affect the results from studies of transplantation immunity. Low temperatures will curtail allograft rejection while high temperatures can prolong it. Valid results are obtained at temperatures comparable to the animal's normal environment. Similarly age is important. Early investigators using amphibians, for example, observed no rejection response; they were primarily embryologists whose major concern was to test the self-differentiative capacities of transplanted embryonic primordia (COOPER, 1975). Thus, most of their experiments were terminated during the late embryonic or early larval life of the host before the immune capability is evident. HILDEMANN and HAAS (1959) were the first to indicate that the tadpole's rejection of tissue allografts is actually an immune reaction characterized by both anamnesis and infiltration of leukocytes. This work, and early studies by HILDEMANN on fish (HILDEMANN, 1956), initiated much of what was to follow dealing with the phylogenesis of transplantation immunity.

Investigators have since performed transplant experiments on and examined the responses of many of the lower vertebrates and invertebrates. Some of the most interesting and intensive studies have resulted from those dealing

* Supported primarily by NIH Grant HD 09333-01 from the National Institute of Child Health and Human Development. I thank Mrs. LOIS GEHRINGER and Mrs. PAMELA KONRAD for assistance in preparation of the manuscript.

with the earthworm (COOPER, 1974; DUPRAT, 1970; VALEMBOIS, 1974). To date earthworms are phylogenetically the most primitive animals to exhibit a cellular immune response resembling that of vertebrates. As this chapter points out, many even more primitive animals, e.g., cnidaria and platyhelminthes, and such advanced groups as the echinoderms also exhibit ancestral immune responses. The complexity of the response depends upon an animal's phylogenetic position.

Continued experimental work will undoubtedly reveal important similarities between transplantation immune phenomena of vertebrates and invertebrates. Perhaps in simpler organisms there is humoral immunity that more closely parallels the antibody response of vertebrates. This review, however, proposes a link between invertebrate and vertebrate cellular immune reactions, i.e., transplantation immunity not humoral immunity.

B. Transplantation Reactions in Invertebrates Other than Annelids and Echinoderms

1. Organelle Transplantation in Protozoans (Sarcodina, Ciliata)

Acceptance or rejection of a foreign organelle in a protozoan is a primitive form of recognition, the primordial attribute of the vertebrate's immune response. The ameba has greatly facilitated organelle transplantation studies, since transplants, especially nuclear transfers, are easily made. The *Amoeba*'s response is characterized by specificity of both nucleus and cytoplasm (GOLDSTEIN, 1970). Allo-or homotransfers, transplants of nuclei to cytoplasms of the same strain, are at least 90% successful in yielding viable mass cultures. Autogeneic transfers, where the nuclei are removed and immediately replaced in the same cytoplasm, are always successful (HAWKINS and COLE, 1964). As a result of his work with ciliates, TARTAR (1970) suggested that protozoan incompatibilities are primordial immune phenomena with evolutionary implications. They may represent "evidence at the unicellular level of an anticipation of those specifities which so sharply limit the interindividual grafting of tissues in man" (TARTAR, 1964).

2. Metazoans—Specificity of Reaggregation in Porifera

The sponge, *Demospongia,* a representative metazoan and diploblastic animal is important to studies of the origins of specific recognition. The behavior of aggregated sponge cells in vitro reveals the inherent capacity of all cells to distinguish between self and not-self. The sponge, thus, has an undisputed role in understanding the phylogenesis of immune reactions. In his classic study on sponge regeneration from dissociated cells, WILSON (1907) observed that cells of a given species aggregate with like kind after mixing of several cell types. GALTSOFF (1925) later showed that cell sorting occurs between different cell types during the reformation of a dissociated sponge, *Microciona prolifera.* More recently the situation in sponges has been reviewed by VAN DE VYVER (1970), TURNER *et al.* (1974), and MACLENNAN (1974).

What causes cell aggregation has not been proven. HUMPHREYS (1967) believes a large glycoprotein molecule, a component of the cell surface coat, is responsible. SPIEGEL (1954) also compared invertebrate recognition reactions to the earliest events of vertebrate immune responses by his analysis of aggregation in sponges. Inspired by TYLER's (1946) autoantibody concept and WEISS's (1946) "molecular ecology", SPIEGEL hypothesizes that cells are held together by specific macromolecules of at least two stereochemically reciprocal types per cell arranged on the cell surface. These early speculations regarding cell binding were important to understanding antigen recognition.

3. Incompatibility in Cnidaria (Hydrozoa, Anthozoa)

LOEB's (1945) account of tissue incompatibilities among the Cnidaria, formerly the Coelenterates, was an important contribution to the study of self, not-self specificity. DU PASQUIER (1974) has recently reviewed the genetic control of histocompatibility reactions from a phylogenetic viewpoint dealing with Cnidarians.

According to CAMPBELL and BIBB (1970) *Hydra* accepts autografts but destroys other types of transplants that are genetically incompatible. One can conclude that reasonably simple allelic differences between animals are sufficient to produce graft incompatibility. In the Anthozoa, THEODOR's studies (1971) of invertebrate tissue recognition contradict the view that allogeneic ectoderm histoincompatibility developed late in evolution. In his work with the arborescent coelenterates, the Gorgonacea, autografts are successful and survive indefinitely, but segments of branches taken from two different individuals fail to fuse. In more distantly related xenogeneic cultures of gorgonian tissue, mutual damage and histotoxicity occur within 1–4 days of contact. In allogeneic combinations a similar disintegration of tissue occurs, but usually after a longer delay. THEODOR refers to histotoxicity in gorgonians as an "induced suicide." This might offer a primitive mechanism to explain cell destruction by cytotoxic or "non immune" reactions in cultures of vertebrate cells. Of considerable potential importance is the recent study of HILDEMANN and his colleagues on corals from the Great Barrier Reef (personal communication).

4. Platyhelminthes and Sipunculida

LINDH (1959) made transplants in flatworms, *Turbellaria,* experiments important initially for concepts related to developmental biology, i.e., induction and regeneration, rather than to origins of immunity. With an immunologic interpretation, the results are significant to the phylogenesis of transplantation immune responses; auto- and allotransplants succeed. This equivocal finding should be reinvestigated with a longer observation period. In some cases heterotransplants, those between the same genus but different species, behave as allotransplants. However, in most instances, such as between *Planaria dorotocephala* and *Planaria maculata,* only temporary regeneration occurs, suggesting the recognition of nonself.

Though the sexes are separate in the sipunculid, *Dendrostomum zostericolum,* each retains its gametes in the coelom for long periods of time; thus, technically, transplantations can be made by injecting the eggs, sperm, into the coelom of another. According to Triplett *et al.* (1958) treatments such as washing, heating, and sonication apparently destroy the capacity for self-recognition and, also, result in encapsulation and death of autogeneic eggs. With another tissue, both auto- and allo-tentacle first-set grafts are encapsulated by host coelomocytes at similar rates. Contrary to a typical immune response involving memory, second-set transplants are not encapsulated at an accelerated rate. This experiment too should be repeated utilizing better controls.

5. Equivocal Incompatibilities in Mollusca (Pelecypoda, Gastropoda, Cephalopoda)

Drew and de Morgan (1910) were among the first to report on the fate of transplanted tissues in molluscs. Transplantations of mantle strips and female gonads in *Pecten irradians* result in healing of most grafts after 49 hours. However, none healed if male gonads were used or if transplantations were performed under the mantle. Well-healed autografts retained eyes, tentacles, and contractibility for over a month. This information is equivocal, because they observed that auto- and allotransplants behaved similarly. Des Voigne and Sparks (1969) made allografts of oyster (*Crassostrea gigas*) mantle to slits in the connective tissue near the palps. Though some implants were rejected by the host, others remained viable and appeared normal. Wound healing at first seems inhibited, but leukocytes eventually delineate the wound and form a union with the implants. Canzonier (1963) reported 50% rejection of both normal and diseased implants of allogeneic tissues in *Crassostrea virginica*. However, once implants become fused to the host, there is no indication of host rejection. The blood spaces join with those of the host, and no cross circulation is apparent.

Cheng (1970) reviewed experiments using other gastropods. Transplants of digestive gland tissues were made from the gastropods *Helisoma duryi normale, Helisoma trivolvis, Tarebia granifera,* and *Melania newcombi* into the cephalopedal sinuses of *Helisoma duryi normale*. Recipients evidently are able to differentiate between allografts and xenografts; host reactions to xenografts are more rapid and generally more severe than their reaction to allografts. In other gastropods, Tripp (1961) found that pedal tissue allografts in the cephalopedal sinus (space between the anterior cerebral region and the foot) of *Australorbis glabratus* are successful if layers of the two tissues are first joined. Though implantation of fresh allogeneic tissue elicits only a transient hemocytic infiltration, formalin-fixed allogeneic tissue is encapsulated; such studies require further confirmation. In cephalopods after transplanting skin between octopus, Cushing (1962) found no differences in the behavior of autografts or allografts. Both survive as long as the hosts except when there are technical failures.

Such equivocal findings among the molluscs point out clearly that our knowledge of mollusc transplantation reactions is still hampered by lack of appropriate techniques. We still have no definitive studies showing specific cell mediated immunity.

6. Arthropoda

a) Diptera

HADORN's (1937) early studies of ovarian transplants in *Drosophila* were done from the viewpoint of the geneticist and embryologist, rather than of the immunologist. HADORN transplanted ovaries and testes into normal larvae and obtained distinct but limited development. This suggests that host factors, perhaps immune, prevent development. KAMBYSELLIS (1968) analyzed genetic differences between populations of *Drosophila* by performing interspecific (xeno-) transplants of larval ovaries. Although his concern was genetic differences, he found it possible to induce tolerance in arthropods if transplants are made during early stages of development, a finding comparable to those of vertebrates.

b) Orthoptera

SCOTT (1971) attempted to determine what constitutes foreignness to an invertebrate by implanting nylon filaments into the American cockroach, *Periplaneta americana*. Hemocytes from the host's body fluid completely encapsulate the filaments, and a multilayered capsule forms that isolates the particle from the circulation. Furthermore, interspecific xenogeneic implants from another insect, *Nauphoeta cineria,* are also recognized as foreign and encapsulated. More distantly related xenoimplants, such as those from *Calliphora,* the blow fly, or even from mice are also encapsulated within 24 hours after implantation.

By contrast, allogeneic transplants, nerve cords exchanged between members of *Periplanata americana*, are not encapsulated. It is, thus, probable that autoimplants would not be encapsulated either. When, however, allogeneic nerve ends are treated with various enzymes so that unknown properties are removed, hemocytes encapsulate the allogeneic particles. This work strongly supports the view that specific recognition is determined by the properties of the antigeneic surface. If the self-recognition sites on the membrane were untreated, the implants would be recognizable as self, and would be "immune" to attack.

BELL (1972) transplanted ovaries in 18 species of cockroaches in studies of insect hormones. Intraspecific allografts resulted in the initiation of yolk formation and oocyte growth rates comparable to controls. Heterotransplants of ovaries led to sequestered host vitellogenins, but the grafts grew to terminal stages only when donor and host were closely related. When ovaries were transplanted between species of different superfamilies or families, yolk formation did not occur. Thus, the fate of endocrine glands can be tested after transplantation, revealing the degree of histocompatibility between donor and host.

7. Genetic Control in Urochordata

FREEMAN (1970) reviewed the results of Japanese workers on the genetic control of transplantation specificity in *Botryllus*, a colonial ascidian. Working with *B. primigenus*, OKA and WATANABE (1960) showed that if two parental nonfusable colonies are mated, four classes of progeny result in the F_1. Each progeny class then fuses with members of its class, those of two other classes, and with both parents. Assuming that the parents are both heterozygous at a locus for colony specificity with genotypes expressed by the notation AB and CD (with each letter representing one allele), the F_1 generation possesses four classes of progeny: AC, AD, BC and BD. Thus, colonies with at least one allele in common at the colony specificity locus will fuse with each other; matings of the F_1 progeny producing F_2 and colony fusion tests established this as a correct scheme. According to a genetic analysis by HILDEMANN and REDDY (1973), these results do not agree with the immunogenetic rules of transplantation established for vertebrates: AD can fuse with BD but not with BC colonies.

In a further analysis of recognition events in *Botryllus,* TANAKA (1973) and WATANABE and TANAKA (1973) arrived at the following conclusions: They view nonfusion reactions (NFR) as a measure of allogeneic inhibition when two incompatible ascidian colonies are placed in mutual contact. The response is irreversible and progresses to completion even if one participating member is removed. Colony specific NFR, according to one possible interpretation, resides in the test matrix and blood that causes death of granular amebocytes. It is noteworthy that the so-called nonimmunologic allogeneic inhibition described by the MÖLLERS (1966) was interpreted as an evolutionary precursor of immune type responses, probably related to the immunologic surveillance system (BURNET, 1970).

8. Summary of Quasi Immunorecognition

The ability to recognize the difference between self and not-self is an attribute observed at the latest in metazoans. Indeed, transplantations of cell organelles in protozoans produce incompatibility reactions that are specific. According to HILDEMANN and REDDY (1973), "*Quasi immuno-recognition* or [the] capacity for non-self recognition of allogeneic tissue followed by incompatibility reactions appears characteristic of coelenterates as shown in colonial hydroids, gorgonians, and hard corals". The term is appropriate, one which they use "because of the apparent specificity of the antagonistic reactions and the compatible lag period preceding manifestations of incompatibility. Absence of a memory component enters this kind of surveillance system unlike the vertebrate response." Thus from simple animals to the most complex, *quasi immunorecognition* is a universal characteristic.

C. Transplantation Reactions in Invertebrates that Reveal Primordial Cell-Mediated Immunity

I. Short-term Immunologic Memory

Echinoderms are important for assessing the phylogeny of transplantation immunity. Echinoderms, according to some taxonomists, are close to the vertebrates ancestrally; thus they are excellent for studying transplantation immune reactivities intermediate between invertebrates and vertebrates. The phylum Echinodermata includes the sea cucumbers (class Holothuroidea), sea stars (Asteroidea), brittle stars (Ophiuroidea), sea urchins and sand dollars (Echinoidea), sea lilies (Crinoidea), and several extinct classes. Earlier studies dealing with allograft recognition in echinoderms are equivocal, mainly due to difficult technique and husbandry. Transplantations were performed to heterotopic sites and the animals maintained in excessively cold sea water, two variables that create difficulty in distinguishing between graft acceptance and rejection (GHIRADELLA, 1965; BRUSLÉ, 1967).

II. Cell and Tissue Responses that Indicate Self Recognition in Echinoderms

To understand cell recognition but not anamnesis, REINISCH and BANG (1971) injected *Arbacia* (sea urchin) cells (some are deeply pigmented), into *Asterias* (sea star) in vivo. The number of circulating amebocytes in the hosts dropped abruptly. The *Arbacia* cells adhered to and were phagocytosed by host cells that clumped consistently within the papulae, outpushings of the body wall. Injection of *Asterias* cells into *Asterias* does not elicit cell clumping, nor is it followed by a drop in circulating amebocytes. These results suggest that *Asterias'* recognition of intact foreign cells evokes a defense mechanism completely different from simple responses to an injected foreign body such as carborundum particles. In fact, this echinoderm response closely resembles the type of self-, not-self cell recognition demonstrable within the vertebrate phylum and is no different from that of other invertebrates not belonging to this evolutionary line.

III. Transplantation in Asteroidea

Despite the difficulty in making echinoderm transplants, GHIRADELLA (1965) found that two starfishes, *Patiria miniata* and *Asterias forbesi,* discriminate between reciprocal allo-, and xenocoelomic implants and heterogeneic pyloric caecum from two other species, *Asterias vulgaris* and *Henricia sanguinolenta.* Normal allografts, although healthy after 5 weeks, are surrounded by connective tissue and amebocyte masses. Although amebocytes are usually associated with damaged allograft areas, amebocytic attack, phagocytosis, and encapsulation are, apparently, not associated with the elimination of xenotransplants. Xeno-grafts are eliminated by the hosts one week after transplantation. *Henricia* caecum is extruded through the dermal branchiae by both hosts; *Patiria* disposes of *Asterias* caecum by transfering it from the host ray to the cardiac stomach where it is digested or extruded through the mouth.

IV. Short-term Memory

Because of the rigid exoskeleton of the echinoderm body, enormous technical difficulties must be surmounted before adequate grafting procedures can be undertaken. Despite this, HILDEMANN and DIX (1972) made substantial progress in defining specific recognition and a memory component in echinoderms. To define the events in allograft destruction, they chose the sea cucumber (*Cucumaria tricolor*) and the horned sea star (*Protoreaster nodosus*) from the Great Barrier Reef. Because of variable colorations, pigment cell destruction, like in other invertebrates and primitive vertebrates, is the easiest external criterion of graft rejection.

Autografts in both genera heal permanently. In *Cucumaria,* three distinct cell layers are evident—the epidermis, an outer muscle layer, and a deep muscle layer. *Protoreaster* integument autografts show an outer epithelium with secretory cells and muscle fiber bundles. Three layers are distinguishable into epidermis, thick dermis with loose connective tissue, and an underlying muscle layer into which crypts extend.

Allograft destruction occurs in both species, and the response is apparently no different from chronic allograft destruction in other invertebrates. Progressive pigment cell destruction heralds allograft rejection. In the sea cucumber, the epidermis initially becomes edematous with vacuolation and loss of cytoplasm in some areas. Macrophages are abundant at 173 days, although they may have appeared earlier. During later rejection stages macrophages and "lymphocytes" were associated with *Cucumaria* grafts. At terminal stages of rejection, *Protoreaster* grafts show less macrophages and more eosinophils in the dermis and loose connective tissue. First-set allograft destruction occurs at 4–6 months at 21° C.

Few second-set grafts were performed, to test for memory, but all showed pronounced accelerated rejection (positive memory). The second-set response was characterized by early inflammatory discoloration and hyperplasia leading to invasive resorption of grafts. This type of response was interpreted as short-term memory or interruption of the induction phase, since repeat test grafts were performed when first-set transplants were only partially rejected. There is no other evidence that long-term memory may exist in echinoderms, demonstrable by positive memory, i.e., accelerated rejection of second transplants performed after first-set transplant destruction. Echinoderms offer a second phylum in addition to the earthworm model that offers evidence of specificity and memory.

V. The Earthworm Model

The earthworm, a complex invertebrate, possesses a coelomic cavity equipped with several types of coelomocytes that effect its immune responses. A comparison of this annelid's coelomocyte system with the vertebrate's lymphomyeloid system reveals some important similarities. Earthworms exhibit an immune response that resembles the vertebrate cellular immune response more than it does humoral mechanisms of other invertebrates studied to date (COOPER, 1965a, b). Its phagocytic organ's source of coelemocytes may be a primitive counterpart of the vertebrate reticuloendothelial system. Coelomocytes are responsible for graft rejection. They infiltrate foreign transplants and are able to transfer the response by a memory mechanism. Humoral immunity, though effective, is nonspecific.

1. First- and Second-Set Allograft Rejection in *Lumbricus terrestris* and *Eisenia foetida*

The technical procedure for performing transplants are easily learned (COOPER, 1968). Autografts are important for showing recognition of self; they heal grossly after 24 hours, microscopically after 48 hours, and survive permanently. Inter-population allografts in *Lumbricus terrestris* survive less well than intrapopulation allografts; the frequency is increased from 5 to 15%, suggesting a greater tissue alloantigen diversity reflected in populations separated by wide geographic barriers. In another earthworm, rejection of first-set allografts in a single population of *Eisenia foetida* also occurs and often requires a maximum of 255 days. The patterns of total rejection time in allogeneic combinations are similar. Comparative immunologists in France led by DUPRAT (1964) also made some of the first attempts to understand graft rejection in earthworms, particularly with regard to the capacity for specificity and anamnesis in allogeneic combinations. DUPRAT (see review CHATEAUREYNAUD-DUPRAT, 1970) found that first-set allografts exchanged between *Eisenia foetida* from the same location heal promptly and remain grossly intact. Initial transplants between worms from different regions are, however, like xenografts, always destroyed, confirming the genetic heterogeneity of worms.

2. Rejection of First- and Second-Set Xenografts Exchanged between *Lumbricus* and *Eisenia*

First-set and second-set xenografts of integument exchanged between *Lumbricus terrestris* and *Eisenia foetida* heal grossly during the first 24 hours, but subsequently are destroyed (COOPER, 1968). Pigment cell breakdown can range from 6 to 148 days (Fig. 1). Soon after an initial graft heals, acidophil phagocytic cells infiltrate the graft-host contact zone. Although most second-set xenografts are destroyed by accelerated reactions, a significant number show the opposite effect, a prolonged survival in comparison to first-set grafts. As there is no apparent donor specificity in the rejection times of repeat grafts, hosts apparently lack precise receptors for detection of differences in donor antigens.

There are several generalities relative to the earthworm's response to xenografts: (1) acute rejection, 11 days or less, of first sets is followed by prolonged survival of second sets; chronic rejection is generally followed by an accelerated destruction of repeat grafts; (2) short intervals, 0–4 days, between first and second-set grafts produce accelerated rejections; extended intervals, 33–71 days, lead to prolonged survival of challenge grafts; (3) early onset of rejection of second-set grafts is usually followed by accelerated breakdown; conversely, late onset of rejection normally precedes prolonged survival. The accelerated second-set response in xenogeneic earthworm combinations supports the view that memory or anamnesis has been induced by first-set transplants.

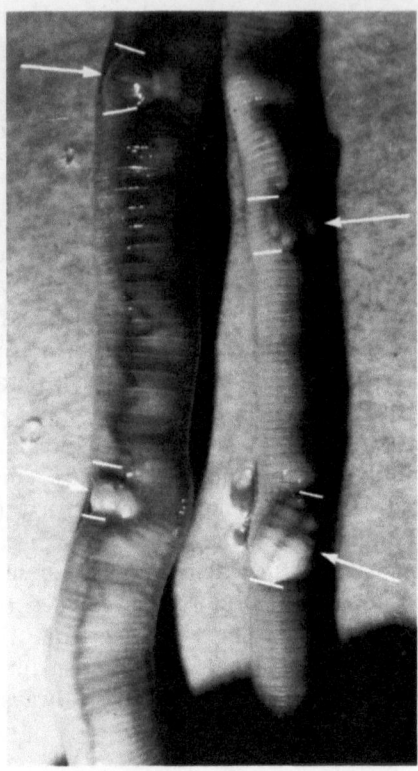

Fig. 1. Earthworms, *Lumbricus terrestris* (*left*) and an *Eisenia foetida* (*right*) host, show autografts (*top*) and xenografts (*bottom*). The autografts are well healed and will survive permanently. The xenografts are healed but show beginning signs of pigment cell destruction, which signals graft rejection

3. Specificity and Anamnesis

Specificity of allo- and xeno- but not autograft rejection supports the hypothesis that earthworms exhibit a "primitive" immune reaction. Furthermore intrafamilial xenogeneic transplants survive longer than infamilial ones, suggesting a refinement of distinction between closely related xenogeneic antigens. Specificity is also apparent when two xenografts are performed simultaneously on a *Lumbricus* host; both exhibit similar survival endpoints (COOPER, 1969). However, if there is a 5-day interval between first and second-set grafts, both the first and second-set transplants undergo an accelerated rejection, indicating the host's heightened reaction. Presumably this occurs because there is an interruption of the inductive phase. A first-set *Allolobophora* transplant grafted to *Lumbricus* simultaneously with a second-set *Eisenia* graft but 5 days after the first-set *Eisenia* graft is destroyed at a time equivalent to a single *Allolobophora* graft; this is, however, different from either of the two *Eisenia* transplants. Although this may not be clearly a memory response, it is specific to the three transplants.

4. The Cellular Response

a) Adoptive Transfer of the Xenograft Reaction

According to BAILEY *et al.* (1971), graft rejection can be produced by transferring immune coelomocytes. They grafted *Lumbricus* with *Eisenia* xenografts and subsequently injected coelomocytes from them into nonimmune hosts. When grafted later with a transplant from the original *Eisenia,* they reject such test grafts faster than first grafts. Coelomic fluid alone does not cause this accelerated reaction, nor does saline or coelomocytes from unsensitized worms. The coelomocyte, therefore, is a prime example of an invertebrate wandering cell that recognizes and reacts to antigen (BURNET, 1968). The coelomocyte provides a model for studying the evolutionary ancestors of vertebrate leukocytes and immunocytes. VALEMBOIS (1963) drew attention to the earthworm as an excellent coelomate invertebrate for studying graft rejection.

b) Quantitation of Coelomocyte Responses

Quantitative differences between the response of earthworm coelomocytes to autogeneic and to xenogeneic grafts provide evidence of an anamnestic reaction (HOSTETTER and COOPER, 1972, 1973). Following second-set grafts there is an increase in numbers of coelomocytes, a heightened reaction. The initial response to autografts is characterized by variable accumulations of basophilic coelomocytes. They usually attach to autografts on or near the lining of the coelom.

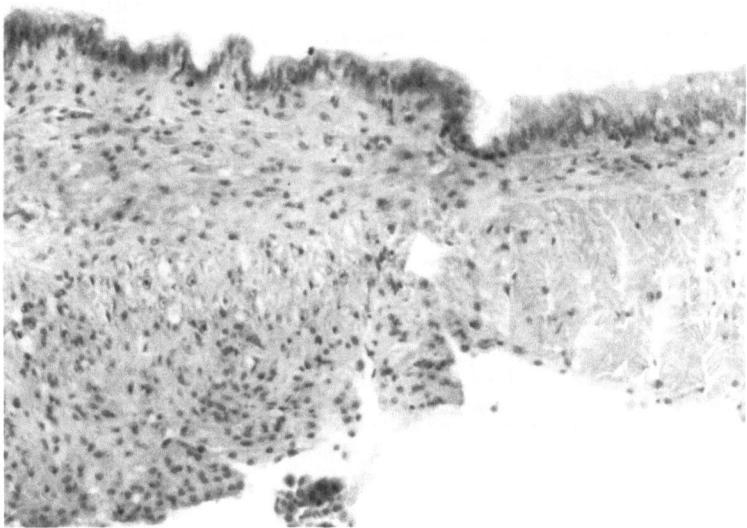

Fig. 2. A composite photomicrograph of an earthworm (*Lumbricus*) xenograft 10 days postgrafting. The graft is at the left and the intact host tissue at the right. Notice the absence of all graft tissue except for a few longitudinal muscle bundles. × 320 (From COOPER, Transplantation **6**, 322 337, 1968)

This cellular response diminishes considerably and terminates between days 6 and 7 postgrafting. Only occasionally are acidophilic coelomocytes found near autografts. Of two muscle layers, it is the longitudinal of autografts that is often reduced to approximately one-half its normal thickness. Basophilic coelomocytes rapidly infiltrate xenografts during the first 2 days postgrafting and destroy the longitudinal muscle layer. Massive accumulations of basophilic coelomocytes line the undersurface of xenografts surrounding loose muscle fibers; acidophilic cells are also present but seem to play a minor role (Fig. 2). After day 6 postgrafting, most grafts become progressively infiltrated with acidophilic and basophilic coelomic cells. By day 8 postgrafting normal graft morphology is totally destroyed, leaving no longitudinal or circular muscular layers, and coelomocyte infiltration extends to the epithelium by day 10 postgrafting.

c) Total and Differential Cell Counts Relative to Auto- and Xenografts

Normal coelomic fluid of *Lumbricus* contains both acidophilic and basophilic coelomocytes. There is no variability in differential cell counts between xenografts, autografts, and normal coelomic fluid during the first 12 hours postgrafting. However the total number of coelomocytes in association with xenografts and autografts increases significantly 24 hours postgrafting. Xenografts contain a higher total number of cells than do autografts but also a slightly lower percentage of acidophilic cells.

d) Second-set Reactions

More than twice as many coelomocytes are associated with second-set than with first-set xenografts 24 hours postgrafting. This increase in response to second-set xenografts is interpreted as an anamnestic response. It results from a re-exposure to a foreign antigen. Coelomocytes proliferate after having been primed by contact with the first-set graft. Thus, a first-set xenograft causes an increase in total coelomocyte numbers, and many may become attached to host tissues. Stimulation by a second-set xenograft may cause mobilization or an increase by mitosis in the total numbers of coelomocytes. Although this study of coelomocytes associated with xenografts requires extension, there is support for immunologic memory in *Lumbricus* in response to tissue transplants.

e) Acid Phosphatase Observations

Although acid phosphatase may not be directly involved in the graft rejection process, it is a good marker for lysosomes that contain enzymes capable of destroying xenografts. The dense deposition of acid phosphatase under xenografts indicates the presence of lysosomal material between xenograft tissues and host coelomocytes. Lysosomal enzymes in invertebrate leukocytes have been demonstrated by Janoff and Hawrylko (1963) and Grimstone et al. (1969). Acid phosphatase activity can be detected in both autografts and xenografts, but is much less apparent in autografts.

5. The Role of Temperature in Earthworm Tissue Graft Rejection

The rejection rate of first-set xenografts exchanged between *Lumbricus* and *Eisenia* is temperature dependent like that of poikilothermic vertebrate immune reactions. WINGER and COOPER (1969) found that xenograft survival is prolonged as the temperature is lowered but that higher temperatures accelerate rejection. Raising the temperature beyond a certain point seems to prolong graft survival. *Eisenia* lives best in a warmer environment than *Lumbricus;* thus, graft rejection in *Eisenia* is fastest at 23° C, and in *Lumbricus* at 20° C. One important consequence of information relative to temperature is the lack of wide-spread distribution of survival times at higher temperatures. This inevitably leads to more accelerated second-set rejections than those at 15° C. Of prime importance is the demonstration of significant increases in the number of accelerated second-set survival times.

6. Summary

The annelid does exhibit the kind of immune response that has been defined for the vertebrate. The annelid's cell-mediated immune response shows both specificity and memory, a cell-dependent process. Though the invertebrate coelomocyte may not be directly related to the vertebrate plasma cell in evolutionary development or capable of producing antibodies, it is considered to be an analogous precursor. The annelid response may, therefore, be prototypic and may represent the earliest, or the most primitive form of immune capability.

D. Transplantation Immunity in Fishes

I. Introduction

HILDEMANN's (1957) work with goldfish first introduced transplantation reactions in poikilothermic vertebrates as mediated by immune mechanisms. He observed a typical inflammatory reaction to scale allografts and determined that the length of time required for both first- and second-set graft rejection varied inversely with temperature. Moreover, there is a clear distinction between a primary and a secondary response to scale allografts. At any temperature second-set scale allografts are destroyed at approximately one-half to two-thirds the survival time of primary grafts from the same donor. These studies were extended and reviewed by HILDEMANN and COOPER (1963).

II. The Hagfish

Cyclostome or jawless agnathan fishes are considered by most systematists to be the most primitive living vertebrates. Under proper laboratory conditions, hagfish are as capable of recognizing and destroying allografts as mammals.

Their immune system readily distinguishes between self tissue and foreign allo-grafts, as revealed by typical delayed type reactions such as lymphocyte infiltra-tion, hemorrhage, and a gross indicator of survival, pigment cell destruction. According to HILDEMANN and THOENES (1969) there is also a memory response characterized by an accelerated rejection (28 days rather than 72 days) of second-set grafts after the destruction of first sets. Furthermore, among the agnathans, the opposite usually occurs, i.e., negative memory; rejection of second-set grafts is usually not accelerated but prolonged.

III. The Lamprey

The lamprey, *Petromyzon marinus,* a close relative of the hagfish, rejects skin allografts, and apparently there is immunologic memory. As shown by PEREY *et al.* (1968) ammocetes or larvae of the sea lamprey exhibit chronic reactions to allografts at about 20° C. Because the survival times recorded range from 7–252 days, rigid criteria for assessing the end points of graft survival may not have been employed. The rejection itself is undoubtedly an immune response, because it is accompanied by inflammation and lymphoid cell infiltration of the graft-host contact zones.

IV. Cartilaginous Fishes

This group, like the previous one, exhibits a chronic rejection of initial allografts; autografts are never destroyed. PERRY *et al.* (1968) also studied the sting ray, *Dasyatus americana,* and found that the onset of first-set graft rejection occurs by 21 days. Second-set grafts have a curtailed survival of less than 12 days, and more severe inflammatory reactions also occur, confirming the existence of a memory component. The horned shark's (*Heterodontis francisci*) progressive development of immunity to skin allografts has been described by BORYSENKO and HILDEMANN (1970). Although the kinetics of its first-set rejections are similar to those of the sting ray, the mean survival time of successive second-, third-, and fourth-set skin allografts decreases significantly. As there is a vigorous, acute destruction of fourth-set grafts, a defective immune system does not explain slow rejections of first-set grafts.

V. Bony Fishes (Holosteans; Teleosts)

A primitive teleost, *Osteoglossum bicirrhosum,* exhibits an immune response to scale allotransplants at 25° C (BORYSENKO and HILDEMANN, 1969). However, pig-ment cell destruction is slower than in higher teleosts. As second-set responses occur at a median survival time (MST) of 17.9 days and first-set at an MST of 51 days, memory is indicated. The range of third-party rejection times from 4.3–15.4 days reveals a diversity of transplantation antigens in this species. In teleost fish studied (HILDEMANN, 1972) and reviewed by HILDEMANN (1970), control autografts are permanently successful and there is acute, complete rejection of scale allografts. Capillary blood flow in first-set allografts is restored when original graft and host vessels are inosculated within 72 hours after transplantation. Circulation persists, however, only for a few days until hemostasis occurs and graft breakdown begins. Blood flow in second-set grafts rarely occurs. If it does, it is only partial, sluggish, and of short duration. Vascular damage, on the other hand, accompanied by extravasation of blood, is generally more intense, appears earlier, and develops more rapidly in second- than in first-set allografts.

E. Transplantation Immunity in Amphibians

Before there is gross discernable appearance of foreign graft destruction, leukocytes infiltrate the host's graft area and participate in graft destruction. As is typical, there is an accelerated response to second-set grafts. The inflammatory response consists of vasodilation, hemostasis, and, finally, destruction. Amphibians generally can be divided into two groups, each with a characteristic immune response to skin allografts. The legless apodans and the urodeles exhibit chronic or slow rejection while the anurans exhibit faster or acute rejection.

I. Adult Apodans

1. Introduction

COOPER and GARCIA-HERRARA (1968) have studied transplantation immunity, lymphoid organs, and blood cells of caecilians. Their initial studies were performed on a species tentatively identified as *Typhlonectes compressicauda,* but later found to be *Nectrocaecilia cooperi* (TAYLOR, 1970). Of the usual lymphoid organs, apodans possess both a thymus and spleen. The spleen and liver are curious grossly, as they appear elongated; otherwise, the histology is similar to other amphibians, and at this level of phylogeny, it is expected that the liver and kidney undoubtedly play a role in immune reactions.

2. General Description of Autografts and Allografts

As in other poikilotherms, pigment cell destruction signals the characteristically chronic rejection of first-set allografts. In addition to this sign of inflammation, one can often grossly identify vasodilation and hemostasis. Apodans also exhibit the phenomenon of negative memory, i.e., second-set grafts are not always destroyed faster than first-set grafts but occasionally are prolonged.

3. Histopathology

The histology of graft rejection in the apodan reveals a sequence of changes characteristic of immune responsiveness. Normal skin consists of an outer epidermis composed of 4–6 layers of stratified squamous epithelial cells; the basement membrane appears beneath the epithelium. In addition, connective tissue fibers, abundant skin glands, and melanocytes are present. A circular muscle layer lies just beneath a longitudinal bundle (Fig. 3). The epithelium of rejected allografts is flattened to about 2–3 cell layers and is more intensely acidophilic than normal skin. Also, the separation between epithelium and underlying dermis disappears, leaving a flattened graft with substantial amounts of connective tissue. Melanocytes, skin glands, and the integrity of the muscle bundles are absent. The presence of lymphocytes and granulocytes is final evidence that caecilians can reject skin allografts by an immune response (Fig. 4).

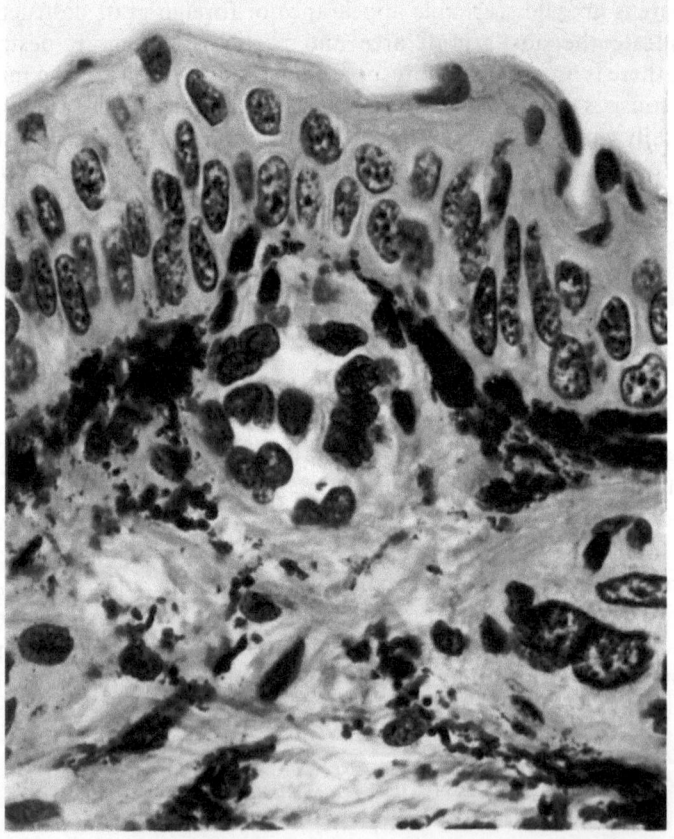

Fig. 3. Normal skin of the caecilian or legless amphibian (*Nectrocaecilia cooperi*). A single layer of dead desquamated cells overlies the stratified squamous epithelial layer. Beneath the epithelium is a basement membrane and a layer of dermal melanophores surrounding multicellular glands. Loose connective tissue, fibroblasts, and capillaries are just beneath the basement membrane. ×200
(From COOPER and GARCIA-HERRERA, Copeia **2**, 224–229, 1968)

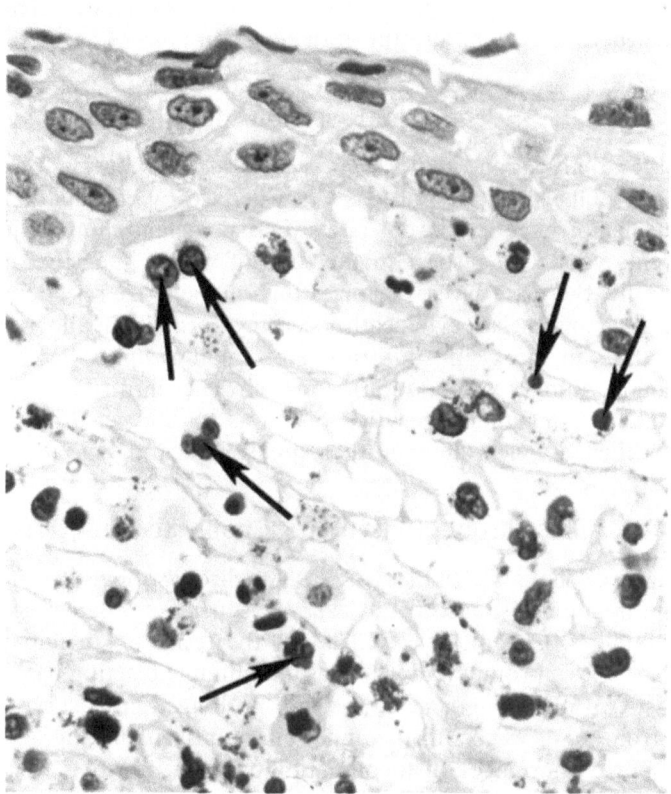

Fig. 4. Section of a first-set allograft from *Nectrocaecilia* after rejection 8–11 days postgrafting. Although the epithelium appears alive, none of the formed elements such as glands, muscle, or melanophores are present in this rejected graft. Many pyknotic nuclei are present (*lower arrow, two arrows to right*) along with lymphocytes (*two upper arrows*) and neutrophils (*middle arrow*). ×640 (From COOPER and GARCIA-HERRERA, Copeia **2**, 224–229, 1968)

II. Adult Urodeles

1. The Latent Phase

Because urodeles, unlike fishes and larval or adult amphibians, display the curious, but still immunologic, prolonged rejection of allografts, embryologists once erroneously attributed fast rejections to poor technical procedures. Such explanations were dispelled, however, by COHEN's immunologic interpretations. COHEN (1966a) observed that when dorsal, pigmented skin is allografted to the throat and flank of adult field-collected *Diemictylus viridescens,* a long latent period of about 16 days occurs if they are maintained at $23 \pm 0.5°$ C. Allografts, in fact, are grossly and histologically indistinguishable from autografts during this period. There is an initial dilation of graft vessels resulting in a honeycomb pattern often comparable to normal skin. Circulation is usually restored in both autografts and allografts between 10 and 11 days after grafting. Furthermore, dermal collagen thickness of all grafts increases fivefold throughout both the latent and the graft rejection phases.

2. The Rejection Phase

COHEN (1966b) also found that *Diemictylus viridescens* begins to reject first-set allografts at 17 days. The response is characterized by vasodilation, hemostasis at day 20, hemorrhage at day 23, and eventual melanophore death at day 40. These events vary with respect to the time of onset, intensity, and duration. Histologically, there are several changes that characterize rejection (hemostasis, hemorrhaging, and melanocyte death) occuring normally in allografts, but never in autografts—an increasing infiltration of small lymphocytes prior to graft destruction (secondary vasodilation), and a stronger infiltration of lymphocytes concommitant with glandular death.—Second-set grafts performed 28 days after first grafts elicited a clear anamnestic response indicating specificity.

3. The Chronic Rejection Response to Xenografts

According to COHEN and HILDEMANN (1968), chronic allograft rejection characterizes the immune response of at least six genera of salamanders from four different families. Chronic rejection is not the result of an impaired immune mechanism, since a prompt and vigorous alloimmune reaction has been reported for at least two of the six genera. Instead, prolonged graft survival is thought to result from: (1) "weak" histocompatibility antigens having additive effects; (2) wide-spread sharing of histocompatibility antigens; (3) a lack of a major *H-2* type complex histocompatibility locus (HILDEMANN and COHEN, 1967).

As an approach to testing this, COHEN (1969) performed reciprocal first-set skin xenografts between four genera of adult urodeles. Chronic rejection occurs in six combinations (MST: 32–50 days) and subacute rejection in two combinations (MST: 19 and 24 days). Several interfamilial xenografts survive indefinitely. As in allograft rejection, xenograft reactions too, are attributed to weak histocompatibility interactions and antigen sharing. Whether these common antigens are exclusively transplantation, species-specific, or tissue-specific remains speculative. This example of chronic xenograft rejection offers additional evidence for the lack of a major histocompatibility locus in urodele amphibians and suggests that weak transplantation antigens function also as weak antigens in xenogeneic hosts.

4. Role of the Thymus in Graft Rejection

Although urodele amphibians exhibit a much slower rate of allograft destruction than even larval anurans, their immune tissues and organs seem to be, in number, type, and bodily distribution, as diverse as those of anurans. Thus, rapidity of graft rejection, as an immunologic criterion, is not dependent entirely upon numbers of foci of lymphocytes. However, there may be differences in morphology inherent in these tissues, which accounts for this prolonged rate of rejection.

HIGHTOWER and ST. PIERRE (1971) found no cortex, medulla, myoid cells, or bodies resembling Hassall's corpuscles in the salamander thymus. Bilateral thymectomy of larvae during the first month posthatching effectively abrogates the development of transplantation immunity to weak alloantigens. If the thymus is removed as late as 2 months posthatching, allograft survival is still prolonged.

CHARLEMAGNE and HOUILLON (1968) and TOURNEFIER (1968) thymectomized 6–8-week-old larvae of *Pleurodeles waltlii* and transplanted allografts from 4 different donors at 12–15 months postthymectomy. In this study, 16 tolerated all 4 of their grafts. Autopsies revealed thymic remnants in 3 of the 8 larvae that rejected transplants; the 5 others had no thymus. By contrast, controls did not accept transplants except for 25% of the larvae with a natural tolerance. This may have been due to a substantial amount of inbreeding in *Pleurodeles* populations.

Some thymectomized larvae succumb to the usual wasting disease and die at approximately 20 months. Aplasia of the reticuloendothelial system, a decrease in spleen size, and complete disappearance of the cortical granulopoietic layer in the liver also occur. One year to 18 months after thymectomy, adults that were thymectomized as 8-week-old (*Triturus alpestris*) larvae just prior to metamorphosis received two skin allografts from different donors. In a group of 39 larvae, 30 tolerated allografts indefinitely (more than 200 days), but 9 rejected them in a typical urodele delayed response. Of the 9, 4 had thymic remnants, but 5 had no thymus.

5. Histologic Differences in Skin

TABAN and CONNELLY (1972) found that histoanatomical differences in skin type influence graft rejection in newts. They labeled host and graft with tritiated thymidine after exchanging reciprocal skin grafts between *Notophtalmus viridescens* and *Ambystoma mexicanum*. The adepidermal membrane, dermal collagen, and activity of host epithelial cells play an important role in graft rejection. An initial latent period at seven days was followed by the establishment of blood circulation. Later, by the end of the second week, a strong secondary vasodilation occurred. Many mitoses were observed in the area surrounding the graft, and the graft dermis was progressively infiltrated with inflammatory cells, mostly lymphocytes, polymorphonuclear leukocytes, and macrophages. Secondary vasodilation was followed by hemostasis and graft destruction. Only a scar and parts of the dermal collagenous membrane were present after one month.

6. Suppression of Transplantation Immunity

In addition to much effort devoted to characterizing transplantation immune responses in amphibians, ways of abrogating this response have also been studied by irradiation and tissue-induced suppression.

a) Irradiation

α) Diemictylus viridescens

Using graded 500–3,000 R doses of irradiation, Cohen (1966c) successfully inhibited destruction of allografts for up to 35 days at $23 \pm 0.5°$ C. The subsequent
lymphocyte concentrations vary according to the dosage of irradiation. Grafts
from hosts receiving 500–1,000 R had 20% more lymphocytes than grafts on
hosts irradiated with 1,500 R, 2,000 R, and 3,000 R. Higher irradiation, apparently, destroyed all lymphocytes.

β) Cyonops pyrrhogaster

Murakawa (1968) showed that 350 R can double the survival time of skin
allografts on the Japanese newt. However, a slightly higher dose of 450 R
produced no signs of graft destruction, even 120 days postirradiation. By contrast, the normal graft rejection response can also be restored. When spleen,
liver, or thymus was removed prior to 450 R irradiation and then autografted,
the newt rapidly recovered the capacity for allograft rejection. There was a
high mortality rate between 35 and 50 days after newts received 450 R irradiation
followed by allogeneic spleen grafts. Survivors, however, seemed to develop
a tolerance to subsequent skin grafts from spleen donors. Newts that received
liver implants had a less intense response to skin allografts than those that
received spleen implants; this suggested absence of participating cells from the
liver.

b) Liver-or Kidney-induced Suppression

Baldwin and Cohen (1970) suppressed allograft immunity in the salamander,
Diemictylus viridescens, by transplanting first the liver and then the skin from
the same original donor. In these instances, both liver and skin survival times
were often prolonged. By contrast, control allogeneic skin grafts and subcutaneous liver fragments were rejected at the same time, chronically, 4–10 weeks
after transplantation. Survival times of first- and second-set control skin grafts
were 42.5 and 21.5 days, while survival times for test grafts transplanted 1,
3, 6, or 9 weeks after liver implantation were 60.5, 79.1, 37.5, and 49.0. Liver
implants did not always effectively suppress transplantation immunity. Instead,
they seemed to sensitize some newts such that they rejected later test skin
grafts below the lower range limit of control first-set skin grafts. Immunosuppression was eliminated and the fate of skin graft rejection increased by removing
the liver implant prior to transplanting the test graft.

Baldwin and Cohen (1972) subsequently found that subcutaneous implants
of Diemictylus viridescens dorsalis liver or kidney fragments significantly delayed
up to 85% of the typically subacute rejections of test skin allografts transplanted
at varying postimplantation intervals. Onset of rejection of some test grafts
was sometimes earlier than that of control skin grafts, but total rejection was
never complete at the accelerated second-set rate. The highest incidence of
prolonged skin graft survival occurred when transplants were made before or

after maximum implant destruction, and the lowest when test grafts were transplanted after implants were heavily infiltrated with small lymphocytes. Hosts carrying viable primary skin grafts rejected no secondary transplants during the two-month observation period, supporting the hypothesis that alloantigenic pretreatment with kidney or liver implants elicited mutually opposing facets of immunological reactivity.

III. Anurans

1. Larvae

a) Introduction

Early studies of transplantation immunity were largely confined to the adult poikilotherm's immune response, but HILDEMANN and HAAS (1959) emphasized the importance of studying immune competence in developmentally immature animals. Since their work, there has been a substantial union between embryology and transplantation immunology involving amphibian eggs, larvae, and histocompatibility (SIMNETT, 1964; VOLPE and MC KINNELL, 1966; VOLPE, 1964, 1970, 1971; VOLPE and GEBHARDT, 1965). HILDEMANN and HAAS found that the bullfrog, *Rana catesbeiana*, developed transplantation immunity to skin allografts during larval stages. Thus, there is a similar MST, e.g., 11.8 ± 1.0 days for first-set allografts at 25° C regardless of larval age from 2 months to 2 years as they approach metamorphosis. Allograft responsiveness, once developed, is essentially the same regardless of stage of development, and despite the larval changes ensuing during metamorphosis. The larval anuran continues to figure prominently in deciphering problems related to the maturation of the self, not-self recognition capacity and the immune response (COOPER *et al.*, 1975).

b) Histopathology

Graft rejection in American bullfrog larvae at $25 \pm 1°$ C is characterized by dissemination of pigment cells throughout the epidermis. BACULI and COOPER (1970) found that breakdown of the epidermis and invasion of the dermis by lymphocytes and fibroblasts begin during the first week. Further breakdown occurs during the second week, and is accompanied by a re-epithelialization of the graft periphery and formation of a new highly cellular dermis. Prior to its destruction, the dermis appears as a thick, homogeneous, eosinophilic, almost acellular mass that is gradually replaced by a cellular connective tissue. During the early stages of rejection, eosinophils are prominent in the epidermis, kidneys, and liver. Increased numbers of mitoses, large lymphocytes, and blast cells appear in the lymph glands, spleen, and liver prior to cellular infiltrations into allografts. Small lymphocytes predominate, indicating again their important role in the rejection mechanism.

HILDEMANN and HAAS (1962) drew particular attention to the importance of the small lymphocytes that appear in the peripheral blood at about 40 days posthatching when larvae become competent to reject allografts. The period before then, when small lymphocytes are absent from the peripheral blood, corresponds to the period when bullfrog tadpoles can be made partially tolerant to allografts. Contrary to the situation in older tadpoles, many newly-hatched immature larvae can be made partially or completely tolerant to allografts. As in immunologic reactions of other species, temperature greatly affects the larval bullfrog's response. Allografts survive about three times as long at 15° C as they do at 25° C. Anamnesis or memory is demonstrable by accelerated rejection of second-set grafts in 5.1 ± 0.3 days at 25° C (HILDEMANN and HAAS, 1959).

c) Histocompatibility in Several Populations of Rana catesbeiana

The specificity of allograft rejection, once it develops, can provide a system for analyzing the immunogenetics of amphibian populations by comparing graft survival between, for example, three geographically isolated populations of bullfrog tadpoles. HILDEMANN and HAAS (1961) exchanged single skin allografts between pairs of unrelated tadpole siblings at 25° C, but observed no destruction until at least 9 days. If related tadpoles serve as both donor and recipient of two successive allografts, there is an accelerated rejection at 7 days or less. This accelerated rejection invariably occurs when the same donor provides both grafts.

An accelerated rejection of a second graft from a different donor indicates that both donors share one or more strong histocompatibility antigens that are absent in the recipient. The percent of antigen sharing is a measure of the genetic diversity in populations. In one population, 58% of known siblings rejected test allografts with accelerated reactions. This indicates a highly significant five- to sixfold increase in common histocompatibility antigens among siblings and suggests that many histocompatibility alleles at various loci can segregate in wild populations. Each tadpole must have at least one antigen different from those existing in any other tadpole.

d) Role of the Thymus in Transplantation Immunity

If the thymus, a central generator of immunocompetent cells, is removed prior to one month of age posthatching in tadpoles (*Rana catesbeiana*), transplantation alloimmune responses can be abrogated in their later life. Subsequent allografts have a significantly prolonged survival time. In addition, thymectomy causes a curious runting syndrome that is similar to that in thymectomized mammals. Runting also occurs in *Alytes obstetricans* (DU PASQUIER, 1965, 1968), but not in *Xenopus laevis* (MANNING, 1971).

The prime role of the thymus in cellular immunity of anurans was established in 1965 by COOPER and HILDEMANN, who thymectomized larvae of the bullfrog, *Rana catesbeiana*. In larvae of the midwife toad, *Alytes obstetricans,* DU PASQUIER (1965, 1968) also observed that thymectomy during larval life produces a state of tolerance to cutaneous allografts. Moreover, a certain number of thymectomized *Alytes* and bullfrog larvae develop serious cachexia accompanied by lymphocytic aplasia, characteristics of the runting syndrome observed in mammals. CURTIS and VOLPE (1971) performed thymectomy on the leopard frog, *Rana pipiens,* to determine the subsequent fate of tail tip and dorsal skin allografts. The most successful early thymectomies, i.e., when no thymic tissue is found in later autopsy of tadpoles, correspond to prolonged survival of allogeneic grafts. Complete or partial extirpation of the thymus after it has differentiated in late larval life, does not lead to a decline in immunologic capacity as measured by allograft survival. The thymus, therefore, exerts its most profound effect during, or shortly after, the time when it is fully differentiated as a lymphoid organ.

HORTON and MANNING (1972) successfully thymectomized *Xenopus laevis* larvae at 23° C as early as 8 days postfertilization when the thymus is only beginning to undergo lymphoid differentiation. Here, too, a complete thymectomy (revealed by gross histologic autopsy) at an early stage of development does impair subsequent alloimmune responsiveness. They believe it unlikely that any prolonged extensive passaging of cells through the thymus could have occurred before its removal at 8 days. It is further unlikely that sufficient thymic-dependent lymphocytes occur in thymectomized toadlets to account for subsequent allograft rejection, unless the special properties of such cells were established by an embryonic thymic influence. Perhaps graft rejection in *Xenopus* involves cooperation of cells from different sources.

2. Bone Marrow Restoration of Transplantation Immunity in Adult Leopard Frogs

After metamorphosis, drastic morphologic changes occur as the adult frog emerges (FRIEDEN and JUST, 1970): A new set of lymphomyeloid (LM) organs develops, bone marrow appears, and IgG becomes another immunoglobulin type. Thus, at this point in evolution, it is possible to examine an animal in which bone marrow does not exist, but will ultimately develop. Also, T and B cells and their interactions can be observed in two different life stages.

COOPER and SCHAEFER (1970) tested the capacity of bone marrow to restore transplantation immunity in three groups of leopard frogs. Control nonirradiated frogs rejected allografts at approximately 14 days at 25° C. Frogs given total body irradiation (5,000 R) began to die 7 days postirradiation and most died with surviving allografts. Graft survival in partially irradiated and reconstituted frogs was only delayed by 2 days and deaths were fewer than in the total body irradiated group. In reconstituted frogs the right hind limb was shielded in the center of a block of lead allowing less than 20 R exposure. Bone marrow is thus apparently capable of restoring transplantation immunity in frogs rendered incompetent by damaging irradiation. It provides a source of lymphocytes or stem cells that can differentiate between self and not-self and that are highly reactive to tissue alloantigens.

F. Transplantation Immunity in Reptiles

I. Introduction

Since MAY's (1924) early work, knowledge of reptilian transplantation immunity has progressed. Though the turtle has yielded much information on the characteristics of allograft destruction, the chameleon, *Anolis carolinensis,* the iguana, *Ctenosaura pectinata,* and the yucca night lizard, *Xanthusia vigilis,* have also been convenient, easily maintained reptiles for study (see review by COHEN, 1971). Transplant survival time in reptiles is longer than it is in anuran amphibians, but much the same as it is in apodans and urodeles.

II. The Chronic Response in Turtles

Although large adult snapping turtles reject allografts and xenografts faster than young snappers do, they still exhibit a chronic rejection pattern (BORYSENKO, 1969a, b, 1970). A purely physical reason could be that the turtle's thick dermal pad slows the rate of lymphoid cell infiltration resulting in a lengthy rejection process. However, turtle skin is actually no thicker than rabbit skin, yet rabbits reject first-set grafts within a week. Furthermore, snappers less than 1 year old reject skin allografts from donors at about the adult rate. Such grafts are much thinner than those of large adult turtles. Thus, rate of rejection is apparently dependent neither on age nor on the physical thickness of the transplant. Like the reaction to foreign transplants in all other vertebrates, the response of the snapping turtle to skin allografts can be divided into two major phases. The latent phase involves several morphologic changes due to the ongoing healing and adjustment. First, mononuclear cells migrate to the wound and to inflammation sites immediately and up to 3 days after transplantation. These cells consist of large and small lymphocytes, monocytes, plasma cells, and, usually, neutrophils. A marked dermal thickening is evident in autografts, allografts, and xenografts in the latter part of the latent phase. The rejection phase follows and is characterized by continued lymphoid cell invasion, vascular breakdown, and, finally, necrosis of foreign tissue. Although vasodilation and hemostasis are usually reported as indicators of the rejection phase, these criteria are often difficult to observe grossly in adult snapping turtles.

III. The Importance of Temperature in Turtles

As confirmed by BORYSENKO (1969a, b) the immune response of the snapping turtle is temperature-dependent. At $25 \pm 1°$ C there is a 10–15-day period when both skin autografts and allografts are well healed and firmly anchored to surrounding host tissue. There is no edema and, except for the still noticeable cuts, graft and host are indistinguishable. During this healing stage, the host's epidermal cells surround the graft, grow across the wound area, and thin out.

A few days after the wound area is covered, mitosis begins and the epidermis thickens. Although autografts remain unchanged grossly and histologically, some mononuclear infiltration does occur initially.

At $10 \pm 1°$ C, however, snapping turtles show a retarded immunologic reaction to skin allografts. There is neither gross nor histologic evidence of skin allograft or xenograft incompatibility. Histologic analysis, in fact, indicates no abnormal lymphoid cell infiltration to grafts from either snapping or painted turtles. Low temperatures evidently inhibit the rejection process, or decelerate it markedly. One interesting event, occurring in both allografts and autografts at this temperature, is aggravated vasodilation in the graft one to three weeks after transplantation. BORYSENKO (1969a, b) noted that when animals kept at $10 \pm 1°$ C for 50 days are transferred to $25 \pm 1°$ C, they develop loose xenografts at 18 and 26 days, and at 23 and 29 days after transfer, the grafts are lost. Elevating the temperature thus releases and augments a latent immune reaction. At $33 \pm 1°$ C snappers reject allografts at approximately 24 days, which is significantly faster than the number of days required at $25 \pm 1°$ C.

IV. The Mexican Iguana

The iguana is an advantageous reptile for studies of graft survival since transplants are relatively easy to perform. Furthermore, the lymphocytic infiltration typical of the vertebrate's inflammatory response is usually observed in destroyed grafts. Sloughing of dead allografts, or the actual dislodging of the outer keratin layer, signals the final stage of graft rejection in the iguana (COOPER and APONTE, 1968).

Chronic rejection may well be the result of low temperature. At $25°$ C the antibody response in iguanas is generally poor. Accordingly, it is possible that a higher temperature might produce an acute allograft response. However, since allograft and xenograft rejection rates in the iguana are slower than those in certain fishes, anuran amphibian larvae and adults, it seems likely that temperature does not play a significant role in the rate of transplant rejection. Of particular interest in the iguana is the phenomenon of *negative memory*. Instead of accelerated rejections of second-set grafts there is also an increased survival time as compared to the first sets. It appears that those animals exhibiting prolonged survival of first-set grafts often show both manifestations of memory (COHEN and BORYSENKO, 1970).

V. The Garter Snake

According to TEREBEY (1972), the garter snake, *Thamnophis sirtalis,* sheds a layer of keratin following transplantation of skin allografts. The shedding cycle is determined by the recipient and not by skin type, since timing of the shedding cycle is dictated by the host animal. The response, furthermore, does not seem to be affected by age, sex, or the stage between sheddings when grafts are taken from donors. In rats, skin allografts initially exhibit timing of the donor's hair growth cycle, but eventually allografts also become synchronized with the recipient. Less complex mechanisms seem to be involved in the shedding cycle in garter snakes than in the hair-growth cycle that evolved in mammals.

References

BACULI, B.A., COOPER, E.L.: Histopathology of skin allograft rejection in larval Rana catesbeiana. J. Exp. Zool. 173, 329–340 (1970).

BAILEY, S., MILLER, B.J., COOPER, E.L.: Transplantation immunity in annelids. II. Adoptive transfer of the xenograft reaction. Immunology 21, 81–86 (1971).

BALDWIN, W.M., COHEN, N.: Liver-induced immunosuppression of allograft immunity in urodele amphibians. Transplantation 10, 530–537 (1970).

BALDWIN, W.M., COHEN, N.: Immunosuppression of subacute skin allograft rejection in the newt, Diemictylus v. dorsalis by alloantigenic pretreatment with kidney and liver implants. Folia Biol. (Praha) 18, 181–188 (1972).

BELL, W.J.: Yolk formation by transplanted cockroach oocytes. J. Exp. Zool. 181, 41–48 (1972).

BORYSENKO, M.: Skin allograft and xenograft rejection in the snapping turtle, Chyledra serpentina. J. Exp. Zool. 170, 341–358 (1969a).

BORYSENKO, M.: The maturation of the capacity to reject skin allografts and xenografts in the snapping turtle, Chelydra serpentina. J. Exp. Zool. 170, 359–364 (1969b).

BORYSENKO, M.: Transplantation immunity in Reptilia. Transpl. Proc. 2, 299–306 (1970).

BORYSENKO, M., HILDEMANN, W.H.: Scale (skin) allograft rejection in the primitive teleost, Osteoglossum bicirrhosum. Transplantation 8, 403–412 (1969).

BORYSENKO, M., HILDEMANN, W.H.: Reactions to skin allografts in the horn shark, Heterodontis francisci. Transplantation 10, 545–551 (1970).

BRUSLÉ, J.: Homogreffs et heterogreffes du tegument et des gonades chez Asterina gibbosa et Asterina pancerii (Echinodermes, Asterides). Cahiers De Biologie Marine 8, 417–420 (1967).

BURNET, F.M.: Evolution of the immune process in vertebrates. Nature (London) 218, 426–430 (1968).

BURNET, F.M.: The concept of immunological surveillance. Progr. Exp. Tumor Res. 13, 1–27 (1970).

BURNET, F.M.: Invertebrate precursors to immune responses. In: Contemporary Topics in Immunobiology, Vol. 4, pp. 13–24. New York: Plenum Press 1974.

CAMPBELL, R.D., BIBB, C.: Transplantation in coelenterates. Transpl. Proc. 2, 202–211 (1970).

CANZONIER, W.J.: Histological observation on the response of oysters to tissue implants. Proc. Nat. Shellfish Assoc. 54, 1 (1963).

CHARLEMAGNE, J., HOUILLON, C.: Effects de la thymectomie larvaire chez l'amphibian urodèle, Pleurodeles waltlii Michah. Production à l'état adult d'une tolérance aux homogreffes cutanées. C.R. Acad. Sci. (Paris) 267, 253–256 (1968).

CHATEAUREYNAUD-DUPRAT, P.: Specificity of allograft reaction in Eisenia foetida. Transpl. Proc. 2, 222–225 (1970).

CHENG, T.C.: Immunity in mollusca with special reference to reactions to transplants. Transpl. Proc. 2, 226–230 (1970).

COHEN, N.: Tissue transplantation immunity in the adult newt, Diemictylus viridescens. I. The latent phase: healing, restoration of circulation, and pigment cell changes in autografts and allografts. J. Exp. Zool. 163, 157–162 (1966a).

COHEN, N.: Tissue transplantation immunity in the adult newt, Diemictylus viridescens. II. The rejection phase: first and second-set allograft reactions and lack of sexual dimorphism. J. Exp. Zool. 163, 173–190 (1966b).

COHEN, N.: Tissue transplantation in the adult newt, Diemictylus viridescens. III. The effects of x-irradiation and temperature on the allograft reaction. J. Exp. Zool. 163, 231–240 (1966c).

COHEN, N.: Chronic skin graft rejection in the urodela. II. A comparative study of xenograft rejection. Transplantation 7, 332–346 (1969).

COHEN, N.: Reptiles as models for the study of immunity and its phylogenesis. J. Amer. Vet. Med. Assoc. 159, 1662–1671 (1971).

COHEN, N., HILDEMANN, W.H.: Population studies of allograft rejection in the newt, Diemictylus viridescens. Transplantation **6**, 208–217 (1968).

COHEN, N., BORYSENKO, M.: Acute and chronic rejection: Possible phylogeny of transplantation antigens. Transpl. Proc. **2**, 333–336 (1970).

COOPER, E.L.: A method of tissue grafting in the earthworm, Lumbricus terrestris. Amer. Zool. **4**, 233 (1965a).

COOPER, E.L.: Rejection of body wall xenografts exchanged between Lumbricus terrestris and Eisenia foetida. Amer. Zool. **5**, 169 (1965b).

COOPER, E.L.: Transplantation immunity in annelids. I. Rejection of xenografts exchanged between Lumbricus terrestris and Eisenia foetida. Transplantation **6**, 322–337 (1968).

COOPER, E.L.: Specific tissue graft rejection in earthworms. Science **166**, 1414–1415 (1969).

COOPER, E.L.: Contemporary Topics in Immunobiology 4. New York: Plenum Press 1974.

COOPER, E.L.: Amphibian Immunity in Physiology of The Amphibia. New York: Academic Press (in press) (1975).

COOPER, E.L., HILDEMANN, W.H.: Allograft reaction in bullfrog larvae in relation to thymectomy. Transplantation **3**, 446–448 (1965).

COOPER, E.L., APONTE, A.: Chronic allograft rejection in the iguana Ctenosaura pectinata. Proc. Soc. Exp. Biol. (N.Y.) **128**, 150–154 (1968).

COOPER, E.L., GARCIA-HERRERA, F.: Chronic skin allograft rejection in the apodan Typhlonectes compressicauda. Copeia **2**, 224–229 (1968).

COOPER, E.L., SCHAEFER, D.W.: Bone marrow restoration of transplantation immunity in the leopard. frog Rana pipiens. Proc. Soc. Exp. Biol. (N.Y.) **135**, 406–414 (1970).

COOPER, E.L., BROWN, B.A., WRIGHT, R.W.: New ideas on amphibian immunity: the lymph gland, a generator of T- and B-cells. Amer. Zool. **15**, 85–92 (1975).

CURTIS, S.K., VOLPE, E.P.: Modification of responsiveness to allografts in larvae of the leopard frog by thymectomy. Develop. Biol. **24**, 177–197 (1971).

CUSHING, J.: Blood groups in marine animals and immune mechanisms of lower vertebrates and invertebrates (comparative immunology). Proc. Conf. on Immuno-Reproduction: La Jolla, Calif. The Population Council; New York (1962).

DES VOIGNE, D.M., SPARKS, A.: The reaction of the Pacific oyster, Crassostrea gigas, to homologous tissue transplants. J. Invert. Pathol. **14**, 293–300 (1969).

DREW, G.H., DE MORGAN, W.: The origin and formation of fibrous tissue produced as a reaction to injury in Pectin maximus, as a type of lamellibranchiata. Quart. J. Micros. Sci. **55**, 595–620 (1910).

DU PASQUIER, L.: Aspects cellulaires et humoraux de l'intolérance l'intolérance homogreffes de tissu musculaire chez le tetard d'Alytes obstetricans. Compt. Rend. **261**, 1144–1147 (1965).

DU PASQUIER, L.: Les proteines seriques et le complex lymphomyeloide chez le tetard d'Alytes obstetricans normal et thymectomise extrait des. Ann. Inst. Pasteur (Paris) **114**, 490–502 (1968).

DU PASQUIER, L.: Ontogeny of the immune response in cold-blooded vertebrates. Current Topics Microbiol. Immunol. **61**, 37–88 (1973).

DU PASQUIER, L.: The genetic control of histocompatibility reactions: phylogenetic aspects. Arch. Biol. (Bruxelles) **85**, 91–103 (1974).

DUPRAT, P.: Evidence de réactions immunitaires dans les homogreffes de paroi du corps chez le Lombricien Eisenia foetida typica. C.R. Acad. Sci. (Paris) **259**, 4177–4180 (1964).

DUPRAT, P.: Specificity of allograft reaction in Eisenia foetida. Transpl. Proc. **2**, 222–225 (1970).

FREEMAN, G.: Transplantation specificity in echinoderms and lower chordates. Transpl. Proc. **2**, 236–239 (1970).

FRIEDEN, E.A., JUST, J.: Hormonal responses on amphibian metamorphosis. In: Biochemical Actions of Hormones, pp. 1–52. New York: Academic Press 1970.

GALTSOFF, P.S.: Regeneration after dissociation (an experimental study on sponges). I. Behavior of dissociated cells of Microciona prolifera under normal and altered conditions. J. Exp. Zool. **42**, 183–222 (1925).

GHIRADELLA, H.T.: The reactions of two starfishes, Patiria miniata and Asterias foresi, to foreign tissue in the coelom. Biol. Bull. **128**, 77–89 (1965).

GOLDSTEIN, L.: Nucleo-cytoplasmic incompatibilities in free-living amoeba. Transpl. Proc. **2**, 191–193 (1970).

GRIMSTONE, A.V., ROTHERAM, S., SALT, G.: An electron-microscope study of capsule formation by insect blood cells. J. Cell. Sci. **2**, 281 292 (1969).

HADORN, E.: Transplantation of gonads from lethal to normal larvae in Drosophila melanogaster. Proc. Soc. Exp. Biol. (N.Y.) **36**, 632–634 (1937).

HAWKINS, S.E., COLE, R.J.: Studies on the basis of cytoplasmic inheritance in amoebae. Exp. Cell Res. **37**, 26 (1964).

HIGHTOWER, J.A., ST. PIERRE, R.L.: Hemopoietic tissue in the adult newt, Notopthalmus viridescens. J. Morphol. **135**, 299–308 (1971).

HILDEMANN, W.H.: Goldfish erythrocyte antigens and serology. Science **124**, 315–316 (1956).

HILDEMANN, W.H.: Scale transplantation in goldfish (Carassius auratus). Ann. N.Y. Acad. Sci. **64**, 775–790 (1957).

HILDEMANN, W.H.: Transplantation immunity fishes: Agnatha, chondrichthyes and osteichthyes. Transpl. Proc. **2**, 253–259 (1970).

HILDEMANN, W.H.: Phylogeny of transplantation reactivity. In: Transplantation Antigens, Markers of Biological Individuality, pp. 3–73. New York-London: Academic Press 1972.

HILDEMANN, W.H.: Transplantation reactions of two species of osteichthyes (Teleostei) from South Pacific coral reefs. Transplantation **14**, 261- 267 (1972).

HILDEMANN, W.H., HAAS, R.: Homotransplantation immunity and tolerance in the bullfrog. J. Immunol. **83**, 478–485 (1959).

HILDEMANN, W.H., HAAS, R.: Developmental changes in leukocytes in relation to immunological maturity. In: Mechanisms of Immunologic Tolerance, pp. 35–49. Czech. Acad. Sci. Prague, New York: Academic Press 1962.

HILDEMANN, W.H., HAAS, R.: Histocompatibility genetics of bullfrog populations. Evolution **15**, 267–277 (1961).

HILDEMANN, W.H., COHEN, N.: Weak histoincompatibilities: emerging rules and generalizations. In: Histocompatibility Testing, pp. 13–20. Munksgaard, Copenhagen 1967.

HILDEMANN, W.H., COOPER, E.L.: Immunogenesis of homograft reactions in fishes and amphibians. Fed. Proc. **22**, 1145–1151 (1963).

HILDEMANN, W.H., DIX, T.G.: Transplantation reactions of tropical Australian echinoderms. Transplantation **15**, 624–633 (1972).

HILDEMANN, W.H., REDDY, A.L.: Phylogeny of immune responsiveness; marine invertebrates. Fed. Proc. **32**, 2188–2194 (1973).

HILDEMANN, W.H., THOENES, G.H.: Immunological responses of Pacific hagfish. Transplantation **7**, 506- 521 (1969).

HORTON, J.D., MANNING, M.J.: Response to skin allografts in Xenopus laevis following thymectomy at early stages of lymphoid organ maturation. Transplantation **14**, 141–154 (1972).

HOSTETTER, R.K., COOPER, E.L.: Coelomocytes as effector cells in earthworm immunity. Immunol. Comm. **1**, 155–183 (1972).

HOSTETTER, R.K., COOPER, E.L.: Cellular anamnesis in earthworms. Cell. Immunol. **9**, 384–392 (1973).

HUMPHREYS, T.: The cell surfaces and specific cell aggregation. In: The Specificity of Cell Surfaces, pp. 199–210. Englewood Cliffs, New Jersey: Prentice-Hall Inc. 1967.

JANOFF, A., HAWRYLKO, E.: Lysosomal enzymes in invertebrate leucocytes. J. Cell. Comp. Physiol. **64**, 267–271 (1963).

KAMBYSELLIS, M.P.: Interspecific transplantation as a tool for indicating phylogenetic relationships. Proc. Nat. Acad. Sci. (Wash.) **59**, 1169–1172 (1968).

LINDH, N.O.: Heteroplastic transplantation of transversal body sections in flatworms. Arkiv. für Zool. **12**, 183–195 (1959).

LOEB, L.: The Biological Basis of Individuality. Illinois: C.C. Thomas 1945.

MACLENNAN, A.P.: The chemical bases of taxon-specific cellular reaggregation and "self"- "not-self" recognition in sponges. Arch. Biol. (Bruxelles) **85**, 53–90 (1974).

MANNING, M.J.: The effect of early thymectomy on histogenesis of the lymphoid organs in Xenopus laevis. J. Embryol. Exp. Morphol. **26**, 219–229 (1971).

MAY, R.M.: Skin grafts in the lizard Anolis carolinensis. Brit. J. Exp. Biol. **1**, 539–555 (1924).

MÖLLER, G., MÖLLER, E.: Interaction between allogeneic cells in tissue transplantation. Ann. N.Y. Acad. Sci. **129**, 735–749 (1966).

MURAKAWA, S.: Studies on the transplantation immunity in the Japanese newt, Cynops pyrrhogaster. Sabco J. **4**, 17–32 (1968).

OKA, H., WATANABE, H.: Problems of colony specificity in compound ascidians. Bull. Biol. Asamushi **10**, 153 (1960).

PEREY, D.Y.E., FINSTAD, J., POLLARA, B., GOOD, R.A.: Evolution of the immune response. VI. First and second-set skin homograft rejection in primitive fishes. Lab. Invest. **19**, 591–597 (1968).

REINISCH, C.L., BANG, F.B.: Cell recognition: Reactions of the sea star Asterias vulgaris to the injection of amebocytes of sea urchin Arbacia punctulata. Cell. Immunol. **2**, 496–503 (1971).

SCOTT, M.T.: Recognition of foreignness in invertebrates. Transplantation studies using the American cockroach, Periplaneta americana. Transplantation **11**, 78–86 (1971).

SIMNETT, J.D.: Histocompatibility in the platanna Xenopus laevis laevis (Daudin) following nuclear transplantation. Exp. Cell Res. **33**, 232–239 (1964).

SPIEGEL, M.: The role of specific surface antigens in cell adhesion. I. The reaggregation of sponge cells. Biol. Bull. **107**, 130–148 (1954).

TABAN, C.H., CONNELLY, T.G.: Histological observations on allografts and reciprocal xenografts in newts Notophthalmus viridescens and axolotls Ambystoma mexicanum. J. Exp. Zool. **182**, 15–30 (1972).

TANAKA, K.: Allogeneic inhibition in a compound ascidian, Botryllus primigenus (Oka). II. Cellular and humoral responses in "non-fusion" reaction. Cell. Immunol. **7**, 429–443 (1973).

TARTAR, V.: Experimental Techniques with Ciliates in Methods and Physiology, Vol. 1, pp. 109–125. New York: Academic Press 1964.

TARTAR, V.: Transplantation in protozoa. In: Transplantation Proceedings **2**, 183. W.H. HILDEMANN and E.L. COOPER (eds.). New York: Grune & Stratton, 1970.

TAYLOR, E.H.: An aquatic caecilian from the Magdalena River. Colombia, S.A. XLVIII, 845–848 (1970).

TEREBEY, N.: The effect of shedding on skin homografts in the garter snake, Thamnophis sirtalis. Amer. J. Anat. **135**, 435–440 (1972).

THEODOR, J.L.: Reconnaissance du "self" et reconnaissance des "not-self". Arch. Zool. Exp. Gen. **112**, 113–116 (1971).

TOURNEFIER, A.: Etude histologique des hétérogreffes embryonnaires de tégument chez les amphibiens urodèles. Bull. Soc. Zool. France **93**, 99–108 (1968).

TRIPLETT, E.L., CUSHING, J.E., DURALL, G.L.: Observations on some immune reactions of the sipunculid worm, Dendrostomum zostericolum. Amer. Nat. **92**, 287–293 (1958).

TRIPP, M.R.: The fate of foreign materials experimentally introduced into the snail Australorbis glabratus. J. Parasitol. **47**, 745–751 (1961).

TURNER, R.S., WEINBAUM, G., KUHNS, W.J., BURGER, M.M.: The use of lectins in the analysis of sponge reaggregation. Arch. Biol. (Bruxelles) **85**, 35–51 (1974).

TYLER, A.: An auto-antibody concept of cell structure, growth and differentiation. Growth (suppl.) **10**, 7–19 (1946).

VALEMBOIS, P.: Recherches sur la nature de la réaction antigreffe chez le lombricien Eisenia foetida. C.R. Acad. Sci. (Paris) **257**, 3489–3490 (1963).

VALEMBOIS, P.: Cellular aspects of graft rejection in earthworms and some other metazoa. In: Contemporaty Topics in Immunobiology **4**, 121–126. New York: Plenum Press 1974.

VAN DE VYVER, G.: La non confluence intraspécifique chez les Spongiaires et la notion d'individu. Ann. Embr. Morph. **3**, 251–262 (1970).

VOLPE, E.P.: Fate of neural crest homotransplants in pattern mutants of the leopard frog. J. Exp. Zool. **157**, 179–196 (1964).

VOLPE, E.P.: Transplantation immunity and tolerance in anurans. Transpl. Proc. **2**, 286–292 (1970).

VOLPE, E.P.: Immunological tolerance in amphibians. Amer. Zool. **11**, 207–218 (1971).

VOLPE, E.P., GEBHARDT, B.M.: Effect of dosage on the survival of embryonic homotransplants in the leopard frog Rana pipiens. J. Exp. Zool. **160**, 11–28 (1965).

VOLPE, E.P., McKINNELL, R.G.: Successful tissue transplantation in frogs produced by nuclear transfer. J. Hered. **57**, 167–174 (1966).

WATANABE, H., TANAKA, K.: Allogeneic inhibition in a compound ascidian Botryllus primigenus Oka. I. Processes and features of "non-fusion" reaction. Cell. Immunol. **7**, 410–426 (1973).

WEISS, P.: The problem of specificity in growth and development. Yale J. Biol. Med. **19**, 235–278 (1946).

WILSON, H.V.: On some phenomena of coalescence and regeneration in sponges. J. Exp. Zool. **5**, 245–258 (1907).

WINGER, L.A., COOPER, E.L.: Effect of temperature on the first-set xenograft rejection in the earthworm Eisenia foetida. Amer. Zool. **9**, 352 (1969).

Ontogenetic Aspects

Osias Stutman and Catherine E. Calkins

With 3 Figures and 3 Tables

A. Introduction

This chapter is a description of the ontogenic aspects of transplantation immunity. "Ontogeny" is defined in *Webster's Dictionary* as "the...course of development of an individual organism". In the context of this chapter we will analyze the course of development of an individual function (i.e., the capacity to reject foreign transplants) in some selected species, including man. This analysis will be done by discussing two interrelated aspects: (1) the development of the ability to reject foreign tissues as a function of age and (2) the development of the probable effector cells responsible for cell-mediated immunity, such as graft rejection, as well as other functions related to competent lymphocytes of the thymus-dependent lineage. Since the exact mechanisms by which foreign tissue grafts are destroyed are still not properly defined, we will describe the ontogenic events mainly as "all-or-none" phenomena. However, we are including descriptions of developmental events of the thymus-dependent cell-mediated immune responses, since the vast bulk of evidence indicates that a major component of graft rejection is mediated by thymus-dependent responses (see Wilson and Billingham, 1967 or Najarian and Foker, 1969 for review). Although humoral antibodies can, under special circumstances, mediate the destruction of allografts (see for example Baldamus et al., 1973) and hyperacute organ rejections are the results of humoral mechanisms (Najarian and Foker, 1969), it is accepted that the main effector mechanism is related to thymus-dependent cell-mediated responses.

Additional evidence for the thymus-dependency of transplantation immunity includes: (1) poor allograft rejection capacity in patients with T-cell deficiencies (Hoyer et al., 1968; Gatti and Good, 1970) while agammaglobulinemic patients (i.e., B-cell deficiency with intact T-cell functions) show in general, normal skin allograft rejection (Schubert et al., 1960; Good et al., 1962); (2) the profound effects of thymectomy (see Miller and Osoba, 1967 for review) or of congenital absence of the thymus in mice (see Wortis, 1974) on the capacity to reject allografts or to generate cell-mediated immune responses; (3) in birds, bursectomy has no effect on allograft rejection while thymectomy impairs cell-mediated immunity including allograft rejection (Aspinall et al., 1963; Szen-

Berg and Warner, 1964) and even intact allograft rejection has been demonstrated in agammaglobulinemic bursectomized chickens (Perey *et al.*, 1967); and (4) lamb embryos are capable of rejecting skin grafts *in utero* at a time when they are incapable of producing antibodies to many antigens (Schinckel and Ferguson, 1953; Silverstein *et al.*, 1963). In summary, it seemed reasonable to analyze ontogeny of transplantation immunity as a thymus-dependent function.

B. Ontogeny of Lymphoid Structures

It is apparent from Table 1 that two main features are characteristic of the development of lymphoid tissues in mammals (as well as in other vertebrates, see Cohen, 1975): (1) the first site of appearance of lymphocytes is within the thymus and (2) although the chronologic events suggest either "seeding out" of cells or a thymic influence for lymphocyte differentiation in the peripheral lymphoid organs, a thymus independent lymphoid differentiation is also apparent (see data on B-cells in liver in Table 1 and also Stutman, 1973; Nossal and Pike, 1973a, b, for B-cells in mouse; Lawton *et al.*, 1972 for B-cells in man and Lawton *et al.*, 1975 for review). It is also apparent from Table 1 that the "tempo" of maturation, even from a morphologic standpoint, differs from species to species. Two main groups can be separated: (1) rodents such as mouse, rat, and hamster with short gestation periods in which maturation proceeds for some days after birth (and thymus appears approximately at the middle point of the gestation period) and (2) species such as lamb, pig, and man, which have longer gestation periods and which are usually immunologically competent at birth (and the thymus appears during the first third of the gestation period). However, there are enough exceptions to these prototypes to caution

Table 1. Comparative development of lympho-hematopoietic tissues in mammals[a]

Time of event (days)	Mouse	Pig	Lamb	Man
Yolk sac hematopoiesis	7–8	15–16	?	21–28
Liver hematopoiesis	11	28	30	42
B-cells in liver	15	?	?	65–68
Spleen hematopoiesis	15	32–36	65	90–100
Spleen lymphopoiesis	17–19	48	65	140–150
B-cells in spleen	17–18	?	?	140
Marrow hematopoiesis	15–16	51	?	140
Epithelial thymus rudiment	10–11	21–22	30	40
Lymphocytes in thymus	12–14	28	43	70
Lymph node lymphopoiesis	18–19	52	45	70–130
Lymphocytes in Peyer's patches	+1	77	75	120?
Lymphocytes in blood	18	38	50	120–130
Gestation period	19–21	114–120	150	220–270

[a] For data on mouse see text and Owen (1972); for pig see Kruml *et al.* (1970); for lamb see Morris (1973); for man see Sabin (1909), Van Furth *et al.* (1965), Stites *et al.* (1972), Lawton *et al.* (1972) and Bailey and Weiss (1974). For general reference see Metcalf and Moore (1971)

against absolute generalizations. For example, studies with marsupial embryos (a species that would fall in the first group, i.e., like the rodents) indicate that although the thymus is the main initial site of lymphoid differentiation, extrathymic nodes may precede (KALMUTZ, 1962; BLOCK, 1964); a similar observation has been made in the cat (ACKERMAN, 1967), a species that probably would fall in the second group. It was proposed (GOOD and PAPERMASTER, 1964) that the degree of immunologic maturity at birth would dictate the effects of neonatal thymectomy, and indeed, while the immune deficiency induced by neonatal thymectomy is most profound in species that complete immunologic maturity after birth, such as mouse and rat (see MILLER and OSOBA, 1967), the effects may be minimal in species such as the lamb (MORRIS, 1973). On the other hand, the effects of removal of the bursa of Fabricius in birds on their capacity to produce immunoglobulins is most apparent when the bursectomy is performed before hatching (VAN ALTEN et al., 1968). In man, adult thymectomy plus additional immunodepression produced profound immunodeficiency, as indicated by delayed skin allograft rejection and inability to produce cell-mediated responses (PIROFSKY et al., 1972). These results are comparable to the effects of combination of adult thymectomy and immunodepression in other species including mice (MONACO et al., 1965).

This early appearance of the thymus during development and the fact that the thymus contained the same "particles" as those found in the lymph, lymph nodes, and blood, prompted HEWSON to conclude that "the thymus exists during the early periods of life when these particles seem to be most wanted" (HEWSON, in FALCONER, 1777). At the turn of this century it was theorized that these cells originated in the thymus and that "...the original leucocytes, starting from their birth place in the thymus, penetrate into almost every part of the body, and there create new centers for growth, for increase and useful work for themselves and for the body..." (BEARD, 1900); and the thymus was even equated with the British Isles, sending worthy citizens to the rest of the Empire! Indeed, some of the present-day morphologic descriptions have not gone beyond these original insights into the functions of the thymus.

The peculiar compartmentalization of cell types presented in Table 1, in a simple chronologic order, will become clearer after the discussion of the possible mechanisms of lymphopoiesis in mammals (see also METCALF and MOORE, 1971; OWEN, 1972, 1973; STUTMAN, 1972; and GREAVES et al., 1974 for comprehensive reviews on development, structure, and function of the lymphoid system).

The notion that there are two broad categories of immune responses, although simplistic in its inception, has been extremely useful for the study of lymphoid physiology. Basically it depends on whether circulating antibody or direct lymphocyte participation is the predominant component in a given immune response; these two main types have been described as "humoral immunity" and "cellular" or "cell-mediated immunity" (see the Introduction). Thus, humoral immunity includes those responses such as antibody production, immediate hypersensitivity, allergic reactions, and some bactericidal reactions against various microorganisms and can usually be passively transferred with serum from immune animals. Cell-mediated immunity includes skin or other tissue graft rejections, graft-versus-host reactions, and delayed hypersensitivity reactions (or some possible in vitro correlates of these responses) and can be transferred with cells but not with serum from immune animals. It is interesting to note that although this division is artificial (i.e., even humoral immunity ultimately depends upon cells, and many responses are actually the sum of complex interactions between both mechanisms), it has been a useful concept. An excellent example of this usefulness is indeed represented by the studies on the ontogeny of immune responses in mammals. By the use of ablation-replacement experiments it became established in a number of species that neonatal thymectomy profoundly affects the capacity to produce cell-mediated responses (see MILLER and OSOBA, 1967 for review) while removal of a lymphoid organ unique to birds, the bursa of Fabricius, interferes with humoral antibody production (GLICK, 1964; COOPER et al., 1966). It is accepted that the thymus and the bursa separately control the maturation of two distinct lymphocyte populations known as T and B lymphocytes, respectively (GREAVES et al., 1974), and that T lymphocytes are essential for cell-mediated responses while B lymphocytes are precursors of the antibody secreting cells (GREAVES et al., 1974). Although there is no organ comparable to the bursa in mammals, and B-cell differentiation may occur throughout the lymphoid tissues from precursors of hematopoietic origin (NOSSAL and PIKE, 1973a, b; STUTMAN, 1973), there is substantial evidence for two main lymphocyte classes in mammals that are probably analogous to those in the avian populations (see OWEN, 1972, 1973; STUTMAN, 1972, 1973; GREAVES et al., 1974; LAWTON et al., 1975).

The definition of these two lymphocyte realms has necessitated a reinterpretation of many immunologic phenomena, especially concerning the interactions between the two lymphocyte systems that seem essential for many immune responses (see GREAVES et al., 1974 for review). Similarly, various new regulatory mechanisms indicate that both lymphocyte populations influence each other and that the overall response may be a complex balance of these regulatory functions (see GERSHON, 1974; WIGZELL, 1974; HELLSTRÖM and HELLSTRÖM, 1972). This need for reinterpretation becomes most apparent when attempting to analyze a problem such as ontogeny of transplantation. It is for this reason that we have somewhat simplified the problem by assuming that transplantation immunity is mediated by a thymus-dependent cell-mediated response. However, we are also obliged to analyze ontogeny of thymus-dependent functions in general, as we presently understand the problem, due to the lack of solid information on the actual ontogeny of transplantation immunity proper.

The origin of the lymphocytes within the thymus had been the cause for considerable debate and will be discussed briefly before describing what we think are the possible steps for T-cell differentiation. Two main theories have been proposed: (1) the lymphocytes in thymus derive from hematopoietic immigrants that colonize the epithelial anlage (MAXIMOW, 1909; SMITH, 1965; MOORE and OWEN, 1967a, b; HOSHINO et al., 1969; MANDEL, 1970; ACKERMAN and HOSTETLER, 1970) and (2) thymic lymphocytes are derived from endodermal epithelial components of the primitive thymus (AUERBACH, 1960, 1961; ACKERMAN and KNOUFF, 1964, 1965; KOSTOWIECKI, 1965; SANEL, 1967). In a series of ablation-replacement experiments in the mouse, using hematopoietic cells with chromosome markers that permit the recognition of the dividing progeny, it was demonstrated that such cells migrated into the thymus and were subsequently exported to the peripheral lymphoid tissues (FORD and MICKLEM, 1963; HARRIS and FORD, 1964; FORD, 1966; MICKLEM et al., 1966; DAVIES et al., 1966, 1968, 1971; STUTMAN, 1970; DOENHOFF et al., 1970; STUTMAN and GOOD, 1971 a, b). These studies were considered a confirmation of the hematopoietic origin, after an intrathymic step of differentiation, of the peripheral T lymphocytes (and will be discussed in more detail in the next paragraphs). However, this interpretation has been questioned by TURPEN et al. (1973, 1975), who showed that in the frog, the main source of thymic cells within the thymus and subsequently exported, seems to be the thymus proper. It appears that species differences, especially differences in mechanisms of early embryonic hematopoiesis, could explain these discrepancies (i.e., in the frog the mesenchyma in the bronchial area may be the source of the hematopoietic cells colonizing the thymus anlage, while yolk sack seeds the periphery, a mechanism that does not exist in mammals). Species differences also seem important since in morphologic studies from one laboratory, images suggesting epithelial origin of the thymic lymphocytes were observed in chicken and hamster (ACKERMAN and KNOUFF, 1964, 1965) but not in the rabbit (ACKERMAN and HOSTETLER, 1970). Although AUERBACH's experiments (1960, 1961) in vitro suggest a direct origin of lymphocytes from thymic epithelium, it has been shown that at day 14 (see Table 1) there are already hematopoietic immigrants present in the thymus. Conversely, when 11–12-day-old mouse embryonic thymuses were cultured either in diffusion chambers in the chick chorioallantois (OWEN and RITTER, 1969) or in organ cultures (MANDEL and RUSSELL, 1971; MANDEL et al., 1972), no lymphoid differentiation within the thymus was observed, while cultures from thymuses at later ages would differentiate into lymphoid cells. It should be indicated that the putative lymphoid stem cells can be identified in the early fetal mouse thymus with light as well as with electron microscopy (MOORE and OWEN, 1967b; HOSHINO et al., 1969; MANDEL, 1970). In earlier studies it was also shown that thymic autografts from adult guinea pigs or rats enclosed in cell-impermeable chambers, lost their lymphoid cells and were incapable of replacing them, provided that the chamber remained impermeable to cells (GREGOIRE, 1958). In summary, most of the experiments in mammalian thymuses in vitro suggest that the origin of the thymic lymphocytes is related to a stream of hematopoietic immigrants. Another possible interpretation of the frog experiments may be related to the apparent susceptibility of thymus traffic to histocompatibility differences in mice (STUTMAN and GOOD, 1969). Although under extreme conditions such as lethal whole body irradiation, the thymus can be repopulated even by xenogeneic cells (see MICKLEM and LOUTIT, 1966 for review) under gentler, albeit nonphysiologic conditions, such as thymus grafts in thymectomized animals, the traffic of hematopoietic cells to thymus proved to be extremely sensitive to even minor histocompatibility differences (STUTMAN and GOOD, 1969), a possibility that cannot be excluded from the studies with outbred frogs. Concerning the possibility of artifacts dependent on thymus grafting in the mammalian experiments, suggested by TURPEN et al. (1975), it should be noted that an afferent stream of immigrating cells has been detected in the undisturbed thymus in situ by the use of parabiosis of syngeneic mice with chromosome markers (Harris *et al.*, 1964; Ford, 1966) and also in synchorial twins of different sexes in marmosets and in freemartins (Ford, 1966). In the last instance, cells of both sexes were detected in thymus (51% of the dividing cells were male) as well as in marrow and spleen (Ford, 1966). It is difficult to interpret these results as anything but the consequence of traffic and seeding of blood-borne hematopoietic cells to the thymus.

There is compelling evidence that hematopoietic tissues are derived from the differentiation of stem cells into specialized blood cells (Till *et al.*, 1964; Lajtha, 1966 and also Metcalf and Moore, 1971 for review). These types of regulatory cytokinetics have been well defined for erythroid differentiation (Till *et al.*, 1964; Lajtha, 1966) and to a certain degree for the myeloid series (Metcalf and Moore, 1971) and are characterized by the generation of a dividing output of progenitor cells (i.e., three main compartments: stem cell, progenitor, and differentiated progeny) as defined by Lajtha (1966). Within this context, "progenitor" is defined as the "ultimate source of a cell population in question" (Lajtha, 1966) while "stem cell" implies a self-maintaining population of cells from which other cell lines originate. In general, stem cell is associated with the idea of a multipotential cell and applies probably to the stem cell that gives rise to the hematopoietic and lymphoid system in mammals and birds (Moore and Owen, 1967a; Wu *et al.*, 1968). The first hematopoietic stem cells of the mammalian and avian embryo are formed in the blood islands of the early yolk sac (see Table 1 and Metcalf and Moore, 1971), probably by differentiation of cells that migrate from the primitive streak (Murray, 1932). In mammals, hematopoiesis in the yolk sac and at various sites within the embryo is succeeded and progressively replaced by blood cell formation in the liver, and finally in bone marrow, where it persists throughout life (see Table 1 for chronology and Metcalf and Moore, 1971 for more detailed description). As was the case for the thymus (see previous paragraphs), this progression gave rise to controversy as to whether each new site was generated by differentiation of new hematopoietic stem cells in situ, or whether stem cells from the already established sites migrate to and populate the new areas (see Metcalf and Moore, 1971 for discussion). It became apparent from studies using chromosome markers (Moore and Owen, 1965), by characterization of the hematopoietic stem cell present in the circulation (Barnes and Loutit, 1967; Metcalf and Moore, 1971) or by in vitro culturing procedures (Moore and Metcalf, 1970) that the most probable interpretation of the sequential differentiation is through migration of hematopoietic stem cells in the blood stream. This was demonstrated in a direct way for erythropoiesis in the mouse: when mouse embryos were cultured with their intact yolk sacs, liver hematopoiesis would proceed as scheduled, while no hematopoiesis occurred in similar embryos cultured in the absence of their yolk sacs (Moore and Metcalf, 1970). However, the validity of some of these experiments has been questioned (for interesting polemic see Harrison and Russell, 1972 and Marks and Rifkin, 1972). In summary, blood-forming islets within the embryo and the yolk sac may be the major sites of origin for hematopoiesis (or for generation of hematopoietic stem cells) and hematopoiesis in other organs is probably initiated by migrant stem cells from this original area (METCALF and MOORE, 1971; OWEN, 1972, 1973). Indeed, yolk sac stem cells have been shown to contain precursors for hematopoietic cells of all the types (MOORE and METCALF, 1970) and lymphoid cells of both the T (STUTMAN and GOOD, 1971 b) and B series (STUTMAN, 1973). Similarly, it has been demonstrated that fetal liver contains hematopoietic stem cells that give rise to erythroid, myeloid, etc. lines (see for example SILINI et al., 1967 or BARKER et al., 1969) as well as the lymphoid series (TYAN and COLE, 1963; TAYLOR, 1965; TYAN et al., 1966; TYAN and COLE, 1966) that can differentiate into functional T (STUTMAN and GOOD, 1971 a, b) or functional B-cells (TYAN and HERZENBERG, 1968; STUTMAN, 1973). Similar studies have been performed with adult bone marrow, showing that the stem cell can generate both hematopoietic and lymphoid progeny (WU et al., 1968). Indeed, bone marrow contains precursor or stem cells that can give rise to T-cells after migration to thymus (FORD and MICKLEM, 1963; FORD, 1966; DOENHOFF et al., 1970; STUTMAN, 1970, 1972) or to B-cells (STUTMAN, 1973) and antibody-forming cells (MITCHELL and MILLER, 1968; NOSSAL et al., 1968). The latter is a thymus-independent differentiation pathway (TYAN and HERZEN-BERG, 1968; STUTMAN, 1973).

Figure 1 shows the aspect of the large basophylic stem cells in the early mouse yolk sac (in this case from a 10–11-day-old embryo). For a detailed morphologic description of these cells see MOORE and OWEN, 1967b; HOSHINO et al., 1969; MANDEL, 1970. Figure 2 shows a section through a 14-day-old

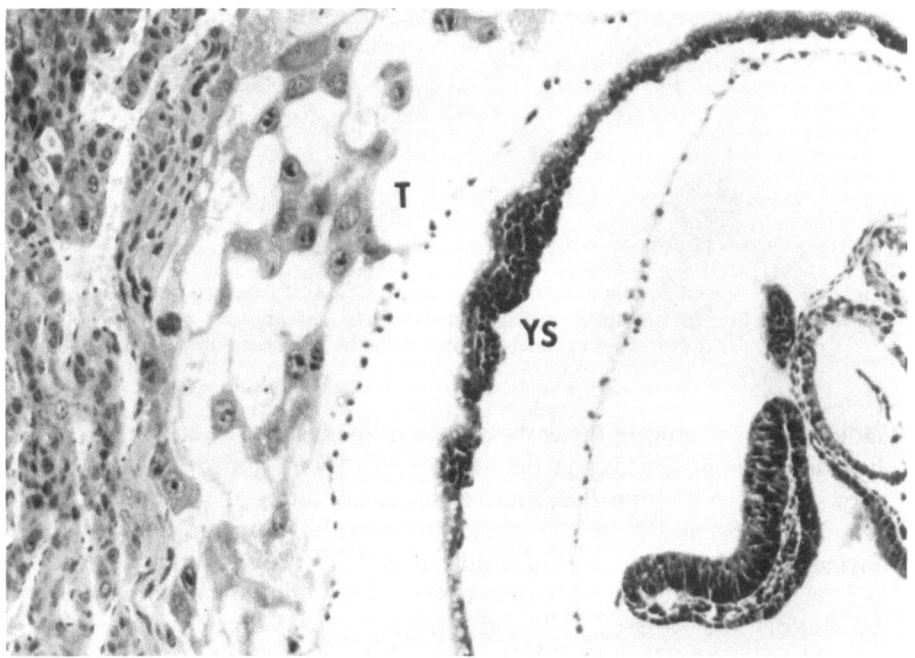

Fig. 1. Blood island in yolk sac (indicated by *YS*) from a 10–11-day-old CBA/H embryo. Dark staining cells are hematopoietic stem cells. *T* indicates trophoblast. H & E, ×40

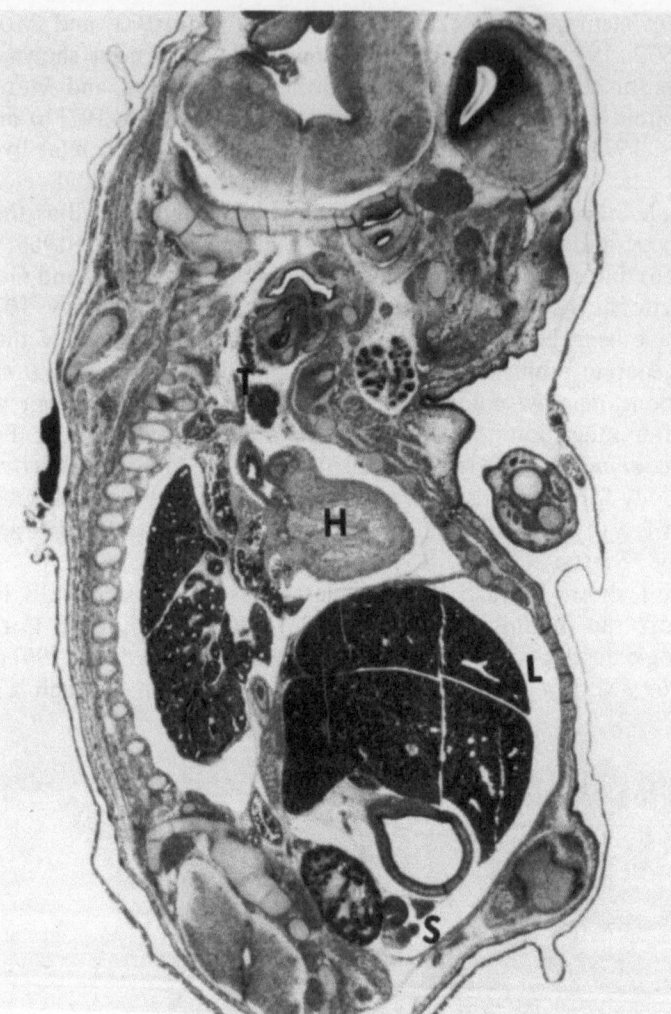

Fig. 2. Section of a 14-day-old CBA/H embryo, showing the first lymphoid thymus (*T*), the large hematopoietic liver (*L*) and the early spleen rudiment (*S*). Also apparent is the absence of bone marrow cavity in sections of vertebrae, ribs and limbs. *H* indicates heart. H & E, ×40

mouse embryo showing the early lymphoid thymus and especially the massive hematopoiesis in the liver in the absence of a bone marrow cavity. Figure 3 shows the thymus from that same embryo, indicating the presence of active lymphopoiesis and the absence of the cortex–medulla organization of the adult thymus (the development of a visible medullary area in the mouse thymus is a relatively late event, approximately at 17 days of embryonation, as shown by MANDEL and RUSSELL, 1971 and MANDEL et al., 1972).

Although the "T and B" terminology proposed by ROITT et al. (1969) has been widely accepted and used, some clarification seems necessary. This terminology attempts to relate the functional capacity of immunocompetent lympho-

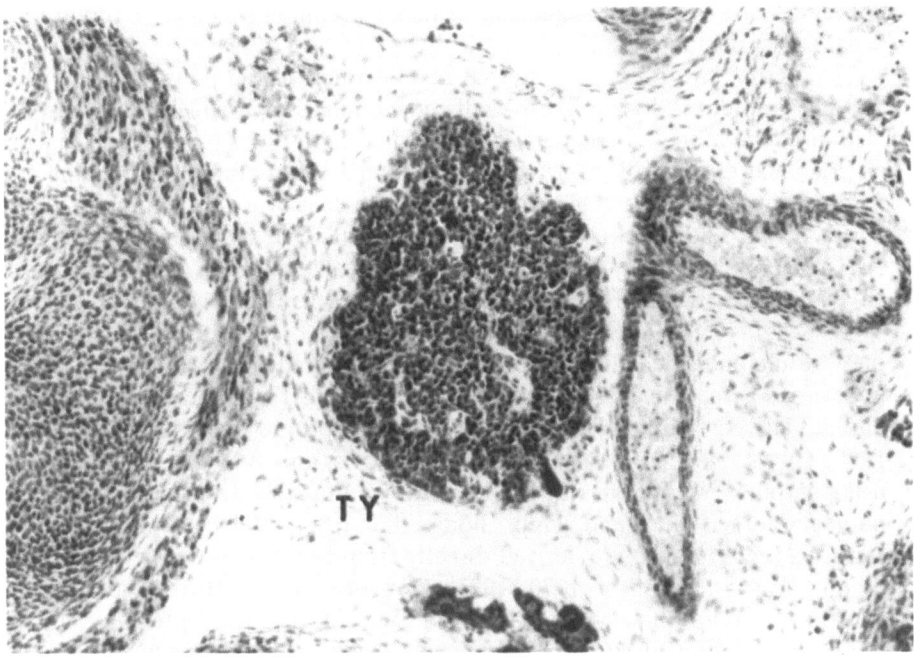

Fig. 3. Larger magnification of the thymus (*TY*) from Figure 2, showing lobulated structure with vasculature and small lymphocytes infiltrating the parenchyma, without delineation of cortex and medulla. H & E, ×40

cytes to their site of differentiation: "T" equals thymus derived, thymus processed or thymus dependent, while "B" equals bursa-equivalent derived, bone marrow derived, nonthymus processed, thymus independent (and actually, bursa derived or bursa processed in birds). The use of "processed" versus "derived" should be encouraged, since, as will be discussed in the next paragraphs, T-cells are actually "derived" from hematopoietic precursors present in the bone marrow in the adult mammal (and in the yolk sack and hematopoietic liver in the embryo). Similarly, "thymus dependency" can be questioned, since the mature T lymphocyte in the peripheral lymphoid tissues is, indeed, thymus-dependent for its development (and renewal) but not for its function, i.e., T lymphocytes do not require additional thymic influence to perform their functional responses.

Although chromosomal analysis has indicated that under certain circumstances the hematopoietic as well as the lymphoid system in mouse chimeras was derived from a limited number of clones (TRENTIN *et al.*, 1967) or from the progeny of a single clone of stem cells (WU *et al.*, 1968), it is not clear at what level stem cell comittment occurs. Based on the hematopoietic model, an attractive hypothesis would be that a single type of circulating stem cell can differentiate into the various types of blood cells, including T and B lymphocytes, depending upon the microenvironment it enters, and occuring as a chance event (TILL *et al.*, 1964; MOORE and OWEN, 1967a; WU *et al.*, 1968). However, although there is enough suggestive evidence accumulated, this possibility still needs direct demonstration.

The term "traffic" has been used several times in the previous paragraphs and needs some clarification, especially concerning its possible role in lympho-cyte differentiation. As was mentioned before, the use of chromosome markers in irradiated mice has demonstrated the existence of migration of dividing cells from bone marrow (or other hematopoietic tissues) via the thymus to lymph nodes (Ford and Micklem, 1963; Ford, 1966; Stutman and Good, 1969, 1971a, b). This journey has a duration of weeks, and the thymus seems to have an instructional effect upon the migrating cells (Harris and Ford, 1964; Stutman, 1970, 1972; Stutman and Good, 1971a, b). The interpretation of these results indicated that the proliferating stem cells of hematopoietic origin underwent a sequence of maturation steps during this process and that the differentiative potential of the stem cells became progressively restricted (Ford, 1966; Owen, 1972, 1973; Stutman, 1972; Boyse and Bennett, 1974). Indeed, using chromosome markers, it has been shown that cells from the recirculating pool in thoracic duct and lymph nodes that react to T-cell mitogens or to allogeneic cells in vitro are derived directly from hematopoietic precursors after thymus traffic (Stutman, 1970, 1972; Doenhoff et al., 1970; Stutman and Good, 1971a, b). In contrast, a second type of traffic's represented by the rapid recirculation of small mature lymphocytes (mainly T-cells) from blood into lymphoid tissues and back to blood, which takes place within hours (Ford and Gowans, 1969). Thus, the first type of traffic is related to maturation of hematopoietic precursors into competent T-cells, under the influence of the thymus, while the second type is related to the functions of the mature small lymphocyte. As a matter of fact, as indicated in a previous paragraph, recircula-tion (i.e., the second type of traffic) is acquired by progeny of stem cell origin after differentiation within the thymus (Stutman, 1972; Stutman and Good, 1971a, b). The property of "recirculation" is a characteristic of the "recirculat-ing pool" of lymphocytes, which in the normal mouse is composed mainly of T-cells (Miller et al., 1971; Sprent, 1973).

These differentiation steps, especially the intrathymic ones, are accompanied by the display on the cell surface of antigens that are characteristic of the T series, such as TL, Thy.1, etc. (see Boyse et al., 1968 for discussion of these antigens and also Boyse and Bennett, 1974). These antigenic changes have been followed during ontogeny (see Owen and Raff, 1970; Owen, 1972, 1973) and are coincident with the appearance of lymphoid cells within the thymus (see Section D and Table 2 for further discussion).

In summary, our present understanding of the mechanism of thymus-depen-dent development is as follows. It seems that two factors are necessary for the normal development and maintenance of thymic function: (1) an intact reticuloepithelial framework in the thymus and (2) a supply of stem cells of hematopoietic origin that are sensitive to the local inductive action of the thymus (Stutman et al., 1970; Dardenne et al., 1974). This particular traffic of cells to the thymus, followed by subsequent export of the post-thymic cells to the periphery, is unidirectional, i.e., the post-thymic cells do not return to thymus under normal conditions (Stutman, 1972). The epithelial framework also seems to be the source of a product of the thymus present in serum that acts like a "poietic" substance favoring T-cell differentiation (DARDENNE et al., 1974; BACH et al., 1975). Using chromosome markers (i.e., precursor cells with chromosome markers and subsequent detection of the same marker in the immunocompetent progeny), it has been demonstrated that as a consequence of traffic a series of post-thymic cells are generated: (1) an immunologically incompetent cell that is sensitive to the humoral activity of the thymus and can further differentiate into competent T-cells (STUTMAN, 1975a); (2) a competent T-cell, which appears to be derived directly from the previous type under the influence of thymic humoral factors (STUTMAN, 1975a, b); (3) T-cells with different functional as well as surface antigen characteristics (see Section D, and CANTOR and BOYSE, 1975); (4) T-cells that are either rapidly or slowly dividing cells, i.e., short- and long-lived lymphocytes (STUTMAN, 1972). The relationship of these subpopulations of T-cells to some of the subpopulations defined in functional studies (GREAVES et al., 1974; CANTOR and BOYSE, 1975) deserves further study. The post-thymic precursor cells described in (1) seem to be the target for the functional effects of at least two small molecular weight products isolated from thymus (TRAININ et al., 1975) and from serum (BACH et al., 1975). Concerning ontogeny, it has been shown that stem cells with the capacity to differentiate into T- or B-cells appear in the mouse embryo in the yolk sac and follow the pattern of hematopoietic development (see Table 1): they are detected after day 12 of embryonation in the hematopoietic liver and after birth in bone marrow and spleen (STUTMAN et al., 1970; STUTMAN and GOOD, 1971a, b; STUTMAN, 1972, 1973). Thus, it seems that there is further maturation of T-cell post-thymic precursors in the periphery and that such maturation may be guided by thymic humoral factors. On the other hand, there is also evidence that a purified extract from thymus may induce antigenic changes in hematopoietic precursors that are characteristic of the intrathymic stage of differentiation (i.e., appearance of TL antigen and Thy.1), indicating that the intrathymic stage may also be mediated by the humoral activity of the thymus (SCHEID et al., 1975). It is still unclear to what degree these different components, i.e., traffic, export, thymic humoral factors, etc. actually occur during ontogeny under physiologic conditions, especially the magnitude of these different components as main contributors for the development and maintenance of the peripheral pool of competent T lymphocytes.

C. Ontogeny of Transplantation Immunity

As was indicated in the Introduction, we will discuss the ontogeny of the capacity to reject foreign grafts, while in Section D we will discuss the ontogeny of other T dependent functions. This is due mainly to the paucity of ontogenic studies on transplantation and to the need for a better understanding of the possible mechanisms of T dependent functions.

In the few mammalian species in which the ability of embryos, newborns, or animals within a few days after birth, to reject foreign tissue grafts was measured, it became apparent that with few exceptions, such capacity was present and usually was as efficient as in the adult. This early maturation of transplantation immunity contrasts with the maturation patterns of a wide variety of other immune responses (see Section D and also STERZL and SILVERSTEIN, 1967 for review). For example, the mean rejection time of newborn A/J mice grafted with C57BL/6 skin was 10.8 ± 0.6 SE days, while in the adults of the same strain combination it was 9.6 ± 0.6 (BORAKER and HILDEMANN, 1965). In general, normal allograft rejection was observed in newborn or young mice (MILLER, 1964; BORAKER and HILDEMANN, 1965), rats (STEINMULLER, 1961), and rabbits (NAJARIAN and DIXON, 1962). In the experiments of BORAKER and HILDEMANN (1965), although the mice could reject the allogeneic skin grafted at birth, they were unable to produce antibodies directed against the allogeneic antigens until 11–15 days of age. In rats, while the ability to reject xenogeneic skin appeared at birth in both Lewis and BN strains, the ability to reject allogeneic rat skin was fully developed at 3 days of age in Lewis and only at 19 days postpartum in BN strains (STEINMULLER, 1961). In the rat the adult levels of allograft rejection are reached at approximately 20 days of age (STEINMULLER, 1961), and this may explain that in some instances, actual tolerance was produced as a consequence of allogeneic skin grafting at birth (RAWLES, 1955; MEDAWAR and WOODRUFF, 1958). However, the histology of graft rejection is essentially comparable between newborn and adults (STEINMULLER, 1961). In the mouse, not only does transplantation immunity appear early in life, but it is also rapidly affected by neonatal thymectomy: mice 3 days after neonatal thymectomy already show the immune deficiency expressed as incapacity to reject allografts (MILLER, 1964). In the lamb it has been shown that 80–117-day-old (SCHINCKEL and FERGUSON, 1953) as well as 120–139-day-old fetuses (SILVERSTEIN et al., 1963) could reject allogeneic skin, when grafted in utero, at a rate comparable to the rejections observed in adults. In the stepwise chronology of immune reactivity in the embryonic lamb fetus, skin graft rejection is one of the first responses to appear (SILVERSTEIN and PRENDERGAST, 1970). Specific transplantation immunity has been induced by immunization during the embryonic or newborn period in mice (measured either as capacity to produce graft-versus-host reactions: HOWARD and MICHIE, 1962; BRENT and GOWLAND, 1963; or as capacity to reject skin or tumor grafts: BORAKER and HILDEMANN, 1965), rats (STEINMULLER, 1961), and rabbits (PORTER, 1960). Similarly, delayed hypersensitivity skin reactions could be induced by immunization of guinea pig embryos (UHR, 1960) and has been detected in premature neonatal humans (UHR et al., 1960). For an extensive discussion concerning the so-called "immunologically neutral" period during early development (quite essential for some of the early interpretations of tolerance induction), see BRENT and GOWLAND (1963).

In summary, it is apparent from the rather limited number of studies actually measuring transplantation immunity in mammals either at birth or shortly after, that: (1) such functions are readily detected and are usually of the same magnitude as the response in adults; (2) that they appear before the full development of many other immune functions such as the capacity to produce antibodies directed to the same alloantigens that elicit transplantation immunity or other

T-dependent functions; (3) the responses are thymus-dependent even at the early age and (4) the young animal also has the capacity to develop specific immunity to transplantation antigens.

D. Ontogeny of Thymus-Dependent Functions

A number of criteria establish the maturity of the thymus-dependent T-cell, the cell or group of cells responsible for cell-mediated immunity. These include the presence of typical cell surface receptors or antigens, responsiveness to certain mitogens and allogeneeic cell stimuli in vitro, ability to initiate graft-versus-host reactions in an unresponsive allogeneic animal, and ability to help in the humoral response to an antigen as well as the ability to destroy specific target cells in vitro and to reject allogeneic tissues in vivo (see GREAVES et al., 1974 for review). Here we will consider only information derived from mouse or human studies, since these represent the most complete picture we have to date of the development of immune responsiveness.

Surface antigens of murine lymphocytes have been studied extensively for their distribution and developmental patterns (Table 2). Thy.1 (theta), an antigen

Table 2. Appearance of T-cell markers and functions in the mouse[a]

	Thymus		Spleen	
	Appear-ance[b]	Adult level[c]	Appear-ance[b]	Adult level[c]
Surface antigens				
Thy.1	16d	18d	17d	+7d
TL	16d	18d	None	None
Ly 1,2,3	?	?	birth[d]	+10 wk (decreased)
1	?	?	+d14	10 wk
2,3	?	?	+d14	10 wk
H-2	17d	17d	15d	+d4
Functions				
Antigen binding	14d	(lost birth)	15d	+d7
PHA responsiveness	15d	(lost, +d4)	+d7	+30–60d
Con A responsiveness	15d	+d21	birth	+30–60d
Allogeneic cell responsiveness	18d	+d21	+d7	+30–60d
Syngeneic spleen cell responsiveness	18d	(lost, +d4)	None	None
GVH activity	birth	birth	birth	+d2
Helper activity	birth	+d2	+d4	+d8

[a] See text for references.
[b] These figures represent the earliest time in gestation at which the antigens or functions have been demonstrated; + designates days after birth.
[c] These figures represent the age at which the developing cells stabilize at normal adult levels; + designates days after birth.
[d] Earliest age tested.

present on ectodermal cells and thymus-derived lymphocytes (REIF and ALLEN, 1964), appears first in development in the 16-day-old embryonic thymus and reaches adult levels by 18 days, well before birth (REIF and ALLEN, 1964; OWEN and RAFF, 1970; STOBO and PAUL, 1972; SPEAR et al., 1973). Thy.1 positive cells appear in the spleen around the time of birth, and adult levels are reached by 7 days of life (SPEAR et al., 1973). The lymph node attains its full complement of these cells by day 4 after birth (OWEN, 1972). Thy.1 positive cells are also present in the blood and in Peyer's patches of newborn mice (RAFF and OWEN, 1971; OWEN, 1972), but at a lower level than in the adult (REIF and ALLEN, 1964).

Similarly, 14-day embryonic mice have no demonstrable thymic TL antigen, one found only on leukemic cells and on the normal thymocytes of certain mouse strains (OLD et al., 1963), yet at 16 days, 45% of the thymus cells of these mouse strains are TL positive and by 18 days, the embryonic thymus contains near adult levels of TL positive cells (82%) (OWEN and RAFF, 1970). Although the 14-day embryonic thymus has no demonstrable Thy.1 or TL positive cells, this organ does contain cells that have the potential for lymphocytic maturation in this microenvironment, since in vitro incubation of such embryonic thymus results in the appearance of lymphocytes that are both Thy.1 (90%) and TL (61%) positive (OWEN and RAFF, 1970).

CANTOR and BOYSE (1975) have recently described 3 classes of peripheral T-cells by their Ly antigens. These antigens are confined to lymphocytes and are present in higher concentrations in the thymus (BOYSE et al., 1968). Three main Ly specificities have been described and numbered 1 to 3, and each has two allelic forms (BOYSE et al., 1971). All newborn splenic T-cells are Ly 1,2,3. By 2 weeks, Ly 1,2,3 cells are decreased considerably and there is an increased number of Ly 1 cells. Ly 2,3 cells increase at a slower rate. Adult proportions (50% Ly 1,2,3, 33% Ly 1, and 8% Ly 2,3 among splenic T-cells) of the 3 Ly classes of T-cells are reached by 10 weeks after birth (CANTOR and BOYSE, 1975).

H-2 alloantigens (the major histocompatibility antigen series of the mouse) have been demonstrated at low levels in the spleen of the 15-day embryonic mouse (SCHLESINGER, 1965), a stage when it is not found in the thymus. H-2 bearing cells are present in small numbers in the spleen until birth when they increase rapidly and are near adult numbers by day 4. Although H-2 antigens are present in all tissues, their amount per cell may be variable and within the ontogeny studies described, "H-2 bearing" cells indicate cells with readily demonstrable antigens using conventional serologic techniques (SCHLESINGER, 1967). The thymus shows no H-2 positive cells until day 17, 2 days later than the spleen (a time coincident with a large relative increase in small lymphocytes in the thymus, Table 1), when they are present in approximately adult numbers. This level of H-2 positivity is maintained with minor fluctuations until 1 month of age. There is then a gradual increase in the relative numbers of these cells until 6 months of age. At this time in its development, the thymus has more H-2 bearing cells than the spleen, which overtakes the thymus only at 4 days after birth. Although H-2 bearing cells have been identified in embryonic life, it is necessary to use much higher concentrations of complement in their demonstration, suggesting that these antigens are present at a lower density in the newborn and fetal cells than in adult cells (SCHLESINGER, 1965, 1967).

Other mouse T-cell antigens, namely MSLA (SHIGENO et al., 1968) and GIX (STOCKERT et al., 1971), remain to be examined in fetal and neonatal tissues.

The presence of receptors on human lymphocytes for sheep erythrocytes seems to mark them as thymus-derived cells although the immunologic function of these receptors is not well understood (STITES et al., 1972). Cells bearing these receptors are present in the 11-week embryonic thymus and reach peak levels of 65% at 15 weeks before they decrease to a fairly constant 30% in the latter weeks of gestation. Erythrocyte binding cells appear first in the fetal spleen at 17 weeks (STITES et al., 1972; see Table 3).

Table 3. Appearance of T-cell characteristics in human fetal development[a]

	Thymus		Spleen	
	Appearance[b]	Level[c]	Appearance[b]	Level[c]
SRBC rosette formation	12 wk	17 wk	16 wk	30 wk
Antigen binding	11 wk[d]	15 wk (lost by 10 yr)	17 wk	?
PHA responsiveness	10 wk	19 wk	13 wk	18 wk
PHA induced cytotoxicity	16 wk[d]	?	?	?
Allogeneic cell responsiveness	13 wk	20 wk	14 wk[d]	16 wk
Ability to stimulate allogeneic cells	11 wk	?	15 wk[d]	18 wk

[a] See text for references.
[b] This column represents the time in fetal development where the function was first demonstrated.
[c] These functions seemed to reach peak levels before birth, decreasing thereafter in the thymus, or stabilizing in the spleen. Appearance of adult levels of these functions is not clearly defined.
[d] Earliest age tested.

Specific antigen binding cells are first identifiable in mice in the 14-day embryonic thymus (DWYER and MACKAY, 1972a; DECKER et al., 1974) and on days 15–17 in the spleen (DWYER and MACKAY, 1972a; SPEAR et al., 1973). The numbers of thymic antigen binding cells reach a peak during fetal development and decrease to the low adult level at birth. In the spleen, the numbers increase rapidly to adult levels at 7 days after birth (SPEAR et al., 1973).

Antigen binding cells are detectable in the human fetal thymus after 12 weeks and reach peak numbers around 17 weeks from which they fall off gradually to almost none at 10 years of age (DWYER and MACKAY, 1972b). Lymphocytes binding antigen in the human spleen appear around 16 weeks of fetal development and steadily increase in number to 30 weeks (DWYER and MACKAY, 1972b). Thus, the human T-cell developmental process seems to be analogous to that of the mouse. It is not possible to draw conclusions from these experiments on the appearance of mature T-cells in the spleen, however, because antigen binding is a property of both B- and T-cells (reviewed by ROELANTS, 1972).

Although capacity to respond to different antigens by antibody formation seems to appear at different times in development (reviewed by STERZL and

SILVERSTEIN, 1967), cells specifically binding each of the antigens tested appear within the same 24-hour embryonic period and in the same relative proportions as they exist in the adult (DECKER *et al.,* 1974; SPEAR *et al.,* 1973).

Quite a different aspect of T-cell maturity is the ability to proliferate in response to mitogens and allogeneic stimuli (GREAVES *et al.,* 1974). It has also been postulated that mitogens differ, i.e., phytohemagglutinin (PHA) triggers a different and probably more highly differentiated class of T-cells than concanavalin A (Con A) (STOBO and PAUL, 1973). Certainly in the adult mouse, unseparated thymocytes are poorly reactive to PHA while they respond well to Con A (STOBO and PAUL, 1973). Peripheral lymphoid organs respond well to both, suggesting that Con A stimulates the undifferentiated thymocyte as well as the mature T-cell, while PHA stimulates only the mature T-cell (STOBO and PAUL, 1973).

Fetal and newborn (15–19 days of gestation to 4 days after birth) murine thymocytes, unlike adult cells, respond vigorously to PHA but poorly to Con A and PWM (MOSIER, 1974; STOBO and PAUL, 1973). Their PHA reactivity has decreased markedly at birth and is at the normal low adult levels by 1 week after birth (MOSIER, 1974; HOWE and MANZIELLO, 1972). The Con A response begins to increase by 8 days after birth and reaches adult high reactivity in the third week (MOSIER, 1974; STOBO and PAUL, 1972).

Appearance of these T-cell activities follows a different pattern in the spleen (see Table 2). Newborn spleen acquires mitogen responsiveness as Thy.1-bearing cells appear and reaches adult levels by 4–7 weeks after birth; Con A reactivity reaches a peak level faster than that of PHA (STOBO and PAUL, 1972).

Similar events occur in human fetal development (see Table 3). As in the mouse, these fetal thymocytes respond well to PHA by 10–14 weeks of gestation and then decrease to lower adult levels after the 18–25 week (KAY *et al.,* 1966; PAPIERNIK, 1970; STITES *et al.,* 1974). This change occurs simultaneously with an increase in the size of the thymus cortex (PAPIERNIK, 1970). Peripheral blood is responsive to PHA by 12 weeks (earlier times were not tested) and spleen becomes responsive after 13 weeks gestation. Adult levels are attained rapidly after birth (KAY *et al.,* 1966; STITES *et al.,* 1974). PHA also induces cytotoxic lymphocytes in human fetal lymphocytes (STITES *et al.,* 1972; HAYWARD and SOOTHILL, 1972). This activity appears in 16-week fetal thymocytes and is maintained (allowing for variability) through fetal development (HAYWARD and SOOTHILL, 1972).

Responsiveness to allogeneic cells in the mouse thymus has a similar pattern to that of PHA. There is a peak of high reactivity near birth (exact timing probably is dependent upon the strain tested). BALB/C thymocytes first react in MLR after 18 days of gestation and are the best responders at birth, decreasing in the first week of life before their responsiveness returns in the third week to adult levels, equal to that existant at birth (MOSIER, 1974). HOWE and MANZIELLO (1972) find peak MLR reactivity in the CBA thymus after birth, which is lost by 15 days of age. Reactivity to allogeneic cells in the spleen does not occur until 2 weeks after birth (ADLER *et al.,* 1970a; HOWE and MANZIELLO, 1972), but it does appear more rapidly than that to PHA, attaining adult levels slightly earlier.

At the same time, these fetal and neonatal thymocytes are responsive in MLR to adult syngeneic spleen cells. BALB/C mice show this activity from 18 days of gestation until shortly after birth (4 days) (MOSIER, 1974), though the response was only about 30% of that to allogeneic spleen cells. CBA mice again are on a delayed time course, the response to syngeneic spleen cells appearing and peaking 2–3 days after birth, decreasing subsequently during the first month of life (HOWE et al., 1970).

Responsiveness to allogeneic cells in the human fetus appears first in the liver at 8 weeks and at 13 weeks in the thymus. Spleen and peripheral blood are responsive by 14 weeks (STITES et al., 1974). Proliferation in response to allogeneic cells seems to be a property of different cells rather than reactivity to PHA, since liver cells never respond to PHA while they respond very early to allogeneic cells (CARR et al., 1973).

Embryonic murine cells are not active in inducing graft-versus-host disease (GVHD) (RITTER, 1971; CHAKRAVARTY et al., 1975). Newborn thymocytes on the other hand are as effective as adult thymus in inducing in vivo or in vitro GVHD (COHEN et al., 1963; SOSIN et al., 1966; CHISCON et al., 1972; RITTER, 1971; CHAKRAVARTY et al., 1975). Newborn splenic lymphocytes were only 1/10 as active as adult cells in GVHD (SOSIN et al., 1966) until reacting at adult levels at about 1 week after birth (CHISCON et al., 1971). Some reports do exist of the reactivity of yolk sac, placenta, liver, lung, and thymus in specifically manipulated GVHD assays (TYAN, 1968; HOFMAN and GLOBERSON, 1973). Studies involving preculture of immature embryonic murine thymus (13–14 days of gestation) prior to injection into foreign hosts (RITTER, 1971) or into in vitro GVHD cultures (CHAKRAVARTY et al., 1975) demonstrate the presence in embryonic tissues of cells with the potential of inducing GVHD, providing they are given a chance to mature.

Care must be taken in interpreting the MLR and GVHD responsiveness (LAFFERTY et al., 1972), as this seems to be a property of hematopoietic cells and is different from response to antigenic stimulation. More significant immunologically is the ability to stimulate cells in MLR. Mouse pleen attains this capacity apparently in parallel with its capacity to respond in an MLR by 1–2 weeks after birth, reaching a peak at 30–60 days (ADLER et al., 1970b). It remains unclear as to why this activity appears so late when H-2 is present well before birth. However, the appearance of the LD and SD determinants of the H-2 complex (those that stimulate in MLR, see SCHENDEL and BACH, 1974) in ontogeny has not been reported. Stimulatory cells are found in human fetal tissues (Table 3) especially in the spleen, bone marrow, and peripheral blood, though thymus and liver also have some activity (STITES et al., 1974).

The ability to act as helper cells in humoral immune responses to thymus-dependent antigens develops after birth in the thymus and days later in the spleen (CLAMAN et al., 1966; CHISCON and GOLUB, 1972; ARRENBRECHT, 1973). Helper activity in the thymus was at about 10% of adult level at birth and up to 30–50% by day 4. It is at this time (from 15 days of gestation to 3 days after birth) that tolerance to soluble protein (TERRES and HUGHES, 1959) and allogeneic antigens (BILLINGHAM et al., 1953; BRENT and GOWLAND, 1963) can most easily be induced. There is a recent report, furthermore, suggesting that neonatal spleen contains suppressor T-cells active in regulating in vitro humoral immune responses (MOSIER and JOHNSON, 1975).

CHAKRAVARTY *et al.* (1975) have reported the ability of 16-day embryonic thymic cells to act as helper cells in the humoral sheep erythrocyte response after a 24-hour incubation in culture with Con A. By 18 days, the prestimulated embryonic thymocytes have the same activity as similarly treated adult thymocytes. Although the differentiation mechanisms of T-cells remain obscure, it is clear that presumptive T-cells exist in the 14–16-day embryonic thymus and that at least some stages of maturation occur there.

E. Concluding Remarks

From this brief review it is apparent that, whether analyzed as the capacity to reject allotransplants or as other T dependent immune functions, cell-mediated immunity can be detected in young mammals. On the other hand, the analysis of the available literature shows that additional detailed information seems to be required for a better understanding of the actual ontogenic steps in immunologic development. The exact mechanisms of lymphopoiesis are still undefined, although a substantial amount of information has been accumulated concerning thymus-dependent steps of differentiation and cell-to-cell interactions, especially interactions necessary for expression of immune reactivity. The development of regulatory mechanisms or regulatory cells is still undefined. The actual steps of early events for B-cell differentiation need clarification and definition. There is almost no information available on the ontogenesis of other accessory cells required for expression of immune reactivity, such as macrophages or "adherent" cells. In addition, the exact mechanism of allograft rejection has not been adequate defined. In summary, the many gaps in our information concerning the ontogeny of transplantation immunity, make this review almost a list of unfulfilled desires, interspersed with the available experimental data on the subject. As further support of this contention, compare the bibliographies (especially on the animal species discussed in this chapter) of the few available reviews on the subject (GOOD and PAPERMASTER, 1964; STERZL and SILVERSTEIN, 1967, and SOLOMON, 1971) with the present review.

Acknowledgement

The experimental work discussed in this review was supported by U.S. Public Health grants CA-08748 and CB-16899. We would like to thank Ms. LINDA STEVENSON for her assistance in the manuscript and Mr. JOHN HLINKA for his help in the photography.

References

ACKERMAN, G.A., KNOUFF, R.A.: Lymphocyte formation in the thymus of the embryonic chick. Anat. Rec. **149**, 191–216 (1964).

ACKERMAN, G.A., KNOUFF, R.A.: The epithelial origin of the lymphocytes in the thymus of the embryonic hamster. Anat. Rec. **152**, 35–54 (1965).

ACKERMAN, G.A.: Developmental relationship between the appearance of lymphocytes and lympho-poietic activity in the thymus and lymph nodes of the fetal cat. Anat. Rec. **158**, 387–400 (1967).

ACKERMAN, G.A., HOSTETLER, J.R.: Morphological studies of the embryonic rabbit thymus: The in situ epithelial versus the extrathymic derivation of the initial population of lymphocytes in the embryonic thymus. Anat. Rec. **166**, 27–46 (1970).

ADLER, W.H., TAKIGUCHI, T., MARSH, B., SMITH, R.T.: Cellular recognition by mouse lymphocytes in vitro. I. Definition of a new technique and results of stimulation by phytohemagglutinin and specific antigens. J. Exp. Med. **131**, 1049–1078 (1970a).

ADLER, W.H., TAKIGUCHI, T., MARSH, B., SMITH, R.T.: Cellular recognition by mouse lymphocytes in vitro. II. Specific stimulation by histocompatibility antigens in mixed cell culture. J. Immunol. **105**, 984–1000 (1970b).

ARRENBRECHT, S.: Normal development of the thymus-dependent limb of humoral immune responses in mice. Europ. J. Immunol. **3**, 506–511 (1973).

ASPINALL, R.L., MEYER, R.K., GRAETZER, M.A., WOLFE, H.R.: Effect of thymectomy and bursec-tomy on the survival of skin homografts in chickens. J. Immunol. **90**, 872–877 (1963).

AUERBACH, R.: Morphogenetic interactions in the development of the mouse thymus gland. Develop. Biol. **2**, 271–284 (1960).

AUERBACH, R.: Experimental analysis of the origin of cell types in the development of mouse thymus. Develop. Biol. **3**, 336–354 (1961).

BACH, J.F., DARDENNE, M., PLEAU, J.M., BACH, M.A.: Isolation, biochemical characteristics and biological activity of a circulating thymic hormone in the mouse and in the human. Ann. N.Y. Acad. Sci. **249**, 186–210 (1975).

BAILEY, R.P., WEISS, L.: Ontogeny of human fetal lymph nodes. Amer. J. Anat. **142**, 15–28 (1974).

BALDAMUS, C.A., McKENZIE, I.F., WINN, H.J., RUSSELL, P.S.: Acute destruction by humoral anti-body of rat skin grafted to mice. J. Immunol. **110**, 1532–1541 (1973).

BARKER, J.E., KEENAN, M.A., RAPHALS, L.: Development of the mouse hematopoietic system. II. Estimation of spleen and liver "stem" cell number. J. Cell. Physiol. **74**, 51–56 (1969).

BARNES, D.W.H., LOUTIT, J.F.: Effects of irradiation and antigenic stimulation on circulating haemopoietic stem cells of the mouse. Nature (London) **213**, 1142–1143 (1967).

BEARD, J.: The source of leucocytes and the true function of the thymus. Anat. Anz. **18**, 550–573 (1900).

BILLINGHAM, R.E., BRENT, L., MEDAWAR, P.B.: Actively acquired tolerance of foreign cells. Nature (London) **1972**, 603–606 (1953).

BLOCK, M.: The blood forming tissues and blood of the newborn oppossum (Didelphys virginiana). Ergebn. d. Anat. u. Entwickl. **37**, 235–366 (1964).

BORAKER, D.K., HILDEMANN, W.H.: Maturation of alloimmune responsiveness in mice. Transplanta-tion **3**, 202–223 (1965).

BOYSE, E.A., MIYAZAWI, M., AOKI, J., OLD, L.J.: Ly-A and Ly-B: Two systems of lymphocyte isoantigens in the mouse. Proc. Roy. Soc. B **170**, 175–193 (1968).

BOYSE, E.A., ITAKURA, K., STOCKERT, E., IRITANI, C.A., MIURA, M.: Ly-C: a third locus specifying alloantigens expressed only on thymocytes and lymphocytes. Transplantation **11**, 351–352 (1971).

BOYSE, E.A., BENNETT, D.: Differentiation and the cell surface: Illustrations from work with T-cells and sperm. In: Cellular Selection and Regulation in the Immune Response, pp. 155–176. New York: Raven Press 1974.

BRENT, L., GOWLAND, G.: Immunological competence of newborn mice. Transplantation **1**, 372–376 (1963).

CANTOR, H., BOYSE, E.A.: Functional subclasses of T lymphocytes bearing different Ly antigens. I. The generation of functionally distinct T-cell subclasses is a process independent of antigen. J. Exp. Med. **141**, 1376–1389 (1975).

CARR, M.C., STITES, D.P., FUDENBERG, H.H.: Dissociation of responses to phytohemagglutinin and adult allogeneic lymphocytes in human fetal lymphoid tissues. Nature New Biol. **241**, 279–281 (1973).

CHAKRAVARTY, A., KUBAI, L., SIDKY, Y., AUERBACH, R.: Ontogeny of thymus cell function. Ann. N.Y. Acad. Sci. **249**, 34–42 (1975).

CHISCON, M.O., FIDLER, J.M., GOLUB, E.S.: Functional development of the interacting cells in the immune system of the mouse to heterologous erythrocytes studied in vivo and in vitro. Fed. Proc. **30**, 526 (1971).

CHISCON, M.O., GOLUB, E.S.: Functional development of the interacting cells in the immune response. I. Development of T-cell and B-cell function. J. Immunol. **108**, 1379–1386 (1972).

CLAMAN, H.N., CHAPERON, E.A., TRIPLETT, R.F.: Immunocompetence of transferred thymus marrow cell combinations. J. Immunol. **97**, 828–832 (1966).

COHEN, M.W., THORBECKE, G.J., HOCHWALD, G.M., JACOBSON, E.B.: Induction of a graft-versus-host reaction in newborn mice by injection of newborn or adult homologous thymus cells. Proc. Soc. Exp. Biol. (N.Y.) **114**, 242–244 (1963).

COHEN, N.: Phylogeny of lymphocyte structure and function. Amer. Zool. **15**, 119–133 (1975).

COOPER, M.D., PETERSON, R.D.A., SOUTH, M.A., GOOD, R.A.: The functions of the thymus system and bursa system in the chicken. J. Exp. Med. **123**, 75–102 (1966).

DARDENNE, M., PAPIERNIK, M., BACH, J.F., STUTMAN, O.: Studies on thymus products. III. Epithelial origin of the serum thymic factor. Immunology **27**, 299–304 (1974).

DAVIES, A.J.S., LEUCHARS, E., WALLIS, V., KOLLER, P.C.: The mitotic response of thymus-derived cells to antigenic stimulus. Transplantation **4**, 438–451 (1966).

DAVIES, A.J.S., FESTENSTEIN, H., LEUCHARS, E., WALLIS, V.J., DOENHOFF, M.J.: A thymic origin for some peripheral-blood lymphocytes. Lancet **I**, 183–184 (1968).

DAVIES, A.J.S., LEUCHARS, E., WALLIS, V., DOENHOFF, M.J.: A system for lymphocytes in the mouse. Proc. Roy. Soc. B **176**, 369–384 (1971).

DECKER, J.M., CLARKE, J., BRADLEY, L.M., MILLER, A., SERCARZ, E.E.: Presence of antigen-binding cells for five diverse antigens at the onset of lymphoid development: lack of evidence for somatic diversification during ontogeny. J. Immunol. **113**, 1823–1833 (1974).

DOENHOFF, M.J., DAVIES, A.J.S., LEUCHARS, E., WALLIS, V.: The thymus and circulating lymphocytes of mice. Proc. Roy. Soc. B **176**, 69–85 (1970).

DWYER, J.M., MACKAY, I.R.: The development of antigen binding lymphocytes in foetal tissues. Immunology **25**, 871–879 (1972a).

DWYER, J.M., MACKAY, I.R.: Validation of autoradiography for recognition of antigen-binding lymphocytes in blood and lymphoid tissues. Clin. Exp. Immunol. **10**, 581–597 (1972b).

FALCONAR, M.: Experimental inquiries into the properties of the blood: Part 3. Containing a description of the red particles of the blood in the human subject and in other animals; with an account of the structure and offices of the lymphatic glands, of the thymus gland, and of the spleen; being the remaining part of the observations and experiments of the late Mr. William Hewson, F.R.S. and Teacher of Anatomy. London, Longman 1777.

FORD, C.E.: Traffic of lymphoid cells in the body. In: The Thymus: Experimental and Clinical studies, pp. 131–152. Boston: Little, Brown & Co. 1966.

FORD, C.E., MICKLEM, H.S.: The thymus and lymph nodes in radiation chimeras. Lancet **I**, 359–362 (1963).

FORD, W.L., GOWANS, J.L.: The traffic of lymphocytes. Seminars in Hematology **7**, 67–83 (1969).

GATTI, R.A., GOOD, R.A.: The immunological deficiency diseases. Med. Clin. North America **54**, 281–307 (1970).

GERSHON, R.K.: T-cell control of antibody production. Contemp. Topics Immunobiol. **3**, 1–40 (1974).

GLICK, B.: The bursa of Fabricius and the development of immunological competence. In: The Thymus in Immunbiology, pp. 343–358. New York: Hoeber 1964.

GOOD, R.A., KELLY, W.D., ROTSTEIN, J., VARCO, R.L.: Immunological deficiency diseases: Agammaglobulinemia, hypogammaglobulinemia, Hodgkin's disease and sarcoidosis. Progr. Allergy **6**, 187–319 (1962).

GOOD, R.A., PAPERMASTER, B.W.: Ontogeny and phylogeny of adaptive immunity. Adv. Immunol. **4**, 1–115 (1964).

GREAVES, M.F., OWEN, J.J.T., RAFF, M.C.: T and B Lymphocytes: Origins, Properties and Roles in Immune Responses. Amsterdam: Excerpta Medica 1974.

HARRIS, J.E., FORD, C.E.: Cellular traffic of the thymus: Experiments with chromosome markers. Evidence that the thymus plays an instructional part. Nature (London) 201, 884–885 (1964).

HARRIS, J.E., FORD, C.E., BARNES, D.W.H., EVANS, E.P.: Cellular traffic to the thymus: Experiments with chromosome markers. Evidence from parabiosis for an afferent stream of cells. Nature (London) 201, 886–887 (1964).

HARRISON, D.E., RUSSELL, E.S.: Fetal liver erythropoiesis and yolk sac cells. Science 177, 187 (1972).

HAYWARD, A.R., SOOTHILL, J.F.: Reaction to antigen by human foetal thymus lymphocytes. In: Ontogeny of Acquired Immunity, pp. 261–273. Amsterdam-London-New York: Elsevier 1972.

HELLSTRÖM, K.E., HELLSTRÖM, I.: The role of serum factors ("blocking antibodies") as mediators of immunological non-reactivity to cellular antigens. In: Ontogeny of Acquired Immunity, pp. 133–143. Amsterdam-London-New York: Elsevier 1972.

HOFMAN, F., GLOBERSON, A.G.: Graft-versus-host response induced in vitro by mouse yolk sac cells. Europ. J. Immunol. 3, 181–183 (1973).

HOSHINO, T., TAKEDA, M., ABE, K., ITO, T.: Early development of thymic lymphocytes in mice, studied by light and electron microscopy. Anat. Rec. 164, 47–66 (1969).

HOWARD, J.G., MICHIE, D.: Induction of transplantation immunity in the newborn mouse. Transpl. Bull. 29, 91–96 (1962).

HOWE, M.L., GOLDSTEIN, A.L., BATTISTO, J.: Isogeneic lymphocyte interaction: Recognition of self antigens by cells of the neonatal thymus. Proc. Nat. Acad. Sci. (Wash.) 67, 613–619 (1970).

HOWE, M.L., MANZIELLO, B.: Ontogenesis of the in vitro response of murine lymphoid cells to cellular antigens and phytomitogens. J. Immunol. 109, 534–539 (1972).

HOYER, J.R., COOPER, M.D., GABRIELSEN, A.E., GOOD, R.A.: Lymphopenic forms of congenital immunologic deficiency diseases. Medicine 47, 201–226 (1968).

KAY, H.E.M., WOLFENDALE, M.M., PLAYFAIR, J.H.L.: Thymocytes and phytohemagglutinin. Lancet II, 804 (1966).

KALMUTZ, S.E.: Antibody production in the opppossum embryo. Nature (London) 193, 851–853 (1962).

KOSTOWIECKI, M.: Primary human lymphocytes as derivatives of the thymic epithelial cords. Z. f. mikr. anat. Forsch. 73, 404–432 (1965).

KRUML, J., KOVARU, F., POSPISIL, M., TREBICHAVSKY, I.: The development of lymphatic tissue during ontogeny. In: Developmental Aspects of Antibody Formation and Structure. Vol. 1, pp. 35–54. New York-London: Academic Press 1970.

LAFFERTY, K.J., WALKER, K.I., SCOLLAY, R.G., KILLEY, V.A.A.: Allogeneic interactions provide evidence for a novel class of immunological reactivity. Transpl. Rev. 12, 198–228 (1972).

LAJTHA, L.G.: Cytokinetics and regulation of progenitor cells. J. Cell. Physiol. 67, Sup. 1, 133–148 (1966).

LAWTON, A.R., SELF, K.S., ROYAL, S.A., COOPER, M.D.: Ontogeny of B-lymphocytes in the human fetus. Clin. Immunol. Immunopath. 1, 84–93 (1972).

LAWTON, A.R., KINCADE, P., COOPER, M.D.: Sequential expression of germ line genes in development of immunoglobulin class diversity. Fed. Proc. 34, 30–33 (1975).

MANDEL, T.: Differentiation of epithelial cells in the mouse thymus. Z. Zellforsch. 106, 498–515 (1970).

MANDEL, T., RUSSELL, P.J.: Differentiation of foetal mouse thymus. Ultrastructure of organ cultures and of subcapsular grafts. Immunology 21, 659–674 (1971).

MANDEL, T., RUSSELL, P.J., BYRD, W.: Differentiation of the thymus in vivo and in vitro. In: Cell Interactions, 3rd. Lepetit Colloquium, pp. 183–191. Amsterdam: North Holland 1972.

MARKS, P.A., RIFKIND, R.A.: Fetal liver erythropoiesis and yolk sac cells. Science 177, 187 (1972).

MAXIMOW, A.: Untersuchungen über Blut und Bindegewebe. Über die Histogenese der Thymus bei Säugetieren. Arch. f. mikr. Anat. 74, 525–621 (1909).

MEDAWAR, P.B., WOODRUFF, M.F.A.: The induction of tolerance by skin homografts on newborn rats. Immunology 1, 27–34 (1958).

METCALF, D., MOORE, M.A.S.: Haemopoietic Cells. Amsterdam-London: North Holland 1971.

MICKLEM, H.S., LOUTIT, J.F.: Tissue Grafting and Radiation. New York-London: Academic Press 1966.

MICKLEM, H.S., FORD, C.E., EVANS, E.P., GRAY, J.: Interrelationships of myeloid and lymphoid cells: Studies with chromosome-marked cells transfused into lethally irradiated mice. Proc. Roy. Soc. B 165, 78–102 (1966).

MILLER, J.F.A.P.: Effects of thymic ablation and replacement. In: The Thymus in Immunobiology, pp. 436–460. New York: Hoeber 1964.

MILLER, J.F.A.P., OSOBA, D.: Current concepts of the immunological function of the thymus. Physiol. Rev. 47, 437–520 (1967).

MILLER, J.F.A.P., BASTEN, A., SPRENT, J., CHEERS, C.: Interaction between lymphocytes in immune responses. Cell. Immunol. 2, 469–495 (1971).

MITCHELL, G.F., MILLER, J.F.A.P.: Cell to cell interaction in the immune response. II. The source of hemolysin-forming cells in irradiated mice given bone marrow and thymus or thoracic duct lymphocytes. J. Exp. Med. 128, 821–837 (1968).

MONACO, A.P., WOOD, M.L., RUSSELL, P.S.: Adult thymectomy: Effect on recovery from immunologic depression in mice. Science 149, 432–434 (1965).

MOORE, M.A.S., OWEN, J.J.T.: Chromosome marker studies on the development of the haemopoietic system in the chick embryo. Nature (London) 208, 956–958 (1965).

MOORE, M.A.S., OWEN, J.J.T.: Stem cell migration in developing myeloid and lymphoid structures. Lancet II, 658–659 (1967a).

MOORE, M.A.S., OWEN, J.J.T.: Experimental studies on the development of the thymus. J. Exp. Med. 126, 715–725 (1967b).

MOORE, M.S.A., METCALF, D.: Ontogeny of the haemopoietic system: Yolk sac origin of in vivo and in vitro colony forming cells in the developing mouse embryo. Brit. J. Haematology 18, 279–296 (1970).

MORRIS, B.: Effect of thymectomy on immunological responses in the sheep. Contemp. Topics. Immunobiol. 2, 39–62 (1973).

MOSIER, D.E.: Ontogeny of mouse lymphocyte function. I. Paradoxical elevation of reactivity to allogeneic cells and phytohemagglutinin in BALB/C fetal thymocytes. J. Immunol. 112, 305–310 (1974).

MOSIER, D.E., JOHNSON, B.M.: Ontogeny of mouse lymphocyte function. II. Development of the ability to produce antibody is modulated by T lymphocytes. J. Exp. Med. 141, 216–226 (1975).

MURRAY, P.D.F.: The development in vitro of the blood of the early chick embryo. Proc. Roy. Soc. B 111, 497–521 (1932).

NAJARIAN, J.S., DIXON, F.J.: Homotransplantation immunity of neonatal rabbits. Proc. Soc. Exp. Biol. (N.Y.) 109, 592–594 (1962).

NAJARIAN, J.S., FOKER, J.E.: Mechanisms of kidney allograft rejection. Transpl. Proc. 1, 184–193 (1969).

NOSSAL, G.J.V., CUNNINGHAM, A., MITCHELL, G.F., MILLER, J.F.A.P.: Cell to cell interaction in the immune response. III. Chromosomal marker analysis of single antibody-forming cells in reconstituted, irradiated and thymectomized mice. J. Exp. Med. 128, 839–853 (1968).

NOSSAL, G.J.V., PIKE, B.L.: Differentiation of B lymphocytes from stem cell precursors. In: Microenvironmental Aspects of Immunity, pp. 11–18. New York-London: Plenum Press 1973a.

NOSSAL, G.J.V., PIKE, B.L.: Studies on the differentiation of B lymphocytes in the mouse. Immunology 25, 33–45 (1973b).

OLD, L.J., BOYSE, E.A., STOCKERT, E.: Antigenic properties of experimental leukemias. I. Serological studies in vitro with spontaneous and radiation-induced leukemias. J. Nat. Cancer Inst. 31, 972–986 (1963).

OWEN, J.J.T.: The origin and development of lymphocyte populations. In: Ontogeny of Acquired Immunity, pp. 35–54. Amsterdam-London-New York: Elsevier 1972.

OWEN, J.J.T.: Anatomy of the lymphoid system. In: Defense and Recognition, pp. 35–64. London: Butterworths 1973.

OWEN, J.J.T., RAFF, M.C.: Studies on the differentiation of thymus-derived lymphocytes. J. Exp. Med. 132, 1216–1232 (1970).

OWEN, J.J.T., RITTER, M.A.: Tissue interactions in the development of thymus lymphocytes. J. Exp. Med. 129, 431–442 (1969).

PAPIERNIK, M.: Correlation of lymphocyte transformation and morphology in the human fetal thymus. Blood 36, 470–479 (1970).

PEREY, D.Y., COOPER, M.D., GOOD, R.A.: Normal second set wattle homograft rejection in agammaglobulinemic chickens. Transplantation 5, 615–623 (1967).

PIROFSKY, B., REID, R.R., RAMIREZ-MATEOS, J.C., BARDANA, E.J., AUGUST, A.: Synergistic immunosuppressive action of antithymocyte antisera and thymectomy in the human. Clin. Exp. Immunol. 12, 89–101 (1972).

PORTER, K.A.: Runt disease and tolerance in rabbits. Nature (London) **185**, 789–790 (1960).

RAFF, M.C., OWEN, J.J.T.: Thymus-derived lymphocytes: Their distribution and role in the development of peripheral lymphoid tissues of the mouse. Europ. J. Immunol. **1**, 27–30 (1971).

RAWLES, M.E.: Pigmentation in autoplastic and homoplastic grafts of skin from foetal and newborn hooded rats. Amer. J. Anat. **97**, 79–127 (1955).

REIF, A.E., ALLEN, J.M.: The AKR thymic antigen and its distribution in leukemias and nervous tissues. J. Exp. Med. **120**, 413–433 (1964).

RITTER, M.A.: Functional maturation of lymphocytes within embryonic mouse thymus. Transplantation **12**, 279–282 (1971).

ROELANTS, G.E.: Antigen recognition by T and B lymphocytes. Current Topics Microbiol. Immunol. **59**, 135–165 (1972).

ROITT, I.M., GREAVES, M.F., TORRIGIANI, G., BROSTOFF, J., PLAYFAIR, J.H.L.: The cellular basis of immunological responses. Lancet **II**, 367–371 (1969).

SABIN, F.R.: On the development of the lymphatic system in human embryos with a consideration of the morphology of the system as a whole. Amer. J. Anat. **9**, 43–91 (1909).

SANEL, F.T.: Ultrastructure of differentiating cells during thymic histogenesis. Z. Zellforsch. **83**, 8–29 (1967).

SCHEID, M.P., GOLDSTEIN, G., HAMMERLING, U., BOYSE, E.A.: Lymphocyte differentiation from precursor cells in vitro. Ann. N.Y. Acad. Sci. **249**, 531–538 (1975).

SCHENDEL, D.J., BACH, F.H.: Genetic control of cell-mediated lympholysis in mouse. J. Exp. Med. **14**, 1534–1546 (1974).

SCHINCKEL, P.G., FERGUSON, K.A.: Skin transplantation in the foetal lamb. Australian J. Biol. Sci. **6**, 533–541 (1953).

SCHLESINGER, M.: Immune lysis of thymus and spleen cells of embryonic and neonatal mice. J. Immunol. **94**, 358–364 (1965).

SCHLESINGER, M.: Expression of antigens in normal mammalian cells. In: Immunity, Cancer and Chemotherapy, pp. 281–306. New York-London: Academic Press 1967.

SCHUBERT, W.K., FOWLER, R., MARTIN, L.W., WESR, C.D.: Homograft rejection in children with congenital immunological defects: agammaglobulinemia and Aldrich syndrome. Transpl. Bull. **26**, 125–128 (1960).

SHIGENO, N., HÄMMERLING, U., ARPELS, C., BOYSE, E.A., OLD, L.J.: Preparation of lymphocyte-specific antibody from anti-lymphocyte serum. Lancet **II**, 320–323 (1968).

SILINI, G., POZZI, L.V., PONS, S.: Studies on the haemopoietic stem cells of mouse foetal liver. J. Embryol. Exp. Morph. **17**, 303–318 (1967).

SILVERSTEIN, A.M., PRENDERGAST, R.A., KRANER, K.L.: Homograft rejection in the fetal lamb: The role of circulating antibody. Science **142**, 1172–1173 (1963).

SILVERSTEIN, A.M., PRENDERGAST, R.A.: Lymphogenesis, immunogenesis and the generation of immunological diversity. In: Developmental Aspects of Antibody Formation and Structure, pp. 69–77. New York-London: Academic Press 1970.

SMITH, C.: Studies on the thymus of the mammal. XIV. Histology and histochemistry of embryonic and early postnatal thymuses of C57BL/6 and AKR strain mice. Amer. J. Anat. **116**, 611–629 (1965).

SOLOMON, J.B.: Fetal Neonatal Immunology. Amsterdam: North Holland 1971.

SOSIN, H., HILGARD, H., MARTINEZ, C.: The immunologic competence of mouse thymus cells measured by the graft-versus-host spleen assay. J. Immunol. **96**, 189–195 (1966).

SPEAR, P.G., WONG, A.L., RUTISHAUSER, U., EDELMAN, G.M.: Characteristics of splenic lymphoid cells in fetal and newborn mice. J. Exp. Med. **138**, 557–573 (1973).

SPRENT, J.: Circulating T and B lymphocytes in the mouse. I. Migratory properties. Cell. Immunol. **7**, 10–39 (1973).

STEINMULLER, D.: Transplantation immunity in the newborn rat. I. The response at birth and maturation of response capacity. J. Exp. Zool. **147**, 233–257 (1961).

STERZL, J., SILVERSTEIN, A.M.: Developmental aspects of immunity. Adv. Immunol. **7**, 337–460 (1967).

STITES, D.P., WYBRAN, J., CARR, M.C., FUDENBERG, H.H.: Development of cellular immune competence in man. In: Ontogeny of Acquired Immunity, pp. 113–129. Amsterdam-London-New York: Elsevier 1972.

STITES, D.P., CARR, M.C., FUDENBERG, H.H.: Ontogeny of cellular immunity in the human fetus. Development of response to phytohemagglutinin and to allogeneic cells. Cell Immunol. **11**, 257–271 (1974).

STOBO, J.D., PAUL, W.E.: Functional heterogeneity of murine lymphoid cells. II. Acquisition of mitogen responsiveness and of θ antigen during the ontogeny of thymocytes and "T" lymphocytes. Cell. Immunol. **4**, 367–380 (1972).

STOBO, J.D., PAUL, W.E.: Functional heterogeneity of murine lymphoid cells. III. Differential responsiveness of T-cells to phytohemagglutinin and Concanavalin A as a probe for T-cell subsets. J. Immunol. **110**, 362–375 (1973).

STOCKERT, E., OLD, L.J., BOYSE, E.A.: The G_{ix} system: A cell surface alloantigen associated with murine leukemia virus; implications regarding chromosomal integration of the viral genome. J. Exp. Med. **133**, 1334–1355 (1971).

STUTMAN, O.: Hemopoietic origin of cells responding to phytohemagglutinin in mouse lymph nodes. In: Proc. Fifth Leukocyte Culture Conference, pp. 671–681. New York: Academic Press 1970.

STUTMAN, O.: Traffic of cells and development of immunity. In: Membranes and Viruses in Immunopathology, pp. 437–450. New York-London: Academic Press 1972.

STUTMAN, O.: Hemopoietic origin of B-cells in the mouse. In: Microenvironmental Aspects of Immunity, pp. 19–26. New York-London: Plenum Press 1973.

STUTMAN, O.: Humoral thymic factors influencing postthymic cells. Ann. N.Y. Acad. Sci. **249**, 89–104 (1975a).

STUTMAN, O.: Characterization of a T-cell precursor in mouse spleen. Transpl. Proc. **7**, 291–293 (1975b).

STUTMAN, O., GOOD, R.A.: Traffic of hemopoietic cells to the thymus: Influence of histocompatibility differences. Exp. Hemat. **19**, 12–15 (1969).

STUTMAN, O., GOOD, R.A.: Immunocompetence of cells derived from hemopoietic liver after traffic to thymus. In: Morphological and Functional Aspects of Immunity, pp. 129–133. New York: Plenum Press 1971a.

STUTMAN, O., GOOD, R.A.: Immunocompetence of embryonic hemopoietic cells after traffic to thymus. Transpl. Proc. **3**, 923–925 (1971b).

STUTMAN, O., YUNIS, E.J., GOOD, R.A.: Studies on thymus function. II. Cooperative effect of newborn and embryonic hemopoietic liver cells with thymus function. J. Exp. Med. **132**, 601–612 (1970).

SZENBERG, A., WARNER, N.L.: Immunological reactions of bursaless fowls to homograft antigens. Ann. N.Y. Acad. Sci. **120**, 150–161 (1964).

TAYLOR, R.B.: Plutipotential stem cells in mouse embryo liver. Brit. J. Exp. Path. **46**, 376–383 (1965).

TERRES, G., HUGHES, W.L.: Acquired immune tolerance in mice to crystalline bovine serum albumin. J. Immunol. **83**, 459–467 (1959).

TILL, J.E., McCULLOCH, E.A., SIMINOVITCH, L.: A stochastic model of stem cell proliferation based on the growth of spleen colonyforming cells. Proc. Nat. Acad. Sci. (Wash.) **51**, 29–36 (1964).

TRAININ, N., KOOK, A.I., UMIEL, T., ALBALA, M.: The nature and mechanism of stimulation of immune responsiveness by thymus extracts. Ann. N.Y. Acad. Sci. **249**, 349–361 (1975).

TRENTIN, J.J., WOLF, N., CHENG, V., FAHLBERG, W., WEISS, D., BONHAG, R.: Antibody production by mice repopulated with limited numbers of clones of lymphoid cell precursors. J. Immunol. **98**, 1326–1337 (1967).

TURPEN, J.B., VOLPE, E.P., COHEN, N.: Ontogeny and peripheralization of thymic lymphocytes. Science **182**, 931–933 (1973).

TURPEN, J.B., VOLPE, E.P., COHEN, N.: On the origin of thymic lymphocytes. Amer. Zool. **15**, 51–61 (1975).

TYAN, M.L.: Studies on the ontogeny of the mouse immune system. I. Cell-bound immunity. J. Immunol. **100**, 535–542 (1968).

TYAN, M.L., COLE, L.J.: Mouse fetal liver and thymus: Potential source of immunologically active cells. Transplantation **1**, 347–350 (1963).

TYAN, M.L., COLE, L.J.: Further observations on potential immunologically competent cells of fetal liver origin. Transplantation **4**, 557–564 (1966).

TYAN, M.L., COLE, L.J., NOWELL, P.C.: Fetal liver and thymus: Roles in the ontogenesis of the mouse immune system. Transplantation **4**, 79–83 (1966).

TYAN, M.L., HERZENBERG, L.A.: Immunoglobulin production by embryonic tissues: Thymus independent. Proc. Soc. Exp. Biol. (N.Y.) **128**, 952–954 (1968).

UHR, J.W.: Development of delayed hypersensitivity in guinea pig embryos. Nature (London) **187**, 957–958 (1960).

UHR, J.W., DANCIS, J., NEWMAN, C.G.: Delayed-type hypersensitivity in premature neonatal humans. Nature (London) **187**, 1130–1132 (1960).

VAN ALTEN, P.J., CAIN, W.A., GOOD, R.A., COOPER, M.D.: Gammaglobulin production and antibody synthesis in chickens bursectomized as embryos. Nature (London) **217**, 358–360 (1968).

VAN FURTH, R., SCHUIT, H.R.E., HIJMANS, W.: The immunological development of the human fetus. J. Exp. Med. **122**, 1173–1188 (1965).

WIGZELL, H.: On the relationship between cellular and humoral antibodies. Contemp. Topics Immunobiol. **3**, 77–96 (1974).

WILSON, D.B., BILLINGHAM, R.E.: Lymphocytes and Transplantation Immunity. Adv. Immunol. **7**, 189–273 (1967).

WORTIS, H.H.: Immunological studies of nude mice. Contemp. Topics Immunobiol. **3**, 243–263 (1974).

WU, A.M., TILL, J.E., SIMINOVITCH, L., McCULLOCH, E.A.: Cytological evidence for a relationship between normal haematopoietic colony-forming cells and cells of the lymphoid system. J. Exp. Med. **127**, 455–464 (1968).

Humoral and Cell-Mediated Mechanisms of Allograft Rejection

K. Theodor Brunner and Jean-Charles Cerottini

A. Introduction

Allograft immunity is generally considered as a manifestation of cell-mediated immunity (CMI). This concept was introduced by MITCHISON (1954) and BILLINGHAM et al. (1954), who showed that allograft immunity could be regularly transferred from immune donors to normal recipients with lymphoid cells, but not with serum. However, the actual mechanism by which transfer of immune lymphoid cells leads to graft destruction is still not entirely elucidated.

Basic investigations of the mechanisms of graft rejection began with in vivo observations of normal tissue or tumor allografts undergoing rejection, and of local and systemic graft-versus-host reactions. The basic event observed was an invasive-destructive lesion of the graft produced by mononuclear cells composed mainly of lymphoid cells and macrophages, similar to those observed in delayed type hypersensitivity reactions. The case in favor of a decisive role of CMI in graft rejection was further strengthened by the demonstration of successful allografts in immunosuppressed or immunodeficient recipients with impairment of CMI, and the lack of success in recipients with a selective deficiency in antibody formation. Similar conclusions were drawn from studies of grafts to privileged sites (eye, brain, hamster cheek pouch), and from the in vivo use of diffusion chambers bearing cell-impermeable membranes. The weight of all these observations was somewhat counterbalanced by occasional reports describing graft rejection following local injection or transfer of large amounts of antiserum, as for instance in skin grafts to rabbits or to nude mice. It was also noted that grafts in the form of cell suspensions such as

---

Abbreviations used in this contribution:

CMI:	cell-mediated immunity	*CL:*	cytotoxic lymphocytes
CMC:	cell-mediated cytotoxicity	*PFC:*	plaque forming cells
T-cells:	thymus-derived lymphocytes	*GVH:*	graft-versus-host
B-cells:	bursa-derived lymphocytes	*ConA:*	concanavalin A
CTL:	cytolytic T lymphocytes	*CB:*	cytochalasin B
K-cells:	killer cells	*AD-CMC:*	antibody-dependent CMC
Fc:	Fc portion of IgG molecules	*AD-LMC:*	antibody-dependent LMC
MLC:	mixed leukocyte culture	*SMAF:*	specific macrophage arming factor
PHA:	phytohemagglutinin	*EDTA:*	ethylene-diamine tetraacetic acid

allogeneic leukemia cells, leukocytes, erythrocytes, and platelets, or grafts to preimmunized recipients appear to be particularly sensitive to antibody.

More recently, the problem of the complexity inherent in in vivo studies has been at least partly overcome by the introduction of in vitro models of allograft immunity. The first of these models was based on the observation that lymphoid cells from immune donors could destroy in vitro target cells carrying surface antigens to which the donors were sensitized. These cytotoxic reactions could be distinguished from those mediated by antibody and complement, and the term cell-mediated cytotoxicity (CMC) was generally adopted to describe them. Based on these results, it was assumed that CMC was an in vitro correlate of CMI to allografts in vivo. As will be discussed below, this is by no means the case.

Further studies of CMC were greatly facilitated by progress in the characterization of cells involved in immune responses. It was shown that lymphocytes could be divided into T- and B-cells, both containing antigen-reactive cells which could proliferate and differentiate when stimulated by specific antigen. Whereas B-cells differentiate into antibody-forming cells, and are thus responsible for humoral immunity, T-cells differentiate into effector cells with various functions, including (a) helper activity in antibody formation, (b) release of various factors mediating delayed hypersensitivity reactions, (c) activation of macrophages in infections with intracellular microorganisms, and (d) cytotoxicity for target cells carrying sensitizing antigens.

Cytolytic T lymphocytes (CTL) are thus the effector cells involved in some in vitro systems of CMC. However, it is now generally recognized that several mechanisms of CMC exist, involving different cell types. In fact, recent studies have shown at least two different pathways by which lymphocytes exert a direct cytotoxic effect on target cells in vitro. The first is mediated by sensitized T-cells which interact directly with membrane-associated antigens via specific receptors. Humoral antibody is not involved and may even inhibit, presumably by competing with the CTL for the same antigenic determinants. The second pathway depends on the presence of IgG antibody bound to target cell antigens, and is mediated by normal lymphoid cells carrying receptors for the Fc portion of IgG molecules. Although present evidence indicates that the effector cells, usually described as K or killer cells, of this antibody-dependent CMC are not T-cells, their exact nature remains to be established. Monocytes and PMN cells also have receptors for Fc, but their cytotoxic activity appears to be restricted to antibody-coated erythrocytes. In addition to lymphocytes, it has been shown that macrophages carrying cytophilic antibodies or specific "arming" factors (receptors?) released by sensitized T-cells may induce specific cytotoxicity in vitro. Depending on the assay system, the source of target cells, the allograft model system or the time of immunization, CMC may thus involve T and non-T lymphoid cells, macrophages, antibody, and soluble factors, which participate alone or in combination. As will be discussed below, an additional complexity has been suggested by the recent demonstration of effector T-cells which act as "memory" cells with no direct lytic activity, but capable of differentiating into highly active cells within a few hours following contact with the appropriate antigenic stimulus.

A further important in vitro model of allograft immunity has been introduced by the recent demonstration that CTL with specificity for alloantigens can be generated in unidirectional mixed leukocyte cultures (MLC). This provided a system in which both induction and effector phase of cell-mediated immunity could be studied. In attempts to characterize the antigenic determinants recognized by T-cells responding to alloantigens in MLC, evidence was obtained suggesting that the complementary structures recognized by CTL in target cell destruction were identical to or closely related with H-2 or HL-A antigens, but that the proliferative response leading to the generation of CTL depended on additional antigenic differences coded by genes located in the major histocompatibility complex. Furthermore, studies of CTL induction in long-term mouse MLC have shown that the same lymphocyte population could be repeatedly stimulated by the same alloantigen, and that each stimulation resulted in a rapid increase in cytotoxicity followed by proliferation. Further studies, based on cell separation techniques, have led to the tentative establishment of a differentiation pathway for CTL (see Section E).

The in vivo significance of the various expressions of CMC in vitro is difficult to evaluate. However, advances in the study of the physicochemical and functional properties of cells involved in immune responses, and the availability of new methods of cell separation and identification based on surface markers and differences in size, density, electrophoretic mobility, adherence, and phagocytic activity, have allowed the design of appropriate experiments. In particular, it has become possible to obtain well-defined cell populations for transfer to immunologically deprived allograft recipients, or to isolate, identify, and study cell populations from grafts undergoing rejection. The limited number of such studies carried out so far have shown that it is possible to transfer allograft immunity to lethally irradiated recipients with purified immune T-cell populations containing CTL induced either in vivo or in vitro. This suggested that CTL alone can be effective in graft rejection. Studies of cells isolated from grafts and tumors undergoing rejection have also demonstrated the presence of CTL, whereas solid evidence for the presence of cytotoxic macrophages is so far lacking. It has also recently been shown that immune cell populations devoid of measurable CTL but containing increased numbers of CTL precursor cells (memory cells?) could transfer immunity. No model system demonstrating the transfer of allograft rejection with cytotoxic macrophages or showing functional in vivo activity of antibody-dependent CMC has, however, so far been described.

Although most in vitro and in vivo studies thus point to the importance of effector mechanisms of cell-mediated immunity (CTL and/or macrophages armed or activated by sensitized T lymphocytes) in graft rejection, it is also clear that humoral immunity (antibody and complement or antibody and macrophages or K-cells) may contribute to or independently mediate graft destruction. The relative importance of the two basic immune mechanisms, both of which may involve amplification by macrophages, appears to depend on the type of graft, the concentration and type of antibody, and the availability of complement, macrophages, and perhaps K-cells.

In attempts to evaluate the relative importance of cell-mediated versus humoral immunity in graft rejection, it has also become increasingly clear that, as in all immune responses, T- and B-cell functions are closely interrelated, and are subject to complex regulatory mechanisms effective both at the induction and effector level. Of particular importance are (a) regulation by antibody (enhancement), (b) tolerance induction and/or blocking by antigen or immune complexes, (c) helper and suppressor activity of subpopulations of T- and B-cells, and perhaps (d) regulation by humoral and cellular antireceptor responses.

In this complex system, mechanisms that protect the graft are opposed to those that destroy it. Knowledge of these mechanisms is therefore of decisive importance if specific unresponsiveness rather than the nonspecific immunodepression presently used in human organ grafting is to be achieved. Prolonged or indefinite survival of organ allografts has already been obtained in experimental animals with various protocols inducing specific unresponsiveness.

In the present review, a number of distinct mechanisms of cell-mediated cytotoxicity which have been described in recent years as a result of in vitro studies of cell-mediated and humoral immunity in allogeneic systems will be presented. The nature of the effector cells, the mechanisms underlying the various pathways of cytotoxicity in vitro, and the relevance of the in vitro findings to the rejection of allografts in vivo will be discussed. Further details can be found in recent reviews (MÖLLER, G., 1973; CEROTTINI, J.-C. and BRUNNER, K.T., 1974).

B. Assay Methods of Cell-Mediated Cytotoxicity (CMC)

Following the first observations of specific in vitro cytotoxicity of lymphocytes from allograft recipients, numerous methods for the quantitative assay of CMC have been proposed. A detailed description of these methods, and a discussion of their applicability and limitations has been presented in recent articles (BLOOM and GLADE, 1971; BLOOM et al., 1973; SMITH and LANDY, 1975). The assay for CMC usually follows two basic approaches. The first measures target cell lysis based on the release of radioactivity (usually ^{51}Cr) from prelabeled target cells. This provides a simple, rapid, and sensitive test which is independent of target cell proliferation, and has proved particularly useful for the quantitative assay of CMC in well-defined model systems of allografts and tumor immunity, and in the analysis of the mechanisms of target cell destruction. The second is based on the evaluation of target cell numbers (by visual counts or postlabeling) following incubation with lymphocytes for 48 hours. This test is usually performed with target cells grown as monolayers in microplates, and viable cell counts at the end of the incubation period may reflect a combination of direct lysis, cell detachment, and growth inhibition and/or stimulation. The test has been widely used in assays of CMC in syngeneic tumor systems.

Contradictory results have occasionally been obtained when CMC of immune cells was tested in parallel with the ^{51}Cr release test and the microplate assay. In studies in rat kidney allograft recipients it was found that the short-term

^{51}Cr release test measured the cytotoxic effect of sensitized T-cells only, whereas the 48-hour microplate assay detected both cytotoxicity of T- and non-T-cells (BIESECKER et al., 1973). Similar observations were made in mouse tumor systems (PLATA et al., 1974). These results have drawn renewed attention to the fact that CMC is the expression of more than one mechanism (see Section H), and that different assay systems may not measure the same one.

In view of the complexity of the factors that can influence the final result of the microplate assay, the present report will be mainly based on results obtained with the ^{51}Cr release test. The sensitivity and precision of this assay allows the detection of CMC in appropriate model systems in a few minutes after incubation of cytotoxic lymphocytes and target cells. Its application may, however, be limited by the high spontaneous release of isotope label ($> 2\%$/hour) from some freshly explanted target cells, which may reach unsuitable levels especially if prolonged incubation times are needed to detect cytotoxicity. Another factor which might be limiting is the relatively high number of lymphocytes required for the test, since a minimum of approx. 3×10^3–10^4 target cells/tube is used to provide sufficient radioactive label, and high lymphocyte/target cell ratios (up to 100:1) may be needed to detect small numbers of CTL.

In general, studies of CMC are severely limited by the lack of assays for detecting individual effector cells. However, the ^{51}Cr release test allows the estimation of the relative frequency of effector cells in different cell populations (CEROTTINI and BRUNNER, 1974). Such an estimate is based on the existence of a quantitative relationship between the number of target cells lysed and the concentration of effector cells. In well-defined systems, in which a constant number of labeled target cells has been exposed to increasing numbers of immune lymphoid cells for a constant period of time, it has been found that specific cytotoxicity varied linearly with the logarithm of the number of lymphoid cells. Moreover, it was observed that the dose-response curves obtained with different cell populations resulted in parallel lines. It is therefore possible to estimate the relative frequency of effector cells by comparing the number of cells required to achieve a fixed value of ^{51}Cr release, for example 50 percent of the releasable isotope. A different approach for the quantitative evaluation of effector cell frequencies has recently been proposed by MILLER and DUNKLEY (1974).

It should perhaps be mentioned here that in contrast to the ^{51}Cr release assay, a simple dose-response curve is usually not obtained in the microplate assay. In fact, a dose-dependent growth stimulating effect, or, at higher concentrations, a growth inhibitory effect of normal control lymphocytes may be observed. Superimposed on this is the specific inhibitory and/or cytotoxic effect of immune lymphocytes, making the quantitative evaluation of cytotoxicity difficult.

The demonstration of specificity of CMC is usually based on the use of target cells bearing related or unrelated membrane antigens. However, for reasons which are still unclear, important differences in susceptibility to lysis of different cells of the same genotype are encountered, and may render the interpretation of results of direct cytotoxicity tests difficult. The selection of appropriate target cells is therefore of great importance. As a rule, lymphoblast or lymphoma cell lines provide more sensitive target cells than adherent cells like fibroblasts or macrophages, although the latter have the advantage of being readily available. Obviously, the choice of highly sensitive target cells of the appropriate genotype may increase the sensitivity of the cytotoxic test manyfold. An example is the use of PHA-induced lymphoblasts instead of lymphocytes in the detection of cytotoxic lymphocytes formed in human mixed leukocyte cultures (LIGHTBODY et al., 1971).

C. Cytotoxicity Mediated by Specifically Sensitized T-Cells

In vitro cytotoxicity of lymphoid cells from allograft recipients was first observed by GOVAERTS (1960) and ROSENAU and MOON (1961), a result which was subsequently confirmed in many similar studies. The cytotoxic effect was originally considered to represent a manifestation of CMI. However, not until 1970 was direct evidence obtained that sensitized T lymphocytes can destroy appropriate target cells independently of antibody, normal T- or B-cells, antibody-forming cells, K-cells, and/or macrophages.

The early studies had shown cytotoxicity of immune lymphoid cells to be specific, to depend on close contact between reacting cells, and to be independent of added complement. Antibody was apparently not involved since addition of alloantibody directed against the target cells inhibited rather than increased cytotoxicity. The first observations had also suggested that target cell destruction was a slow process of several hours or days, but the subsequent development of improved assay methods, the availability of cell populations containing a high frequency of effector cells, and the use of highly sensitive target cells allowed the demonstration that target cell killing can take place within minutes.

The first direct evidence for mediation of cytotoxicity by sensitized T-cells was provided by studies of the formation of cytotoxic lymphocytes (CL) and of alloantibody plaque forming cells (PFC) in inbred mice (CEROTTINI et al., 1970a; CEROTTINI et al., 1970b; CEROTTINI et al., 1971). Based on methods allowing the independent assay of both types of effector cells against the same target cells in vitro, it was successively shown that (a) spleen cells transferred into lethally irradiated allogeneic recipients produced both CL and PFC, whereas transferred thymus cells produced CL only, and (b) specific elimination of T lymphocytes from immune spleen cells with anti-θ serum and complement abrogated CMC without reducing the number of PFC, whereas treatment of the same cells with rabbit antiserum against mouse B-cells or plasma cells and complement completely inhibited the formation of PFC without affecting CL.

These results, which were confirmed in several other studies (CEROTTINI and BRUNNER, 1974), showed that sensitized T-cells were responsible for CMC in allograft responses and GVH reactions in mice. Similar conclusions were drawn from subsequent studies of CL formation in mixed leukocyte cultures, where both spleen and thymus cells produced CL in response to allogeneic stimulation (WAGNER et al., 1973; HÄYRY et al., 1972).

D. In Vivo Formation of Cytotoxic T Lymphocytes

With the development of quantitative in vitro assays for CMC, it has become possible to follow the appearance of cytotoxic T lymphocytes (CTL) during the primary and secondary response to histoincompatible grafts. In a limited number of studies in mice and rats, the appearance of CTL was measured with the ^{51}Cr-release test following allogeneic skin grafts or intraperitoneal, subcutaneous, or intravenous injection of normal or malignant allogeneic cells, and (in rats) following kidney allografts. After skin grafts in mice, CTL were first detected on day 6 in the regional lymph nodes, and subsequently in the spleen and contralateral nodes (DEGIOVANNI, 1972). Following intraperitoneal injection of allogeneic tumor cells, comparative studies of CTL appearance in spleen and blood showed a delay between formation in the spleen and release into the circulation (BRUNNER et al., 1970). Depending on the type and site of graft, cytotoxic activity in general reaches a peak between days 6–12, and then drops first rapidly and then gradually to very low levels over a period of weeks or months. Highest activities are observed at the rejection site, that is, following intraperitoneal injection in the peritoneal cavity, after skin grafts in the regional lymph nodes, and after intravenous injection in the spleen. Activities are also high in the blood and thoracic duct, but negligable in the thymus. These observations indicate that at least some of the CTL belong to the circulating pool of lymphocytes.

A close correlation between peak CTL activity and allograft rejection was usually observed in these studies, a result which is in support of a definite role of these cells in graft destruction. It should be noted, however, that cytotoxic antibody is also produced in allograft immunity, and the peak of cytotoxic activity has been found to coincide closely with the peak of IgM alloantibody.

Another important aspect of CTL formation in response to allografts concerns the question of memory. Accelerated rejection of second grafts of the same specificity had suggested the existence of a secondary type of cell-mediated immune response, based on the presence of increased numbers of antigen-reactive lymphocytes or memory cells. However, persistence of effector cells in the primed host could also have accounted for accelerated graft rejection. Recent studies in vivo and in vitro have now provided strong evidence in favor of the concept of memory T-cell formation in response to allogeneic stimulation (BRUNNER and CEROTTINI, 1971; CEROTTINI et al., 1974b; WILSON, 1974). It was first shown that in the absence of measurable CTL, mice preimmunized with allogeneic cells responded to a second stimulation by the same alloantigen with an earlier appearance, accelerated formation, and higher peak of CTL. Subsequent studies showed that a typical secondary formation of CTL could also be demonstrated in vitro with spleen cells from immunized mice, suggesting the presence of increased numbers of CTL precursor (memory) cells (see Section E). In addition, in both instances a qualitative difference between primary and secondary (memory) CTL precursor cells was suggested by the almost identical response of the latter to particulate antigen and intact cells, whereas adequate primary responses could only be elicited with intact cells (ENGERS et al., 1975).

E. In Vitro Formation of Cytotoxic T Lymphocytes

Important progress in the understanding of the formation and of the differentiation pathway of cytotoxic T lymphocytes (CTL) has been provided by studies of in vitro induction. The first demonstration of in vitro formation of CL was made in a xenogeneic system using rat lymphocyte cultures on mouse fibroblast monolayers (Ginsburg, 1968; Berke et al., 1969). Häyry and Defendi (1970) then made the important observation in the mouse that CTL were generated in unidirectional mixed leukocyte cultures (MLC). Cytotoxicity of the effector cells was specifically directed against histocompatibility antigens carried by target cells syngeneic to the stimulating cells, whereas target cells of the responder genotype or cells carrying other unrelated antigens were not affected.

Of the several systems of in vitro induction of CTL described in various species, including man, the culturing of normal (responding) lymphocytes with allogeneic, mitomycin, or x-ray treated (stimulating) lymphocytes in MLC appear to be the most effective, that is, lymphoid cells were found to stimulate better than nonlymphoid cells. It was also shown that both T- and B-cells could induce CTL formation and that the ratio of stimulator to responder cells and the presence of adherent cells was important for optimal responses.

In the mouse, conclusive evidence was obtained that the precursors of CTL formed in MLC are thymus-derived cells (Wagner et al., 1973; Häyry et al., 1972). Nearly pure populations of T-cells such as thymus cells or spleen cells depleted of B-cells were able to generate CL in MLC. These results were confirmed by the demonstration that the cytotoxic activity of the effector cells could be abolished by the selective destruction of T-cells with anti-θ serum and complement. Removal of B-cells from the responding cell population had no effect on CTL generation in MLC, suggesting the absence of B-T cooperation in the induction phase. On the other hand, cooperation between two T-cell subpopulations has been suggested (Wagner et al., 1974).

Improvements in culture conditions of mouse MLC, depending in particular on the addition of 2-mercaptoethanol, have resulted in increased cytotoxic activities, and have allowed the analysis of CTL formation in long-term cultures (Cerottini et al., 1974a; Macdonald et al., 1974; Macdonald et al., 1975a; Macdonald et al., 1975c). In such a system, cytotoxic activity was first detected on day 2, rose rapidly to a peak on days 4–5, and then declined slowly. Cell separation studies showed that at the peak of the response, cytotoxicity was associated with medium to large cells, while residual activity was found in the small lymphocyte region. When spleen cells from mice previously immunized with the same alloantigen were stimulated in MLC, a typical secondary type of response was observed, characterized by the accelerated formation of higher levels of CTL. This suggested the presence of increased numbers of CTL precursor (or memory) cells in the immune cell population. Further analysis showed that the same MLC population could be repeatedly stimulated in vitro over a period of several weeks by reexposure to the same alloantigen. Kinetic studies revealed that a rapid increase in cytotoxicity occurred in the first 24 hours after restimulation, and that this increase was independent of DNA synthesis (or proliferation), but associated with a concomitant increase in cell size. This apparent differentiation step was regularly followed by proliferation and a parallel increase in cytotoxic activity. Since cell fractions showing the highest response upon restimulation also contained the residual CTL generated during the earlier MLC, it was tempting to speculate that the same cell can be stimulated repeatedly, that is, that CTL differentiate into precursors or memory cells.

The CTL induced by repeated stimulation in MLC proved to be highly active in vitro and in vivo, that is, they led to target cell destruction at ratios of effector to target cells as low as 0.3:1, and protected lethally irradiated mice against subcutaneous growth of allogeneic tumor cells when injected intravenously (CEROTTINI et al., in preparation).

F. Mechanism of T-Cell Cytotoxicity

In recent years, the study of the mechanism of target cell destruction by cytotoxic lymphocytes has been greatly facilitated by the availability of highly active effector cells, and the use of quantitative in vitro assay systems, in particular the ^{51}Cr release test. The subject has been reviewed in detail elsewhere (CEROTTINI and BRUNNER, 1974 and 1976).

Early studies had shown that cytotoxicity was specific, needed no added complement, and depended on close contact between viable CTL and the relevant target cells. Thus, initiation and rate of lysis was considerably accelerated when the reacting cells were centrifuged to a pellet, or when Petri dishes containing the dispersed cells were rocked on a platform. On the other hand, lymphocytes and target cells suspended in semisolid or viscous media did not interact.

Following contact mediated by specific receptors, irreversible changes of the membrane permeability of target cells occur very rapidly. The actual pathway of this lethal event is, however, unknown. The demonstration of specificity of the cytotoxic effect does not necessarily imply the presence of specific effector molecules. By analogy with antibody-dependent, complement-mediated lysis, cytotoxicity of CTL may be considered as a two-step phenomenon involving specific recognition followed by nonspecific lysis. This concept is also supported by the observation that lymphocytes stimulated with PHA, ConA, or specific staphylococcal antigen exert a nonspecific cytotoxic effect if close contact or bridging to target cells is provided for. The nonspecific step is not, however, mediated by a diffusible nonspecific factor, such as lymphotoxin, since it could be shown that unrelated target cells added to a system of CTL and relevant target cells were not affected. On the other hand, it cannot be excluded that such factors are released at the site of contact and are active at short range.

Using lymphocyte populations containing high relative frequencies of CTL, it has been possible to show that lysis may proceed at a rate almost as fast as that induced by antibody and complement, that is, to become measurable within minutes (MACDONALD, 1975). The data also indicate that one lymphocyte can kill several target cells, since the number of target cells lysed may exceed the number of lymphocytes added, and two successive populations of target cells may be destroyed with undiminished efficiency by the same effector cell population.

It is well established that cytotoxic lymphocytes must be alive and metabolically active to be effective. Inhibitors of energy metabolism and of RNA and protein synthesis, but not of DNA synthesis, were shown to reduce or abolish cytotoxicity. To what extent these inhibitors affected the target cells is, however, not clear. Total but reversible inhibition of cytotoxicity was also noted with EDTA and with cytochalasin B, a drug which might act either by disrupting the microfilament system, or by affecting transport of glucose and glucosamine. Evidence has finally been obtained that drugs which increase the intracellular cAMP level inhibit cytotoxicity, and the involvement of secretory processes modulated by intracellular cAMP and cGMP has been suggested.

Several groups of investigators have attempted to resolve the lytic process into discrete steps, based mainly on the analysis of specific attachment and differential dependence on temperature and calcium and magnesium ions (Henney, 1973; Berke and Amos, 1973; Martz, 1974). It was generally agreed that the first step was characterized by the establishment of a physical adhesion between effector and target cell, which, according to one study (Martz, 1975) is quite firm and takes place within one minute at 37° C. In the same study it was shown that formation of adhesions could be prevented, and adhesions could be disrupted, by EDTA. If CTL were separated from target cells immediately after adhesions had formed, the lytic process was prevented. If, however, the aggregates were incubated for a few minutes at 37° C under conditions which prevented further interactions (addition of 10% dextran), lysis occurred during the next 2–3 hours, even in the presence of EDTA, or when effector cells were destroyed with specific antiserum and complement, or were inactivated by heating at 45° C. In summary, target cell lysis was resolved into three steps, namely (1) physical adhesion, (2) lethal interaction, and (3) effector cell independent lysis. Since lysis leading to release of radioactivity from ^{51}Cr-labeled target cells is a slow process, the ^{51}Cr release test underestimates the rate of target cell killing. On the other hand, since at high effector cell to target cell ratios significant lysis can be demonstrated within a few minutes, it seems possible that multiple lethal interactions may occur and lead to accelerated release of ^{51}Cr.

G. Specificity of Target Cell Destruction by Cytotoxic T Lymphocytes

Specificity of target cell destruction by CTL has been convincingly demonstrated in a great many experiments. Specificity, that is, lysis of target cells carrying transplantation antigens identical to or cross reacting with the sensitizing antigen and not of target cells carrying unrelated antigens is, however, relative, since cytotoxicity depends on the sensitivity of the particular target cell used. It may thus be important to consider the ratio between the minimal number of lymphocytes required for significant lysis, and the maximal number of normal or irrelevant immune lymphocytes producing no lysis of the same target cell.

Specificity suggests the presence of specific receptors on the surface of CTL, complementary to antigenic determinants on the target cell surface. Support for the existence of such receptors has been provided by experiments showing specific adsorption of CTL on appropriate target cell monolayers, and by inhibition of cytotoxicity by antisera directed against the appropriate transplantation antigens. Attempts to inhibit target cell destruction by CTL with soluble, serologically active antigen preparations have, however, so far not been successful.

In attempts to define more accurately the specificity of the antigenic determinants recognized by cytotoxic T lymphocytes, an inhibition assay using a mixture of ^{51}Cr-labeled and unlabeled target cells was proposed (ORTIZ-LANDAZURI and HERBERMAN, 1972). Competitive inhibition of lysis of labeled target cells by immune lymphoid cells was noticed in the presence of unlabeled target cells bearing the sensitizing antigens, whereas lysis was unaffected by the addition of target cells lacking the relevant antigens. The general applicability of this method to different systems remains to be established.

H. Antibody-Dependent Cytotoxicity Mediated by Normal Lymphoid Cells

Following the original observation by MÖLLER (1965), it has been shown that target cells coated with small amounts of specific IgG antibody may be lysed in vitro by certain thymus-independent lymphoid cells from normal donors as well as by normal nonlymphoid cells such as monocytes, macrophages, and polymorphonuclear (PMN) cells (PERLMANN and HOLM, 1969; MACLENNAN, 1972; PERLMANN et al., 1972). A common feature of these effector cells is their surface receptors for the Fc portion of the IgG molecule, by virtue of which they interact with the antibody-coated target cells. Cytotoxicity is independent of added complement, and will operationally be referred to as antibody-dependent cell-mediated cytotoxicity (AD-CMC), or when mediated by lymphoid cells as AD-LMC. The antibody involved in this phenomenon is also referred to as lymphocyte-dependent antibody (LDA).

A certain amount of confusion has been caused by the fact that reports concerning AD-CMC have often described results obtained with a heterogenous combination of target cells (including erythrocytes), antibody, and lymphoid cells from different species. It is now generally agreed, however, that although effector cells from different species may have somewhat different properties, they can tentatively be separated into two types. The first is a lymphoid cell, usually referred to as K (or killer) cell, able to lyse most IgG antibody-coated target cells with the exception of erythrocytes (but including chicken erythrocytes). The second is represented by nonlymphoid cells (monocytes, PMN cells) which are strongly active against sensitized erythrocytes (including chicken erythrocytes), and much less so against other cells.

In man, AD-LMC has been particularly well studied. It was shown that human peripheral blood lymphocytes from which most PMN cells and monocytes had been removed had pronounced cytotoxic activity for antibody-coated chicken erythrocytes or human cell lines. The active cells, usually designated as K-cells, were found to be nonadherent, nonphagocytic, small to medium size lymphocyte-like cells which could not be classified as either T- or B-cells. For the investigation of human K-cells, ^{51}Cr-labeled Chang liver cells (a human cell line) or cultured mouse leukemia cells (L 1210 or EL4 cell lines) coated with rabbit antibody have been used as target cells. In addition, human lymphocytes sensitized with anti-HL-A antibodies, chicken erythrocytes, and other cell types were shown to be adequate target cells.

A nonlymphoid effector cell of AD-CMC in human peripheral blood has the characteristics of a monocyte, and is cytotoxic for human group A or Rh-positive red blood cells sensitized with appropriate IgG isoantibody (HOLM, 1972). Human monocytes are also found to be cytotoxic for sensitized chicken erythrocytes, a cell which is also sensitive to human K-cells, certain B-cells, and neutrophils (CHESS et al., 1974; MACDONALD et al., 1975).

In the mouse, both lymphoid effector cells which have physical characteristics similar to those of human K-cells, and myeloid cells which are glass-adherent have been described (GREENBERG et al., 1973; GREENBERG et al., 1975). These cells are active against sensitized chicken erythrocytes, but appear to be less effective against other cell types. In different species, macrophages, monocytes, and PMN cells, in addition to causing extracellular lysis of sensitized erythrocytes, were observed to cause some damage to unsensitized Chang cells and cause nonspecific detachment of fibroblast monolayers.

The mechanisms of target cell lysis by effector cells of AD-CMC and of cytotoxic T lymphocytes (CTL) have certain similarities. Both are independent of complement, depend on direct contact between viable effector and target cells, and are inhibited by EDTA and CB. Both reactions are specific, depending for AD-CMC on specific anti-target cell antibody, and for CTL on specific T-cell receptors (CEROTTINI and BRUNNER, 1976).

As reviewed by MACLENNAN (1972) and PERLMANN et al. (1972), an important festure of the AD-CMC mechanism relates to the interaction between effector cell receptors and the complementary structures on the Fc portion of the sensitizing IgG molecule. This interaction appears to be rather weak, since IgG antibody in its monomeric form is not cytophilic for the effector cell. On the other hand, the avidity of lymphocyte receptors for IgG molecules tied together by free or cell-bound antigen or by heat aggregation is sufficient for binding. It is therefore not surprising that pretreatment of target cells with antibody induces cytotoxicity, while pretreatment of effector cells does not. Similarly, while it is unlikely that certain lymphocytes from immune donors adsorb enough antibody in vivo to exert cytotoxicity in vitro, they may adsorb antigen-antibody complexes formed in vitro or in vivo and thereby acquire specific cytotoxicity. It is obvious that such an effect would depend critically upon the relative proportions of antigen and antibody.

For similar reasons, AD-CMC is readily inhibited by the presence of unrelated antigen-antibody complexes or heat-aggregated IgG. The formation of such complexes may also explain the inhibitory effect of antisera directed against membrane constituents of cells present in the effector cell population, like anti-

IgG and anti-θ sera. Since soluble antigen-antibody complexes are known to circulate in the blood without being removed by the reticuloendothelial system, it appears important to further investigate their inhibitory activity, especially in vivo.

In view of the fact that antibody-coated target cells may be lysed by normal lymphoid cells, the question arises whether in vitro cytotoxicity of immune lymphocytes from allograft recipients could also be mediated by such a mechanism. Such immune cell populations would have to contain non-T lymphoid cells with Fc receptors, and cells producing IgG antibody to the target cells. In fact, several studies have shown T- and non-T-cell cytotoxicity of immune lymphoid cells in allograft and tumor systems (MACLENNAN and HARDING, 1970; LAMON et al., 1973; BIESECKER et al., 1973; PLATA et al., 1974; O'TOOLE et al., 1974). Removal of Ig and/or Fc receptor carrying cells on Ig-anti-Ig columns abolished the non-T-cell mediated effect, a result which is compatible with an AD-CMC mechanism. More studies are, however, needed to formally resolve this question.

Destruction of target cells in vitro by AD-CMC is a highly efficient mechanism. Only very small amounts of antibody are needed, and lytic titers which were 100–1,000-fold higher than those obtained with the complement mediated assay were observed. The question of the in vivo significance of AD-CMC is, however, still open. Further characterization of K-cells, and cell transfer studies in appropriately depleted recipients might help to resolve it.

I. Cytotoxicity Mediated by Macrophages

In recent years, the role of macrophages in graft rejection has been extensively studied for a number of reasons. Apart from the fact that monocytes and macrophages accumulate in grafts which undergo rejection, it has been realized that macrophages may cooperate with sensitized T-cells in the effector phase of cell-mediated immune responses. Thus, convincing evidence has been obtained that acquired resistance to intracellular parasites involves a two-step mechanism, whereby sensitized T-cells interacting with specific antigen release nonspecific mediator substances which activate macrophages (MACKANESS, 1974). As a consequence of this activation, macrophages acquire increased nonspecific microbicidal activity. In allograft and tumor immunity, a similar mechanism was suggested by studies demonstrating specific or nonspecific cytotoxicity of macrophages in vitro. A certain amount of contradictory or incomplete data makes it difficult, however, to establish a definite pathway for cytotoxic macrophages at this time. In the following, some of the pertinent results and problems will be briefly outlined.

In a number of studies, it has been convincingly demonstrated that macrophages can acquire nonspecific cytotoxic activity in vivo and in vitro, leading to growth inhibition or lysis of target cells KELLER (1976). Thus, macrophages activated in vivo by chronic infection with protozoa, metazoa, or intracellular bacteria, or by injection of BCG or complete Freund's adjuvant were cytotoxic in vitro, in particular for target cells with abnormal growth patterns like tumor cells. Other studies showed that normal macrophages became nonspecifically cytotoxic after exposure in vitro to agents such as endotoxin, double-stranded RNA, and poly I-poly C. Normal macrophages exposed in vitro to immune lymphoid cells (from mice immunized with BCG or with antigens in complete Freund's adjuvant) and specific antigen also acquired nonspecific cytotoxic activity. Finally, supernatants of sensitized lymphocytes and specific antigen, or supernatants from mixed leukocyte cultures appear to induce nonspecific (or specific) cytotoxicity to macrophages in vitro. The latter observations suggested a phenomenon similar to the two-step mechanism in acquired resistance to intracellular parasites, that is, release of a nonspecific macrophage activating factor from specifically stimulated, sensitized T lymphocytes.

Specific cytotoxicity of macrophages has recently been reported by several authors. This implied the involvement of specific recognition structures on the surface of the macrophages. However, the nature of these receptors has not been clearly established. Earlier studies in mice had suggested the involvement of cytophilic antibody on the macrophage membrane. As mentioned in Section H, macrophages have surface receptors for the Fc portion of IgG molecules (in the mouse also for IgM molecules and an α-globulin having the characteristics of a cytophilic antibody) and, as is the case for K-cells, the avidity of these receptors is very much increased for antibody which is complexed to antigen. In these studies in mice, cytotoxicity was abrogated by trypsin treatment, and antibody could be eluted by incubation at 56° for 30 min. Trypsin-treated macrophages also regained activity after exposure to immune serum or heat eluate. Although suggestive, experiments demonstrating cytophilic antibody on macrophages do not provide conclusive evidence for its involvement in macrophage cytotoxicity, since in a different report, growth inhibition by immune macrophages was found to be unaffected by anti-Ig serum.

In subsequent studies, again in mice, Evans and Alexander (1972) and Lohmann-Matthes and Fischer (1973) described specific "arming" of macrophages with what appeared to be T-cell receptors. In the most pertinent of these experiments, the potential role of contaminating T-cells was circumvented by incubating normal macrophages with cell-free supernatants from cultures consisting of in vivo or in vitro sensitized T-cells and specific target cells. Such supernatants were found to render the macrophages specifically cytotoxic. The factor responsible for this effect was called specific macrophage arming factor (SMAF); it was shown to possess a cytophilic moiety for macrophages as well as a specific recognition site for target cells, and to consist of two major components with molecular weights of > 300,000 and 50,000–60,000. The factor appeared to be produced by T-cells, since no factor was generated when target cells were incubated with immune spleen cells from which T-cells had been selectively removed by treatment with anti-θ serum and complement. On the other hand, SMAF was produced in supernatants from MLC consisting of thymus cells and relevant target cells. In view of these results, it was tempting to assume that SMAF corresponded to specific T-cell receptors shed during incubation of immune T-cells with antigen.

A problem often encountered in attempts to demonstrate specificity of macrophage-mediated cytotoxicity is related to the fact that interaction with specific antigens appears to activate the macrophages and thereby render them nonspecifically cytotoxic for unrelated target cells. In addition, as mentioned above, nonspecific macrophage activating factors like endotoxin or factors released from T-cells stimulated by the pertinent or unrelated antigens may superimpose their effect and thereby mask a specific phase of interaction. This may explain negative results obtained recently in attempts to demonstrate SMAF in MLC supernatants (PFIZENMAIER et al., 1975).

K. Relevance of CMC to Allograft Rejection

Following the basic observation that allograft rejection can be transferred from immune donors to normal recipients with cells, and not or only rarely with serum, much effort has been devoted to the in vitro study of cell-mediated cytotoxicity (CMC). From the various models just discussed, it is clear, however, that CMC is the expression of several mechanisms, including direct cytotoxicity of sensitized T-cells, antibody-dependent cytotoxicity of non-T lymphoid and non-lymphoid cells, and cytotoxicity of armed and/or activated macrophages. In view of the complexity of these mechanisms, some of which may in fact have no counterpart in vivo, it appears difficult to decide how transfer of immune lymphocytes leads to graft destruction.

However, recent developments in the knowledge of the physicochemical and antigenic characteristics of cells involved in immune responses have permitted the design of experiments in which in vitro function can be put under test in vivo. One approach is the study of well-defined cell populations following transfer into animals which are normally or artificially depleted of a given cell type. Such a transfer should reproduce the in vitro function, the effect should be dose-dependent and abolished by selective removal of the effector cell, and it should be possible to identify the effector cells at the target site. A different approach is the separation, identification, and functional in vitro analysis of effector cells isolated from grafts undergoing rejection. A limited number of such studies has been undertaken, and the available evidence points to a major role of cytotoxic T lymphocytes in allograft destruction, at least in the mouse. Macrophages appear not always to be a requisite, but they may amplify the activity of immune T-cells in certain instances.

In experiments designed to analyze the role of defined cell populations transferred into immunologically deprived recipients, SPRENT and MILLER (1972) were the first to demonstrate activity of immune T-cells. They observed accelerated skin allograft rejection in neonatally thymectomized mice following intravenous injection of a pure population of syngeneic T-cells sensitized against the alloantigens of the graft. The immune T-cell population, obtained by transfer of thymus cells into irradiated recipients of the donor genotype, contained highly active cytotoxic lymphocytes as determined in vitro, and it was thus tempting to attribute graft rejection to their direct cytolytic activity. However, the experiments did not exclude a helper effect of T-cells in antibody production, or mediation of graft rejection by macrophages armed or activated by factors released by the immune T-cells. Such an effect was suggested in a study in mice in which immune T-cells failed to cause rapid rejection of skin grafts when injected at the time of irradiation, whereas the same population was effective when skin grafts and T-cell transfer were made in thymectomized, irradiated recipients 4 weeks after bone marrow reconstitution. This suggested participation of both immune T-cells and monocytes in the rejection process.

In a different study, defined immune cell populations were injected into lethally irradiated recipients of tumor allografts (FREEDMAN et al., 1972). Complete protection was observed with syngeneic thymus or spleen cell populations previously sensitized by transfer into irradiated allogeneic recipients. When, however, T-cells were selectively removed from the immune spleen cells by treatment with anti-θ serum and complement prior to transfer, no protection was obtained, indicating that the B-cells including antibody-forming cells contained in the transferred population were ineffective.

Recent studies have shown that T-cells sensitized in vitro are also able to prevent allogeneic tumor growth, or to induce skin allograft rejection in immunologically deprived mice (ROUSE et al., 1972; CEROTTINI et al., in preparation). In these studies, as well as in those using immune T-cells induced in vivo, the transferred immunity was specific, a fact which speaks against the participation of nonspecific factors or effector cells.

Several successful attempts to transfer tumor allograft immunity with peritoneal cells from immune animals were also reported (NELSON, 1972). They were considered evidence in favour of a predominant role of macrophages in graft rejection. However, in these studies no attempt was made to rule out the participation of T lymphocytes, which have been shown to be particularly active in peritoneal cell populations following intraperitoneal immunization with allogeneic cells. When purified immune macrophages were transferred, these cells showed an inhibitory effect only on tumor cells injected at the same, but not at a different site (TSOI and WEISER, 1968). Similarly, in tumor allografts in hamsters, the protective effect of lymph node cells given systemically or locally was little affected by reduction of available macrophage precursors through radiation, or local introduction of large numbers of nonspecifically induced peritoneal exsudate cells (NOMOTO et al., 1970).

L. The Role of Antibody in Allograft Rejection

There is no doubt that antibody may mediate or contribute to allograft rejection (CARPENTER et al., 1976). The role of antibody in allograft destruction has been particularly evident in certain well-defined clinical situations and experimental model systems, in particular those involving the presence of preformed antibody or the transfer of antibody to normal or immunodeficient recipients with impairment of CMI. The pathologic manifestations of antibody-mediated graft destruction are characterized by a predominance of vascular lesions involving formation of immune complexes, activation of complement, and aggregation of platelets and PMN-cells.

A representative example of antibody-mediated allograft destruction is the hyperacute (white graft) rejection of renal allografts observed in recipients previously sensitized to the donor's histocompatibility antigens by skin grafts or blood transfusions or in ABO incompatible situations (KISSMEYER-NIELSEN et al., 1966). In the presence of preformed antibody, grafts were rejected within hours. Antibody could be eluted from such grafts, and immunofluorescent studies revealed IgG and C deposition on endothelial cells of glomerular capillaries. Electron micrographs showed platelet adherence to capillary endothelial cells, PMN cell accumulation in the lumen, endothelial cell swelling, and destruction of the basement membranes. Similar observations were made in rat and rabbit renal and heart allografts in immune animals.

The effect of transfer of antibody into recipients of skin and tumor allografts has also been extensively investigated. In recent studies, the use of immunodeficient recipients with impairment of CMI has allowed the dissociation of antibody-mediated effects from those of CMI. Thus, in ALS-treated, adult thymectomized mice that received rat skin xenografts, it was found that intraperitoneal injection of mouse anti-rat serum caused acute graft rejection within 1 day. The studies suggested involvement of complement and PMN-cells (WINN et al., 1973). Similar findings were made in rat recipients of skin allografts. The possible involvement of complement was also confirmed in nude mice (KOENE et al., 1974). In these studies, recipients of skin allografts treated with alloantiserum and rabbit complement rejected grafts within 4 days. Rabbit complement alone, however, also caused rejection, suggesting that nude mice may form alloantibody directed against allografts, but that murine complement is not capable of mediating rejection.

Finally, in rat and mouse allograft recipients attempts were made to characterize antibodies that inhibited or facilitated tumor growth or graft rejection. In a study in rats, IgG_{2a} was cytotoxic in vitro but had no in vivo effect on tumor growth, whereas IgG_{2b} appeared to cause enhancement (FELDMAN). In mice, it was shown that sera containing cytotoxic antibodies (IgG_2) could cause enhancement as well as rejection of skin allografts, a prerequisite for the latter being the simultaneous administration of rabbit complement. On the other hand, IgG_1, which lacks complement-mediated cytotoxic activity, but is (like other IgG subclasses) active in antibody-dependent CMC in vitro, had only enhancing activity (KOENE et al., 1973; JANSEN et al., 1975).This showed that opposite biological activities can be present within a single subclass, and that enhancing activity cannot be assigned to either IgG_1 or IgG_2 exclusively.

From these and other studies it can be concluded that antibody of the appropriate type either preformed or injected may, depending on the type of graft, the timing of immunization or injection, and the immune state of the host, contribute to graft rejection or protect the graft.

References

Berke, G., Ax, W., Ginsburg, H., Feldman, M.: Graft rejection in tissue culture. II. Quantification of the lytic action on mouse fibroblasts by rat lymphocytes sensitized on mouse embryo monolayers. Immunology 16, 643–657 (1969).

Berke, G., Amos, D.B.: Mechanism of lymphocyte-mediated cytolysis. The LMC cycle and its role in transplantation immunity. In: Transpl. Rev. 17, 71–107. Copenhagen: Munksgaard 1973.

Biesecker, J.L., Fitch, F.W., Rowley, D.A., Scollard, D., Stuart, F.P.: Cellular and humoral immunity after allogeenic transplantation in the rat. II. Comparison of a ^{51}Cr release assay and modified microcytotoxicity assay for detection of cellular immunity and blocking serum factors. Transplantation 16, 421–431 (1973).

Billingham, R.E., Brent, L., Medawar, P.B.: Quantitative studies on tissue transplantation immunity. II. The origin strength and duration of activity and adoptively acquired immunity. Proc. Roy. Soc. Ser. B. 143, 58–80 (1954).

Bloom, B.R., Glade, P.R., eds.: In: In vitro methods in cell-mediated immunity. New York: Academic Press 1971.

Bloom, B.R., Landy, M., Lawrence, H.S., eds.: In vitro methods in cell-mediated immunity: A progress report. Cell. Immunol. 6, 331–347 (1973).

Brunner, K.T., Cerottini, J.-C.: Cytotoxic lymphocytes as effector cells of cell-mediated immunity. In: Progress in Immunology I, 385–398. Academic Press, Inc. New York and London, 1971.

Brunner, K.T., Mauel, J., Rudolf, H., Chapuis, B.: Studies of allograft immunity in mice. I. Induction, development and in vitro assay of cellular immunity. Immunology 18, 501–515 (1970).

Carpenter, C.B., d'Apice, A.J.F., Abbas, A.K.: The role of antibodies in the rejection and enhancement of organ allografts. In: Advances in Immunology 22, 1–55, New York: Academic Press 1976.

Cerottini, J.-C., Nordin, A.A., Brunner, K.T.: In vitro cytotoxic activity of thymus cells sensitized to alloantigens. Nature 227, 72–73 (1970a).

Cerottini, J.-C., Nordin, A.A., Brunner, K.T.: Specific in vitro cytotoxicity of thymus-derived lymphocytes sensitized to alloantigens. Nature 228, 1308–1309 (1970b).

Cerottini, J.-C., Nordin, A.A., Brunner, K.T.: Cellular and humoral response to transplantation antigens. I. Development of alloantibody-forming cells and cytotoxic lymphocytes in the graft-versus-host reaction. J. Exp. Med. 134, 553–564 (1971).

Cerottini, J.-C., Brunner, K.T.: Cell-mediated cytotoxicity, allograft rejection, and tumor immunity. In: Advances in Immunology, Vol. 18, 67–132. New York: Academic Press 1974.

Cerottini, J.-C., Brunner, K.T.: Mechanism of T and K cell-mediated cytolysis. In: B and T cells in Immune Recognition (F. Loor and G.E. Roelants, eds.), Wyley and Sons, Chichester, England. In press 1976.

Cerottini, J.-C., Engers, H.D., Macdonald, H.R., Brunner, K.T.: Generation of cytotoxic T lymphocytes in vitro. I. Response of normal and immune mouse spleen cells in mixed leukocyte cultures. J. Exp. Med. 140, 703–717 (1974a).

Cerottini, J.-C., Macdonald, H.R., Engers, H.D., Brunner, K.T.: Differentiation pathway of cytolytic T lymphocytes: In vivo and in vitro studies. In: Progress in Immunology II, Vol. 3, 153–160. New York: North Holland, 1974b.

Chess, L., Macdermott, R.P., Sondel, P.M., Schlossman, S.F.: Separation of cells involved in human cellular hypersensitivity. In: Progress in Immunology II, Vol. 3, 125–132. New York: North Holland 1974.

Degiovanni, G.: Evaluation quantitative in vitro de la réponse cellulaire à l'allogreffe cutanée chez la souris. C.R. Soc. Biol. 166, 722–727 (1972).

Engers, H.D., Thomas, K., Cerottini, J.-C., Brunner, K.T.: Generation of cytotoxic T lymphocytes in vitro. V. Response of normal and immune mouse spleen cells to subcellular alloantigens. J. Immunol. in press (1972).

Evans, R., Cox, H., Alexander, P.: Immunologically specific activation of macrophages armed with the specific macrophage arming factor (SMAF). Proc. Soc. Exp. Biol. Med. 143, 256–259 (1973).

FELDMAN, J.D.: Personal communication.

FREEDMAN, L.R., CEROTTINI, J.-C., BRUNNER, K.T.: In vivo studies of the role of cytotoxic T-cells in tumor allograft immunity. J. Immunol. **109**, 1371–1378 (1972).

GINSBURG, H.: Graft versus host reaction in tissue culture. I. Lysis of monolayers of embryo mouse cells from strains differing in the H-2 histocompatibility locus by rat lymphocytes sensitized in vitro. Immunology **14**, 621–635 (1968).

GOVAERTS, A.: Cellular antibodies in kidney homotransplantation. J. Immunol. **85**, 516–522 (1960).

GREENBERG, A.H., HUDSON, L., SHEN, L., ROITT, I.M.: Antibody-dependent cell-mediated cytotoxicity due to a "Null" lymphoid cell. Nature New Biol. **242**, 111–113 (1973).

GREENBERG, A.H., SHEN, L., WALKER, L., ARNAIZ-VILLENA, A., ROITT, I.M.: Characteristics of the effector cells mediating cytotoxicity against antibody-coated target cells. Eur. J. Immunol. **5**, 474–480 (1975).

HÄYRY, P., DEFENDI, V.: Mixed lymphocyte cultures produce effector cells: Model in vitro for allograft rejection. Science **68**, 133–135 (1970).

HÄYRY, P., ANDERSSON, L.C., NORDLING, S., VIROLAINEN, M.: Allograft response in vitro. Transplant. Rev., Vol. **12**, 91–140 (1972).

HENNEY, C.S.: On the mechanism of T-cell mediated cytolysis. In: Transpl. Rev. **17**, 37–70. Copenhagen: Munksgaard 1973.

HOLM, G.: Lysis of antibody treated human erythrocytes by human leukocytes and macrophages in tissue culture. Int. Arch. Allergy **43**, 671–682 (1972).

JANSEN, J.L.J., KOENE, R.A.P., V. KAMP., G.J., TAMBOER, W.P.M., WIJDEVELD, P.G.A.B.: Isolation of pure IgG subclasses from mouse alloantiserum and their activity in enhancement and hyperacute rejection of skin allografts. J. Immunol. **115**, 387–391 (1975).

KELLER, R.: Cytostatic and cytocidal effects of activated macrophages. In: Immunobiology of the Macrophage. pp. 487–508, New York: Academic Press 1976.

KISSMEYER-NIELSEN, F., OLSEN, S., POSBORG PETERSEN, V., FJELDBORG, O.: Hyperacute rejection of kidney allografts, associated with pre-existing humoral antibodies against donor cells. Lancet II, 662–665 (1966).

KOENE, R.A.P., GERLAG, P.G.G., HAGEMANN, J.F.H.M., VAN HAELST, U.J.G., WIJDEVELD, P.G.A.B.: Hyperacute rejection of skin allografts in the mouse by the administration of alloantibody and rabbit complement. J. Immunol. **111**, 520–526 (1973).

KOENE, R.A.P., GERLAG, P.G.G., JANSEN, J.J., HAGEMANN, J.F.H., WIJDEVELD, P.G.A.B.: Rejection of skin grafts in the nude mouse. Nature **251**, 69–70 (1974).

LAMON, E.W., WIGZELL, H., KLEIN, E., ANDERSSON, B., SKURZAK, H.M.: The lymphocyte response to primary moloney sarcoma virus tumors in Balb/c mice. Definition of the active subpopulations at different times after infection. J. Exp. Med. **137**, 1472–1493 (1973).

LIGHTBODY, J., BERNOCO, D., MIGGIANO, V.C., CEPELLINI, R.: Cell mediated lympholysis in man after sensitization of effector lymphocytes through mixed leukocyte cultures. G. Batteriol. Virol., Immunol. Ann. Osp. Maria Vittoria Torino **64**, 243–254 (1971).

LOHMANN-MATTHES, M., FISCHER, H.: T-cell cytotoxicity and amplification of the cytotoxic reaction by macrophages. In: Transpl. Rev. Vol. 17, pp. 149–171. Copenhagen: Munksgaard 1973.

MACDONALD, H.R., ENGERS, H.D., CEROTTINI, J.-C., BRUNNER, K.T.: Generation of cytotoxic T lymphocytes in vitro. II. Effect of repeated exposure to alloantigens on the cytotoxic activity of long-term mixed leukocyte cultures. J. Exp. Med. **140**, 718–730 (1974).

MACDONALD, H.R.: Early detection of potentially lethal events in T-cell-mediated cytolysis. Eur. J. Immunol. **5**, 251–254 (1975).

MACDONALD, H.R., CEROTTINI, J.-C., BRUNNER, K.T.: Generation of cytotoxic T lymphocytes in vitro. III. Velocity sedimentation studies of the differentiation and fate of effector cells in long-term mixed leukocyte cultures. J. Exp. Med. **140**, 1511–1521 (1975a).

MACDONALD, H.R., BONNARD, G.D., SORDAT, B., ZAWODNIK, S.A.: Antibody-dependent cell-mediated cytotoxicity: Heterogeneity of effector cells in human peripheral blood. Scand. J. of Immunol. in press (1975b).

MACDONALD, H.R., SORDAT, B., CEROTTINI, J.-C., BRUNNER, K.T.: Generation of cytotoxic T lymphocytes in vitro. IV. Functional activation of memory cells in the absence of DNA synthesis. J. Exp. Med. in press (1975c).

MACKANESS, G.: The immunological basis of acquired cellular resistance. J. Exp. Med. **120**, 105–120 (1964).

MACLENNAN, I.C.M., HARDING, B.: The role of immunoglobulins in lymphocyte-mediated cell damage in vitro. II. The mechanism of target cell damage by lymphoid cells from immunized rats. Immunology 18, 405–412 (1970).

MACLENNAN, I.C.M.: Antibody in the induction and inhibition of lymphocyte cytotoxicity. Transplant. Rev. 13, 67 (1972).

MARTZ, E.: Interruption of the sequential release of small and large molecules from tumor cells by low temperature during cytolysis mediated by immunt T-cells or complement. Proc. Nat. Acad. Sci. 71, 177–181 (1974).

MARTZ, E.: Early steps in specific tumor cell lysis by sensitized mouse T-lymphocytes. I. Resolution and characterization. J. Immunol. in press (1975).

MITCHISON, N.A.: Passive transfer of transplantation immunity. Proc. Roy. Soc., Ser B. 142, 72–87 (1954).

MILLER, R.G., DUNKLEY, M.: Quantitative analysis of the ^{51}Cr release cytotoxicity assay for cytotoxic lymphocytes. Cell. Immunol. 14, 284–302 (1974).

MÖLLER, E.: Contact-induced cytotoxicity by lymphoid cells containing foreign isoantigens. Science 147, 873–879 (1965).

MÖLLER, G., ed.: Effector cells in cell-mediated immunity. In: Transplant. Rev. vol. 17. Copenhagen: Munksgaard 1973.

NELSON, D.S.: Macrophages as effector cells of cell-mediated immunity. Crit. Rev. Microbiol. Vol. I, pp. 353–384 (1972).

NOMOTO, K., GERSHON, R.K., WAKSMAN, B.H.: Role of nonimmunized macrophages in the rejection of an allotransplanted lymphoma. J. Nat. Cancer Inst. 40, 23–30 (1968).

ORTIZ DE LANDAZURI, M., HERBERMAN, R.B.: Specificity of cellular immune reactivity to virus-induced tumours. Nature New Biol. 238, 18–19 (1972).

O'TOOLE, C., STEJSKA, V., PERLMANN, P., KARLSSON, M.: Lymphoid cells mediating tumor-specific cytotoxicity to carcinoma of the bladder. Separation of the effector population using a surface marker. J. Exp. Med. 139, 457–466 (1974).

PERLMANN, P., HOLM, G.: Cytotoxic effects of lymphoid cells in vitro. Advan. Immunol. 11, 117–193 (1969).

PERLMANN, P., PERLMANN, H., WIGZELL, H.: Lymphocyte-mediated cytotoxicity in vitro. Induction and inhibition by humoral antibody and nature of effector cells. Transplant. Rev. 13, 91–114 (1972).

PFIZENMAIER, K., TROSTMANN, H., RÖLLINGHOFF, M., WAGNER, H.: Cell-mediated allograft responses in vitro: VI. Studies on macrophage-mediated cytotoxicity. Immunology 29, 961–976 (1975).

PLATA, F., GOMARD, E., LECLERC, J.-C., LEVY, J.-P.: Comparative in vitro studies on efffector cell diversity in the cellular immune response to murine sarcoma virus (MSV)-induced tumors in mice. J. Immunol. 112, 1477–1487 (1974).

ROSENAU, W., MOON, H.D.: Lysis of homologous cells by sensitized lymphocytes in tissue culture. J. Nat. Cancer Inst. 27, 471–483 (1961).

ROUSE, B.T., WAGNER, H., HARRIS, A.W.: In vivo activity of in vitro immunized lymphocytes. I. Tumor allograft rejection mediated by in vitro activated mouse thymocytes. J. Immunol. 108, 1353–1361 (1972).

SMITH, R.T., LANDY, M., eds.: Immunobiology of the tumor-host relationship. Proc. of an Int. Conference, Milan, Italy, New York: Academic Press 1975.

SPRENT, J., MILLER, J.F.A.P.: Interaction of thymus lymphocytes with histoincompatible cells. III. Immunological characteristics of recirculating lymphocytes derived from acrivated thymus cells. Cell. Immunol. 3, 213–230 (1972).

TSOI, M.S., WEISER, R.S.: Mechanisms of immunity to sarcoma. I. Allografts in the C57BL/Ks mouse. I. Passive transfer studies with immune peritoneal macrophages in X-irradiated hosts. J. Nat. Cancer Inst. 40, 23–30 (1968).

WAGNER, H., RÖLLINGHOFF, M., NOSSAL, G.J.V.: T-cell mediated immune response induced in vitro: A probe for allograft and tumor immunity. In: Transplant. Rev. Vol. 17, 3 36. Copenhagen: Munksgaard 1973.

WAGNER, H., RÖLLINGHOFF, M., SHORTMAN, K.: Evidence for T-T-cell synergism during in vitro cytotoxic allograft responses. In: Progress in Immunology II, Vol. 3, 111–120. New York: North Holland 1974.

WILSON, D.B.: Immunologic reactivity to major histocompatibility alloantigens: HARC, effector cells and the problem of memory. In: Progress in Immunology II, Vol. 2, pp. 145–156. New York: North-Holland 1974.

WINN, H.J., BALDAMUS, C.A., JOOSTE, S.V., RUSSELL, P.S.: Acute destruction by humoral antibody of rat skin grafted to mice. The role of complement and polymorphonuclear leukocytes. J. Exp. Med. **137**, 893–910 (1973).

WINN, H.: The mechanisms of immunological enhancement. In: Progress in Immunology II, Vol. 3, 207–216. New York: North-Holland 1974.

Cell Systems Participating in Graft Rejections

J. HAGMANN, M.W. HESS, H.U. KELLER, and H. COTTIER

A. Introduction

The present short chapter on cell lines participating in graft rejection may be considered as an addendum to other chapters contained in this volume. Since the latter have in part been written as long as 2 years ago, it seemed appropriate to include in the collection of review papers on transplantation a short summary covering the essentials of more recent findings in the field of cellular immunology. This domain of research is now rapidly expanding, and the following text is an attempt to summarize experimental observations published in 1975 and the first half of 1976, however, some earlier reports will also be referred to.

B. Lymphocytes

I. Development of the Immune System and Lymphocyte Subclasses

1. Early Ontogenesis of Lymphoid Organs and Cells

Lymphoid cells appear in the embryonic mouse thymus on the 12th day of gestation (MOORE and OWEN, 1967). They are large, basophilic, have a prominent nucleolus and are negative for the TL and the Thy-1 antigens. In human embryos, thymic lymphoid cells are first seen around the 9th week of gestation (HAMMAR, 1910).

Cells of similar morphologic appearance were found, e.g., in the yolk sac of mice (MOORE and METCALF, 1970), and these yolk sac cells can be recovered in the bone marrow, spleen, Peyers patches, and mesenteric lymph node after injection into 800 R-irradiated adult mice.

There are two theoretical possibilities with regard to the origin of these first thymic lymphocytes in embryonic life:

1. de novo formation from epithelial cells in the embryonic thymus;
2. an external source.

The results of most recent studies strongly support the latter hypothesis, i.e., the population of the thymus by blood-borne stem cells (for reviews see OSOBA, 1974; OWEN, 1974). In the mouse, these stem cells were reported to originate from the yolk sac (METCALF and MOORE, 1971), and, in latter developmental stages, from the liver and the bone marrow (MOORE and METCALF, 1970). However, convincing evidence was presented indicating that the chick and the quail intraembryonic blood-islands and not the yolk sac are the major source of stem cells (LE DOUARIN, personal communication). In these latter two species, interphase cells can be distinguished by their morphologic appearance, and embryonic chimeras may be produced which permit full identification of cell traffic from one part of the kyema to another. In this system, it was also shown that the embryonic thymus experiences so-called attractivity periods during which a massive influx of blood lymphoid cells into the organ occurs, while the magnitude of this process prior to and after this phase is small (LE DOUARIN and JOTEREAU, 1975). Studies on chimeric frogs, on the other hand, were interpreted in the sense that thymic lymphocytes may originate in the thymus itself and, from this site, seed into bone marrow and spleen (VOLPE and TURPEN, 1975). More work is needed to confirm or dismiss this notion. HOFMAN and GLOBERSON (1976) tried to evaluate the immunologic potential of yolk sac cells in the mouse and found 9-day-old embryonic yolk sac cells able to elicit a Graft-versus-Host (GvH) reaction (splenomegaly assay) in 4 out of 17 cases, whereas these cells didn't stimulate nor respond in a mixed lymphocyte reaction (MLC), and were not stimulated by PHA and ConA.

In fetal mice, cells with surface Ig can be found almost as early as lymphoid cells in the thymus, however, the former do not seem to be mature B cells in the sense that they would be able to differentiate into antibody-producing elements upon culture in vitro with bacterial lipopolysaccharide (LPS) (ROSENBERG and CUNNINGHAM, 1975).

2. Postnatal Development of the Lymphocytic Systems

In postnatal life, precursor cells are still immigrating into the thymus, although at a low rate (BRAHIM and OSMOND, 1970). This influx, however, can increase after peripheral antigenic stimulation (MICKLEM et al., 1972). Since at about the time of birth in mice, and already before birth in humans, the bone marrow becomes the major hematopoietic organ, we can assume it to be also the main source of the thymic precursor cells in postnatal life.

There is evidence for a pluripotential thymic cell precursor giving rise to myeloid cells in spleen colonies and lymphocytes in the thymus (for review see OSOBA, 1974). But recent studies indicate that the immediate thymic precursor cell actually entering the thymus is already precommitted to the T-pathway, i.e., a "prethymocyte": Nude (congenitally athymic) and thymectomized mice have a population of lymphocytes which is surface Ig-negative, low-Thy-1, Ly-negative, and TL-positive. They are further characterized by low electrophoretic mobility, no propensity for recirculation and a short life span (1–2 days). These prethymocytes are produced in the BM: They represent 75–95% of all lymphocytes in the 13-day-old embryonic thymus and only 1–2% in the liver at the same age. The appearance of these cells may be controlled by a thymic humoral factor: their number increases after thymectomy and falls again after the implantation of thymic tissue, even if enclosed in a millipore chamber (LOOR and ROELANTS, 1975; ROELANTS *et al.,* 1975, 1976a and b).

Further support for the existence of precommitted prethymic progenitor cells came from experiments where the phenotypic expression of the alloantigens Thy-1, TL, and Ly was induced by an extract of mouse thymus named "thymosin" (KOMURO and BOYSE, 1973; KOMURO *et al.,* 1975), as well as by various agents which are known to increase cellular cAMP (SCHEID *et al.,* 1973; COHEN and PATTERSON, 1975; SINGH and OWEN, 1975).

EL-ARINI and OSOBA (1973) tried to characterize precursor cells by equilibrium density centrifugation of mouse bone marrow cells (which, in their system, are not susceptible to anti-Thy-1-serum and complement and do not respond in MLR and GVH-reactions). Cells giving rise to MLR and GVH-positive lymphocytes peaked at 1.064 gcm^{-3}, whereas hematopoietic colony-forming cells were less dense (1.060 gcm^{-3}).

The origin of the B cell is less well known. An observation analogous to the one where Thy-1-negative lymphocytes differentiated into Thy-1-positive cells under the influence of thymic extracts and of agents rising the intracellular cAMP has been made by HAEMMERLING *et al.* (1975). These authors were able to convert a certain population of Ia-negative murine lymphocytes from bone marrow and spleen into Ia-positive cells exposing them to catecholamines, prostaglandin PGE$_1$, cAMP, bacterial endotoxin, lipid A, ubiquitin, and thymopoietin. The Ia-negative precursor cell bears already surface immunoglobulin. In this context, the discovery of the Th-B antigen is also of interest (YUTOKU *et al.,* 1976). The Th-B antigen is present on mouse B cells, plasma cells, and immature thymocytes and studies on its nature gave rise to the hypothesis that it may appear early in the development of lymphoid cells on a precursor cell for both T and B cells, and that subsequently it may be lost during the differentiation of the T, but not the B cells.

3. The Central Role of the Thymus

In recent years, the application of a host of different methods has led to the division of thymic lymphocytes into subpopulations. These methods detect physical properties (size, density, electrophoretic mobility), surface antigens (Thy, Ly, TL, etc.), susceptibility to drugs and irradiation, and functions (mitogen-responsiveness, GvH-activity, response to alloantigens, helper and suppressor activity). The physiologic roles of these subpopulations are not yet fully understood, nor do we have sufficient knowledge with regard to the way they are related to each other, i.e., whether they represent sequential stages in a maturing process, or rather parallel lines. Reviews on the subject may be found in DYMINSKI and SMITH, 1974; SHORTMAN *et al.,* 1975; and CANTOR and WEISSMAN, 1976.

Thymic lymphocytes can be divided into those populating the cortex ("thymocyte" sensu strictiori) and those populating the medulla. Cortical lymphocytes represent the major population in the young mouse (approx. 85%, as compared to about 15% medullary lymphocytes). Conventional smears reveal the presence of small (5–7 μ), and medium to large (8–12 μ) lymphocytes in both the cortex and the medulla (26% of medium to large cells in the medulla, 11% in the cortex of the young mouse) (Bryant, 1972). Large cells of both regions are mitotically active (Potmesil and Goldfeder, 1973).

In the following section we will summarize the characteristics of thymocyte subpopulations related to these two (major and minor) groups.

Hydrocortisone treatment—except for a small corticosteroid-resistant fraction—eliminates the cortical thymocyte population, while in the medulla only larger lymphoid cells seem to be affected (Droege and Zucker, 1975). In mice, LPS seems to have a similar effect (Uccini et al., 1976). Medullary lymphocytes are also more radioresistant than cortical cells (Blomgren and Andersson, 1971).

Hetero- and alloantisera reveal several surface antigens confined to thymocytes or thymocytes and peripheral T cells (for review see Schlesinger, 1972).

TL antigens (TL 1.2.3.4) can be detected on the surface of thymocytes in TL-positive strains of mice. Leukemic cells may also carry the antigen, even in otherwise TL-negative strains. In TL positive strains the major (cortical) thymocyte population is TL+, whereas the antigen is absent from the minor, medullary population (Konda et al., 1973).

Thy 1.1 (θAKR) and Thy 1.2 (θC3H) antigens are expressed on thymocytes and peripheral T cells of the mouse. However, differential quantitative cytotoxic assays on mouse thymic lymphocytes can distinguish between a major population (80–85%) with a high Thy-1-concentration and a minor, low-Thy-1 population representing the medullary lymphocytes (Shortman and Jackson, 1974).

The reverse is true for the antigens of the major histocompatibility complex in the mouse (H-2 complex): high levels of H-2 antigens are present on the minor, predominantly medullary population, low levels are characteristic of the major population (Konda et al., 1973). Finally, the Ly and G_{Ix} antigens were shown to be present on the major population of cortical thymocytes, whereas they couldn't be detected on cells of the minor population (Konda et al., 1973).

Cytochemical staining for nonspecific acid esterase, which, in peripheral lymphocytes, does distinguish (positive) T-cells from (negative) B-cells, shows mainly positive cells in the medulla and predominantly negative ones in the cortex (Mueller et al., 1975). Ruuskanen et al. (1975) studied the ultracytochemical appearance of alkaline phosphatase (AP) on the cell membrane of guinea pig thymic lymphocytes. They found a small population of AP-negative lymphocytes which was located in the medulla. Furthermore, AP negative cells appeared to be lymph node–seeking, whereas AP-positive (mainly cortical) thymocytes, upon artificial peripheralization, were found predominantly in the spleen and the liver from which sites they disappeared after 3 days (Ruuskanen, 1975).

Several workers showed the cortisone-resistant, low-Thy-1 thymocytes to be of faster electrophoretic mobility than normal thymocytes (Shortman et al., 1975). An even better separation of the two populations may be obtained by equilibrium density gradient centrifugation: low-Thy-1 cells are light in density, cortical high-Thy-1 cells are denser. However, both high-Thy-1 and low-Thy-1 categories show a marked heterogeneity with many density peaks (SHORTMAN, 1971). In addition, examination of dividing thymocytes revealed low-Thy-1 and high-Thy-1 cells in the light fraction and predominantly high-Thy-1 cells in the dense fraction (SHORTMAN *et al.,* 1975). Finally, sedimentation velocity studies, which are not useful in separating low-Thy-1 from high-Thy-1 thymocyte populations, are very effective in distinguishing between larger, dividing and smaller, nondividing cells (SHORTMAN *et al.,* 1975).

DROEGE *et al.* (1974) combined size distribution with preparative cell electrophoresis and bovine serum albumin (BSA) density gradient centrifugation. The resulting "fingerprints" (two-dimensional distribution patterns) allowed the discrimination of four thymocyte populations in the mouse and the chicken: two cortical populations (early and late population) of small lymphocytes, a medullary population of small lymphocytes, and a population of medium-sized lymphocytes ("prolymphocytes"). The significance of these findings in relation to T cell development will be discussed below.

In summary, we can distinguish two broad categories of thymic lymphocytes:

1. a major population comprising approximately 85% of all thymic lymphocytes, which are high-Thy-1, low H-2, TL-positive, corticosteroid-sensitive, and located mainly in the cortex, and

2. a minor population (10–20%), consisting of low-Thy-1, high-H-2, TL-negative, corticosteroid-resistant cells located predominantly in the medulla.

Considering the functional capacities of the different thymocyte subpopulations, one generally finds that the minor, medullary subpopulation is immunologically active and—in this respect—resembles the peripheral T-cells.

Mitogen-responsiveness. PHA, a T-cell stimulating lectin, is mitogenic for the minor subpopulation in mouse, rat, and man (for references see DYMINSKI and SMITH, 1974), whereas its effectiveness on the whole thymic lymphocyte population is only minimal. ConA, on the other hand, does stimulate both the minor and, although to a lesser degree, the major subpopulation (STOBO *et al.,* 1972). SHORTMAN *et al.* (1975) found a differential responsiveness of low-Thy-1 cells to the two mitogens: cells lighter than 1.072 g/cm^3 responded predominantly to PHA, whereas ConA-responsiveness was found both in the former (< 1.072 g/cm^3) as well as in a denser (1.074 g/cm^3) region.

Mixed lymphocyte culture and cytotoxic lymphocytes. Thymic lymphocytes are able to respond to allogeneic peripheral lymphocytes and to generate cytotoxic activity. Responsible for these two properties is the minor, i.e., predominantly medullary population (SHORTMAN *et al.,* 1972).

The prevailing opinion is that I-region gene products, which are expressed mainly on B-lymphocytes, are responsible for the stimulating effect in mixed lymphocyte reactions (MLR) (see below). BERMAN *et al.* (1976), studying a one-way MLR in mice, showed that spleen lymphocytes could stimulate both allogeneic splenic lymphocytes and thymic lymphocytes, whereas thymic lymphocytes could stimulate only peripheral, but not thymic lymphocytes. Column-purification of thymic lymphocytes led them to the conclusion that medullary B-cells and/or a subpopulation of stimulating T-cells were responsible for the stimulation of splenic lymphocytes by thymic cells. HAN *et al.* (1976) got similar results in a human system, in which they found no activity in a thymus-thymus combination and a weak reaction in only 11 out of a total of 21 experiments where peripheral blood lymphocytes were the responding cells and thymic lymphocytes the stimulating population. Lause *et al.* (1976), on the other hand, studied BSA-gradient purified mouse thymic lymphocyte subpopulations and showed a significant stimulatory activity in the lighter cell fractions, whereas the denser cells, as well as the unseparated population did not stimulate peripheral lymphocytes.

Boehmer and Shortman (1975), exploring an MLR-system, tried to draw conclusions regarding the differentiation of T-lymphocytes. Using allogeneic or syngeneic B-lymphocytes as stimulators, they showed that (1) adult CBA thymus cells responding to *allogeneic* cells were enriched in the light density region, which was also low-Thy-1. With the same stimulatory cells, they found responding splenic T-cells in both light and dense regions; and (2) that adult CBA thymus cells responding in a *syngeneic* MLR were located in the light and dense zones, whereas there was no such activity in a spleen cell population. Finally, in 4-day-old mice, cells reacting to syngeneic lymphocytes were present in the light zone only. Immature cells being generally lighter than mature ones, these experiments suggest that there is a cell line, responding in the syngeneic system, which undergoes a complete maturation process in the thymus.

Graft-versus-host reaction. Cells responsible for GVH-reactivity are residing in the minor thymic subpopulation: they are characterized by low density, resistance to cortisone, low-Thy-1, and high H-2 concentration (Leckband and Boyse, 1971; Levey and Burleson, 1972). Cantor and Asofsky (1972), studying the synergy between T-cell subsets in GVH-reaction, found a subset located mainly in the spleen and the thymus, which was resistant to treatment with antithymocyte serum (ATS) in vivo, and which co-operated with a second subset of cells in peripheral blood and lymph nodes, susceptible to in vivo ATS treatment.

Helper cells. Helper activity appears to be a function of the minor thymic lymphocyte subpopulation (reviewed in Dyminsky and Smith, 1974).

Suppressor cells. The thymus appears to contain cells suppressing immune responses. Suppressor cells were found, e.g., in mice bearing tumors (Fujimoto *et al.*, 1976a and b; Takei *et al.*, 1976). These cells regulating negatively the immune response against the tumor are located predominantly in the thymus and the spleen, are hydrocortisone resistant, of low density, and reach their peak activity at late stages of progressive tumor growth (Takei *et al.*, 1976). By injecting thymic lymphocytes into irradiated hosts, Rich and Rich (1976) noted the appearance in the host spleen of cells suppressing a MLR at 4 days. Precursors of antigen-specific suppressor cells induced in vitro have been described by Kontiainen and Feldman (1976). They seem to be enriched in the spleen and the cortisone-resistant thymic lymphocyte population. Furthermore, there are some reports concerning radiosensitive suppressor cells of thymic origin (McCullagh, 1975c; Gaag and McCullagh, 1975). McCullagh and coworkers found such cells in neonatal, but not in adult thymuses of rats. These cells were able to suppress tumor rejection and an adaptive response to SRBC. Droege (1976) examined antigen-inexperienced thymic suppressor cells inhibiting antibody production and cell-mediated immunity in young chicken. Characteristics of this thymic cell population are, apart from radiosensitivity, bursa-dependency, spleenseeking behavior, and loss of activity after standing for 1–2 h on ice without bovine serum albumin.

Taking into consideration the results reported above, the following concepts of T-cell development are emerging:

According to one theory, the high-Thy-1, cortisone-sensitive, dense lymphocytes (major population) are the precursors of medullary lymphocytes.

Based on kinetic evidence and examination of cell density, cell size and cell lability, on the other hand, a second theory has appeared more recently. This alternative theory favors the concept of two different T-cell lines, one undergoing complete maturation in the thymus (major population), the second one completing maturation in the periphery (discussed by SHORTMAN et al., 1975).

Finally, one should add a note of caution. The thymus is generally considered to be a "primary" organ, i.e., an organ functioning independently from exterior (antigenic) influence. Studies performed by BRYANT et al. (1975), however, clearly show that antigenic stimulation changes the kinetic behavior within the thymus and that hence the thymus may respond to peripheral stimuli in one way or another.

II. Peripheral Lymphocytes

1. Lymphocyte Subclasses

Although there is considerable interaction between T- and B-lymphocytes and uncertainty about the ultimate origin of B-cells, it is still helpful to retain the concept of duality of the immune system, and we will consider subpopulations of the T- and the B-cell line separately. Differences and separation methods of T- and B-cells have been reviewed extensively (GREAVES et al., 1973), the following sections will thus deal with the heterogeneity within these subpopulations only.

a) T Cells

α) Surface Antigens

Surface antigens on different peripheral murine lymphocyte subpopulations can be demonstrated by immunofluorescence, immunoferritin labeling, cytotoxicity, mixed agglutination, or complement fixation. The various antigens were reviewed by RAFF (1971) and SCHLESINGER (1972). They include the antigen of the major histocompatibility complex, Thy-1, Ly (BOYSE et al., 1968, 1971; CANTOR and BOYSE, 1975a, b; SHIKU et al., 1975), as well as antigens detected by heteroantisera raised against different T-cell populations [mouse-specific lymphocyte antigen (MSLA, SHIGENO et al., 1968); MPLA, RAFF and CANTOR, 1971].

A comparison of autoradiographic results following local thymus labeling in vivo with immunofluorescence findings on Thy-1-positive cells of mice revealed that T-cells may lose at least some of this surface antigen shortly after peripheralization (CHANANA et al., 1974). After treating murine peripheral T-cells with fluorescein-labeled anti-Thy-1.2-serum, dull (low Thy-1) cells could be separated from bright (high-Thy-1) cells using the fluorescein-activated cell sorter (Cantor *et al.*, 1975). Low-Thy-1 cells were damaged by antilymphocyte serum (ALS) in vivo to a greater extent, homed to lymph nodes in higher proportions than high-Thy-1 cells, and were not affected shortly after adult thymectomy. High-Thy-1 cells, in contrast, were less decreased in number by ALS-treatment in vivo, homed preferentially to the spleen, and were reduced in number shortly after adult thymectomy. The former cells are usually referred to as T2-cells, the latter ones as T1-cells. Similarly, treatment of T-cells with antimouse-thymo-cyte serum and complement did distinguish between a sensitive and a more resistant population with characteristics analogous to the high-Thy-1 and low-Thy-1-cells, respectively (Araneo *et al.*, 1975).

Recently attempts to detect an antigen defining the subpopulation of cytotox-ic mouse T-cells seem to have been successful: the "Mouse-Killer-T-Cell-Anti-gen" (MKTCA) is revealed by a heteroantiserum raised against nu/nu spleen cells containing T-cell precursors and absorbed with erythrocytes, thymic leuke-mia cells, thymocytes, and fetal liver cells. MKTCA appears to be present on T-cells responsible for cell-mediated cytotoxicity and absent from helper cells (Kisielow *et al.*, 1976).

Ia antigens, which are products of I-region genes in the mouse (for review see Shreffler and David, 1975), play a role in graft-versus-host reactivity and the mixed lymphocyte reaction. Although Ia-antigens are found predomi-nantly on B-cells (Sachs and Cone, 1973; Haemmerling *et al.*, 1974; Hauptfeld *et al.*, 1975; Niederhuber *et al.*, 1975; Abbas *et al.*, 1976), they are also expressed on a T-cell subpopulation (Frelinger *et al.*, 1974). By treating splenic T-cells with a specific anti-Ia serum and complement, Niederhuber *et al.* (1976) could remove the subpopulation responding to ConA, whereas the response to PHA was not affected.

Finally, although immunoglobulins can be detected on the surface of T-cells, it is still unclear whether all of them are attached by means of Fc-receptors, or whether they are produced by T-cells themselves (Marchalonis, 1975).

β) Receptors

Spontaneous rosette formation by peripheral T-cells with sheep red blood cells (E-rosettes) is the most widely used assay for T-cells in the human (Jondal *et al.*, 1972). However, a subpopulation of active peripheral blood T-lympho-cytes, characterized by especially rapid rosette formation with sheep erythrocytes, was found to increase in individuals developing delayed cutaneous hypersensitiv-ity to microbial antigens (Felsburg *et al.*, 1976).

Receptors for activated complement (CR) and the Fc-portion of immuno-globulin (FcR) have been described in detail for B-lymphocytes of several species (see below). However, not all T-cells are completely devoid of these surface structures, and T-cell subclasses may consequently be distinguished by the pres-ence or absence of Fc- and—possibly—C-receptors (for review see Parish, 1975).

Most workers were unable to detect complement receptors on T-cells, al-though some groups published positive results (Arnaiz and Hay, 1975; Chiao and Good, 1976).

Fc-receptors, on the other hand, are present on functional subgroups of antigen-activated T-cells. In the mouse spleen, 10–30% of Thy-1-positive cells carry the receptor (ANDERSON and GREY, 1974; BASTEN *et al.,* 1975b; PARISH, 1975; STOUT and HERZENBERG, 1975a). Fc-receptors of mouse T-cells have been shown to bind aggregated mouse IgG (ANDERSON and GREY, 1974), aggregated human IgG (SANTANA and TURK, 1975), and complexes with mouse IgM (LAMON *et al.,* 1975), whereas human T-cells bind erythrocytes coated with rabbit IgM (McCONNEL and HURD, 1976b) and IgG (FERRARINI *et al.,* 1975). LAMON *et al.* (1976) found IgMFc-receptors to be different from IgGFc- as well as C-receptors. Using a modified rosetting technique, KRAMMER *et al.* (1975) could detect Fc-receptors on parental lymph node T-cells activated by injection into irradiated F_1 hybrid mice, but not on normal lymph node T-cells. Activated T-cells from the thoracic duct lymph also lacked the receptor. IgM demonstrable by surface immunofluorescent staining on H-2–activated cells seem to be B-cell–derived alloantibodies passively fixed on the cells' surface and Fc-receptors may play a role in this phenomenon (HUDSON and SPRENT, 1976). Finally, it has been shown that ConA-responsive cells are enriched in the Fc+ T-cell population (STOUT and HERZENBERG, 1975b).

γ) Activation by Polyclonal Stimulators

Several mitogens are known to stimulate T-cells nonspecifically. Extensive recent reviews of the subject were given by LING and KAY (1975), OPPENHEIM and ROSENSTREICH (1976), and WEDNER and PARKER (1976). The plant lectins phytohemagglutinin (PHA) and Concanavalin A (ConA) as well as sodium periodate (NaIO4) are apparently more or less T-cell specific. Pokeweed mitogen (PWM) and antilymphocyte serum (ALS), on the other hand, activate both T- and B-cells.

There is some evidence for differential responsiveness of T-cells to ConA and PHA, and this phenomenon may be used for distinguishing between T-cell subpopulations.

STOBO and PAUL (1973) determined the ratio between the PHA- and the ConA-responsiveness (PHA: ConA ratio) in different lymphocyte suspensions and found high ratios in populations enriched for lymph node–seeking lymphocytes, low ratios in low-Thy-1, cortisone-resistant thymocytes, and in splenic lymphocytes compared to lymph node cells. Other workers confirmed and extended these findings, showing that PHA-responsive splenic T-cells are enriched in the high-density, very low Thy-1 population, whereas they found ConA-responsiveness in both the high-density as well as in a second, short-lived and tissue-fixed population with lesser density and somewhat higher Thy-1 concentration (SHORTMAN *et al.,* 1973; MUGRABY *et al.,* 1975a; RAWSON and HUANG, 1975; SCHLESINGER *et al.,* 1976).

δ) Physical Properties

Mouse T-cells are of higher electrophoretic mobility than B-cells, a property which can be used for preparative cell separation (ANDERSSON *et al.,* 1973; v. BOEHMER *et al.,* 1974; DUMONT, 1975). However, this result was not achieved with human peripheral blood lymphocytes, which displayed no bimodal electro-phoretic distribution of fast T-cells and slow B-cells (VASSAR et al., 1976). SHORT-MAN et al. (1975) also found the method not promising for separating mature mouse T-cell subclasses.

Equilibrium density gradient centrifugation does not distinguish between mouse T- and B-cells, but is particularly suitable for separating peripheral T-cell subclasses (SHORTMAN et al., 1972). The surviving T-cells were found predomi-nantly in the high density fraction 2 weeks after adult thymectomy. Moreover, in normal CBA mice, thoracic duct lymphocytes were mainly dense cells. These observations show dense cells to be long-lived and recirculating, whereas the lighter splenic T-cells are short-lived (SHORTMAN et al., 1975).

As in the thymus, velocity sedimentation analysis of splenic mouse lympho-cytes resulted in a complex heterogeneous pattern (SHORTMAN et al., 1975).

In summary, we are confronted with essentially two main subclasses of peripheral murine T-cells, i.e., T1- and T2-cells. T1-cells are short-lived, nonrecir-culating, rapidly dividing cells homing preferentially to the spleen. T2-cells are long-lived, recirculating cells attaining high concentrations in thoracic duct lymph, and, to some extent, in blood and lymph nodes. As we have seen above, these two subclasses may be further characterized by their surface anti-gens, mitogen-responsiveness, and physical properties. It is still an open question whether these subclasses represent sequential stages in one line of development or if, as the more recent data appear to indicate, there are at least two parallel T-cell lines which may be traced back to the thymus itself.

b) B-cells

Antibodies, and hence B-lymphocytes—as plasma cell precursors—play a role in the rejection of transplants (for review see CARPENTER et al., 1976). Division of B-cells into subclasses is based mainly on their physical characteristics, recep-tors for the Fc-portion of Ig, and for activated complement components, surface Ig, and responsiveness to polyclonal activators.

α) Receptors

Receptors for C3b (BIANCO et al., 1970; GELFAND et al., 1976), C3d (ROSS et al., 1973), and C4b (ROSS et al., 1973; BOKISCH and SOBEL, 1974) have been shown to be present on B-lymphocytes of different species, including man (for review see NUSSENZWEIG, 1974). These receptors seem to represent surface structures independent from each other. SIMONIAN et al. (1976) could demonstrate that not only complement components bound to antigen-antibody complexes, but also fluid phase C3b can bind to the receptor. About 40% of splenic B-cells of the 6-week-old CBA mouse are C-receptor positive (CR+) (PARISH, 1975). Several authors tried to shed light on the function of the C-receptor. Some of these experiments suggest a role in cell-activation, either directly by C3b (HARTMANN and BOKISCH, 1975), or by passive focusing in the induction of a polyclonal antibody response (MOELLER and COUTINHO, 1975). PARISH and CHILCOTT (1975) found that all antigens tested could activate CR+-cells, whereas only antigens possessing repeating determinants did activate CR−-cells. Other studies demonstrate a change in the presence of the receptor during different maturation stages of B-cells. Results suggesting the loss of CR have been reported after stimulation with B-cell mitogens (MOELLER, 1974) and after antigenic stimulation of precursors of IgM-secreting cells (RAMASAMY and WILLIAMS, 1975). The relative fall in number of CR+-cells during the first 72 h after LPS-stimulation may, on the other hand, also be interpreted as being due to stimulation and proliferation of CR−-cells (GORMUS and SHANDS, 1975). McCONNEL and HURD (1976a) found no C3b-receptors on any antibody-secreting cells. Separation into CR− and CR+ lymphocyte subpopulations finally showed the precursors of 7S-antibody forming cells to occur in both fractions, whereas the C-receptor seemed to be required for the 19S-AFC precursors (MASON, 1976).

Fc-receptors for aggregated Ig, antibody, and antibody-antigen complexes involving Ig of different classes (e.g., in the mouse: IgG1 ≫ IgG2b, IgM; BASTEN et al., 1972b) have been demonstrated on the majority of B-cells of various species (BASTEN et al., 1972; DICKLER et al., 1972; PARASKEVAS et al., 1972; HALLBERG et al., 1973; ANDERSON et al., 1974; THEOFILOPOULOS et al., 1974; LAMON et al., 1976); for reviews, see WARNER (1974) and PARISH (1975). About 80% of B-cells of adult mice are Fc+ (ANDERSON et al., 1974). Although aggregated IgG does bind more efficiently, monomeric IgG also binds to Fc-receptors (RAMASAMY et al., 1976). The latter seem to be closely related to Ia-antigens. In fact, several workers could demonstrate that anti-Ia-Fab is able to block FcR of mouse B-cells (BASTEN et al., 1975, 1976; SCHIRRMACHER et al., 1975), and SOLHEIM et al. (1976) showed the same phenomenon in human lymphocytes using anti-HLA-D-Fab (but not using anti HLA-A-, anti-HLA-B-, or anti-HLA-C-Fab). Moreover, independence of FcR from CR and surface Ig has been proven (ABBAS and UNANUE, 1975; RAMASAMY and LAWSON, 1975; BASTEN et al., 1976). In contrast to the C-receptor, Fc-receptors were also detected on IgM-antibody-secreting cells, but not on IgG-secreting cells (McCONNEL and HURD, 1976b).

In summary, based on the presence or absence of these two receptors, it is possible to distinguish four B-cell subpopulations: Fc+CR+, Fc+CR−, Fc−CR+, and Fc−CR−.

β) Surface Immunoglobulin

Surface immunoglobulin (SIg), detectable by conventional methods, represent the most salient feature of B-lymphocytes (for review see MARCHALONIS, 1975).

In man, the majority of surface-Ig positive lymphocytes carry both IgM and IgD, minor populations being positive for IgM or IgD only (KNAPP et al., 1973; ROWE et al., 1973). Using anti-IgG-F(ab′)$_2$ sera to avoid binding of immune complexes to Fc-receptors, the number of SIgG+ cells detected was, however, very low (WINCHESTER et al., 1975).

Recently, the discovery of an IgD-like molecule on murine B-cells (VITETTA et al., 1975; PARKHOUSE et al., 1976) has led to a better characterization of different B-cell subclasses, although FINKELMANN et al. (1976) proposed that this "δ"-chain, having a different electrophoretic mobility, may not be a true homologue of human IgD. However, 20–30% of splenic B-cells have been found to carry IgM only, 30–40% to carry the IgD-like molecule ("IgD") only, and 40–50% to carry both "IgD" and IgM (Lisowska-Bernstein and Vasalli, 1975; Parkhouse and Abney, 1975; Parkhouse *et al.*, 1976). With an antiserum recently prepared against "IgD," as many as 90% of splenic B-cells were IgD + IgM + (Knight and Pernis, 1975). Moreover, whereas newborn mice possess only surface-IgM positive lymphocytes, surface IgD is appearing at 10–15 days and is predominant at 3 months (Vitetta *et al.*, 1975). These results suggest an IgM − IgD switch. Further support for this theory came from experiments showing that (1) in young mice large splenic B-cells carry IgM only, small ones both IgM and IgD and that (2) in older animals both large and small cells are IgM + IgD + although large cells possess relatively more IgM (Goodman *et al.*, 1975). Thus IgM +-cells seem to give rise to small lymphocytes bearing both IgM and IgD.

γ) Physical Properties

Physical separation methods have been applied to distinguish between different antibody-forming cell precursors.

The results show that antibody-forming cell precursors in unprimed mice (virgin AFC-P) are "atypical," i.e., fast sedimenting, not very dense B-cells with high electrophoretic mobility. Progenitor activity for a memory IgG response in hapten-primed animals, on the other hand, was found among the slowly sedimenting, dense, electrophoretically slowest "typical" B-cells. IgM-AFC-P in primed animals, finally, exhibit intermediate characteristics. It should be noted that in neonatal animals the virgin AFC-P are also slowly sedimenting, dense B-cells (Schlegel *et al.*, 1975a, b; Fidler *et al.*, 1976). In addition, IgMAFC-progenitors are more adherent, and IgGAFC-progenitors from hapten-primed animals less adherent to glass-bead columns than the majority of spleen cells (Schlegel and Shortman, 1975).

δ) Polyclonal B Cell Activators (PBAs)

Stimulation with PBAs has increased our understanding of B-cell heterogeneity as well as B-cell maturation. The most widely used PBA in mice is bacterial lipopolysaccharide (LPS). After stimulation with LPS, two parallel events may be observed (Askonas *et al.*, 1976): (1) generation of a large number of small B-cells with high density of surface Ig, but no internal Ig-pool and (2) development of a small number of Ig-secreting cells with a large internal pool of Ig. Vitetta *et al.* (1976) also obtained a heterogeneous pattern after LPS-treatment: lymphocytes carrying surface IgD only, did enlarge and proliferate, but did not give a polyclonal response nor did they synthesize and secrete IgM, whereas cells with surface IgM and IgD did enlarge and became IgM-secreting plasma cells. According to one hypothesis, IgD-only cells are memory cells becoming IgG-secreting plasma cells.

Considerable insight into B-cell maturation and B-cell heterogeneity has been provided by studies comparing the effects of different PBAs, namely dextran-sulphate (DxS), LPS, and purified protein derivative from tubercle bacteria

(PPD). Measuring DNA synthesis and the number of plaque-forming cells, the following pattern of response was obtained: DxS stimulated DNA synthesis to a high degree, but very few PFCs were produced. PPD, on the other hand, induced the development of a large number of antibody-secreting cells, but DNA synthesis remained relatively low. LPS finally stimulated both DNA-synthesis and PFC-generation to a high degree. Furthermore, an age dependency of PBA-induced responses has been noted. In fact, fetal bone marrow cells are stimulated by DxS only, whereas bone marrow cells from adult mice respond to DxS and LPS. Besides, fetal liver cells acquire PBA responsiveness in the order DxS, LPS, and PPD. A picture is thus emerging, where at least three partially overlapping B-cell subsets of increasing differentiation level are stimulated sequentially first by DxS, which may stimulate precursor B-cells, then LPS, and finally PPD, leading to antibody-secreting end cells (GRONOWICZ and COUTINHO, 1975).

c) Null Cells

About 15% of mouse spleen cells are devoid of both the Thy-1 antigen and surface Ig. These cells have been termed "null cells." A small fraction (<6%) of these cells carry the Fc-receptor and are killer (K) cells. The remaining null cells probably comprise hemopoietic stem cells and some immature forms of B-cells (RYSER and VASALLI, 1974). More than 50% of the null cells found in human peripheral blood will develop surface Ig by 3 days of culture (CHESS et al., 1975).

2. The Functions of Peripheral Lymphocytes

a) Helper and Suppressor Activity

Immunologic responses seem to be regulated by helper and suppressor lymphocytes. Suppressor cells (SC) appear to form a heterogeneous population comprising specific and nonspecific T suppressor lymphocytes as well as nonspecifically suppressing B-cells. Best known among the SC populations are T-lymphocytes, which seem to act mainly on other T-cells (for review see MOELLER, 1975). These suppressor T-cells have been characterized by different methods.

Some of the more recent results may be summarized as follows:

1. Neonatal splenic T-cells (McCULLAGH, 1975b, 1976; MOSIER and JOHNSON, 1975) and peripheral blood T-cells from human newborns (OLDING and OLDSTONE, 1976) are able to suppress a response to sheep red blood cells (SRBC) and a mixed lymphocyte reaction (MLR), respectively.

2. Precultured lymphocytes contain a population of nylon-adherent T-cells which suppress a subsequent MLR (HODES and HATHCOCK, 1976).

3. Adherent T-cells in the peritoneal exudate of mice inhibit the in vitro response of purified T-cells to ConA (MUGRABY et al., 1975b).

4. Radiosensitive T-cells can suppress a response to tumor transplants (ROTTER and TRAININ, 1975) or an adoptive immune response to SRBC (McCULLAGH, 1975a).

FELDMAN and KONTIAINEN (1976) showed that T-cell–T-cell interaction is necessary for the induction of antigen-specific suppressor activity in vitro: whereas the latter could not be obtained with lymphocytes from either ALS-treated or adult thymectomized animals, a combination of the two populations was able to reconstitute the ability to induce suppressor cells. The direct SC precursor was resistant to adult thymectomy, but sensitive to antilymphocyte serum.

Recently, evidence has accumulated indicating that helper function on the one hand, and suppressor and/or cytotoxic activity on the other hand, are mediated by different T-cell subpopulations (IGARASHI *et al.*, 1975). By applying a velocity sedimentation gradient, TSE and DUTTON (1976) were able to separate ConA-induced helper and suppressor T-cells. The helper cells were recovered in the top pool and were relatively radioresistant, whereas the radiosensitive suppressor cells were confined to the bottom pool of the gradient. Even more pertinent results with regard to functional definition of T-lymphocytes have been achieved by Ly-phenotyping of cells mediating the respective activities. Antisera against the products of genes located on two unlinked loci (Ly-1 and Ly-2/Ly-3) distinguish three classes of murine peripheral T-cells: 50% are Ly-123+, 33% Ly-1+, and 6–8% Ly-23+. Ontogenetically Ly-123+ cells appear before the cells of the two other classes. Moreover, the number of Ly-123+ cells is reduced shortly after adult thymectomy, whereas Ly-1+ and Ly-23+-cells show no numerical changes in the early phases after this treatment (CANTOR and BOYSE, 1975a). Furthermore, experimental results favor the hypothesis that Ly-1+-cells are programmed to initiate delayed type hypersensitivity and helper function, Ly-23+ to generate killer activity and suppressive function (CANTOR and BOYSE, 1975a; HIRST *et al.*, 1975; SHIKU *et al.*, 1975; HUBER *et al.*, 1975). It is also interesting to note that the maturation of Ly-23-+-cells to killer cells can be amplified by Ly-1+-cells, due to selective recognition of I-regionantigens by Ly-1+-cells which, in contrast to Ly-23+-cells, are activated by Ia differences (CANTOR and BOYSE, 1975b). The findings of JANDINSKI *et al.* (1976) also explain the inability of ConA-stimulation to generate helper activity, because in this system the helper effect is masked by the activation of Ly-23+-cells which in turn exhibit suppressor activity. We are, thus, confronted with a situation where the original $TL+Ly-123+$ T-cell differentiates either to become a precommitted $TL-Ly-1+$ potential helper cell (T_H) or a precommitted $TL-Ly-23+$ potential suppressor/cytotoxic cell ($T_{C,S}$). It is not yet established where this differentiation step takes place—i.e., in the thymus or in the periphery—and it is an equally open question if suppressive and cytotoxic activity can be separated from each other (CANTOR *et al.*, 1976).

b) Cell-Mediated Cytotoxicity

Various cell types appear to be involved in cell-mediated cytotoxicity: cytotoxic T-cells, non-T-lymphocytes, macrophages, and polymorphonuclear granulocytes.

Cytotoxic lymphocytes (CTL) are generated after in vivo or in vitro (e.g., mixed lymphocyte culture) sensitization. ZAGURY *et al.* (1975) studied the ultrastructural appearance of these cells at a single-cell level and found them to be small to medium size lymphocytes with an indented nucleus and cytoplasm containing one-membrane-bound, lysosomelike granules, no rough endoplasmatic reticulum and a well-developed Golgi apparatus. With regard to the Fc- and C-receptor, ARNAIZ-VILLENA et al. (1975) lost the cytotoxic activity of a spleen cell population sensitized against allogeneic mouse cells after depletion of C3-receptor bearing (CR+) cells and concluded that CR+ T-cells may play a role in the effector phase of specific cell-mediated cytotoxicity. KRAMMER et al. (1975) injected parental T-cells into irradiated F_1 hybrids and collected the spleen cells after 5 days. These cells were 100% donor derived, 80% Ia+, 1% Ig+, 30–40% FcR+; thoracic duct T-cells, on the other hand, were all FcR-negative. After separation of FcR+ and FcR− spleen cells by depletion of EA-rosettes, they found cytotoxic activity in both the FcR+ and the FcR− population.

There is evidence for T-cell–T-cell interaction taking place in the generation of CTL. CANTOR and coworkers (CANTOR and SIMPSON, 1975; SIMPSON and CANTOR, 1975) characterized the populations involved and could show (1) prekiller cells, which were enriched in lymph node T-cell suspensions, sensitive to in vivo ATS-treatment and relatively radiosensitive; and (2) a population of regulatory (amplifying or suppressing) cells in the spleen, which was ATS-resistant, but affected by adult thymectomy. Moreover, suppressing regulatory cells were more radiosensitive than amplifying cells. The nature of human CTL is less well defined, but it seems established that both the afferent and efferent phases of cell-mediated cytotoxicity are—at least predominantly—T-cell functions (SONDEL et al., 1975a). There may exist a heterogeneity of CTL precursors and/or of differentiation into effector cells. In fact, ALTMAN and COHEN (1975) found an enhanced antifibroblast reaction, but an impaired MLR in both the proliferation and the cytotoxic phase after hydrocortisone administration in vivo.

Several workers compared the CTL system with other forms of cell-mediated cytotoxicity. KIESSLING et al. (1976) examined (1) the "naturally occurring killer cell" (NK-cell) active against Moloney leukemia virus (MLV)-induced lymphoma cells (KIESSLING et al., 1975a, b); (2) the antibody-dependent cytotoxic cell (ADCC-cell) killing sensitized chicken erythrocytes (CRBC); and (3) CTL-killing P815 mastocytoma cells. Whereas NK-cells were insensitive to EAC-rosette-depletion, not inhibited by aggregated γG, trypsin sensitive, and Thy-1-negative, ADCC was abolished after EAC-rosette-depletion or treatment with aggregated γG, but trypsin-resistant, and CTLs were trypsin-sensitive and Thy-1-positive. Differences between CTL and ADCC-cells exist also in the mechanism of cytolysis, where the two systems are characterized by different cation requirements (GOLDSTEIN and SMITH, 1976).

These results lead us to another category of cytotoxic lymphocytes, the nonphagocytic, "non-T" cytotoxic cells active mainly in the ADCC system. Most workers describe these cells as FcR+ lymphocytes (mouse: GREENBERG and SHEN, 1973; GREENBERG et al., 1975; RAMSHAW et al., 1976; human: DE-BRACCO et al., 1976; SANDILANDS et al., 1976). More conflicting results concern the complement receptors: According to some authors, depletion of CR+ lymphocytes abolishes or diminishes ADCC (v. BOXEL et al., 1973; GREENBERG et al., 1975; PERLMAN et al., 1975); other workers found no cytotoxic activity in cell populations enriched for CRL (DEBRACCO et al., 1976; RAMSHAW et al., 1976). Conflicting results may be due in part to differences in the assay systems used. GHAFFAR et al. (1976) reported an elevated ADCC in mice bearing a tumor and a concomitant rise in Fc+ lymphocytes. Finally, it should be noted that T-cells may also be active in an ADCC-system: LAMON et al. (1975) used IgM-coated MSV-sarcoma cells as targets and found them to be killed by T-cells which they think are IgMFc+.

c) Mixed Lymphocyte Cultures

The mixed lymphocyte culture (MLC) is a widely used in vitro model reflecting allograft responses. In a mixed lymphocyte reaction (MLR), both cell proliferation and the generation of cytotoxic effector cells may be observed.

The course of events in a primary MLR comprises first the appearance of blast cells, which then revert to small, resting, primed T-cells. Upon reexposure to the same antigen, these primed cells react in a secondary MLC, characterized by the following features: specificity, acceleration, and greater amplitude of the response (3H-thymidin-incorporation) (FRADELIZI and DAUSSET, 1975). Furthermore it has been shown that primary blast CTL revert to clonally restricted nonlytic T-cells which, upon reexposure, generate secondary CTL in the absence of cell proliferation (WAGNER and ROELLINGHOFF, 1976). HAEYRY and ANDERSSON (1975) separated activated (blast) cells primed in a one-way MLC by Ig-velocity sedimentation and studied the properties of the reverted secondary T-cells. These cells responded promptly in a secondary MLC, were nonresponsive to PHA and ConA, displayed specific cytotoxicity, were long-lived, and homed preferentially to the spleen.

Several studies indicate that lymphocyte-defined (LD) antigens are responsible for the proliferative response, whereas the classical, serologically defined (SD) H-2K, and H-2D antigens lead to the generation of CTL (BEVAN, 1975; ROELLINGHOFF et al., 1975). In accord with this theory are studies showing that, in comparison with T-cells, murine B-cells, which express the Ia-antigens, stimulate preferentially in a MLR. It should be noted, though, that SONDEL et al. (1975b), using human purified lymphocyte subpopulations, found both T- and B-cells to stimulate in a MLR and to generate CTL. This could mean that human T-cells bear LD-antigens. However, from the above results it has been found that two T-cell subclasses are involved in MLCs: (1) T_1 (helper) cells activated by LD antigens and (2) T_2 (cytotoxic) cells activated by SD antigens (ROELLINGHOFF and WAGNER, 1975; SIMPSON, 1975). In this context it is interesting to note that whereas UV-treated allogeneic cells (HAEYRY and ANDERSSON, 1975; ROELLINGHOFF and WAGNER, 1975; WAGNER and ROELLINGHOFF, 1976) and subcellular antigen preparations (ENGERS et al., 1975) are unable to generate a proliferative or a cytotoxic response in a primary MLC, they generate a strong CTL response in a secondary MLC. This again is interpreted in the sense that SD-antigens are sufficient for secondary CTL-stimulation. Using another approach for studying T-cell–T-cell interaction, HOWE and COHEN

(1975 a, b) showed that a mixed responding population consisting of lymph node cells and thymocytes or lymph node cells and spleen cells led to an enhanced MLR.

d) Graft-Versus-Host Reaction (GVHR)

Compared with the MLR, the GVHR involves very complex mechanisms which are still poorly understood. It seems clear that donor T-cells are responsible for initiating the whole sequence of events, but it is still a matter for debate what role the host-derived, proliferating lymphocytes play in the effector arc of the reaction. An extensive review of GVHR may be found in GREBE and STREILEIN, 1976.

As in MLR and the generation of CTL, there is evidence for T-cell–T-cell interaction taking place between donor T-cell subclasses in GVHR. Combinations of thymocytes with peripheral blood lymphocytes or peripheral lymph node cells give enhanced GVHR. Treatment of thymocytes with anti-TL-serum and complement prior to injection into semiallogeneic F_1 hybrids leaves the GVHR of thymocytes alone unchanged, but abolishes the synergistic effect in combination with lymph node cells (TIGELAAR et al., 1975). The results of these studies suggest that lymphocytes supply the precursors of cells inflicting the injuries in the host, and that the lymph node or peripheral blood T-cells contain a subpopulation amplifying their activity. Further characterization of the two interacting populations revealed that amplifier cells are most abundant in peripheral blood and lymph nodes, rapidly recirculating and highly sensitive to in vivo treatment with antithymocyte serum (ATS), whereas precursor cells are more abundant in thymus and spleen, less ATS-sensitive, and slowly recirculating. Moreover, the two populations are recovering independently after ATS-treatment in vivo (MORSE and ASOFSKY, 1976).

Recently, the importance of host-derived lymphocytes in the generation of many features of GVHR has been given renewed emphasis, ROLSTAD (1976) studied the cell composition of popliteal lymph nodes of normal and T-depleted (B) F_1 hybrid rats after injection of parental lymphocytes.

The results lead to the conclusion that donor T-cells are stimulated by host non-T-cells, but that the following increase in cellularity of the popliteal lymph node involves primarily host cells, and that trapping cannot be the main cause of this phenomenon. CLANCY and coworkers (1976) also tried to characterize the cell populations taking part in the GVHR. After injecting immunoincompetent neonatal rats with allogeneic lymphocytes, they found increased levels of FcR+-cells in the spleen and lymph nodes. The increase occurred earlier in the spleen, but was more marked in lymph nodes. Moreover, FcR+-cells were of host origin. Histologic examination of the spleen and lymph nodes revealed a depleted white pulp and cortex, respectively, containing cell debris. In the medulla, many plasma cells of host origin were seen. The known occurrence of autoantibodies in GVH-disease and the involvement of Fc-receptors in antibody-dependent cytotoxicity may lead to speculations concerning the function of these FcR+-cells.

C. Macrophages

A compilation of what was known until a year ago about biochemistry, functional morphology, cellular kinetics, and roles of mononuclear phagocytes has been published in van Furth (1975). More recent reports indicate the following:

Macrophages seem to be involved in many immunologic functions, directly or via soluble factors. For instance, strong evidence points to their role in immune induction (reviewed by Unanue and Calderon, 1975; Rosenthal et al., 1975), the induction of tolerance (Lukic et al., 1975), the generation of helper cells (Erb and Feldman, 1975), and T-lymphocyte activation by mitogens (Rosenstreich et al., 1976). Cells with the characteristics of macrophages have been found in rabbit peripheral blood suppressing a secondary response to sheep red blood cells (Luzzati and Lafleur, 1976) and in the spleen of tumor-bearing mice suppressing a response to mitogens (Pope et al., 1976).

Data obtained by Lafferty et al. (1976) suggest that macrophages might play a role in the activation of host T-lymphocytes by an allograft. Culturing thyroid allografts in vitro for prolonged periods increased their survival time in the recipient. Furthermore, adherent cells ingesting latex particles were found to modify human lymphocyte proliferation in a MLC (Berlinger et al., 1976). In the guinea pig, on the other hand, the macrophage seems to be the predominant stimulator in a MLC (Greineder and Rosenthal, 1975).

Nabarra and Descamps (1976) studied the cells infiltrating human renal allografts in vivo by electron microscopy and found a high percentage of macrophages (about 30%).

Based on studies in vitro, considerable evidence has accumulated suggesting that these macrophages may have nonspecific effector functions in allograft rejection. Cytotoxic activity of macrophages has been reported in an antibody-dependent cellular cytotoxicity (ADCC) system using erythrocytes (Cohen et al., 1975; Kovithavongs et al., 1975; Walker and Demus, 1975; Pollack et al., 1976) or tumor cells (Evans and Alexander, 1972a, b; Piessens et al., 1975; Boyle and Ormerod, 1976), as targets. Consequently, macrophages from mice grafted with allogeneic skin became cytotoxic for donor target cells (Dimitriu et al., 1975).

In analogy to the situation in lymphocyte-mediated ADCC, surface receptors have been thought essential in the mechanisms involved. Fc-receptor-carrying macrophages have been detected by various workers (Rabellino and Metcalf, 1975; Ramshaw and Parish, 1976). Monomeric IgG2a did bind strongly, IgG2b weakly, and IgM, IgA, and IgG1 were not bound significantly to these receptors (Unkeless and Eisen, 1975). Fc-receptor activity was found to change depending on conditions, being increased on macrophages in inflammatory exudates as compared to normal, unstimulated macrophages, and on peritoneal as compared to alveolar macrophages (Rhodes, 1975). In addition, receptors for C3b, but not for C3d, were described (Griffin et al., 1975; Rabellino and Metcalf, 1975; Ramshaw and Parish, 1976). These C-receptors appear to be independent from the Fc-receptors (Griffin et al., 1975), but closely related to the H-2 antigens on mouse macrophages (Schlesinger and Chaouat, 1975).

D. Neutrophilic Granulocytes

Present knowledge (until 1974) about the role of polymorphonuclear granulo-cytes (PMN) in graft rejection has been compiled by JERUSALEM and JAP (this volume). Although it is known since the 1960s that neutrophils can play an important role in the rejection of skin grafts, little additional information has appeared in the last 2 years.

NABARRA and DESCAMPS (1976) found only 2% PMNs among the cells infiltrating human renal allografts. PMNs carry receptors for both C3 and IgG. In agar colonies, 50–60% of all neutrophils did bind erythrocytes coated with antibody and complement or with antibody alone (RABELLINO and MET-CALF, 1975). Moreover, neutrophils are able to lyse antibody-coated target cells at very low PMN: target cell ratios (GALE and ZIGHELBOIM, 1975).

E. Other Cells and Structures

ANDERSON et al. (1975) described microvascular changes in lymph nodes draining skin allografts. They observed contracted venous sphincters, dilated segmental veins, and increased vascular permeability in the first 48 h. At the same time, an increased number of lymphocytes crossed the high endothelial venules. More-over, increased length and arborization of high endothelial venules was due to focal proliferation of endothelial cells in transition zones from high to low endothelium. High endothelial cells showed an increase in cytoplasmic basophilia and acid hydrolase activity as well as numerous polyribosomes, RER cysternae, and lysosomes.

To the best of our knowledge, no major advances concerning the role of eosinophils, mast cells, and reticulum cells in graft rejection have been made during the last 2 years.

References

ABBAS, A.K., UNANUE, E.R.: Interrelationships of surface immunoglobulin and Fc receptors on mouse B lymphocytes. J. Immunol. **115**, 1665-1671 (1975)

ABBAS, A.K., DORF, M.E., KARNOWSKY, M.J., UNANUE, E.R.: The distribution of Ia antigens on the surfaces of lymphocytes. J. Immunol. **116**, 371–378 (1976)

ALTMAN, A., COHEN, I.R.: Heterogeneity in the development of cytotoxic T lymphocytes in vitro revealed by sensitivity to hydrocortisone. J. exp. Med. **142**, 790–795 (1975)

ANDERSON, C.L., GREY, H.M.: Receptors for aggregated IgG on mouse lymphocytes. Their presence on thymocytes, thymus-derived, and bone marrow-derived lymphocytes. J. exp. Med. **139**, 1175-1188 (1974)

ANDERSON, N.D., ANDERSON, A.O., WYLLIE, R.G.: Microvascular changes in lymph nodes draining skin allografts. Amer. J. Path. **81**, 131–153 (1975)

ANDERSSON, L.C., NORDLING, S., HAEYRY, P.: Fractionation of mouse T and B lymphocytes by preparative cell electrophoresis. Cell. Immunol. **8**, 235–248 (1973)

ARANEO, B.A., MARRACK, P.C., KAPPLER, J.W.: Functional heterogeneity among the T-derived lymphocytes of the mouse. II. Sensitivity of subpopulations to antithymocyte serum. J. Immunol. **114**, 747-751 (1975).

Arnaiz-Villena, A., Hay, F.C.: Complement receptor lymphocytes. Analysis of immunoglobulin on their surface and further evidence of heterogeneity. Immunology **28**, 719–729 (1975)

Arnaiz-Villena, A., Jones, B., Roitt, I.M.: Allograft cytotoxicity. Role of T lymphocytes bearing a receptor for complement. Immunology **29**, 903–908 (1975)

Askonas, B.A., Roelants, G.E., Mayor-Withey, K.S., Welstead, J.L.: Dual pathway of B lymphocyte differentiation in vitro. Europ. J. Immunol. **6**, 250–256 (1976)

Basten, A., Miller, J.F.A.P., Sprent, J., Pye, J.: A receptor for antibody on B lymphocytes. I. Method of detection and functional significance. J. exp. Med. **135**, 610–626 (1972a).

Basten, A., Warner, N.L., Mandel, T.: A receptor for antibody on B lymphocytes. II. Immunochemical and electron microscopy characteristics. J. exp. Med. **135**, 627–642 (1972b)

Basten, A., Miller, J.F.A.P., Abraham, R.: Relationship between Fc receptors, antigen-binding sites on T and B cells, and H-2 complex-associated determinants. J. exp. Med. **141**, 547–560 (1975a)

Basten, A., Miller, J.F.A.P., Warner, N.L., Abraham, R., Chia, E., Gamble, J.: A subpopulation of T cells bearing Fc receptors. J. Immunol. **115**, 1159–1165 (1975b)

Basten, A., Miller, J.F.A.P., Abraham, R., Gamble, J., Chia, E.: A receptor for antibody on B lymphocytes. III. Relationship of the receptor to immunoglobulin and Ia determinants. Int. Arch. Allergy **50**, 309–321 (1976)

Berlinger, N.T., Lopez, C., Good, R.A.: Facilitation or attenuation of mixed leukocyte culture responsiveness by adherent cells. Nature (Lond.) **260**, 145–146 (1976)

Berman, M., Puryear, K., Argyris, B.F.: In vitro recognition of alloantigens: nature of responding and stimulating cells. Cell. Immunol. **23**, 126–139 (1976)

Bevan, M.J.: Alloimmune cytotoxic T cells: evidence that they recognize serologically defined antigens and bear clonally restricted receptors. J. Immunol. **114**, 316–319 (1975)

Bianco, C., Patrick, R., Nussenzweig, V.: A population of lymphocytes bearing a membrane receptor for antigen-antibody-complement complexes. 1. Separation and characterization. J. exp. Med. **132**, 702–720 (1970)

Blomgren, H., Andersson, B.: Characteristics of the immunocompetent cells in the mouse thymus: cell population changes during cortisone-induced atrophy and subsequent regeneration. Cell. Immunol. **1**, 545–560 (1971)

Boehmer, H. v., Shortman, K.: The differentiation of T lymphocytes. Density characterization of thymic and peripheral T cells responding in syngeneic and allogeneic mixed lymphocyte reactions. Aust. J. exp. Biol. med. Sci. **53**, 281-295 (1975)

Boehmer, H. v., Shortman, K., Nossal, G.J.V.: The separation of different cell classes from lymphoid organs. X. Preparative electrophoretic separation of lymphocyte subpopulations from mouse spleen and thoracic duct lymph. J. cell. Physiol. **83**, 231–242 (1974)

Bokisch, V.A., Sobel, A.T.: Receptor for the fourth component of complement on human B lymphocytes and cultured lymphoblastoid cells. J. exp. Med. **140**, 1336 (1974)

Boxel, J.A. van, Paul, W.E., Frank, M.M., Green, I.: Antibody-dependent lymphoid cell-mediated cytotoxicity: role of lymphocytes bearing a receptor for complement. J. Immunol. **110**, 1027–1036 (1975)

Boyle, M.D.P., Ormerod, M.G.: Destruction of allogeneic tumour cells by peritoneal macrophages. Production of lytic effectors by immune mice. Transplantation **21**, 242–246 (1976)

Boyse, E.A., Miyazawa, M., Aoki, T., Old, L.J.: Ly-A and Ly-B. Two systems of lymphocyte isoantigens in the mouse. Proc. roy. Soc. B **170**, 175–193 (1968)

Boyse, E.A., Hakura, K., Stockert, E., Iritani, C.A., Miura, M.: Ly-C. A third locus specifying alloantigens expressed only on thymocytes and lymphocytes. Transplantation **11**, 351–353 (1971)

Bracco, M.M. de E. de, Isturiz, M.A., Manni, J.A.: Cell-mediated cytotoxicity. Characterization of the effector cells. Immunology **30**, 325–333 (1976)

Brahim, F., Osmond, D.G.: Migration of bone marrow lymphocytes demonstrated by selective bone marrow labeling with thymidine-H^3. Anat. Rec. **168**, 129 (1970)

Bryant, B.J.: Renewal and fate in the mammalian thymus: mechanisms and inference of thymocytokinetics. Europ. J. Immunol. **2**, 38–45 (1972)

Cantor, H., Asofsky, R.: Synergy among lymphoid cells mediating the graft-versus-host response. III. Evidence for interaction between two types of thymus-derived cells. J. exp. Med. **135**, 764–779 (1972)

CANTOR, H., BOYSE, E.A.: Functional subclasses of T lymphocytes bearing different Ly antigens. I. The generation of functionally distinct T-cell subclasses is a differentiative process independent of antigens. J. exp. Med. **141**, 1376–1389 (1975a)

CANTOR, H., BOYSE, E.A.: Functional subclasses of T lymphocytes bearing different Ly antigens. II. Cooperation between subclasses of Ly+ cells in the generation of killer activity. J. exp. Med. **141**, 1390–1399 (1975b)

CANTOR, H., SIMPSON, E.: Regulation of the immune response by subclasses of T lymphocytes. I. Interaction between pre-killer T cells and regulatory T cells obtained from peripheral lymphoid tissues of mice. Europ. J. Immunol. **5**, 330–336 (1975)

CANTOR, H., WEISSMAN, I.: Development and function of subpopulations of thymocytes and T lymphocytes. In: Progress in allergy, KALLOS, P., WAKSMAN, B.H., DE WECK, A. (eds.), Vol. 20, pp. 1–64. Basel: Karger 1976

CANTOR, H., SIMPSON, E., SATO, V.L., FATHAM, C.G., HERZENBERG, L.A.: Characterization of subpopulations of T lymphocytes. I. Separation and functional studies of peripheral T cells binding different amounts of fluorescent anti-Thy 1.2 (Theta) antibody using a fluorescence-activated cell sorter (FACS). Cell. Immunol. **15**, 180–196 (1975)

CANTOR, H., SHEN, F.W., BOYSE, E.A.: Separation of helper T cells from suppressor T cells expressing different Ly components. II. Activation by antigen after immunization, antigen-specific suppressor and helper activities are mediated by distinct T-cell subclasses. J. exp. Med. **143**, 1391–1401 (1976)

CARPENTER, C.B., D'APICE, A.J.F., ABBAS, A.K.: The role of antibodies in the rejection and enhancement of organ allografts. Advanc. Immunol. **22**, 1–65 (1976)

CHANANA, A.D., SCHAEDELI, J., HESS, M.W., COTTIER, H.: Variations in the expressions of θ-C3H alloantigen on thymic and peripheral lymphocytes of newborn and adult mice. Cell. Immunol. **13**, 216–229 (1974)

CHESS, L., LEVINE, H., MACDERMOTT, R.P., SCHLOSSMAN, S.F.: Immunologic functions of isolated human lymphocyte subpopulations. IV. Further characterization of the surface Ig negative, E rosette negative (null cell) subset. J. Immunol. **115**, 1483–1487 (1975)

CHIAO, J.W., GOOD, R.A.: Studies of the presence of membrane receptors for complement, IgG and the sheep erythrocyte rosetting capacity on the same human lymphocytes. Europ. J. Immunol. **6**, 157–162 (1976)

CLANCY, J., TONDER, O., BOETTCHER, C.E.: The effect of neonatal rat graft-vs-host disease (GVHD) on Fc receptor lymphocytes. J. Immunol. **116**, 210–217 (1976)

COHEN, J.J., PATTERSON, C.K.: Induction of theta-positive lymphocytes and lymphoblasts in mouse bone marrow by mitogens. J. Immunol. **114**, 374–376 (1975)

COHEN, S.A., EHRKE, M.J., MIHICH, E.: Mouse effector functions involved in the antibody-dependent cellular cytotoxicity to xenogeneic erythrocytes. J. Immunol. **115**, 1007–1012 (1975)

DICKLER, H.B., KUNKEL, H.G.: Interaction of aggregated gamma-globulin with B lymphocytes. J. exp. Med. **136**, 191–196 (1972)

DIMITRIU, A., DY, M., THOMSON, N., HAMBURGER, J.: Macrophage cytotoxicity in the mouse immune response against a skin allograft. J. Immunol. **114**, 195–199 (1975)

DOUARIN, N.M. LE, JOTEREAU, F.V.: Tracing of cells of the avian thymus through embryonic life in interspecific chimeras. J. exp. Med. **142**, 17–40 (1975)

DROEGE, W.: The antigen-inexperienced thymic suppressor cells: a class of lymphocytes in the young chicken thymus that inhibits antibody production and cell-mediated immune responses. Europ. J. Immunol. **6**, 279–287 (1976)

DROEGE, W., ZUCKER, R.: Lymphocyte subpopulations in the thymus. Transplant. Rev. **25**, 3–25 (1975)

DROEGE, W., ZUCKER, R., JAUKER, U.: Cellular composition of the mouse thymus: Developmental changes and the effect of hydrocortisone. Cell. Immunol. **12**, 173–185 (1974)

DUMONT, F.: Electrophoretic mobility and surface immunoglobulin of albumin gradient fractionated mouse spleen cells. Immunology **28**, 731–739 (1975)

DYMINSKI, J.W., SMITH, R.T.: Immunological activities of thymus cell subpopulations. Ser. Haematol. **7**, 524–547 (1974)

EL-ARINI, M.O., OSOBA, D.: Differentiation of thymus-derived cells from precursors in mouse bone marrow. J. exp. Med. **137**, 821–837 (1973)

ENGERS, H.D., THOMAS, K., CEROTTINI, J,-C., BRUNNER, K.D.: Generation of cytotoxic T lymphocytes in vitro. V. Response of normal and immune spleen cells to subcellular alloantigens. J. Immunol. **115**, 356–360 (1975)

ERB, P., FELDMAN, M.: The role of macrophages in the generation of T helper cells. III. Influence of macrophage-derived factors in helper cell induction. Europ. J. Immunol. **5**, 759–766 (1975)

EVANS, R., ALEXANDER, P.: Role of macrophages in tumour immunity. I. Cooperation between macrophages and lymphoid cells in syngeneic tumour immunity. Immunology **23**, 615–626 (1972a)

EVANS, R., ALEXANDER, P.: Role of macrophages in tumour immunity. II. Involvement of a macrophage cytophilic factor during syngeneic tumour growth inhibition. Immunology **23**, 627-636 (1972b)

FELDMAN, M., KONTIAINEN, S.: Suppressor cell induction in vitro. II. Cellular requirements of suppressor cell induction. Europ. J. Immunol. **6**, 302–305 (1976)

FELSBURG, P.J., EDELMAN, R., GILMAN, R.H.: The active E rosette test: correlation with delayed cutaneous hypersensitivity. J. Immunol. **116**, 1110–1114 (1976)

FERRARINI, M., MORETTA, L., ABRILE, R., DURANTE, M.L.: Receptors for IgG molecules on human lymphocytes forming spontaneous rosettes with sheep red cells. Europ. J. Immunol. **5**, 70–72 (1975)

FIDLER, J.M., HOWARD, M.C., SHORTMAN, K.: Antigen-initiated B-lymphocyte differentiation. VIII. Sedimentation velocity and buoyant density characterization of virgin antibody-forming cell progenitors in the adoptive immune response of unprimed CBA mice to 4-hydroxy-3-iodo-5-nitrophenylacetic acid-polymerized bacterial flagellin antigen. J. exp. Med. **143**, 1220–1238 (1976)

FINKELMAN, F.D., BOXEL, J.A. VAN, ASOFSKY, R., PAUL, W.E.: Cell membrane IgD: demonstration of IgD on human lymphocytes by enzymecatalyzed iodination and comparison with cell surface Ig of mouse, guinea pig, and rabbit. J. Immunol. **116**, 1173–1181 (1976)

FRADELIZI, D., DAUSSET, J.: Mixed lymphocyte reactivity of human lymphocytes primed in vitro. I. Secondary response to allogenic lymphocytes. Europ. J. Immunol. **5**, 295–301 (1975)

FRELINGER, J.A., NIEDERHUBER, J.E., DAVID, C.S., SHREFFLER, D.C.: Evidence for the expression of Ia (H-2-associated) antigens on thymus-derived lymphocytes. J. exp. Med. **140**, 1273–1284 (1974)

FUJIMOTO, S., GREENE, M.I., SEHON, A.H.: Regulation of the immune response to tumour antigens. 1. Immunosuppressor cells in tumourbearing hosts. J. Immunol. **116**, 791–799 (1976a)

FUJIMOTO, S., GREENE, M.I., SEHON, A.H.: Regulation of the immune response to tumour antigens. II. The nature of immunosuppressor cells in tumour-bearing hosts. J. Immunol. **116**, 800–806 (1976b)

FURTH, R. VAN (ed.): Mononuclear phagocytes in immunity, infection, and pathology. Oxford: Blackwell Scientific Publications 1975

GAAG, R. V. D., MCCULLAGH, P.: Facilitation of the growth of an allogeneic tumour by suppressor cells in newborn rats. Aust. J. exp. Biol. med. Sci. **53**, 421-429 (1975)

GALE, R.P., ZIGHELBOIM, J.: Polymorphonuclear leukocytes in antibody-dependent cellular cytotoxicity. J. Immunol. **114**, 1047–1051 (1975)

GELFAND, J., FAUCI, A.S., GREEN, I., FRANK, M.M.: A simple method for the determination of complement receptor-bearing cells. J. Immunol. **116**, 595–599 (1976)

GHAFFAR, A., CALDER, E.A., IRVINE, W.J.: K cell cytotoxicity against antibody-coated chicken erythrocytes in tumor-bearing mice: its development with progressively growing tumor and the effect of immunization against the tumor. J. Immunol. **116**, 315-318 (1976)

GOLDSTEIN, P., SMITH, E.T.: The lethal hit stage of mouse T and non-T cell-mediated cytolysis: differences in cation requirements and characterization of an analytical "cation pulse" method. Europ. J. Immunol. **6**, 31-37 (1976)

GOODMAN, S.A., VITETTA, E.S., MELCHER, U., UHR, J.W.: Cell surface immunoglobulin. XIII. Distribution of IgM and IgD-like molecules on small and large cells of mouse spleen. J. Immunol. **114**, 1646–1648 (1975)

GORMUS, B.J., SHANDS, J.W.: Endotoxin-stimulated spleen cells: characterization of the responding cells. J. Immunol. **115**, 118-123 (1975)

GREAVES, M., OWEN, J.J.T., RAFF, M.C.: T and B lymphocytes. New York: American Elsevier Publ. Co. 1973

GREBE, S.C., STREILEIN, J.W.: Graft-versus-host reactions: a review. Advanc. Immunol. **22**, 120–221 (1976)

GREENBERG, A.H., SHEN, L.: A class of specific cytotoxic cells demonstrated in vitro by arming with antigen-antibody complexes. Nature (New Biol.) **245**, 282–285 (1973)

GREENBERG, A.H., SHEN, L., WALKER, L., ARNAIZ-VILLENA, A., ROITT, I.M.: Characteristics of the effector cells mediating cytotoxicity against antibody-coated target cells. II. The mouse nonadherent K cell. Europ. J. Immunol. **5**, 474–480 (1975)

GREINEDER, D.K., ROSENTHAL, A.S.: Macrophage activation of allogeneic lymphocyte proliferation in the guinea pig mixed leukocyte culture. J. Immunol. **114**, 1541–1547 (1975)

GRIFFIN, F.M., BIANCO, C., SILVERSTEIN, S.C.: Characterization of the macrophage receptor for complement and demonstration of its functional independence from the receptor for the Fc portion of immunoglobulin G. J. exp. Med. **141**, 1269–1277 (1975)

GRONOWICZ, E., COUTINHO, A.: Functional Analysis of B cell heterogeneity. Transplant. Rev. **24**, 3–40 (1976)

HAEMMERLING, G.J., DEAK, B.D., MAUVE, G., HAEMMERLING, U., MCDEVITT, H.O.: 'B' lymphocyte alloantigens controlled by the I region of the major histocompatibility complex in mice. Immunogenetics **1**, 68 (1974)

HAEMMERLING, U., CHIN, A.F., ABBOTT, J., SCHEID, M.P.: The ontogeny of murine B lymphocytes. I. Induction of phenotypic conversion of Ia − to Ia + lymphocytes. J. Immunol. **115**, 1425–1431 (1975)

HAEYRY, P., ANDERSSON, L.C.: Generation of T memory cells in one-way mixed lymphocyte culture. III. Homing and lifetime of "secondary" lymphocytes. Cell. Immunol. **17**, 165–180 (1975)

HALLBERG, T., GURNER, B.W., COOMBS, R.A.: Opsonic adherence of sensitized ox red cells to human lymphocytes as measured by rosette formation. Int. Arch. Allergy **44**, 500–513 (1973)

HAMMAR, J.A.: Fünfzig Jahre Thymusforschung. Kritische Übersicht der normalen Morphologie. Ergebn. Anat. Entwickl.-Gesch. **19**, 1–274 (1910)

HAN, T., MINOWADA, J., SUBRAMANIAN, S., SINKS, L.F.: Human thymus cells. Excellent responders but poor stimulators in one-way mixed lymphocyte reactions. Immunology **30**, 361–366 (1976)

HARTMANN, K.-U., BOKISCH, V.A.: Stimulation of murine B lymphocytes by isolated C3b. J. exp. Med. **142**, 600–610 (1975)

HAUPTFELD, M., HAUPTFELD, U., KLEIN, J.: Ia and H-2 antigens on blast cells. Transplantation **19**, 528–530 (1975)

HIRST, J.A., BEVERLEY, P.C.L., KISIELOW, P., HOFFMANN, M.K., OETTGEN, H.F.: Ly antigens: markers of T cell function on mouse spleen cells. J. Immunol. **115**, 1555–1557 (1975)

HODES, R.J., HATHCOCK, K.S.: In vitro generation of suppressor cell activity: suppression of in vitro induction of cell-mediated cytotoxicity. J. Immunol. **116**, 167–177 (1976)

HOFMAN, F., GLOBERSON, A.: Immunological potential of yolk sac cells. In: Advances in experimental medicine and biology, FELDMAN, M. and GLOBERSON, A. (eds.), Vol. 66, pp. 51–57. New York: Plenum Press 1976

HOWE, M.L., COHEN, L.: Lymphoid cell subpopulations. I. Synergy between lymph node cells and thymocytes in response to alloantigens and mitogens. J. Immunol. **115**, 1227–1232 (1975a)

HOWE, M.L., COHEN, L.: Lymphoid cell subpopulations. II. Characterization of cell populations responsible for synergy in the mixed lymphocyte interaction. J. Immunol. **115**, 1233–1238 (1975b)

HUBER, B., DEVINSKY, O., GERSHON, R.K., CANTOR, H.: Cell-mediated immunity: delayed-type hypersensitivity and cytotoxic responses are mediated by different T-cell subclasses. J. exp. Med. **143**, 1534–1539 (1976)

HUDSON, L., SPRENT, J.: Specific adsorption of IgM antibody onto H-2-activated mouse lymphocytes. J. exp. Med. **143**, 444–449 (1976)

IGARASHI, T., OKADA, M., KISHIMOTO, S., YAMAMURA, Y.: The relation between the T cells responsible for cell-mediated cytotoxic killing of mastocytoma cells and the helper-cell effect. Immunology **28**, 37–47 (1975)

JANDINSKI, J., CANTOR, H., TANAKUMA, T., PEAVY, D.L., PIERCE, C.W.: Separation of helper T cells from suppressor T cells expressing different Ly components. I. Polyclonal activation: Suppressor and helper activities are inherent properties of distinct T-cell subclasses. J. exp. Med. **143**, 1382–1390 (1976)

JONDAL, M., HOLM, G., WIGZELL, H.: Surface markers on human B and T lymphocytes. I. A large population of lymphocytes forming nonimmune rosettes with SRBC. J. exp. Med. **136**, 207–215 (1972)

KIESSLING, R., KLEIN, E., WIGZELL, H.: Natural killer cells in mouse. I. Cytotoxic cells with specificity for mouse Moloney leukemia cells. Specificity and distribution according to genotype. Europ. J. Immunol. **5**, 112–117 (1975a)

KIESSLING, R., KLEIN, E., PROSS, H., WIGZELL, H.: Natural killer cells in the mouse. II. Cytotoxic cells with specificity for mouse Moloney leukemia cells. Characteristics of the killer cell. Europ. J. Immunol. **5**, 117–121 (1975b)

KIESSLING, R., PETRANYI, G., KAERRE, K., JONDAL, M., TRACEY, D., WIGZELL, H.: Killer cells: a functional comparison between natural, immune T-cell and antibody-dependent in vitro systems. J. exp. Med. **143**, 772–780 (1976)

KISIELOW, P., SHIKU, H., HIRST, J.A.: A new differentiation antigen defining a subpopulation of mouse T cells. Nature (Lond.) **261**, 137–139 (1976)

KNAPP, W., BOLHUIS, R.L.H., RADL, J., HIJMANS, W.: Independent movement of IgD and IgM molecules on the surface of individual lymphocytes. J. Immunol. **111**, 1295–1298 (1973)

KNIGHT, K., PERNIS, B.: Preparation of an antiserum against mouse IgD. In: Annual report 1975, Basel Institute for Immunology, p. 42 (1975)

KOMURO, K., BOYSE, E.A.: Induction of T lymphocytes from precursor cells in vitro by a product of the thymus. J. exp. Med. **138**, 479–482 (1973)

KOMURO, K., GOLDSTEIN, G., BOYSE, E.A.: Thymus-repopulating capacity of cells that can be induced to differentiate to T cells in vitro. J. Immunol. **115**, 195–198 (1975)

KONDA, S., STOCKERT, E., SMITH, R.T.: Immunologic properties of mouse thymus cells: membrane antigen patterns. Associated with various cell subpopulations. Cell. Immunol. **7**, 275–289 (1973)

KONTIAINEN, S., FELDMAN, M.: Suppressor cell induction in vitro. I. Kinetics of induction of antigen-specific suppressor cells. Europ. J. Immunol. **6**, 296–301 (1976)

KOVITHAVONGS, T., RICE, G., THONG, K.L., DOSSETOR, J.B.: Effector cell activity in antibody-mediated cell dependent immune lysis. II. Evidence for different populations of effector cells for different targets. Cell. Immunol. **18**, 167–175 (1975)

KRAMMER, P.H., HUDSON, L., SPRENT, J.: Fc-receptors, Ia-antigens, and immunoglobulin on normal and activated mouse T lymphocytes. J. exp. Med. **142**. 1403–1415 (1975)

KRAMMER, P.H., ELLIOTT, B.E., BOEHMER, H. V.: Fc-rosetting and nonrosetting T cells are killer cells. Europ. J. Immunol. **6**, 138–139 (1976)

LAFFERTY, K.J., BOOTES, A., DART, G., RADOVICH, G., TALMAGE, B.W.: Is a specialized stimulator cell required for the induction of allograft immunity? In: Advances in experimental medicine and biology, FELDMAN, M. and GLOBERSON, A. (eds.), Vol. 66, pp. 87–93. New York: Plenum Press 1976

LAMON, E.W., WHITTEN, H.D., LIDIN, B., FUDENBERG, H.H.: IgM-induced tumor cell cytotoxicity mediated by normal thymocytes. J. exp. Med. **142**, 542–547 (1975a)

LAMON, E.W., WHITTEN, H.D., SKURZAK, H.M., ANDERSSON, B., LIDIN, B.: IgM antibody-dependent cell-mediated cytotoxicity in the Moloney sarcoma virus system: the involvement of T and B lymphocytes as effector cells. J. Immunol. **115**, 1288–1294 (1975b)

LAMON, E.W., ANDERSSON, B., WHITTEN, H.D., HURST, M.M., GHANTA, V.: IgM complex receptors on subpopulations of murine lymphocytes. J. Immunol. **116**, 1199–1203 (1976)

LAUSE, D.B., WAKSAL, S.D., WAKSAL, H.W., ST. PIERRE, R.L.: Thymocyte subpopulations as stimulators in the mixed lymphocyte reaction. In: Advances in experimental medicine and biology, Vol. 66, FELDMAN, M. and GLOBERSON, A. (eds.), pp. 123–127. New York: Plenum Press 1976

LECKBAND, E., BOYSE, E.A.: A minor population of immunocompetent cells among mouse thymocytes. Science **172**, 1258–1260 (1971)

LEVEY, R.H., BURLESON, R.: Studies on the isolation of lymphocytes active in cell-mediated immune responses. II. Identification and recovery of an immunocompetent subpopulation of mouse thymocytes. Cell. Immunol. **4**, 316–332 (1972)

LING, N.R., KAY, J.E.: Lymphocyte stimulation. Amsterdam: North-Holland Publ. Co. 1975

LISOWSKA-BERNSTEIN, B., VASALLI, P.: The surface immunoglobulins of mouse spleen B lymphocytes: radioiodination, biosynthetic labeling and immunofluorescent studies. In: Membrane receptors of lymphocytes, SELIGMAN, M., PREUD'HOMME, J.L., KARILSKY, F.M. (eds.). Amsterdam: North-Holland Publ. Co. 1975

LOOR, F., ROELANTS, G.E.: Immunofluorescence studies of a possible prethymic T-cell differentiation in congenitally athymic (nude) mice. Ann. N. Y. Acad. Sci. **254**, 226 (1975)

LUKIC, M.L., COWING, C., LESKOWITZ, S.: Strain differences in ease of tolerance induction to bovine gamma-globulin: dependence on macrophage function. J. Immunol. **114**, 503–506 (1975)

LUZZATI, A.L., LAFLEUR, L.: Suppressor cells in rabbit peripheral blood. Europ. J. Immunol. **6**, 125–129 (1976)

MARCHALONIS, J.J.: Lymphocyte surface immunoglobulins. Science **190**, 20–29 (1975)

MASON, D.W.: The requirement for C3 receptors on the precursors of 19S and 7S antibody-forming cells. J. exp. Med. **143**, 1111–1121 (1976)

MCCONNEL, I., HURD, C.M.: Lymphocyte receptors. I. Receptors for Fc of IgG and complement (C3b) on immunoglobulinbearing, antigenbinding and antibody-secreting cells. Immunology **30**, 825–833 (1976a)

MCCONNEL, I., HURD, C.M.: Lymphocyte receptors. II. receptors for rabbit IgM on human T lymphocytes. Immunology **30**, 835–839 (1976b)

MCCULLAGH, P.: Radiosensitivity of suppressor cells in newborn rats. Aust. J. exp. Biol. med. Sci. **53**, 399–411 (1975a)

MCCULLAGH, P.: Role of the thymus in suppression of immune responses in newborn rats. Aust. J. exp. Biol. med. Sci. **53**, 413–420 (1975b)

MCCULLAGH, P.: Suppressor cells in homograft tolerant rats. Aust. J. exp. Biol. med. Sci. **53**, 431–436 (1975c)

MCCULLAGH, P.: Modification of the tolerant state by neonatal thymectomy. Immunology **31**, 39–45 (1976)

METCALF, D., MOORE, M.A.S.: Haemopoietic cells: their origin, migration and differentiation. Frontiers of Biology, Vol. 24. Amsterdam: North-Holland Publ. Co. 1971

MICKLEM, H.S., OGDEN, D.A., PRITCHARD, H.: Influence of cutaneous sensitization with oxazolone on recruitment of myelogeneous stem cells in the thymus. Clin. exp. Immunol. **12**, 103–110 (1972)

MOELLER, G.: Effect of B-cell mitogens on lymphocyte subpopulations possessing C′3 and Fc receptors. J. exp. Med. **139**, 969–982 (1974)

MOELLER, G. (ed.): Suppressor T Lymphocytes. Transpl. Rev. **26** (1975)

MOELLER, G., COUTINHO, A.: Role of C′3 and Fc receptors in B-lymphocyte activation. J. exp. Med. **141**, 647–663 (1975)

MOORE, M.A.S., OWEN, J.J.T.: Experimental studies on the development of the thymus. J. exp. Med. **126**, 715–726 (1967)

MOORE, M.A.S., METCALF, D.: Ontogeny of the haemopoietic system. Yolk sac origin of in vivo and in vitro colony forming cells in the developing mouse embryo. Brit. J. Haemat. **18**, 279 (1970)

MORSE, H.C., ASOFSKY, R.: Effects of antithymocyte serum on lymph node cells participating in the graft-versus-host reaction. Cell. Immunol. **24**, 69–78 (1976)

MOSIER, D.E., JOHNSON, B.M.: Ontogeny of mouse lymphocyte function. II. Development of the ability to produce antibody is modulated by T lymphocytes. J. exp. Med. **141**, 216–226 (1975)

MUELLER, J., BRUN DEL RE, G., BUERKI, H., KELLER, H.U., HESS, M.W., COTTIER, H.: Non-specific acid esterase activity: a criterion for differentiation of T and B lymphocytes in mouse lymph nodes. Europ. J. Immunol. **5**, 270–274 (1975)

MUGRABY, L., GERY, I., SULITZEANU, D.: Subpopulations of mouse spleen lymphocytes. II. Immunological reactivity of spleen cells fractionated on BSA density gradients. Immunology **28**, 589–596 (1975a)

MUGRABY, L., GERY, I., SULITZEANU, D.: Subpopulations of mouse spleen lymphocytes. III. Cellular interactions in the response to Concanavalin A. Immunology **28**, 1123–1133 (1975b)

NABARRA, B., DESCAMPS, B.: Ultrastructure of cells infiltrating human kidney allografts. Clin. exp. Immunol. **24**, 300–309 (1976)

NIEDERHUBER, J.E., FRELINGER, J.A., DUGAN, E., COUTINHO, A., SHREFFLER, D.C.: Effects of anti-Ia serum on mitogenic responses. I. Inhibition of the proliferative response to B cell mitogen, LPS, by specific anti-Ia sera. J. Immunol. **115**, 1672–1676 (1975)

NIEDERHUBER, J.E., FRELINGER, J.A., DINE, M.S., SHOFFNER, P., DUGAN, E., SHREFFLER, D.C.: Effects of anti-Ia sera on mitogenic responses. II. Differential expression of the Ia marker on phytohemagglutinin- and Concanavalin A–reactive T cells. J. exp. Med. **143**, 372–381 (1976)

NUSSENZWEIG, V.: Receptors for immune complexes on lymphocytes. Advanc. Immunol. **19**, 217–258 (1974)

OLDING, L.B., OLDSTONE, B.A.: Thymus-derived peripheral lymphocytes from human newborns inhibit division of their mothers lymphocytes. J. Immunol. **116**, 682–686 (1976)

Oppenheim, J.J., Rosenstreich, D.L.: Signals regulating in vitro activation of lymphocytes. Progr. Allergy **20**, 65–194 (1976)

Osoba, D.: Precursors of thymus lymphocytes. Ser. Haematol. **7**, 446–463 (1974)

Owen, J.J.T.: Ontogeny of the immune system. In: Progress in immunology II, vol. 5, Brenz, L. and Holborow, J. (eds.), pp. 163–173. Amsterdam: North-Holland Publ. Co. 1974

Paraskevas, F., Lee, S.-T., Orr, K.B., Israels, L.G.: A receptor for Fc on mouse B-lymphocytes. J. Immunol. **108**, 1319–1327 (1972)

Parish, C.R.: Separation and functional analysis of subpopulations of lymphocytes bearing complement and Fc receptors. Transplant. Rev. **25**, 98–120 (1975)

Parish, C.R., Chilcott, A.B.: Functional significance of the complement receptors on B lymphocytes. Cell. Immunol. **20**, 290–303 (1975)

Parkhouse, B., Abney, E.R.: Heterogeneity of surface immunoglobulins of murine B lymphocytes. In: Membrane receptors of lymphocytes, Seligman, M., Preud'Homme, J.L., Karilsky, F.M. (eds.). Amsterdam: North-Holland Publ. Co. 1975

Parkhouse, R.M.E., Hunter, I.R., Abney, E.R.: Heterogeneity of surface immunoglobulin on murine B lymphocytes. Immunology **30**, 409–412 (1976)

Perlman, P., Perlman, H., Mueller-Eberhard, H.J.: Cytolytic lymphocytic cells with complement receptor in human blood. Induction of cytolysis by IgG antibody but not by target cell-bound C3. J. exp. Med. **141**, 287–296 (1975)

Piessens, W.F., Churchill, W.H., David, J.R.: Macrophages activated in vitro with lymphocyte mediators kill neoplastic but not normal cells. J. Immunol. **114**, 293–299 (1975)

Pollack, S.B., Nelson, K., Grausz, J.D.: Separation of effector cells mediating antibody-dependent cellular cytotoxicity (ADC) to erythrocyte targets from those mediating ADC to tumor targets. J. Immunol. **116**, 944–946 (1976)

Pope, B.L., Whitney, R.B., Levy, J.G., Kilburn, D.G.: Suppressor cells in the spleen of tumor-bearing mice: enrichment by centrifugation on hypaque-ficoll and characterization on the suppressor population. J. Immunol. **116**, 1342–1346 (1976)

Potmesil, M., Goldfeder, A.: Nuclear morphology and cell proliferation kinetics of thymic lymphocytes. Exp. Cell Res. **77**, 31–40 (1973)

Rabellino, E.M., Metcalf, D.: Receptors for C3 and IgG on macrophages, neutrophil and eosinophil colony cells grown in vitro. J. Immunol. **115**, 688–692 (1975)

Raff, M.C.: Surface antigenic markers for distinguishing T and B lymphocytes in mice. Transplant. Rev. **6**, 52–80 (1971)

Raff, M.C., Cantor, H.: Subpopulations of thymus cells and thymus-derived lymphocytes. In: Progress in immunology, Amos, B. (ed.), p. 83–93. New York: Academic Press 1971

Ramasamy, R., Lawson, Y.: Independent movement of surface immunoglobulin from Fc receptors on lymphocyte membranes. Immunology **28**, 301–304 (1975)

Ramasamy, R., Williams, H.: C3 receptors on direct plaque-forming cells. Immunology **28**, 577–580 (1975)

Ramasamy, R., Richardson, N.E., Feinstein, A.: The specificity of the Fc receptor on murine lymphocytes for immunoglobulins of the IgG and IgM classes. Immunology **30**, 851–858 (1976)

Ramshaw, I.A., Parish, C.R.: Surface properties of cells involved in antibody-dependent cytotoxicity. Cell. Immunol. **21**, 226–235 (1976)

Rawson, A.J., Huang, T.C.: The response to phytohemagglutinin or to concanavalin A as a probe for subpopulations of human peripheral blood lymphocytes. Cell. Immunol. **17**, 310–314 (1975)

Rhodes, J.: Macrophage heterogeneity in receptor activity: the activation of macrophage Fc receptor function in vivo and in vitro. J. Immunol. **114**, 976–981 (1975)

Rich, R.R., Rich, S.S.: Suppression of mixed lymphocyte reactions by alloantigen-activated spleen-localizing thymocytes. Cell. Immunol. **22**, 358–368 (1976)

Roelants, G.E., Loor, F., Boehmer, H. v., Sprent, J., Haegg, L.-B., Mayor, K.S., Ryden, A.: Five types of lymphocytes (Ig$-\theta-$, Ig$-\theta+$weak, Ig$-\theta+$strong, Ig$+\theta-$ and Ig$+\theta+$) characterized by double immunofluorescence and electrophoretic mobility organ distribution in normal and nude mice. Europ. J. Immunol. **5**, 127–131 (1975)

Roelants, G.E., Mayor, K.S., Haegg, L.B., Loor, F.: Immature T lineage lymphocytes in athymic mice; Presence of TL, lifespan and homeostatic regulation. Europ. J. Immunol. **6**, 75–81 (1976a)

ROELANTS, G.E., MAYOR, K.S., HAEGG, L.B., LOOR, F.: Ontogeny of T lymphocytes studied in athymic and foetal mice. In: Advances in experimental medicine and biology, vol. 66, FELDMAN, M. and GLOBERSON, A. (eds.), p. 59–62. New York: Plenum Press 1976b

ROELLINGHOFF, M., WAGNER, H.: Secondary cytotoxic allograft response in vitro. I. Antigenic requirements. Europ. J. Immunol. 5, 875 879 (1975)

ROELLINGHOFF, M., PFIZENMEIER, K., TROSTMANN, H., WAGNER, H.: T cell proliferation in the mixed lymphocyte culture does not necessarily result in the generation of cytotoxic T effector cells. Europ. J. Immunol. 5, 560–564 (1975)

ROLSTAD, B.: The host component of the graft-versus-host reaction. Transplantation 21, 117–123 (1976)

ROSENBERG, Y.L., CUNNINGHAM, A.J.: Ontogeny of the antibody-forming cell lines in mice. I. Kinetics of appearance of mature B cells. Europ. J. Immunol. 5, 444–447 (1975)

ROSENSTREICH, D.L., FARR, J.J., DOUGHERTY, S.: Absolute macrophage dependency of T lymphocyte activation by mitogens. J. Immunol. 116, 131–139 (1976)

ROSENTHAL, A.S., LIPSKY, P.E., SHEVACH, E.M.: Macrophage-lymphocyte interaction and antigen recognition. Fed. Proc. 34, 1743–1748 (1975)

ROSS, G.D., POLLEY, M.J., RABELLINO, E.M., GREY, H.M.: Two different complement receptors on human lymphocytes. One specific for C3b and one specific for C3b inactivator cleaved C3b. J. exp. Med. 138, 798–811 (1973)

ROTTER, V., TRAININ, N.: Inhibition of tumor growth in syngeneic chimeric mice mediated by a depletion of suppressor T cells. Transplantation 20, 68–74 (1975)

ROWE, D.S., HUG, K., FORNI, L., PERNIS, B.: Immunoglobulin D as a lymphocyte receptor. J. exp. Med. 138, 965–972 (1973)

RUUSKANEN, O.: Subpopulations of guinea pig thymocytes. Different distribution patterns of alkaline phosphatase positive and negative autologous thymocytes. Cell. Immunol. 15, 246–254 (1975)

RUUSKANEN, O.J., PELLINIEMI, L.J., KOUVALAINEN, K.E.: Alkaline phosphatase in differentiating guinea pig thymocytes: an ultracytochemical study. J. Immunol. 114, 1611–1615 (1975)

RYSER, J.-E., VASALLI, P.: Mouse bone marrow lymphocytes and their differentiation. J. Immunol. 113, 719–728 (1974)

SACHS, D.H., CONE, J.L.: A mouse B-cell alloantigen determined by gene(s) linked to the major histocompatibility complex. J. exp. Med. 138, 1289–1304 (1973)

SANDILANDS, G., GRAY, K., COONEY, A., FROEBEL, K., ANDERSON, J.R.: Human lymphocyte subpopulations and K cells. Int. Arch. Allergy 50, 416–426 (1976)

SANTANA, V., TURK, J.L.: Binding of aggregated human immunoglobulin to murine thymocytes and T cells through receptors for the Fc region. Immunology 28, 1173–1178 (1975)

SCHEID, M.P., HOFFMANN, M.K., KOMURO, K., HAEMMERLING, U., ABBOTT, J., BOYSE, E.A., COHEN, G.H., HOOPER, J.A., SCHULOF, R.S., GOLDSTEIN, A.L.: Differentiation of T cells induced by preparations from thymus and by nonthymic agents. The determined state of the precursor cell. J. exp. Med. 138, 1027–1032 (1973)

SCHIRRMACHER, V., HALLORAN, P., DAVID, C.S.: Interactions of Fc receptors with antibodies against Ia antigens and other cell surface components. J. exp. Med. 141, 1201–1209 (1975)

SCHLEGEL, R.A., SHORTMAN, K.: Antigen-initiated B lymphocyte differentiation. IV. The adherence properties of antibody-forming cell progenitors from primed and unprimed mice. J. Immunol. 115, 94–99 (1975)

SCHLEGEL, R.A., BOEHMER, H. V., SHORTMAN, K.: Antigen-initiated B lymphocyte differentiation. V. Electrophoretic separation of different subpopulations of AFC progenitors for unprimed IgM and memory IgG responses to the NIP determinant. Cell. Immunol. 16, 203–217 (1975a)

SCHLEGEL, R.A., SHORTMAN, K., STOCKER, J.W., ODGERS, M.: Antigendependent B-lymphocyte differentiation. A comparison of the electrophoretic mobilities of AFC-progenitors, induced AFC and background AFC specific for several antigens. Aust. J. exp. Biol. med. Sci. 53, 117–127 (1975b)

SCHLESINGER, M.: Antigens of the thymus. Progress in Allergy 16, 214 (1972)

SCHLESINGER, M., ISRAEL, E., GERY, I.: Antigenic properties of subsets of splenic T lymphocytes responding to lectins. Immunology 30, 865–872 (1976)

SHIGENO, N., HAEMMERLING, U., ARPELS, C., BOYSE, E.A., OLD, W.J.: Preparation of lymphocyte-specific antibody from anti-lymphocyte serum. Lancet 1968 II, 320–323 (1968)

Shiku, H., Kisielow, P., Bean, M.A., Takahashi, T., Boyse, E.A., Oettgen, H.F., Old, L.J.:
Expression of T-cell differentiation antigens on effector cells in cell-mediated cytotoxicity in
vitro. Evidence for functional heterogeneity related to the surface phenotype of T cells. J. exp.
Med. 141, 227–241 (1975)

Shortman, K.: The density distribution of thymus, thoracic duct and spleen lymphocytes. J.
cell. Physiol. 77, 319–330 (1971)

Shortman, K., Jackson, H.: The differentiation of T lymphocytes. I. Proliferation kinetics and
interrelationships of subpopulations of mouse thymus cells. Cell. Immunol. 12, 230–246 (1974)

Shortman, K., Brunner, K.T., Cerottini, J.-C.: Separation of stages in the development of
the "T" cells involved in cell-mediated immunity. J. exp. Med. 135, 1375–1391 (1972)

Shortman, K., Byrd, W.J., Cerottini, J.-C., Brunner, K.T.: Characterization and separation
of mouse lymphocyte subpopulations responding to phytohemagglutinin and pokeweed mitogen.
Cell. Immunol. 6, 25–40 (1973)

Shortman, K., Boehmer, H. v., Lipp, J., Hopper, K.: Subpopulations of T lymphocytes. Transplant.
Rev. 25, 163–210 (1975)

Shreffler, D.C., David, C.S.: The H-2 major histocompatibility complex and the I immune
response region: genetic variation, function, and organization. Advanc. Immunol. 20, 125–195
(1975)

Simonian, S., Molenaar, J.L., Zeijlemaker, W.P., Knape, J.T.A., Bakker, S., Ponsman, K.W.:
Interaction of human lymphocytes with fluid phase human C3b detected by immunofluorescence.
Europ. J. Immunol. 6, 52–56 (1976)

Simpson, E.: Stimulation of mixed lymphocyte cultures and cytotoxic responses: evidence that
T cells express SD but not LD antigens, whereas B cells express both. Europ. J. Immunol.
5, 456–461 (1975)

Simpson, E., Cantor, H.: Regulation of the immune response by subclasses of T lymphocytes.
II. The effect of adult thymectomy upon humoral and cellular responses in mice. Europ. J.
Immunol. 5, 337–343 (1975)

Singh, U., Owen, J.J.T.: Studies on the effect of various agents on the maturation of thymus
stem cells. Europ. J. Immunol. 5, 286–288 (1975)

Solheim, B.G., Thorsby, E., Moeller, E.: Inhibition of the Fc receptor of human lymphoid
cells by antisera recognizing determinants of the HLA system. J. exp. Med. 143, 1568–1574
(1976)

Sondel, P.M., Chess, L., MacDermott, R.P., Schlossmann, S.F.: Immunologic functions of
isolated human lymphocyte subpopulations. III. Specific allogeneic lympholysis mediated by
human T cells alone. J. Immunol. 114, 982–987 (1975a)

Sondel, P.M., Chess, L., Schlossmann, S.F.: Immunologic functions of isolated human lymphocyte
subpopulations. IV. Stimulation of MLC and CML by human T cells. Cell. Immunol. 18, 351–359
(1975b)

Stobo, J.D., Paul, W.E.: Functional heterogeneity of murine lymphoid cells. III. Differential responsiveness of T cells to phytohemmagglutinin and concanavalin A as a probe for T cell subsets.
J. Immunol. 110, 362–375 (1973)

Stobo, J.D., Rosenthal, A.S., Paul, W.E.: Functional heterogeneity of murine lymphoid cells.
I. Responsiveness to and surface binding of concanavalin A and phytohemagglutinin. J. Immunol. 108, 1–17 (1972)

Stout, R.D., Herzenberg, L.A.: The Fc receptor on thymus-derived lymphocytes. I. Detection
of a subpopulation of murine T lymphocytes bearing the Fc receptor. J. exp. Med. 142, 611–621
(1975a)

Stout, R.D., Herzenberg, L.A.: The Fc receptor on thymus-derived lymphocytes. II. Mitogen
responsiveness of T lymphocytes bearing the Fc receptor. J. exp. Med. 142, 1041–1051 (1975b)

Takei, F., Levy, J.G., Kilburn, D.G.: In vitro induction of cytotoxicity against syngeneic mastocytoma and its suppression by spleen and thymus cells from tumour-bearing mice. J. Immunol.
116, 288–293 (1976)

Theofilopoulos, A.N., Dixon, F.J., Bokisch, V.A.: Binding of soluble immune complexes to
human lymphoblastoid cells. I. Characterization of receptors for IgGFc and complement and
description of the binding mechanism. J. exp. Med. 140, 877–894 (1974)

Tigelaar, R.E., Gershon, R.K., Asofsky, R.: Graft-versus-host reactivity of mouse thymocytes:
effect of in vitro treatment with anti-TL serum. Cell. Immunol. 19, 58–64 (1975)

TSE, H., DUTTON, R.W.: Separation of helper and suppressor T lymphocytes on a ficoll velocity sedimentation gradient. J. exp. Med. **143**, 1199–1210 (1976)

UCCINI, S., RUCO, L., SORAVITO, G., ADORINI, L., DORIA, G., BARONI, C.D.: Cell selection in the thymus of mice treated with Escherichia coli lipopolysacchararide (LPS). In: Advances in experimental medicine and biology, vol. 66, FELDMAN, M. and GLOBERSON, A. (eds.), pp. 95–99. New York: Plenum Press 1976

UNANUE, E.R., CALDERON, J.: Evaluation of the role of macrophages in immune induction. Fed. Proc. **34**, 1737–1742 (1975)

UNKELESS, J.C., EISEN, H.N.: Binding of monomeric immunoglobulins to Fc receptors of mouse macrophages. J. exp. Med. **142**, 1520–1533 (1975)

VASAR, P.S., LEVY, E.M., BROOKS, D.E.: Studies on the electrophoretic separability of B and T human lymphocytes. Cell. Immunol. **21**, 257–271 (1976)

VITETTA, E.S., MELCHER, U., McWILLIAMS, M., LAMM, M.E., PHILLIPSQUAGLIATA, J.M., UHR, J.W.: Cell surface immunoglobulin. XI. The appearance of an IgD-like molecule on murine lymphoid cells during ontogeny. J. exp. Med. **141**, 206–215 (1975)

VITETTA, E.S., FORMAN, J., KETTMAN, J.R.: Cell surface immunoglobulin. XVIII. Functional differences of B lymphocytes bearing different surface immunoglobulin isotypes. J. exp. Med. **143**, 1055–1066 (1976)

VOLPE, E.P., TURPEN, J.B.: Thymus: central role in the immune system of the frog. Science **190**, 1101–1103 (1975)

WAGNER, H., ROELLINGHOFF, M.: Secondary cytotoxic allograft responses in vitro. II. Differentiation of memory T cells into cytotoxic T lymphocytes in the absence of cell proliferation. Europ. J. Immunol. **6**, 15–21 (1976)

WALKER, W.S., DEMUS, A.: Antibody-dependent cytolysis of chicken erythrocytes by an in vitro-established line of mouse peritoneal macrophages. J. Immunol. **114**, 765–769 (1975)

WARNER, N.L.: Membrane immunoglobulins and antigen receptors on B and T lymphocytes. Advanc. Immunol. **19**, 67–216 (1974)

WEDNER, H.J., PARKER, C.W.: Lymphocyte Activation. Progr. Allergy **20**, 195–300 (1976)

WINCHESTER, R.J., FU, S.M., HOFFMAN, T., KUNKEL, H.G.: IgG on lymphocyte surfaces; technical problems and the significance of a third cell population. J. Immunol. **114**, 1210–1212 (1975)

YUTOKU, M., GROSSBERG, A.L., STOUT, R., HERZENBERG, L.A., PRESSMAN, D.: Further studies on Th-B, a cell surface antigenic determinant present on mouse B cells, plasma cells and immature thymocytes. Cell. Immunol. **23**, 140–157 (1976)

ZAGURY, D., BERNARD, J., THIERNESS, N., FELDMAN, M., BERKE, G.: Isolation and characterization of individual functionally reactive cytotoxic T lymphocytes: conjugation, killing and recycling at the single cell level. Europ. J. Immunol. **5**, 818–822 (1975)

General Tolerance Phenomena[1]

T. Hraba

A. Introduction

In 1953, Medawar and his collaborators (Billingham et al., 1953) succeeded in inducing experimentally transplantation tolerance in mice and chickens. Intraembryonic injections of allogeneic cells produced in the recipients permanent or at least prolonged survival of skin grafts of the same genotype as that of the intraembryonically injected cells. Independently, Hašek (1953b, 1956) at the same time induced tolerance to alloantigens in chickens. He described a technique for producing embryonic parabiosis in birds (Hašek, 1953a; Hraba, 1968) by the connection of chorioallantoic blood vessels. This parabiosis ended naturally at hatching. He observed that chickens joined during embryonic life lost the ability to form antibodies to the erythrocytes of their partner.

Experimental induction of transplantation tolerance by Medawar's group constitutes a further development of their earlier findings in cattle twins (Anderson et al., 1951; Billingham et al., 1952). Because the genetic analysis of inheritance based on mating experiments in cattle is expensive, twin studies are very important for this purpose. In order to evaluate the observations in twins, it is necessary to know their zygosity. The determination of zygosity by skin transplants seems a simple method: there are no antigenic differences in monozygotic twins, and consequently there is no reason for graft rejection. On the other hand, antigenic differences in dizygotic twins are the same as in siblings of separate birth, and graft rejection should occur regularly. However, Medawar and his collaborators found that skin grafts usually surviced in cattle twins. Skin graft survival was observed even in twins that were definitely diagnosed as dizygotic by other criteria.

This unexpected graft survival results from the frequent occurrence of vascular placental anastomosis in dizygotic twins of cattle. The anastomosis causes a sexual disbalance in the female partners of the heterosexual twin pairs in cattle, so-called freemartinism. Another effect of the anastomosis is the transfer of hematopoietic stem cells from one twin to the other, which leads to permanent erythrocyte chimerism. The presence of two antigenically different populations of erythrocytes in most dizygotic cattle twins was observed by Owen et al. (1945).

---

[1] This contribution is dedicated to Prof. Dr. Milan Hašek on the occasion of his 50th birthday.

Erythrocyte chimerism and the resulting skin graft survival and freemartinism have also been observed in sheep (STORMONT *et al.*, 1953; HRABA *et al.*, 1956; MOORE and ROWSON, 1958), but the frequency is much lower than in cattle. Furthermore, the exceptional occurrence of red cell chimerism has been reported in man (DUNSFORD *et al.*, 1953; BOOTH *et al.*, 1957; NICHOLAS *et al.*, 1957; SANGER and RACE, 1971; RACE and SANGER, 1972). In other species, erythrocyte chimerism resulting from natural embryonic parabiosis has been described in chickens from double-yolked eggs (BILLINGHAM *et al.*, 1956a) and in minks (RAPACZ *et al.*, 1965); in primates, it occurs as a regular phenomenon in marmosets (BENIRSCHKE *et al.*, 1962; GENGOZIAN *et al.*, 1969).

The finding of erythrocyte chimerism in cattle was an important stimulus to BURNET and FENNER (1949) in the formulation of their theory of antibody formation. They realized that the duration of erythrocyte chimerism, even in immunologically mature animals, was possible only because the chimeric twins had lost the ability to develop transplantation immunity to the intraembryonically transferred hematopoietic cells of the partner twin. In order to explain the nonreactivity to self components, they postulated for the early stages of development a different reactivity to the antigenic stimuli than in later stages. The antigen that induces antibody formation in immunologically mature animals should elicit the specific suppression of immune reactivity in the early stages of development. This process had to be brought about in a way analogous or identical to that of the induction of the adaptive enzymes. At that time the structure of the adaptive enzymes was not known to be genetically determined; it was thought to be induced by a process in which the enzymes became gradually adapted to the new substrate. BURNET and FENNER hypothesized that the antigen induces a specific enzyme in the embryo. Later in life, the antigen is handled by that adaptive enzyme in a way that precludes the initiation of antibody formation. In normal development, when the embryo is isolated from infectious and other antigenic factors, the specific nonreactivity should be induced only by the antigens of the own body and would be the basis of the recognition of "self" and "nonself". However, when in cattle twins the partner's cells are transferred by vascular anastomosis, their antigens should also induce specific nonreactivity in their host. The consequences would be the permanent survival of the partner's hematopoietic stem cells, leading to erythrocyte chimerism, and the ability to accept the twin's skin grafts, because of the sharing of individual transplantation antigens between different tissues.

The theory of BURNET and FENNER influenced the work of MEDAWAR and his collaborators and also the term they used to describe the phenomenon they observed: actively acquired tolerance. This term was descriptive in stressing the important nature of the phenomenon — tolerance of the graft by the host. Stating that this tolerance was actively acquired implied its relation to actively acquired immunity; it meant that it also was a specific outcome of the encounter with the antigenic stimulus, though a diametrically opposite one.

The finding of MEDAWAR and his collaborators (BILLINGHAM *et al.*, 1956a) that transplantation tolerance can be abolished by the adoptive transfer of normal lymphoid cells has been of particular importance for further development in this field of research. They concluded that in the tolerant organism those cells that are able to produce an immune reaction to the tolerated graft are absent. This finding has influenced their definition of immunologic tolerance (BILLINGHAM *et al.,* 1956a): "Tolerance represents the specific and systemic failure of the mechanism of immunological response which is brought about by exposing embryos or very young animals to 'antigenic' stimuli, i.e., to stimuli which would have caused older animals to have become sensitive or immune. It is due to a primary central failure of the mechanism of the immunological reaction, and not to some intercession at a peripheral level."

This finding has also decisively influenced the explanation of the mechanism of immunologic tolerance in BURNET's clonal selection theory of antibody formation, which takes into account the genetic determination of the structure of the proteins, including adaptive enzymes and antibodies (BURNET, 1959). According to this theory, the encounter with the antigen of young lymphoid cells, belonging to the cell clone reactive to the antigen injected, results in the death of those cells. Only mature cells are stimulated by the antigen to proliferate and later to differentiate into antibody-producing cells. Immunologic tolerance would be the result of an antigen-induced elimination of the cell clones reacting with the respective antigen. New cells with the immunocompetence of the eliminated clones can arise by somatic mutation any time during the life. Tolerance can therefore be permanent only when the antigen is present in the body and eliminates the new immunocompetent cells. This is the case in tolerance to own antigens. The nonreactivity to self components is induced by eliminating the cell clones capable of reacting with them (so-called forbidden clones).

Thus far, BURNET's clonal selection theory is the dominant theory not only of antibody formation but also of immunologic tolerance.

B. Tolerance Phenomena and Other Specific Inhibitions of Immune Reactions

BURNET and FENNER, and MEDAWAR considered immunologic tolerance to be a general immunologic phenomenon. In this sense, the term immunologic tolerance was later used to designate other states of specific inhibition of immune reactions that seemed to be due to the same mechanism as actively acquired tolerance to allografts. For the latter, the term transplantation tolerance is used. Sometimes the terms immunologic paralysis or immunologic unresponsiveness, originally used to designate the specific states of immunologic tolerance, are used for all tolerance phenomena. Because the term immunologic tolerance is currently more widely used and is preferred by the WHO Scientific Group on Factors Regulating the Immune Response (1969), I will use it here.

Some of the phenomena of specific inhibition were already known before BURNET and FENNER formulated their hypothesis. These included the Sulzberger-Chase phenomenon, immunologic paralysis, and immunologic enhancement. However, the discovery and analysis of most of these phenomena were made in parallel or were stimulated by the development of transplantation tolerance studies.

In general, I accept the definition of immunologic tolerance formulated by BILLINGHAM *et al.* (1956a) with the modification that the antigen for tolerance induction need not be injected during the embryonic or early postnatal period. Some of the tolerance phenomena are induced in adult individuals; this has also been shown to be possible even in transplantation tolerance (MARIANI *et al.*, 1959; SHAPIRO *et al.*, 1961). Immunologic immaturity of young animals is not a precondition, but a facilitating factor, in tolerance induction, as is nonspecific depression of immune reactivity by x-irradiation or immunosuppressive drugs in adults. This point in the heuristically invaluable theory of antibody formation of BURNET and FENNER was incorrect because of insufficient evidence at that time.

I. Inhibition States Classified as Immunologic Tolerance

In addition to transplantation tolerance, which has been briefly characterized in the Introduction, the following phenomena are generally classified as belonging to the category of immunologic tolerance.

1. The Sulzberger-Chase Phenomenon

As early as 1928 this inhibition phenomenon was described in humans by FREI and shortly thereafter analyzed in guinea pigs by SULZBERGER (1929a, b). They observed that the intravenous injection of neosalvarsan prevented the later induction of cutaneous sensitivity to this drug. Independently, CHASE (1946) prevented the sensitization to simple chemicals in guinea pigs by administering them perorally before the cutaneous sensitization. He demonstrated that the cutaneous sensitivity could not be transferred with serum, but he succeeded in doing it by adoptive transfers of lymphoid cells. CHASE (1949) also proved that the nonreactivity induced by the peroral administration of a contact allergen could be overcome by adoptive transfers of cells from immune animals. This actually was the first abolition of tolerance by the adoptive transfer of cells from nontolerant animals. This and the finding that neither blocking nor inhibiting antibodies could be detected in unresponsive animals (CHASE, 1963) strongly supported the view that this inhibition state was effected by a central failure of the immune mechanism. Hence, it could be classified as one of the states of immunologic tolerance.

2. Immunologic Paralysis

FELTON and OTTINGER (1942) observed in mice that large doses of purified pneumococcal polysaccharides specifically suppressed the ability to form antibody to the type of pneumococcal polysaccharide used. Pneumococcal polysaccharides are known to persist in the tissues for long periods of time (FELTON *et al.*, 1955; STARK, 1955). It has been hypothesized that antibody formation in paralyzed mice is not suppressed but masked by an excess of antigen (KAPLAN *et al.*, 1950; STARK, 1955). However, immunologic paralysis could be abrogated by passively transferred immune cells (BROOKE and KARNOFSKY, 1961; NEEPER and SEASTONE, 1963). Furthermore, no cells forming antibodies against the paralyzing pneumococcal polysaccharide in suppressed mice were detected by the immunofluorescence technique (SERCARZ and COONS, 1959, 1963) or later, by the more sensitive method of localized hemolysis in gel (MEDLÍN et al., 1969). Using the latter technique, HOWARD et al. (1970) found that the increase in the immunizing dose at first led to an increase of plaque-forming cells and at the same time to a decrease of circulating antibodies. This was probably due to the persisting higher concentrations of antigen in the tissues and the resulting neutralization of the antibodies. However, when even larger doses of the polysaccharide were injected, the antibody-forming cells were no longer detectable (HOWARD et al., 1971). The foregoing findings have proved that immunologic paralysis can be considered as a phenomenon belonging to the category of immunologic tolerance.

3. Tolerance to Heterologous Serum Proteins

The first evidence of this inhibition phenomenon was obtained at about the same time as transplantation tolerance was induced experimentally. In rabbits, perinatal injections of heterologous serum proteins led to the suppression of antibody formation when the treated rabbits were challenged with the same protein after reaching immunologic maturity (HANAN and OYAMA, 1954; DIXON and MAURER, 1955; CINADER and DUBERT, 1955). A similar effect was obtained by multiple injections of large doses of these antigens in adult rabbits (DIXON and MAURER, 1955). Later, this type of inhibition was induced in many other species. It was termed acquired immunologic tolerance by CINADER and DUBERT (1955), whereas DIXON and MAURER (1955) coined the term immunologic unresponsiveness. The latter is still used by some authors.

In immunologic tolerance to heterologous serum proteins, the amount of antigen injected can be exactly measured. This is also true for pneumococcal polysaccharides with the difference that heterologous serum proteins are catabolized relatively quickly. This enabled SMITH and BRIDGES (1958) to determine that the duration of tolerance to serum proteins was limited and that its length increased with the amount of antigen used for tolerance induction. Their original view (SMITH and BRIDGES, 1958; SMITH, 1961) that tolerance was terminated when the injected protein had disappeared from the circulation had to be abandoned because the rate of catabolism of different heterologous proteins did not correlate with the duration of tolerance to them (DIETRICH and WEIGLE, 1963), and because in some cases tolerance to heterologous proteins persisted even when the antigen had been eliminated from the circulation of the tolerant animals (BUSSARD, 1962; HUMPHREY, 1964; MITCHISON, 1965). It seems that the persistence of antigen in a location other than in the serum is crucial for the maintenance of tolerance. Because additional small doses of the tolerated protein could maintain tolerance (SMITH and BRIDGES, 1958), it has been hypothesized that transplantation tolerance, which persists in the absence of further inoculation of antigen, is maintained by continuous secretion of the antigen either from the test graft or from cells of the inoculum used for tolerance induction. The observation of MITCHISON (1962) that the persistence of tolerance to the nonrepopulating cells, i.e., allogeneic erythrocytes in chickens, depends on continuous supply of a new antigen, supports this hypothesis.

It was established very early that tolerance can also be induced to low molecular haptens conjugated to heterologous serum proteins (CINADER and PIERCE, 1958), and such conjugates have often been used in the study of tolerance. The fact that challenge of animals, tolerant to a heterologous serum protein, with a conjugate formed between this protein and a hapten can bring about the termination of tolerance (CINADER and DUBERT, 1955, 1956; WEIGLE, 1962) has proved to be an important finding. Immunization with a natural antigen crossreacting with the tolerated one, for example, the challenge of rabbits tolerant to bovine serum albumin with human serum albumin (WEIGLE, 1961), has the same effect.

DRESSER (1961 b) observed that a solution of bovine serum globulin, freed of aggregated material by ultracentrifugation, lost its antigenicity unless it was administered with an adjuvant (DRESSER, 1961 a), but it was able to induce tolerance. This preparation exerted its tolerogenic effect even when administered in very low doses (DRESSER, 1962). The term tolerogen is used for the antigenic substances that lack immunogenicity but are capable of inducing tolerance.

The first case of low-dose tolerance was described with bovine serum albumin (MITCHISON, 1964). This protein induces in mice tolerance in two zones of antigen concentration: one higher and one lower than the zone of the concentrations eliciting an immune response. Low-zone tolerance was induced mainly by heterologous serum proteins, but it was also achieved by *Salmonella* flagellin (NOSSAL and ADA, 1964; NOSSAL *et al.,* 1965; SHELLAM and NOSSAL, 1968) and by bacteriophage fd (WEBER and KÖLSCH, 1972).

The central nature of the inhibition of immune response in tolerance to heterologous serum proteins has been suggested in the early experiments with the adoptive transfer of lymphoid cells in rabbits (WEIGLE and DIXON, 1959; SMITH, 1960) and confirmed in extensive experiments in syngeneic mice (WEIGLE, 1973). Another proof is the absence of antibody-forming cells in animals tolerant to heterologous proteins, which is well documented by the sensitive methods for their detection (CHILLER *et al.,* 1970; BELL and SHAND, 1973). In addition to the suppression of antibody formation, the absence of cell-mediated immunity has been found in guinea pigs (HUMPHREY and TURK, 1961; TURK and HUMPHREY, 1961) and rabbits (CHUTNÁ and HRABA, 1962) tolerant to heterologous serum proteins. It can be said that in this tolerance phenomenon the mechanism of the inhibition state has been analyzed in greatest detail.

In concluding this section, I would like to emphasize that tolerance to heterologous proteins is not limited to serum proteins. The first findings of tolerance to defined heterologous nonserum proteins were obtained by BUSSARD (1957) with yeast glucose-6-phosphate dehydrogenase and by CINADER *et al.* (1958) with bovine ribonuclease, both in newborn rabbits. Tolerance to *Salmonella* flagellin (NOSSAL and ADA, 1964) belongs to the best analyzed cases of tolerance states (NOSSAL *et al.,* 1965).

4. Tolerance to Other Antigens

In addition to the antigens mentioned in the preceding paragraphs, heterologous cells were often used for the induction of tolerance. In the first experiments of this type with chicken–duck embryonic parabionts (HAŠEK and HRABA, 1955a, b) and with intraembryonic injections of turkey erythrocytes into chickens (SIMONSEN, 1955), the tolerance induced was only partial, i.e., the antibody formation was decreased but not completely suppressed. Tolerance to sheep erythrocytes in rats (NOSSAL, 1958) and in mice (FRIEDMAN, 1965) was often used to analyze the mechanism of tolerance (HRABA, 1974/5).

Also, bacteria and viruses were used successfully for tolerance induction (for references, see HRABA, 1968), but the tolerance achieved was only partial. The incomplete tolerance was probably due to the antigenic complexity of the whole viruses or bacteria, as was the case in the tolerance to heterologous cells.

Other antigens, which do not fit in any of the preceding categories, are bacterial lipopolysaccharides and nucleic acids. Tolerance to lipopolysaccharide has been induced in adult mice (BRITTON, 1969). This tolerance is short-lived, and relatively large doses of antigen are necessary for its induction.

The interest in blocking antinuclear autoantibody production in New Zealand Black (NZB) mice led to the induction of tolerance to polyinosinic-polycytidylic acid (STEINBERG et al., 1970), calf thymus DNA (PARKER et al., 1974), and ribonucleosides (ESHHAR et al., 1975).

II. Other Antigen-induced States of Specific Inhibition of the Immune Response

Two inhibition phenomena elicited by the antigen, which are supposed to be effected by mechanisms different from immunologic tolerance, are classified under this heading.

1. Immunologic Enhancement

This phenomenon was known before transplantation tolerance had been induced experimentally (CASEY, 1932). It was found that in some cases injections of killed allogeneic tumors were not only ineffective in inducing immunity against the tumor transplants; they in fact decreased it. The observed inhibition of transplantation immunity was specific for the tumor that had been used for the pretreatment.

At the time when transplantation tolerance was described, SNELL (1954) hypothesized that immunologic enhancement was effected by the same mechanism. However, KALISS and KANDUTSCH (1956) found that the serum of animals injected with killed allogeneic tumor tissue could transfer the suppression of transplantation immunity to the untreated control animals. The effective factor in the serum was an antibody directed against alloantigens of the donor. Evidently, injection of the alloantigenic material led to an immune reaction manifested by antibody production, and the antibody was operative in bringing about the inhibition of tumor graft rejection. BILLINGHAM *et al.* (1956b) therefore concluded that immunologic enhancement is a phenomenon other than immunologic tolerance.

2. Immune Deviation

This unresponsive state is characterized by the inhibition of cellular immunity and of some classes of antibodies directed against the antigen used for its induction, with persisting or even enhanced production of other classes of antibodies (ASHERSON and STONE, 1965; ASHERSON, 1966; LOEWI *et al.*, 1966; DVO-RAK *et al.*, 1966). Immune deviation is induced by relatively small doses of antigen, incorporated mostly into incomplete Freund's adjuvant, alum precipitated, or injected even in a soluble form. The antigen used for challenge is incorporated into complete Freund's adjuvant. The inhibitory effect cannot be transferred with serum of the pretreated animals. The type of the inhibition present in immune deviation resembles some states of partial immunologic tolerance (TURK and HUMPHREY, 1961; BOREL *et al.*, 1966; BOREL and DAVID, 1970). However, it differs from tolerance (ASHERSON, 1968) in that (1) it is induced by injection of small amounts of antigen in adult animals; (2) the antigen can be injected in a highly immunogenic form (alum precipitated or incorporated in incomplete Freund's adjuvant); and (3) x-irradiation, which favors the induction of immunologic tolerance, prevents induction of immune deviation.

It is of general interest that the immune deviation type suppression of immune reactions has been achieved in some experimental autoimmune syndromes by the injection of a tissue antigen in saline before injection of the same antigen in complete Freund's adjuvant (JANKOVIĆ and FLAX, 1963; CHUTNÁ and RYCHLÍ-KOVÁ, 1964a, b; CHUTNÁ, 1970). Because cellular immunity is primarily responsible for tissue damage in these autoimmune syndromes, this pretreatment, which suppresses the cell-mediated reactions, prevents their development.

C. Mechanisms of Immunologic Tolerance

I. The Relation of Antibody-Induced Suppression to Immunologic Tolerance

The first serious challenge to the concept of immunologic tolerance was provided by the data on specific suppression of the immune response by antibodies. The adverse effect of a mixture of antigen with an excess of antibody on active antibody formation in the recipients has been studied since the discovery of this effect in the 1890's (for references, see UHR and MÖLLER, 1968). A new aspect was introduced by the observations of UHR and BAUMANN (1961) that antibody administered separately from antigen, even as late as 5 days after immunization, can suppress the immune response. The view has been expressed that this is a feedback mechanism regulating the immune response. The phenomenon has been thoroughly analyzed in the immune response to sheep erythrocytes (ROWLEY and FITCH, 1964; MÖLLER and WIGZELL, 1965). In this system, it has also been found that antibody produced in small quantities can effect the suppression of the immune response. Rats given only a single injection of antibodies and injected with sheep red blood cells for the first time one day later, and then at weekly intervals, show a low antibody response as long as antigen injections are continued (NEIDERS et al., 1962). Active antibody production, not passively administered antibody, accounts for the maintenance of the suppression of antibody formation in this system.

A simple neutralization of the antigen could not explain all the phenomena described, since even small amounts of antibody could exert the suppressive effect in some cases. It seems probable that the antibody affects the immune response in a more subtle way and that relatively small amounts of antibody at critical sites depress the immune response. Furthermore, it has even been assumed that the action of antibody is directed immediately at immunocompetent cells (ROWLEY and FITCH, 1964; CHAN and SINCLAIR, 1971). Although some evidence points to the macrophage as the target of the inhibitory effect of antibodies (PIERCE, 1969; RYDER and SCHWARTZ, 1969; HAUGHTON and ADAMS, 1970; ABRAHAMS et al., 1973), other experiments suggest that lymphocytes may be the target of this action (GERSHON et al., 1974; HOFFMANN et al., 1974).

Taking into account that the suppression of immune response is incomplete in many states of immunologic tolerance and that transient antibody production accompanies induction of tolerance in some cases, it has been natural to hypothesize that immunologic tolerance phenomena are also effected by the action of antibodies produced in low quantities in tolerant animals rather than by a direct action of the antigen (ROWLEY and FITCH, 1965; SINCLAIR and CHAN, 1971).

Data are available that do not agree with the preceding view. In the inhibition states mediated by the weak immune response, antibody-producing cells are present in detectable quantities (ROWLEY and FITCH, 1965). On the other hand, these cells could not be demonstrated, even by very sensitive techniques, in some cases of immunologic tolerance, especially to heterologous serum proteins (CHILLER et al., 1970; BELL and SHAND, 1973). Moreover, no antibody-producing cells were detectable even during induction of tolerance to bovine serum albumin in newborn rabbits (CHILLER et al., 1973). Evidently, tolerance could be induced without antibody production in this case.

As mentioned previously, some antigens lacking immunogenicity are able to induce tolerance. They cannot be expected to evoke production of antibodies that might be responsible for the inhibition of immune response observed after the administration of these antigens.

II. Cellular Processes in Immunologic Tolerance

Clarification of the mechanisms of immunologic tolerance requires identification of the type of cells responsible for it. There is strong evidence that small lymphocytes are the critical target cells in tolerance induction. This evidence comes mainly from experiments with the transfers of thoracic duct cells (GOWANS et al., 1962; MCGEGOR and GOWANS, 1963; BILLINGHAM et al., 1963). While cells of normal animals can abolish the tolerant state in the recipients, or restore the immune responsiveness of x-irradiated recipients, thoracic duct cells of tolerant animals are unable to do it. On the other hand, the macrophages of tolerant animals generally have been found to be able to fulfil their functions normally (HARRIS, 1967; FORBES, 1969).

During the last decade, two classes of lymphoid cells, T- and B-cells, have been described. Much effort has been aimed at clarifying the role of these two types of cells in immune tolerance (GERSHON et al., 1968; TAYLOR, 1968; MILLER and MITCHELL, 1970; PLAYFAIR, 1969; CHILLER et al., 1970, 1971; RAJEWSKI, 1971). The data obtained agree in general with the conclusion that tolerance can be induced in both types of cells. However, tolerance in T-cells is induced faster, with smaller doses of antigen, and persists longer than in the B-cells. This leads to tolerance states where only the T-cell population is tolerant and the B-cell population is immunologically reactive. In these situations, the lack of T-cell cooperation with B-cells prevents antibody production by the reactive B-cells and causes the maintenance of immunologic tolerance.

Best evidence for the nature of cellular processes leading to tolerance induction comes from tolerance induction to flagellin in vitro (DIENER and ARMSTRONG, 1967, 1969). Polymerized flagellin is very effective in inducing tolerance in vitro, though it is a very potent immunogen both in vivo and in vitro. On the other hand, the monomeric flagellin and even the smaller unit of flagellin, Fragment A, though tolerogenic in vivo, lack tolerogenic capacity in vitro, and are weak immunogens both in vivo and in vitro. It seems that the effective tolerogens in vitro are the substances that, due to their repetitive determinants, can cross link surface receptors to an extent that is beyond the optimum for the induction of immune response. This view is supported by the observation that Fragment A, which alone is not tolerogenic, induces tolerance in vitro, when bound with an adequate amount of antibody (FELDMAN and DIENER, 1970; DIENER and FELDMAN, 1970, 1972). This finding raises the question whether the antigen-antibody complexes cannot act as tolerogenic stimuli also in other situations. If this were the case, the difference between the unresponsive states induced directly by the antigen and at least some cases of unresponsiveness induced by the antibodies would be obliterated.

The major question posed by the clonal selection theory, as to whether the cell clones reactive to the tolerated antigen are eliminated in tolerant animals, has not yet been answered. The possibility remains that the respective cell clones are only inhibited. Because tolerant cells would exist in such cases, it would be easier to demonstrate them than to prove the elimination of the respective cell clones. In the latter case, no positive signs would be expected to signal the situation. On the other hand, if tolerant cells would exist, they could be detected on the basis of some positive signs. The most effective way of visualizing them would be to reverse their unresponsiveness and to render them immunologically reactive.

A very efficient way of terminating tolerance is the immunization with certain antigens that cross react with the tolerated antigen. However, it seems that this can be achieved only when the reactive B-cells are present in tolerant animals and when tolerance is maintained by the absence of the reactive T-cells. The cross-reacting antigens activate the T-cells reacting with the determinants of the injected antigen, which are different from determinants of the tolerated antigen. These activated T-cells can then effect antibody production to the tolerated antigen by cooperating with B-cells reactive to the determinants shared by the tolerated and cross-reacting antigens (BENJAMIN and WEIGLE, 1970).

Probably a similar mechanism is involved in situations where the injection of the tolerated antigen with bacterial lipopolysaccharide (CHILLER and WEIGLE, 1973; MADAR et al., 1973) or polyanions (DIAMANTSTEIN and WAGNER, 1973) breaks tolerance. Also in this case, probably only T-cells are tolerant, and the lipopolysaccharide or the polyanions substitute for the missing cooperative stimulus, which activates the reactive B-cells. The antibody-producing cells of the tolerant animals are therefore not the tolerant cells that have lost tolerance but the already reactive cells visualized in these circumstances. The same might be true for the termination of tolerance by allogeneic cells, capable of mounting the graft-versus-host reaction, in the tolerant recipients (McCULLAGH, 1970, 1972).

Another approach to the problem of eliminating the immunocompetent cells in tolerant animals is the detection of antigen-binding cells in unresponsive animals. In some cases, essentially the same numbers of such cells are found in tolerant and in normal, nonimmune animals (ADA and COOPER, 1971; MADAR et al., 1971; COOPER et al., 1972). In other cases, the numbers of antigen-binding cells are reduced in tolerant animals (NAOR and SULITZEANU, 1969; KATZ et al., 1971; ARGYRIS et al., 1972). However, the cells detected could have been reactive B-cells, which are present in some cases of immunologic tolerance. The number of antigen-binding cells indeed correlates well with the reactivity of B-cells in tolerance to human gamma globulin in mice (WEIGLE et al., 1974). The finding that no significant numbers of antigen-binding cells can be detected in these mice at a time when both T- and B-cell populations are tolerant, is very important for the problem discussed. However, before concluding that this proves the elimination of the cell clones reactive to the tolerated antigen, it should be clarified whether the absence of antigen-binding cells is not just simulated by a blockade of their receptors with tolerogen, as has been observed in the case of tolerance induced by the DNP hapten bound to isogeneic globulin (ALDO-BENSON and BOREL, 1974). The number of cells with tolerogen attached to their surface is in the tolerant mice even higher than the number of antigen-binding cells in control animals, but the tolerogen bound to their surface prevents them from binding the labeled antigen that has been used for the detection of antibody-binding cells.

Other findings also point to the possibility that the tolerated antigen, or the hapten, remains attached to the surface of immunocompetent cells and probably is instrumental in causing unresponsiveness (Biro and Arroyave, 1970; Gronowicz and Coutinho, 1975). Blockade of the receptors of immuno-competent cells by the tolerated antigen or hapten, causing their functional inhibition, is an attractive and verifiable hypothesis.

The existence of reversibly inhibited cells was described in tolerance to pneu-mococcal polysaccharides (Howard et al., 1972) and to bacterial lipopolysaccha-ride (Sjöberg, 1972). In both these states the transfer of lymphoid cells from tolerant donors to normal syngeneic irradiated recipients led to the termination of tolerance. This recovery from tolerance was so fast that it could hardly be explained by the recruitment of reactive cells from a pool of newly maturing immunocompetent cells. Also, the findings of increased numbers of antigen-binding cells in animals tolerant to pneumococcal polysaccharide (Howard et al., 1969, 1971) and to bacterial lipopolysaccharide (Sjöberg and Möller, 1970; Sjöberg, 1971) pointed to the reversible inhibition of immunocompetent cells in these tolerant animals. Evidently, there exists an antigen-effected blocking of differentiation of cells immunocompetent to the tolerated antigen that pre-vents their maturation from antigen-binding into antibody-secreting cells. How-ever, such a situation is not a rule. In other states of immunologic tolerance, the transfer of cells of the tolerant animals into normal animals does not break their unresponsiveness (Stastny, 1964; Shellam, 1971; Bell and Shand, 1973; Hamilton et al., 1974; Mitchell et al., 1974).

It is probable that different levels of the differentiation process are affected in various states of immunologic tolerance. This view is supported by the finding that an excess of antigen can block the maturation of memory cells into antibody-forming cells (Byers and Sercarz, 1970; Rittenberg and Bullock, 1972) and even depress actively, not by simple neutralization, antibody production in individual antibody-forming cells (Schrader and Nossal, 1974). It is improb-able that in these situations the inhibitory effect is obtained in the same manner as in the unstimulated lymphoid cells, which are the target of tolerance induction in other situations (Chiller et al., 1973; Fidler and Golub, 1974).

III. Suppressor Cells

In some experimental systems in which tolerance seems to be involved, it has been observed that the adoptive transfer of nonimmune allogeneic cells does not abrogate the unresponsive state, although immune cells are able to do it. In most of these cases, it has been possible to transfer the unresponsiveness to normal recipients with lymphoid cells or with serum of "tolerant" animals (Crowle and Hu, 1969; Tong and Boose, 1970; Terman et al., 1973a, b). Antibody-mediated suppression of the immune response, alone or in combina-tion with immunologic tolerance, was clearly responsible for the inhibition observed. So far, these findings are warning against accepting any inhibition state as a tolerance phenomenon unless sufficient evidence is available.

Still another category of active suppression phenomena has been described. The first observations of this kind were made by Gershon and Kondo (1971). Using the transfer of thymus and bone marrow cells to irradiated recipients, they provided evidence that in their experimental model the T-cells from tolerant donors were not only incapable of cooperating with normal B-cells, but that they prevented the cooperation of normal T- and B-cells. The available evidence pointed against the involvement of antibody in this phenomenon, which the authors have called "infectious tolerance." According to their view, the inhibition was caused by suppressor T-cells.

Suppressor cells were observed first in mice immunized with pneumococcal polysaccharide after treatment with antilymphocyte serum (BAKER et al., 1970a). The treatment enhanced antibody formation, and this enhancement could be abrogated by infusing syngeneic thymocytes (BAKER et al., 1970b). This finding was interpreted as enhancement of antibody formation by eliminating suppressor cells. Suppressor cells were later found in other systems, too (DROEGE, 1971; KERBEL and EIDINGER, 1972). OKUMURA and TADA (1971) observed that the transient production of IgE homocytotropic antibody in rats could be prolonged by x-irradiation and that this prolonged production was depressed by the transfer of thymus or spleen cells. Later, they succeeded in isolating a humoral factor derived from T-lymphocytes that exerted the suppressive effect. This factor possessed the specificity and affinity for the carrier part of the antigen but, though it was a protein, it lacked immunoglobulin determinants, and its molecular weight was approximately 50,000 (TADA et al., 1973; OKUMURA and TADA, 1974).

All cases of suppressor cells mentioned previously concern suppressor T-cells. In some other systems, the B-cells suppressing cellular immunity have been described (KATZ et al., 1974a; KERCKHAERT et al., 1974). Circulating antibody can also depress cellular immunity, but at least in one of the foregoing systems in which the suppressor B-cells were operative, the suppressor effect could not be proved to be mediated by the antibody (KATZ et al., 1974b).

The involvement of suppressor cells in the states of immune unresponsiveness has been studied extensively in the Sulzberger-Chase phenomenon. Suppressive cells, preventing sensitization of normal recipients, were found in mice rendered unresponsive to dinitrobenzene (ASHERSON et al., 1971; ZEMBALA and ASHERSON, 1973). Suppressor cells responsible for this effect are T-cells. In this system the suppressive effect can be transferred by a humoral factor (ZEMBALA et al., 1975). This factor can bind the antigen, and its effect is specific. It has a maximal molecular weight of 50,000. The factor loses its activity when incubated with macrophages, and because the macrophages become suppressive after such incubation, the factor is obviously adsorbed to them.

Probably a similar situation exists in guinea pigs rendered unresponsive to contact hypersensitivity (POLAK and TURK, 1974; POLAK, 1975). Cyclophosphamide treatment, which is known to inactivate suppressor cells thereby enhancing contact hypersensitivity, breaks the unresponsiveness of the guinea pigs.

Similarly, in tolerance to fowl gamma globulin induced in adult mice, evidence was provided for the inclusion of suppressor cells in the category of T-cells (BASTEN et al., 1974). On the other hand, investigators working with tolerance to human gamma globulin in adult mice were not able to detect suppressor cells (WEIGLE et al., 1974). The conclusions as to the role of suppressor cells in the unresponsive states should be made with caution. It should be determined whether the activity of suppressor cells can fully explain the inhibition of the immune response observed in situations where these cells have been detected, or whether other mechanisms are also operating, which might be even more important. In any event, in view of the existence of suppressor cells, the available data on the mechanisms of immunological tolerance should be re-evaluated and re-examined.

IV. Transplantation Tolerance

Transplantation tolerance was considered to be an inhibition state caused by deletion or inactivation of the respective immunocompetent cell clones because it could have been abrogated by the adoptive transfer of nonimmune lymphoid cells (BILLINGHAM et al., 1956a). However, by the end of the 1950's VOISIN (1960) hypothesized that immunologic tolerance and immunologic enhancement (for the latter he coined the term facilitation reaction) are caused by the same mechanism, i.e., by an immune reaction that counteracts the immune reaction responsible for graft rejection. Together with his collaborators he obtained a considerable body of data showing that antibodies are produced in animals considered to be tolerant and that these antibodies may enhance the growth of allogeneic tumors (VOISIN, 1962, 1971; VOISIN et al., 1968, 1972). However, these data could not refute an alternative explanation that these were the cases of incomplete tolerance and that the enhancement mechanism cooperated with the mechanism of immunologic tolerance in effecting the graft survival. On the other hand, it cannot be denied that cases of transplantation tolerance, in which circulating antibodies are present, are no exception.

At least one state of transplantation tolerance cannot be explained by assuming that it is mediated by circulating antibodies. Two groups of investigators succeeded in inducing transplantation tolerance in bursectomized chickens (ROUSE and WARNER, 1972; CRONE, 1973). Because bursectomy removes the primary lymphoid organ responsible for the maturation of B-cells, which are the producers of circulating antibodies, antibody responses are suppressed in these birds. Therefore, it cannot be expected that circulating antibody responses against the donor's antigens effected the inhibition of transplantation immunity observed in these chickens.

Furthermore, the extent to which immunologic enhancement is caused only by circulating antibodies is not clear. CHUTNÁ (1968a, b, 1971) obtained a prolongation of allogeneic skin grafts in the recipients treated with lyophilized spleen cells in saline, particularly after incorporation of the antigen into incomplete or complete Freund's adjuvant. She was unable to achieve a comparable effect by serum from the pretreated mice, so she suspected that mechanisms other than circulating antibodies took part in the observed prolongation of graft survival.

Of particular importance for the clarification of the mechanism of immunologic tolerance were the findings of the HELLSTRÖMs and their collaborators (HELLSTRÖM et al., 1970, 1971; WEGMANN et al., 1971). They observed in different systems of transplantation tolerance that the tolerant animals possessed lymphoid cells exhibiting in vitro cytotoxicity toward cells syngeneic with the tolerated graft. This finding was difficult to explain by weak tolerance because these cells were also detected in tetraparental mice. Although, in the meantime, evidence has accumulated that lymphoid cell chimerism, which seems to be decisive for the induction of transplantation tolerance, varies considerably in tetraparental animals (GORNISH et al., 1972; DEOL, 1973; TUFFREY et al., 1973), the finding of the cytotoxic cells in these animals should be taken as a serious memento.

It was further observed by the HELLSTRÖM group that serum of the "tolerant" animals, possessing leukocytes cytotoxic to the tolerated cells, contained specific factors suppressing this cytotoxic reaction. Also, a blocking factor was detected in the serum of tetraparental chimeras. They concluded that transplantation tolerance was an inhibition phenomenon in which cellular immunity to the transplantation antigens was present, but its manifestation was suppressed by a blocking factor present in the body fluids. The available evidence points to the conclusion that this blocking factor is an antigen-antibody complex (WRIGHT et al., 1973, 1974).

These findings contradict the view that the mechanism causing immunologic tolerance is a central failure of the immune mechanism induced by the direct, unmediated action of the antigen, and they have stimulated naturally a vigorous discussion (ATKINS and FORD, 1972; BRENT et al., 1972; MEDAWAR, 1973). Blocking activity in the serum of most of the tolerant animals has also been found by other investigators (CHUTNÁ et al., 1973). However, cytotoxically active lymphocytes were detected in only about 50% of the tolerant rats tested. These authors (HAŠEK et al., 1975) could not demonstrate that the blocking factors played any role in the induction of tolerance.

In contrast to the presence of cytotoxic cells, cells causing graft-versus-host reactions and reactive in vitro in the mixed lymphocyte reaction are mostly absent in tolerant animals (SILVERS et al., 1970; ATKINS and FORD, 1972; ELKINS, 1973). The immune processes underlying graft rejection are complex. Whether cells showing cytotoxicity in vitro are also active in vivo in graft rejection is not yet known. Nor has the in vivo role of cells responsible for the mixed lymphocyte and graft-versus-host reactions been determined. In the relatively well-known system of the in vitro reactions it has been found that different antigens, or at least different antigenic determinants, are responsible for the mixed lymphocyte reactions and for the cytotoxicity induced in vitro. It is possible that tolerance to some of these antigens and at the same time immunity to others may be present.

In any event, it cannot be denied that cells displaying cytotoxicity in vitro, factors blocking this cytotoxicity, and circulating antibodies with enhancing capacity, all of them being specific for alloantigens of the tolerated graft, occur almost regularly in tolerant animals. What remains to be elucidated is whether they are the decisive factors in graft survival or secondary factors that cooperate or compete with the primary ones. At present, it can only be guessed whether the decisive factor is immunologic tolerance, i.e., a central inhibition of the transplantation reaction induced directly by the antigen. Even if the deletion or inactivation of immunocompetent cell clones were responsible for transplantation tolerance, it might be caused by a mechanism other than the direct action of antigen on immunocompetent cells. On the basis of their experiments, Ram-seier (1973) and Rowley *et al.* (1973) suggest that anti-idiotypic antibodies may eliminate lymphocytes carrying receptors for the tolerated antigens in chimeric animals. Further, enhancing antibodies may act by peripheral blockade of transplantation antigens (Möller, 1963a) or by competing with the effector cells at the target cell level (Möller, 1963b), but their major effect seems to be at the level of lymphoid tissue (Winn, 1974). The possibility is not excluded that this effect involves inactivation of the cell clones responsible for graft rejection.

As in other inhibition systems, the situation in transplantation tolerance is further complicated by the recent findings of suppressor cells. Elkins (1972) found that rats in which transplantation tolerance was adoptively terminated displayed reduced reactivity in mixed lymphocyte and graft-versus-host reactions. When their cells were mixed with normal lymphocytes, the reactivity of normal cells was strikingly inhibited. A similar situation was observed in allograft-tolerant chickens (Rouse and Warner, 1974; Droege and Mayor, 1975). Droege (1974) showed that the transfer of thymocytes of normal young donors prolonged significantly the survival of allogeneic skin grafts in chickens. Silvers (1974) observed that the excision of lymphoid tissue in mice tolerant to skin grafts impaired the duration of tolerance. He suspected that this impairment was caused by the removal of suppressor cells. Kilshaw *et al.* (1975) proved by cell transfers in mice unresponsive to skin allografts that suppressor cells were operative. However, their experimental system seems to differ in its mechanism from other cases of transplantation tolerance (Kilshaw *et al.*, 1974).

V. Mechanism of Unresponsiveness to Self Components

It is generally accepted that autotolerance is the mechanism ensuring nonreactivity to self components, although there is very little unambigous evidence for this view. When tolerance was at first considered to be a complete absence of reactivity to the tolerated antigen, there were two groups of findings that were difficult to reconcile with the mechanism of autotolerance. One was the frequent detection of autoantibodies in normal individuals (for references, see Hraba, 1968). The other was a relatively easy and reliable induction of autoimmune syndromes in experimental animals immunized with homologous or heterologous tissue antigens incorporated into complete Freund's adjuvant.

A satisfactory explanation for at least some of these findings has been provided by the termination of tolerance to heterologous proteins by challenge with cross-reacting antigens. Autoantibodies are often elicited by contact with microorganisms (Asherson, 1968). It was proved for some of the microorganisms provoking the production of autoantibodies that they share antigenic determinants with the autoantigen reacting with the corresponding autoantibodies. It was suspected that the cross-reacting external agent or denatured self components might terminate autotolerance in the same manner as cross-reacting antigens break tolerance to heterologous proteins. This explanation was corroborated by WEIGLE (1965). He succeeded in inducing autoimmune thyroiditis in rabbits by injecting hapten-conjugated homologous thyroglobulin without adjuvant. Similar results were obtained with testicular antigens (POKORNÁ and VOJTÍŠ-KOVÁ, 1964).

As has been discussed previously, the termination of tolerance by cross-reacting antigens seems to be possible only when B-cells of the tolerant animal regain spontaneously immune reactivity while T-cells still are unresponsive (WEIGLE, 1971). The results of CLAGGET and WEIGLE (1975) indicate that this may be the case with autoantigens. These investigators proved by transfers of thymocytes and bone marrow cells in mice that T-cells were required for the production of antibodies to autologous thyroglobulin elicited by immunization with heterologous thyroglobulin. When looking for antigen-binding cells they found that few, if any, thymocytes reacted with autologous thyroglobulin. On the other hand, significant numbers of thymocytes bound heterologous thyroglobulin. In the spleens of athymic nude and normal mice, comparable numbers of cells binding homologous thyroglobulin were present; this led to the conclusion that cells binding autologous thyroglobulin were B-cells. This conclusion is supported by the finding of BANKHURST et al. (1973) that in human peripheral blood the number of cells binding homologous thyroglobulin is drastically reduced after the removal of cells becoming attached to antihuman immunoglobulin coated beads.

In experimental autoimmune syndromes induced by immunization with antigens incorporated into complete Freund's adjuvant, the tissue injury is often brought about by cell-mediated immunity. According to the foregoing view, T-cells are supposed to be unreactive to self components. Apparently, the explanation of the break of tolerance, used for autoantibody production, is not applicable here. It might be explained by the "sequestration" of the responsible autoantigens, if these substances would not leave the organ of their origin in sufficient amounts. Therefore, they would not induce tolerance at all, or they would induce only partial tolerance.

However, other evidence points to the existence of T-cells reactive with self components that can hardly be considered sequestered. COHEN et al. (1971) observed that rat spleen cells or thymocytes, when cultivated in vitro with syngeneic fibroblasts, acquired cytotoxicity to them. It was further proved that in this situation lymphocytes might become cytotoxic to reticulum cells of the thymus (COHEN and WEKERLE, 1972). Some lymphocytes possess the capacity to recognize self components before being explanted. The cells that are self-recognizing do not become cytotoxic, but recruit other T-cells to become the effector cytotoxic cells (COHEN, 1973 a, b). Cells activated by in vitro cultivation with syngeneic fibroblasts cause a considerable enlargement of the draining lymph nodes when injected into the footpads of syngeneic animals.

Apparently, lymphocytes capable of recognizing self antigens exist in normal animals. This raises the question of how they are prevented from becoming activated and from causing the development of cytotoxic cells. It has been found that normal serum contains a factor that inhibits the recognition of self antigens by these lymphocytes. COHEN and WEKERLE (1973) assume that this factor is the antigen recognized by the self reacting lymphocytes. According to their hypothesis, it is present in the serum in a tolerogenic form. In this form it blocks lymphocytes from binding with the immunogenic form of the same antigen on tissue cells.

Suppressor cells also seem to be involved in the unresponsiveness to self components CUNNINGHAM (1975) observed in normal mice relatively large numbers of cells producing antibodies against autologous erythrocytes. These cells are most easily detected by hemolytic plaque formation with syngeneic erythrocytes treated with bromelain. The injection of bromelain-treated erythrocytes does not increase the number of these cells. On the other hand, bacterial lipopolysaccharide enormously increases their number, as does antilymphocyte serum. The simplest explanation of these findings is that a large number of cells capable of forming these antibodies are present in the body but that these cells are blocked by suppressor cells. This system may be atypical, because the responsible antigen becomes exposed when erythrocytes degenerate.

Other evidence for the involvement of suppressor cells in the unresponsiveness to self components comes from findings in NZB mice. These mice develop spontaneously an autoimmune disease (HOWIE and HELYER, 1968) characterized by hemolytic anemia, lymphocyte infiltration of different organs, and a renal disease caused by antigen-antibody complexes. In young NZB mice high antibody production and difficult induction of immunologic tolerance are observed (PLAYFAIR, 1968; WEIR et al., 1968; STAPLES and TALAL, 1969a, b). These anomalies seem to be caused by the loss of thymic suppressor function (BARTHOLD et al., 1974), which occurs before other thymic functions are impaired (GHAFFAR et al., 1970; GELFAND and STEINBERG, 1973).

In any event, it does not seem that only one mechanism is involved in bringing about the nonreactivity to self components. The share of the different mechanisms in effecting this unresponsiveness is impossible to estimate on the basis of the data known at present.

D. Conclusions

The past 25 years have witnessed unprecedented interest in the phenomena of specific inhibition of immune reactions that far exceeded the general increase of interest in immunologic problems. It has been aroused mainly by the successes of reconstructive surgery requiring the suppression of transplantation immunity. Immunologic incompatibility, not problems of the surgical technique, limits the therapeutic possibilities of organ transplantation. Although the studies of immunologic tolerance to defined antigens have contributed more to the knowledge of the mechanisms of unresponsive states, the discovery and analysis of transplantation tolerance have been major factors initiating changes in the attitudes of the immunologic community, which has not reacted in a similar manner to any of the preceding discoveries of inhibition phenomena. Another important influence upon this change has been the development of immunology itself. It is well reflected and formulated in BURNET's theories, which are an attempt to integrate immunology into the framework of the new biology, shaped mainly by the discoveries in the field of molecular biology, and, at the same time, to consider the specific problems posed by the development of immunologic knowledge. Proved or disproved, the theories put forth by BURNET and MEDAWAR to elucidate tolerance have served fully the purpose by giving an orientation and stimulation to successful research.

At present it is clear that, in addition to immunologic tolerance, other mechanisms are in play in the states of specific unresponsiveness. This has led some authors to the proposal of a new classification of unresponsiveness, or tolerance:

1. The classical form of tolerance, in which unresponsiveness is due to the direct action of antigen on the corresponding clones of immunocompetent cells leading to their deletion or inactivation. This form of tolerance is called passive, negative, direct, or inactive.

2. Unresponsive states in which antigen acts on one set of cells and these cells inhibit the activity of another set of cells either by their products or by direct interaction. This form is called active, positive, or indirect unresponsiveness or tolerance. GERSHON and KONDO (1971) used the term "infectious tolerance" for one of these unresponsive states.

Both of these categories may include unresponsive states effected by different mechanisms. Active unresponsive states are mediated either by antibodies or by suppressor cells, and inside of each of these groups different mechanisms may operate. It is also probable that the classical form of tolerance may be brought about by different types of interaction of antigen with immunocompetent cells. In addition, different mechanisms may operate at the same time in individual inhibition states, as seems to be the case in transplantation tolerance. Evidently, the phenomena of specific unresponsiveness reflect the complexity of immune response not only in the plurality of immune reactions but also in the complexity of interactions of the participating cells.

If the elucidation of the mechanism of immunologic tolerance has been considered necessary for the understanding of the mechanism of immune reactions earlier, now the suppressive processes are becoming an integral part of the different mechanisms effecting and regulating the immune responses.

References

ABRAHAMS, S., PHILLIPS, R.A., MILLER, R.G.: Inhibition of the immune response by 7S antibody. J. Exp. Med. 137, 870–892 (1973)

ADA, G.L., COOPER, M.G.: The in vivo localization patterns and the in vitro binding to lymphocytes of normal and tolerant rats by Salmonella flagellin and its derivatives. Ann. N.Y. Acad. Sci. 181, 96–107 (1971)

ALDO-BENSON, M., BOREL, Y.: The tolerant cell; direct evidence for receptor blocade by tolerogen. J. Immunol. 112, 1793–1803 (1974)

ANDERSON, D., BILLINGHAM, R.E., LAMPKIN, G.H., MEDAWAR, P.B.: The use of skin grafting to distinguish between monozygotic and dizygotic twins in cattle. Heredity 5, 379–397 (1951)

ARGYRIS, B.F., HARITOU, H., COONEY, A.: Density gradient fractionation of mouse lymphoid tissues, I. Plaque-forming and rosette-forming cells in normal, sensitized and tolerant spleen. Cell. Immunol. 3, 101–112 (1972)

ASHERSON, G.L.: Selective and specific inhibition of 24 h skin reactions in the guinea-pig. II. The mechanism of immune deviation. Immunology 10, 179–186 (1966)

ASHERSON, G.L.: Autoantibody production as a breakdown of immune tolerance. In: Regulation of the Antibody Response, pp. 68–69. Springfield: C.C. Thomas 1968

ASHERSON, G.L., STONE, S.H.: Selective and specific inhibition of 24 h skin reactions in the guinea pigs. I. Immune deviation: description of the phenomenon and the effect of splenectomy. Immunology **9**, 205–217 (1965)

ASHERSON, G.L., ZEMBALA, M., BARNES, R.M.R.: The mechanism of immunological unresponsiveness to picryl chloride and the possible role of antibody mediated depression. Clin. Exp. Immunol. **9**, 111–121 (1971)

ATKINS, R.C., FORD, W.L.: The effect of lymphocytes and serum from tolerant rats on the graft-versus-host activity of normal lymphocytes. Transplantation **13**, 442–444 (1972)

BAKER, P.J., BARTH, R.F., STASHAK, P.W., AMSBAUGH, D.F.: Enhancement of the antibody response to type III pneumococcal polysaccharide in mice treated with antilymphocyte serum. J. Immunol. **104**, 1313–1315 (1970a)

BAKER, P.J., STASHAK, P.W., AMSBAUGH, D.F., PRESCOTT, B., BARTH, R.F.: Evidence for the existence of two functionally distinct types of cells which regulate the antibody response to type III pneumococcal polysaccharide. J. Immunol. **105**, 1581–1583 (1970b)

BANKHURST, A.D., TORRIGIANI, G., ALLISON, A.C.: Lymphocytes binding human thyroglobulin in healthy people and its relevance to tolerance for autoantigens. Lancet **1**, 226–230 (1973)

BARTHOLD, D.B., KYSELA, S., STEINBERG, A.D.: Decline in suppressor T cell function with age in female NZB mice. J. Immunol. **112**, 9–16 (1974)

BASTEN, A., MILLER, J.F.A.P., SPRENT, J., CHEERS, C.: Cell-to-cell interaction in the immune response. X. T-cell-dependent suppression in tolerant mice. J. Exp. Med. **140**, 199–217 (1974)

BELL, E.B., SHAND, F.L.: Cellular events in protein tolerant inbred rats. I. The fate of thoracic duct lymphocytes and memory cells during tolerance induction to human serum albumin. Europ. J. Immunol. **3**, 259–267 (1973)

BENIRSCHKE, K., ANDERSON, J.M., BROWNHILL, L.E.: Marrow chimerism in marmosets. Science **138**, 513–515 (1962)

BENJAMIN, D.C., WEIGLE, W.O.: The termination of immunological unresponsiveness to bovine serum albumin in rabbits. I. Quantitative and qualitative response to cross-reacting albumin. J. Exp. Med. **132**, 66–76 (1970)

BILLINGHAM, R.E., LAMPKIN, G.H., MEDAWAR, P.B., WILLIAMS, H.L.: Tolerance to homografts, twin diagnosis and the freemartin condition in cattle. Heredity **6**, 201–212 (1952)

BILLINGHAM, R.E., BRENT, L., MEDAWAR, P.B.: Actively acquired tolerance of foreign cells. Nature (London) **172**, 603–605 (1953)

BILLINGHAM, R.E., BRENT, L., MEDAWAR, P.B.: Quantitative studies on tissue transplantation immunity. III. Actively acquired tolerance. Philos. Trans. (A/B) **239**, 357–414 (1956a)

BILLINGHAM, R.E., BRENT, L., MEDAWAR, P.B.: "Enhancement" in normal homografts with a note on its possible mechanism. Transpl. Bull. **3**, 84–88 (1956b)

BILLINGHAM, R.E., SILVERS, W.K., WILSON, D.B.: Further studies on adoptive transfer of sensitivity to skin homografts. J. Exp. Med. **118**, 397–420 (1963)

BIRO, C.E., ARROYAVE, C.: On the existence of a live immunologically unresponsive lymphoid cell. Immunology **18**, 387–391 (1970)

BOOTH, P.B., PLAUT, G., JAMES, J.D., IKIN, E.W., MOORES, P., SANGER, R., RACE, R.R.: Blood chimerism in a pair of twins. Brit. Med. J. II, 1456–1458 (1957).

BOREL, Y., FAUCONNET, M., MIESCHER, P.A.: Selective suppression of delayed hypersensitivity by the induction of immunologic tolerance. J. Exp. Med. **123**, 585–598 (1966)

BOREL, Y., DAVID, J.R.: In vitro studies of the suppression of delayed hypersensitivity by the induction of partial tolerance. J. Exp. Med. **131**, 603–610 (1970)

BRENT, L., BROOKS, C., LUBLING, N., THOMAS, A.V.: Attempts to demonstrate an in vivo role for serum blocking factors in tolerant mice. Transplantation **14**, 382–387 (1972)

BROOKE, M.S., KARNOVSKY, M.J.: Immunological paralysis and adoptive immunity. J. Immunol. **87**, 205–208 (1961)

BRITTON, S.: Regulation of antibody synthesis against Escherichia coli endotoxin. II. Specificity, dose requirements and duration of paralysis induced in adult mice. Immunology **16**, 513–526 (1969)

BURNET, F.M.: The Clonal Selection Theory of Acquired Immunity. London: Cambridge University Press, 1959

BURNET, F.M., FENNER, F.: The Production of Antibodies. Melbourne: Macmillan Company 1949

BUSSARD, A.: Tolérance immunologique provoqué chez le lapin envers certains antigènes de la levure. C.R. Acad. Sci. (Paris) **245**, 2430–2433 (1957)

BUSSARD, A.E.: Immunological behaviour of rabbits towards human serum albumin two years after neonatal injection of the same antigen. In: Mechanisms of Immunological Tolerance, pp. 85–94. Prague: Publishing House of the Czechoslovak Academy of Sciences 1962

BYERS, V.S., SERCARZ, E.E.: Induction and reversal of immune paralysis in vitro. J. Exp. Med. **132**, 845–857 (1970)

CASEY, A.E.: Experimental enhancement of malignancy in the Brown-Pierce rabbit tumor. Proc. Soc. Exp. Biol. (N.Y.) **29**, 816–818 (1932)

CHAN, P.L., SINCLAIR, N.R.STC.: Regulation of the immune response. V. An analysis of the function of the Fc portion of antibody in suppression of an immune response with respect to inter-action with components of the lymphoid system. Immunology **21**, 967–981 (1971)

CHASE, M.W.: Inhibition of experimental drug allergy by prior feeding of the sensitizing agent. Proc. Soc. Exp. Biol. (N.Y.) **61**, 257–259 (1946)

CHASE, M.W.: Studies on the mechanism of inhibition of experimental drug allergy by prior feeding of the sensitizing agent. Abstr. 49th Gen. Meeting Soc. Amer. Bact., p. 75 (1949)

CHASE, M.W.: Tolerance towards chemical allergens. In: Tolérance acquise et la Tolérance naturelle à l'égard de Substances antigéniques définies, pp. 139–160. Paris: Editions du C.N.R.S. 1963

CHILLER, J.M., HABICHT, G.S., WEIGLE, W.O.: Cellular sites of immunologic unresponsiveness. Proc. Nat. Acad. Sci. (Wash.) **65**, 551–556 (1970)

CHILLER, J.M., HABICHT, G.S., WEIGLE, W.O.: Kinetic differences in unresponsiveness of thymus and bone marrow cells. Science 171, 813–815 (1971)

CHILLER, J.M., WEIGLE, W.O.: Termination of tolerance to human gamma globulin in mice by antigen and bacterial lipopolysaccharide (endotoxin). J. Exp. Med. **137**, 740–750 (1973)

CHILLER, J.M., ROMBALL, C.G., WEIGLE, W.O.: Induction of immunological tolerance in neonatal and adult rabbits. Differences in the cellular events. Cell. Immunol. **8**, 28–39 (1973)

CHUTNÁ, J.: Enhancement of skin homografts and dissociation of immune responses in mice immunized with lyophilized tissues in Freund's adjuvant. Nature (London) **217**, 175–177 (1968a)

CHUTNÁ, J.: Prolonged survival of H-2 different skin allografts in mice specifically immunized with lyophilized spleens in Freund's adjuvant. Folia Biol. (Praha) **14**, 140–147 (1968b)

CHUTNÁ, J.: Study of mechanism of specific inhibition of delayed sensitivity and IgM antibodies in guinea pigs immunized with organ-specific antigen. Int. Arch. Allergy **37**, 278–292 (1970)

CHUTNÁ, J.: The mechanism of immunological enhancement of H-2-incompatible skin grafts in mice. Transplantation **12**, 28–35 (1971)

CHUTNÁ, J., HRABA, T.: Attempt to induce immunological tolerance in rabbits by antigen (HSA)-antibody precipitate. In: Mechanisms of Immunological Tolerance, pp. 95–102. Prague: Publishing House of the Czechoslovak Academy of Sciences 1962

CHUTNÁ, J., RYCHLÍKOVÁ, M.: Prevention and suppression of experimental autoimmune aspermatogenesis in adult guinea pigs. Folia Biol. (Praha) **10**, 177–187 (1964a)

CHUTNÁ, J., RYCHLÍKOVÁ, M.: A study of the biological effectiveness of antibodies in the development and prevention of experimental autoimmune aspermatogenesis. Folia Biol. (Praha) **10**, 188–197 (1964b)

CHUTNÁ, J., HAŠEK, M., SLÁDEČEK, M., VIKLICKÝ, V., BUBENÍK, J.: Analysis of immunological reactivity in skin-allograft tolerating rats. Folia Biol. (Praha) **19**, 252–260 (1973)

CINADER, B., DUBERT, J.M.: Acquired immune tolerance to human albumin and the response to subsequent injections of diazoalbumin. Brit. J. Exp. Path. **36**, 515–529 (1955)

CINADER, B., DUBERT, J.M.: Specific inhibition of reponse to purified protein antigens. Proc. Roy. Soc. B. **146**, 18–33 (1956)

CINADER, B., PEARCE, J.H.: The specificity of acquired immunological tolerance to azo proteins. Brit. J. Exp. Path. **39**, 8–29 (1958)

CINADER, B., PEARCE, J.H., CARTER, B.G.: Acquired immunological tolerance to bovine ribonuclease. Nature (London) **181**, 1208–1209 (1958)

CLAGETT, J.A., WEIGLE, W.O.: Roles of T and B lymphocytes in the termination of unresponsiveness to autologous thyroglobulin in mice. J. Exp. Med. **139**, 643–660 (1974)

COHEN, I.R.: Cell-mediated auto-immunity: antigen reactive lymphocytes recruit specific effector lymphocytes. Nature New Biol. **242**, 60–61 (1973a)

Cohen, I.R.: The recruitment of specific effector lymphocytes by antigen-reactive lymphocytes in cell-mediated autosensitization and allosensitization reactions. Cell. Immunol. **8**, 209–220 (1973b)

Cohen, I.R., Globerson, A., Feldman, M.: Autosensitization in vitro. J. Exp. Med. **133**, 834–845 (1971)

Cohen, I.R., Wekerle, H.: Autosensitization of lymphocytes against thymus reticulum cells. Science **176**, 1324–1326 (1972)

Cohen, I.R., Wekerle, H.: Regulation of autosensitization. The immune activation and specific inhibition of self-recognizing thymus-derived lymphocytes. J. Exp. Med. **137**, 224–238 (1973)

Cooper, M.G., Ada, G.L., Langman, R.E.: The incidence of hemocyanin-binding cells in hemocyanin-tolerant rats. Cell. Immunol. **4**, 289–303 (1972)

Crone, M.: Tolerance to allogeneic cells induced in bursectionized chickens. Scand. J. Immunol. **2**, 349–355 (1973)

Crowle, A.J., Hu, C.C.: Adoptive transfer of immunologic tolerance into normal mice. J. Immunol. **103**, 1242–1247 (1969)

Cunningham, A.J.: Active suppressor mechanism maintaining tolerance to some self components. Nature (London) **254**, 143–144 (1975)

Deol, M.S.: Chimaeras and the forbidden-clone theory of self-tolerance. Nature (London) **242**, 469 (1973)

Diamantstein, T., Wagner, B.: The use of polyanions to break immunological tolerance. Nature New Biol. **241**, 117 (1973)

Diener, E., Armstrong, W.D.: Induction of antibody formation and tolerance in vitro to a purified protein antigen. Lancet **2**, 1281–1284 (1967)

Diener, E., Armstrong, W.D.: Immunological tolerance in vitro: kinetic studies at the cellular level. J. Exp. Med. **129**, 591–603 (1969)

Diener, E., Feldmann, M.: Antibody-mediated suppression of the immune response in vitro. II. A new approach to the phenomenon of immunological tolerance. J. Exp. Med. **132**, 31–43 (1970)

Diener, E., Feldmann, M.: Relationship between antigen and antibody-induced suppression of immunity. Transpl. Rev. **8**, 76–103 (1972)

Dietrich, F.M., Weigle, W.O.: Induction of tolerance to heterologous proteins and their catabolism in C57B1/6. J. Exp. Med. **117**, 621–631 (1963)

Dixon, F.J., Maurer, P.H.: Immunological unresponsiveness induced by protein antigens. J. Exp. Med. **101**, 245–257 (1955)

Dresser, D.W.: The effectiveness of lipid and lipidophilic substances as adjuvants. Nature (London) **191**, 1169–1171 (1961a)

Dresser, D.W.: Acquired immunological tolerance to a fraction of bovine gamma-globulin. Immunology **4**, 13–23 (1961b)

Dresser, D.W.: Specific inhibition of antibody production. II. Paralysis induced in adult mice by small quantities of protein antigen. Immunology **5**, 378–388 (1962)

Droege, W.: Amplifying and suppressive effect of thymus cells. Nature (London) **234**, 549–551 (1971)

Droege, W.: Suppressive effect of thymus cells on the allograft rejection. Z. Immunitätsfsch. **147**, 294 (1974)

Droege, W., Mayor, H.: Graft versus host reactivity and inhibitory serum factors in allograft tolerant chickens. Transplantation **19**, 517–520 (1975)

Dunsford, I., Bowley, C.C., Hutchinson, A.M., Thompson, J.S., Sanger, R., Race, R.R.: A human blood-group chimera. Brit. Med. J. **II**, 81 (1953)

Dvorak, H.F., Billote, J.B., McCarthy, J.S., Flax, M.H.: Immunologic unresponsiveness in the adult guinea pig. III. Variation of the antigen and vehicle of suppression. Induction of unresponsiveness in the adult rat. J. Immunol. **97**, 106–111 (1966)

Elkins, W.L.: Cellular control of lymphocytes initiating graft vs. host reactions. Cell. Immunol. **4**, 192–196 (1972)

Elkins, W.L.: The cellular basis of transplantation tolerance. Transpl. Proc. **5**, 685–689 (1973)

Eshhar, Z., Benacerraf, D.H., Katz, D.H.: Induction of tolerance to nucleic acid determinants by administration of a complex of nucleoside d-glutamic acid and d-lysine (D-GL). J. Immunol. **114**, 872–876 (1975)

FELDMANN, M., DIENER, E.: Antibody-mediated suppression of the immune response in vitro. I. Evidence for a central effect. J. Exp. Med. **131**, 247–274 (1970)

FELTON, L.D., OTTINGER, B.: Pneumococcus polysaccharides as a paralysing agent on the mechanism of immunity in white mice (abstract). J. Bact. **43**, 94–95 (1942)

FELTON, L.D., PRESCOTT, B., KAUFMANN, G., OTTINGER, B.: Pneumococcal antigenic polysaccharide substances from animal tissues. J. Immunol. **74**, 205–213 (1955)

FIDLER, J.M., GOLUB, E.S.: Immunological tolerance to a hapten. III. Induction of tolerance to trinitrophenyl in B cells in various differentiation states. J. Immunol. **112**, 1891–1899 (1974)

FORBES, I.J.: Analysis in vitro of tolerance. Immunology **16**, 699–706 (1969)

FREI, W.: Über willkürliche Sensibilisierung gegen chemisch definierte Substanzen. I. Mitteilung: Untersuchungen mit Neosalvarsan am Menschen. Klin. Wschr. **7**, 539–542 (1928)

FRIEDMAN, H.: Failure of spleen cells from immunologically tolerant mice to form antibody plaques to sheep erythrocytes in agar gel. Nature (London) **205**, 508–509 (1965)

GELFAND, M.C., STEINBERG, A.D.: Mechanisms of allograft rejection in New Zealand mice. I. Cell synergy and its age-dependent loss. J. Immunol. **110**, 1652–1662 (1973)

GENGOZIAN, N., BATSON, J.S., GREENE, C.T., GOSSLEE, D.G.: Hemopoietic chimerism in imported and laboratory-bred marmosets. Transplantation **8**, 633–652 (1969)

GERSHON, R.K., WALLIS, V., DAVIES, A.S.J., LEUCHARS, E.: Inactivation of thymus cells after multiple injections of antigen. Nature (London) **218**, 380–381 (1968)

GERSHON, R.K., KONDO, K.: Infectious immunological tolerance. Immunology **21**, 903–914 (1971)

GERSHON, R.K., MOKYR, M.B., MITCHELL, M.S.: Activation of suppressor T cells by tumour cells and specific antibody. Nature (London) **250**, 595–597 (1974)

GHAFFAR, A., KRSIAKOVA, M., PLAYFAIR, J.H.L.: Deficient cell-mediated immunity in adult NZB mice. Transplantation **10**, 432–433 (1970)

GORNISH, M., WEBSTER, M.P., WEGMANN, T.G.: Chimaerism in the immune system of tetraparental mice. Nature (London) **237**, 249–251 (1972)

GOWANS, J.L., McGREGOR, D.D., COWEN, D.M., FORD, C.E.: Initiation of immune responses by small lymphocytes. Nature (London) **196**, 651–655 (1962)

GRONOWICZ, E., COUTINHO, A.: Hapten induced B cell paralysis. II. Evidence for trivial mechanisms of tolerance. Europ. J. Immunol. **5**, 413–420 (1975)

HAMILTON, J.A., MILLER, J.F.A.P., KETTMAN, J.: Hapten-specific tolerance in mice. II. Adoptive transfer studies and evidence for unresponsiveness in the B cells. Europ. J. Immunol. **4**, 268–276 (1974)

HANAN, R., OYAMA, J.: Inhibition of antibody formation in mature rabbits by contact with antigen at an early age. J. Immunol. **73**, 49–53 (1954)

HARRIS, G.: Macrophages from tolerant rabbits as mediators of a specific immunological response in vitro. Immunology **12**, 159–163 (1967)

HAŠEK, M.: Parabiosis of birds during embryogenesis (in Czech). Čs. biol. **2**, 25–31 (1953a)

HAŠEK, M.: Vegetative hybridization of animals by joining their blood circulations during embryonic development (in Czech). Čs. biol. **2**, 265–277 (1953b)

HAŠEK, M.: Tolerance phenomena in birds. Proc. Roy. Soc. B **146**, 67–77 (1956)

HAŠEK, M., HRABA, T.: Immunological effects of experimental embryonal parabiosis. Nature (London) **175**, 764–765 (1955a)

HAŠEK, M., HRABA, T.: The significance of phylogenetic kinship in immunological approximation during embryogenesis. Folia Biol. (Praha) **1**, 1–10 (1955b)

HAŠEK, M., CHUTNÁ, J., SLÁDEČEK, M., MACHÁČKOVÁ, M., BUBENÍK, J., MATOUŠEK, V.: Attempts to compare the effectiveness of blocking factors and enhancing antibodies in vivo and in vitro. Transplantation **20**, 95–100 (1975)

HAUGHTON, G., ADAMS, D.O.: Specific immunosuppression by minute doses of passive antibody. II. The site of action. J. Reticuloendothelial Soc. **7**, 500–517 (1970)

HELLSTRÖM, I., HELLSTRÖM, K.E., STORB, R., THOMAS, E.D.: Colony inhibition of fibroblasts from chimeric dogs mediated by the dogs' own lymphocytes and specifically abrogated by their serum. Proc. Nat. Acad. Sci. (Wash.) **66**, 65–71 (1970)

HELLSTRÖM, I., HELLSTRÖM, K.E., ALLISON, A.C.: Neonatally induced allograft tolerance may be mediated by serum-borne factors. Nature (London) **230**, 49–50 (1971)

HOFFMANN, M.K., KAPPLER, J.W., HIRST, J.A., OETTGEN, H.F.: Regulation of the immune response. V. Antibody mediated inhibition of T and B cell cooperation in the in vitro response to red cell antigens. Europ. J. Immunol. **4**, 282–286 (1974)

HOWARD, J.G., ELSON, J., CHRISTIE, G.H., KINSKY, R.G.: Studies on immunological paralysis. II. The detection and significance of antibody-forming cells in the spleen during immunological paralysis with type III pneumococcal polysaccharide. Clin. Exp. Immunol. 4, 41–53 (1969)

HOWARD, J.G., CHRISTIE, G.H., COURTENAY, B.M.: Treadmill neutralization of antibody and central inhibition. Transplantation 10, 351–353 (1970)

HOWARD, J.G., CHRISTIE, G.H., COURTENAY, B.M.: Studies in immunological paralysis. IV. The relative contributions of continuous antibody neutralization and central inhibition to paralysis with type III pneumococcal polysaccharide. Proc. Roy. Soc. B 178, 417–438 (1971)

HOWARD, J.G., CHRISTIE, G.H., COURTENAY, B.M.: Studies on immunological paralysis. VII. Rapid reversal of Felton's paralysis as evidence for 'tolerant' cells. Proc. Roy. Soc. B 180, 347–361 (1972)

HOWIE, J.B., HELYER, B.J.: The immunology and pathology of NZB mice. Adv. Immunol. 9, 215–266 (1968)

HRABA, T.: Mechanism and Role of Immunological Tolerance. Basel–New York: S. Karger, 1968

HRABA, T.: Tolerance to sheep red blood cells. Allergie u. Immunologie 20/21, 137–144 (1974/5)

HRABA, T., HAŠEK, M., ČUMLIVSKI, B.: Immunological approximation of sheep triplets, natural embryonic parabionts. Folia Biol. (Praha) 2, 276–283 (1956)

HUMPHREY, J.H.: Immunological unresponsiveness to protein antigens in rabbits. I. The duration of unresponsiveness following a single injection at birth. Immunology 7, 449–461 (1964)

HUMPHREY, J.H., TURK, J.L.: Immunological unresponsiveness in guinea pigs. I. Immunological unresponsiveness to heterologous serum proteins. Immunology 4, 301–309 (1961)

JANKOVIĆ, B.D., FLAX, M.H.: Alterations in the development of experimental allergic thyroiditis induced by injection of homologous thyroid extract. J. Immunol. 90, 178–184 (1963)

KALISS, N., KANDUTSCH, A.A.: Acceptance of tumor homografts by mice injected with antiserum. I. Activity of serum fractions. Proc. Soc. Exp. Biol. (N.Y.) 91, 118–121 (1956)

KAPLAN, M.H., COONS, A.H., DEANE, H.W.: Localization of antigen in tissue cells. III. Cellular distribution of pneumococcal polysaccharides types II and III in the mouse. J. Exp. Med. 91, 15–30 (1950)

KATZ, D.H., DAVIE, J.M., PAUL, W.E., BENACERRAF, B.: Carrier function in anti-hapten antibody responses. IV. Experimental conditions for the induction of hapten-specific tolerance or for the stimulation of anti-hapten anamnestic responses by "nonimmunogenic" hapten-polypeptide conjugates. J. Exp. Med. 134, 201–223 (1971)

KATZ, S.I., PARKER, D., SOMMER, G., TURK, J.L.: Suppressor cells in normal immunization as a basic homeostatic phenomenon. Nature (London) 248, 612–614 (1974a)

KATZ, S.I., SOMMER, G., PARKER, D., TURK, J.L.: B-cell suppression of delayed hypersensitivity reactions. Nature (London) 251, 550–552 (1974b)

KERBEL, R.S., EIDINGER, D.: Enhanced immune responsiveness to a thymus-independent antigen early after adult thymectomy: Evidence for short-lived inhibitory thymus-derived cells. Europ. J. Immunol. 2, 114–118 (1972)

KERCKHAERT, J.A.M., VAN DEN BERG, G.J., WILLERS, J.M.N.: Influence of cyclophosphamide on the delayed hypersensitivity of the mouse. Ann. Immunol. (Inst. Pasteur) 125, 415–426 (1974)

KILSHAW, P.J., BRENT, L., THOMAS, A.V.: Specific unresponsiveness to skin allografts in mice. II. The mechanism of unresponsiveness induced by tissue extracts and antilymphocytic serum. Transplantation 17, 57–69 (1974)

KILSHAW, P.J., BRENT, L., PINTO, M.: An active suppressor mechanism preventing skin allograft rejection in mice. Transpl. Proc. 7, 225–228 (1975)

LOEWI, G., HOLBOROW, E.J., TEMPLE, A.: Inhibition of delayed hypersensitivity by pre-immunization without complete adjuvant. Immunology 10, 339–347 (1966)

MADAR, J., SLÁDEČEK, M., BALCAROVÁ, J., HRABA, T.: Rosette forming cells in partial tolerance. Folia biol. (Praha) 17, 204–208 (1971)

MADAR, J., HRABA, T., SEDLÁK, J.: The influence of lipopolysaccharide on immunological tolerance. Folia Biol. (Praha) 19, 289–292 (1973)

MARIANI, T., MARTINEZ, C., SMITH, J.M., GOOD, R.A.: Induction of immunological tolerance to male skin isografts in female mice subsequent to neonatal period. Proc. Soc. Exp. Biol. (N.Y.) 101, 596–599 (1959)

MCCULLAGH, P.J.: The abrogation of sheep erythrocyte tolerance in rats by means of the transfer of allogeneic lymphocytes. J. Exp. Med. 132, 916–925 (1970)

McCullagh, P.J.: The abrogation of immunological tolerance by means of allogeneic confrontation. Transpl. Rev. **12**, 180–197 (1972)

McGregor, D.D., Gowans, J.L.: The antibody response of rats depleted of lymphocytes by chronic drainage from the thoracic duct. J. Exp. Med. **117**, 303–320 (1963)

Medawar, P.B.: Tolerance reconsidered – A critical survey. Transpl. Proc. **5**, 7–9 (1973)

Medlín, J., Říha, I., Šterzl, J.: The antibody response preceding immunological paralysis. Folia biol. (Praha) **15**, 309–312 (1969)

Miller, J.F.A.P., Mitchell, G.F.: Cell to cell interaction in the immune response. V. Target cells for tolerance induction. J. Exp. Med. **131**, 675–699 (1970)

Mitchell, G.F., Lafleur, L., Anderson, K.: Evidence for readily induced tolerance to heterologous erythrocytes in nude mice. Scand. J. Immunol. **3**, 39–49 (1974)

Mitchison, N.A.: Tolerance of erythrocytes in poultry: Loss and abolition. Immunology **5**, 359–369 (1962)

Mitchison, N.A.: Induction of immunological paralysis in two zones of dosage. Proc. Roy. Soc. B **161**, 275–292 (1964)

Mitchison, N.A.: Recovery from immunological paralysis in relation to age and residual antigen. Immunology **9**, 129–138 (1965)

Möller, G.: Studies on the mechanism of immunological enhancement of tumor homografts. II. Effect of isoantibodies on various tumor cells. J. Nat. Cancer Inst. **30**, 1177–1203 (1963a)

Möller, G.: Studies on the mechanism of immunological enhancement of tumor homografts. III. Interaction between humoral isoantibodies and immune lymphoid cells. J. Nat. Cancer Inst. **30**, 1205–1226 (1963b)

Möller, G., Wigzell, H.: Antibody synthesis at the cellular level. Antibody-induced suppression of 19S and 7S antibody response. J. Exp. Med. **121**, 969–989 (1965)

Moore, N.W., Rowson, L.E.: Freemartins in sheep. Nature (London) **182**, 1754–1755 (1958)

Naor, D., Sulitzeanu, D.: Binding of ^{125}I-BSA to lymphoid cells of tolerant mice. Int. Arch. Allergy **36**, 112–113 (1969)

Neeper, C.A., Seastone, C.V.: Mechanisms of immunologic paralysis by pneumococcal polysaccharide. I. Studies on adoptively acquired immunity to pneumococcal infection in immunologically paralyzed and normal mice. J. Immunol. **91**, 374–383 (1963)

Neiders, M.E., Rowley, D.A., Fitch, F.W.: The sustained suppression of hemolysin response in passively immunized rats. J. Immunol. **88**, 718–724 (1962)

Nicholas, J.W., Jenkins, W.J., Marsh, W.L.: Human blood chimeras. A study of surviving twins. Brit. Med. J. I, 1458 (1957)

Nossal, G.J.V.: The induction of immunological tolerance in rats to foreign erythrocytes. Australian J. Exp. Biol. Med. Sci. **36**, 235–244 (1958)

Nossal, G.J.V., Ada, G.L.: Recognition of foreignness in immune and tolerant animals. Nature (London) **201**, 580–582 (1964)

Nossal, G.J.V., Ada, G.L., Austin, C.M.: Antigens in immunity. X. Induction of immunological tolerance to Salmonella adelaide flagellin. J. Immunol. **95**, 665–672 (1965)

Okumura, K., Tada, T.: Regulation of homocytotropic antibody formation in the rat. VI. Inhibitory effect of thymocytes on the homocytotropic antibody response. J. Immunol. **107**, 1682–1689 (1971)

Okumura, K., Tada, T.: Regulation of homocytotropic antibody formation in the rat. IX. Further characterization of the antigen-specific inhibitory T cell factor in hapten-specific homocytotropic antibody response. J. Immunol. **112**, 783–791 (1974)

Owen, R.D.: Immunogenetic consequences of vascular anastomoses between bovine twins. Science **102**, 400–402 (1945)

Parker, L.P., Hahn, B.H., Osterland, K.: Modification of NZB/NZW F$_1$ autoimmune disease by development of tolerance to DNA. J. Immunol. **113**, 292–297 (1974)

Pierce, C.W.: Immune responses in vitro. II. Suppression of the immune response in vitro by specific antibody. J. Exp. Med. **130**, 365–379 (1969)

Playfair, J.H.L.: Strain differences in the immune response of mice. I. The neonatal response to sheep red cells. Immunology **15**, 35–50 (1968)

Playfair, J.H.L.: Specific tolerance to sheep erythrocytes in mouse bone marrow cells. Nature (London) **222**, 882–883 (1969)

Polak, L.: Suppressor cells in different types of unresponsiveness to DNCB contact sensitivity in guinea-pigs. Clin. Exp. Immunol. **19**, 543–549 (1975)

POLAK, L., TURK, J.L.: Reversal of immunological tolerance by cyclophosphamide through the inhibition of suppressor cell activity. Nature (London) **249**, 654–655 (1974)

POKORNÁ, Z., VOJTÍŠKOVÁ, M.: Autoimmune damage of the testes induced with chemically modified organ specific antigen. Folia Biol. (Praha) **10**, 261–267 (1964)

RACE, R.R., SANGER, R.: Blood group mosaics. Haematologia **6**, 63–71 (1972)

RAJEWSKY, K.: The carrier effect and cellular cooperation in the induction of antibodies. Proc. Roy. Soc. B **176**, 385–392 (1971)

RAMSEIER, H.: Immunization against abolition of transplantation tolerance. Europ. J. Immunol. **3**, 156–164 (1973)

RAPACZ, J., SHACKELFORD, R.M., JAKÓBIEC, J.: Blood group studies in the domestic mink. In: Blood Groups of Animals, pp. 211–215. Prague: Publishing House of the Czechoslovak Academy of Sciences 1965

RITTENBERG, M.B., BULLOCK, W.W.: In vitro initiated secondary anti-hapten response. III. Separable roles of hapten and carrier in immune paralysis. Immunochemistry **9**, 491–504 (1972)

ROUSE, B.T., WARNER, N.L.: Induction of T cell tolerance in agammaglobulinemic chickens. Europ. J. Immunol. **2**, 102–104 (1972)

ROUSE, B.T., WARNER, N.L.: The role of suppressor cells in avian allogeneic tolerance: implications for the pathogenesis of Marek's disease. J. Immunol. **113**, 904–909 (1974)

ROWLEY, D.A., FITCH, F.W.: Homeostasis of antibody formation in the adult rat. J. Exp. Med. **120**, 987–1005 (1964)

ROWLEY, D.A., FITCH, F.W.: The mechanism of tolerance produced in rats to sheep erythrocytes. II. The plaque-forming cell and antibody response to multiple injections of antigen begun at birth. J. Exp. Med. **121**, 683–695 (1965)

ROWLEY, D.A., FITCH, F.W., STUART, F.P., KÖHLER, H., COSENZA, H.: Specific suppression of immune responses. Science **181**, 1133–1141 (1973)

RYDER, R.J.W., SCHWARTZ, R.S.: Immunosuppression by antibody: localization of site of action. J. Immunol. **103**, 970–978 (1969)

SANGER, R., RACE, R.R.: Some contributions of blood groups to human genetics. Amer. J. Clin. Path. **55**, 635–645 (1971)

SCHRADER, J.W., NOSSAL, G.J.V.: Effector cell blockade. A new mechanism of immune hyporeactivity induced by multivalent antigens. J. Exp. Med. **139**, 1582–1598 (1974)

SERCARZ, E., COONS, A.H.: Specific inhibition of antibody formation during immunological paralysis and unresponsiveness. Nature (London) **184**, 1080–1082 (1959)

SERCARZ, E., COONS, A.H.: The absence of antibody producing cells during unresponsiveness to BSA in the mice. J. Immunol. **90**, 478–491 (1963)

SHAPIRO, F., MARTINEZ, C., SMITH, J.M., GOOD, R.A.: Tolerance of skin homografts induced in adult mice by multiple injections of homologous spleen cells. Proc. Soc. Exp. Biol. (N.Y.) **106**, 472–475 (1961)

SHELLAM, G.R.: Mechanism of induction of immunological tolerance. VII. Studies of adoptive tolerance to flagellin. Int. Arch. Allergy **40**, 507–519 (1971)

SHELLAM, G.R., NOSSAL, G.J.V.: Mechanism of induction of immunological tolerance. IV. The effects of ultra-low doses of flagellin. Immunology **14**, 273–284 (1968)

SILVERS, W.K.: The influence of removing lymphoid tissue on the persistence of tolerance of skin allografts in mice. J. Immunol. **113**, 804–809 (1974)

SILVERS, W.K., LUBAROFF, D.M., WILSON, D.B., FOX, D.: Mixed lymphocyte reactions and tissue transplantation tolerance. Science **167**, 1264–1266 (1970)

SIMONSEN, M.: Induced tolerance to heterologous cells and induced susceptibility to virus. Nature (London) **175**, 763–764 (1955)

SINCLAIR, N.R.STC., CHAN, P.L.: Relationship between antibody-mediated immunosuppression and tolerance induction. Nature (London) **234**, 104–105 (1971)

SJÖBERG, O.: Antigen-binding cells in mice immune or tolerant to Escherichia coli polysaccharide. J. Exp. Med. **133**, 1015–1025 (1971)

SJÖBERG, O.: Rapid breaking of tolerance against Escherichia coli lipopolysaccharide in vivo and in vitro. J. Exp. Med. **135**, 850–859 (1972)

SJÖBERG, O., MÖLLER, E.: Antigen binding cells in tolerant animals. Nature (London) **228**, 780–781 (1970)

SMITH, R.T.: Studies on the mechanism of immune tolerance. In: Mechanisms of Antibody Formation, pp. 313–328. Prague: Publishing House of the Czechoslovak Academy of Sciences 1960

SMITH, R.T.: Immunological tolerance of non-living antigens. Adv. Immunol. **1**, 67–127 (1961)

SMITH, R.T., BRIDGES, R.A.: Immunological unresponsiveness in rabbits produced by neonatal injection of defined antigens. J. Exp. Med. **108**, 227–250 (1958)

SNELL, G.D.: Enhancing effect (or actively acquired tolerance) and the histocompatibility-2 locus in the mouse. J. Nat. Cancer Inst. **15**, 665–678 (1954)

STAPLES, P.J., TALAL, N.: Rapid loss of tolerance induced in weanling NZB and B/W F_1 mice. Science **163**, 1215–1216 (1969)

STAPLES, P.J., TALAL, N.: Relative inability to induce tolerance in adult NZB and NZB/NZW F_1 mice. J. Exp. Med. **129**, 123–139 (1969)

STARK, O.K.: Studies on pneumococcal polysaccharide. II. Mechanism involved in production of "immunological paralysis" by type I pneumococcal polysaccharide. J. Immunol. **74**, 130–133 (1955)

STASTNY, P.: Persistence of acquired tolerance in cells transferred to an antigen-free environment. J. Immunol. **92**, 626–629 (1964)

STEINBERG, A.D., DALEY, G.G., TALAL, N.: Tolerance to polyinosinic-polycytidylic acid in NZB/NZW mice. Science **167**, 870–871 (1970)

STORMONT, C., WEIR, W.C., LANE, L.L.: Erythrocyte mosaicism in a pair of sheep twins. Science **118**, 695–696 (1953)

SULZBERGER, M.B.: Zur Frage der experimentellen Salvarsan Überempfindlichkeit. Klin. Wschr. **8**, 253–254 (1929 a)

SULZBERGER, M.B.: Hypersensitiveness to neoarphenamine in guinea pigs: experiments in prevention and in desensitization. Arch. Derm. Syph. (Berlin) **20**, 669–697 (1929 b)

TADA, T., OKUMURA, K., TANIGUCHI, M.: Regulation of homocytotropic antibody formation in the rat. VIII. An antigen-specific T cell factor that regulates anti-hapten homocytotropic antibody response. J. Immunol. **111**, 952–961 (1973)

TAYLOR, R.B.: Immune paralysis of thymus cells by bovine serum albumin. Nature (London) **220**, 611 (1968)

TERMAN, D.S., MINDEN, P., CROWLE, A.J.: Resistance of neonatal tolerance in mice to abrogation by normal immunocytes. Cell. Immunol. **6**, 273–283 (1973 a)

TERMAN, D.S., MINDEN, P., CROWLE, A.J.: Adoptive transfer of neonatally induced tolerance into normal mice. Cell. Immunol. **6**, 284–291 (1973 b)

TONG, J.L., BOOSE, D.: Immunosuppressive effect of serum from CBA mice made tolerant by the supernatant from ultracentrifuged bovine γ-globulin. J. Immunol. **105**, 426–430 (1970)

TUFFREY, M., BARNES, R.D., EVANS, E.P., FORD, C.E.: Dominance of AKR lymphocytes in tetraparental AKR↔CBA-T6T6 chimaeras. Nature (London) **243**, 207–208 (1973)

TURK, J.L., HUMPHREY, J.H.: Immunological unresponsiveness in guinea pigs. II. The effect of unresponsiveness on the development of delayed type hypersensitivity to protein antigens. Immunology **4**, 310–317 (1961)

UHR, J.W., BAUMANN, J.B.: Antibody formation. I. The suppression of antibody formation by passively administered antibody. J. Exp. Med. **113**, 935–957 (1961)

UHR, J.W., MÖLLER, G.: Regulatory effect of antibody on the immune response. Adv. Immunol. **8**, 81–127 (1968)

VOISIN, G.A.: Discussion. In: Symposium on Mechanism of Antibody Formation, pp. 222–224. Prague: Publishing House of the Czechoslovak Academy of Sciences, 1960

VOISIN, G.A.: Immunological tolerance to living cells, homologous disease and immunological facilitation (enhancement phenomenon). A working hypothesis allowing a unified concept. In: Mechanism of Immunological Tolerance, pp. 435–455. Prague: Publishing House of the Czechoslovak Academy of Sciences, 1962

VOISIN, G.A.: Immunity and tolerance: a unified concept. Cell. Immunol. **2**, 670–689 (1971)

VOISIN, G.A., KINSKY, R., MAILLARD, J.: Réactivité immunitaire et anticorps facilitants chez des animaux tolérant aux homogreffes. Ann. Inst. Pasteur **115**, 855–879 (1968)

VOISIN, G.A., KINSKY, R.G., DUC, H.T.: Immune status of mice tolerant of living cells. II. Continuous presence and nature of facilitation-enhancing antibodies in tolerant animals. J. Exp. Med. **135**, 1185–1203 (1972)

WEBER, G., KÖLSCH, E.: Low zone tolerance: a possible defect in the switch from IgM to IgG production. Europ. J. Immunol. **2**, 191–193 (1972)

WEGMANN, T.G., HELLSTRÖM, I., HELLSTRÖM, K.E.: Immunological tolerance: "Forbidden clones" allowed in tetraparental mice. Proc. Nat. Acad. Sci. (Wash.) **68**, 1644–1647 (1971)

WEIGLE, W.O.: The immune response of rabbits tolerant to bovine serum albumin to the injection of other heterologous serum albumins. J. Exp. Med. **114**, 111–125 (1961)

WEIGLE, W.O.: Termination of acquired immunological tolerance to protein antigens following immunization with altered protein antigens. J. Exp. Med. **116**, 913–928 (1962)

WEIGLE, W.O.: The induction of autoimmunity in rabbits following injection of heterologous or altered homologous thyroglobulin. J. Exp. Med. **121**, 289–308 (1965)

WEIGLE, W.O.: Recent observations and concepts in immunological unresponsiveness and autoimmunity. Clin. Exp. Immunol. **9**, 437–447 (1971)

WEIGLE, W.O.: Immunological unresponsiveness. Adv. Immunol. **16**, 61–122 (1973)

WEIGLE, W.O., CHILLER, J.M., LOUIS, J.A.: Tolerance: central unresponsiveness or peripheral inhibition. Progr. Immunol. **3**, 187–196 (1974)

WEIGLE, W.O., DIXON, F.J.: The antibody response of lymph node cells transferred to tolerant recipients. J. Immunol. **82**, 516–519 (1959)

WEIR, D.M., McBRIDE, W., NAYSMITH, J.D.: Immune response to a soluble protein antigen in NZB mice. Nature (London) **219**, 1276 (1968)

WINN, H.: The mechanisms of immunological enhancement. Progr. Immunol. **3**, 207–216 (1974)

WRIGHT, P.W., HARGREAVES, R.E., BANSAL, S.C., BERNSTEIN, I.D., HELLSTRÖM, K.E.: Allograft tolerance: presumptive evidence that serum factors from tolerant animals that block lymphocyte-mediated immunity in vitro are soluble antigen-antibody complexes. Proc. Nat. Acad. Sci. (Wash.) **70**, 2539–2543 (1973)

WRIGHT, P.W., HARGREAVES, R.E., BERNSTEIN, I.D., HELLSTRÖM, I.: Fractionation of sera from operationally tolerant rats by DEAE cellulose chromatography; evidence that serum blocking factors are associated with IgG. J. Immunol. **112**, 1267–1270 (1974)

ZEMBALA, M., ASHERSON, G.L.: T cell suppression of the T cell phenomenon of contact sensitivity. Nature (London) **244**, 227–229 (1973)

ZEMBALA, M., ASHERSON, G.L., MAYHEW, B., KREJČÍ, J.: In vitro absorption and molecular weight of specific T-cell suppressor factor. Nature (London) **253**, 72–74 (1975)

Transplantation of Cells: Experimental and Clinical Observations

GERHARD R.F. KRUEGER

With 44 Figures and 3 Tables

A. Introduction

This chapter deals with the general physiologic, pathophysiologic, and anatomic characteristics of cell transplantation. Like all other types of tissue transplantation, the outcome of cell engraftment is controlled by histocompatibility and MLC antigens (see Chapters 1 and 3); the major systems are summarized again in Figure 1. Each system is composed of antigen groups which vary from individual to individual. They are controlled by genetic loci on the chromosome (autosome), and since we are dealing with chromosome pairs, there are two alleles for each gene locus. The possible allelic (haplotype) combinations for a simple genetic locus in the offspring of two parents are shown in Figure 2. It may be seen from this figure to what extent tissue typing is necessary in a family to obtain not only the antigenic phenotype of an individual but also the genotypic penetration of a certain antigen combination within the family. According to the antigenic relatedness (HLA system) between donor and recipient we refer to autotransplantation of cells, isotransplantation, allotransplantation, and xenotransplantation. Autotransplantation refers to grafting within one individual, isotransplantation to grafting within two individuals of the same species who are practically isogenic (such as identical twins), allotransplantation to grafting between two nonidentical individuals from the same species, and xenotransplantation to grafting between two individuals from different species. In addition, blood group antigens must be considered when blood is transfused. Unlike tissue and organ transplantation, engrafted cells are more or less deprived of

MAJOR HISTOCOMPATIBILITY SYSTEM (MHS) REGION

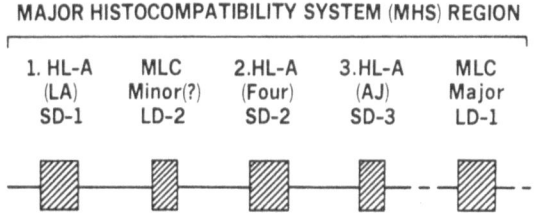

Fig. 1. Gross summary of major histocompatibility systems

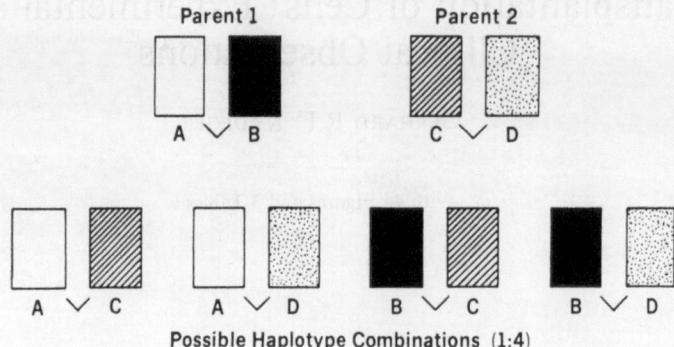

Fig. 2. Summary of possible haplotype combinations

their natural environment. Thus the selective and destructive mechanisms of the recipient can become more readily effective. Such mechanisms are both immunogenic and nonimmunogenic. Furthermore, the influence of engrafted cells upon the recipient organism varies from that of transplanted tissues, since cells circulate through the body and may actively support or attack it at locations distant from the initial site of implantation or infusion.

Therefore, although cell transplantation seems simple technically as compared to tissue and organ transplantation, its sequelae in terms of graft-host interrelationships are more complex and difficult to elucidate.

We will concentrate on the transplantation of intact cells and not of parts of cells although the latter has been attempted and in some cases with favorable clinical results. In addition, we will consider primarily the transplantation of bone marrow cells, since this procedure is today the most important cell transplantation procedure (disregarding blood transfusion).

It should be mentioned here, that this communication is based primarily on practical experience by the author as a member of the Cooperative Bone Marrow Transplantation Group of the National Cancer Institute, NIH, USA, under the leadership of DR. ROBERT G. GRAW, JR.[1]

B. Historical Notes

Sporadic reports of cell transplantation performed in ancient times date back to the 30th century before Christ. At that time as well as in the Middle Ages blood of young persons was infused into older ones for rejuvenation (for a review, see SAUNDERS, 1972). One such recipient was (in all probability) Pope Innocent VIII, who in 1492 received blood from three young men. Besides

[1] The cooperation of all members of this group is gratefully acknowledged: R.A. YANKEE, B.G. LEVENTHAL, G.N. ROGENTINE, G.P. HERZIG, J.O. NEEFE, R.H. HALTERMAN, C.B. MERRITT, R.L. COROLLA, J. WHANG-PENG, E.S. HENDERSON, H.R. GRALNICK, M.I. BULL, J.M. BULL, C.H. KIRKPATRICK, M.H. MCGINNIS, J. DECTER.

human blood, blood from animals was perfused, preferably from sheep which were supposed to have a symbolic relationship to Christ's blood. Although the medical literature of those days (CARDANO, 1556) stressed the high risk of mortality of such procedures, nevertheles quite a number of blood transfusion were done through the centuries. This may indicate the extent to which overzealous physicians and experimentalists can influence the interpretation of unfavorable results.

It was not until the turn of this century when LANDSTEINER and others laid the scientific basis for blood group isoantigens. And it was not until 40–50 years later that the antigenic conditions were determined to allow successful transplantation of various tissues including white blood cells (GORER, 1937; MEDAWAR, 1945; SNELL, 1948). A historical landmark in bone marrow transplantation was the first successful suppression of acute radiation death by grafting marrow cells into lethally irradiated mice as done by LORENZ, CONGDON, and DELTA UPHOFF (LORENZ et al., 1951). Such investigations were without doubt markedly boosted by the threat of nuclear warfare and its consequences. The experiments in mice done by this group greatly influenced research in cell transplantation, and initiated extensive investigations of the immunological conditions influencing bone marrow take or rejection, and graft-versus-host reactions (for a review, see BEKKUM and DE VRIES, 1967). Besides bone marrow cells, cells from various other sources were tested for their capacity to reconstitute deficient hematopoiesis.

Table 1. Bone Marrow Transplantation in Acute Leukemia up to 1971[a]

Year	Leukemic status	Bone marrow graft	No of patients	Takes (%)	No. of remissions	Duration of remissions
Before 1964	Relapse	Allograft	168	2	27	—
	Remission	Allograft	13	30	7	3–10 mos.
	Relapse	Isograft	9	?	8	2–12 mos.
1964–1968	Relapse	Allograft	24	70	3	8–20 mos.
1969–1971 Paris	Remission	Allograft	10	50	0	0
Seattle	Relapse	Allograft	5	60	3	85–200 days
	Relapse	Isograft	9	100	9	48–342 days
Holland	Remission	Allograft	3	100	2	43–56 days
Baltimore	Relapse	Allograft	7	85	5	32–215 days
Bethesda	Relapse	Allograft	9	89	7	10–132 days
	Relapse	Isograft	4	100	4	10–365 days
	Remission	Allograft	1	100	1	69 days
Other	Relapse	Allograft	3	0	1	30 days

[a] From GRAW et al., Exp. Hematol. **22**, 118 (1972)

In man, bone marrow transplantation under scientific conditions, has been done since 1956, when a group of scientists around GEORGE MATHÉ at Paris treated some physicists who were accidentally exposed to a lethal dose of ionizing radiation. In 1959 MATHÉ published the first technical procedure for engrafting bone marrow in man. Since that time, a number of collaborative groups engaged in human bone marrow transplantation have been established, the collective results of which are shown in Table 1. In order to limit the available data, Table 1 summarizes the results of bone marrow transplantation for one clinical indication—acute leukemia. Transplantation of cells other than from blood and bone marrow in man need not be considered here. However, brief mention of other cell transplantations will be made here and there throughout this paper.

C. Cell Types Used for Transplantation and Indications for the Respective Procedure

The number of cell types used for transplantation is limited, basically, to those cells that may be able to stimulate or substitute a decreased hematologic or immunologic function. Such cells include lymphoreticular and hematopoietic cells (leukocytes, erythrocytes, platelets). Although several cell systems have been successfully transplanted under experimental conditions, only a few can be used in man: clinical use is determined by the availability of the respective cells, the ease of engraftment, cell survival with functional activity, and the degree of immune response initiated by the engrafted cells.

I. Experimental Transplantation

Experiments in cell transplantation are legion and new publications appear nearly daily in the literature. In this review, therefore, only a limited number of references can be discussed so as to outline the general state of knowledge and the conclusions that can be drawn from such knowledge. Essentially, mature hematopoietic and immunocompetent cells as well as their immature precursors were transplanted. Representative collected data are shown in Table 2. As seen from this table, the various cell types were transplanted to *reconstitute lethally irradiated animals,* to study the effect of immunologically incompatible cells on the recipient organism (that is, graft-versus-host reaction; see HOBIK in this handbook), and to transfer immune competence (passive or adoptive immunity). The survival time of the engrafted cells varies with the mode of cell procurement, with the type of cell engrafted, with the degree of immunologic relatedness of host and donor, and with the state of immunologic competence of host and donor cells. Measuring the survival time of lethally irradiated animals as an indicator for a functioning graft provides the following data: isogenic fetal liver cells up to 100% at 90 days (mice); allogenic fetal liver cells up to 65% at 90 days (mice); xenogenic fetal liver cells up to 12% at 90 days (rat cells to

Table 2. Cell Transplantation in Experimental Animals

Types of cells	Animal	Immunological relatedness	Indications for transplantation	References
Fetal liver cells	Mice	Isogeneic	Hematopoietic	JACOBSEN et al., 1954; DUPLAN, 1956; UPHOFF, 1958
	Mice-Rats Rabbits	Xenogeneic Allogeneic	Reconstitution	LENGEROVA, 1959; URSO et al., 1959; PORTER, 1959
Fetal liver and thymus cells	Mice-Rats	Xenogeneic	Induction of GVHR	BLESSING, 1972
Embryonic liver and spleen cells	Mice	Allogeneic	Hematopoietic Reconstitution	BARNES et al., 1958
Fetal hemato-poietic stem cells from liver tissues	Mice	Allogeneic	Hematopoietic Reconstitution	LÖWENBERG et al., 1973
Fetal hemato-poietic cells from bone marrow	Mice	Isogeneic	Hematopoietic Reconstitution	CONGDON and URSO, 1957
Fetal spleen cells	Mice-Rats	Xenogeneic	Hematopoietic Reconstitution	URSO et al., 1959
Adult bone marrow	Mice	Isogeneic	Hematopoietic	SCHWARTZ et al., 1957; ASHWOOD-SMITH, 1961
	Mice	Allogeneic	Reconstitution	KRUEGER, 1961; CONGDON et al., 1952
	Mice-Rat	Xenogeneic		VOS et al., 1961
	Rabbits	Allogeneic		PORTER and MURRAY, 1951
	Guinea Pig	Allogeneic		SHAW and VERMUND, 1961
	Dogs	Allogeneic Autogeneic		STORB et al., 1973; BULL et al., 1975
	Rhesus monkeys	Allogeneic Autogeneic		WOODRUFF et al., 1969; MERRITT et al., 1972; SCHAEFER et al., 1972; VAN BEKKUM et al., 1969; KRUEGER et al., 1975
Adult spleen cells	Mice	Isogeneic	Hematopoietic	COLE et al., 1952; BARNES and LOUTIT, 1955
			Reconstitution	JACOBSON et al., 1955
Thymus cells	Mice	Isogeneic	Repopulation studies	TAYLOR, 1963; PARROTT et al., 1966

Table 2 (continued) see p. 280

Table 2 (continued)

Types of cells	Animal	Immunological relatedness	Indications for transplantation	References
Thoracic duct cells	Mice	Isogeneic	Repopulation studies	GENSER and GOWANS, 1962; DELORME, 1961
	Rats	Allogeneic Xenogeneic		ANDERSON and WHITELAW, 1960
Macrophages	Mice		Transfer of Immune Competence	WEISER et al., 1965; PEARSALL and WEISER, 1968; TSOI and WEISER, 1968
Lymph node cells	Mice			MITCHISON, 1955
	Rats	Allogeneic	Studies of GVHR	SILVERS and BILLINGHAM, 1969
Cultured hemato-poietic cells	Mice			BILLEN, 1957a and b BILLEN, 1959
Leukemoid blood	Mice	Isogeneic		CONGDON et al., 1956; SMITH and CONGDON, 1957
Leukocytes	Rat		Cell distribution studies;	HOLLINGSWORTH et al., 1951
	Rabbit	Allogeneic	Agranulocytosis, Anti-Infection	NYE and BARRS, 1932; MUNSTER et al., 1974

mice). Cells from fetal liver include a large number of hematopoietic stem cells, which explains the effectiveness of this procedure (LURIA et al., 1971). Accordingly, selective enrichment by gradient centrifugation of such hemato-poietic cells from liver cell suspensions enhances the repopulating efficiency upon subsequent transplantation (LÖWENBERG et al., 1973). Similar results can be obtained when adult hematopoietic cells are transplanted either from the spleen (rodent) or from the bone marrow. The survival time of adult hemato-poietic cells is less favorable when derived from an immunologically incompatible donor (allograft or xenograft). When mice received transplants of isogenic bone marrow cells after lethal irradiation, their survival amounted up to 100% at 30 days postgrafting; allogenic bone marrow grafts, however, were followed by 40% 30-day survivals, and xenogenic grafts (rat) by 0–10% survival over the same period. Besides the degree of immunologic relationship, the cell number engrafted influences the duration of survival as well as the dose rate of pretrans-plant x-irradiation and the time interval between radiation and bone marrow transplantation. A 24-h delay of marrow engraftment after irradiation proved to be optimal.

Macrophages, lymph node cells, and thymocytes were primarily transplanted to transfer immunity, especially antitumor immunity, and to induce graft-versus-host reactions (see HOBIK in this handbook). Accordingly, the effectiveness of cell transplantation was determined by antitumor cytotoxicity or by observing lesions indicative of graft-versus-host reactions. Long-lived small lymphocytes from the thoracic duct as well as from other sources proved effective in initiating graft-versus-host reactions (GOWANS, 1962; HILDEMAN, 1964; PORTER and COOPER, 1962); all of these cells, however, were not immunologically compatible, but allogenic. The results, therefore, indicate immunocompetence of transplanted cells rather than their ability to reconstitute the host.

Macrophages, upon engraftment, can not *initiate graft-versus-host* disease intrinsically; however, they may participate in such a reaction when initiated by lymphocytes (WEISER *et al.*, 1965). In an immunologic reaction, therefore, macrophages probably exert primarily a helper function; this can also be concluded from the results of studies of antitumor cytotoxicity (TEVETHIA and ZARLING, 1972). Such a helper function is part of the host response that should be reconstituted by cell transplantation. The complete spectrum of macrophage functional activity is too complex to be discussed in detail here. The interested reader is referred to specialized texts such as ROOS (1970) and to the monograph of PEARSALL and WEISER (1970).

Bone marrow cells in various animal species are rich in cells that can initiate graft-versus-host reactions, and thus prove immunologically competent (VAN BEKKUM and DE VRIES, 1967). Again, successful engraftment with hematologic and immunologic reconstitution of the host depends upon the degree of relatedness between host and donor. It appears that also in bone marrow transplantation, the number of immunocompetent lymphoid cells defines both the degree of subsequent immunologic reconstitution and the risk of developing graft-versus-host reaction. HILGARD (1970) stressed that the cooperation of thymic and nonthymic cells (e.g., bone marrow cells) is necessary for the production of the graft-versus-host reaction. More specific data will be found in HOBIK later in this volume.

Transplantation of isogenic and allogenic spleen cells, bone marrow cells, and lymph node cells served in various animals to *transfer immunity* against infectious organisms and malignant neoplasms; both antibody producing cells and immune competent lymphocytes (adoptive immunization) were transplanted (HARRIS *et al.*, 1954; MAKINODAN *et al.*, 1958; WUNDERLICH *et al.*, 1972; MUNSTER *et al.*, 1974). The number of viable mononuclear cells transferred varied usually between 10^6 and 10^9 (in rodents). The anti-infectious effect of transfused leukocytes appears somewhat limited, however, since these cells remain usually 30 minutes to 12 hours in the circulation after which most of them are sequestered in extracirculatory compartments as well as in pulmonary capillaries (LAWRENCE *et al.*, 1945; ROSSE and GURNEY, 1959; HOLLINGSWORTH *et al.*, 1957; BIERMAN *et al.*, 1955; NYE and BARRS, 1932). Figure 3 shows the organ distribution of infused bone marrow cells during the first week postengraftment. In some cases, leukocytes are detected for even longer times (up to 12 days) in the peripheral blood (KLINE and CLIFFTON, 1952); they may also recirculate to some extent after their initial disappearence. In any case, the benificial anti-infectious effect of transfused leukocytes can only be expected when large quantities are administered, and when compatibility with the recipient allows good survival of the cells. The antitumor effectiveness of the graft appears closely

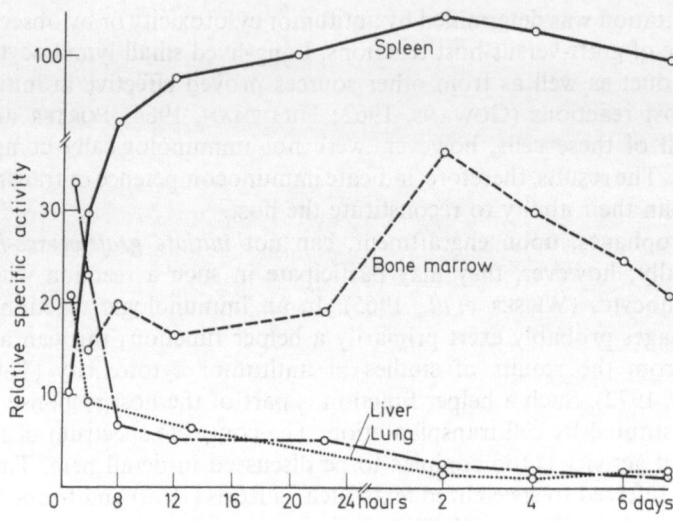

Fig. 3. Organ distribution of infused bone marrow cells

related to its absolute content in T-lymphocytes (thymus-dependent lymphocytes). A variation of cell transplantation for antitumor immunotherapy was
attempted by Mathé et al. (1965), Denton and Symes (1969) and others (Boranic, 1968 and 1971); these authors transplanted intentionally immunologically
incompatible cells (allogenic bone marrow) to induce a graft-versus-host reaction
and to make use of it as graft-antitumor reaction. Such treatment was usually
combined with chemotherapy. The reports of an antitumor effect, however,
are controversial. Positive results probably depend upon the presence and density
of transplantation antigens on the surface of the tumor cells.

Besides the indications for experimental cell transplantation mentioned so
far, two more should be discussed: cell transfer for the *induction of tolerance*
and cell transfer for inhibition of graft-versus-host reactions. Transfer of lymph
node cells, spleen cells, and bone marrow cells to recipients in the absence
of specific antigens may cause sustained specific tolerance (Zaalberg, 1953;
van Bekkum and de Vries, 1967; Sercarz and Coons, 1962; Friedman, 1964a
and b). Cell suspensions from different components of the lympho- and hemoreticular tissues differ in their capacity to confer tolerance, and the cell dose
is a factor of equal importance; although lymph node cells adapt less readily
to a foreign environment than bone marrow cells and thus become less readily
tolerant, they tend to maintain immunologic tolerance for longer periods than
bone marrow cells (van Bekkum and de Vries, 1967). The small lymphocyte,
which carries immunologic memory and is present in the various preparations
in different quantity appears to be responsible for the different effectiveness
of both cell preparations.

Billingham et al. (1962) induced tolerance towards second antigens by transferring nonisogenic cells to newborn hosts (allogenic cells and cells from one
parental strain to F_1 hybrids). These cells carried the antigenic characteristics

against which tolerance was to be induced. In this model in addition, cell suspensions from the various types of lympho- and hemoreticular tissues showed a different activity. Bone marrow cells are more effective than spleen cells, lymph node cells, and leukocytes. Spleen cells from an infant donor, however, proved as effective as adult bone marrow cells. This can be explained by the fact that rodent spleens are rich in hematopoietic cells and therefore resemble bone marrow cells more closely than do spleen cells from normal adult donors.

BORTIN et al. (1969) could *suppress the clinical signs of graft-versus-host reactions* by mixing and incubating at 37° C for 1 hour parental C57B1/6J spleen cells with neonatal C57B1/6J liver cells and injecting them into B6D2F$_1$ mice. Preincubation at 4° C had no protective effect with respect to developing graft-versus-host reaction. Since cell viability after incubation was not significantly decreased, the results appear to indicate that the immune competence of transplanted cells was probably selectively impaired whereas the hematopoietic restorative activity (in terms of colony-forming units and survival time of engrafted mice) was unaffected. Similar observations were published earlier by COSGROVE et al. (1959). Presumably, the inactivation of immune competence by this procedure is enzymatic in nature, although the exact mechanism remains to be elucidated.

A protective effect of a somewhat different nature against the development of lethal graft-versus-host disease was observed by SILVERS and BILLINGHAM (1969), who administered allogenic lymph node cells simultaneously with normal host cells (at a similar dose of 10^7 cells in rats). Timing in this experiment appears to be quite critical: a time difference of only 4 hours between the injection of allogenic and autogenous cells nearly eliminates the protective effect. It appears that immediate confrontation between the two immunologically incompatible cells types is necessary for rendering the allogenic cells less dangerous for the recipient.

A third protective procedure to avoid lethal graft-versus-host reaction is to transplant bone marrow cells or lymphoid cells after selective elimination of immunocompetent cells by gradient centrifugation (DICKE et al., 1968, 1970). The method leads to enrichment of large hematopoietic and lymphoid cells (probably stem cells) which upon transfer to the respective recipient (mice and monkey) appear less likely to be followed by acute severe graft-versus-host reaction (DICKE, 1970). Similar effects were observed by transplanting hematopoietic cells from the spleen of animals in which stem cells were increased by prior exposure to phenylhydrazine (TOYA et al., 1972).

Finally, another aspect of experimental bone marrow transplantation, which was recently outlined by THIERFELDER (1975), is to *differentiate between hematopoietic stem cell defects* of the recipient and *microenvironmental defects*. When compatible bone marrow is transplanted into animals with stem cell defects (as in cyclic neutropenia of dogs or congenital macrocytic anemia of certain mice), the underlying disease is likely to be cured; however, bone marrow engraftment into animals with microenvironmental defects (as the hematopoietic stem cell deficiency in mice of SlSld genotype) is not followed by cure.

II. Human Transplantation

As indicated above, the number of cell types transplanted in man is limited compared to animal experiments. As experimental studies indicate, only isogenic and well-matched allogenic cells can be expected to reconstitute the recipient hematologically or immunologically and thus justify the clinical indications for cell transplantation. Also, since a large number of cells needs to be transplanted, availability of such cells represents another serious limitation. In practice, the therapeutic use of cell transplantations is restricted in man to the transfusion of blood and its separated cellular components, or to the transplantation of bone marrow.

1. Indications for Transplantation of Blood and its Components

The clinical indications for the transplantation of blood are diverse and so generally known that they need not be repeated here. The essential requirement for the blood transfusion is the compatibility of major blood groups (primarily ABO) between donor and recipient. Pathologic sequelae after transfusion of incompatible blood (ABO incompatibility) due to hemolysis have been extensively investigated and described by MASSHOFF (1949). The predominant lesions consist in a generalized hyperpermeability of capillaries which is most prominent in liver and kidney ("serous inflammation" of RÖSSLE), followed by sequestration and excretion of blood products with subsequent degenerative organ changes ("hemoglobulinuric nephropathy").

Isolated cellular blood components are used therapeutically to make up for specific deficiencies such as thrombocytes in thrombocytopenia, packed leukocytes in leukocytopenia or agranulocytosis, and erythrocytes in severe anemia. Among the engrafted leukocytes for supportive care of agranulocytotic patients were cells from patients with chronic myelogenous leukemia (CML). It was felt that blood from such patients was rich enough in leukocytes to correct the granulocytic deficiency of the host (SCHWARZENBERG et al., 1965; GRAW et al., 1970). This technique, however, which carries a considerable risk, became obsolete after the development of newer devices to collect normal granulocytes such as the NCI-IBM Continuous Flow Blood Cell Separator (Celltrifuge AIC, GRAW et al., 1971 and 1972).

2. Indications for Transplantation of Bone Marrow

Similarly, bone marrow transplantation is indicated in certain deficiencies of the hemoreticular and lymphoreticular tissues, inherited and inborn, or acquired. Such conditions include radiation accidents, immune deficiency syndromes, aplastic anemia, and acute leukemia (FERREBEE and THOMAS, 1960; BACH, ALBERTINI et al., 1968; GATTI et al., 1968; BUCKLEY et al., 1971; DUPONT et al., 1973; HILGARTNER et al., 1970; SPECK, 1973; STORB et al., 1974; THOMAS and EPSTEIN, 1965; GRAW et al., 1972; RUDOLPH et al., 1973). In certain cases of immune deficiency disease, bone marrow infusion was combined with transplantation of thymic tissue to support recovery of cellular immunologic activity (DE

KONING *etal.*, 1969; LEVEY *et al.*, 1971). The indication for bone marrow transplantation in *accidents with ionizing (lethal) irradiation* is easy; ultimately there is no other therapeutical regimen. The limitations of therapy in this group of patients arise primarily from the availability of compatible donors and from coping with the adverse sequelae of allografting (see Section F).

More difficult to determine is the exact indication for bone marrow transplantation in *immune deficiency syndromes*. In fact, the transplantation in the various types of immune defects is still in the experimental stage. It appears that severe combined immune deficiency syndromes of common variable types, especially Swiss-type agammaglobulinemia, constitutes one indication for bone marrow transplantation (RUBINSTEIN *et al.*, 1971; DE KONING *et al.*, 1969; LEVEY *et al.*, 1971; BACH *et al.*, 1968; BUCKLEY *et al.*, 1971; DUPONT *et al.*, 1973). The outcome of this procedure will depend largely upon the recurrence of cellular immune reactivity which is not always guaranteed. It would seem, therefore, that an ideal indication for immunologic reconstitution by bone marrow engraftment are isolated humoral immune deficiency syndromes (Table 3).

Similarly difficult is the decision to transplant bone marrow in *aplastic anemia*, especially with respect to a given case. In contrast to patients with immune deficiency syndromes, those with aplastic anemia need careful pretransplant immunosuppression, a procedure not without danger. The decision for

Table 3. WHO Classification of Primary Immune Deficiency Disorders[a]

Type	Suggested Cellular Defect		
	B cells	T cells	Stem cells
Infantile X-linked agamma-globulinemia	+		
Selective immunoglobulin deficiency (IgA)	+[b]		
Transient hypogammaglobulinemia of infancy	+		
X-linked immunodeficiency with hyper-IGM	+[b]		
Thymic hypoplasia (pharyn. pouch syndrome. DIGEORGE)		+	
Episodic lymphopenia with lymphocytotoxin		+	
Immunodeficiency with normal or hyperimmunoglobulinemia	+	+[c]	
Immunodeficiency with ataxia telangiectasia	+	+	
Immunodeficiency with thrombocytopenia and eczema (WISKOTT-ALDRICH)	+	+	
Immunodeficiency with thymoma	+	+	
Immunodeficiency with short-limbed dwarfism	+	+	
Immunodeficiency with generalized hematopoietic hypoplasia	+	+	+
Severe combined immunodeficiency			
(a) autosomal recessive	+	+	+
(b) X-linked	+	+	+
(c) sporadic	+	+	+
Variable immunodeficiency (largely unclassified)	+	+[c]	+

[a] From KUNKEL *et al.*, 1972
[b] Involve some but not all B cells
[c] Encountered in some but not all patients

bone marrow transplantation, therefore, should be made with the utmost caution. Only those cases with a dismal prognosis should be considered, and only those that seem to be based upon a hematopoietic stem cell incompetence, not upon a deficiency of the matrix (see Section CI); it is rather difficult, however, to differentiate both types. SPECK (1973a and b) listed the following prognostically unfavorable parameters that justify bone marrow therapy; progressive pancytopenia with a progressively empty marrow (verified by repeated biopsies); a decreased number of hematopoietic stem cells in the bone marrow (as estimated by in vitro counting of colony-forming units); and an unfavorable course of reticulocyte counts. When such criteria suggest radical therapeutic intervention, bone marrow transplantation should be done at the earliest possible date, since delays lead to complications such as the development of agranulocytosis with septicemia, and presensitization of the patient by repeated blood transfusions. The importance of bone marrow transplantation in aplastic anemia is stressed by SPECK (1973a) who stated that 65% of the cases diagnosed in the 5-year period of 1967–1972 died despite intensive conservative therapy including blood cell transfusions, and only 4 out of 31 patients showed partial or complete remission within 1–3 months of corticosteroid treatment. In contrast, of the 23 patients with aplastic anemia of STORB et al. (1974) with a duration of the aplastic phase of 1.5–15 months prior to transplantation, 10 have returned to normal activity with normal stem cells repopulating the marrow postengraftment. The survival time at the time of publication is up to 2.3 years.

Bone marrow transplantation in patients with *acute leukemia* [acute lymphoblastic leukemia (ALL) and acute myeloblastic leukemia (AML)] is reserved for advanced stages of the disease who show no significant response to conventional (chemotherapeutic) treatment.

Transplantation can be done both in remission as well as in relapse, but remission is, of course, favored.

Although many publications on bone marrow transplantation in acute leukemia do not cite specific criteria for indication, it can be deduced from the various case histories that there is general agreement about whom and when to transplant. As in the cases of aplastic anemia, it is advisable not to attempt bone marrow engraftment too late, that is, in the late stage of the disease when host resistence is poor and the patients may already undergone courses of septicemia. Also, at this time presensitization of the bone marrow recipient may have occurred through multiple transfusions of blood or its components. Recently, bone marrow transplantation was even used as a primary therapeutic approach in patients with AML (SANTOS et al., 1974).

Besides transplantation of collective bone marrow cells, DICKE et al. (1973) used stem cell concentrates as bone marrow grafts in man. Lymphocyte-poor stem cell concentrates obtained by density gradient centrifugation appear to ameliorate subsequent graft-versus-host disease.

Finally, it should be mentioned that besides adult bone marrow, fetal bone marrow transplantation has been attempted in leukemic patients (although in combination with adult allogenic marrow; THOMAS and EPSTEIN, 1965). The results, however, were apparently not promising and no further experiments were carried out.

D. Technique of Cell Transplantation

Knowledge of the technique of cell transplantation is necessary for every patholo- gist involved in the morphologic evaluation of transplantation sequelae. In the following paragraphs, the procedure of bone marrow grafting is described as it is performed by the NCI Cooperative Bone Marrow Transplantation Group (Pamphlet No. 70-4). It serves as a representative example of cell transplantation.

I. Details of Patient Selection

Patients with malignancies, immune deficiency diseases, and others with bone marrow or lymphoreticular hypofunction have a high mortality caused primarily by infection and hemorrhage secondary to thrombocytopenia. Supportive care of such patients with transfusion of blood components has been employed to alleviate temporarily the primary hematologic defect and, in certain cases, the lymphoreticular defect. However, long-term support in this manner is not feasible because of difficulties in obtaining the necessary quantities of leukocytes and other blood cells, their short survival time in the host, and alloimmunization following multiple transfusions. Attempts to transplant bone marrow for he- matologic and immunologic reconstitution appears, therefore, to be indicated in such patients; the task is to produce a stable chimerism with more or less functioning foreign hemo- and lymphoreticular cells in the defective host. This, however, is hampered by three main obstacles: recurrence of malignancy after incomplete eradication, failure to obtain engraftment, and the attack of host cells by the infused immunocompetent cells, that is, the graft-versus-host reac- tion. Avoidance of these complications will influence the decision as to which type of patient should be selected for bone marrow transplantation as well as pre- and posttransplant treatment.

In all patients selected for bone marrow therapy, a close immunologic related- ness (compatibility) is necessary for both engraftment and avoidance of the lethal graft-versus-host reaction. This compatibility is expressed in terms of similarity of HL-A antigens (phenotypical and genotypical) as well as in terms of stimulatory activity of host and donor cells in mixed leukocyte culture (MLC tests). Ideally, bone marrow donors should represent identical twins (syngenic transplantation), but such a situation is so rare that nonidentical donors must be used (allogenic transplantation). The requirements for an allogenic marrow donor are that he posses identical HL-A haplotypes with the recipient in terms of two identified HL-A specificities at the first and second subloci (see Chapters 1 and 3), and that the MLC tests are nonstimulatory. Transplantation across an ABO blood group barrier, however, seems to be possible (in the case of preexisting blood group isoantibodies against donor erythrocytes absorption of these antibodies is advised; GRAW et al., 1972).

In addition to cell typing, all bone marrow graft recipients without immune defects need pretransplant immunosuppression, and patients with malignancies need pretransplant cytotoxic or radiologic tumor eradication.

1. Selection of the Host

The patient and his entire family will have had HL-A typing and MLC tests, both done at least twice by independent laboratories. Complete erythrocyte phenotyping and estimation of isohemagglutinin titers are performed. All evidence of infections must be cleared (no temperature above 38° C). Complications of the primary disease must be under full therapeutic control (e.g., in leukemia of the central nervous system). The patient and/or responsible members of his family must be informed as to the nature of the therapeutic procedure, its risk, and its prognostic significance. The patient and/or his closest relative (wife, parent) must agree to the procedure.

2. Selection of the Donor

HL-A typing of the patient and his entire family must be performed and repeated until a final decision can be made as to a possible matched donor within his family. No bone marrow transplantation will be attempted unless there is evidence of identity between donor and recipient as determined by HL-A serotyping and haplotype analysis. Nonstimulatory MLC tests are necessary to support the evidence for a match, and complete ABO phenotyping is done. All tests are performed at least twice. The donor must be free of disease and fully agree to the procedure.

II. Preevaluation and Pretreatment of Host and Donor

The NCI Cooperative Bone Marrow Transplantation Group prepared a list of studies that should be done on donors as well as hosts. These studies define the current physiologic status of donor and recipient, the limitations and complications of bone marrow transplantation, and define possible markers for a positive engraftment. Besides such laboratory investigations, the therapeutic regimen (primarily for the recipient) is designed to prepare the organism for bone marrow allografting. Both are briefly outlined in the following paragraphs.

1. Pretreatment of the Donor

The donor must be hospitalized for at least 24 hours preceding the procedure, and a consent form must be signed for multiple bone marrow aspirations. A complete case history and physical examination is performed including the following:

  a) Chest x-ray.
  b) Ekg.
  c) Urea nitrogen, glucose, SGOT, bilirubin, prothrombin time, partial thromboplastin time, fibrinogen, elctrophoresis, routine urine analysis.
  d) Serologic tests: Australia antigen, toxoplasmosis titer, cytomegalovirus complement fixation titer, Candida titer, Aspergillus precipitate titer.
  e) Complete blood counts including reticulocytes.

f) Bone marrow aspirate for cytogenetics.

g) Skin testing (requires at least 3 weeks for completion of studies): tuberculin test, mumps, brucella, trichophyton, histoplasmosis, streptokinase-streptodornase. These tests should be done after confirmatory HL-A and MLC tests are performed. The skin tests serve to demonstrate later adoptive immunity in the marrow recipient.

h) Storage of blood products: donor platelets should be frozen for posttransplant support of the patient. One unit of blood will be kept for reinfusion into the donor post marrow donation. Peripheral blood lymphocytes are obtained by plasmapheresis and kept frozen for future studies. Leukocytes are obtained from the donor for infusion to the patient 1 day prior to immunosuppression (in recipients without immune deficiency syndroms).

1. Urine and saliva are cultured for cytomegalovirus. The donor tests as outlined serve as a control of his disease-free status. In addition, immunologic studies are performed for demonstration of adoptive immunity in the marrow recipient secondary to positive engraftment, that is, the host's acquiring immunologic reactivity against antigens which he did not recognize before transplantation, but against which the donor was immunized.

2. Pretreatment of the Recipient

The bone marrow recipient is placed in an unmodified hospital room with reverse isolation precautions (gown, mask, hat, and gloves) on the day preceding immunosuppression. The consent form for bone marrow transplantation is signed. Daily physical examinations including weight are continued.

The following laboratory tests and therapeutic measures are done prior to transplantation:

a) Chest x-ray in the week preceding pretransplant immunosuppression (or preceding transplantation in patients with immune deficiency syndromes).

b) EKG in the week prior to immunosuppression or transplantation.

c) Serum is obtained for the serum bank over a period of several days.

d) Peripheral blood lymphocytes are tested for their response to phytohemagglutinine (PHA).

e) Skin testing is done as outlined for the donor.

f) Skin punch biopsy is performed for comparison with later biopsies.

g) Baseline cultures are done when the patient is placed in the isolation room (fifth day prior to transplant): blood, stool, urine, throat, and perineal skin cultures for aerobic bacteria and fungi; in addition, urine, throat washings, and saliva are tested for cytomegalovirus.

h) Stools are checked for occult blood.

i) Serologic tests are done as outlined for the donor.

j) Bone marrow is aspirated for cytogenetic studies.

k) Complete erythrocyte phenotyping is done as well as determination of isohemagglutinin titers.

l) Saliva is tested for secretor status.

m) Patient is transfused to get hemoglobin values of 12–14 mg%.

n) Patient is placed in reverse isolation room and daily disinfective baths are initiated (Phisohex baths).

o) Peripheral blood lymphocytes are obtained by plasmapheresis and are frozen (initiated several weeks prior to transplantation).

Similar to the donor, these tests are performed in the prospective marrow recipient to control his current stable status with regard to his disease, to make sure that he is free of subclinical infections, and to check his state of immunologic reactivity.

Besides the foregoing investigative and preparatory procedures, patients with aplastic anemia and acute leukemia need pretransplant immunosuppression, combined with a tumor-eradicating regimen in leukemics.

p) Classic techniques.

Pretransplant immunosuppression in aplastic anemia is achieved by administration of cyclophosphamide (Cytoxan, Endoxan) according to the SANTOS regimen (SANTOS et al., 1971; BUCKNER et al., 1973): donor antigen (500 ml whole blood) is given i.v. to stimulate immunocompetent cell clones. Bone marrow transplantation is performed 24 hours after the last administration of cyclophosphamide. This scheme has been modified by other investigators who administer 60 mg/kg/day cyclophosphamide on 4 subsequent days, and, to avoid cardiopulmonary complications, reduce the dosage to 45–50 mg/kg/day cyclophosphamide (GRAW et al., 1972; Fig. 4).

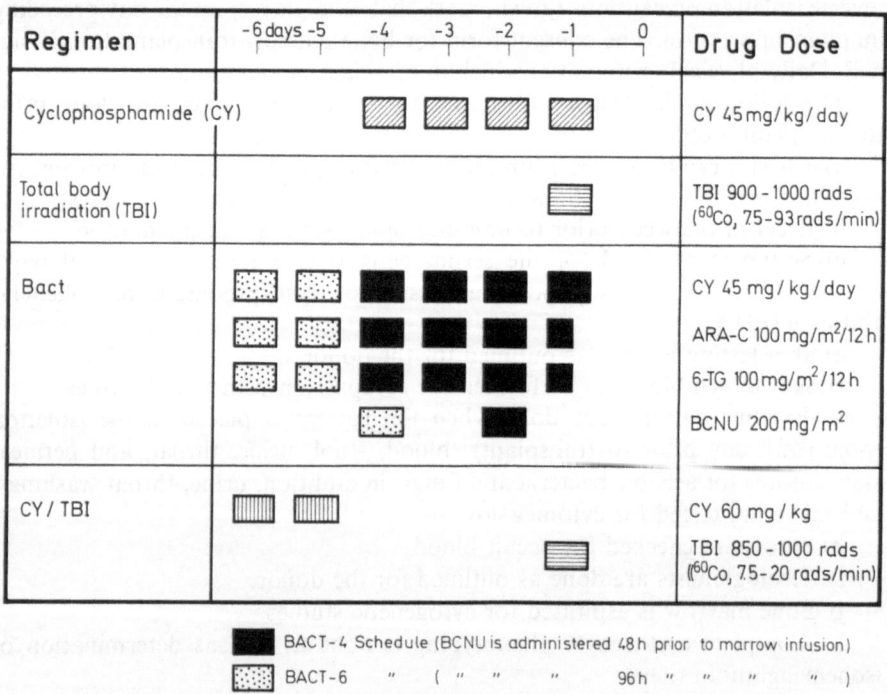

Fig. 4. Schedule of pretransplant immunosuppression and chemotherapy

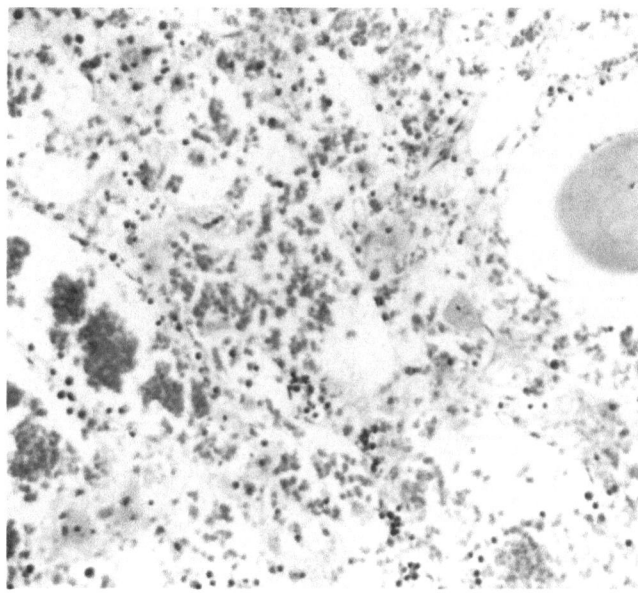

Fig. 5. Severe acute bone marrow aplasia post cyclophosphamide, 45 mg/kg/day × 4. H & E, × 150

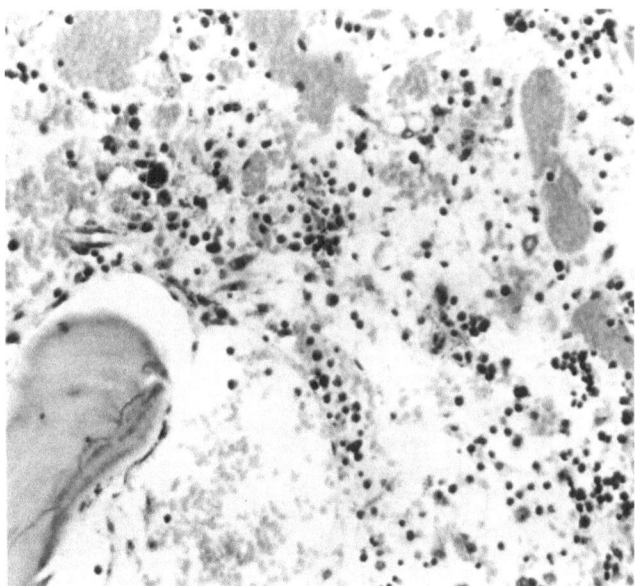

Fig. 6. Severe acute bone marrow aplasia after total body irradiation, 1,000 rads. H & E, × 150

Another immunosuppressive regimen consists of total body irradiation (TBI) at 100-rad midline tissue exposure, exposure rate: 5.0–5.7 R/min at midpoint. Patients are placed between two opposing 1,500 Ci-^{60}Co sources (STORB *et al.*, 1974). Other groups vary the exposure rate and total body dose.

The immunosuppressive effect as well as the ablation of hematopoiesis by both cyclophosphamide and TBI can be seen in Figures 5–10, which show severe atrophy, edema, and hemorrhage of lymph nodes, spleen, and bone marrow.

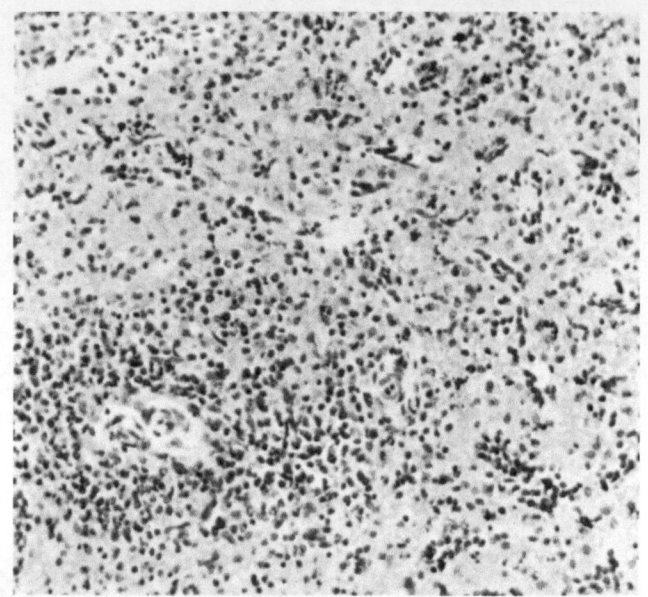

Fig. 7. Severe splenic atrophy post cyclophosphamide, 45 mg/kg/day × 4. H & E, × 150. Note small follicular remnant

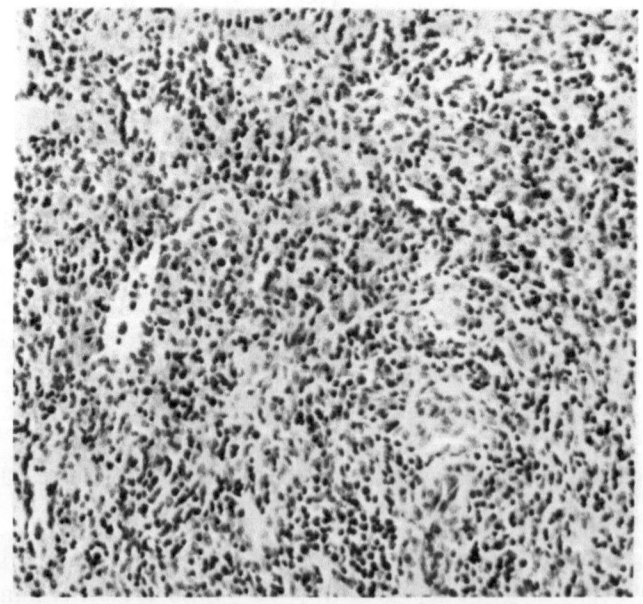

Fig. 8. Severe splenic atrophy after total body x-irradiation, 1,000 rads. H & E, × 150. Remaining are primarily stromal cells

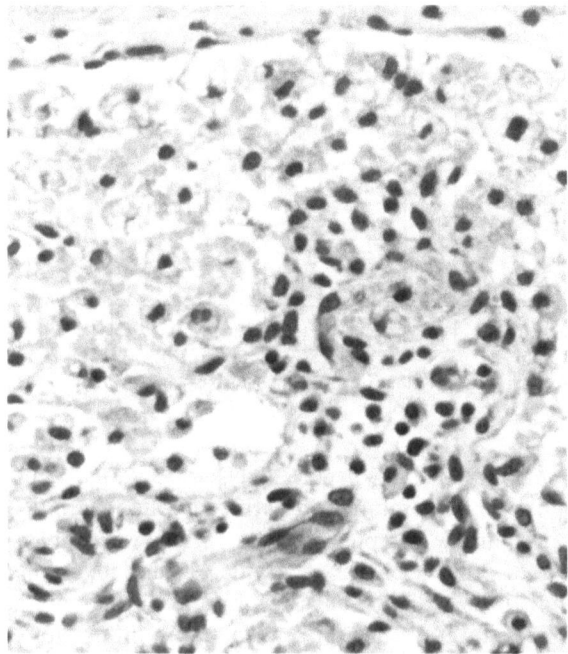

Fig. 9. Severe diffuse lymph node atrophy post cyclophosphamide, 45 mg/kg/day × 4. H & E, × 375

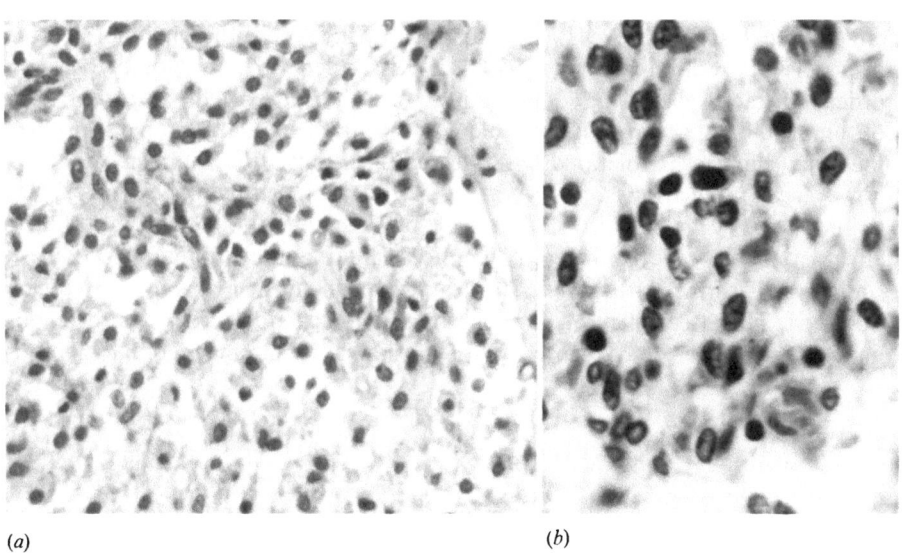

(a)   (b)

Fig. 10. (a) Severe diffuse lymph node atrophy after total body irradiation, 1,000 rads. H & E, × 375. (b) Note residual stromal cells, macrophages, and occasional pyknotic lymphoid cell. H & E, × 600

Regimen	#	Engraft-ment (%)		Remission (%)		Remission Duration (days)	
						Median	Range
CY	9	6/9	(67)	4/8	(50)	92	48 - 140
TBI	2	1/2	(50)	1/2	(50)	37	-
BACT	6	4/6	(67)	4/4	(100)	115	32 - 1095+
CY/TBI	5	5/5	(100)	5/5	(100)	41	16 - 113
CY+TBI	11	7/11	(64)	5/10	(50)	65	37 - 140
BACT+CY/TBI	11	9/11	(82)	9/9	(100)	78	16 - 1095+
Total	22	16/22	(73)	14/16	(74)	71	16 - 1095+

Fig. 11. Effect of pretransplant therapy on bone marrow engraftment and remission of leukemia (Courtesy of Dr. Robert G. Graw, Jr., NCI-NIH)

Mathé *et al.* (Mathé and Schwarzenberg, 1974) used antilymphocyte glob-ulin (ALG), alone or in combination with cyclophosphamide, for pretransplant conditioning of marrow recipients; 4–8 g ALG were given 4–12 days prior to transplantation. When cyclophosphamide was added, 45 mg/kg/day was given an 4 subsequent days ending 6 days prior to bone marrow grafting. Although some destructive effect of such pretransplant immunosuppressive therapy on leukemic cells can be observed, it apparently is no guaranty that leukemia will not recur.

q) Newer techniques.

A combination of pretransplant immunosuppression with an optimal anti-leukemic effect is achieved by a four-drug combination protocol; the 4–6-day cyclophosphamide regimen is supplemented by two agents considered to be effective against cells of AML (cytosine arabinoside and 6-thioguanine); a fourth drug, bis-chloroethyl-nitrosurea (BCNU), is added on day 3 of cytostasis in order to attack cells in the G–O resting phase. Because of the apparent return of tumor in one patient, this schedule was recently extended to 6 days, provided the 4-day therapy is tolerated without complications. In a number of patients, however, complications of this rather aggressive therapy might be expected (Buja *et al.*, 1974; see also Chapter 6.3 of this handbook). The morphologic effect of the BACT regimen on lymphoreticular and hemoreticular tissues is similar, as is shown in Figures 5–10, except that hemorrhage is more frequently observed. The effect of the various pretreatment schedules with regard to bone marrow graft take and recurrence of leukemia is summarized in Figure 11.

III. Procurement of Bone Marrow Cells

Bone marrow is obtained from multiple aspiration sites on both anterior and posterior iliac crests and sternum. Other possible sites are the acromium, ribs, and spinal bone. The donor is kept under general anesthesia. Five to 10 ml of blood with marrow is aspirated through trocars into heparinized syringes, placed in sterile beakers containing a mixture of heparin and tissue culture media (TC-199), and thoroughly mixed. Subsequently the marrow is filtered through 300-, 200μ mesh stainless steel sieves to remove particles. Samples of the final aspirate are compared with the peripheral blood cell count for correction of the total number of nucleated bone marrow cells. The marrow will then be directly infused intravenously without a filter. Altogether, from 300–400 ml of the blood/bone marrow mixture about 10^{10} nucleated cells can be obtained. MATHÉ et al. (1972) give the following concentrations of nucleated cells in bone marrow aspirates from the various sites: sternum (manubrium and body) 15,000–50,000/mm^3; posterior iliac crest and posterior surface 20,000–80,000/mm^3; iliac crest 10,000–40,000/mm^3; anterior superior iliac spine 10,000–45,000/mm^3.

Although leukocytes may persist for several hours in the bone marrow after the death of a patient (PERRY et al., 1960), no adequate information is available concerning the proliferative capacity of such cells, and no cadaver bone marrow was been used yet for transplantation.

Frozen marrow cells as used in animal experiments have not yet found broad application in man. However, frozen autogenous marrow taken during the remission phase of leukemia may be used if the bone marrow allograft does not take or if a life-threatening graft-versus-host reaction (GVHR) makes destruction of the allograft advisable. In general, several 10^5 cells/ml suspended in physiologic salt solution (e.g., Hanks solution, tissue culture media 199, NCTC 109, or CMRI 1450) with the additive of 4–10% serum and glycerol (12%) dimethyl sulfoxide (DMSO, 7.5–12%) with or without polyvinyl pyrrolidone (PVP) are frozen to $-80°$ C in a liquid nitrogen freezer. Freezing is done at a rate of 1–2° C per minute and thawing by rapid immersion of the marrow containers in a 37–40° C water bath (O'GRADY, 1970; MALININ, 1973). Freezing and storage of bone marrow suspensions is done in glass ampulles or plastic transfer packs. The ratio of air-to-fluid in the container should be 2:1. This is necessary to assure adequate oxygen for the maintenance of viable cells, which even at low temperatures probably retain a baseline metabolism. Small separate samples of bone marrow serve bacteriologic and morphologic studies including viability tests prior to engraftment. According to MALININ (1973), human bone marrow cells frozen at low temperature with the addition of a cryoprotective agent (such as DMSO) can stay viable without critical loss of cell numbers even under longterm storage.

In some instances concentrated hematopoietic stem cells are used for transplantation instead of complete bone marrow according to the method of DICKE et al. (1969 and 1973). The cells are separated by discountinuous albumin density gradient centrifugation. A 35% stock solution of bovine serum albumin (BSA) is prepared at room temperature in 0.155 M Tris buffer pH 7.2, at an osmolarity of 375 mosmols. The different BSA concentrations are obtained by dilution with 0.154 M NaCl, 0.01 M sodium phosphate buffer, pH 7.2 (osmolarity of sodium phosphate buffer: 300 mosmols). The fraction with an osmolarity of 15 mosmols below the stock solution contains a large number of hematopoietic stem cells; this fraction is refractionated subsequently from a stock solution of 370 mosmols, and fractions 2 and 3 of it contain the largest numbers of hematopoietic stem cells and the lowest numbers of phytohemagglutinine-responsive lymphocytes. The gradients are centrifuged at 2,000 (1,000 g at tube bottom) and 10° C for 30 minutes.

IV. Cell Grafting

Bone marrow with contaminating blood (heparinized) is infused intravenously into the recipient immediately after donation. This is done slowly using a syringe and a needle of about 1.2 mm in diameter. Previously frozen marrow may be washed in physiologic salt solution to remove the preservative (glycerol of DMSO). Besides the intravenous route, which is used commonly today, intraperitoneal and intracardial injections have been attempted; the intraperitoneal transfer of bone marrow is still quite commonly used by the Minnesota transplant group (PARK et al., 1974). The intramuscular, subcutaneous, and intrathoracic routes, however, have proved to be rather ineffective in animal experiments (cited by VAN BEKKUM and DE VRIES, 1967). Similarly ineffective experimentally were injections of bone marrow cells into testis and brain.

The nucleated cell dose transplanted varies in general from 7×10^5/kg (3-months-old baby with combined immune deficiency syndrome (IDS) to 9×10^9/kg (10-year-old female with CLL), with an average of 10^7 in IDS and 10^8 in leukemia, suspended in a volume of 200–400 ml. It is estimated that a total of 4×10^9 nucleated cells is necessary for repopulation of human bone marrow 7–14 days after engraftment.

V. Cells other than Bone Marrow Cells used for Transplantation in Man

PARK et al. (1974) transplanted thymus cells from one fetus in combination with liver cells from three fetuses in a total dose of 10^8 nucleated cells per kg i.p. into an 8-month-old male with Swiss type immune deficiency syndrome. The patient died 15 days postengraftment with transient restoration of humoral and cellular immune reactivity.

As indicated above, transfusion of concentrated blood cell components is done to reconstitute patients with specific quantitative or qualitative defects of the respective cell system. Candidates for granulocyte transfusion are patients with agranulocytosis, acute leukemia, aplastic anemia, and solid tumors showing less than 500 circulating leukocytes per cubic millimeter. Such patients are prone to develop septicemia caused by gram-negative organisms, fungi, and viruses. Donors are usually ABO-compatible family members not necessarily matched for HL-A antigens. Unmatched white blood corpuscles (WBC) are x-irradiated with 1,500 rads prior to infusion to avoid GVHR. Donor leukocytes are collected by the NCI-IBM Continous Flow Blood Cell Separator, as mentioned above, or by continous flow filtration leukopheresis (GRAW et al., 1971 and 1972; HERZIG et al., 1972). Granulocytes are usually collected at 20 g (about 500 rpm) or below, lymphocytes at 70 g (about 1,000 rpm), and thrombocytes in a second centrifugation at 275 g (about 2,000 rpm). Besides the two procedures mentioned, other methods of separating leukocytes have been tried such as filtration through glass particles, selective hemolysis, phytohemagglutinine administration, and density gradient centrifugation with high molecular weight substances (albumin, fibrinogen, gamma globulin, dextran, and polybrene) (FLEMING, 1926; VALLEE et al., 1974; MINOR and BURNETT, 1948; SKOOG and BECK, 1956; GARVIN, 1961; LALEZARI, 1962; FREIREICH et al., 1964).

Recipients are examined for the presence of preformed leukocyte antibodies against donor cells. No donor is used to whom the recipient has preformed antibodies. Selected samples of leukocytes to be transfused are studied for their phagocytic potential using the activity of the hexose monophosphate shunt and their bactericidal capacity is measured by the ingestion and destruction of bacteria (e.g., *Staphylococcus albus*) (GRAW et al., 1972). The number of transfused WBC averaged 14×10^9 initial dose with daily compatible transfusions for the period of infection and granulocytopenia. Granulocyte recovery in a patient is calculated according to the following formula (GRAW et al., 1972):

$$\text{Recovery (WBC \%)} = \frac{\text{WBC increment/ml} \times \text{Blood vol. (ml)} \times 100}{\text{Total WBC transfused}}$$

The WBC increment is expressed for a standard body surface area of 1 m^2 and a standard dose of 1×10^{10} WBC. The corrected WBC increment is then given as follows:

$$\text{Corr. increment WBC} = \frac{\text{WBC increment/ml}^3 \times \text{surface area (m}^2)}{\text{Total number of WBC infused (}10^{10})}$$

Like bone marrow, separated WBC can be transfused fresh or after frozen storage. Freezing is done in TCM-199 or Tyrode's solution with 12% DMSO or 15% glycerol, and storage at $-78°$ C or $-196°$ C (SCHWARZENBERG et al., 1965).

VI. Posttransplant Clinical Investigation of Bone Marrow Recipient

For adequate monitoring of the patient during the immediate (5 weeks) posttransplant period a number of clinical tests is indicated which shall be briefly outlined (thereafter the tests are usually performed on a weekly basis):

1) Complete blood counts are done daily.

2) Renal and liver function tests are done every other day for 10 days, then once a week.

3) The clotting status is done every other day for 2 weeks, then once weekly.

4) EKG is done on days 2, 4, and 6, and chest x-ray on day 1 and when necessary.

5) Bone marrow status including cytogenetics is checked on days 5, 10, and 15 and subsequently once a week.

6) Stools for occult blood are checked on days 1, 3, and 6, then twice a week.

7) Serology (toxoplasmosis, cytomegalovirus, fungi) is done weekly.

8) Erythrocyte phenotype, isohemagglutinin titer, and saliva for secretor status are tested weekly.

9) Cultures (throat, urine, stool, perineal skin) are done on days 3, 7, 11, 15, and 20, then weekly.

10) Skin biopsy is taken 48 hours after skin rash is obsserved; similarly liver biopsies are taken when enzymes are elevated.

11) The immunolgic capacity of the patient is checked by repeating the pretransplant tests 3 weeks after bone marrow engraftment.

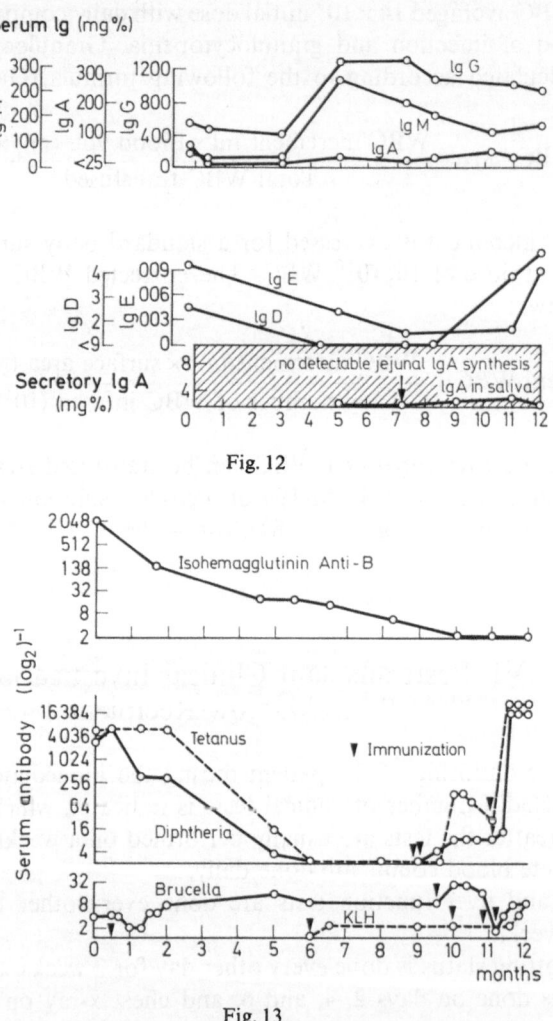

Fig. 12

Fig. 13

Fig. 12 and 13. Serum immunoglobulins and antibodies in patient T.G. with AML, BACT (4) therapy, and bone marrow allografting

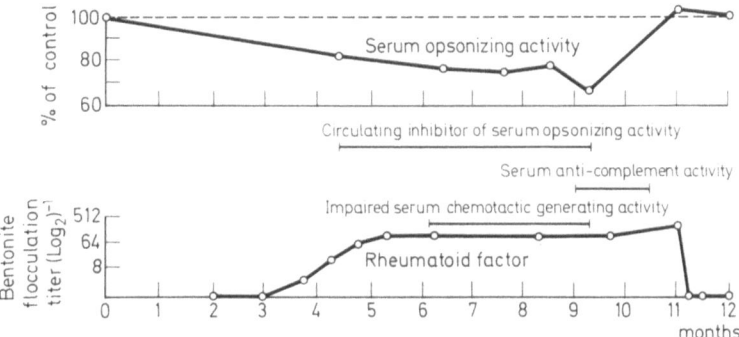

Fig. 14. Serum opsonizing activity and chemotaxis after bone marrow allografting in patient T.G.

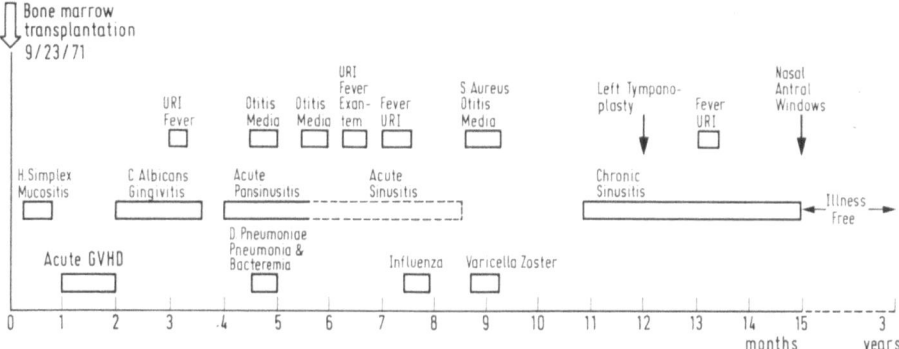

Fig. 15. Course of infectious complications following bone marrow allografting in patient T.G.
(Figs. 12–15 courtesy of Dr. ROBERT G. GRAW, JR., NCI-NIH)

The tests outlined are performed to control hematopoietic recovery of the patient, prove positive engraftment of allogenic bone marrow cells, and to determine his degree of hematopoietic cell chimerism. In addition, some of the investigations serve to detect incipient infections, graft-versus-host reaction, and defective blood coagulation. Finally, tests to define immunologic reactivity of the patient also serve as a check on adoptive immunity. Figures 12–15, which exhibit the clinical course of a patient after bone marrow allografting, underscore the necessity to perform tests as outlined above. All figures are from the same patient, an 18-year-old male with AML who received an HL-A and MLC-matched bone marrow graft after BACT (4 days) pretransplant chemotherapy. He acquired immunologic competence 1 year postgrafting at which time his repeated infections terminated. After more than $3^1/_2$ years after bone marrow transplantation, he shows no signs of recurrent leukemia, is healthy, and works full time.

E. Demonstration and Localization
of Engrafted Cells

There are various methods to demonstrate the engraftment and the distribution of transplanted cells in the host organism; some of these methods are applicable only under experimental conditions, others are used clinically to prove graft take. The easiest method to study cell distribution in the experimental animal is to transplant cells labeled with radioactive substances such as ^{51}Cr or ^3H-thymidine. The latter marker is somewhat less recommended because label leaks from the cell into its environment and may be taken up by bystander cells. It may be used, however, for brief experiments.

Using these isotopic cell markers, it was demonstrated in rats and mice (NOWELL et al., 1957; BALNER et al., 1962; FLIEDNER, 1960) that about 15 minutes after intravenous infusion large numbers of these cells localize in the *lung* as well as in the *liver*. By 24–48 hours later, infused cells are detected primarily in *spleen* and *bone marrow*, that is, in the hematopoietic tissues in the rodent. After 3 hours postinfusion, cells start to shift from the lungs to the hematopoietic organs, and there they can be traced throughout a period of 8 days (Fig. 3).

For *histologic investigations* of the localization of infused hematopoietic cells into a lethally irradiated recipient or into a recipient with extensive hemo- and lymphoreticular atrophy post chemotherapy, *enzyme reactions* can be used such as the phosphatase, esterase, and peroxidase tests. We used, for example, the chloroacetate esterase reaction to demonstrate hematopoietic cell colonies in histologic sections. In dogs and rhesus monkeys investigated at various intervals postallotransplantation, as well as in man, hematopoietic cells are demonstrated to a significant extent in small vessels of *lungs* and *kidney*, as well as in *sinuses of lymph nodes* and *spleen* up to 3–4 days after marrow infusion (Figs. 16–18). Thereafter, hematopoietic cell colonies are observed with increasing frequency and increasing size in the *lymph node, spleen*, and *bone marrow*.

The extent of hematopoietic cell proliferation depends upon the dose of transplanted cells, and also varies somewhat with the species investigated. In lymph nodes, these cells localize primarily in medullary cords and in the cortex (Figs. 19 and 20). In the spleen, the follicular remnant and the peritrabecular region show similar hematopoietic stem cell colonies (Figs. 21 and 22). The time and extent of ultimate morphologic regeneration of lymphoreticular tissues depends upon the number of lymphoid cells present in the bone marrow graft. In this respect it is of interest, that apparently bone marrow from adult individuals (at least in rodents) contains more lymphoid cells (B-lymphocytes) than bone marrow from young ones (FARRER et al., 1974). The extent of morphologic regeneration of lymphoreticular tissues, however, does not necessarily reflect the degree of functional recovery of immune reactivity. This pertains especially to the regeneration of cellular immune reactivity (T-cell response) which rarely recovers completely (URSO and GENGOZIAN, 1973). In our experience, one out of 36 allografted patients regained T-cell function 1 year after he was engrafted. Cell suspensions from bone marrow aspirates are poor in thymus-dependent

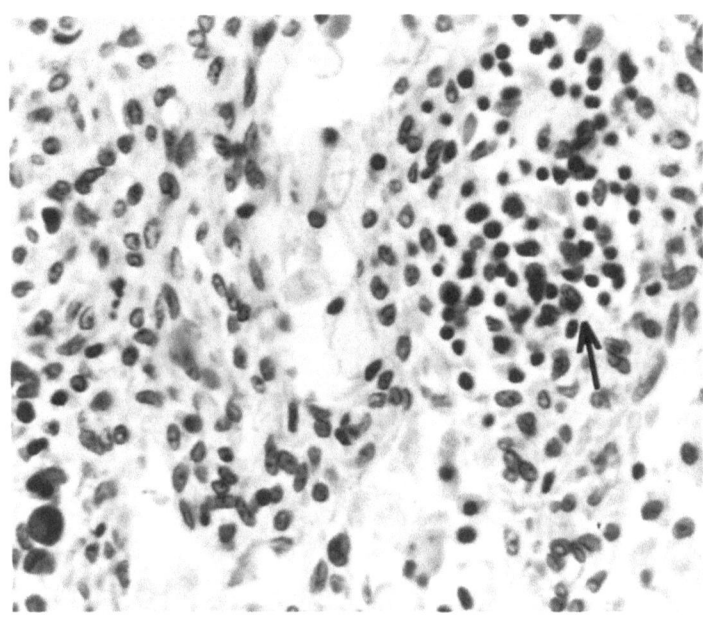

Fig. 16. Early recolonization after bone marrow allografting. Note hematopoietic cells accumulating in small capillaries with subsequent emigration (*arrow*). The hematopoietic origin of these cells was confirmed by chloroacetate esterase stain. H & E, × 375

lymphocytes (PARK *et al.*, 1972), and although such paucity of T-cells may decrease the risk of developing graft-versus-host disease, it may also represent a considerable obstacle to reconstitution of cell-mediated immunity in the marrow recipient.

Since recovery of immunologic reactivity in the host appears to depend upon the number of immunocompetent cells infused with the bone marrow, cell separation methods prior to bone marrow transplantation are still open for discussion, and may be even contraindicated.

The bone marrow is repopulated first concentrically around small vessels with subsequent growth of individual colonies (Fig. 23). Whereas erythropoietic colonies localize preferentially around capillaries and sinuses, granulocytopoietic cells tend to home along bone spicules. Megakaryocytes may be found to proliferate occasionally in small clusters (Fig. 24).

The findings at serial autopsies of experimental animals with bone marrow engraftment suggest that certain morphologic changes in the host's bone marrow stroma precede the settling of erythropoietic and granulocytopoietic colonies (see also Section FI). Such early changes consist in resorption of radiologically or chemotherapeutically caused debris. One observes phagocytosis of cellular debris including erythrocytes from hemorrhages (a picture similar to that observed in lymph nodes and spleen). Capillaries start to proliferate, partially at the site of fibrinous fiber stars (Fig. 25), and apparently initiate the reconstruction of the reticular stroma in which infused cells will later reside. Foci of osteoclasia are noted (Fig. 26) associated with new bone formation. Such bone

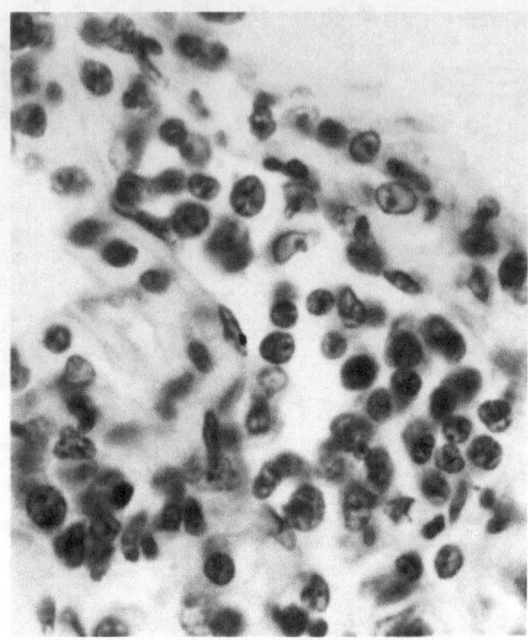

Fig. 17. Hematopoietic cells in splenic capillary during early posttransplant period. H & E, ×600

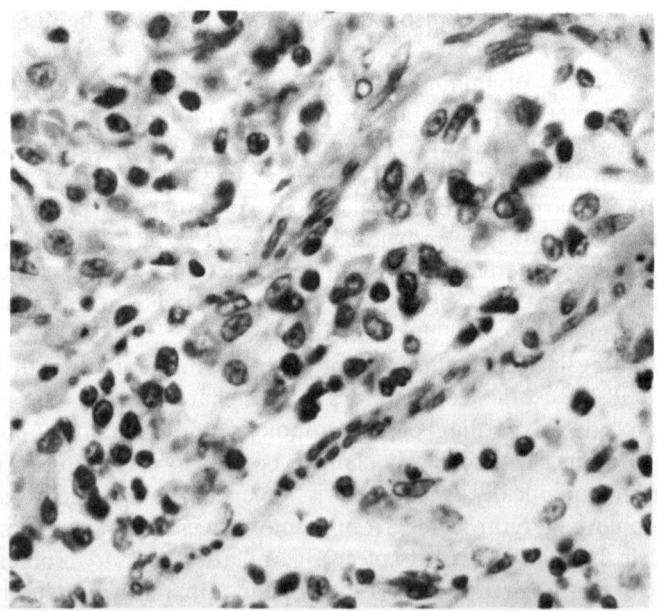

Fig. 18. Hematopoietic cells in lung vessels during early posttransplant period. H & E, ×600

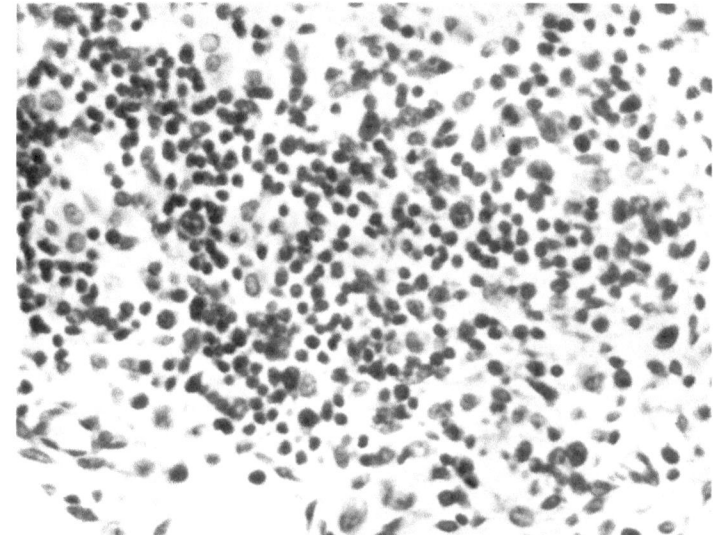

Fig. 19. Lymphoid stem cell colonies in lymph node cortex during the first week after bone marrow allografting. H & E, × 375

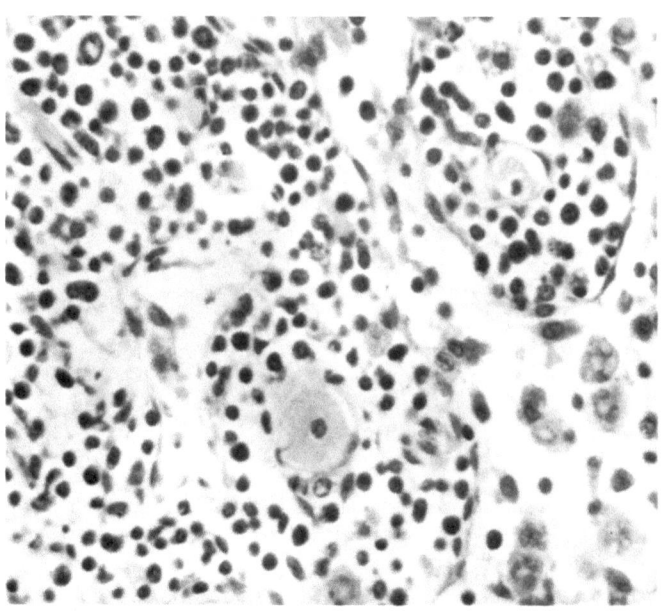

Fig. 20. Stem cell colonies in medullary cords of lymph node during the first week after bone marrow allografting. H & E, × 375

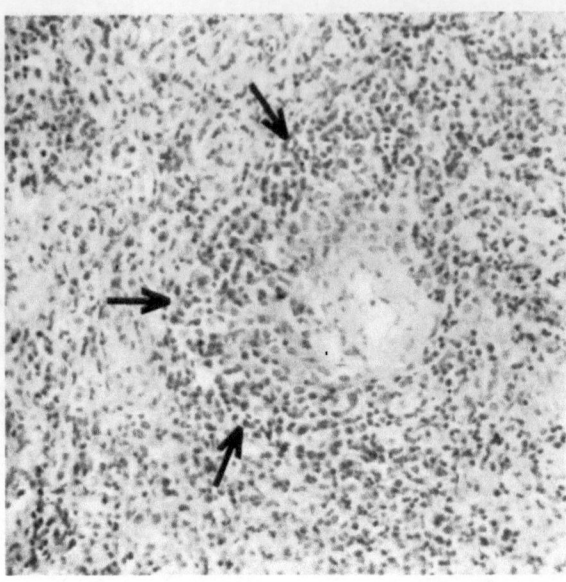

Fig. 21. Perifollicular lymphoid stem cell colonies in the spleen during the early posttransplant period (*arrows*). H & E, ×150

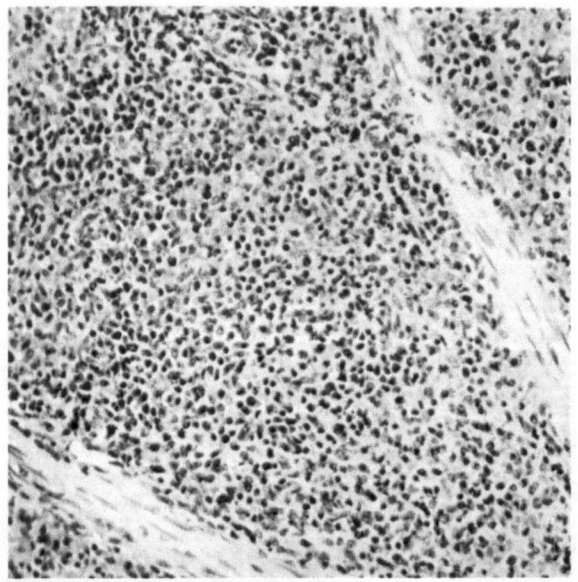

Fig. 22. Peritrabecular lymphoid stem cell colonies in the spleen during the early posttransplant period. H & E, ×375

changes together with the formation of new capillaries appear to represent an important microinductive factor for the subsequent homing and proliferation of hematopoietic colonies. The described stromal changes in the severely atrophic

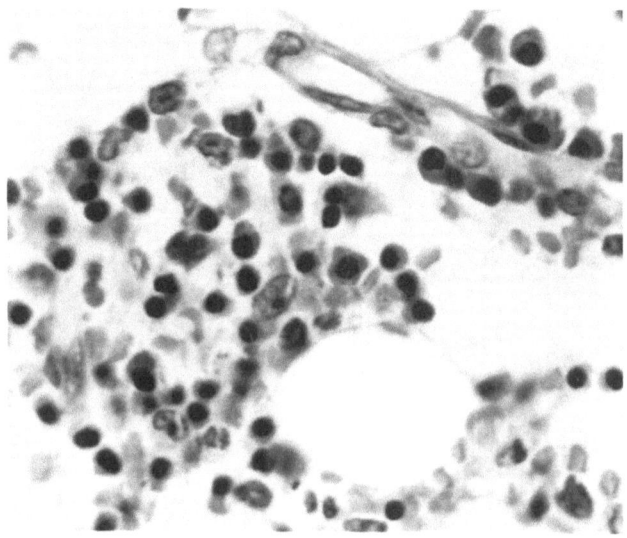

Fig. 23. Pericapillary hematopoietic colonies in the bone marrow during early posttransplant period.
H & E, ×600

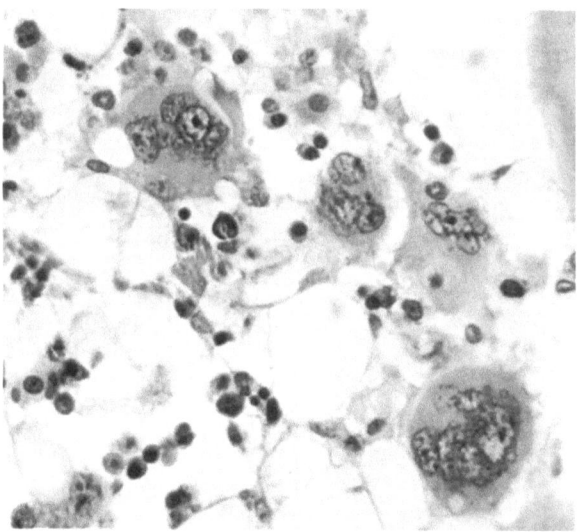

Fig. 24. Proliferating young megakaryocyte in the bone marrow during early posttransplant period.
H & E, ×600

marrow spaces occur within the first few days after radiation or chemotherapy and bone marrow engraftment. Their intensity depends upon the extent of the pretransplant damage to the bone marrow and its stroma. It remains to be elucidated, however, whether the primary disease (e.g., aplastic anemia as compared with acute leukemia) also affected the marrow which may influence

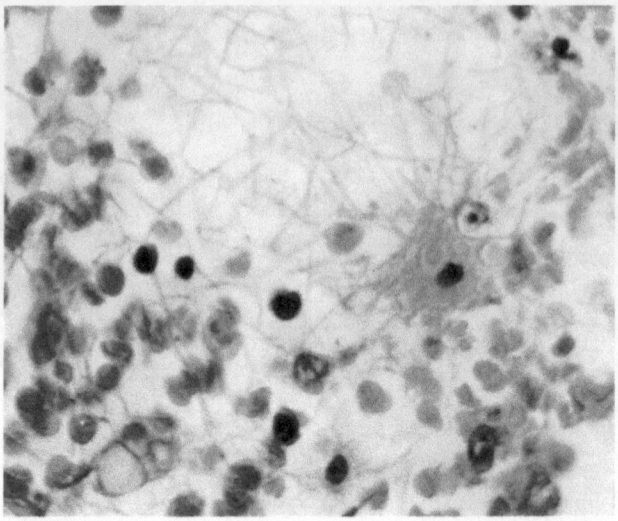

Fig. 25. Fibrinous star in bone marrow post irradiation. At this site early capillary proliferation is partly initiated. H & E, ×600

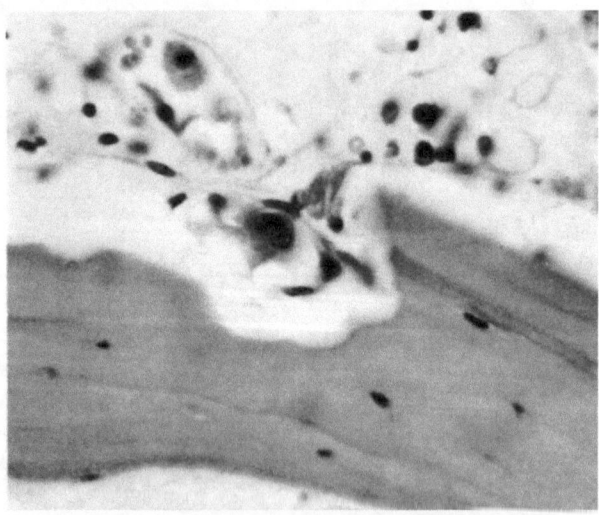

Fig. 26. Focal bone resorption and capillary proliferation preceding homing of hematopoietic colonies after bone marrow allografting. H & E, ×375

later the homing of infused hematopoietic cells. Eight to 10 days after transplantation of an adequate bone marrow dose, extensive *focal to diffuse repopulation* of the host bone marrow is observed histologically (sternum, ribs, and iliac crest); however, the number of megakaryocytes is variable, sometimes

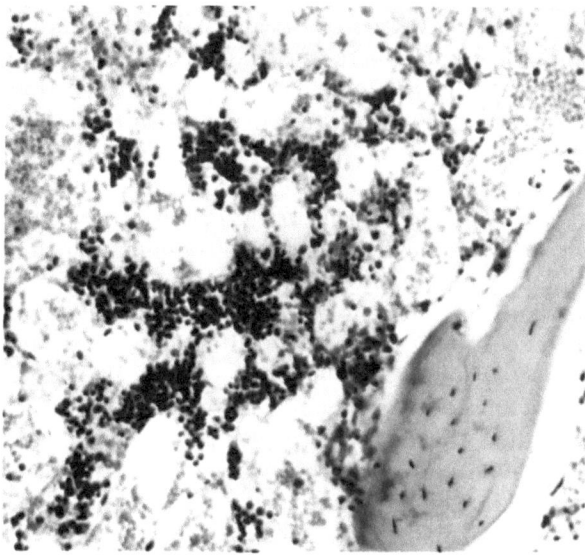

Fig. 27. Focal bone marrow recolonization during the first week after bone marrow allografting. H & E, × 150

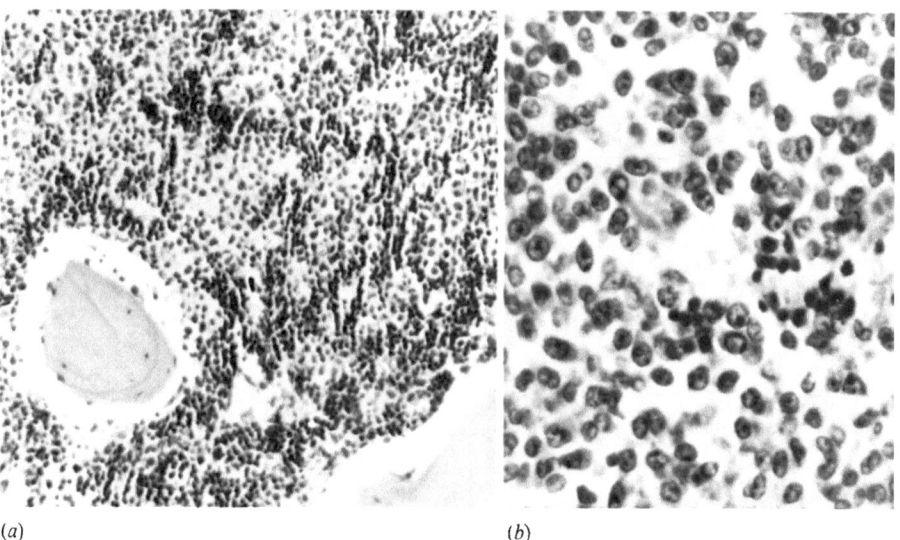

(a)   (b)

Fig. 28. (a) Diffuse bone marrow recolonization 10 days after bone marrow allografting. H & E, × 150. (b) Cytologic details of cell population in recolonized bone marrow 10 days after transplantation. Note diffuse myeloblastic hyperplasia with focal erythropoiesis. H & E, × 375

quite low, and no significant maturation of granulocytopoiesis is histologically impressive (Figs. 27 and 28). It would appear that maturation occurs insofar as cells are able to respond to leukotactic stimuli; this is suggested by morphologically immature cells accumulating at foci of bacterial infection. VAN BEKKUM and DE VRIES (1967), however, observed a normally mature bone marrow 7 days after transplantation. There appears to be no significant time difference in marrow repopulation when autogenous or allogenic marrow cells are infused, although in some instances it seemed that allogenic marrow cells led slightly faster to the recolonization of marrow spaces. Interestingly enough this was observed especially in animals suffering severe acute graft-versus-host disease (KRUEGER et al., 1975). It is open for further investigation whether a certain (slight) degree of foreignness stimulates cell proliferation. If, however, the immunologic difference between host and donor is too pronounced (e.g., in xenogenic transplantation), engraftment and repopulation is inhibited (xenogenic resistence). In the rodent this appears to affect initially splenic recovery more than bone marrow reconstitution (RAUCHWERGER et al., 1973a). Hypercellular marrow can often be observed for about 1 month after grafting as a consequence of rapid proliferation of hematopoietic stem cells. Extramedullary hematopoiesis in spleen, lymph node, and liver also usually persists during this time. Recovery of hematopoiesis after bone marrow transplantation in other species than the ones observed by us follows a similar course (VAN BEKKUM and DE VRIES, 1967).

The *thymus* is not reconstituted after bone marrow grafting to any significant extent, which may account for the long-standing defect in cell-mediated immunity in marrow recipients. Infused marrow cells rarely proliferate in the thymus, and when it was demonstrated, proliferation was rather short-lived (up to 3%

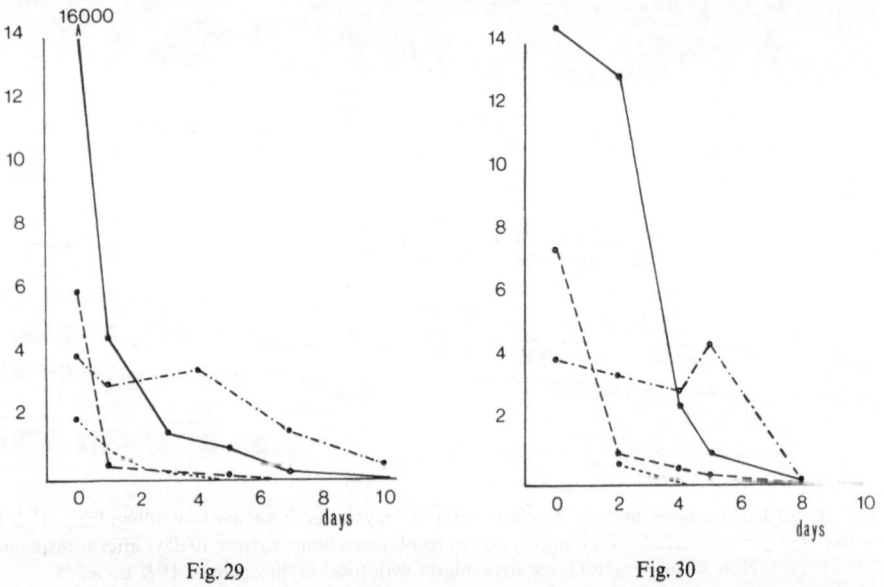

Fig. 29   Fig. 30

Fig. 29. Circulating blood cell values after total body irradiation, rhesus monkey, 860 rads. · — · total white cells $\times 10^3$, · · lymphocytes $\times 10^3$, · · · · · · thrombocytes $\times 10^5$, · · · · · · reticulocytes ($^0/_{00}$)

Fig. 30. Circulating blood cell values after total body irradiation, rhesus monkey, 860 rads, and bone marrow allografting. No graft take. · — · total white cells $\times 10^3$, · — · lymphocytes $\times 10^3$, · · · · · · thrombocytes $\times 10^5$, · · · · · · reticulocytes ($^0/_{00}$)

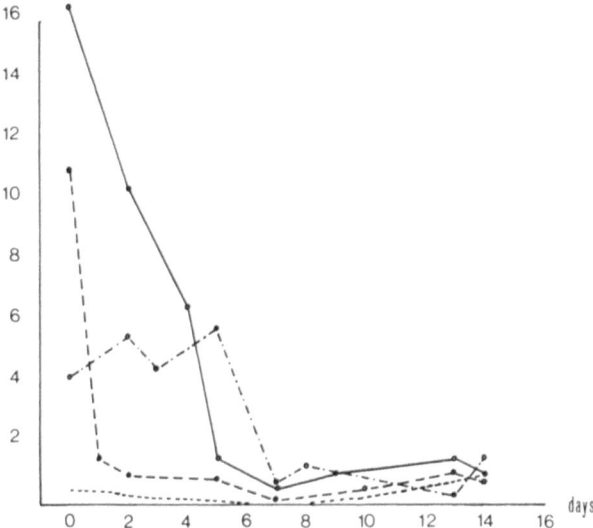

Fig. 31. Circulating blood cell values post total body irradiation, rhesus monkey, 860 rads, and bone marrow allografting. Acute graft-versus-host disease. $\cdot - \cdot$ total white cells $\times 10^3$, $\cdot - \cdot \cdot$ lymphocytes $\times 10^3$, $\cdot \cdot \cdot \cdot \cdot$ thrombocytes $\times 10^5$, $\cdot \cdot \cdot \cdot \cdot$ reticulocytes ($^0/_{00}$)

of infused marrow cells for no more than 3 weeks: FORD and MICKLEM, 1963; TAKADA and TAKADA, 1973). There is also experimental evidence that thymus tissue does not recover spontaneously (BORUM, 1969). Morphologic increase in thymic lymphoid cell population does not necessarily represent functional recovery. The time distribution of infused marrow cells is summarized for the mouse in Figure 3, and the average cellular recovery of peripheral blood is given in Figures 29–32. FORD and MICKLEM (1963) used chromosome markers of cells from bone marrow and lymphoid tissues to localize infused cells in coisogenic mice. Both bone marrow and lymphoid cells recolonized host lymph nodes and thymus, yet bone marrow cells caused the larger part of it and appeared to provide the more permanent cell population. Regeneration of bone marrow, however, as STODTMEISTER and FLIEDNER (1973) demonstrated in rat experiments, does not exclude later development of myelofibrosis and myelopoietic insufficiency (see late rejection). Thus ultimate reconstitution of the marrow can definitely be proved only after a long period of time.

There are several indicators to prove bone marrow grafts in man. The most general indicator of engraftment is a rising peripheral blood count during the third week after transplantation. Figures 29–33 show examples of such values in rhesus monkeys after bone marrow transplantation. Demonstration of donor-type *sex chromatin* in leukocytes when grafting was done across sexes (sex-linked granulocyte appendages, mononuclear cell sex chromatin, sex chromosomes: MATHÉ *et al.*, 1960 and 1963; SEMAN, 1961; HELLRIEGEL *et al.*, 1974); determination of red cell antigens, of immunoglobulin allotypes (MATHÉ *et al.*, 1963; GRAW *et al.*, 1974), as well as the demonstration of specific tolerance based on chimerism or donor-type immune reactions are used. Tolerance in a chimeric

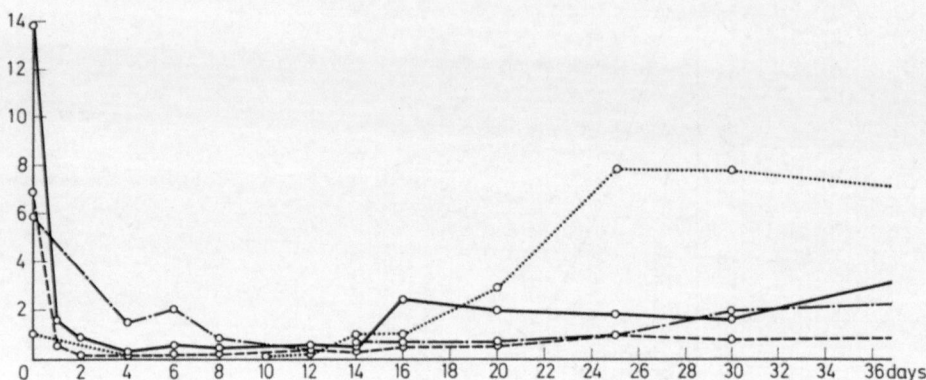

Fig. 32. Circulating blood cell values post total body irradiation, rhesus monkey, 860 rads, and bone marrow allografting. Acute graft-versus-host disease treated with anti-lymphocyte serum. · —· total white cells ×10³, ·—·· lymphocytes ×10³, ······· thrombocytes ×10⁵, ······ reticulocytes (⁰/₀₀)

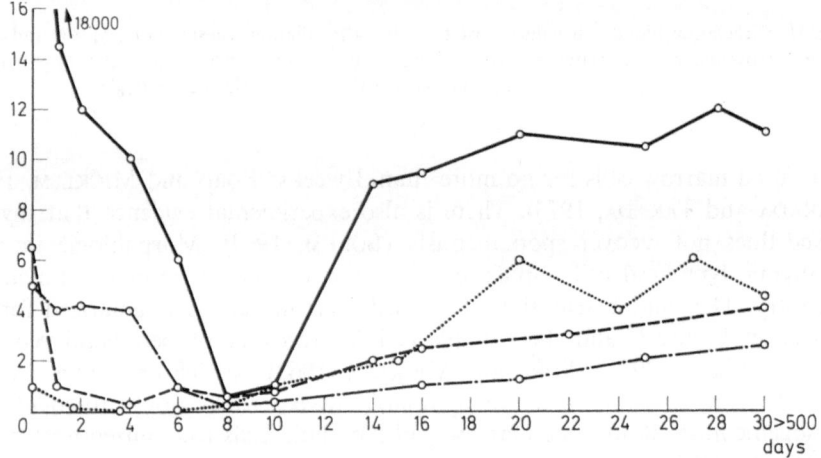

Fig. 33. Circulating blood cell values post total body irradiation, rhesus monkey, 860 rads, and bone marrow autografting with complete recovery. · —· total white cells ×10³, ·—· lymphocytes ×10³, ······· thrombocytes ×10⁵, ······ reticulocytes (⁰/₀₀)

state can be proved by donor-type skin transplants. Donor-type immune reactivity is demonstrated by stimulation of the graft recipient with antigens against which the marrow donor was sensitized but not the host. In the case of transplantation across certain HL-A antigens, such antigens can be determined in circulating host cells to estimate engraftment. Finally, the secretor status in fresh saliva specimens when different in donor and host may be used as an indicator for a functioning graft. Replacement of hematopoietic cells by bone marrow allografting is not complete as a rule; instead, peripheral blood cells show a chimerism with 50–100% donor cells whereas in the bone marrow the content in donor cells is even less (sometimes 10–20%) (KERSEY et al., 1971; GRAW et al., 1972; SANTOS et al., 1974; STORB et al., 1974).

TAKADA *et al.* (1971a and b) presented evidence from mouse experiments, that the extent of cellular depletion of the recipient's bone marrow (by radiation) determines the degree of donor cell proliferation. The results of GRAW *et al.* (1974) are similar: the incidence of graft take was increased when more aggressive chemotherapy was applied. Also, the degree of donor chimerism was markedly improved. There appears to exist a competition of stem cell proliferation in the bone marrow in favor of the the host cell. Also, cells appear to proliferate and settle permanently more easily in their natural environment; in the mouse, for instance, proliferation of splenic cells in the bone marrow was less persistent than marrow cells.

Of special interest is the observation of a split chimerism affecting lymphoreticular tissues; whereas B-cells were shown to be of donor origin, T-lymphocytes usually possess the characteristics of the host (MATHÉ and SCHWARZENBERG, 1974). This appears to pertain, however, primarily to graft recipients treated with antilymphocyte globulin. This is especially astonishing since it was expected, that after atrophy of the thymus no T-cell recovery will occur. The fact that recovery may indeed occur probably points to the presence of residual (thymically primed) T-stem cells despite extensive chemotherapy.

F. Graft-Host Interactions

I. Microenvironmental Influences

In addition to the antigenic differences between host and donor that influence graft take with subsequent proliferation and differentiation, microenvironmental influences appear to play a major role in effective marrow reconstitution. Such microenvironmental influences probably originate from nonhematopoietic cells transplanted together with hematopoietic cells, as, for instance, in stromal elements including cells supporting bone formation. Besides these cells of donor origin, host stromal cells, surely contribute to the microenvironment necessary for bone marrow cell proliferation. This can be deduced from the fact that infused hematopoietic cells tend to colonize pre-existent hematopoietic structures in the same way as infused lymphoid cells populate the respective T- and B-cell regions in lymphoreticular tissues. FRIEDENSTEIN *et al.* (1974) showed that fibroblasts can exert such necessary microenvironmental influences. They separated these cells from bone marrow or splenic cell suspensions by transient tissue cultures, and upon retransplantation, fibroblastic cells showed formation or production of reticular stroma depending upon their tissue origin. Hemoreticular and lymphoreticular cells tended to aggregate at these locations.

Earlier, TRENTIN (1971) presented data that the differentiation of a pluripotent hematopoietic stem cell is induced and directed by stromal components of bone marrow and spleen. Under their influence, differentiation occurs along the erythroid, neutrophil granulocytic, eosinophil granulocytic, and megakaryocytic lines, although splenic stroma in the experiment appears to favor erythroid differentiation while bone marrow stroma favors granulocytic differentiation. TRENTIN calls this the stromal "hemopoietic inductive microenvironment" (HIM). As mentioned above, defects in this inductive microenvironment with subsequent hematopoietic insufficiency cannot be cured by bone marrow cell infusion; transplantation of intact stromal cells in addition would be necessary. Influence exerted by the HIM appear not to be strongly species specific (RAUCH-WERGER et al., 1973).

Possible interrelations between autochthonous bone and bone marrow were recently briefly outlined by BURKHARDT (1974), and the importance of the vascular system was stressed; it appears reasonable to assume that HIM will vary with the type of pre-existent disease ultimately leading to bone marrow transplantation (e.g., leukemia versus aplastic anemia), and will vary also with the type of pretransplant therapy (e.g., x-irradiation versus the administration of antilymphocyte sera). Diseases and treatment causing destruction of the normal vascular-mesenchymal framework of the bone marrow spaces may also interfere with the positive effects of HIM on engrafted marrow cells. Such parameters, however, need more extensive investigation. In the context of microenvironmental influences, mention shall be made of the phenomenon of *genetic resistance* (allogenic resistance, hybrid resistance), which accounts for the proliferation inhibitory effect exerted by the host upon infused incompatible bone marrow and lymphoid cells (TRENTIN et al., 1973; URSO and GENGOZIAN, 1973). Its mechanism is not yet well understood, and it is assumed to be nonimmunologic in nature, or a type of immune response so far undefined.

II. Graft Rejection

Graft rejection can be differentiated from the failure of a graft take by initial signs of marrow recovery. Unlike the rejection of organ transplants (e.g., kidney transplants) where we know four types or phases of rejection (peracute, acute, subchronic, and late rejection), in bone marrow rejection we usually define only two types: the *early rejection* and the *late rejection*. Adequate immunologic pretransplant testing should preclude peracute rejection, which may have occurred in a few instances during the early transplantation era when knowledge of the antigenic status of donor and recipient was scanty. In the latter case distinction between failure of engraftment and peracute rejection is not possible on morphologic grounds alone; Instead immunologic evidence for an antigraft immune reaction is necessary. In both situations – peracute rejection and failure of engraftment – the bone marrow remains histologically empty, although in some cases of experimentally induced peracute rejections, small vessels contain platelet and fibrinous thrombi occasionally admixed with nuclear debris and accompanied by degenerative vacular lesions. Similar vascular changes, however, can be observed secondary to lethal irradiation or extensive chemotherapy as well as in endotoxemia. The course of peripheral blood cell counts in failure of bone marrow graft take is shown in Figure 30.

Early bone-marrow-graft rejection is characterized clinically by a peripheral blood cell picture similar to the one shown in Figure 30, but with an initial

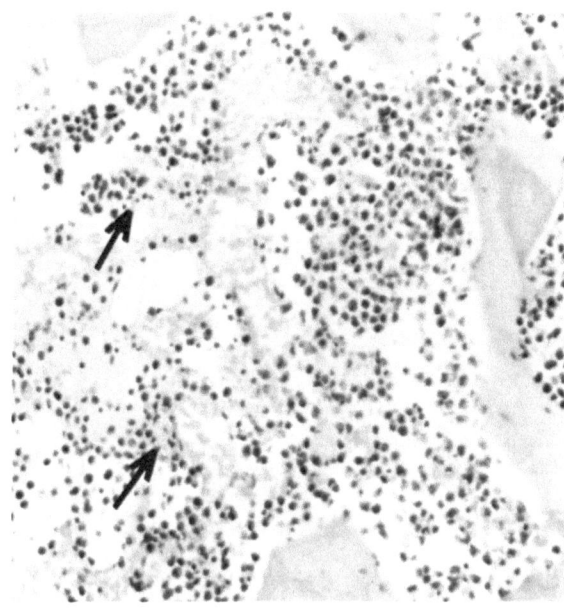

Fig. 34. Early bone marrow allograft rejection. Note edematous stroma and focal cellular pyknosis
(*arrow*). H & E, × 150

rise in granulocytes and in platelets as well as a slight rise in lymphocytes.
Animals and patients usually die within 4–6 weeks secondary to such infectious
complications as gram-negative sepsis, generalized mycoses, or viral diseases
(cytomegalovirus, herpes simplex virus). Without adequate supportive care
(granulocyte and thrombocyte transfusions), death in early rejection may occur
even earlier.

The *bone marrow* shows a decreased to moderate cellularity with maturation
arrest; it is not empty as in failure of graft take. There may be foci of hematopoietic cell necrosis with nuclear debris and edema (Fig. 34). In *lymph nodes*
and *spleen* focal follicular necrobiosis with karyorhexis and lymphoid cells is
observed. In extracortical regions of the lymph node small foci of necrosis
occur around small blood vessels. Deposition of fibrinoid substances (exudate)
is noted within secondary follicles of spleen and lymph nodes as well as at
other sites of extramedullary hematopoiesis with necrobiotic changes (Figs. 35–
36). Cellular necrobiosis initiates reactive phagocyte hyperplasia. In the further
course of rejection, fibroblast proliferation will start at these sites if the patient
has not already died. This pertains primarily to individuals in whom the rejection
crisis is treated with immunosuppressive drugs. Some of these drugs support
fibroplasia per se (see Chapter 7.3) and thus enhance rejection-initiated fibrosis.
Focal necrobiotic changes in lympho- and hemoreticular tissues need to be
differentiated in each case from similar lesions secondary to septicemia and
toxemia which is usually a consequence of graft rejection. In such cases, however,
we may see foci of bacteria associated with microfocal necrosis, and the lesions
are observed also in other organs, primarily in the liver. A peculiar reaction

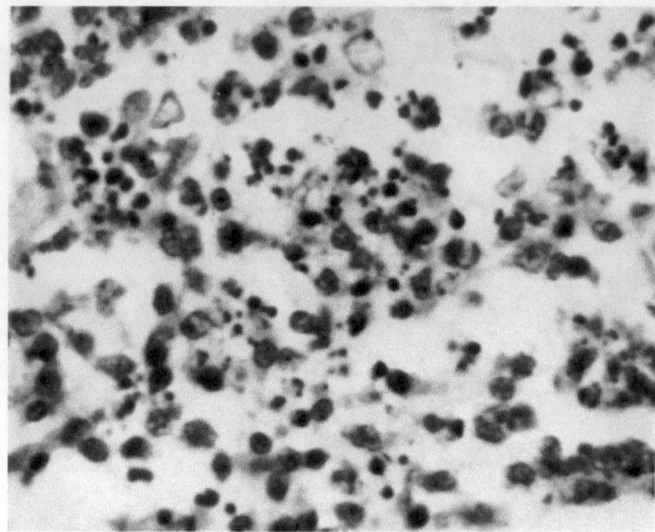

Fig. 35. Early rejection after bone marrow allografting. Note focal cellular disruption in lymph node. H & E, ×600

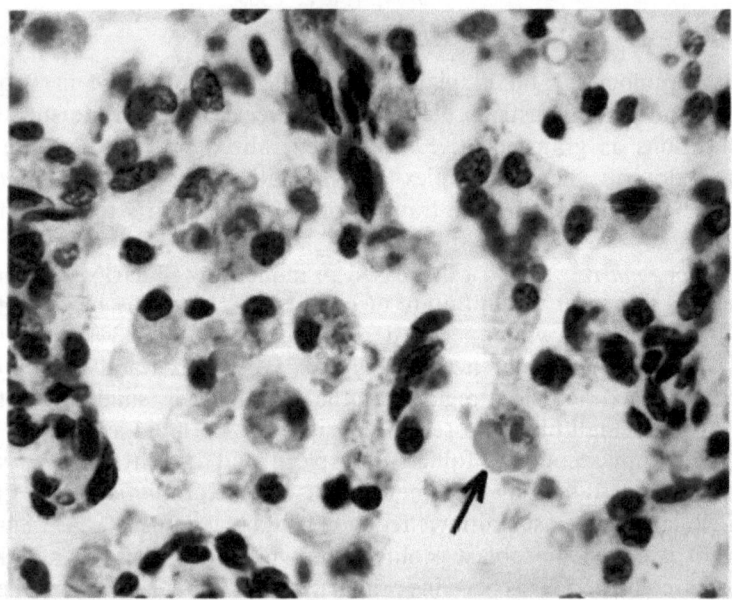

Fig. 36. Early rejection after bone marrow allografting. Note sinus histiocytosis and erythrophagocytosis (*arrow*), lymph node. H & E, ×600

observed in lymphoreticular tissues in protracted acute rejection or in chemotherapeutically suppressed acute rejection is the development of reticulohistiocytic granulomas. Such changes can also be observed in late rejection of bone marrow

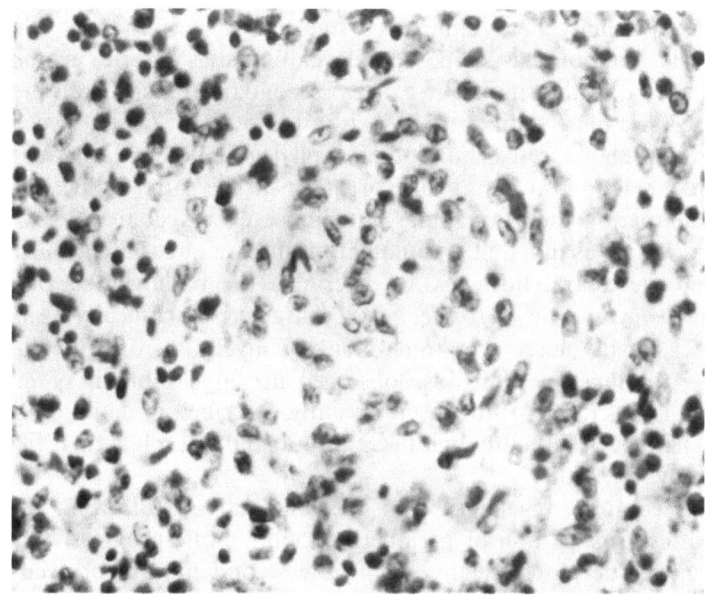

Fig. 37. Nodular lymphoreticular cell proliferate ("Granuloma") in lymph node during protracted
bone marrow allograft rejection. H & E, × 375

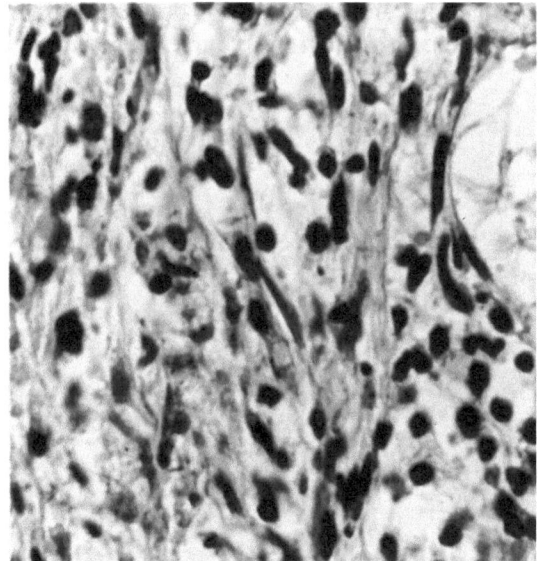

Fig. 38. Focal bone marrow cell pyknosis, necrobiosis, and early fibroblast proliferation in late
allograft rejection (initial lesion). H & E, × 600

allografts. Histiocytic granulomas with epithelioid cells and occasional foreign-
body giant cells occur in lymph nodes (primarily cortical), spleen (primarily
intrafollicular), and occasionally in the bone marrow (Fig. 37). They contain

scattered plasma cells, lymphocytes, and activated blast cells which are hard to classify. Granulomas supposedly develop at sites of prior lymphoid cell destruction (e.g., at the site of pre-existent secondary follicles) and probably represent excessive phagocytic activity. It is not known yet whether such granulomas are directly related to rejection-induced cell destruction or rather to a secondarily impaired reaction to extraneous organisms. The latter impression may arise from comparing the granulomas with those observed in cases of granulocyte deficiency such as in lethal granulomatous disease of children. Further investigations are necessary, however, to determine the pathogenesis of such lesions.

Late bone marrow graft rejection is characterized clinically a slowly developing, occasionally acute symptomatology of myelofibrosis. Histologically, bone marrow findings parallel those observed in "myelofibrosis of immunological type" (Lennert, 1964); they were recently described in detail by Stodtmeister and Fliedner (1973), although these authors did not relate their findings closely to marrow rejection.

After complete regeneration of the bone marrow following allotransplantation with normalization of peripheral blood counts, progressive hematopoietic insufficiency develops usually during the second month (or even later). Early lesions consist in maturation arrest of bone marrow cells with focal degeneration and necrobiosis (Fig. 38). Nuclear pyknosis and fragmentation of hematopoietic cells with cytoplasmic degeneration occurs. Scattered proliferation (mitoses) of lymphoid cells are found in the bone marrow. At sites of cellular disintegration a faint eosinophilic intercellular material is observed with subsequent fibroblast proliferation (Fig. 39). In the further course, a patchy myelofibrosis develops

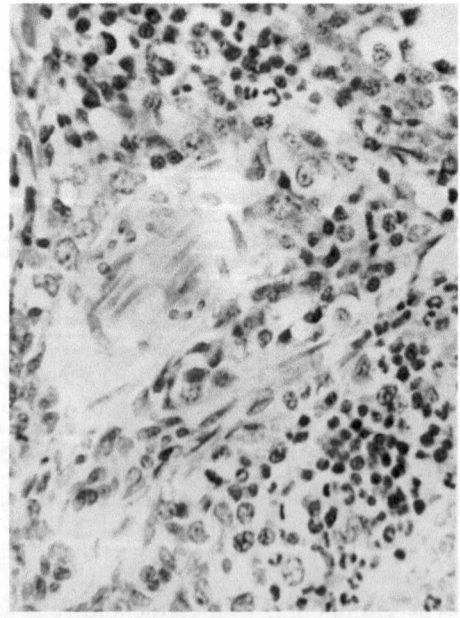

Fig. 39. Vascular sclerosis and perivascular fibroblasia in the bone marrow during late rejection.
H & E, × 375

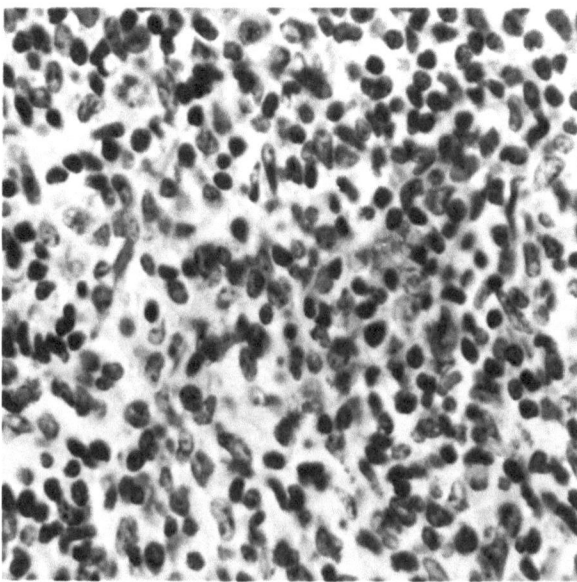

Fig. 40. Lymph node paracortex in late rejection; note depletion of small lymphocytes with increase in fibroreticular cells. H & E, a) ×374, b) ×675

in such areas, which are distributed uniformly throughout the hematopoietically active bone marrow.

Changes observed in *lymphoreticular tissue* resemble those in acquired immune deficiency syndromes. Lymph node paracortex and cortex become irregularily depleted of lymphocytes; paracortical pathology is usually more pronounced than cortical (Fig. 40). Secondary follicles contain necrobiotic cells and nuclear debris with phagocytosis, and a granulomatous reaction may be observed as described in acute rejection. Foci of activated (blastic) lymphoreticular stem cells appear primarily in the paracortex so that the resulting picture may be difficult to distinguish from chronic graft-versus-host reaction. Similar atrophic changes can be seen in the follicular white pulp of the spleen. Besides a generalized lymphocytic depletion with occasional granulomas, the peripheral follicular zone and the centrifollicular zone (periarterial sheath) become fibrotic. In addition occasional blast cell aggregates may be noted in this area. Peyer's patches participate in the generalized lymphoreticular atrophy. Nonlymphoreticular and nonhematopoietic tissues are initially not effected; they may show secondary lesions caused by septicemia or disseminated viral infections (Fig. 41).

In certain instances the term "host-versus-graft rejection" (HVGR) has been used instead of graft rejection (HARD and KULLGREN, 1970). We concur with CONGDON (1971) that there is no difference between HVGR and graft rejection, and therefore do not use the term. In experimental HVGR, as described by HARD and KULLGREN, a proliferative response, especially of the spleen, was described which exceeded the one observed in our case material, and which clinically caused the syndrome of hypersplenism. It appears that this response

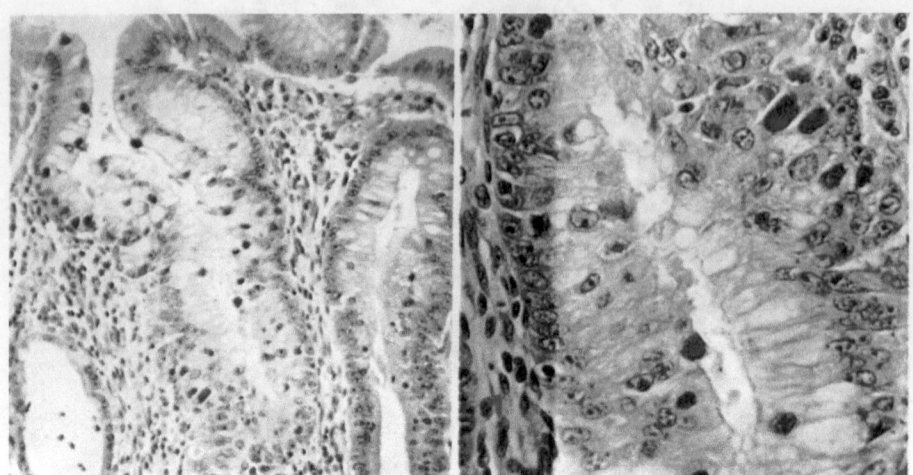

Fig. 41. Complication of chronic GVHR: Herpes enteritis and colitis; note multiple inclusion bodies in crypt epithelia. H & E, ×375

depended upon the selective genetic relationship between host and donor and upon the failure of immunosuppressive treatment before transplantation.

III. Graft-Versus-Host Reaction (GVHR)

This subject is discussed in detail by HOBIK in Chapter 11 of this handbook, and therefore need not be repeated here. It may be stated, however, that GVHR, brought about by a reaction of immunocompetent donor cells against the immunoincompetent host, constitutes one of the major obstacles to successful bone marrow transplantation in many instances. As we have learned from our human and experimental case material, it may be rewarding to separate graft-versus-host reaction (GVHR) from graft-versus-host disease (GVHD). A patient can experience mild and transient GVHR without really suffering clinically from it, that is, without developing GVHD. On the other hand, a patient may succumb clinically from severe GVHD without much histologically proven evidence for GVHR. It appears to us now, that mild persistant GVHR, not diagnostic by histology since its specific lesions are missing, may retard or inhibit the recovery from lesions induced by mechanisms other than GVHR. For instance, radiation-induced vascular or intestinal damage may persist or even be enhanced by "subhistologic" GVHR (Figs. 42 and 43). Furthermore, although GVHR appears primarily to be a cellular immune reaction, it is hard to exclude at least histologically humoral mechanisms. Although for therapeutic and prognostic reasons, a histologic differential diagnosis of GVHR should be attempted (Fig. 44; KRUEGER et al., 1972), clinical GVHD without histologic proof of GVHR does not exclude interference of donor cells with the host recovery.

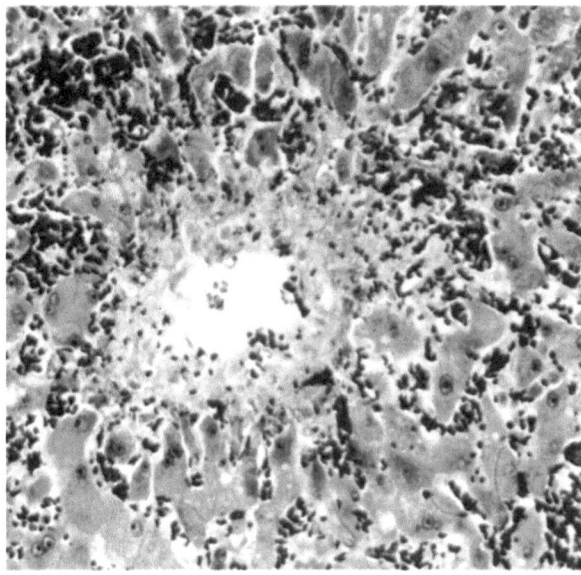

Fig. 42. Complication of subclinical GVHR: failure of repair of radiation-induced vascular damage; note intimal thickening with cellular infiltration and mild hemorrhage of central vein, liver. Masson's trichrome stain, ×150

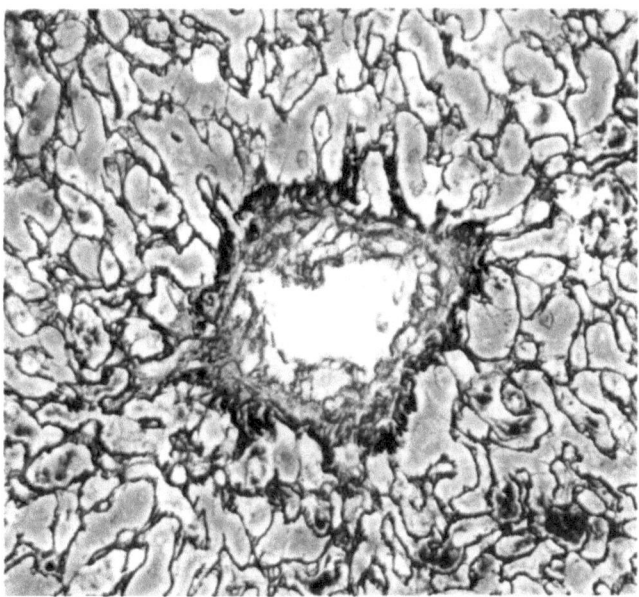

Fig. 43. Same lesion as shown in Figure 42; note increase in reticulin fiber in vascular intima. Wilder's reticulin stain, ×150

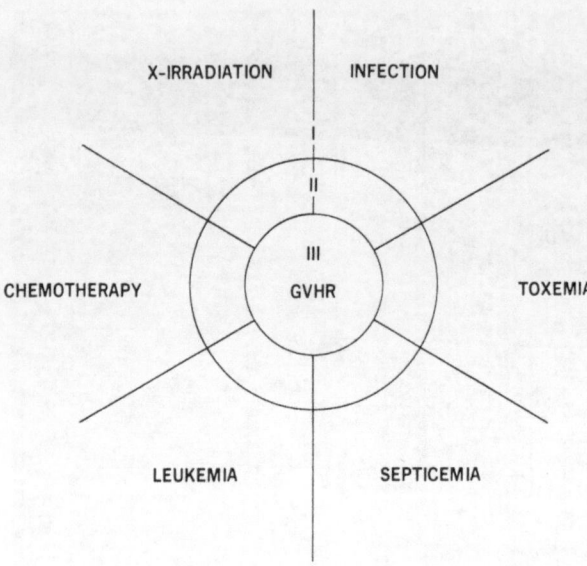

Fig. 44. Spectrum of tissue lesions observed in bone marrow allografted individuals. I: Tissue lesions not induced by GVHR (graft-versus-host reaction). II: Tissue lesions induced by GVHR as well as by other mechanisms. III: Tissue lesions induced by GVHR

IV. Therapeutic Intervention of Postengraftment Disease

There are several indications for therapeutic intervention during the early and late posttransplantation period; they arise from disturbances of the host caused by immediate host-graft interactions, or from adverse effects of pregrafting treatment. Such disturbances consist primarily of lymphoreticular and hematopoietic incompetence of the host followed by infection and hemorrhage as well as graft rejection or GVHR (GVHD). [In addition, in dog experiments, we observed initially severe hemoglobulinuric nephropathy following transplantation of frozen bone marrow cells (with the cryoprotective agent DMSO). It was thought that erythrocytes lysed rapidly during this procedure and caused the disease; elimination of erythrocytes before freezing abolished this side effect.] To cope with the hematologic and lymphoreticular incompetence a scheme of posttransplantation supportive care has been devised which is briefly outlined here. Its knowledge to the pathologist is necessary in order to consider morphologic variations of the sequelae of host-graft interaction caused by supportive treatment. Essentially, the patient will receive in the immediate posttransplantation period:

1. Red blood cell (RBC) support from ABO-matched random blood donors. It is preferable to use erythrocytes of a blood type that will not confuse the RBC marker followed in the transplant recipient. Also, the freshest blood available should be used (less than 2 days old) in order to avoid significant RBC deterioration. Otherwise, the pathologist may expect lesions secondary to hemolysis.

2. Platelets from a HL-A matched donor or, if necessary from a random donor will be given after irradiation of the thrombocytes with 1,500 R. Consequently, the pathologist will have to search for signs of a bleeding tendency or of unusual platelet coagulation.

3. Granulocyte support will serve as prophylaxis against infection. Cell concentrates irradiated with 1,500 R will be given from a matched donor on days 1, 3, 5, 6, 7, or 8 posttransplantation, and whenever necessary thereafter. Exessive granulocyte disintegration during the early postinfusion period may cause pulmonary pathology (occlusion of multiple capillaries by cellular debris with subsequent pulmonary edema).

4. For the prevention of GVHR, immunosuppressive drugs (e.g., methotrexate, 10 mg/m^2 on days, 1, 3, and 6, and 5 mg/m^2 i.v. weekly thereafter) or antilymphocyte sera will be given (10–15 ml/day). Such substances influence the morphology, especially of lymphoreticular tissues (KRUEGER, 1972), by causing an irregular atrophy with or without focal stem cell proliferation. They also may mask a still ongoing GVHR if the latter is not completely suppressed.

5. Systemic or local (nonabsorbable) antibiotics may be given.

6. Plasma infusion or hyperalimentation are administered when necessary.

Adverse effects of such drug therapy with its morphologic sequellae are discussed by HENDERSON and KRUEGER in this handbook.

G. Conclusions

Similar to the transfusion of blood, transfer of selected blood cells possesses its sound clinical indications and can be regarded as "post-experimental". No serious adverse effects are expected under certain precautions such as adequate matching of donor and host, pretransfusion irradiation of white cells and thrombocytes, and use of fresh materials. Transplantation of bone marrow, however, has not yet progressed beyond the experimental phase. There are still many specific topics that need extensive investigation, both immunologic and nonimmunologic. Investigation of microenvironmental influences (HIM) upon the engrafted marrow, study of allogeneic competition (AC; i.e., allogeneic inhibition and enhancement) among host and donor stem cells, and investigation of influences of therapeutic measures upon both HIM and AC need to be intensified. Besides, immunologic parameters of graft rejection and graft-versus-host reaction are still not known well enough. Furthermore, the exact pathogenetic relationship between graft-versus-host reaction (GVHR) and graft-versus-host disease (GVHD) needs elucidation. In this area especially we may gain from exact pathomorphologic investigations in combination with functional studies. Many of these studies will have to be done in experimental animals with adequate control groups that are not available from human case material. In evaluating the results, species-specific reactions need to be assessed more extensively. Despite all of this, however, there is ample practical evidence that bone marrow transplantation is justified in certain cases, even with our present state of knowledge, and that it may result in cure of the sick patient.

Transplantation of cells other than from blood and bone marrow is done to answer various questions experimentally. In man, however, we are still in the "pre-experimental" or early experimental phase, and no clear-cut clinical indication exists yet for such procedures.

Finally, it might be mentioned that, as with any other new therapeutic regimen, new adverse effects can be expected as a consequence of cell allotransplantation. There is sound experimental evidence, for instance, that malignant lymphomas occur to a significant degree in individuals suffering chronic (subclinical) graft-versus-host reaction (HIRSCH, 1973; ARMSTRONG et al., 1970). Longstanding immunosuppressive chemotherapy in connection with persistant antigeneic stimulation by engrafted cells may result in lymphoreticular neoplasia (KRUEGER, 1974 and 1975). Finally, the incidence of de novo cancers of various other types appears to be increased under such conditions, as we known from kidney allotransplantation in man (PENN and STARZL, 1972).

References

ARMSTRONG, M.Y.K., GLEICHMANN, E., GLEICHMANN, H., BELDOTTI, L., ANDRE-SCHWARTZ, J., SCHWARTZ, R.S.: Chronic allogenic disease. II. Development of lymphomas. J. Exp. Med. **132**, 417–439 (1970)

ASHWOOD-SMITH, M.J.: Preservation of mouse bone marrow at −79° C with dimethyl sulphoxide. Nature (London) **190**, 1204–1205 (1961

BACH, F.H., ALBERTINI, R.J., ANDERSON, J.L., JOO, P., BORTIN, M.M.: Bone marrow transplantation in a Patient with the Wiskott-Aldrich-Syndrome. Lancet II, 1364–1366 (1968)

BALNER, H., SIMMEL, E.B., CLARKE, D.A.: Proliferation and rejection of transplanted Tritium labeled bone marrow cells in mice. Transpl. Bull. **29**, 427–435 (1962)

BARNES, D.W.H., LOUTIT, J.F.: The radiation recovery factor: Preservation by the Polge-Smith-Parkes technique. J. Nat. Cancer Inst. **15**, 901–905 (1955)

BARNES, D.W.H., ILBERY, P.L.T., LOUTIT, J.P.: Avoidance of secondary disease in radiation chimeras. Nature (London) **181**, 488 (1953)

BIERMAN, H.R., K.H., CORDES, F.L.: The sequestration and visceral circulation of leukocytes in man. Ann. N.Y. Acad. Sci. **59**, 850–862 (1955)

BILLINGHAM, R.E., DEFENDI, V., SILVERS, W.K., STEINMÜLLER, D.: Quantitative studies on the induction of tolerance of skin homografts and on runt disease in neonatal rats. J. Nat. Cancer Inst. **28**, 365–435 (1962)

BLESSING, J.: Graft-versus-host disease induced by fetal thymus and liver cells. Transplant. **14**, 512–514 (1972)

BORANIC, M.: Transient graft-versus-host reaction in the treatment of leukemia in mice. J. Nat. Cancer Inst. **41**, 421–433 (1968)

BORANIC, M.: Time pattern of antileukemic effect of graft-versus-host reaction in mice. Transplant. Proc. **3**, 394–396 (1971)

BORTIN, M.M., RIMM, A.A., SALTZSTEIN, E.C.: Graft-versus-host inhibition I. Incubated parental strain spleen and liver cells administered to F1-mice. J. Immunol. **102**, 1042–1049 (1969)

BORUM, K.: Lack of restoration of thymic tissue following partial surgical thymectomy in the mouse. Acta path. microbiol. Scand. **76**, 515–519 (1969)

BUCKNER, C.D., CLIFT, R.A., FEFER, A., FUNK, D.D., GLUCKSBERG, H., RAMBERG, R.E., STORB, R., THOMAS, E.D.: Aplastic anemia treated by marrow transplantation. Transpl. Proc. **5**, 913–916 (1973)

BURKHARDT, R.: Interrelations between bone marrow and bone. Verh. dtsch. Ges. Path. **58**, 205–218 (1974)

BUJA, L.M., FERRANS, V.J., GRAW, R.G.: Cardiac pathologic findings in patients treated with bone marrow transplantation. Human Path. **7**, 17–45 (1976)

BULL, M.: Canine allogenic bone marrow transplantation. Study of variables influencing reproducible engraftment. Submitted for publication.

CARDANO, G.: De Rerum Varietate, Chapter 44 Lib. VIII. Basel: 1556 (cited by SAUNDERS)

COLE, L.J., FISHLER, M.C., ELLIS, M.E., BOND, V.P.: Protection of mice against X-irradiation by spleen-homogenates administered after exposure. Proc. Soc. Exp. Biol. Med. **80**, 112–117 (1952)

CONGDON, C.C., URSO, I.S.: Homologous bone marrow in the treatment of radiation injury in mice. Amer. J. Path. **33**, 749–767 (1957)

CONGDON, C.C., UPHOFF, D.E., LORENZ, E.: Modification of acute irradiation injury in mice and guinea pigs by injection of bone marrow: a histopathologic study. J. Nat. Cancer Inst. **13**, 73–107 (1952)

COSGROVE, G.E., UPTON, A.C., POPP, R.A., CONGDON, C.C.: Inhibition of foreign spleen reaction by inactivation of donor cells with recipient antisera. Proc. Soc. Exp. Biol. Med. **102**, 525–527 (1959)

DE KONING, J., VAN BEKKUM, D.W., DICKE, K.A., DOOREN, L.J., VAN ROOD, J.J., RADL, J.: Transplantation of bone-marrow cells and fetal thymus in an infant with lymphopenic immunological deficiency. Lancet I, 1223–1227 (1969)

DENTON, P.M., SYMES, M.O.: Attemps to induce a graft-versus-tumor reaction against AKR lymphomata in isogenic mice, by injection of melphalan and foreign immunologically competent cells. Brit. J. Cancer **23**, 95–102 (1969)

DICKE, K.A.: Results of monkey bone marrow cell fractionation to prevent acute secondary disease after transplantation. In: Annual Rep. Radiobiological Institute TNO, Rijswijk, Netherlands, 1970, pp. 108–110

DICKE, K.A., VAN BEKKUM, D.W.: Avoidance of acute secondary disease by purification of hemopoietic stem cells with density gradient centrifugation. Exp. Hematol. **20**, 126–130 (1970)

DICKE, K.A., VON HOOFT, J.I.M., VAN BEKKUM, D.W.: The selective elimination of immunologically competent cells from bone marrow and lymphatic cell mixtures. II. Mouse spleen cell fractionation on a discontinuous albumin gradient. Transplantation **6**, 562–570 (1968)

DICKE, K.A., TRIDENTE, G., VAN BEKKUM, D.W.: The selective elimination of immunologically competent cells from bone marrow and lymphocyte cell mixtures. Transplant. **8**, 422–434 (1969)

DICKE, K.A., SCHAEFER, U.W., VAN BEKKUM, D.W.: The use of stem cell concentrates as bone marrow grafts in man. Transplant. Proc. **5**, 909–916 (1973)

DUPLAN, J.F.: Restauration des radiolésions par le foie foetal: influence de l'âge du donneur et du nombre des cellules injectées. C.R. Soc. Biol. **150**, 949–951 (1956)

DUPONT, B., ANDERSON, V., ERNST, P., FAVER, V., GOOD, R.S., HANSEN, G.S., HENRIKSEN, K., JENSEN, K., JUHL, F., KILLMAN, S.A., KOCH, C., MULLER-BERAT, N., PARK, B.H., SVEJGAARD, A., THOMSEN, M., WIIK, A.: Immunologic reconstitution in severe combined immunodeficiency with HL-A-incompatible bone marrow graft: Donor selection by mixed lymphocyte culture. Transplant. Proc. **5**, 905–908 (1973)

EBBELL, B.: The papyrus ebers. Munksgaard, Copenhagen, 1937 (cited by SAUNDERS)

FARRAR, J.L., LOUGHMAN, B.E., NORDIN, A.A.: Lymphopoietic potential of bone marrow cells from aged mice: Comparison of the cellular constituents of bone marrow from young and aged mice. J. Immunol. **112**, 1244–1249 (1974)

FERREBEE, J.W., THOMAS, E.D.: Transplantation of marrow in man. Arch. Int. Med. **106**, 523–531 (1960)

FLEMING, A.: A simple method of removing leukocytes from blood. Brit. J. Exp. Path. **7**, 281–286 (1926)

FLIEDNER, T.M.: Die Transfusion von H^3 thymidin-markierten homologen Knochenmarkzellen in ganzkörperbestrahlte Ratten. Nucl. Med. I, 299–313 (1960)

FORD, C.E., MICKLEM, H.S.: The thymus and lymph nodes in radiation chimeras. Lancet I, 359–362 (1963)

FREIREICH, E.J., LEVIN, R.H., WHANG, J., CARBONE, P.P., BRONSON, W., MORSE, E.E.: The function and fate of transfused leukocytes from donors with chronic myelocytic leukemia in leukopenic patients. Ann. N.Y. Acad. Sci. **113**, 1081–1089 (1964)

FRIEDENSTEIN, A.J., CHAILAKHYAN, R.K., LATSINIK, N.V., PANASYUK, A.F., KEILISS-BOROK, I.V.: Stromal cells responsible for transferring the microenvironment of the hemopoietic tissues. Transplant. **17**, 331–340 (1974)

FRIEDMAN, H.: Adoptive tolerance to shigella antigen in irradiated mice receiving spleen cell transplants from unresponsive donors. J. Immunol. **94**, 352–357 (1965a)

FRIEDMAN, H.: Transfer and maintenance of adoptive immunologic tolerance to shigella antigens in irradiated mice. Transplant. **3**, 465–477 (1965b)

GARVIN, J.: Factors affecting the adhesiveness of human leukocytes and platelets in vitro. J. Exp. Med. **114**, 51–73 (1961)

GATTI, R.A., ALLEN, H.D., MEUWISSEN, H.J., HONG, R.H., GOOD, R.A.: Immunological reconstitution of sex-linked lymphopenic immunological deficiency. Lancet **II**, 1366–1369 (1968)

GORER, P.A.: The genetic and antigenic basis of tumor transplantation. J. Path. Bact. **44**, 691–697 (1937)

GOWANS, J.L.: Fate of parental strain small lymphocytes in F_1 hybrid rats. Ann. N.Y. Acad. Sci. **99**, 432–455 (1962)

GRAW, R.G., BUCKNER, C.D., WHANG-PENG, J., LEVENTHAL, B.G., KRUEGER, G., BERARD, C.W., HENDERSON, E.S.: Complication of bone marrow transplantation. Graft-versus-host disease resulting from chronic-myelogenous leukemia leukocyte transfusions. Lancet **I**, 338–341 (1970)

GRAW, R.G., HERZIG, G.P., EISEL, R.J., PERRY, S.: Leukocyte and platelet collection from normal donors with the continuous flow blood cell separator. Transfusion **II**, 94–101 (1971)

GRAW, R.G., HERZIG, G., PERRY, S., HENDERSON, E.S.: Normal granulocyte transfusion therapy-treatment of septicemia due to gram-negative bacteria. N. Engl. J. Med. **287**, 367–371 (1972)

GRAW, R.G., JR., LOHRMANN, H.-P., BULL, M.I., DECTER, G.P., HERZIG, G.P., BULL, J.M., LEVENTHAL, B.G., YANKEE, R.A., HERZIG, R.H., KRUEGER, G.R.F., BLEYER, W.A., BUJA, M.L., McGINNIS, M.H., ALTER, H.J., WHANG-PENG, J., GRALNICK, H.R., KIRKPATRICK, C.H., HENDERSON, E.S.: Bone-Marrow transplantation following combination chemotherapy immunosuppression (B.A.C.T.) in patients with acute leukemia. Transpl. Proc. **6**, 349–354 (1974)

GRAW, R.G., YANKEE, R.A., LEVENTHAL, B.G., ROGENTINE, G.N., HERZIG, G.P. *et al.*: Bone marrow transplantation in acute leukemia employing cyclophosphamide. Exp. Hematol. **22**, 118–125 (1972)

GRAW, R.G., YANKEE, R.A., ROGENTINE, G.N., LEVENTHAL, B.G., HERZIG, G.P., HALTERMAN, R.H., MERRITT, C.B., McGINNIS, M.H., KRUEGER, G.R.F., WHANG-PENG, J., CAROLLA, R.L., GULLION, D.S., LIPPMAN, M.E., GRALNICK, H.R., BERARD, C.W., TERASAKI, P.I., HENDERSON, E.S.: Bone marrow transplantation from HL-A-matched donors to patients with acute leukemia. Transplant. **14**, 79–90 (1972)

HARD, R.C., KULLGREN, B.: Etiology, pathogenesis, and prevention of a fatal host-versus-graft syndrome in parent/F1 mouse chimeras. Amer. J. Path. **59**, 203–224 (1970)

HARRIS, T.N., HARRIS, S., BEALE, H.D., SMITH, J.J.: Studies on the transfer of lymph node cells. IV. Effect of X-irradiation of recipient rabbits on the appearance of antibody after cell transfer. J. Exp. Med. **100**, 289–300 (1954)

HELLRIEGEL, K.P., BORBERG, H., REITZ, H., GROSS, R.: Evaluation of the efficiency of leukocyte transfers by Y-chromatin studies. Transpl. Proc. **6**, 399–403 (1974)

HERZIG, G.P., ROOT, R.K., GRAW, R.G.: Granulocyte collection by continuous-flow filtration leukapheresis. Blood **39**, 554–567 (1972)

HILDEMAN, W.H.: Immunological properties of small blood lymphocytes in the graft-versus-host reaction in mice. Transplant. **2**, 38–47 (1964)

HILGARD, H.R.: Synergism of thymus and bone marrow the production of graft-versus-host splenomegaly in x-irradiated hosts. J. Exp. Med. **132**, 317–328 (1970)

HILGARTNER, M.W., LANZKOWSKI, P., NACHMAN, R.L., WEKSLER, M.B.: Bone marrow transplantation for aplastic anemia following hepatitis. In: Proc. 80th Ann. Meet. Amer. Pediat. Soc., 1970, p. 468

HIRSCH, M.S.: Immunological activation of oncogenic viruses. In: Virus Tumorigenesis and Immunogenesis (Ceglowski, W.S., Friedman, H., eds.). New York: Academic Press, 1973, pp. 131–139

HOBIK, H.P.: Graft-Versus-Host-Reactions. In this handbook

HOLLINGSWORTH, J.W., BIREND, J.A., SILBERT, D.A., FINCH, S.C.: Leukocyte mobilization in normal spenectomized and leukemic rats after replacement transfusions. J. Lab. Clin. Med. **50**, 36–44 (1957)

HONG, R., KAY, H.E.M., COOPER, M.D.: Immunologic restitution in lymphopenic immunological deficiency syndrome. Lancet **I**, 503–506 (1968)

JACOBSON, L.O., MARKS, E.K., GASTON, E.O.: Observations on the effect of spleen shielding and the injection of cell suspensions on survival following irradiation. In: Radiobiology Symposium Liége. Bacq, Z.M., Alexander, P. (eds.). London: Butterworths, 1955, pp. 122–133

KERSEY, J.H., MEUWISSEN, H.J., GOOD, R.A.: Graft-versus-host reactions following transplantation of allogenetic hematopoieic cells. Human Path. 2, 389–402 (1971)

KLINE, D.L., CLIFFTON, E.E.: The life span of leukocytes in man. Science 115, 9–11 (1952)

KRUEGER, G.: Preliminary study in micro- and immunoelectrophoresis on the serum of mice with postirradiation treatment. Fellowship Report to EURATOM, Mol, Belgium (1961)

KRUEGER, G.: Morphology of chemical immunosuppression. Adv. Pharmacol. Chemother. 10, 1–90 (1972)

KRUEGER, G.R.F.: Lymphoreticular neoplasia in immunosuppression: Facts and fancies. Beitr. Path. 151, 221–233 (1974)

KRUEGER, G.R.F.: The significance of immunosuppression and antigenic stimulation for the development of malignant lymphomas. (With special reference to cancer chemotherapy.) Rec. Res. Cancer Res. 52, 88–95 (1975)

KRUEGER, G.R.F., BERARD, C.W., DELELLIS, R.A., GRAW, R.G., YANKEE, R.A., LEVENTHAL, B.G., ROGENTINE, G.N., HERZIG, G.P., HALTERMAN, R.H., HENDERSON, E.S.: Graft-versus-host disease. Morphologic variation and differential diagnosis in 8 cases of HL-A matched bone marrow transplantation. Amer. J. Path. 63, 179–202 (1971)

KRUEGER, G.R.F., GRAW, R.G., ROGENTINE, G.N., DARROW, C.C., NEEFE, J.R., LUETZELER, J.: Pathology of modified graft-versus-host disease in bone marrow allografted monkeys treated with antilymphocyte serum. Blut 30, 19–30 (1975)

KUNKEL, H.G., YOUNT, W.J., SIEGAL, F.P.: The varied nature of the immune deficiency states. Trans. Amer. Clin. Climatol. Assoc. 83, 57–62 (1972)

LALEZARI, P.: A new technique for separation of human leukocytes. Blood 19, 109–114 (1962)

LANDSTEINER, K.: Ueber Agglutinationserscheinungen normalen menschlichen Blutes. Wien. klin. Wschr. 14, 1132–1134 (1901)

LANDSTEINER, K., STURLI, A.: Über die Hämagglutinine normaler Sera. Wien. klin. Wschr. 15, 38 40 (1902)

LAWRENCE, J.S., ERVIN, D.M., WETRICH, R.M.: Life cycle of white blood cells; rate of disappearance of leucocytes from peripheral blood of leucopenic rats. Amer. J. Physiol. 144, 284–296 (1945)

LENGEROVA, A.: Comparison of the therapeutic efficiency of homologous and heterologous embryonic haematopoietic cells administered to lethally irradiated mice. Folia Biol. 5, 18–22 (1959)

LENNERT, K.: Akute Osteomyelosklerose. Congress of the German Society of Hematology, Tübingen 1964

LEVEY, R.H., GELFAND, E.W., BATCHELOR, J.R., KLEMPERER, M.R., SANDERSON, A.R., BERKEL, A.I., ROSEN, F.S.: Bone-marrow transplantation in severe combined immunodeficiency syndrome. Lancet II, 571–575 (1971)

LORENZ, E., UPHOFF, D.E., REID, T.R., SHELTON, E.: Modification of irradiation injury in mice and guinea pigs by bone marrow injection. J. Natl. Cancer Inst. 12, 197 201 (1951)

LÖWENBERG, B., DICKE, K.A., DE GROOT, H., VAN BEKKUM, D.W.: Fetal liver hemopoietic grafting and repopulation. In: Annual Rep. Radiobiological Institute TNO, Rijswijk, Netherlands, 1973, pp. 151–152

LURIA, E.A., SAMOYLINA, N.L., GERASIMOV, Y.V., CHERTKOV, J.L.: Proliferation of hematopoietic stem cells in culture of embryonal liver in mice. J. Cell Physiol. 78, 461- 464 (1971)

MAKINODAN, T., PERKINS, E.H., SHEKARCHI, J.C., GENGOZIAN, N.: Use of lethally irradiated isologous mice as in vivo tissue cultures of antibody forming cells. In: Proc. Sympos. Mechanisms Antibody Formation. Prague: Czechosl. Acad. Sci. Publ. House, 1960, pp. 187-189

MALININ, T.I.: Storage and transplantation of bone marrow in the treatment of malignant diseases. J. Surg. Oncol. I, 45–52 (1973)

MASSHOFF, W.: Studien über die Hämolyse. Frankf. Z. Path. 61, 1–41 (1949)

MATHÉ, G.: Transfusion et greffe de cellules myeloides chez l'Homme. In: Biological Problems of Grafting. Oxford: Blackwell, 1959, p. 314

MATHÉ, G., SCHWARZENBERG, L.: Bone-marrow transplantation in France, 1958–1973. Transpl. Proc. 6, 335–343 (1974)

MATHÉ, G., SCHWARZENBERG, L., AMIEL, J.-L.: Bone marrow. In: Transplantation. NAJARIAN, J.S., SIMMONS, R.L. (eds.). Philadelphia: Lea & Febiger, 1972, Chap. 17

MATHÉ, G., BERNARD, J., DEVRIES, M.J., SCHWARZENBERG, L., LARRIEU, M.J., LALANNE, C.M., DUTRIEUX, A., AMIEL, J.L., SURMONT, J.: New trials with homologous bone marrow grafts after total irradiation in children with acute leukemia in remission. The problem of the secondary syndrome in man. Rev. Hematol. 15, 115–161 (1960)
MATHÉ, G., AMIEL, J.L., SCHWARZENBERG, L., CATTAN, A., SCHNEIDER, M.: Haemopoietic chimera in man after allogenic (homologous) bone marrow transplantation. Brit Med. J. 2, 1633–1635 (1963)
MATHÉ, G., AMIEL, J.L., SCHWARZENBERG, L., CATTAN, A., SCHNEIDER, M.: Adoptive immunotherapy of acute leukemia: experimental and clinical results. Cancer Res. 25, 1525–1531 (1965)
MEDAWAR, P.B.: The behaviour and fate of skin autografts and skin homografts in rabbits. J. Anat. 78, 176–199 (1944)
MERRITT, C.B., DARROW, C.C., VAAL, L., ROGENTINE, G.N.: Bone marrow transplantation in thesus monkeys following irradiation modification of acute graft-versus-host disease with antilymphocyte serum. Transplant. 14, 9–20 (1972)
MINOR, A.M., BURNETT, L.: A method for abtaining living leukocytes from human peripheral blood by acceleration of erythrocyte sedimentation. Blood 3, 199–802 (1948)
MUNSTER, A.M., LEARY, A.G., SPICER, S.S., FISHER, M.W.: Effect of lymphocytotherapy on the course of experimental pseudomonas sepsis. Ann. Surg. 179, 482–488 (1974)
NOWELL, P.C., COLE, L.J., ROAN, P.L., HABERMEYER, J.G.: The distribution and in situ growth pattern of injected rat marrow in X-irradiated mice. J. Nat. Cancer Inst. 18, 127–144 (1957)
NYE, R.N., BARRS, V.R.: Distribution of granular leukocytes in normal rabbits. Folia haemat. 47, 402 (1932)
O'GRADY, L.F.: Viability of frozen and stored marrow. Transplant. 9, 181–184 (1970)
PARK, B.H., BIGGAR, W.D., GOOD, R.A.: Paucity of thymus-dependent cells in human marrow. Transplant. 14, 284–286 (1972)
PARK, B.H., BIGGAR, W.D., GOOD, R.A.: Minnesota experience in bone-marrow transplantation in man, 1968 to June 1973. Transplant. Proc. 6, 379–383 (1974)
PEARSALL, N.N., WEISER, R.S.: The Macrophage. Philadelphia: Lea & Febiger, 1970
PENN, I., STARZL, T.E.: A summary of the status of de novo cancer in transplant recipients. Transplant Proc. 4, 719–732 (1972)
PERRY, V.P., STEVENSON, R.E., McFARLAND, W., ZINK, G.A.: Motility studies of human postmortem bone marrow. Blood 16, 1020–1028 (1960)
PORTER, K.A.: Use of foetal haemopoietic tissue to prevent late deaths in rabbit radiation chimaeras. Brit. J. Exp. Path. 40, 273–280 (1959)
PORTER, K.A., COOPER, E.H.: Transformation of adult allogeneic small lymphocytes after transfusion into newborn rats. J. Exp. Med. 115, 997–1008 (1962)
PORTER, K.A., MURRAY, J.E.: Successful homotransplantation of rabbit bone marrow after preservation in glycerol at −70° C. Cancer Res. 18, 117–119 (1958)
RAUCHWERGER, J.M., GALLAGHER, M.T., TRENTIN, J.J.: Xenogeneic resistance to rat bone marrow transplantation. II. Relationship of hemopoietic regeneration and survival. Biomedicine 19, 109–111 (1973a)
RAUCHWERGER, J.M., GALLAGHER, M.T., TRENTIN, J.J.: Role of the hemopoietic inductive microenvironments (HIM) in xenogeneic bone marrow transplantation. Transplant. 15, 610–613 (1973b)
ROOS, B.: Makrophagen: Herkunft, Entwicklung und Funktion. In: Handb. allg. Path., ALTMANN, H.W. et al. (eds.). Berlin: Springer Verlag, 1970, Vol. III, 3
ROSSE, W.F., GURNEY, C.W.: The Pelger-Huet anomaly in three families and its use in determining the disappearance of transfused neutrophils from peripheral blood. Blood 14, 170–186 (1959)
RUDOLPH, R.H., FEFER, A., THOMAS, E.D., BUCKNER, C.D., CLIFT, R.A., STORB, R.: Isogeneic marrow grafts for hematologic malignancy in man. Arch. Int. Med. 132, 279–285 (1973)
SANTOS, G.W., SENSENBRENNER, L.L., BURKE, P.J., COLVIN, M., OWENS, A.H., BIAS, W.B., SLAVIN, R.E.: Marrow transplantation in man following cyclophosphamide. Transplant. Proc. 3, 400–404 (1971)
SANTOS, G.W., SENSENBRENNER, L.L., BURKE, P.J., MULLINS, G.M., ANDERSON, P.N., TUTSCHKA, P.J., BRAINE, H.G., DAVIS, T.E., HUMPHREY, R.L., ABELOFF, M.D., BIAS, W.B., BORGOANKAR, D.S., SLAVIN, R.E.: Allogeneic marrow grafts in man using cyclophosphamide. Transplant. Proc. 6, 345–348 (1974)
SAUNDERS, J.B. DE C.M.: A conceptual history of transplantation. In: Transplantation. NAJARIAN, J.S., SIMMONS, R.L. (eds.). Philadelphia: Lea & Febiger, 1972, Chapter 1

SCHAEFER, U.W., DICKE, K.A., VAN BEKKUM, D.W.: Recovery of haemopoiesis in lethally irradiated monkeys by frozen allogeneic bone marrow grafts. Rev. Europ. Etudes Clin. et Biol. **17**, 483–488 (1972)

SCHWARTZ, I.R., REPPLINGER, E.F., CONGDON, C.C., TOCANTIS, L.M.: Transplantation of bone marrow after preservation at −70° Celsius. J. Appl. Physiol. **II**, 22–23 (1957)

SCHWARZENBERG, L., MATHÉ, G., DE GROUCHY, J., DE NAVA, C., DE VRIES, M.J., AMIEL, J.L., CATTAN, A., SCHNEIDER, M., SCHLUMBERGER, J.R.: White blood cell transfusions. Israel J. Med. Scis. **I**, 925–956 (1965)

SEMAN, G.: Technic for the staining of heterochromatic lobules of leukocytes (especially mononuclear cells). Value of this technic for sex determination. Rev. Franc. Étud. Clin. Biol. **6**, 161–165 (1961)

SERCARZ, E.E., COONS, A.H.: The exhaustion of specific antibody-producing capacity during a secondary response. In: Proc. Sympos. Mechanisms of Immunol. Tolerance (HAŠEK, M., LENGEROVA, A., VOMTISKOSA, M.) (eds.). New York: Academic Press, 1962

SHAW, D.H., VERMUND, H.: Modifications of irradiation effects in the pigeon, Columbia livia. II. Effects of delayed bone marrow implantation. Proc. Soc. Exp. Biol. Med. **107**, 414–420 (1961)

SILVERS, W.K., BILLINGHAM, R.E.: Studies on the immunotherapy of runt disease in rats. J. Exp. Med. **129**, 647–661 (1969)

SKOOG, W.A., BECK, W.S.: Studies on fibrinogen, dextran, and phytohemagglutinin methods of isolating leukocytes. Blood **II**, 436–454 (1956)

SNELL, G.D.: Methods for the study of histocompatibility genes. J. Genetics **49**, 87 (1948)

SPECK, B.: Indikationen zur Knochenmarktransplantation bei Patienten mit aplastischer Anämie und akuter myeloischer Leukämie. Schweiz. med. Wschr. **103**, 508–511 (1973a)

SPECK, B.: Bone marrow transplantation—clinical results and problems. Blut **27**, 297–301 (1973b)

STORB, R., RUDOLPH, R.H., KOLB, H.J., GRAHAM, I.C., MICKELSON, E., ERICKSON, V., LERNER, K.G., KOLB, H., THOMAS, E.D.: Marrow grafts between DL-A-matched canine littermates. Transplant. **15**, 92–100 (1973)

STORB, R., THOMAS, E.D., BUCKNER, C.D., CLIFT, R.A., JOHNSON, F.L., FEFER, A., GLUCKSBERG, H., GIBLETT, E.R., LERNER, K.G., NEIMAN, P.: Allogenic marrow grafting for treatment of aplastic anemia. Blood **43**, 157–180 (1974)

STODTMEISTER, R., FLIEDNER, T.M.: Morphological aspects of myelofibrosis, observed in rats following sublethal whole body irradiation and subsequent allogeneic bone marrow cell transfusion. Folia Haematol. **100**, 23–50 (1973)

TAKADA, Y., TAKADA, A.: Proliferation of donor hematopoietic cells in irradiated and unirradiated host mice. Transplant. **12**, 334–337 (1971)

TAKADA, A., TAKADA, Y.: Proliferation of donor marrow and thymus cells in the myeloid and lymphoid organs of irradiated syngeneic host mice. J. Exp. Med. **137**, 543–546 (1973)

TAKADA, A., TAKADA, Y., AMBRUS, J.L.: Proliferation of donor spleen and bone-marrow cells in the spleens and bone marrows of unirradiated and irradiated adult mice. Proc. Soc. Exp. Biol. Med. **136**, 222–226 (1971)

TEVETHIA, S.S., ZARLING, J.M.: Participation of macrophages in tumor immunity. Natl. Cancer Inst. Monogr. **35**, 279–282 (1972)

THIERFELDER, S.: Experimental bone marrow transplantation. Blut **30**, 1–18 (1975)

THOMAS, E.D., EPSTEIN, R.B.: Bone marrow transplantation in acute leukemia. Cancer Res. **25**, 1521–1524 (1965)

THOMAS, E.D., FERREBEE, J.W.: Prolonged storage of marrow and its use in the treatment of radiation injury. Transfusion **2**, 115–117 (1962)

TOYA, R.E., SMITH, L.H., CONGDON, C.C.: Modification of acute graft-versus-host disease in mice by pretreatment of the donor with phenyl-hydrazine. Exp. Hematol. **22**, 62–63 (1972)

TRENTIN, J.J.: Determination of bone marrow stem cell differentiation by stromal hemopoietic inductive microenvironment (HIM). Amer. J. Path. **65**, 621–628 (1971)

TRENTIN, J.J., RAUCHWERGER, J.M., GALLAGHER, M.T.: Genetic resistance to marrow transplantation. Biomedicine **18**, 86–88 (1973)

UPHOFF, D.E.: Preclusion of secondary phase of irradiation syndrome by inoculation of fetal hematopoietic tissue following lethal total body X-irradiation. J. Natl. Cancer Inst. **20**, 625–632 (1958)

Urso, P., Gengozian, N.: T cell deficiency in mouse allogeneic radiation chimeras. J. Immunol. III, 712–719 (1973)

Urso, I.S., Congdon, C.C., Owen, R.D.: Effect of foreign fetal and newborn blood-forming tissues on survival of lethally irradiated mice. Proc. Soc. Exp. Biol. Med. 100, 395–399 (1959)

Vallee, B.L., Hughes, W.L., Gibson, J.A.: A method for the separation of leukocytes from whole blood by flotation on serum albumin. Blood I, 82–87 (1947)

van Bekkum, D.W., de Vries, M.J.: Radiation chimaeras. New York: Academic Press 1967

van Bekkum, D.W., Balner, H., Dicke, K.A., van Putten, L.M.: Experimental aspects of bone marrow transplantation in primates. Transplant. Proc. I, 25 (1969)

Vos, O., Crouch, B.G., van Bekkum, D.W.: The interval between irradiation and bone marrow transplantation. Int. J. Rad. Biol. 3, 337–349 (1961)

Weiser, R.S., Granger, G.A., Brown, W., Baker, P., Jutila, J., Holme, S.R.: Produce of allogeneic disease in mice. Transplant. 3, 10–21 (1965)

Woodruff, J.M., Eltringham, J.R., Casey, H.W.: Early secondary disease in the rhesus monkey. I. A comparative histopathologic study. Lab. Invest. 20, 499–511 (1969)

Wunderlich, J.R., Martin, W.J., MacDonald, J., Fletcher, F.: Functional capacity of cytotoxic lymphoid cells. Natl. Cancer Inst. Monogr. 35, 243–249 (1972)

Zaalberg, O.G.: Studies in immunological tolerance in radiation chimeras. Int. J. Rad. Biol. 6, 484–488 (1963)

Skin Grafts in Animals and Man

ZOLTAN J. LUCAS

With 4 Figures and 3 Tables

A. Introduction

Techniques for grafting skin were developed in the mid-sixteenth century. Three surgical principles were considered essential: preparation of the graft bed, adequate nutrition of the graft, and good hemostasis to permit graft contact with the host bed. These were rapidly abandoned, however, as crushing gunshot wounds that often necessitated amputation replaced sword slashes as the major form of injury. With the scientific renaissance of biologic sciences in the mid-nineteenth century and the success with use of aseptic free skin grafts permitted by the discovery of antiseptics, experimental and clinical skin grafting were revived. However, physicians did not recognize the biologic fact that grafting from one individual to another almost uniformly produced graft failure (CONVERSE and CASSON, 1968). Losses continued to be attributed to poor surgical technique resulting in inadequate graft nutrition (THIERSCH, 1886).

MURPHY (1926) provided an anatomic basis for the host response to a skin graft, describing accumulations of lymphoid cells at the junction of the skin graft and host. Twenty years later MEDAWAR (1944) confirmed the presence of infiltrating cells at the interface between graft and host, but also localized such cells in the graft itself. The predominance of mononuclear cells in the infiltrate, the more rapid rejection of second-set grafts, and the transfer of sensitivity by living cells from regional lymph nodes but not by immune serum established the rejection or homograft[1] reaction as a form of cellular immunity.

It was soon appreciated that host lymphocytes responded to graft contact by marked proliferation and blastogenesis, occurring predominantly in the local draining lymph nodes, and that such sensitized lymphocytes comprised a circulating pool of lymphocytes which migrated to the graft through the arterial blood (GOWANS et al., 1963). The subsequent, almost explosive, expansion of trans-

Acknowledgments. The assistance of Ms. Judy Whitsell in the preparation of this manuscript is gratefully acknowledged.

[1] Duplicate terminology for the relationship of a donor to a recipient exists: if the graft is from the recipient himself, it is *isogeneic,* or an *autograft;* from a genetically identical individual, *syngeneic,* or an *isograft;* from a member of the same species, *allogeneic,* or an *allograft* or *homograft;* and if from another species, *xenogeneic,* or a *xenograft* or *heterograft.*

plantation immunity knowledge was coupled with its almost immediate clinical application. Induction of neonatal tolerance, and then tolerance in immuno-suppressed adult rodents was achieved. Clinically applicable methods, immuno-suppression with azathioprine and methylprednisolone, were developed. Renal transplantation, formerly an experimental alternative to a lingering death, be-came a reality. The almost emotional fervor of the transplant surgeons, for whom there existed apparently no obstacles to the complete replacement of man's constituent parts, reached a peak with the successful heart transplant in 1968. The public's imagination was captivated and research monies for immu-nologists became available as never before. Knowledge of cellular immunology increased exponentially; lymphocytes were differentiated into T- and B-cells; tissue typing based on serologically defined or lymphocyte-defined antigens was minutely detailed; the Ia system of immune regulatory genes was discovered. Yet, despite these accomplishments during the last 20 years, little has been learned about the specific pathophysiology of skin graft rejection. Many ques-tions posed in the 1960's remain unanswered. What mechanism induces sensitiza-tion of skin grafts? What is the mechanism of rejection? What are the roles of the various infiltrating cells? Why are skin grafts rejected more vigorously than grafts of other organs? Conversely, why do several procedures prolong vascularized organ grafts, yet not skin grafts?

This chapter will present first the basic morphologically established patterns observed in skin allograft rejections; second, a detailed description of the immu-nopathologic processes induced by the infiltrating cells; and third, a contrast of these events in conventional skin grafts having delayed vascularization with immediately vascularized skin grafts.

B. Operational Definition of Transplant Antigens

The concept of *histocompatibility* is derived from the fate of tumor or skin grafts exchanged between *inbred strains* of animals. After brother-sister matings for 20 or more consecutive generations, a homogenous strain showing permanent acceptance of grafts from each other may be obtained. The strain is then assumed to show complete *genetic identity*. Mating two inbred lines results in a first generation offspring (F_1 hybrid) which accepts skin from either parental strain yet whose tissues are rejected by both parents. Rejection represents the recipient's recognition that the graft is foreign. The F_1 hybrid, possessing each of its parents' genes, cannot recognize either parental antigen as "nonself". Both parents, recognizing the foreignness of each other's genes, reject such graft combinations. The occurrence of histocompatibility phenomena presupposes two factors: one, *histocompatibility molecules or antigens* on donor cells; and *recognition structures* on recipient cells which perceive that these antigens are foreign.

Antigens are considered histocompatibility antigens if they can be related to graft rejection. In its original definition, the term *histocompatibility* referred to the growth or failure of growth of tumor or tissue transplants (SNELL and STIMPFLING, 1966). Graft survival or growth is determined by *H-structures* and is under the control of *H-genes* or *H-loci*.

It is estimated that a minimum of 29–32 histocompatibility loci are involved in the rejection of allogeneic skin in the mouse (BAILEY and MOBRAATEN, 1964). Fifteen H-loci have been identified: 13 autosomal loci, an X-chromosome linked locus and a Y-chromosome linked locus. Inbred strains produced by brother-sister matings differ from each other in the number of H-loci differences. The effects of individual H-loci could be studied only after the breeding of *congenic resistant* mouse strains—strains identical except for a single chromosomal segment. Different forms of a single segment or genetic locus are called *alleles*. Since each chromosomal segment is made up of two complementary DNA strands, two possible alleles may occur in one chromosome. If they are identical, the animal is homozygous for that gene; if different, *heterozygous*.

Studies with single H-gene-mismatches result in markedly different graft survival times. Mismatches at the H-2 locus result in rejection in 9.9 days. Mismatches at other H-loci yield mean survival times (MST) of 21 to >400 days. A "strong" antigen has been arbitrarily defined as resulting in rejection in 14 days. By this criterion, as shown in Table 1, the H-2 gene is the major

Table 1. Correlation of mean survival times of skin grafts with histocompatibility differences in mice[a]

Single H-locus incompatibility			Two H-loci incompatibility		
Locus	MST (days)	95% Cont. limits	Locus	MST (days)	95% Cont. limits
H-1	25	23–27	H-1 & H-Y	13	12.8–13.9
H-2	9.9	9.5–10.3	H-4 & H-11	58	49–69
H-3	21	20–23	H-4	164	101–267
H-4	120	46–309	H-11	153	100–236
H-7	23	21–25			
H-8	32	26–39			
H-9	>400	–			
H-10	91	67–122	H-2 plus various non-H-2 incompatibilities		
H-11	78	63–97			
H-12	259	132–510	H-2 & H-4	8.6	8.0–9.2
H-13	38	33–45	H-2	9.9	9.5–10.3
H-Y	15	14.4–15.4	H-4	25	22–27

Multiple (seven or more) non H-2 H-loci incompatibilities					
Loci	MST	95% Cont. limits	Locus	MST	95% Cont. limits
H-1 ⎫			H-1	>200	–
H-3			H-3	36	22–58
H-4			H-4	25	22–27
H-10 ⎬	11	10.5–11.3	H-10	71	46–110
H-11			H-11	164	101–267
H-12			H-12	>300	
H-13 ⎭			H-13	73	23–239

[a] Data abstracted from GRAFF et al. (1966b)

histocompatibility gene in the mouse. Moderate-strength antigens (rejection in 21–38 days) are H-1, H-3, H-7, H-8, H-13, and H-Y; intermediate antigens (rejection in 78–120 days) are H-4, H-10, and H-11; weak antigens (>120 days) are H-9 and H-12 (GRAFF et al., 1966a; GRAFF et al., 1966b).

Fundamental laws governing histocompatibility were initially defined in mice because of the availability of inbred and congenic strains with precisely known genetic disparity. A wealth of detailed knowledge on relating genetic disparity and graft survival exists. There are multiple H-loci, with multiple allelic forms for each H-locus. Where both alleles are present, both phenotypes are equally expressed; the alleles are codominant. Antigenic "strength", operationally defined as the speed or vigor of rejection of grafts mismatched at only that antigenic locus, varies markedly. It is unknown whether molecular structure, cellular distribution of the antigen, or some other factor is responsible for antigenic strength.

The interallelic combination, rather than the particular H-locus, determines the intensity of histocompatibility. This has been decisively demonstrated for "weak" antigens. Thus, grafts mismatched for different alleles of the H-1 locus show graft rejection varying from 15 to over 250 days. [H-1^c→H-1^b (15 days) > H-1^b→H-1^a (25 days) > H-1^a > H-1^b (100 days) > H-1^b→H-1^c (>250 days)] (HILDEMANN, 1970). A similar relationship has been suggested for alleles of the major histocompatibility locus for man.

Multiple histocompatibility differences exhibit additive effects leading to shorter MST only when the constituent antigens of the grafts are similar in strength (HILDEMANN, 1970). For example, differences at H-4 or H-11 (refer to Table 1) result in rejection in about 150 days; mismatch at both, 58 days. Multiple weak incompatibilities can yield survival times similar to those of strong antigenic differences. In the example in Table 1, 7 non-H-2 incompatibilities result in graft rejection in 11 days. Also, when a recipient exhibits its maximum response against a given antigenic disparity, adding more antigenic differences to that graft does not further accelerate graft rejection. (Table 1, H-2 plus non-H-2 incompatibilities.)

The weaker the histocompatibility, the later the time of onset of graft rejection and the greater is the interval between onset and complete rejection. Reports on skin grafts in man (AMOS et al., 1969) show that their survival similarly depends on the genetic relationship between donor and recipient. These findings, not surprising considering the experimental evidence with animals, are of particular importance because genetic relationships in man cannot be controlled. Isografts in man occur only with monozygotic twins; there may be *syngeneic grafts* with certain sibling grafts, but the majority of sibling, almost all parent-child and all nonrelated donor grafts are between *nonidentical* individuals. These allogeneic grafts have varying incompatibilities in the major H-locus alleles and in the numbers and alleles of minor H-loci.

C. Morphologic Changes Occurring in Skin Allografts

Placing a skin graft on an allogeneic host initiates a complex response which results in specific immunity in the host and destruction of the graft. Although much descriptive information on graft rejection is available, knowledge of the mechanisms involved is limited.

I. Sequential Changes in Gross and Microscopic Appearance

The acceptance of autografted skin and its integration into the graft site occurs in three phases: initial primary healing, and the most important re-establishment of vascular and lymphatic connections; a period of general hyperplasia in which all the cellular elements of the graft participate; and a period of restructuring during which the graft returns to the condition of the normal skin, as modified by the geometric and physical conditions imposed by its location. Allografted skin goes through the primary healing process and into the period of hyperplasia with little evidence of an immune response. Thereafter, an inflammatory process engulfs the graft. Lymphocytes and monocytes massively invade through the newly established vascular connections. Edema may be severe. The inflammation proceeds to necrosis; the vascular system is obliterated and the cellular elements of the graft die. The intensity of the cellular response and its rate of development vary inversely with the survival time of the graft. New capillaries from the graft bed revascularize the necrotic area. A second population of granulocytes, lymphocytes, and monocytes invade the disintegrating eschar and convert it to a granulating surface. Epithelial coverage ultimately occurs by growth from the edges of the contracting wound. The entire breakdown process may require only four days (WIENER et al., 1964). The three stages of skin graft rejection almost imperceptively merge into one other.

1. Stage of primary healing. The newly created recipient bed converts into granulating tissue, remaining relatively aseptic as long as the surface is covered by a skin graft. The surface tension of extracellular fluid "sticks" the graft to the host. Fibroblasts and numerous granulocytes accumulate at the interface; collagen fibers and capillaries connect across the interface so that the graft is revascularized and firmly stuck to the host by five days. During the same period, epithelial cells proliferate so that the epidermis becomes thicker. The lymphatic channels are reconstituted before the vascular channels. Microangiograms show that both autografts and allografts are in extensive vascular continuity with the host within 48 hours.

2. Stage of mononuclear cell infiltration. A change unique to allografts is first noted within and adjacent to dermal capillaries when small numbers of mononuclear cells appear. Later, they extend into the dermis and epidermis, initially only to the basal layer, but ultimately to the stratum corneum. Both monocytes and lymphocytes are present. In nonimmunosuppressed hosts, the process from early to dense infiltration takes about two days.

3. Stage of graft necrosis. Cellular degeneration progresses from the basal cell layer to the most superficial layer paralleling the progression of the mononuclear cells. There is relatively little destruction of collagen at this stage. Blood vessels develop stagnation and ultimately obliterate, leading to initially random areas of ischemia which eventually coalesce. The ischemic area forms a hard dehydrated eschar which finally sloughs off, leaving a clean granulating bed

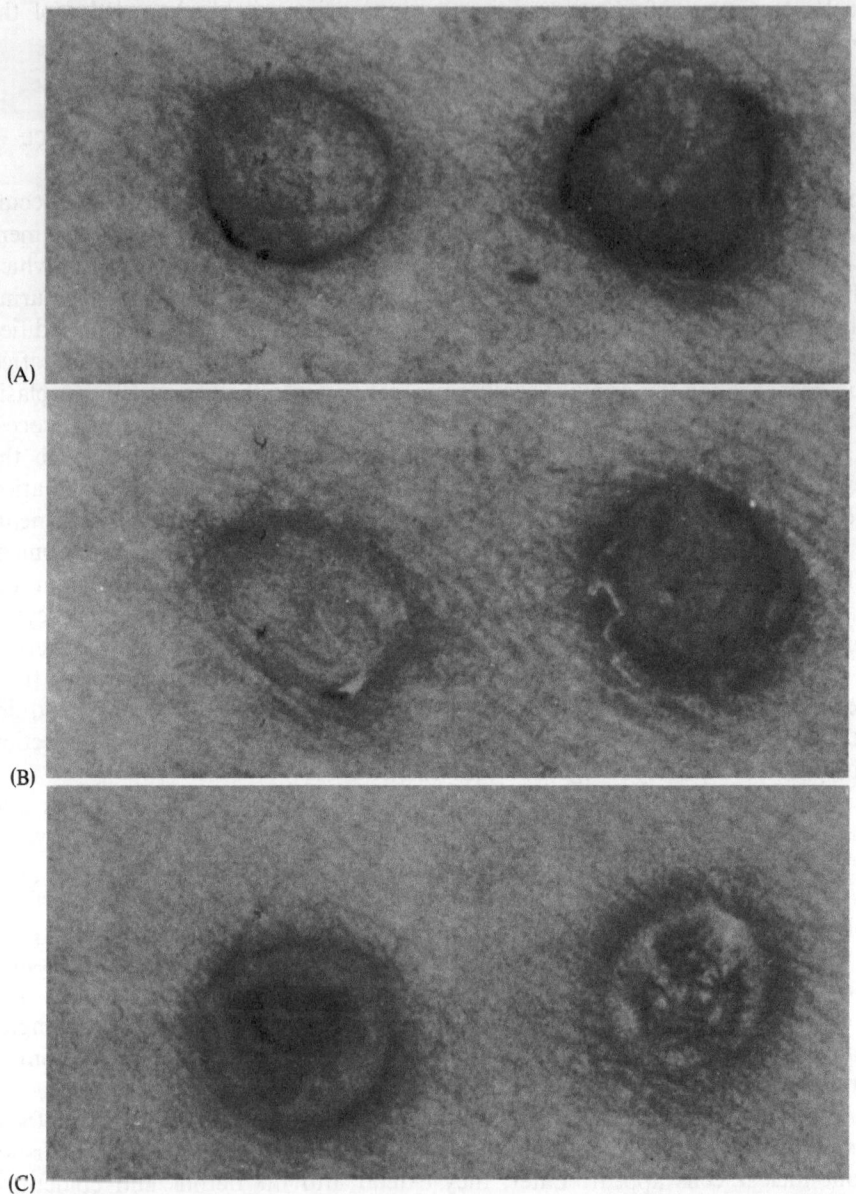

Fig. 1. Serial photographs of human skin grafting. Donor *1* is recipient's father; Donor *2* is his mother. There is one HL-A haplotype incompatibility for each graft. Grafts are ABO compatible. Fig. 1A taken on day 11, Fig. 1B on day 22 and Fig. 1C on day 32 following skin grafting. Using 50% viability as end point, rejection was scored as day 30 for *1* and day 32 for *2*. Fig. 1A shows the halo of erythema involving edges of graft *1*, proceeding faster than graft *2*. Fig. 1B shows dark red discoloration of graft *1* secondary to stagnation of bloodflow and beginning necrosis of lower circumference. Fig. 1C shows eschar on graft *2*, with beginning wound contracture; graft *1* shows 50% graft necrosis and venous stagnation. Photos by courtesy of Drs. F.E. Ward and D.B. Amos, Department of Immunology, Duke University, Durham, No. Carolina

that then undergoes closure by wound contracture and circumferential epithelial migration. Plates showing certain gross features of rejection in human parental to child skin grafts are shown in Figures 1A–C. Histologic patterns of the sequential development of skin graft rejection in the rat are illustrated in Figures 2A–D.

II. Characterization and Quantitation of the Infiltrating Cells

Various methods have been employed to quantitate and characterize the infiltrating cells. JAKOBIAK (1971) isolated and stained cells from 14 mm diameter pieces of grafted mouse skin by trypsinization. A 4 day allograft contained about 157,000 cells, 73% of which were macrophage-like. Background numbers in surrounding nontraumatized skin were only one-third (44,000; 81% macrophage-like). On the sixth day, total recovered cells increased to 1.3×10^6, with all cellular components increased. Macrophages (44%) and lymphocytes (38%) predominated, but both neutrophils (10%) and basophils (8%) were markedly increased relative to the background counts. At 8 days, although total cell count was unchanged, the granulocytes had doubled and the lymphocytes had decreased. Most of the graft infiltrating cells are just under the dermis, in the panniculus adiposus, as well as between the latter and the panniculus carnosus of the graft. There are also many cells between the panniculus carnosus of the graft and the abdominal muscles of the recipient. POULTER et al. (1971) examined a histochemically active population of macrophage in the cellular infiltrates of grafted mice, staining for particulate acid phosphatase activity. They observed two waves of increased activity, an initial ten fold increase from days 6–8, and a secondary twenty-five fold increase occurring between days 10–12. They concluded that on days 7–12 increased permeability of the lysosomal membranes takes place, allowing for leakage of hydrolytic enzymes into the extracellular tissue fluid, and leading to lysis of the surrounding cells.

The stimulus for the increased granulocytes in the infiltrate is unknown, but presumed to result from chemotactic factors released by lymphocytes, activation of the complement reaction or necrosing tissue cells. There is little evidence to implicate bacterial infection, likely to occur with experimental animals. Skin grafts in germ-free animals destroy the allografted skin faster in three of four rat strain combinations tested. The histology of the reaction is similar, except for the rapidity, to that in conventional animals (McDONALD et al., 1971).

III. Comparison of Morphologic Events
in the Homograft Reaction and in other Hypersensitivity Reactions

The skin may be the milieu for other delayed hypersensitivity reactions, some occurring naturally, others after experimental manipulation. These reactions are contrasted in Table 2. Four major types of allergic reactions may elicit skin lesions. An *anaphylactic* type occurs with the local injection of antibody to circulating antigen which passively sensitizes the tissues (passive cutaneous

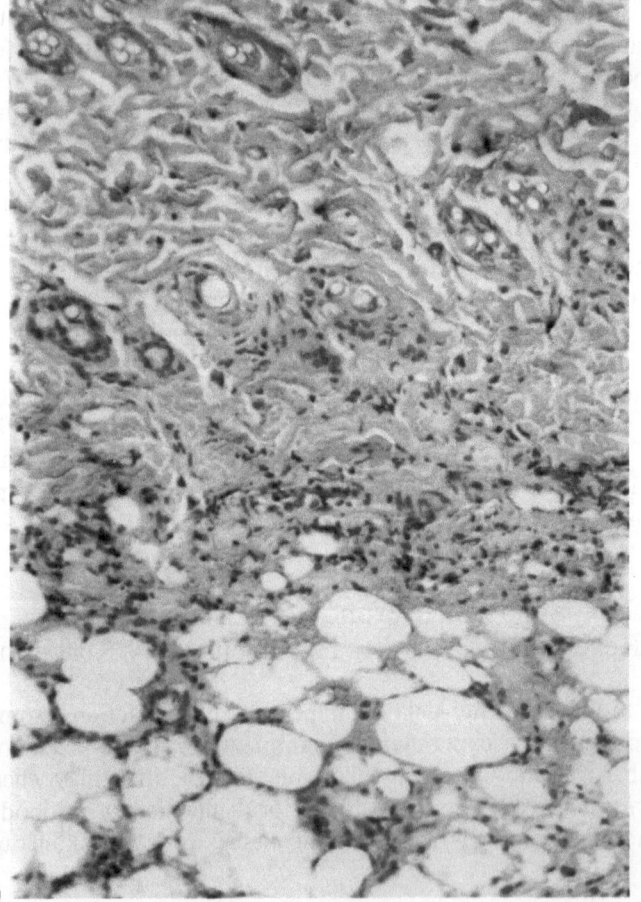

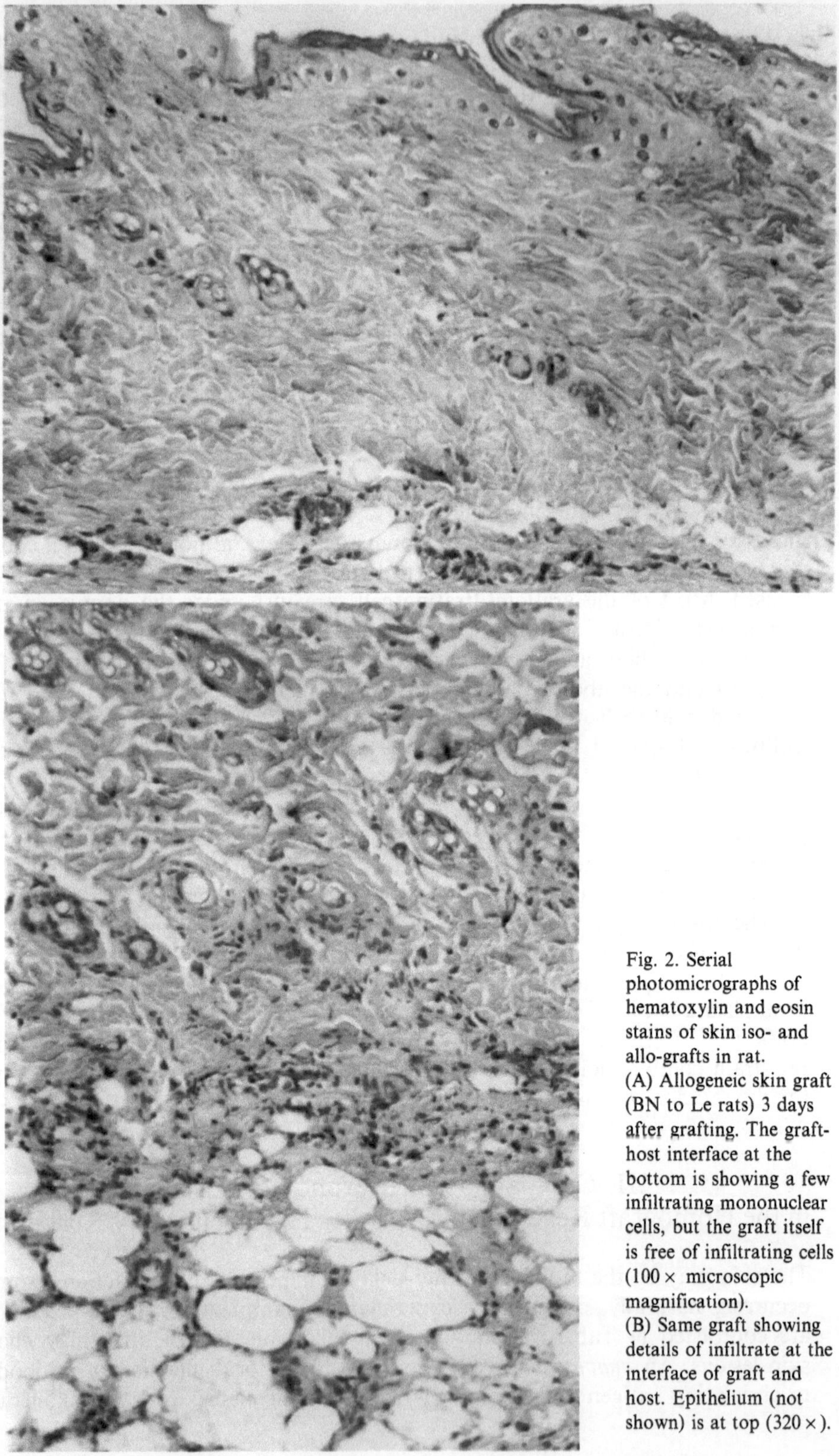

Fig. 2. Serial photomicrographs of hematoxylin and eosin stains of skin iso- and allo-grafts in rat.
(A) Allogeneic skin graft (BN to Le rats) 3 days after grafting. The graft-host interface at the bottom is showing a few infiltrating mononuclear cells, but the graft itself is free of infiltrating cells (100× microscopic magnification).
(B) Same graft showing details of infiltrate at the interface of graft and host. Epithelium (not shown) is at top (320×).

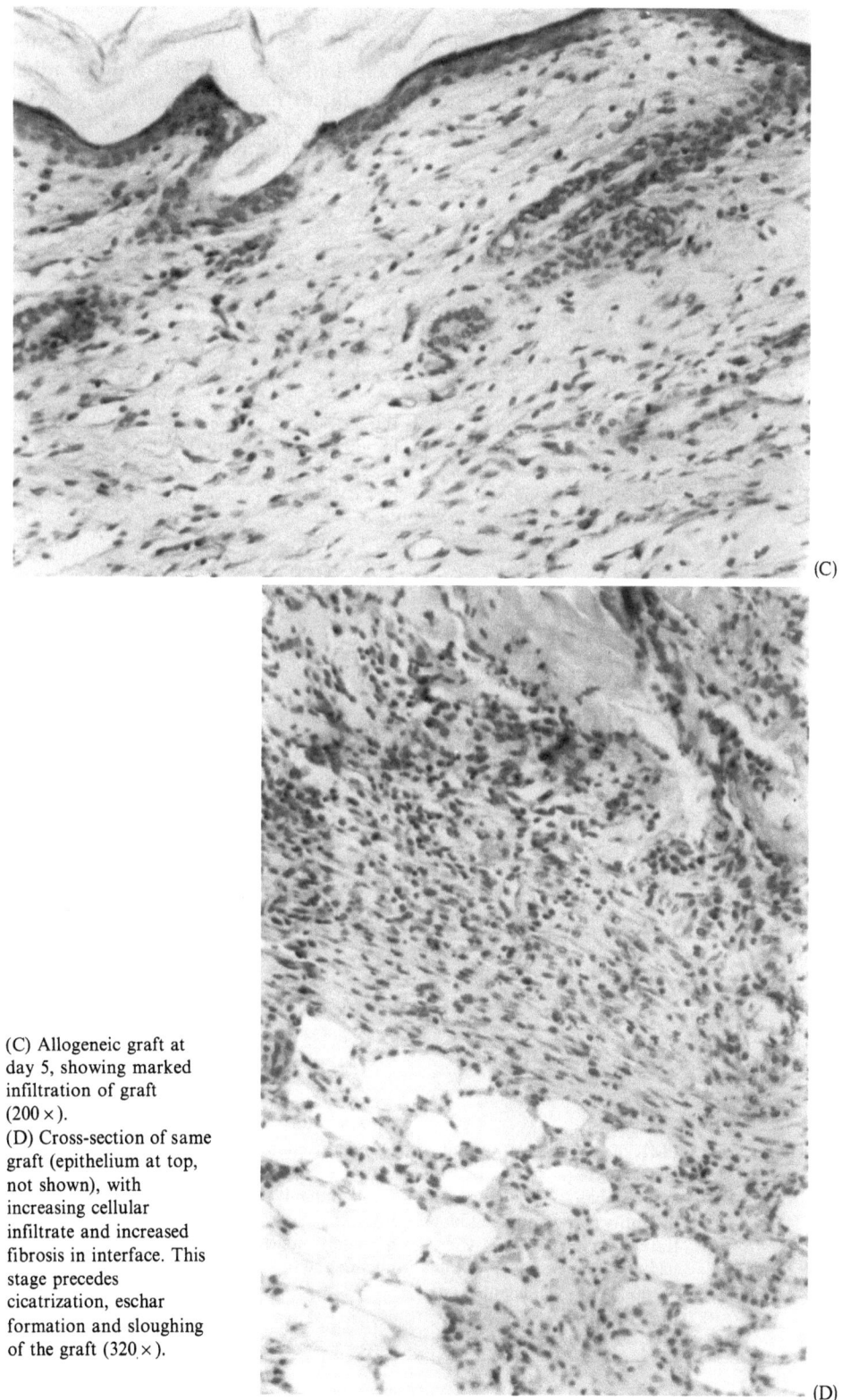

(C) Allogeneic graft at day 5, showing marked infiltration of graft (200 ×).

(D) Cross-section of same graft (epithelium at top, not shown), with increasing cellular infiltrate and increased fibrosis in interface. This stage precedes cicatrization, eschar formation and sloughing of the graft (320 ×).

(C)

(D)

anaphylaxis). Hyperemia of small vessels causes a local erythematous patch; edema may be variable. Polymorphonuclear leukocytes (PMN) rapidly adhere to the endothelium and penetrate to the basement membrane, which, however, remains uninjured. Few PMN penetrate into the intercellular spaces. Damaged endothelial cells slough off. Sometimes the intravascular infiltrate is predominantly eosinophils.

Table 2. Histologic features of allergic skin reactions

	Anaphylaxis (passive cutaneous anaphylaxis)	Arthus (passive Arthus reaction)	Delayed hypersensitivity (tuberculin reaction)	Homograft reaction	
				1st set	"white graft"
Method of induction:	Local injection of antibody, followed by i.v. injection of antigen in nonsensitized host	i.v. injection of antiserum and antigen into skin of nonsensitized host	Intradermal injection of antigen into sensitized host	Allogeneic graft into virgin recipient	Allogeneic graft into presensitized recipient
Responding serum factors	Complement	Complement	None	None	Complement; antigraft antibody
Responding cells	PMN leukocytes	First PMN leukocytes, then macrophages	Mononuclear cells	Initially mononuclear	PMN leukocytes
Rate of response	Within minutes	First noted in 1-2 h	1–2 days	After latent period of 5–7 days	May be catastrophically rapid (minutes to 2 days)
Gross description	Hyperemic patch	Erythematous indurated swelling with punctate hemorrhages	Erythematous wheal of varying induration	Graft becomes pink on days 3–5, develops erythematous halo 2 days later, followed by cyanosis of venous stagnation and necrosis	Graft never becomes pink
Microscopic description	PMN rapidly adhere to endothelium, but do not penetrate beyond basement membrane	Massive infiltration by PMN within and surrounding blood vessels. After 8 hr, PMN disintegrate and macrophages appear	Diffuse reaction with dense multifocal accumulation of mainly mononuclear cells	Mononuclear infiltrate, initially around vessels, then diffuse into interstitium	Dense PMN accumulation at interface of graft and host

An *Arthus reaction* occurs when antibody forms a precipitating complex with antigens in the local tissues, taking place 2–4 hours after the injection of antigen. An erythematous indurated swelling with punctate hemorrhages appears. PMN cells massively infiltrate within and around the blood vessels. Eight hours later, the basement membrane is disrupted and the PMN cells disintegrate and are replaced by macrophages and histiocytes. Large numbers of plasma cells appear after 12 hours. *Delayed sensitivity reactions* take place when sensitized lymphocytes react with soluble, particulate or cellular antigen. Contact sensitivity or tuberculin-type delayed skin reactions are classic examples. In addition, these reactions are considered the major effector mechanism in allograft rejection. The *tuberculin reaction* in man appears in 48–72 hours as an erythematous wheal, with varying degrees of induration at the injection site. There is a dense multifocal accumulation of mainly mononuclear cells around thin-walled blood vessels. From here, cells diffusely infiltrate the surrounding tissue.

Experimental cutaneous analogues of the homograft reaction have been described in the last 10 years. Lymphocytes injected into the dermis give rise to the *direct hypersensitivity reaction,* the *immune lymphocyte transfer reaction* (ILT), the *normal lymphocyte transfer reaction* (NLT), and the mixed lymphocyte reaction in irradiated hamsters. Direct hypersensitivity reactions occur in syrian hamsters, guinea pigs, and man when foreign cells are injected into the skin of presensitized animals. A flare-and-wheal begins in 5–8 hours, reaching maximum intensity in 24–48 hours. An ILT occurs when lymphoid cells from sensitized recipients are injected intradermally into the graft donors. Edema, induration, and erythema occur, and if intensive, may lead to necrosis and scarring. Irradiating hamsters before injecting the cells markedly suppresses the phenomenon, suggesting that the reactions are to circulating hemopoietic cells transiently coursing through the skin rather than to fixed epidermal or fibroblast components of skin. A NLT reaction occurs with the intradermal injection of nonsensitized allogeneic lymphocytes. The NLT reaction is similar to the ILT reaction, but at a much reduced rate. In man it occurs after a latent period of 24–48 hours, reaching peak intensity in 72–96 hours. The mixed lymphocyte reaction (MLR) in irradiated hamsters utilizes the skin as a passive milieu for the interactions of two allogeneic lymphocyte populations. Although these reactions were designed as assays of immunocompetence of reactant cells, their value in the context of pathophysiologic processes in the homograft reaction lies in insights gained in mechanisms of tissue destruction.

D. The Immune Responses Induced by Skin Grafting

The described gross and microscopic changes in the graft are manifestations of the effector phase of the host's immune response. Immunologic events, however, preceed, are concurrent, and occur subsequent to these visual changes. The immune response may be divided into four sequential phases: the *afferent,* where antigen recognition occurs; the *central,* where cell differentiation and

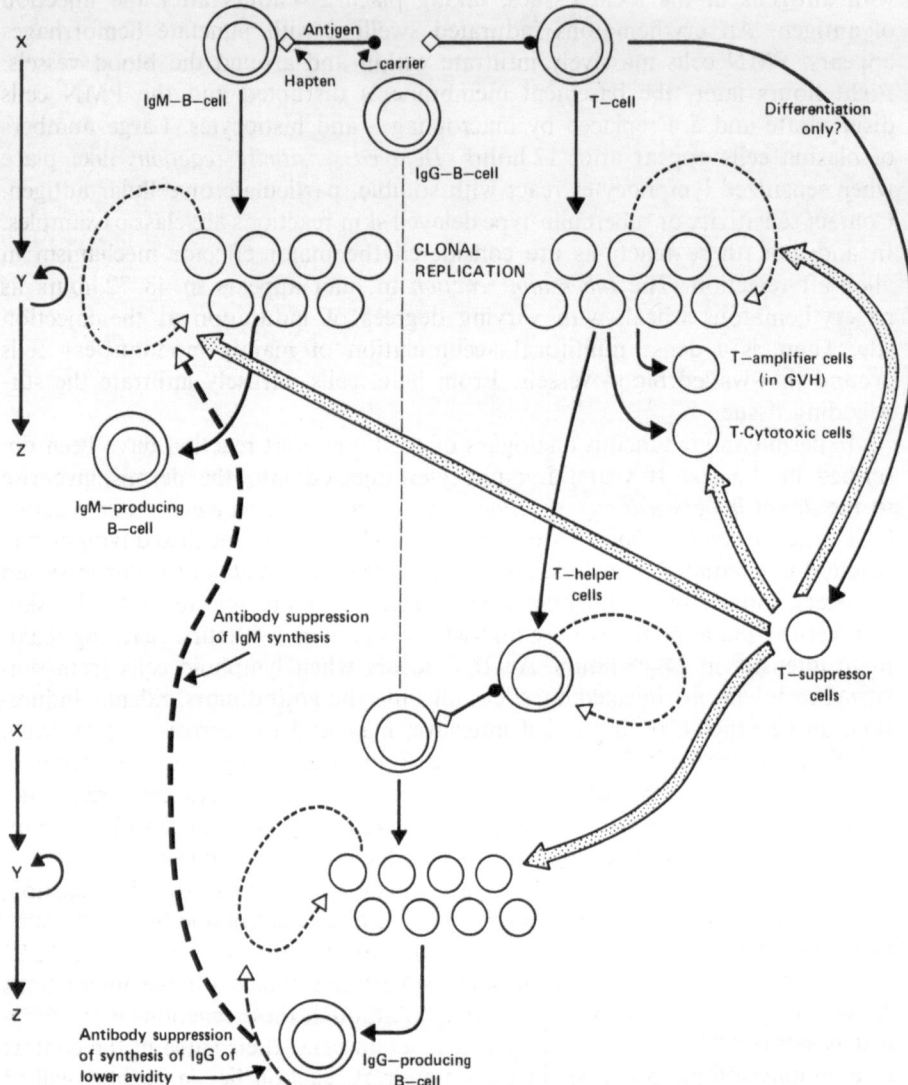

PRIMORDIAL ANTIGEN-SENSITIVE CELLS

Fig. 3. Current summary of immune responses to complex antigen. IgM-producing antigen-sensitive B-cells and antigen-sensitive T-cells recognize different determinants on antigen and undergo clonal replication. IgG-B cells, although present, do not respond until subpopulation of T-helper cells has differentiated from replicating T-cells. Differentiated B-cells produce IgM antibodies; differentiated T-cells fall into several categories, among them, T-amplifier cells, T-cytotoxic cells, and T-helper cells. When stimulated, IgG-producing B-cells similarly undergo clonal replication, differentiating into IgG producing cells. IgG specifically suppresses IgM antibody synthesis and also acts to inhibit replication of T-effector cells (immunologic enhancement). Another subpopulation of T-cells, called suppressor cells, arises late in immune cycle, may not require replication from primordial antigen-sensitive T-cell, and inhibits conversion of memory to effector T- and B-cells. This is similar to an X-Y-Z scheme of maturation where X-cells are multipotential cells, Y-cells are replicating cells of restricted potential and Z-cells are fully differentiated, unipotential effector cells with short half-lives

clonal multiplication for both immediate effector cells and replicating memory cells takes place; the *effector,* where the products of the differentiated immune cells neutralize or eliminate the foreign antigen; and the *autoregulatory,* where feedback inhibition by specific IgG antibody, unique cellular suppression mechanisms and the decreasing amount of antigen regulate the magnitude and form of the residual immune response. These divisions are schematized in Figure 3.

I. Afferent Phase — Antigen Recognition

Contact of antigeneic determinants with antigen-sensitive cells (ACS) begins the immune response. The initial contact is mediated through surface receptors on the lymphocytes.

1. Peripheral or central sensitization. Sensitization may occur peripherally (i.e., ASC migrate to the graft) or centrally (i.e., immunogen released from the graft into the venous or lymphatic circulation contact ASC in the spleen or lymph nodes). STROBER and GOWANS (1965) demonstrated the importance of peripheral sensitization in immediately vascularized renal grafts. Allogeneic sensitization occurred within one hour of recyclic perfusion of thoracic duct lymphocytes through a rat kidney *in situ.* The experiment did not clarify whether contact of circulating lymphocytes with the allogeneic endothelial cells was sufficient, whether antigen escaped into the host circulation, or whether host lymphocytes actually migrated through the renal parenchymal interstitial tissues to effect sensitization.

Two mechanisms create central sensitization. In one, donor lymphocytes existing in the graft as *passenger cells* leave the graft and colonize in lymph nodes and spleen. The major route of exit from immediately vascularized grafts like the kidney is venous; isolation of renal grafts from lymphatic connection by placing the graft in a plastic sac except for the blood vessels does not alter rejection time (HUME and EGDAHL, 1955). Removing passenger leukocytes by irradiation or treating the grafts with cortisone does delay rejection for both skin and renal grafts; however, rejection does ultimately occur.

The pathologic importance of interacting allogeneic lymphocytes in the skin is best illustrated by graft-versus-host (GVH) disease. Here, the lymphohematopoietic organs or tissues are most damaged (lymph nodes, spleen, thymus, bone marrow) and almost equally, the skin. The liver and the GI tract show slight damage, whereas muscle, bone, gonads, endocrine glands, kidney, lung, and nervous tissue are little affected. The skin is probably attacked so vigorously because of its content of leukocytes (BILLINGHAM, 1968). There are other considerations, however, why passenger leukocytes could not explain the entire process of sensitization by skin grafts. Split thickness skin grafts evoke an antibody response in recipients, detected by both hemagglutinating and cytotoxic assays. However, so do pure epidermal grafts which lack blood vessels and "contaminating" leukocytes (AMOS *et al.,* 1954).

The other method of central sensitization results from graft antigens reaching host lymphoid organs by being shed into venous or lymphatic channels. Transplantation antigens are not tightly bound to cell membranes; HL-A antigens have been detected in blood of healthy people (BILLING *et al.*, 1973) and in urine and blood of renal transplant recipients.

2. Privileged sites. A privileged site is one where allografts survive for long periods either because absent lymphatics or avascularity prevents the usual access of isoantigens to the antigen-sensitive cells of the host, or because avascularity prevents sensitized host lymphocytes from reaching the graft. These sites are the brain, the anterior chamber of the eye, the cheek pouch of the hamster, and perhaps the uterus. These sites offer no advantage if the host is presensitized. It has been assumed that these locations do not permit adequate primary sensitization. However, recent studies purporting to show lymphocyte infiltration of nonrejecting implants in the anterior chamber of the eye suggest the importance of other factors (RAJU and GROGAN, 1971).

3. Differences in rates of rejection between delayed and immediately vascularized grafts. Allografted skin is more rapidly rejected than other organs, such as kidney and heart, and its survival is less easily prolonged by modifying the immune response. There are many explanations for this phenomenon. Firstly, the rate of vascularization, slow in skin, may result in ischemic damage with greater vulnerability to immunologic attack. Secondly, skin has a relatively rich lymphatic drainage system which is rapidly established after grafting, Indeed, BARKER and BILLINGHAM (1968) have demonstrated that the lymphatics are a prime pathway of sensitization in skin. If skin grafting is performed so as to prevent re-establishment of the lymphatic drainage, survival is prolonged 20–50 days. As stated earlier, however, similar isolation of kidney grafts do not alter rejection rates. Thirdly, accumulating evidence indicates quantitative and/or qualitative differences in the antigenicity of skin and other organs (LANCE *et al.*, 1971). Finally, organs with immediate vascularization may evoke more of a humoral than a cellular reaction and such interactions of humoral and cellular immunity may autoregulate the immune response.

GRUBER and LUCAS (1972) attempted to differentiate between the effects of lymphatic and vascular connections by performing four types of skin grafts differing in the rates of re-establishing vascular or lymphatic connections. A schematic summary of the types of grafts is presented in Figure 4. The conventional skin graft has immediate re-establishment of lymphatic drainage, but vascularization occurs later, on the fourth or fifth day. When an allograft is placed on an isolated island pedicle flap, with lymphatics stripped from the sole artery and vein, the interposition of a silicone sheet between the flap and its bed prevents lymphatic re-establishment and constitutes a condition that has both delayed lymphatic and delayed vascular connections (Barker-Billingham technique). A skin graft pedicle with its central blood vessels anastomosed to the femoral vessels of the recipient creates both immediate lymphatic and vascular connections. Lastly, an allogeneic pedicle directly anastomosed to recipient vessels but with other contact prevented by interposition of the silicon sheet represents immediate vascularization and delayed lymphatic connection. The mean survival of skin grafted from (Lewis × Brown Norway) F_1 hybrid to Lewis (parental) rats by these four techniques is shown in Table 3. Rejection is delayed only if the rates of both vascular and lymphatic reconstitution are delayed, as with the Barker-Billingham technique. This suggests that the lym-

DELAYED VASCULAR IMMEDIATE LYMPHATIC (DV–IL)

DELAYED VASCULAR DELAYED LYMPHATIC (DV–DL)

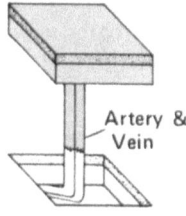

Epithelium

Subcutaneous Tissue

Silicone Rubber Sheet

IMMEDIATE VASCULAR IMMEDIATE LYMPHATIC (IV–IL)

IMMEDIATE VASCULAR DELAYED LYMPHATIC (IV–DL)

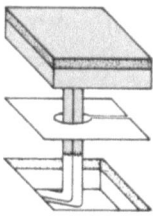

Artery & Vein

Fig. 4. Schematic summary of 4 skin graft models differing in rates of vascular and lymphatic reconstitution. (WUSTRACK *et al.*, 1975; by courtesy of the Williams and Wilkins Co.)

Table 3. Survival of four different skin graft models with enhancing alloimmune serum

Treatment	DV–IL	DV–DL	IV–IL	IV–DL	
				no serum	nonimmune serum
No additives	6, 7, 8, 8, 8, 8, 8, 8 7.6 ± 0.7	12, 12, 16, 16, 17, 22 15.8 ± 3.7	6, 7, 7, 7, 7, 8, 9, 9, 9, 9, 9 7.9 ± 1.1	8, 8, 8, 8, 8, 9, 9 8.3 ± 0.5	6, 7, 8, 8, 9
EAS[a]	7, 8, 8, 9, 11 8.6 ± 1.5 NS[b]	14, 17, 19, 20 17.5 ± 2.7 NS	9, 9, 9, 10, 10 9.4 ± 0.6 NS	11, 11, 12, 14, 14, 17 13.2 ± 2.3 $P = 0.001$[c]	

[a] EAS, enhancing alloimmune serum
[b] NS, not statistically significant
[c] P values compared with untreated grafts of each skin graft model

phatic and vascular routes are both equally effective in inducing sensitization. The relative importance of vascular lymphatic connections relating to immunologic enhancement will be discussed shortly.

II. Central Phase—Clonal Proliferation, Yielding both Memory and Differentiated Effector Cells

Four to six days are required to mount an effective immunologic response to an allograft. During this time, antigen-sensitive cells, small lymphocytes which are metabolically inactive, undergo proliferation. Since only the specific cells bearing receptors for the antigen replicate, this is termed *clonal* proliferation. Some cells differentiate into effector T-cells, others into effector B-cells (antibody-secreting cells); others "regress" into memory T- or B-cells. The molecular process whereby a membrane event, the combination of specific antigen with the specific membrane receptor, is translated into gene derepression or activation remains a mystery.

BILLINGHAM *et al.* (1954) first noted that after skin grafting, the regional lymph nodes undergo proliferative reactions. Simultaneously, MITCHISON (1954) showed that cells in the regional lymph nodes were capable of transmitting memory by adoptive immunization much earlier than cells in other lymphoid tissue. The efferent lymph carries both the cells that carry memory to other organs (CHANANA *et al.*, 1969) as well as the differentiated effector cells which "home" to the target organs and proceed to destroy the graft (CHANANA *et al.*, 1969; WILSON, 1963).

The blastogenic and proliferative response in the local lymph nodes does not yield information as to the mechanism of sensitization. Either allogeneic passenger leukocytes or circulating host lymphocytes sensitized by passage through the graft can enter the reconstituted efferent lymphatics, as can solubilized antigen from the host bed (ELVES, 1970).

III. Effector Phase—the Expression of Immunity

The aim of the immune response is to dispose of a foreign substance. This is accomplished by several different mechanisms: firstly, clonal proliferation of a specifically sensitized T-lymphocyte cytotoxic to target cells; secondly, clonal proliferation of specifically sensitized lymphoid cells that produce antibodies reacting with the antigen; thirdly, recruitment of a nonspecific cellular inflammatory response by lymphokines secreted by activated specific lymphocytes; and fourthly, activation of a general humoral inflammatory response involving four cascading systems normally present in blood: coagulation, fibrinolysis, complement, and kinin generation. Each category will be discussed as it applies to destruction of skin grafts.

1. Specific Immune Cytotoxic Mechanisms

a) Cell-mediated Cytotoxicity (T-cell). Histocompatibility antigen sensitive T-lymphocytes upon contact with allogeneic cells, proliferate and differentiate into cytotoxic T-cells. T-cell mediated cytotoxicity (T-CMC) is considered to be the major immunopathic process during acute allograft rejection. Methods for *in vitro* detection of specific cytotoxic cells have only recently been developed (BRUNNER *et al.*, 1968; LUCAS and WALKER, 1974). The microcytotoxicity assay, the most frequently used technique, observes the difference in target cell number when immune or nonimmune lymphocytes are cultured with target cells. *In vitro* studies have established two phases of cell lysis; one, lymphocyte-dependent; the other, lymphocyte-independent. Subsequently, specific contact occurs between lymphocyte and target, followed by a lymphocyte process that requires cAMP (perhaps indicating the secretion of a toxin) (BOURNE *et al.*, 1974). Thereafter, the lymphocyte detaches from the target in which during the next several minutes to hours, progressively larger osmotic defects occur. Although it is now clear that a cytotoxic cell may kill more than one target and is itself not consumed in the lytic reaction, the fate of a cytotoxic cell remains unknown. Its half-life appears to be only 2–3 days. Antigen is required for its continued generation from memory cells. Such generation may be inhibited by another subpopulation of T-cells, called *suppressor* cells (KUPERMAN *et al.,* 1975).

A current view of the mechanism of skin graft rejection is that cytotoxic cells are generated by proliferation of ASC in the local lymph node and reach the graft through the blood and proceed to destroy it. A pertinent question is whether sufficient numbers of cytotoxic lymphocytes ever enter the skin graft to account for its destruction. Recent findings that many of the mononuclear cells in the rejecting skin graft are of recent bone marrow origin, probably belonging to the monocyte-macrophage series prompt this question (GIROUD *et al.,* 1970). In addition, experiments a decade earlier showed that lymphocytes generated in response to a certain allogeneic graft do not accumulate any more preferentially in that specific graft than in a third party graft (NAJARIAN and FELDMAN, 1962; PRENDERGAST, 1964; HALL, 1962). Such experiments suggest that lymphocytes accumulating in the graft are a random selection of the types present in blood. More recent experiments do show a slight preferential localization of sensitized lymphocytes in specific skin allografts (LANCE and COOPER, 1972; TILNEY and FORD, 1974). The differences, however, are small and their significance may not be related to their direct cytotoxic activity. These cited experiments leave little doubt that the majority of the cells infiltrating a skin graft have *not* been produced specifically in response to the skin graft.

b) Antibody-mediated Cytotoxicity. Antibodies belonging mainly to the IgG and IgM classes bind to cell surface antigens and destroy the target cell by one of four separate mechanisms. *Opsonic adherence,* the major defense against bacteria, is mediated through either IgG or IgM antibodies adhering to the cell surface, thereby altering the net surface electric charge and permitting contact with phagocytes (either PMN or macrophage). *Immune adherence* utilizes receptors on effector cells for the Fc portion of the antibody for linkage to the target. PMN, macrophages, and certain classes of lymphocytes have such surface receptors. Cell destruction occurs either by digestion by lysosomal enzymes from the degranulating macrophages and PMN or by an unknown mechanism utilizing nonsensitized k-lymphocytes (antibody-dependent cell cytotoxicity, ADCC). Lymphocytes are defined by their surface antigens; T-cell membranes contain a specific T-cell antigen (θ in the mouse) and little or no surface immuno-globulin; B-cells contain immunoglobulins and no T-cell antigen; k-cells or null-cells contain neither. Presumably all contain Fc receptors.

Macrophages and PMN cells adhere to targets by still another method. They have membrane receptors for the C3 component of complement. The combination of IgG and IgM with antigen induces a conformational change in the Fc portion, which causes activation and binding of the complement system. When C3 is added to the cellular antigen-antibody-complement complex, PMN or macrophages bind and cause lysis. Lastly, the continued sequential addition of complement ultimately results in the fixation and activation of the terminal C9 component; this ultimately disrupts the target membrane. IgM, having five Fc fragments, is more efficient than IgG in binding complement, and hence, in cytolysis.

The role of antibodies in the accelerated rejection of skin grafts is generally undisputed. However, their role in the acute homograft rejection, if any, is still uncertain. Allogeneic skin grafts are indefinitely accepted by genetically *nude* mice, which have either no or only a rudimentary thymus and do not make antibodies to T-dependent antigens. However, there is histologic evidence of rejection. RYGAARD reported that at seven days, grafts in nude mice were markedly edematous and showed a mild to moderate granulocyte and histiocytic infiltration. In some areas, epidermolysis and re-epithelialization occurred. One week later, the graft edema had decreased, but sporadic areas of superficial necrosis appear with re-epithelialization from the deeper hair follicles (RYGAARD, 1974a, b, c).

BN rats immunosuppressed with rabbit anti-rat thymocyte serum and receiving allogenic (Lewis) skin offer still another model of the ability of antibody to mediate rejection. Such rats having a successfully accepted graft at eleven days reject in accelerated manner if given alloantiserum (BN anti-Le). Histologic studies show vascular dilatation with packing of the blood vessels with erythrocytes and PMN. The tissue spaces are densely infiltrated with PMN. Patchy disruption of blood vessels occur throughout the graft (OLUWASANMI, 1973).

2. Recruitment of Nonsensitized Effector Cells by Lymphokines Secreted by Sensitized T-Cells

The histologic hallmark of a rejecting graft is the dense mononuclear cell infiltrate. However, as described above, the cells are microscopically heterogeneous and contain large numbers of basophils, granulocytes, and macrophage-like cells as well as lymphocytes. In addition, few of the lymphocytes are specifically sensitized to graft antigens. What then, are the mechanisms by which cells accumulate in skin allografts? Several pathways are proposed. Specifically, sensitized lymphocytes could recognize the transplantation antigens in the endothelium of the graft blood vessels, stick, and then pass through or between the endothelial cells to gain entry to the interstitial spaces. The other cells randomly enter the graft, but are then retained by factors generated by the sensitized lymphocytes. Activated lymphocytes do secrete nonimmunoglobulin factors into supernatants which have a variety of biologic effects. These have been given

the generic term *lymphokines*. Among them are chemotactic factors for granulocytes, eosinophils, monocytes, and lymphocytes and migratory inhibition factors
(MIF) for macrophages. Alternatively, even the sensitized lymphocyte could
enter the graft randomly and be inhibited from migrating upon recognition
of antigens on nonendothelial cells (DUMONDE, D.C., 1970).

The similarity between the sequential histologic events during graft rejection
and delayed hypersensitivity skin reactions, in which over 90% of the infiltrating
cells are nonspecific, suggests the importance of recruitment in cellular immune
reactions. In the local area, the accumulated cells are "instructed" by other
lymphokines or antibody to kill the target specifically. Such factors, detected
by biologic assays (specific macrophage activating factor), have not been characterized (ALEXANDER and EVANS, 1971).

The importance of nonspecific cell processes in skin graft destruction is
indicated by the fate of returned skin allografts (LAMBERT and FRANK, 1970).
Skin grafts returned to the untreated skin donor after a four day period on
an intermediate host were reaccepted but only after an intense reaction in
the graft which causes spotty epithelial destruction. The reaction resembles
an induced transfer reaction (DVORAK, 1963). The epithelial destruction was
due to granulocytic and histiocytic infiltration and occurred only if the intermediate host were immunologically competent.

3. Local Activation of the Host's General Inflammatory Response

Two pivotal reactions determine the direction, the intensity, and the speed
with which inflammatory processes are superimposed on the immunologic attack
against a graft. One is the activation of complement; the other, the extent
of vascular endothelial cell injury. The attachment of complement factors to
antigen-antibody complexes occur by removing polypeptides from the inactive
forms present in serum. The larger portions are incorporated into the growing
complex, but the smaller polypeptide split products also have biologic activities.
Thus, anaphylatoxins, split products of C3 and C5, cause histamine release
and local vascular permeability changes. Other complement split products act
as chemotactic factors leading to influx of PMN leukocytes. Such reactions
at the endothelial interface between donor and recipient cause clotting via at
least three mechanisms: one, anaphylatoxin, either directly or indirectly through
vasospasm, activates Hageman factor present in endothelial cells; this permits
thrombin synthesis and the conversion of fibrinogen to fibrin. Two, massive
endothelial cell damage directly activates Hageman factor. The result may be
catastrophic, with total thrombosis and immediate infarction. This is the cause
of the hyperacute rejection syndrome in renal transplants. Last, immune complexes on the endothelial surface aggregate platelets, releasing vasoactive amines,
and forming microthrombi. In addition, activated Hageman factor induces kinin
generation which further decreases tissue perfusion and promotes tissue edema.
Into this increased extracellular fluid space the chemotactic factors draw the
mononuclear cells and PMN leukocytes from the locally slowed circulation.

The liberated Hageman factor simultaneously evokes a counter reaction,
plasminogen activation. Plasmin has two major actions: inactivating Hageman

factor, which stops further fibrin deposition; and enzymatically digesting the fibrin already deposited. In acute homograft rejection these events occur at a slow rate; thrombosis occurs only at a microscopic level, the fibrinolytic reaction keeping pace with the rate of fibrin deposition. This can be readily detected by the marked increase in fibrin-split products in the urine of patients undergoing renal rejection.

4. Correlation of Immunologic and Pathophysiologic Events with Clinical Skin Graft Rejection Syndromes

a) First Set Skin Graft Rejection. Studies of human skin grafts confirm the observations made in animals. The gross or stereomicroscopic appearance of microvasculature of autografts or allografts shows no detectable difference for several days. Each remains blanched for 24 hours, becoming pink by days 3–4. Initially, superficial capillaries are dilated and filled with blood. Flow begins on the third or fourth day, becoming generalized in two more days. Autografts have desquamation of the superficial epithelium, with simultaneous regeneration; by day 6–7 the graft and host epidermis merge.

With allografts a halo of erythema and edema becomes increasingly prominent on the day 6–7 (Fig. 1B). The color becomes cherry red, then cyanotic. Allografts become progressively more edematous. Cyanosis is followed by hemorrhage, dessication, and ultimately escharification (Fig. 1C). These changes relate to alterations in the new blood supply; the superficial capillaries progressively dilate, blood flow stops by day 8–9 and the vessels thrombose shortly thereafter.

Histologic changes similar to those in acutely rejecting kidneys occur, with one exception. Mononuclear cell infiltration is distributed in two layers: in the graft, somewhat localized in the subdermal area; and in the top of the host bed, the true interface between donor and host.

b) Second Set Rejection. The interval between the first and second grafts profoundly affects the survival of second set grafts. A second graft from the same donor performed less than seven days following removal of the rejected first graft, induces a *white graft* reaction. The graft never becomes vascularized. Twenty-four hours after placement, a prominent band of edema fluid filled with PMN leukocytes separates the graft from the underlying host tissues. Twenty-four hours later, the graft necroses with dense infiltration of PMN cells, migrating upwards from the host bed. This corresponds to the hyperacute rejection syndrome in renal grafts. Clotting in the graft does not occur because revascularization does not occur.

Extending the interval between consecutive allografts in mice beyond 12 days causes an *accelerated* type of response. Such grafts show the usual characteristics of an early take, but the rejection process is telescoped into 5–7 days, about four days faster than first set grafts. The histologic features, similar to acute rejection, occur more rapidly in *accelerated rejection*. Lastly, if the interval between the two grafts is extended to 80 days, the graft rejects as a first set graft.

White graft and accelerated graft rejections are mediated by all four effector mechanisms discussed in the previous section, and occurs in presensitized individuals. Placing a kidney into a presensitized recipient almost invariably results in rapid graft destruction. This may be catastrophically rapid, within minutes of grafting (xenograft rejection or hyperacute rejection in allografts) or it may evolve over one to two days of progressive oliguria (accelerated rejection) (LUCAS *et al.,* 1970). The *forme fruste* of this syndrome is seen in skin grafts only under certain experimental conditions because it requires a vascularized state. Such situations are created when animals are immunosuppressed to permit graft survival and then infused with alloantibody (BALDAMUS *et al.,* 1973; KOENE *et al.,* 1973; OLUWASANMI, 1973; WINN *et al.,* 1973). Grafts were rejected within 24–48 hours and require the participation of complement and PMN leukocytes. BALDAMUS *et al.* (1973) were able to prolong rat skin grafted onto mouse for 23–62 days by immunosuppression by thymectomy and rabbit anti-mouse lymphocyte serum. Intravenous administration of mouse anti-rat serum resulted in edema and margination of PMN leukocytes within 5–10 minutes. The PMN's rapidly increased in number and migrated into the interstitial spaces. By 4–6 hours, vessels had become greatly diluted, congested and variously filled with fibrin thrombi. Shortly thereafter, many vessels ruptured and widespread interstitial hemorrhage occurred. These features are similar to those of Arthus reactions.

IV. Autoregulatory Phase

Under ordinary conditions an animal does not develop effector cells or antibodies reacting with its own antigens. In the last twenty years the concept has emerged that the host has lost its capacity to react against itself and instead, has acquired a "natural tolerance to self-antigens". The termination of "natural tolerance" results in *autoimmunity.* BURNET and FENNER (1949) postulated that exposing primitive antigen-sensitive cells to antigen in early fetal life would render those cells incapable of clonal multiplication. The continuous presence of self-antigens forever prevents the emergence of cells responding to self-antigens; such cells are "forbidden clones". The essential validity of this prediction was established when BILLINGHAM *et al.* (1956) induced *tolerance* in mice to histocompatibility antigens by neonatal injection of viable lymphocytes. Since then, immunologic unresponsiveness has been induced to a variety of antigens in neonatal animals, and under certain conditions, in adult animals. Its initiation is dependent on the nature of the antigen, its dose, and the immunocompetence of the animal.

Another state of unresponsiveness, *immunologic enhancement,* is mediated by antibody reacting with the specific antigen. FLEXNER and JOBLING (1906) observed that tumor injected simultaneously with immune serum from animals dying of the same tumor grew much faster than in animals injected with tumor alone. Enhanced tumor growth was subsequently found to result from inhibition of an already ineffectual immune response, leading to earlier death of the animal. This section presents basic concepts concerned with two types of immunologic unresponsiveness to skin grafts: the induction and maintenance of states of either complete or partial tolerance and states of enhancement.

1. Complete or Partial Tolerance

a) Conditions Affecting Induction, Maintenance, and Reversal of Immunologic Tolerance

In the last two decades, a great deal of work has been expended in defining the tolerant state induced not only by neonatal exposure to antigen, but also by manipulations of the immune system in adult animals. The induction of tolerance depends on (1) the immunocompetence of the host, (2) the species and strain of animals, and (3) the nature, dose, and route of administering the antigen. The following general facts have emerged:

(1) It is easier to induce tolerance in immunologically incompetent animals than in normal adults. Methods utilized to abolish or to interfere with the immunocompetence of the host just prior to the administration of antigens are irradiation, immunosuppressive drugs, thoracic duct drainage, or treatment with antilymphocyte globulin (WOODRUFF and ANDERSON, 1963).

(2) The ease of immunologic tolerance depends upon the species and strain of animal. Completely unresponsive states of long duration can be induced in rabbits and mice; similar shorter states in guinea pigs and only hyporesponsive states in chickens (WEIGLE, 1973). Even greater variation occurs among various strains within a species. C57B6/6J mice are rendered tolerant by 0.1 mg deaggregated human gamma globulin; A/J mice required 1 mg; and Balb/CJ mice do not become tolerant with even 10 mg. Cross-mating these strains suggests that unresponsiveness is inherited.

(3) The nature, dose, and route of administration of antigen are major factors in the degree and the duration of tolerance. Antigen rapidly equilibrating between vascular and extravascular spaces are likely to induce tolerance. This is presumably because the antigen comes in contact with all antigen-reactive cells. Heterologous serum proteins, contrasting with bacterial and viral antigens or heterologous erythrocytes, are examples of substances to which tolerance is readily induced. Erythrocytes are rapidly removed from blood, do not equilibrate between the vascular and extravascular compartments, and usually induce only hyporesponsive states. Intravenous administration of antigen is required to obtain rapid distribution of the antigens to all ASC.

Many protein antigens can aggregate in concentrated solution to form polymers. In general, the aggregated or polymeric forms are excellent *immunogens* (a form of a substance that induces immunity); deaggregated or monomeric forms of the same antigen are more likely to induce unresponsiveness to a subsequent injection of the immunogenic form. These are called *tolerogens* (form of antigen that induces tolerance). Examples of immunogens and tolerogens are aggregated and deaggregated gamma globulins and serum albumins.

In general, the larger the dose of tolerogen injected, the more complete and the longer duration of unresponsiveness. With certain antigens, there appear to be two dosage ranges which induce tolerance, one high and one low, and an intermediate dose of antigen which induces immunity. This does not occur when a completely deaggregated antigen is used and may reflect a competition between antigen-sensitive cells and the tolerogenic and immunogenic forms of the antigen (WEIGLE, 1973). Although induced tolerance is often maintained for long periods, immunity returns without further administration of tolerogen. Spontaneous termination of tolerance coincides with the disappearance of antigen from tissue fluids.

b) The Absence of Reactive Cells or the Presence of Nonreactive Cells

Burnet's clonal selection theory suggested that animals develop a specific unresponsiveness to their own body components during early life before maturation of the immune process. The mechanism of how this is done is unknown. Presumably, antigen combines with the receptors of primitive antigen-sensitive cells and causes their elimination before ASC become immunocompetent. These ASC are "forbidden clones". BILLINGHAM et al. (1953) subsequently found that exposure of immunologically immature animals (fetuses or neonates) to foreign antigens would render them unresponsive to that antigen in adult life. Thus, the intrauterine injection of A-line tissue cells into pregnant CBA hosts resulted in offspring which many months after birth were able to accept A-line skin grafts for over 100 days (normal rejection time of A→CBA grafts is 11 ± 0.3 days). Tolerance to accepted skin grafts was broken by the transfer of cells from CBA mice previously sensitized by A-skin grafts.

The findings that antibody response is most readily explained by the mode in which the antigen was presented require modification of the "forbidden clone" theory. Thus, an antigen-sensitive lymphocyte, upon contact with an antigen, has essentially two courses of action: to become unresponsive (tolerant) or to become responsive (activated). The course taken is a property of the antigen (MITCHISON, 1970) rather than the ASC (WEIGLE, 1973). One must realize that experimentally it is very difficult to distinguish between the absence of reactive cells or the presence of nonreactive cells.

c) The Presence of Immunologically Active Lymphocytes Blocked by Serum Factors

The HELLSTROMS (1971) challenged views of essentially absent or nonreactive lymphocytes. Pioneers in the development of sensitive in vitro assays for cytotoxic lymphocytes, they detected such cells in mice rendered tolerant by neonatal injection of allogeneic lymphoid cells. Furthermore, sera from these "tolerant" animals prevented the cytotoxic cells from destroying the targets. Their experiments suggested that tolerance was a variant of immunologic enhancement and mediated by antibody.

BEVERLEY et al. (1973) re-examined the Hellstroms' murine system and found their animals only partially tolerant. By varying the numbers of injected cells into the newborn mice, they induced different degrees of partial or complete tolerance as assessed by duration of skin graft survival. Cytotoxic cells were detected only where tolerance was partial; blocking factors were seen only with very minimal states of unresponsiveness, and then solely as a transient phenomenon.

d) Other Alternatives: Suppressive or Regulatory Events Mediated by Lymphocytes on Immune Reactions

The general observation that every tolerant system yet studied has *some* immune response, although it may be very little, indicates the presence of at least *some* functioning cells. For example, the antibody response of a "completely" tolerant animal is not zero, but a low 2–5% of the normal level (WEIGLE, 1973). In addition, other findings suggest the possibility of a lymphocyte population involved in actively promoting tolerance or in *suppressing* the normal immune response. Thus, if an animal made tolerant to an antigen is irradiated before being challenged with the antigen, tolerance can be terminated, suggesting that perhaps an X-ray-sensitive cell maintains the tolerant state. "Suppressor" cell activity has been found in antigen competition systems, tolerance to soluble and cellular antigens, allotype suppression, nonreactivity to auto-antigens and in the "immunosuppression" accompanying GVH reactions. GERSHON and KONDO (1970) showed that one population of T-cells made in response to sheep red blood cells (SRBC) can block antibody formation against SRBC. Thymectomized irradiated mice repopulated with syngeneic bone marrow cells need T-lymphocytes to obtain maximal antibody levels. Substitution of spleen cells from a donor previously made unresponsive to SRBC prevents antibody formation. Unresponsiveness occurs with a failure of lymphocyte replication and cannot be broken by transfer of normal or even immune syngeneic cells. Thus, one subpopulation of T-cells is required for helper function and another for suppressing antibody formation. Nonreactivity is dominant over reactivity.

2. Immunologic Enhancement

The concept that passive immunity can block active immunization was established about 70 years ago (SMITH, 1909). The term *immunologic enhancement* is restricted to the indefinitely prolonged survival or the delayed rejection of allografts resulting from the presence of specific antigraft antibody in the host (KALISS, 1962). The mechanism is unknown except that it is mediated by antibody. This is a *conditio sine qua non,* separating enhancement from immunologic unresponsiveness (tolerance).

a) General Features of Graft Survival

Enhancement was first observed with tumor grafts, where much of the initial work was done. Accelerated growth of strain-specific tumors occurs in allogeneic recipients which have been pretreated with an antiserum directed against the tumor (passive enhancement) or with injection of antigenic material derived from the tumor genotype (active enhancement). Accelerated tumor growth represents a more successful "take" of the tumor graft. Different tumor cell types show a large variability in their response to enhancing antibodies *in vivo*. In general, the more sensitive the cell is to lysis by cytotoxic antibodies *in vitro*, the more difficult the attainment of enhancement *in vivo*.

Until recently the application of passive immunity to tissue grafts other than tumor cells has been only partially successful. BRENT and MEDAWAR (1962) increased skin graft survival by pretreating incompatible hosts with either passively administered antibodies or with lyophilized tissue.

Enhancement is an interplay between the antigen, the antibody it elicits and the host cellular immune response. The type of antigen and the route by which it is administered largely determine the optimal timing for grafting. Sensitization by allogeneic lymphocytes or solubilized antigen given intravenously does not elicit a cytotoxic cellular response. Kidneys will have prolonged survival if placed 3–6 days after one i.v. injection, or seven days after two i.v. injections 14 days apart. Sera obtained at those times from the sensitized animals (early phase sera) will passively confer indefinite enhancement (ENOMOTO and LUCAS, 1973). In this system transferable enhancing activity is detected before cytotoxic antibody.

Other methods of immunization (e.g., repeated intradermal inoculations of lymphocytes with or without Freund's adjuvant, primary skin or kidney graft) generate cytotoxic lymphocytes and a hyperimmune humoral response with high titers of hemolytic, cytolytic, and agglutinating antibodies. A test graft placed too soon after such stimulation experiences accelerated rejection, but as the time interval between sensitization and grafting increases, enhancement occurs.

b) Relationship Between Organ Vascularity and Immunologic Enhancement

Skin grafts are much more difficult to enhance than either kidney or heart grafts in the same experimental model. JEEKEL et al. (1972) demonstrated the importance of suppressing specifically the host response to all antigens in the skin graft. If the passively administered antisera did not contain antibodies to other H-2 or non-H-2 antigens not present in the recipient mice, prolonged survival was not attained.

The question of how skin grafts are revascularized is still unresolved. The major question is whether the endothelial cells of the regenerated vessels of the graft are derived from the host (and therefore, not antigenically different) or from the graft itself. LAMBERT (1971) showed that in the rabbit the vessels are of donor (graft) origin for at least the period up to and including acute rejection. Microangiographs showed the "regenerated" vessels to be preformed. Furthermore, autoradiography of donor skin prelabeled with ^{3}H-thymidine showed the label to be retained by the endothelial cells, whereas unlabeled skin placed on a labeled recipient's graft bed do not contain any appreciably labeled endothelial cells.

The importance of the rate at which the graft was vascularized was indicated by WARREN et al. (1973) who found that Lewis rats injected at birth with $(L \times BN)F_1$ hybrid lymph node cells accept vascularized heart organ grafts indefinitely, but reject 50% of heart tissue fragment grafts and all skin grafts. Results with skin graft models varying in the rates of lymphatic and vascular reconstitution are identical (WUSTRACK et al., 1975). Immunologic enhancement of skin graft survival resulted only when vascular reconstitution occurred before lymphatic reconstitution. Thus, as shown in table 3, a single injection of alloimmune serum increased mean survival of isolated anastomised pedicle grafts from 7.6 to 13.2 days. The treatment did not prolong survival of grafts with early lymphatic reconstitution even if vascularization was immediate (9.4 days).

There are several reports indicating that an intact spleen is necessary for inducing both active and passive enhancement for tumor and kidney grafts (ENOMOTO and LUCAS, 1973). Splenectomy before or up to 6 days after renal grafting completely blocked the effect of alloimmune serum administered at the time of grafting. The same situation occurs with the passive enchanceability of isolated surgically vascularized pedicle skin grafts (WUSTRACK et al., 1975).

The observation that passive enhancement is effected only in immediately vascularized allografts in recipients with intact spleen suggests the following hypothesis. Passively administered antibody combines with endothelial antigen, is released into the blood as an antigen-antibody complex, and is then processed by the spleen in a manner different from antigen processing in the local lymphatics. There is evidence for each of these processes. Radiolabeled alloimmune globulin, prepared from alloimmune serum, specifically binds to renal (MORRIS and LUCAS, 1971) and skin graft (JONES et al., 1972) antigens. Histocompatibility antigen-antibody complexes are shed off cell surfaces (FAANES et al., 1973; FINE et al., 1973) and circulate in the blood (ROLLEY and MARCHALONIS, 1972). KAPLAN and STREILEIN (1974) have recently made a similar suggestion. They find that when allogeneic skin is grafted into the anterior chamber of the eye, a privileged site, graft survival is prolonged only if the spleen has not been removed. They interpret the critical feature of a privileged site to be the ability to allow antigen direct access to the blood vasculative without first encountering a peripheral lymph node. The initial antigen encounter thus occurs in the spleen, which differ from lymph nodes in its rapid antibody response and in its contents of suppressor T-cells.

The views expressed here suggest that the end result of a graft is determined by a quantitative seesaw battle between cytotoxic lymphocytes and various blocking factors and suppressor cells (FELDMAN, 1972). Early vascularization and an intact spleen promote the production of humoral or cellular blocking factors. Lymphatic reconstitution promotes specific cellular cytotoxic mechanisms. Long-term survival is achievable in renal grafts, but not in skin grafts where the degree of lymphatic reconstitution ultimately attained is greater.

References

ALEXANDER, P., EVANS, R.: Endotoxin and double-stranded RNA render macrophages cytotoxic. Nature [New Biol.] 232, 76–78 (1971)

AMOS, D.B., GORER, P.A., MIKULSKA, B.M., BILLINGHAM, R.E., SPARROW, E.M.: An antibody response to skin homografts in mice. Br. J. Exp. Pathol. 35, 203–208 (1954)

AMOS, D.B., SEIGLER, H.F., SOUTHWORTH, J.G., WARD, F.E.: Skin graft rejection between subjects genotyped for HL-A. Transplant. Proc. 1, 342–346 (1969)

BAILEY, D.W., MOBRAATEN, L.H.: Estimates of the number of histocompatibility loci at which the Balb/c and C57BL/G strain of mice differ. (Abstract) Genetics 50, 233 (1964)

BALDAMUS, CA.A., McKENZIE, I.F.C., WINN, H.J., RUSSELL, P.S.: Acute destruction by humoral antibody of rat skin grafted to mice. J. Immunol. 110, 1532–1541 (1973)

BARKER, C.E., BILLINGHAM, R.E.: The role of afferent lymphatics in the rejection of skin homografts. J. Exp. Med. 128, 197–221 (1968)

BEVERLEY, P.C.L., BRENT, L., BROOKS, C., MEDAWAR, P.B., SIMPSON, E.: *In vitro* reactivity of lymphoid cells from tolerant mice. Transplant. Proc. **5**, 679–684 (1973)

BILLING, R.J., MITTAL, K.K., TERASAKI, P.: Isolation of soluble HL-A antigens from normal human sera by ion exchange chromatography. Tissue Antigens **3**, 251–256 (1973)

BILLINGHAM, R.E., BRENT, L., MEDAWAR, P.B.: Activity acquired tolerance to foreign cells. Nature (Lond.) **172**, 603–606 (1953)

BILLINGHAM, R.E., BRENT, L., MEDAWAR, P.B., SPARROW, E.M.: Quantitative studies on tissue transplantation immunity. II. The origin, strength and duration of actively and adoptively acquired immunity. Proc. R. Soc. Lond. (Biol.) **143**, 58–80 (1954)

BILLINGHAM, R.E., BRENT, L., MEDAWAR, P.B.: Quantitative studies on tissue transplantation immunity. III. Actively acquired tolerance. Phil. Trans. R. Soc. Lond. (Biol.) **239**, 357–412 (1956)

BILLINGHAM, R.E.: The biology of graft-versus-host reactions. Harvey Lectures **62**, 21–78 (1968)

BOURNE, H.R., LICHTENSTEIN, L.M., MELMON, K.L., HENNEY, C.S., WEINSTEIN, Y., SHEARER, G.M.: Modulation of inflammation and immunity by cyclic AMP. Science **184**, 19–28 (1974)

BRENT, L., MEDAWAR, R.B.: Quantitative studies on transplantation immunity. V. The role of antiserum in enhancement and desensitization. Proc. R. Soc. Lond. (Biol.) **155**, 392–416 (1962)

BRUNNER, K.T., MAUEL, J., CEROTTINI, J.-C., CHAPUIS, B.: Quantitative assay for the lytic action of immune lymphoid cells on ^{51}Cr-labelled allogeneic target cells *in vitro*. Inhibition by isoantibody and by drugs. Immunology **14**, 181–196 (1968)

BURNET, F.M., FENNER, T.: The Production of Antibodies. Melbourne: MacMillan and Co., Ltd. 1949

CHANANA, A.D., CRONKITE, E.P., JOEL, D.D., SCHIFFER, L.M., SCHNAPPAUF, H.: Studies on lymphocytes. XII. The role of immunologically committed lymphocytes in rejecting skin allografts. Transplantation **7**, 459–467 (1969)

CONVERSE, J.M., CASSON, P.R.: The historical background of transplantation. In: Human Transplantation. RAPAPORT and DAUSSET (eds.). New York-London: Grune and Stratton 1968, p. 3–10

DUMONDE, D.C.: Lymphokines: Mediators and regulators of cellular immunity. In: Immunopathology, VIth Int. Symposium. MIESCHER (ed.). Basel-Stuttgart: Schwabe and Co. 1970, pp. 289–295

DVORAK, H.C., KOSUNEN, T.U., WAKSMAN, B.H.: The "transfer reaction" in the rabbit: A histologic study. Lab. Invest. **12**, 58–68 (1963)

ELKINS, W.L., HELLSTROM, I., HELLSTROM, K.E.: Transplantation tolerance and enhancement. Transplantation **18**, 38–45 (1974)

ELVES, N.W.: Migration of small lymphocytes from the skin to the regional lymph nodes. Nature **227**, 725–727 (1970)

ENOMOTO, K., LUCAS, Z.J.: Immunologic enhancement of renal allografts in the rat. III. Role of the spleen. Transplantation **15**, 8–16 (1973)

FAANES, R.B., CHOI, Y.S., GOOD, R.A.: Escape from isoantiserum inhibition of lymphocyte-mediated cytotoxicity. J. Exp. Med. **137**, 171–182 (1973)

FELDMAN, J.D.: Immunologic enhancement: A study of blocking antibodies. Adv. Immunol. **15**, 167–214 (1972)

FINE, R.N., BATCHELOR, J.R., FRENCH, M.E.: The uptake of ^{125}I-labelled rat alloantibody and its loss after combination with antigen. Transplantation **16**, 641–648 (1973)

FLEXNER, S., JOBLING, S.W.: On the promoting influence of heated tumor emulsions on tumor growth. Proc. Soc. Exp. Biol. Med. **4**, 156–157 (1906)

GERSHON, R.K., KONDO, K.: Cell interactions in the induction of tolerance; the role of thymic lymphocytes. Immunology **18**, 723–737 (1920)

GIROUD, J.P., SPECTOR, W.G., WILLOUGHBY, D.A.: Bone marrow and lymph node cells in the rejection of skin allografts in mice. Immunology **19**, 857–863 (1970)

GOWANS, J.L., McGREGOR, D.D., COWEN, D.M.: The role of small lymphocytes in the rejection of homograft skin. In: The Immunologically Competent Cell. Ciba Foundation Study Group No. 16. WALSTENHOLME and KNIGHT (eds.). London-Boston: Little, Brown and Co. 1963, pp. 20–38

GRAFF, R.J., HILDEMANN, W.A., SNELL, G.D.: Histocompatibility genes of mice. VI. Allografts in mice congenic at various non-H-2 histocompatibility loci. Transplantation **4**, 425–437 (1966a)

GRAFF, R.J., SILBER, W.K., BILLINGHAM, R.E., HILDEMANN, W.H., SNELL, G.D.: The cumulative effect of histocompatibility antigens. Transplantation **4**, 605–617 (1966b)

GRUBER, R.P., LUCAS, Z.J.: The effect of lymphatic interruption and immediate vascularization on the afferent arc of skin graft rejection. In: Microenvironmental Aspects of Immunity. JANKOVIC and ISAKOVIC (eds.). New York: Plenum Publishing Co. 1972, pp. 545–551

HALL, J.G.: Studies of the cells in the afferent and efferent lymph of lymph nodes draining the site of skin homografts. J. Exp. Med. **115**, 1083–1093 (1962)

HELLSTROM, K.E., HELLSTROM, I., ALLISON, A.C.: Neonatally induced allograft tolerance may be mediated by serum-borne factors. Nature (Lond.) **230**, 49–50 (1971)

HILDEMAN, W.H.: Components and concepts of antigenic strength. Transplant. Rev. **3**, 5–21 (1970)

HUME, D.M., EGDAHL, R.H.: Progressive destruction of renal homografts isolated from the regional lymphatics of the host. Surgery **38**, 194–214 (1955)

JAKOBIAK, M.: Quantitative data concerning the development of the cellular infiltrates of skin allograft in mice. Transplantation **12**, 364–367 (1971)

JEEKEL, J.J., McKENZIE, I.F.C., WINN, H.J.: Immunologic enhancement of skin grafts in the mouse. J. Immunol. **108**, 1017–1024 (1972)

JONES, J.M., PETER, H.H., FELDMAN, J.D.: Binding *in vivo* of enhancing antibodies to skin allografts and specific allogeneic tissues. J. Immunol. **108**, 301–309 (1972)

KALISS, N.: The elements of immunologic enhancement; a consideration of mechanism. Ann. N.Y. Acad. Sci. **101**, 64–79 (1962)

KAPLAN, H.J., STREILEIN, J.W.: Do immunologically privileged sites require a functioning spleen? Nature (Lond.) **251**, 553–554 (1974)

KOENE, R.A.P., GERLAQ, P.G.G., HAGEMANN, J.F.H.M., VAN HAELST, U.J.G., WIJDEVELD, P.G.A.B.: Hyperacute rejection of skin allografts in the mouse by the administration of alloantibody and rabbit complement. J. Immunol. **111**, 520–526 (1973)

KUPERMAN, O., FORTNER, G.W., LUCAS, Z.J.: Immune response to a syngeneic mammary adenocarcinoma. III. Development of memory and suppressor functions modulating cellular cytotoxicity. J. Immunol. **115**, to be published in November 1975

LAMBERT, P.B., FRANK, H.A.: Cellular and vascular components of the allograft reaction. Evidence from returned skin allografts. J. Exp. Med. **132**, 868–884 (1970)

LAMBERT, P.B.: Vascularization of skin grafts. Nature **232**, 279–280 (1971)

LANCE, E.M., BOYSE, E.A., COOPER, S., CARSWELL, E.A.: Rejection of skin allografts by irradiation chimeras: Evidence for skin-specific transplantation barrier. Transplant. Proc. **3**, 864–868 (1971)

LANCE, E.M., COOPER, S.: Homing of specifically sensitized lymphocytes to allografts of skin. Cell. Immunol. **5**, 66–73 (1972)

LUCAS, Z.J., COPLON, N., KEMPSON, R., COHN, R.: Early renal transplant failure associated with subliminal sensitization. Transplantation **10**, 552–529 (1970)

LUCAS, Z.J., WALKER, S.M.: Cytotoxic activity of lymphocytes. III. Standardization of measurement of cell-mediated lysis. J. Immunol. **113**, 209–224 (1974)

McDONALD, J.C., ZIMMERMAN, G., BOLLINGER, R.R., PIERCE, W.A. JR.: Immune competence in germ-free rats. Proc. Soc. Exp. Biol. Med. **136**, 987–993 (1971)

MEDAWAR, P.B.: The behavior and fate of skin autografts and skin homografts in rabbits. J. Anat. **78**, 176–199 (1944)

MITCHISON, N.A.: Passive transfer of transplantation immunity. Proc. R. Soc. Lond. (Biol.) **143**, 72–87 (1954)

MITCHISON, N.A.: Cell cooperation in the immune response: The hypothesis of an antigen presentation mechanism. In: Immunopathology VIth Symposium, MIESCHER (ed.). Basel-Stuttgart: Schwabe and Co. 1970, pp. 52–63

MORRIS, R., LUCAS, Z.J.: Immunologic enhancement of rat kidney grafts: Evidence for peripheral action of homologous antiserum. Transplant. Proc. **3**, 697–700 (1971)

MURPHY, J.B.: Lymphocyte in resistance to tissue grafting, malignant disease and tuberculocis infection. Rockefeller Inst. for Med. Res. Monogr. **21**, 168 (1926)

NAJARIAN, J.S., FELDMAN, J.D.: Passive transfer of transplantation immunity; I. Tritiated lymphoid cells; II. Lymphoid cells in millipore chambers. J. Exp. Med. **115**, 1083–1093 (1962)

OLUWASANMI, J.O.: The role of hyperimmune alloantiserum in allograft survival. Immunology **25**, 881–889 (1973)

PRENDERGAST, R.A.: Cellular specificity in the homograft reaction. J. Exp. Med. **119**, 377–387 (1964)

POULTER, L.W., BRADLEY, N.J., TURK, J.L.: The role of macrophages in skin allograft rejection. I. Histochemical studies during first set rejection. Transplantation 12, 40–44 (1971)

RAJU, S., GROGAN, J.B.: Immunology of anterior chamber of the eye. Transplant. Proc. 3, 605–608 (1971)

ROLLEY, R.T., MARCHALONIS, J.J.: Release and assay of antigen-binding immunoglobulin from the surfaces of lymphocytes of unsensitized mice. Transplantation 14, 734–741 (1972)

RYGAARD, J.: Skin grafts in nude mice. I. Allografts in nude mice of three genetic backgrounds (Balb/c, C3H, C57/BL). Acta Pathol. Microbiol. Scand. [A] 82, 80–92 (1974a)

RYGAARD, J.: Skin grafts in nude mice. II. Rat skin grafts in nude mice of three genetic backgrounds (Balb/c, C3H, C57/BL). The effects after preparation by thymus grafts. Acta Pathol. Microbiol. Scand. [A] 82, 93-104 (1974b)

RYGAARD, J.: Skin grafts in nude mice. III. Fate of grafts from man and donors of other taxonomic classes. Acta Pathol. Microbiol. Scand. [A] 82, 105–112 (1974c)

SMITH, T.: Active immunity produced by so-called balanced or neutral mixtures of diphtheria toxin and antitoxin. J. Exp. Med. 11, 241–256 (1909)

SNELL, G.D., STIMPFLING, J.H.: Genetics of tissue transplantation. In: Biology of the Laboratory Mouse. GREEN, E.L. (ed.). New York: McGraw-Hill 1966, p. 457

STROBER, S., GOWANS, J.L.: The role of lymphocytes in the sensitization of rats to renal homografts. J. Exp. Med. 122, 347–360 (1965)

THIERSCH, C.: Über Hautverpflanzung. Verh. Dtsch. Ges. Chir. 15, 17 (1886)

TILNEY, N.L., FORD, W.L.: The migration of rat lymphoid cells into skin grafts. Some sensitized cells localize preferentially in specific allografts. Transplantation 17, 12-21 (1974)

WARREN, R.P., LOFGREEN, J.S., STEINMULLER, D.: Factors responsible for the differential survival of heart and skin allografts in inbred rats. Transplantation 16, 458–465 (1973)

WEIGLE, W.O.: Immunologic unresponsiveness. Adv. Immunol. 16, 61–122 (1973)

WEINER, J., SPIRO, D., RUSSELL, P.S.: An electron microscopic study of the homograft reaction. Am. J. Pathol. 44, 319-345 (1964)

WILSON, D.B.: The reaction of immunologically activated lymphoid cells against homologous target tissue in vitro. J. Cell. Comp. Physiol. 62, 273–286 (1963)

WINN, H.J., BALDAMUS, C.A., JOOSTE, S.U., RUSSELL, P.S.: Acute destruction by humoral antibody of rat skin grafted to mice: The role of complement and polymorphonuclear leucocytes. J. Exp. Med. 137, 893–910 (1973)

WOODRUFF, M.F.A., ANDERSON, N.D.: Effect of lymphatic depletion by thoracic duct fistula and administration of anti-lymphocyte serum on the survival of skin homografts in rats. Nature (Lond.) 200, 702 (1963)

WUSTRACK, K.O., GRUBER, R.P., LUCAS, Z.J.: Immunologic enhancement of skin allografts in the rat. Transplantation 19, 156-165 (1975)

Transplantation of Connective Tissue

(Tendon, cutis, fascia, and dura)

M. JÄGER and C.J. WIRTH

With 16 Figures

A. Introduction

Until recently the transplantation of native and preserved connective tissue from various sources was based on work done around the turn of the century. HELFERICH (1894) used fascia and GLUCK (1902) skin grafts in treating ankylosis of the jaw.

In addition to their use for the replacement of tendons and ligaments, connective-tissue grafts have currently been used as joint liners in arthroplasty, to close defects in body walls (thorax, abdomen, skull, etc.), for suture material, and as anchoring material. The grafts used for such purposes are fascia, skin, dura and tendon.

Fascia. Since KIRSCHNER (1909; 1913) carried out animal experiments and the first clinical application, fascia has had a firm place in reconstructive surgery. The reason is that clinical needs can usually be supplied from the autologous depot (fascia lata). Although there are several disadvantages in using autologous fascia material, such as the additional area to be operated on, the occurrence of muscle hernias, and the exhaustion of depot if several operations are necessary, only sporadic attempts have been made to use preserved homologous fascia (CRASSELT, 1967; DETHLOFF, 1967).

Skin. The first use of skin, pioneered by LOEWE in 1913 in place of free fascia grafting, was also as an autograft. The tendency for pockets of epithelium and cysts to form in skin grafts not under tension (JOKINEN, 1958; ELO, 1960) and the unreliability of the sterilization of skin autografts by disinfecting the skin surface (JUNGHANNS and JUZBASIC, 1940; HEMPEL, 1952; JUDET and JUDET, 1960) led a number of authors to use skin grafts preserved in Cialit (GSCHWEND, 1958; FRANCILLON, 1959; JUDET, 1960; SCHREIBER, 1967 and others).

Dura. Preservation also made it possible to use dura as a homograft. Taking a cue from neurosurgery, where dura was used orthotopically after brain operations (CAMPBELL, 1958; WEICKMANN, UNGER, MASON, RAAF, all 1961; NASTEFF, 1965), preserved dura was introduced in general surgery for closing large defects in the abdominal wall (FLEMMING, 1963) and thoracic wall (BORNEMISZA, 1965), to replace joint ligaments (FLEMMING, 1965; JÄGER, 1969a, b; 1971a, b; 1973, 1974, 1975), and as an alternative to fascia (FLEMMING, 1961). Dura is used in urology and gynecology for repair of the bladder and vagina. The results so far available show that in a large percentage of cases (HACKENSELLNER: 94.6%) healing was free from complications.

The grafting of pedicle and free autologous tendon was done from an early date, whereas the transplantation of homologous tendons preserved in formalin or alcohol was first successfully applied in animal experiments by NAGEOTTE (1921). NAGEOTTE and SENCERT (1918) also claimed success in man using tendon homografts preserved in alcohol, as did JALIFIER (1920) with heterografts of preserved animal tendons.

In view of their reduced tendency to form adhesions, tendons preserved in Cialit were used in hand surgery by ISELIN et al. (1963), HERZOG (1965), and SEIFFERT (1967) for repair of the flexor tendons.

B. General Section

I. Anatomic Structure of Connective-Tissue Types as it Affects Suitability for Transplantation

Anatomically, two types of connective tissue are distinguished, the dense, nonfibrillar type and the fibrillar type. Skin belongs to the first type and tendons, fascia, and ligaments to the second; dura mater lies somewhere between the two. What chiefly determines the mechanical behavior of grafts of the various connective-tissue types is the density and orientation of the collagen fibers and, to a lesser extent, their content of elastic fibers.

Skin consists of epidermis (ectodermal) and corium (mesodermal). Its mechanical properties are determined by the corium, not the epidermis (ROLLHÄUSER, 1950a, 1950b, 1950c; authors' own research). The collagenous fiber field of corium includes numerous structural elements such as hair follicles and sebaceous glands. The pars papillaris in particular displays a dense, elastic network of fibers. Skin with the epithelium removed is well suited for the plastic repair of fistulas and thoracic wall defects but less suited for the replacement of ligaments and fascia because it stretches too easily.

The *dura mater* forms the outer covering of the brain and spinal cord. Structurally, the dura of the cranium consists mainly of collagenous fibers interwoven in four directions so as to form a three-dimensional network. Elastic fibers are rare in cranial dura but more common in the dura mater of the spinal cord, where the collagenous fibers have a more longitudinal orientation. The latter type is not thick enough to withstand mechanical stresses. Cranial dura, when available as preserved homologous transplant material, thus has the same range of indications as skin but with the additional advantage of stretching less and having less tendency to form adhesions.

Fascia falls into the fibrillar type of connective tissue because the majority of its collagenous fibers run longitudinally (BÖHM and DAVIDOFF, 1898; STÖHR, 1918; SCHAFFER, 1920; WALLRAFF, 1954). Human fascia lata is particularly suitable for grafting because the longitudinal arrangement of its collagenous fibers is well adapted to mechanical stress (GRATZ, 1931). It has very few elastic fibers (VALENTIN, 1912). Because of their good mechanical properties, fascia auto- or homografts are used in reconstructive surgery for the replacement of ligaments, tendons, or capsules, in vascular surgery to wrap around aneurysms and to reinforce vessel sutures, and to strengthen large defects in the abdominal and thoracic walls.

Tendon is the prototype of a fibrillar connective-tissue structure, consisting for the most part of stiff, parallel collagenous fibers and having a low content of cells and ground substances. It is designed for tensile strength and hence is not very elastic (SEIFFERT, 1967); it is the collagen that determines its resistance to tensile stress (ARNOLD, 1972). For this reason tendon is ideal not only for the repair of damaged tendons but also for the plastic replacement of ligaments.

II. Viability and Nonviability: Denaturation of the Graft as it Affects Primary Healing and Restructuring

The concept of the viability of tissues has never been clearly defined. In parenchymatous organs the restoration of physiologic function after reimplantation can be regarded as evidence of vital capacity, but viability in supporting tissues is difficult to assess since they consist mainly of fibrous material and ground substances.

KIRSCHNER (1909), REHN and MIYAUCHI (1914), KLEINSCHMIDT (1914b), and SCHWARTZ (1922) based their ideas on histologic studies of connective-tissue autografts and assumed that vital capacity was present, otherwise the operation would not have been successful.

For homografts LONGMIRE (1954) established a new subdivision into *homovital* and *homostatic*. With homovital transplants (endocrine organs, kidney, muscle, liver, heart, gastrointestinal tract and nerve cells) function depends on the viability of the constituent cells, whereas in homostatic transplants (bone, cartilage, blood vessels, tendons, fascia, and ligaments, as well as other mesenchymal tissues) mechanical function is the all-important factor.

It follows that healing with the ability to function does not depend on the viability of the cells in the tissue (PATE, 1954); however, preservation should not cause too great a change in the physical and chemical structure of connective tissue.

REHN noted the strong inflammatory response often elicited by connective tissue autografts, and their tendency to form adhesions with the surrounding tissue. Even fresh homografts induce inflammatory changes in the graft bed. Thus, VALENTIN (1912) was able to observe a strong inflammatory response following homografting of fresh fascia into corresponding defects in the abdominal skin of dogs and rabbits. HERZOG (1965) and SEIFFERT (1967) observed following transplantation of Cialit-preserved, fresh homologous, and autologous tendons in rabbits that the smallest inflammatory response was obtained with the Cialit material. We confirmed (JÄGER, 1970) in animal experiments that Cialit-preserved homologous dura implanted in the fascia lata of sheep healed with some delay and that the transplant was surrounded by a rim of inflamed cells. The studies of Brüchle (1969) suggest that the factor responsible for this difference is the concentration of the Cialit solution.

The information obtained from experimental studies forms the basis of indications and limitations given for the clinical use of various types of connective tissue preserved in different ways. Note, however, that, when it comes to orthopedic surgery, the advantages and disadvantages of the various types of material as determined by experiment have to be modified in consideration of the clinical requirements of the area of indication in question.

In very general terms, it may be said that in view of the various disadvantages of autografts—additional operative procedures, danger of muscle hernias, additional cosmetic disfigurement, and the exhaustion of depot when several operations are needed—preference should be given to preserved homografts of connective tissue. Here too, for various reasons such as reliability of sterilization and more rapid healing and restructuring, lyophilization is to be preferred to Cialit preservation.

III. Biological and Mechanical Merits of Auto-, Homo-, and Heterologous Transplants

In order to assess the biological and mechanical properties of connective-tissue transplants, it is essential to observe cells and intercellular substances separately (Seiffert). We have already mentioned 'viability' in relation to the merits of free grafts of autologous or homologous, fresh or preserved supporting tissues. The debate on this subject is still going on. For clinical purposes, Longmire's concept of homostatic (i.e. not dependent on the viability of the tissue) transplants of homologous supporting tissues is crucial, since their real function is to act as a structural substitute (Pate), and when in the preserved state they simply take over the mechanical functions (Weidenreich, 1924; Seiffert et al., 1967; Herzog, 1965 and others).

A knowledge of the mechanical characteristics of the various types of connective tissue is of paramount importance for the surgeon replacing tendons and ligaments. For example, failure to anticipate irreversible primary extension may lead to complete functional insufficiency.

Testing of the mechanical properties of supporting tissues has made enormous progress in range and precision, thanks to the application of biomechanics and technology. The following mechanical properties are now determined for supporting tissue: tensile strength, elasticity, extensibility, viscosity, plasticity, relaxation and mechanical recovery (Arnold, 1973).

Skin in particular has repeatedly been the object of testing for mechanical properties. Thus Langer (1861) studied the elongation and elasticity of cadaveric skin and found that elongation along the cleavage lines was less than at right angles to them. A few hours after stress loading all skin strips had returned to their original length. Triepel in 1902 laid down three points for the tensile strength of composite tissues, based on his own research. He stated that tensile strength is a function of the mechanical properties of the strongest component of the tissue, the proportion in which it is present, and its structural type.

His results were confirmed by ROLLHÄUSER in 1950c. As part of a general study of the elasticity of animal and human tissues WÖLISCH et al. (1927) determined the mean tensile strength of human skin as 180 kg/cm². ROLLHÄUSER (1950b) in tests of human abdominal skin found that tensile strength increased with increasing age and was accompanied by a decline in elasticity. DICK (1951) obtained similar results with cadaveric skin. R. and J. JUDET (1960) found no difference in the breaking strength of living and preserved skin. SCHREIBER (1967) studied the elongation and residual elongation of preserved cadaveric skin as it might affect practical applications. KIVILAAKSO (1955) during animal experiments involving whole-skin replacement of portions of Achilles tendon found that breaking strength was reduced in the area of the graft suture. JOKINEN (1958) performed animal experiments to determine the breaking strength of autologous whole-skin grafts and found that operated tendons after only 2 months had approximately normal values for breaking strength. Our tests of the mechanical behavior of living and preserved fascia, dura, and skin (JÄGER and ANDERS, 1969; JÄGER, 1970) showed fascia to be superior to dura and skin in its mechnical characteristics (tensile strength, extension at max. load, and shear modulus).

Fascia grafts are in common use in general surgery, yet there is extraordinarily little information available on the mechanical behavior of fascia. KIRSCHNER (1909) in his first paper on autoplastic transplantation of fascia merely reported a simple test of strength. He clamped a 1-cm wide strip of the iliotibial tract of a newly dead cadaver and subjected it to a load of 25 kg; this caused no damage. In a later study comparing a strip of fascia with a strip of periosteum of the same width he was unable to break it. When the load reached 45 kg, the end of the fascia strip was merely pulled out of the clamp. GRATZ (1931), in studies of the tensile strength of human fascia, determined that its tensile strength is greatest when traction is applied in the longitudinal direction. Conversely, the tensile strength of fascia is very low when the load is applied at right angles to the direction in which the fibers run. He put the mean maximum tensile strength of fascia at 7,000 psi. If we accept the physical definition that a material may be termed elastic if after removal of the load it returns without appreciable delay to the state it was in before deformation, then we cannot accept either KLEINSCHMIDT's (1914a) statement that fascia has very slight elasticity or METZE's (1965) description of lyophilized fascia as inelastic. FLEMMING (1963) also failed to recognize the mechanical properties of fascia when, in reference to REHN's work, he stated that the mechanical loading capacity of fascia was much lower than that of cutis.

The parallel alignment of the fibers in fascia, in contrast to the meshlike arrangement of the fibers in dura and corium, is responsible for poor suture holding (CRASSELT, 1967; DETHLOFF, 1967; METZE, 1965 and others). We carried out mechanical tests on th primary suture holding of the various types of connective tissue (JÄGER, 1970). We had to develop a special technique before the suture holding of fascia could equal or exceed that of dura and skin. The mechanical characteristics we tested fo this purpose were max. breaking strain of the sample, and the ratio of max. breaking strain of the sample to the thickness of the material.

There is still very little known about the mechanical behavior of *dura*. In 1967 Schnell, Plenio, Pauli, Braun and Korb reported that the tensile strength of dura mater is materially reduced when it has been sterilized by gamma irradiation. They gave the range of tensile strength of nonirradiated human dura as 4.5 to 7.7 kg. Our own experimental work (Jäger, 1970) showed that the tensile strength of dura is lower than that of fascia and skin, its shear modulus lies between that of fascia and skin, and its extensibility is slightly less than that of fascia and significantly less than that of skin.

The mechanical properties of *tendon* were first investigated by Wertheim in 1847. Since then a number of authors have studied the biomechanical properties of tendons, especially tensile strength (Cronkite, 1936; Rollhäuser, 1950b; Stucke, 1950; the team of Walker, Harris and Benedict, 1964; Benedict *et al.*, 1968; Ellis, 1965; Elliot, 1967; Viidik, 1967; 1969; Blanton and Biggs, 1970; Welsh *et al.*, 1971; Diamant, 1972; Minns *et al.*, 1973; K. Wilhelm, 1972; Arnold *et al.*, 1972; 1973; Bowitz and Nemetschek, 1974; G. Hirsch, 1974). According to the work of Cronkite (1936) and Stucke (1950), the tensile strength of native tendons lies within the range of 4.69 to 12.75 kp/mm^2. K. Wilhelm (1972) found that human Achilles tendon has an age-dependent static tensile strength of 6.8 to 8.6 kg/mm^2 and a dynamic tensile strength of 9.04 to 11.6 kv/mm^2. Preserved tendons behave differently from fresh tendons (Blanton and Biggs, 1970). The tensile strength of juvenile collagen as against adult collagen is increased more by drying and decreased more by soaking in acetic acid (Rollhäuser, 1950b). According to the work of Benedict, Walker and Harris (1968) and Blanton and Biggs (1970), the tensile strength of human extensor tendons of the lower extremities is greater than that of the flexor tendons. Other biochemical properties of tendon, such as the relationship between tension and extension, rheological features, relaxation, and retardation, have been the object of very little work (Viidik, 1966; Wöhlisch, Mesnil de Rochemont and Gerschler, 1927; Rigby, 1964; van Brocklin and Ellis, 1965). Arnold and his group in 1972, 1973, and 1974 made a series of technical studies of the biomechanical properties of tendons, using 300 tendons taken from the feet of cadavers. Some of this work confirmed reports by earlier authors and some represented new data. In particular, they established that tendons have good elastic and viscous properties but very little plasticity. Thus, when plotting load against elongation, they regularly found that the lower portion of the curve was nonlinear, the next part practically linear, and the short upper portion nonlinear. Tendon relaxation depends upon the speed of the preceding extension. It also depends to some extent on tendon cross-section and length, and the initial tensile stress. Furthermore, tendons have the capability to increase their tension (recover) after they are released from a higher level of stress. Here again, this depends to some extent on speed of extension, duration of relaxation, and stress intensity and thrust. In addition, the viscous properties of tendons induce damping phenomena.

G. Hirsch (1974) did some research on suture holding in severed peronaeus brevis tendons in rabbits. He found that during the first two weeks of the healing period the Bunnell suture gave the best mechanical holding but that from week 4 onward tensile strength was the same for single-tie sutures and

BUNNELL sutures. After 24 weeks the breaking strength of the sutured tendons was still 50% below that of comparable intact tendons in the same individual. Moreover, the BUNNELL suture caused stronger adhesions than the single-tie suture. The author concluded that tendons should be stitched with single-tie sutures, provided adequate relaxation of the tendons could be effected during the operation.

IV. Changes with Age in Connective Tissue as they Affect Transplantation

Changes that occur with age in the various connective-tissue types are important in grafting, particularly when they alter the mechanical properties.

Changes due to aging in the collagenous fibers were first revealed by electron-optic, biochemical, and physicochemical examinations. The electron microscope supplied proof that the structural elements of collagenous fibers, the fibrils and the cement substance, are not the same in the various connective-tissue fiber types nor at different stages of maturity. It became possible to classify the fibers with respect to changes due to aging and organ specificity, both by GÖMÖRI'S silver impregnation method, applied by PAHLKE (1954) to human Achilles tendon, and by determining the thickness of the fibrils (SCHWARZ et al., 1953; 1957).

In addition to the changes visible in the electron microscope, it was possible to detect biochemical and physicochemical changes due to aging in collagenous connective tissue. It is quite generally true that the strength of collagen increases with age. Consolidation occurs at the molecular level through a continuing increase in internal bonding (VERZAR, 1963), due to hydrogen bonding between three amino-acid chains, electrostatic bonding during the fashioning of several of these chain structures into fibrils and, as maturity increases, cross-linking by means of ester bridges (also called 'covalent bridging' by GRASSMANN et al., 1965). A reliable index of aging is the rise in heat resistance or in denaturing temperature. There is relatively little metabolic activity in connective tissue under physiological conditions. Connective tissue does not undergo physiological regeneration but possesses stable cells that multiply only until they achieve specific properties. When this stage is reached at the conclusion of growth, the cells become incapable of dividing and metabolic intensity declines (MASS-HOFF, 1955).

The tensile strength of the collagenous fibrils is determined by the intermolecular bounds — hydrogen bonds, ester bridges, and salt-type bonds (VERZAR, 1963; GRASSMANN, 1955; HÖRMANN, 1966). As one regards the tensile strength of the fibers, which represent the higher structural unit, GUSTAVSON (1956) believes that some importance should also be assigned to the interfilamentary cement.

For *skin* SCHREIBER (1967) and DICK (1951) established that resistance to stretching changes with age. Max. elongation falls in older individuals; the reason for this is said to be, that the elastic fibers of the corium change with age. Our studies (JÄGER, 1970) led to similar conclusions. Samples of the various connective-tissue types (skin, fascia, and dura) were taken from persons in two age groups (about 60 and about 30 years) and tested for three characteristics of mechanical behavior, tensile strength shear modulus, and extension at max. load. In the older group skin, with and without preliminary stretching, gave a high value for shear modulus, but lower values for tensile strength and elongation. This is due to the fact that older persons have lost some of the elastic fibers responsible for the ability of skin to stretch. Fascia gave significantly higher values for tensile strength and shear modulus in the older group. Dura showed no significant difference with age in any of the three mechanical characteristics; we may, however, assume a tendency toward consolidation in the older group. Supplementary studies (Jäger together with Anders, Becker and Krüger, 1971) were undertaken to determine the mechanical behavior of living human fascia over a much broader range of ages (from 2 months before birth to 80 years). This work showed that the principal increase in tensile strength and shear modulus is completed before the end of the third month of age. The sector between the 4th and 7th decades showed only a slight rise in mechanical characteristics in the direction of consolidation (Fig. 1). Similar conclusions werde reached by Rollhäuser (1951) from a survey of the tensile strength of human tendon and skin. Wilhelm (1972) on the other hand, in experimental testing of the mechanical properties of human Achilles tendon, was able to show that loading capacity for both static and dynamic stress declines with age and that the max. loading capacity is found in the third decade of life.

The lesson to be drawn relative to homologous transplants of the various connective-tissue types is, that fascia and dura may be derived from both age groups (around 30 and around 60 years) without any special disadvantages, whereas donors for skin transplants should preferably be selected from the older age group.

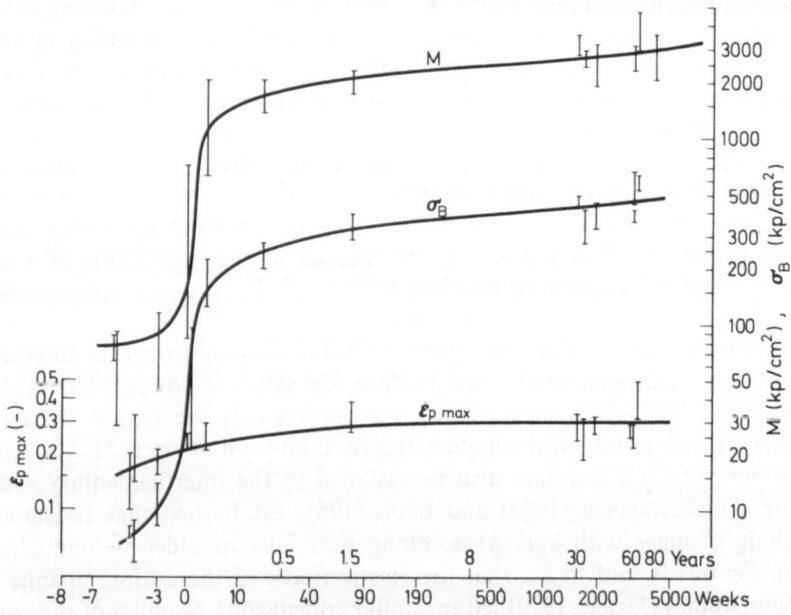

Fig. 1. Mechanical properties of human fascia as a function of age. M shear modulus, σ_B tensile strength, ε_p^{max} percentage elongation

V. Immune Reactions in the Transplantation of Living and Preserved Connective Tissue

The degree of intensity of immune reactions depends primarily on the fine structure of the transplanted tissue, although other factors are involved. The degree of antigenicity is mainly determined by the cell content of the tissue (HUMPHREY and WHITE, 1971 and others).

Dura and fascia have a high proportion of fibers but few cells; for this reason alone, they have low antigenicity. Skin, on the other hand, is very rich in cells, particularly in the epithelial layer. This is why orthotopic skin grafting is well adapted to the study of immunologic phenomena (MEDAWAR, 1958). The rejection of a particular foreign skin graft triggers the immunobiologic defence mechanism in the host organism and for a time confers upon it an enhanced sensitivity to skin grafts from the same donor. With the first transplantation (first set) severe inflammation usually occurs after 1 or 2 weeks as a result of immunobiological events, the outcome being necrosis of the transplant. However, if after the first set the host receives a second transplant, a second reaction, again with necrosis of the graft, occurs much sooner because of the antibodies already present. The occurrence of the second reaction with premature necrosis thus provides proof of the antigenic effect of the first transplant. It is obvious from these findings that preservation must always reduce tissue antigenicity (MEDAWAR, 1954a; 1958; BILLINGHAM et al., 1956; PATE, 1954; HYATT, 1952 and others). This applies equally to preserved skin.

Preservation thus constitutes 'mechanical deantigenization'. SCHREIBER (1967) and ourselves established that the epithelial layer can readily be peeled off from skin preserved in Cialit. We found that lyophilized skin behaved in the same way. This means that the graft can consist mainly of corium and so is rich in fibers and depleted in cells.

SEIFFERT (1967) carried out some experiments that have a bearing upon homografting of skin preserved in different ways. He studied the second reaction of orthotopically transplanted homologous skin in rats, the host animals having been sensitized 14 days before by skin grafts from donor animals that had been preserved in different ways. SEIFFERT found that only Cialit-preserved skin grafts never triggered premature necrosis of the second set. Survival time of the orthotopic second grafts in this case was about the same as that of fresh homografts, i.e. 7 to 10 days. All skin grafts preserved by other methods induced a premature second reaction.

These results were in contradiction to the observations of BILLINGHAM (1952) and MEDAWAR (1958), who found no host sensitization after freeze-drying.

It is clear that preservation reduces the antigenicity of the tissue. The degree to which the reduction of antigenicity is expressed appears to depend upon the method of preservation and the manner in which this influences the antigenic viability of the tissue and of the cells in particular. The residual fibrillar and amorphous ground substance of the supporting tissues is generally regarded as being immunologically inert. STEFFEN et al. (1967), however, succeeded in showing that antibodies to collagen are present under special experimental conditions. This meant that the older view, that collagen possesses little or no antigenicity, had to be revised. Steffen found that soluble and not too strongly denatured collagen preparations, particularly in the presence of adjuvants, possessed adequate immunogenicity.

It seems that the more insoluble and the more purified the material for a collagenous transplantis, the less likely it is to mount an immune reaction. With the methods of preservation in common use today (Cialit and freeze-drying) there is no need to fear antigenicity in connective-tissue transplants. We have used lyophilized connective-tissue transplants (dura, skin, and fascia) in more than 80 patients without a single rejection incident.

VI. Preservation

In preserving the flexible type of connective tissue the aim must be to retain its functional structures, the collagenous fibers. In practical applications of the preservation of homologous connective tissue, such as skin, tendon, dura, or fascia, the requirement is for the mechanical properties of the collagenous fibers to remain largely unchanged. A simple manipulation is to be carried out. Sterility is essential for both clinical purposes and animal experiments. It is therefore highly desirable to employ a method of preservation that sterilizes at the same time.

Chemical preservatives like alcohol or formalin (Nageotte, 1927; Weiden-reich, 1924) are hardly ever used today for preserving clinical transplants because thy hygroscopicity of high-percentage alcohols induces severe shrinkage of the tissue, while formalin causes collagenous fibers to move toward a higher shrinkage temperature, among other things.

In addition to preservation by cold, both above and below freezing point, and embedding in plastics (Idelberger, 1955), two procedures have proved well adapted to the preservation of collagenous connective tissue, freeze-drying and preservation in Cialit.

Freeze-drying (lyophilization). Freeze-drying of homostatic transplants is widely used for clinical purposes. It is a particularly gentle process, involving evaporation of moisture from frozen preparations under high vacuum, which prevents the water from forming aggregates. Experimental and clinical testing was carried out principally by Kreuz et al. (1951), Marrangoni and Ceccini (1951), Turner (1952), Pate (1954), and Neumann (1955).

Freeze-drying is effected in various ways. The object is to combine the preservative action of both drying and deep-freezing. Living tissues are devitalized by lyophilization, but it fails to kill certain microorganisms that are resistant to both freezing and drying. Additional sterilization is needed, usually by means of gamma irradiation or gaseous ethylene oxide. The advantage of preserving tissues by freeze-drying is that they are easy to handle and can be stored at room temperature for a minimum of five years (Metz, 1965). After lyophilization, tissues may be stored in airtight glass jars, light-metal foils, or plastic bags. The use of airtight containers prevents any unintentional rehydration or contamination. Drying must be taken to very low residual moisture, as quite a low percentage of moisture can promote chemical reactions that induce changes in enzyme structure (Neumann, 1955).

Shortly before it is to be used, the lyophilized tissue is removed from its container and rehydrated by soaking for 15 min in Ringer's solution.

Preservation in Cialit. Cialit is a mercury salt with a high affinity for the thio groups of proteins. Its preservative action is due primarily to a blocking of enzymes, which interferes with proteolysis (MARQUARDT). Cialit, even in very dilute form, has a strong bactericidal and fungicidal action (GRÜTER, 1933).

Cialit has been used in a number of ways to preserve flexible tissue types. For preserving *skin*, SANCHIS-OLMOS (1954) was the first to use an organomercury compound, Merthiolate. This compound proved optically unstable, so that he later changed to the chemically more stable Cialit. Further reports on the use of Cialit for preserving skin, particularly for grafting purposes, have been published by JUDET and JUDET (1960; 1961), and the Balgrist Clinic in Zürich (FRANCILLON, 1959; SPIRIG, 1961; SCHREIBER, 1967). There are other reports on experience with Cialit preservation, especially of homologous tendons, by SEIFFERT and coworkers (1964; 1967), HERZOG (1965), and ISELIN *et al.* (1963). These authors are unanimous in praising the good qualities of Cialit: it is optically stable, preserves and sterilizes simultaneously, and is easy and cheap to use.

GRÜTER (1933) did in vitro tests on the bactericidal and fungicidal action of Cialit, but found that tissue samples preserved in Cialit were not always sterile. There is particular difficulty in preserving cadaveric skin. SCHREIBER (1968) recorded no bacterial growth 14 days after storing human cadaveric skin in a 1:2500 solution of Cialit; after 4 weeks, however, he found enterococci and *Pseudomonas fluorescens,* and after 8 weeks again *P. fluorescens.* We had cultures made from a piece of cadaveric skin prepared for mechanical testing after it had been preserved for 4 weeks (3 weeks in a 1:1000 Cialit solution, and 1 week in a 1:3000 Cialit solution). Staphylococci with weak hemolysis and coliform bacteria were found. HERZOG established that Cialit has low toxicity. ADAM *et al.* (1968) were able to demonstrate that mercury compounds react chemically with collagen in vivo. BRÜCHLE (1969) used a Cialit dilution of 1:10,000 in his studies on the healing of native and preserved tendons in rabbits. He saw no infected wounds or symptoms of nontolerance, and all preserved tendons were sterile.

PATE (1954) established that, although viability is not essential in homostatic transplants, the method of preservation must not unduly change the physical and chemical structure of the transplant. SEIFFERT (1967) made macro- and microscopic examinations of rat skin in order to determine what changes resulted from the method and duration of preservation. He found that freeze-dried skin on removal from sealed glass tubes was hard and had the consistency of cardboard, but that on rehydration the skin swelled and regained its natural flexibility. Deep-frozen skin after thawing was barely distinguishable from fresh skin samples. Skin preserved in Cialit soon became pale gray and swollen, and after a time the epidermis could be peeled off. Even after 4 years, no disintegration of the corium was observed.

In histological section, apart from a slight loosening of the corium, rehydrated freeze-dried skin and thawed deep-frozen skin could not be distinguished

from the native preparation. While the slightly shrunken cells of freeze-dried
and deep-frozen skin remained readily recognizable throughout the observation
period, the color of the cells in the Cialit preparation faded progressively and
after a few months they were identifiable only by granular chromatin residues.
Studies of similarly preserved tendons from man, dog, and rabbit gave similar
results over periods of time ranging from the start of preservation to up to
4 years and longer. It was thus concluded that the structural changes seen
in preserved specimens as against fresh tissue were generally least in the deep-
frozen transplants; some structural changes were seen in the freeze-dried tissue
and rather more in the Cialit-preserved tissue. The changes described were
thought to be due less to the duration than to the method of preservation.

The influence of lyophilization with simultaneous sterilization by means
of ethylene oxide or gamma irradiation on the structure of dura was microscopically investigated by KORB, RUNGE and ARKENAU (1967). The only observed
difference between treated and fresh dura was that the former showed a loosening
and coarsening of the structure that was independent of duration of rehydration
or method of sterilization. The collagenous fibers could not readily be distinguished from one another; they formed irregular bundles enclosing optically
empty spaces of different sizes. The nuclei of the fibrocytes were either not
visible or only shadowy. These claims were supported by our own histological
studies (JÄGER, 1970).

Our mechanical studies, however, led us to the conclusion that the mechanical
characteristics depend not only on fiber orientation (particularly in fascia) but
also on changes in the cement substance. We therefore undertook comparative
electron-microscopic studies of dura: fresh, lyophilized, gamma-irradiated
(2.5 Mrad), and Cialit-preserved (3 weeks in 1:1000 Cialit solution followed
by 3 weeks in 1:3000 solution). Submicroscopically, the Cialit-preserved material
showed no significant morphological differences as against fresh dura (Figs. 2
and 4).

The spatial distribution of the interfibrillar cement and the fibrils was unchanged. The cross-striation of the fibrils was the same as in fresh dura. On
the other hand, the lyophilized and gamma-irradiated dura had clearly undergone structural changes (Fig. 3). There was some loss of interfibrillar cement
with swelling of the fibers. Fresh and Cialit-preserved dura did not display
such changes. Mechanical behavior reflected physical condition, with the Cialit-
preserved dura showing mechanical characteristics that were similar to or better
than those of the fresh material. The inferior mechanical characteristics of
lyophilized and gamma-irradiated dura could presumably be attributed to the
submicroscopically visible structural changes.

The mechanical behavior of connective tissue is also influenced by preservation. We investigated the mechanical properties (tensile strength, percentage
elongation, and shear modulus) of human fascia, dura, and skin, both in native
state and preserved in various ways, as a function of the age of the transplant
donor. In general, the decline in the values for shear modulus and tensile
strength due to lyophilization was striking in all samples tested, regardless
of tissue type. Cialit preservation usually caused an increase in shear modulus
and tensile strength with lower elongation values. This difference was apparent

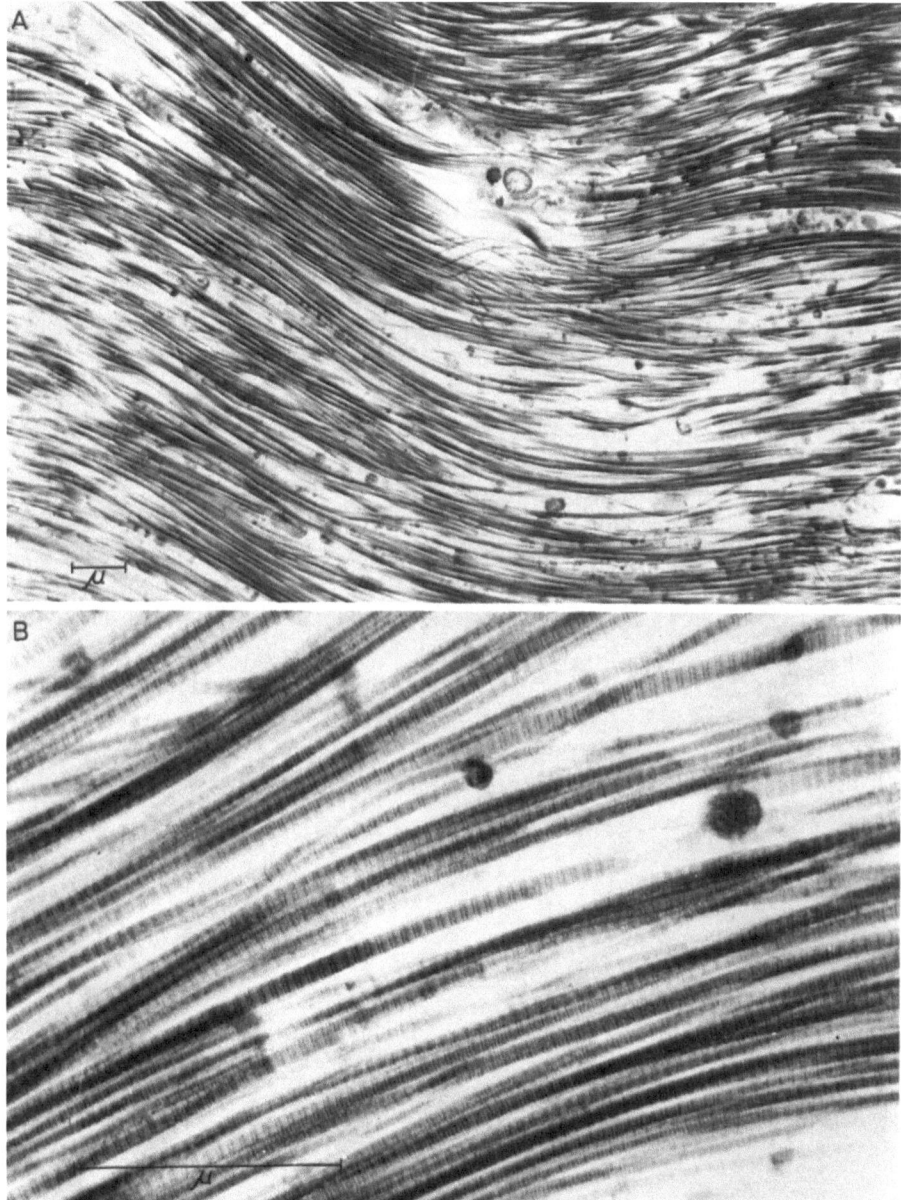

Fig. 2A and B. Fresh dura fixed in glutaraldehyde/osmium tetroxide. Normal spatial distribution of the interfibrillary cement substance and fibrils. Cross-striation of fibrils clearly visible. (A) × 10,000; (B) × 50,000

only in comparison with the lyophilized samples; shear modulus and tensile strength were generally better than in the fresh samples (Figs. 5 to 7).

Fascia with its parallel fibers did not show such pronounced differences due to preservation, especially in Age Group II (around 60 years) whereas in

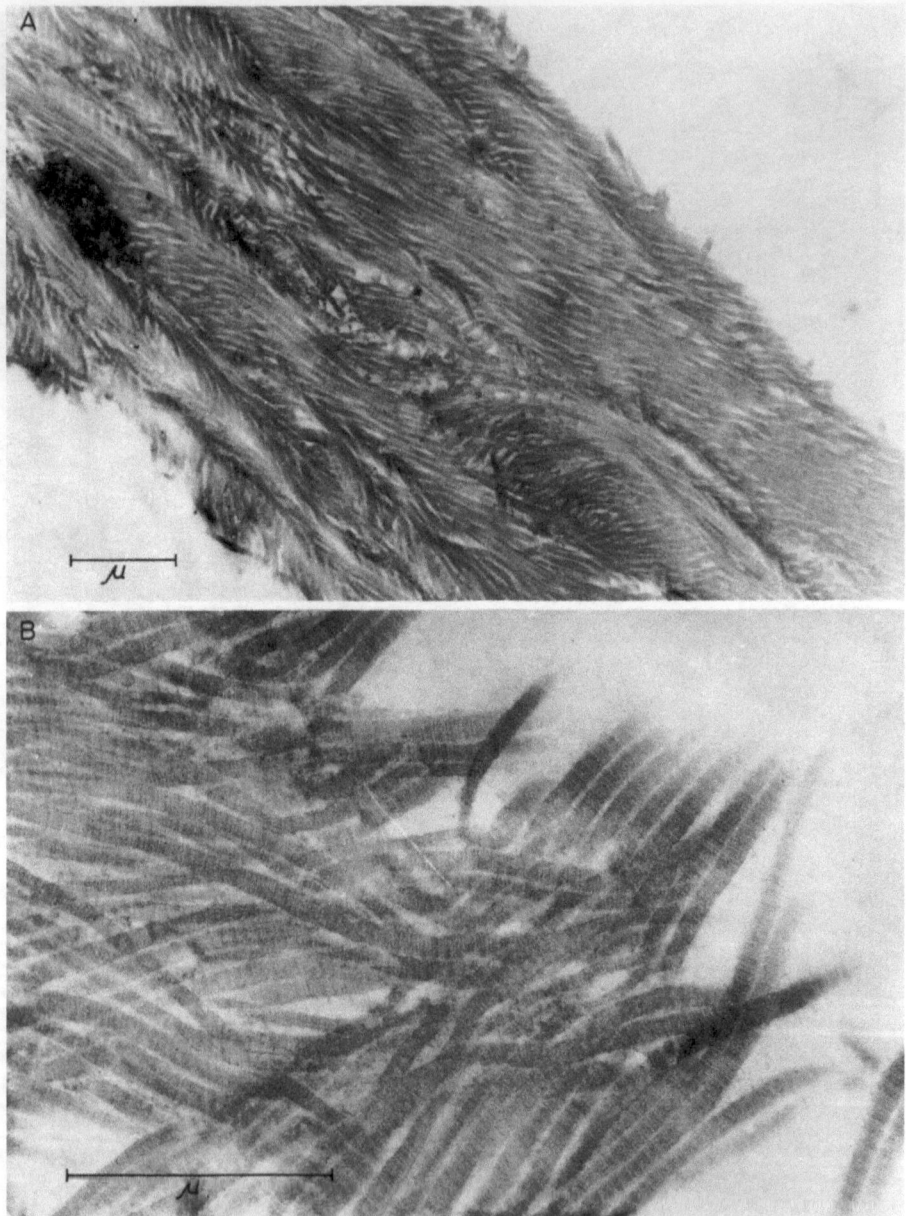

Fig. 3A and B. Lyophilisized dura. Loss of interfibrillary substance with swelling of fibrils.
(A) × 10,000; (B) × 50,000

Age Group I (around 30 years) the differences were significant except for shear modulus.

With dura the values for shear modulus and tensile strength in fresh, lyophilized and Cialit-preserved tissue were in the ratio 2:1:3. In Group I elongation

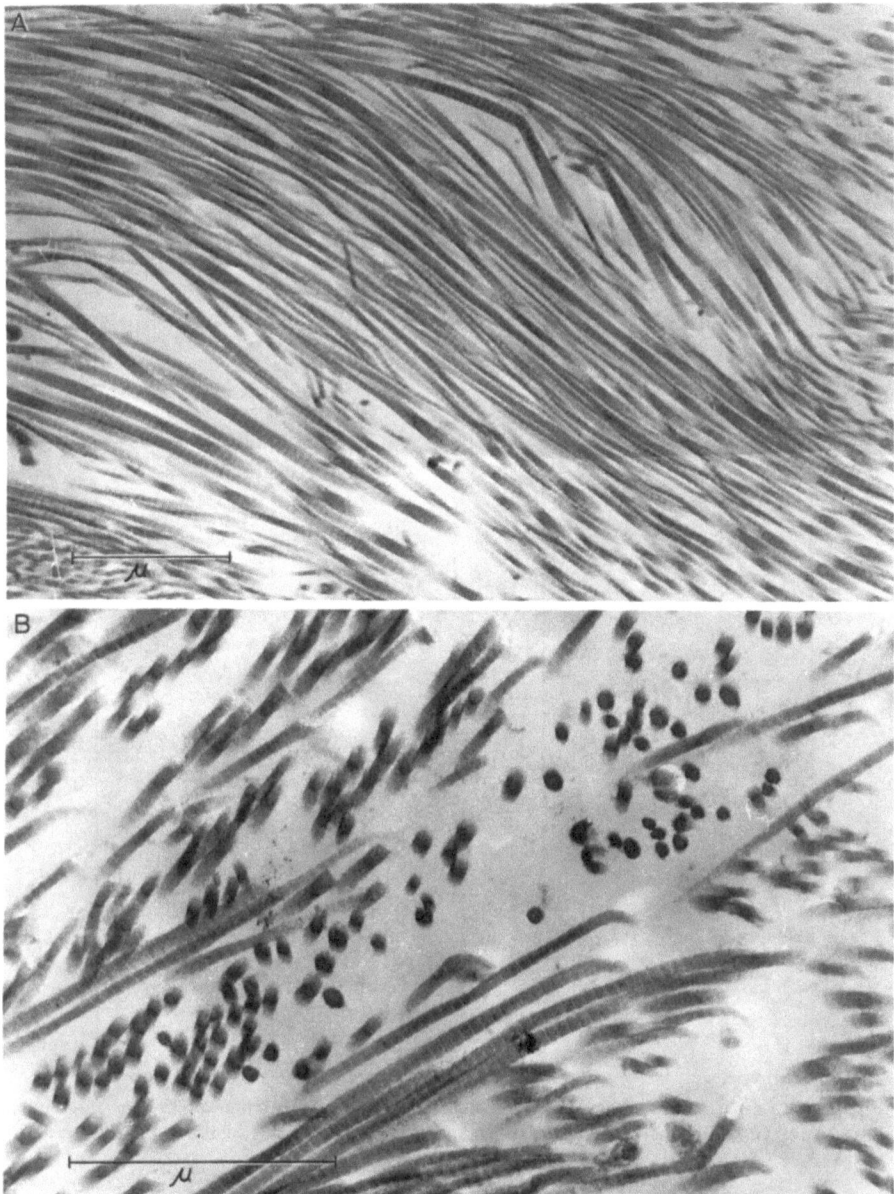

Fig. 4A and B. Cialit-preserved dura. No significant difference from the norm. Cross-striation clearly visible. (A) × 30,000; (B) × 50,000

was significantly increased by lyophilization. The effect of preservation on the mechanical properties of skin was similar to that found with dura. The difference in behavior was always significant, independent of age group.

Thus, lyophilization and sterilization by gammy irradiation almost always lowered the values for shear modulus and tensile strength but increased elonga-

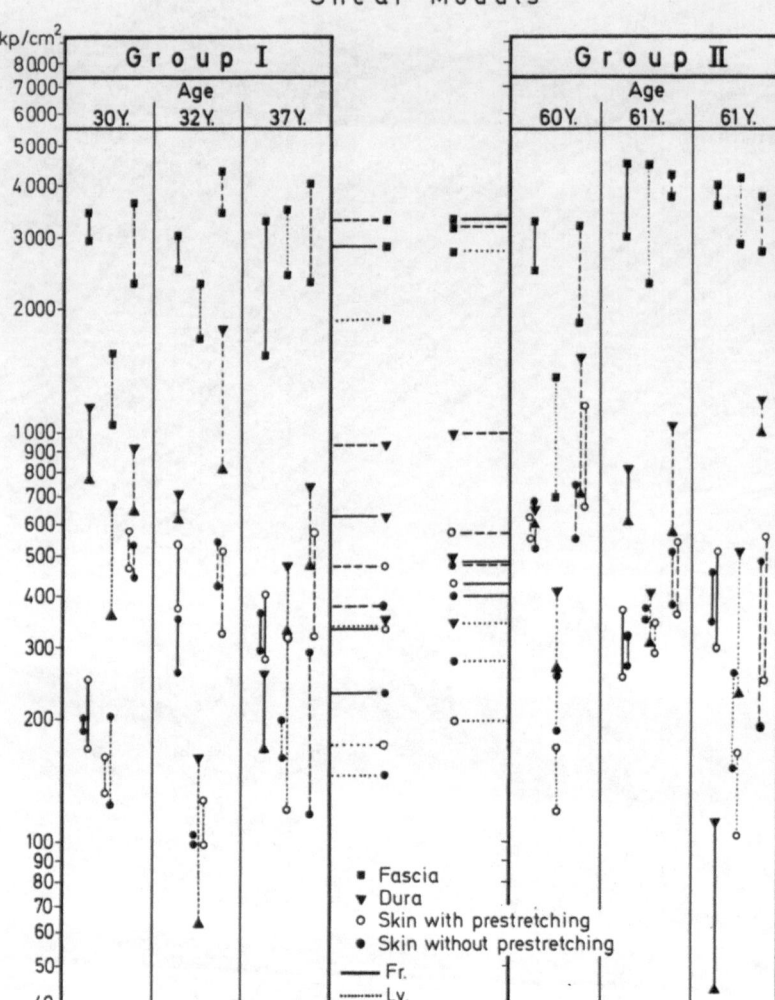

Figs. 5–7. Comparison of mean, min., and max. values for the mechanical properties of human fascia, dura, and skin in native and preserved condition. *FR* fresh, *LY* lyophilized, *CI* Cialit-preserved

tion. Our work failed to show to what extent one or the other of these treatments influenced mechanical behavior. Schnell *et al.* (1967) undertook some research with lyophilized and gamma-irradiated dura in order to settle this question. They found that tensile strength fell with increasing radiation dose. It may thus be assumed that type of sterilization and the radiation dose in radiosterilization both exert a significant influence on the mechanical properties of all types of lyophilized connective tissue. Cialit preservation on the other hand often improves the mechanical strength of all types of connective tissue as compared with the values obtained for native samples.

Tensile Strength

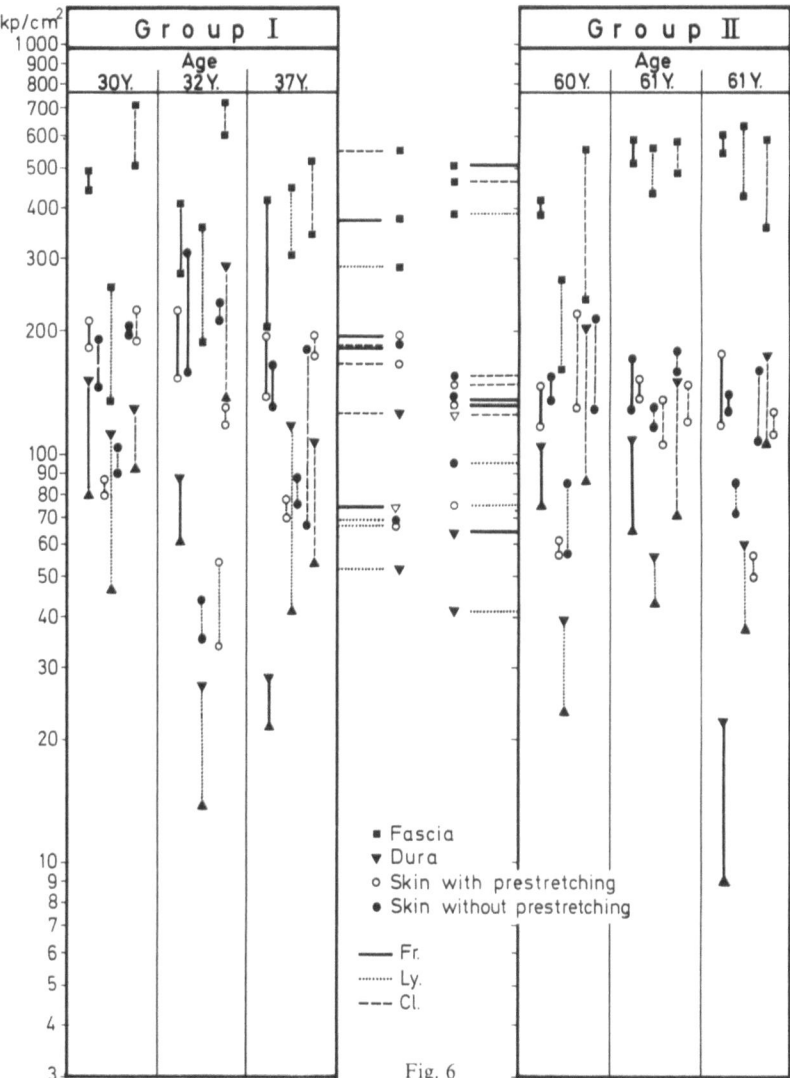

Fig. 6

We carried out animal experiments to study the influence on healing and restructuring and the functional adaptation of the connective-tissue graft of the various methods of preservation (JÄGER, 1970). Lyophilized and Cialit-preserved dura was implanted in the fascia lata of sheep under moderate tension. Homológous lyophilized gamma-irradiated dura healed without significant inflammatory phenomena and was rapidly consolidated. Cialit-preserved dura grafts on the other hand showed a distinct delay in healing and restructuring, and the inflammatory reactions were clearly more severe than with the lyophilized transplants. The rapid penetration of the host fibroblasts and the early

Percentage Elongation

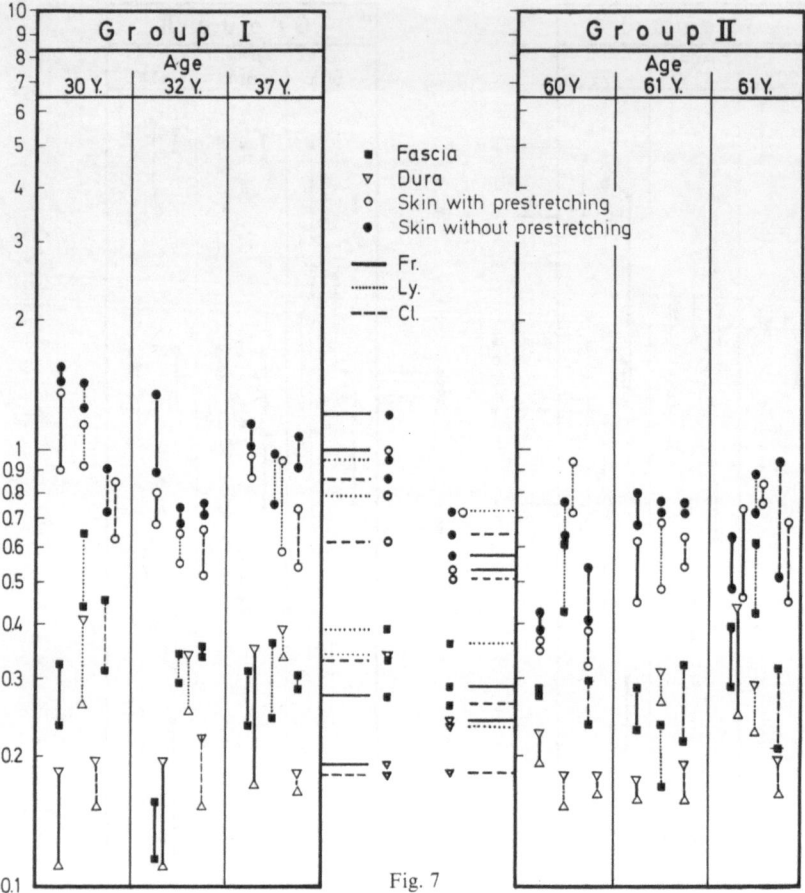

Fig. 7

consolidation of the suture by granulation tissue in the lyophilized samples gave significantly higher maximum values than were recorded for the Cialit-preserved transplants 14 days after implantation. After 12 weeks the Cialit-preserved grafts also showed signs of gradual conversion into orthotopic, functionally appropriate connective tissue. However, the long period required for healing and restructuring is a severe disadvantage in clinical applications. Conversely, the rapid healing followed by functional adaptation of the lyophilized transplants by the 6th week after grafting is, despite the initially lower mechanical values, the decisive factor in clinical applications. Jokinen (1958) observed a similar time course of consolidation with autologous whole-skin replacement of Achilles tendon in rabbits. Breaking strength increased rapidly after week 2, then levelled out at the end of the 2nd month and remained unchanged up to the 4th month. Over the remainder of one year a gradual slight increase was observed. After only 2 months the author recorded approximately the same breaking strength in the tendon grafts as in control tests with normal rabbit Achilles tendon. However, it was not until between the 4th and 8th months that he detected a longitudinal orientation appropriate to function in the region of the transplant. We, however, found a longitudinal orientation corresponding to the tensile strength in lyophilized transplants between the 9th and 12th weeks after implantation. The reason for this difference may have been that our experimental setup included a functional stimulus, designed to promote the longitudinal fiber orientation that determines tensile strength (REHN and MIYAUCHIE, 1914; SALOMON, 1922).

SEIFFERT (1967), after implanting skin homografts preserved in different ways in the dorsal fascia of rabbits, observed that Cialit-preserved transplants showed delayed healing and restructuring. Like us, he noted that in the course of healing the Cialit preparation became encapsulated as if it were a foreign body. Freeze-dried transplants, on the other hand, were organized and interpenetrated without any appreciable inflammatory response. BRÜCHLE (1969), in contrast to SEIFFERT and HERZOG, used tendons preserved in a 1:10,000 Cialit solution in his animal experiments. He observed that the tendon grafts were readily integrated into the host organism. SIEBER (1956) on the basis of animal experiments and biochemical and clinical tests established that the substitution process in a Cialit-preserved bone chip is very much slower than in a deep-frozen chip. His research led him to the belief that the delay in healing and restructuring in Cialit preparations is due to the protein-degrading activity of the preservation medium.

VII. Healing

Today it is universally accepted that only host body tissues heal properly in the biological sense and become integrated after transplantation. Functionally appropriate restructuring of non-host tissues following homo- or heterotransplantation has not yet been reliably achieved, despite partial suppression of the immune reaction. Cell survival is not necessary for function where the effect of connective-tissue transplants is homostatic (PATE, 1954; LONGMIRE, 1954). Here they merely serve as guide rails for the substitution of functionally appropriate host connective tissue. The outcome of connective-tissue grafting, i.e. healing, is dependent upon the structure, preservation, and functional adaptation of the transplant, the graft bed, and the graft anchorage.

While skin after grafting undergoes the classic inflammatory response of rejection, directed primarily against the cell-rich epidermal elements of the skin, it is also necessary, e.g. on transplantation of skin into Achilles tendon or ligaments, for the three-dimensional fiber network of the corium to be transformed into linear structures or fascia-type tissue. What is involved here is a heterotopic transplantation as opposed to e.g. homotopic or orthotopic tendon grafting. LOEWE (1913) suggested implanting skin instead of fascia in the belief, based upon histologic findings, that the implanted skin would lose its specific character and be transformed into a connective-tissue structure. REHN and MIYAUCHIE (1914) demonstrated in animal experiments that both cutaneous and subcutaneous connective-tissue autografts could be transformed under the influence of a functional stimulus, i.e. traction, into the tendon or fascia type of connective tissue. Salomon (1920) reached similar conclusions, although he regarded the functional stimulus as just one link in the chain of positive and negative stimuli. He distinguished two completely different phases after transplantation. In the first, immediately following phase he considered a functional stimulus to be harmful, whereas in the second phase it was a positive factor of ever-increasing importance for ultimate function. However, if skin is transplanted without tension or traction, the result is desquamation of the epithelium, taking the form of epithelial cysts and cysts containing epithelium and hair (Zimches, 1931; Eitner, 1920; Elo, 1960).

During the last decade three groups of authors have reported in detail on their experimental and clinical experience with native and preserved skin grafts, Kallio's group (Kallio, 1955, 1956, 1957, 1964; Jokinen, 1958; Kettunen, 1958; Kivilaakso, 1955; Elo, 1960), the Balgrist Clinic (Francillon, 1958; Gschwend, 1958; Spirig, 1961; Schreiber, 1967), and Judet and Judet (1960). They unanimously recommend three areas of indication: whole-skin arthroplasty, ligament replacement, and repair of the large tendons. Observations made in animal experiments, clinical trials, and histological studies have shown that in ligament replacement and tendon repair both native autografts and preserved homografts undergo gradual restructuring into firm connective tissue with parallel fibers (Judet and Judet, 1960; Jokinen, 1958; Schreiber, 1967).

Fascia has been used almost exclusively in experimental and clinical applications in the form of autografts for the repair of tendons, ligaments, and body walls. Being made up of parallel fibers running in the desired direction, it is morphologically similar to tendon. Many authors prefer it to tendon for the repair of tendons and ligaments. Kirschner (1909) considered fascias the ideal material for tendon replacement.

There is not much information on the transplantation of homologous preserved fascia. Koontz, Haas and Peer all report good, uncomplicated healing of fascia preserved in alcohol. Metze (1965) had a case of secondary traumatic hernia of the thoracic wall, which he closed with homologous lyophilized fascia. Healing and repair of the hernia occurred despite the growth of fibers in the direction of the suture, which had to be cut. Dethloff (1967) and Crasselt (1967) obtained good results respectively with torn fascia and the use of lyophilized dura and fascia for the repair of cruciate and lateral ligaments and ruptured Achilles tendon. Both authors assert that for grafting purposes lyophilized homologous fascia is inferior to lyophilized homologous dura, the reasons being the poor suture holding of fascia due to its longitudinal fiber structure, its extreme elasticity, and its tendency to hyperplasia.

We confirmed (Jäger, 1970) clinical reports of poor suture holding in fascia as compared to dura and corium. We were able to demonstrate that suture holding in fascia could be much improved by doubling the ends of the grafts to be stitched. The resulting increase in thickness is negligible and is usually less than the thickness of normal skin; furthermore, the thick part does not extend beyond the graft insertion. We were unable to discern any influence of method of conservation on suture holding in the various tissue types (Figs. 8 and 9).

Suture Tests

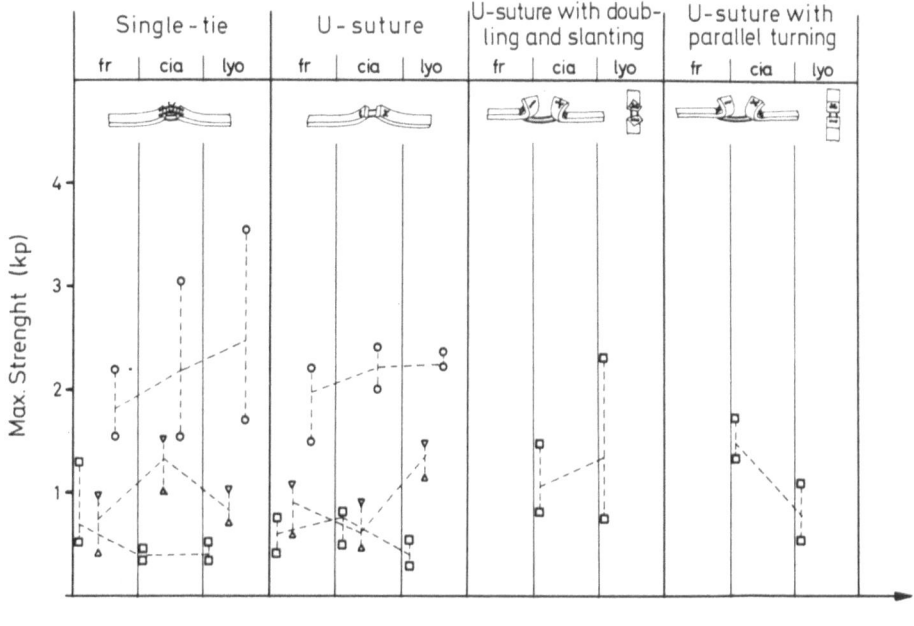

Fig. 8   □ = Fascia   ▽ = Dura   ○ = Skin

Suture Tests

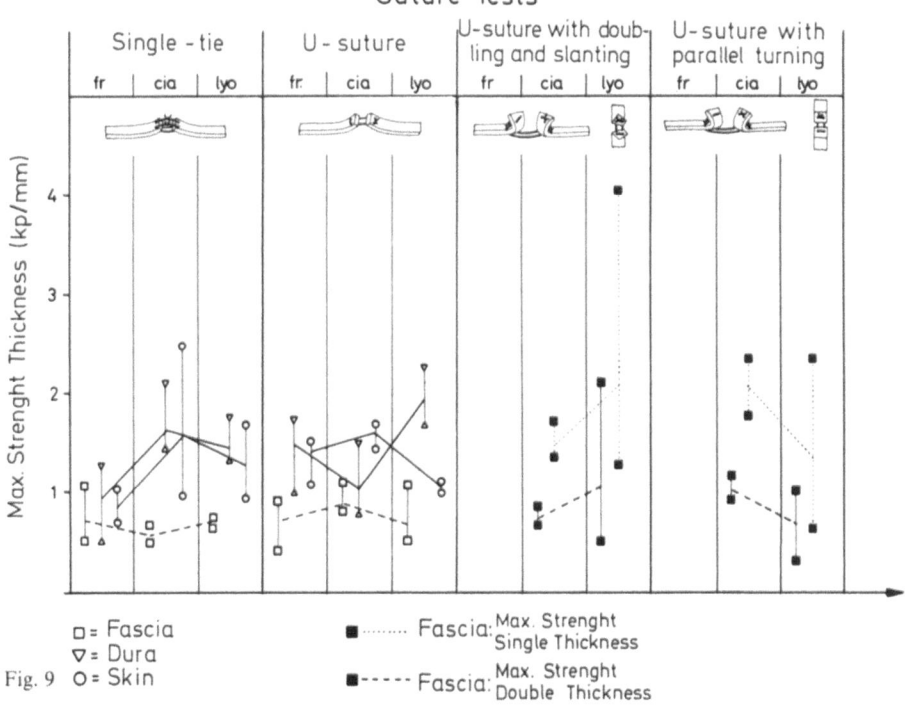

Fig. 9

□ = Fascia
▽ = Dura
○ = Skin

■ ········· Fascia: Max. Strenght Single Thickness

■ ----- Fascia: Max. Strenght Double Thickness

Figs. 8 and 9. Dependence of suture holding on tissue type and suture technique

The information available on the healing and restructuring of preserved homologous dura is based on clinical and histological data obtained from animal experiments. Unger (1965) detected no difference between host and donor dura after 5 months. Bornemisza (1965) after inserting freeze-dried homo- and heterologous dura into pleura defects found that after only one week the graft looked like normal dura, that from weeks 2 to 5 proliferative processes occurred, and at the end of 4 months the cell content of the tissues was almost normal again. There were no adhesions in the direction of the lung.

Dura resembles skin in that its collagenous fibers are arranged in a three-dimensional network. When a dura graft is used in reconstructive surgery, its connective-tissue structure must also undergo transformation. There are no reports in the literature of experimental work in this field. Flemming (1963), however, was able to obtain histological proof of healing 8 months after repairing a hernia of the abdominal wall with lyophilized dura, when the patient died of the primary disease, carcinoma of the stomach. Overlying the muscles was a broad section of anuclear, almost tendinous sclerosed tissue, from which several capillaries had penetrated into the lower sclerosed layers. There was no particular resorptive-cell reaction along the edges. In contrast to findings with orthotopic dura grafting, the transplant had formed adhesions with the bed. Flemming concluded from this that the tendency of dura to form adhesions with the surrounding tissues made it quite unsuitable for tendon replacement.

As mentioned above, we were able to demonstrate experimentally that dura implanted in sheep fascia lata healed without significant inflammatory response and by week 6 already displayed functionel restructuring with longitudinally orientated fibers. Dura grafts preserved in Cialit, however, showed considerably slower healing and restructuring.

Seiffert (1967) conducted detailed animal experiments on the healing of auto-, homo-, and heterologous tendons in both native and preserved state. He concluded, in contrast to Peacock's observations, that the strongest inflammatory response was seen in fresh homologous tendon grafts. Even autologous tendon grafts often gave stronger inflammatory reactions than preserved ones. Here again, the least inflammatory response occurred with Cialit-preserved tendons. Morphologic and autoradiographic studies of rat tail tendon showed that the rate of restructuring in the tendon declined in the order: fresh homologous, fresh autologous, and deep-frozen, freeze-dried, Cialit-preserved, and formalin-preserved homologous tendons. Herzog (1965) also confirmed the uncomplicated functional healing of orthotopically transplanted Cialit-preserved homologous tendons in rabbits. Similar results were obtained in clinical practice when Cialit-preserved homologous tendons were used as free flexor tendon grafts in man (Seiffert, 1967).

C. Specific Section

I. Tendon

The use of free or pedicle tendon autografts has a secure place in reconstructive surgery. Large sheathless tendons have very little tendency to form adhesions and can be securely anchored to soft tissues and bones because their suture holding is good. Tendons are used as free or pedicle grafts to replace ligaments (cruciate ligament, lateral knee ligaments, outer foot ligaments) or as anchoring material for slipping ulna or aplasia of the hand. In combined muscle-tendon grafts they supply strength, for instance in the replacement operation after irreversible paralysis of the radial nerve.

The transplantation of small sheathed tendons, on the other hand, is problematical, especially in the hand, mainly because adhesions of the tendon graft prevent gliding. This problem has not yet been satisfactorily solved, despite much research and many suggestions for treatment. One approach was to perfect suture technique so that primary tendon sutures or tendon grafts would heal without forming adhesions (BUNNELL, 1918; MASON and SHEARON, 1932; KOCH, 1944; VERDAN, 1960; POTENZA, 1964). Another approach was to bring the sutures into positions outside the tendon sheaths by the use of free native or preserved autologous, homologous, or heterologous tendon grafts (BUNNELL, 1918; BOYES, 1950; PULVERTAFT, 1948; 1956; MAX LANGE, 1962; A.N. WITT, 1953; 1957; ISELIN, 1957; RANK and WAKEFIELD, 1960; HERZOG, 1965; SEIFFERT, 1967; SAKELLARIDES, 1973). Attempts to use alloplastic materials to isolate the tendon suture of tendon graft from the tendon sheath (WHEELDON, 1939; GONZALES, 1949; GUEUKDJIAN, 1956; ASHLEY et al., 1959) failed because either the area around the tendon suture failed to heal, or necrosis set in the isolated tendon.

A more promising technique is the preformation of the gliding bed by the temporary insertion of synthetic material or alloplastic tendons (BIESALSKI, 1910; MAYER and RANSOHOFF, 1936; BASSET and CARROLL, 1963; HUNTER, 1965; 1969; 1971; 1973; NICOLLE, 1969; URBANIAK, 1974). SARKIN (1973) demonstrated that even a nylon thread, inserted as a permanent replacement for a flexor tendon and kept under observation for 15 years, guaranteed full performance with free movement of the finger joint and no foreign-body reaction.

Experimental studies have shown that the transplantation of native and preserved homologous tendons gives results as good as or better than those obtained with autologous tendons. Even in 1881, GLUCK noted uncomplicated healing of fresh homografts of gastrocnemius tendons in chicken. PEACOCK found that fresh homologous tendons implanted under the abdominal skin of dogs also healed without complications; he concluded from this that the state of the donor cells does not affect the healing of homologous tendons. Moreover, the preservation of tendon homografts has no adverse effect on the healing process (NAGEOTTE and SENCERT, 1918; WEIDENREICH, 1924; HERZOG, 1965; SEIFFERT, 1967).

SEIFFERT made orthotopic transplants of Cialit-preserved homologous tendons in rabbits and found uncomplicated functional healing of the grafts, a very slight inflammatory response being caused in the graft bed by the Cialit-preserved homologous transplants. These results encouraged him to use Cialit-preserved homologous tendons in free tendon grafting on the human hand. All the Cialit tendon grafts healed without complications. Our own trials indicated an initial capsule-like ensheathing of the homograft with Cialit preservation. SEIFFERT may have succeeded in creating a tendon sheath by means of this effect; some histological data in his monograph suggest that this was the case.

We cannot say with certainty whether adhesions will ultimately occur, or whether they can be prevented, because no satisfactory long-term results have been reported.

There is, of course, sufficient autologous and homologous tendon material available for transplantation, yet it would be interesting to do some research on heterologous tendon grafts, if only to discover the biological fate of collagenous fiber tissue. PEACOCK, however, has shown that when dog tendons are implanted under the abdominal skin of rabbits, uncomplicated healing occurs after destruction of donor cells and ground substance and penetration of host fibroblasts. Even heterologous grafting of the flexor tendons of human fingers, together with the intact tendon sheath, under the abdominal skin of dogs and rabbits showed on examination at intervals up to 12 months that the transplant was firmly bonded to the surrounding tissue. Normal synovial fluid was found in the tendon sheaths and there were no adhesions between the sheath and the tendon within it. Even the clinical use of 'composite-tissue tendon grafts' gave good functional results in certain cases (PEACOCK, 1967; HUESTON et al., 1967).

STERNEMANN and VOORHOEVE (1973) reported good results from repairing the cruciate ligaments of the knee joint with preserved heterologous tendons.

Summing up, it may be said that replacement surgery can in principle be carried out with fresh or preserved homologous or heterologous tendons. In every case the transplanted tendon is used by the host as a 'guide rail' for vitalization, i.e. penetration of cells, and 'individualization' of the ground substance. There are problems with the replacement of sheathed tendons where adhesions may inhibit or prevent gliding. There is probably a gradient in the reaction of the host tissue to native autologous, homologous, and heterologous tendons in that order. Method of preservation, if any, also plays a part here, as mentioned above. Replacement of large tendons without sheaths is less problematical as regards the tendency to form adhesions. Here native autologous tendon material may be expected to provoke the smallest host reaction.

II. Cutis

Indications for the use of autologous or homologous implants of cutis include whole-skin arthroplasty, ligament replacement, plastic replacement of the larger tendons, and repair of the walls of body cavities (LOEWE, 1913; REHN and MIYAUCHI, 1914; EITNER, 1920; PEER, 1955; 1959; KIVILAAKSO, 1955; KALLIO, JOKINEN, KETTUNEN, FRANCILLON, GSCHWEND, all 1958; ELO, 1960; JUDET and JUDET, 1960; SPIRIG, 1961; SCHREIBER, 1967; MÜLLER et al., 1970; BEZOUGLIS and ELIOPOULOS, 1973; ROESCH, 1973). Autologous skin grafting did not establish itself because of the various possible complications, such as the formation of pockets of epithelium or cysts and the unreliability of sterilization. Research by JOKINEN (1958) showed that the formation of pockets of epithelium and cysts depended upon the tension of the graft. Thus, he found that, only 2 weeks after implantation of skin in Achilles tendon under strong traction, vestiges of epithelium were seen only in the region of a few hair follicles. Dermatodeses and long-tendon repairs still showed pockets of epithelium after one month, but no cysts. ELO (1960) transplanted fresh whole skin subperiosteally on the tibia without either fixing or stressing it. This produced epithelial cysts, which continued to grow until the 6th month and thereafter remained stationary. No malignant degeneration of the cysts was observed. Sterility in an autoplastic skin graft is not guaranteed by disinfecting the surface of the skin (HEMPEL, 1952; JUZBASIC, 1940). Consequently, R. and J. JUDET (1960) observed septic incidents in 13% of 23 cases of fresh skin grafts, most of them for the repair of tendons and ligaments. The time and trouble involved in taking autologous skin grafts is also seen as a disadvantage (REHN, 1911a, b; BLÜMER, 1948; HEMPEL, 1952; GIESE, 1953; BAUMGART, 1955; SCHEIBE, 1956; DIEHL, 1959; WESSELHÖFT, 1959 and others).

If whole skin or corium is transplanted heterotopically beneath the surface of the body, the transplant undergoes a structural change, determined by the nature and direction of the mechanical forces to which it is exposed. Thus, a free implant of cutis inserted under tension into a gap in the abdominal wall is transformed into a solid tendinous plate, whereas when the three-dimensional fiber network of corium is implanted into an Achilles tendon defect of used to replace ligaments, its structure becomes that of a tissue with parallel fibers. Skin inserted without function into subcutaneous fatty tissue is in time completely assimilated into the host tissue.

The length of time needed for the healing and restructuring of heterotopically transplanted cutis varies according to different authors. REHN (1914) and later SCHWARTZ (1922) inserted autologous skin into Achilles tendon defects in dogs and found that after 70 days the graft had been transformed into tendon. SWENSON (1950) and HENNEBERT et al. (1962), using the same experimental setup, quoted respectively 152 and 124 days for the restructuring of whole-skin grafts into tendon tissue. MAIR (1945) replaced a piece of lumbodorsal fascia in rabbit with strips of shaven skin inserted under strong traction. After 5 months it was impossible to distinguish with the naked eye between the transplant and normal fascia. KIVILAAKSO (1955) noted that whole skin implanted into a defect in the abdominal skin adapted to its new position within 60 days. Ninety days after repair of an Achilles tendon defect in rabbit by a whole-skin implant its gross appearance was indistinguishable from that of normal tendon. JOKINEN (1958) after whole-skin replacement of Achilles tendon in rabbit saw no function-dependent longitudinal orientation of the fibers in the region of the transplant until between 4 and 8 months. There is clearly a significant dependence of the time required for healing and restructuring upon the early application and strength of the functional stimulus.

Because of the disadvantages of native skin grafts, i.e. formation of pockets of epithelium or cysts and difficulty of sterilization, preserved cutis is now used almost exclusively in reconstructive surgery. However, even Cialit cannot always ensure absolute sterility in skin transplants. Both SCHREIBER (1967) and ourselves (JÄGER, 1970) were able to culture microorganisms after 4 weeks of preservation. R. and J. JUDET (1960) noted that when preserved skin was used for clinical purposes sepsis still occurred in 6% of cases, as opposed to 13% with fresh skin. SEIFFERT (1967) studied the healing of skin grafts preserved in different ways in animal experiments. He was able to show that both autologous skin and homologous skin preserved in different ways (deep-freezing, freeze-drying, Cialit 1:5,000, ethylene oxide with deep-freezing) transplanted subcutaneously in rats were always gradually resorbed. Foreign-body type encapsulation occurred with the preserved homografts. Inflammation was generally more severe with deep-frozen transplants than with freeze-dried and Cialit-preserved preparations. Similar results were obtained with autologous, fresh homologous, and preserved homologous whole-skin transplants, attached under tension to the dorsal fascia of rabbits with the epithelial side down. While the fresh homograft showed the strongest inflammatory changes during week 2, the preserved transplants had only slight inflammation and proliferative attack of the wound bed. The Cialit preparation in particular showed delayed healing and was encapsulated in the manner of a foreign body during the course of healing. In contrast, the deep-frozen and freeze-dried grafts were organized and intergrown by the host. The whole-skin autograft formed large epithelial cysts and was resorbed at an early stage.

Cialit-preserved skin grafts have performed well in clinical applications. Kallio's clinic in Helsinki and the Balgrist Clinic in Zürich have a great deal of experience in this field. Schreiber (1967) has reviewed the case material of the Balgrist Clinic, comprising 104 patients. Cialit-preserved skin was used for replacement surgery. Strips of skin were usually taken for the Cialit skin bank form the thighs of patients undergoing hip surgery; cadaveric skin was never used. They used a Cialit solution of 1:2,500 for preserving the material. In his discussion of the results Schreiber concludes that skin is an excellent plastic material, both mechanically and biologically. The chief proven indications are ligament repair (particularly of the fibular ligament of the foot), and the repair of tears in large tendons (Achilles tendon, tendons effecting extension of the knee). Dermatodeses and skin arthroplasty, on the other hand, have in Schreiber's opinion not given good results, and only a few indications can be justified, e.g. elbow arthroplasty, and dermatodeses for tendon realignment or extension. No complications had ever occurred with fresh skin taken from a living donor and preserved at once in Cialit.

Summarizing, it may be said that native autologous cutis has not performed well as a replacement material because its removal is time-consuming, it is difficult to sterilize, and prone to form pockets of epithelium and cysts. It is better to use preserved homologous or heterologous cutis, although even here sterility cannot be guaranteed. Cutis must be prestretched to improve its mechanical properties.

III. Fascia

Kirschner (1909; 1913) introduced fascia autografts into plastic surgery, and this material has remained deservedly popular. It has three main indications: as replacement of ligaments and large sheathless tendons in traumatic or degenerative defects; as anchoring material in the operative treatment of congenital or acquired anomalies of the postural or motor apparatus; as interposition material in reconstructive surgery of the joints of the upper extremities. Fascia is used almost exclusively as autografts. Its advantages are that it is available in adequate amounts (fascia lata) and, unlike skin, can be taken under absolutely sterile conditions and without time-consuming procedures; furthermore, it does not stretch unduly. Its disadvantages are poor suture holding, the need for additional extension of the operation and the exhaustion of depot if repeated operations are required, additional cosmetic disfigurement, the danger of muscle hernias, and the possibility that the patient may refuse the additional operation.

Research into the healing and restructuring of ortho- and heterotopically transplanted fascia was begun at an early date. The histologic details of the healing process were thoroughly investigated by KIRSCHNER (1909; 1913), KLEINSCHMIDT (1914), VALENTIN (1912; 1913), and SCHWARTZ (1922). It may therefore be accepted as fact that free fascia autografts heal in the living state, as demonstrated by KLEINSCHMIDT using vital staining. After transplantation the fascia graft is first surrounded by a leukocyte-rich layer of fibrin, which organizes so that after a few days the fascia is surrounded by a dense, cell-rich granulating tissue. The nuclear coloration is retained in the fascia along with most of the elastic fibers. SCHWARTZ repaired Achilles tendon defects in rabbit with fascia and was able to demonstrate that, as a result of the functional stimulus, the longitudinal fibers persisted while the crosswise bundles of fascia vanished. When fascia was implanted without function under the skin, all three fiber layers could be detected during the observation period.

There is generally no urgent practical reason to use homologous fascia, for autologous fascia is usually readily available for tissue repair. However, as mentioned above, the fascia lata is sometimes exhausted so that in a few cases lyophilized homologous fascia has also been used. The applications were for a thoracic wall hernia (METZE, 1965), small muscle hernias (DETHLOFF, 1967), cruciate and lateral ligament repairs and ruptured Achilles tendon (CRASSELT, 1967), defects in the abdominal wall (BUCSINA *et al.,* 1972), and elbow and wrist arthroplasty in rheumatoid arthritis sufferers (GRISCHIN, 1970). Only DETHLOFF reported complications. His case material comprised 14 patients in whom lyophilized homologous fascia was used to cover muscle hernias. In 2 cases it was necessary to lance a seroma, and in one case the graft became detached 6 weeks after transplantation. All the authors mentioned as a disadvantage of fascia grafting the poor suture holding due to the longitudinal direction of the fibers. As already stated, we were able to demonstrate that suture holding in fascia can be much improved by doubling the ends of the graft.

Thanks to the adequate supply of the patient's own fascia lata, the material principally used for replacement purposes in reconstructive surgery is native autologous fascia. The disadvantages are the additional extension of the operation and danger of muscle hernias. The poor suture holding due to the longitudinal fiber structure may be improved by doubling the ends of the grafts, which causes the fibers to lie crosswise.

IV. Dura

Since 1958, when CRAWFORD, DUNN and HEARD used preserved dura to close a hernia in an abdominal scar, preserved homologous dura has found increasing application in general surgery as well as in neurosurgery. Dura has certain advantages like low extensibility and good suture holding which make it appear very suitable for replacement of ligaments, capsules, and tendons in the postural and motor apparatus. We (JÄGER, 1970) therefore initiated animal experiments to determine the extent to which healing and restructuring depend upon the preservation and retention time of the dura implant. A total of 27 2-year-old Merino sheep were operated in both hind legs. Homologous sheep dura was used, one half being preserved in Cialit, and one half freeze-dried and sterilized by gamma irradiation, and implanted in the fascia lata under moderate tension. The transplants were removed 2, 6, 9, 12, and 24 weeks after implantation.

Mechanical studies of the excised implants showed that after 2 weeks max. load values were clearly superior in the lyophilized dura grafts as compared with the Cialit-preserved material. At 12 and 24 weeks the mechanical properties of the differently preserved dura grafts showed very little difference. The distinct increase in max. load values between weeks 2 and 6 is worthy of note. It is during this period that the graft becomes consolidated, and this determines the outcome. The clinical significance of this observation is that it affects the length of time for which the graft needs to be rested to allow healing and restructuring to take place. The max. load hardly varies form week 6 to week 24, and this value already matches the max. load of the fascia it has replaced after only 6 weeks. There are no significant differences attributable to method of preservation in elasticity or tensile strength.

Macro- and microscopic studies were made when the graft was excised after 2 weeks, and the histological picture of the lyophilized grafts showed that connective tissue rich in blood vessels and cells had penetrated into the fibrous network of the dura. No inflammatory cells were seen.

The Cialit-preserved grafts (Fig. 10a and b) presented much the same appearance after 2 and 6 weeks but with much stronger and tougher encapsulation of the transplant. No adhesions were seen when lengthwise cuts were made in the sac of connective tissue surrounding the graft. Microscopically, a wide

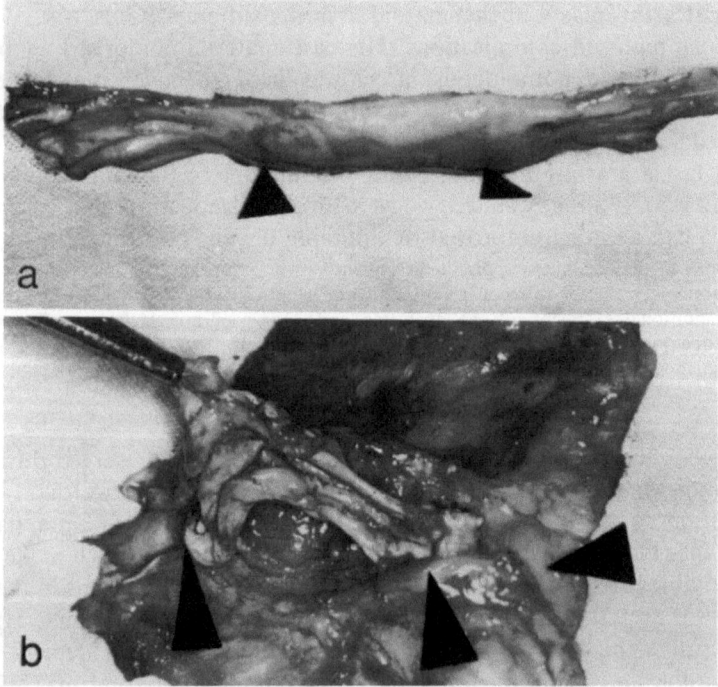

Fig. 10. (a) Cialit-preserved dura graft after 6 weeks. Sac-like, compact covering of connective tissue round graft. Arrows: upper and lower sutures. (b) Sac of connective tissue opened up. Graft covered with fibrous tissue; no adhesions within bed. Arrows: at side: fascia; below: location of sutures

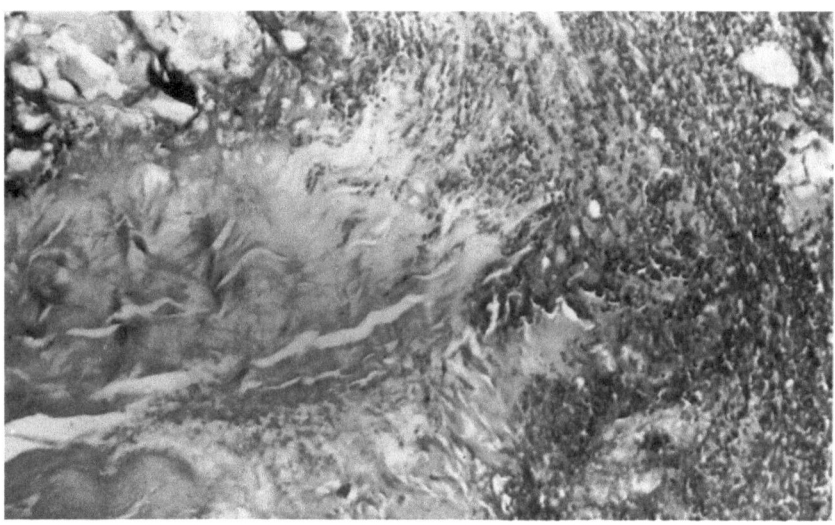

Fig. 11. Cialit-preserved graft after 6 weeks. Obvious demarcating inflammatory reaction. Slight penetration of connective-tissue cells visible in cross-section of edge. Formalin fixation, hematoxylin-eosin staining. × 235

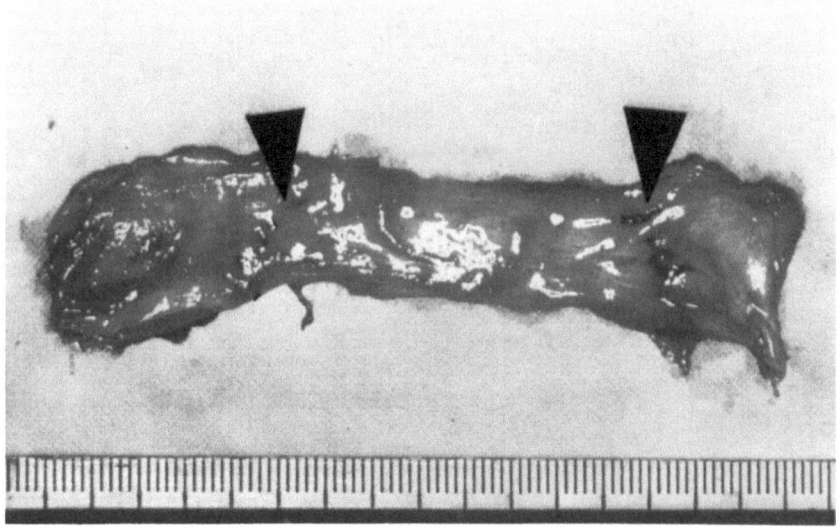

Fig. 12. Gross preparation of a lyophilized homologous dura graft 6 weeks after implantation. Arrows: upper and lower sutures

rim of inflammatory cells was seen between graft bed and graft, resembling a demarcating inflammation. There was no sign of fibroblasts penetrating the fibrous network of the dura (Fig. 11).

After 6 weeks, and much more obviously after 12 weeks, the excised grafts already displayed macroscopically clear characteristics of fascia (Fig. 12); micro-

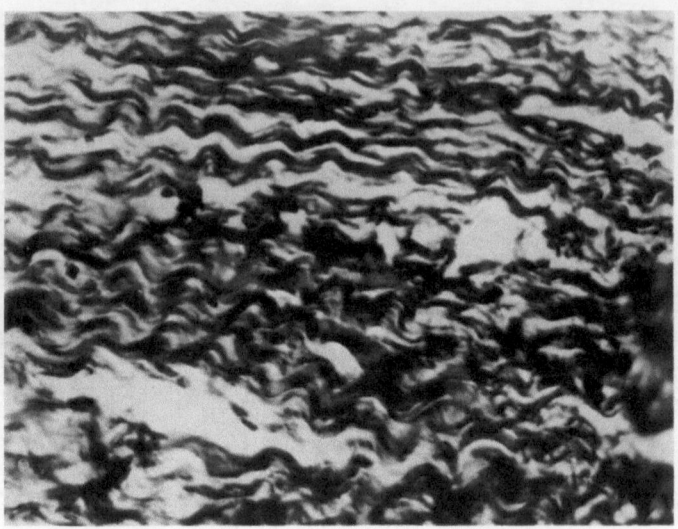

Fig. 13. Lyophilized graft after 12 weeks. Obvious reduction in number of fibroblasts. Oriented fiber structure. Formalin fixation, van Gieson staining. × 588

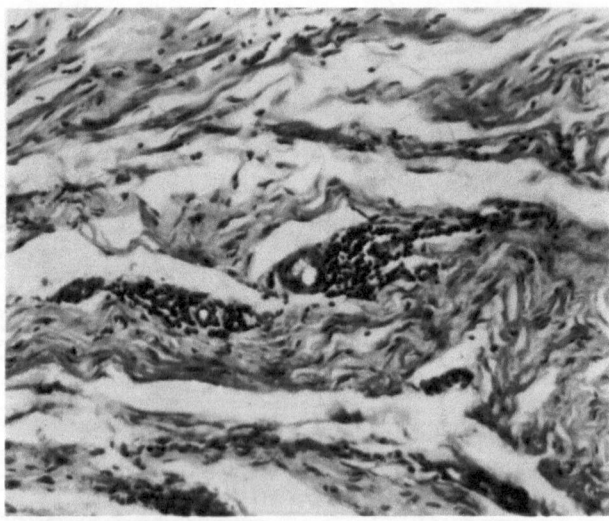

Fig. 14. Cialit-preserved graft after 12 weeks. Beginning of loose longitudinal orientation of fibers. Numerous young fibrocytes. Perivascular infiltrates. Formalin fixation, hematoxylin-eosin staining. × 235

scopically, vascularization was already seen to be diminished, as was the number of fibroblasts, too (Fig. 13). The Cialit-preserved transplants were the first to show fibroblasts being incorporated into the dura network. Perivascular round-cell infiltrates provided proof that the inflammation was subsiding (Fig. 14).

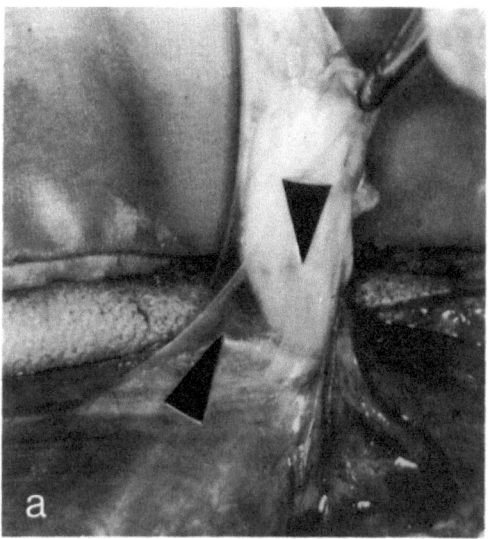

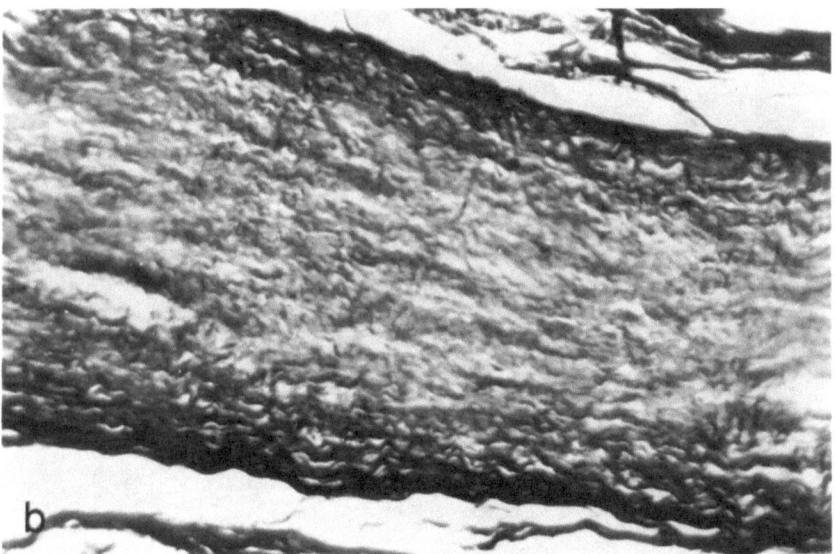

Fig. 15. (a) Lyophilisized graft after 24 weeks. Transparent layer of connective tissue (lower arrow) between bed and graft (upper arrow). (b) Fascia structure of lyophilisized graft after 24 weeks. Formalin fixation, van Gieson staining. ×235

After 24 weeks the lyophilized graft was separated from the bed only by a transparent layer of connective tissue, and some thickening of the fibrous strands was apparent microscopically. The graft had very much the character of fascia (Fig. 15a and b). The Cialit-preserved transplant, on the other hand, showed strong adhesion to the bed, and the graft itself had no rigid fibers like those seen in the lyophilized grafts (Fig. 16a and b).

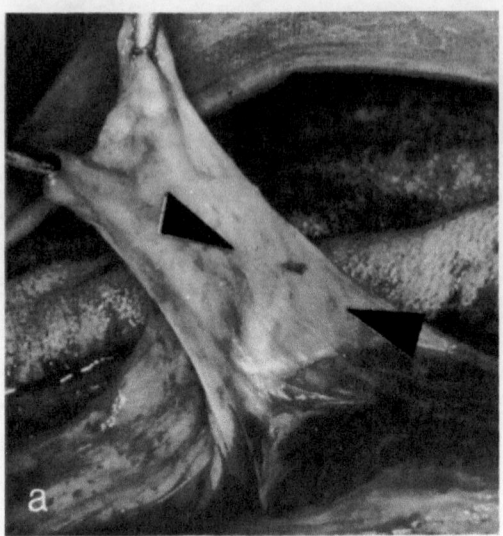

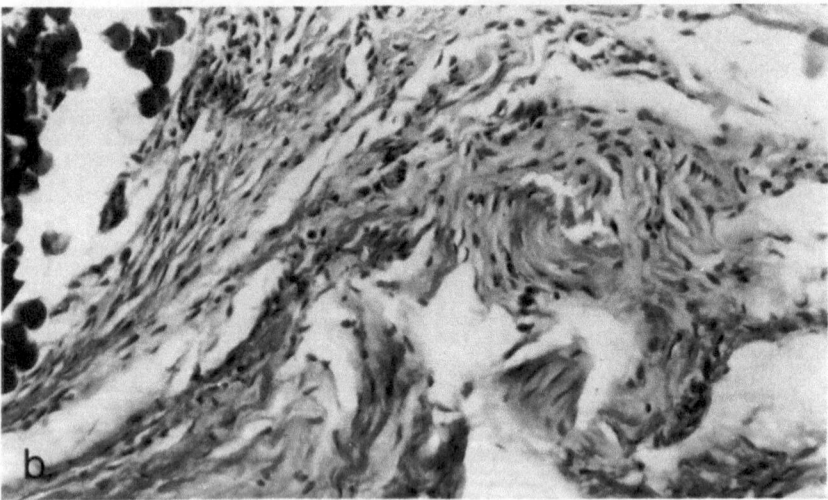

Fig. 16. (a) Cialit-preserved graft after 24 weeks. Strong adhesion (lower arrow) between graft and bed (upper arrow: turning of graft end). (b) Cialit-preserved graft after 24 weeks. No rigid oriented fiber structure. Suture on left. Formalin fixation, hematoxylin-eosin staining. ×235

In the light of these and earlier comparative studies of the mechanical properties of native and preserved connective-tissue types in order to determine their suitability as transplants (JÄGER and ANDERS, 1969), it may be said that lyophilized connective tissue homografts, despite their initially lower values for tensile strength, should be preferred to Cialit-preserved material on account of their faster healing and restructuring into functionally appropriate connective tissue.

The shorter time needed for healing and restructuring is important in orthopedic surgery, as it allows the patient to become mobile sooner, thus shortening the post-operative period of enforced rest and hence the period of sickness.

MATIS and SCHÄFFER (1973) tested the suitability of lyophilized human dura as a replacement for the cruciate ligament in 21 dogs. They found that at 2 weeks restructuring and 'healing in' of the transplants had begun, at 4 weeks they had made good progress, and after 9 weeks were practically complete. After 14 weeks, when the inflammatory cell infitrates had disappeared and the fibers had assumed the desired orientation due to traction, the implanted strip of dura could hardly be distinguished from the normal ligament tissue of the control

SCHMELZLE and SCHMIDT (1974) conducted animal experiments to test the potential of Cialit-preserved human dura grafts in maxillary-facial surgery. Cialit-preserved dura was implanted in the facial region of 18 rabbits, both subperiostally and subcutaneously. The dura samples could still be identified after 241 days. Microscopic studies showed that the dura structure remained intact for the whole of the observation period. The authors, however, think that the fiber structure of the dura would eventually be replaced by the formation of new connective tissue, detectable between the 99th and 205th postimplantation days.

Little is known about the healing and restructuring of preserved homologous dura in man. As mentioned above, FLEMMING (1963) was able to show that, unlike orthotopic dura transplants, lyophilized dura used to repair a hernia of the abdominal wall had formed adhesions with the bed after 8 months. HYOFF and HACKENSELLNER (1965) followed up the healing and restructuring of 28 orthotopically transplanted preserved dura grafts in 22 patients by means of histological sections and 4 biopsy samples. The life of the preserved dura grafts ranged from a few hours to 23 months. The authors were able to establish that the healing and restructuring of orthotopically transplanted dura depends mainly upon the host dura. The graft is surrounded and strengthened in the early months by granulation tissue, which is rapidly converted into a compact plaque of connective tissue. Actual substitution of the graft occurs extremely slowly; vestiges of the original graft were still visible after 2 years.

Reports on clinical experience with the use of preserved homologous dura are generally encouraging. The field of application has been much extended in recent years. Lyophilized dura is used surgically to close body cavities (closure of abdominal wall, thoracic wall, or dura), in arthroplasty (collar bone or shoulder dislocation, repair of cruciate and lateral ligaments in the knee joint), to replace heart valves, also in urology and gynecology for the repair of bladder and vagina (FLEMMING, SERFLING, UNGER, WEICKMANN, CRASSELT).

The range of application for lyophilized gamma-irradiated dura mater in reconstructive surgery is restricted by the natural limitation on the size of the graft. Joining of several pieces cannot be recommended because the sutures represent weak spots. Nevertheless, dura is superior to other materials, particularly for the replacement of ligaments, because it has low elasticity and good suture holding, and is not very thick. The reduction in mechanical strength due to preservation is compensated for by its more rapid healing and restructuring in comparison with Cialit-preserved tissue.

From an orthopedic viewpoint, we give on the basis of our own experience the following range of indications for the various types of preserved homologous connective tissue. *Cutis* is suitable for interposition arthroplasty in large joints of the upper extremity, as anchoring material, and for the replacement of ligaments and tendons, although we have some reservations concerning the last of these indications. *Dura* may be used for interposition arthroplasty in the smaller joints of the upper extremity (finger joints), for the replacement of tendons and ligaments, for the closure of defects in fascia, and as anchoring material. We use preserved *fascia* with certain reservations for the replacement of ligaments and tendons. In exceptional cases preserved *tendons* may be used to replace ligaments in small joints (joint at base of thumb).

D. Future Prospects

Even today, only a theoretical answer can be given to an enquiry as to the biological fate of autologous, homologous, and heterologous connective-tissue transplants. The reason for this is that both the healing process and the functional outcome of *autologous* transplants are greatly influenced among others by mechanical forces, whereas with *homologous* and *heterologous* transplants the healing and restructuring also depend upon inflammatory processes, resorption, and the reconstitution of the graft.

There are basically two theories that attempt to explain the biological fate of *autologous* transplants of supporting tissues.

1. *Survival theory*. Cells survive in autologous grafts of cartilage, fascia, tendon, skin, fat, and bone (PEER, 1955).

2. *Substitution theory*. After transplantation the supporting tissue is gradually resorbed and simultaneously built up again (LEXER, 1919; 1924; AXHAUSEN, 1962).

The primary healing processes of autologous cartilage and skin can be explained by the survival theory, and those of bone by the substitution theory. Neither hypothesis is strictly applicable to the collagenous connective tissues we are discussing here, but it is quite possible that there is partial substitution with simultaneous survival of the transplanted structure.

Similarly, there are only theories to explain the biological fate of fresh or preserved *homologous* and *heterologous* connective-tissue grafts.

1. *Regeneration theory*. The dead connective-tissue structure is regenerated by penetration of new cellular elements from the host (NAGEOTTE, 1927).

2. *Foreign-body theory*. The foreign supporting tissues, whether fresh or preserved, are encapsulated in the host organism like foreign bodies during healing, and are either tolerated (cornea, cartilage) or resorbed (MARCHAND, 1901).

3. *Guide-rail theory*. The graft serves as a guide rail or space occupier for the host's own regenerating tissue. This process requires functional tension of the graft to maintain the characteristic structure of, fascia or tendon (WEIDENREICH, 1924; LONGMIRE, 1954; PATE, 1954).

The guide-rail theory is today generally accepted as the basis of the healing processes in both fresh and preserved homo- and heterologous grafts, and by many authors also for autologous grafts.

The functional outcome of the grafting of autologous, homologous, or heterologous connective tissue ultimately depends not only upon the mechanical orientation of the regenerating tissue but also upon the nature, extension, severity, and duration of the inflammatory response, the resorption, and the reconstitution of the graft. It is therefore not surprising that the possibility of using alloplastic materials is now being explored. Synthetic prostheses are being used with good results for both temporary and long-term replacement of flexor tendons, the aim being to produce adhesion-free gliding within the tendon sheath. Attempts have been made to close large gaps in the abdominal wall with nylon net, in the hope that the holes in the mesh would later be filled in by growth of host tissue. This method was abandoned because the nylon nets did not have a satisfactory resistance to tearing. Successful experiments have been done in animals and in man on the replacement of cruciate ligaments with plastic materials of various kinds (JOHNSON, 1960; OMROD, SINGLETON, VAUGHAN, all 1963; BUTLER, 1964; LÖFFLER, 1964; SALAMON et al., 1970). The range of applications of such materials seems rather restricted. The extent to which synthetic materials can replace connective-tissue grafts has yet to be studied on a long-term basis.

References

ADAM, M., FIETZEK, P., DEYL, Z., ROSMUS, J., KÜHN, K.: Investigations on the reaction of metals with collagen in vivo. 3. The effect of bismuth, copper and mercury compounds. Europ. J. Biochem. 3, (1968) 415.

ANDERS, K., BECKER, G.W., JÄGER, M., KRÜGER, O.: Die Abhängigkeit mechanischen Verhaltens menschlicher Fascie von Faserverlauf, Alter und Konservierung. Arch. orthop. Unfall-Chir. 69, (1971) 246.

ARNOLD, G.: Mechanische Eigenschaften von Sehnen. Verh. Anat. Ges., Zagreb 1971, Anat. Anz., Ergänzungsh. Bd. 130, 499–504 (1972).

ARNOLD, G.: Festigkeit und Kraft-Längenänderungs-Verhalten der Strecksehnen des menschlichen Fußes. Res. exp. Med. 164, 123 (1974a).

ARNOLD, G.: Biomechanische und rheologische Eigenschaften menschlicher Sehnen. Z. Anat. Entwickl.-Gesch. 143, 263 (1974b).

ARNOLD, G., BLUME, C., SASSE, D.: Zur Histomechanik des menschlichen Peritoneum parietale. Anat. Anz. 134, 298–508 (1973).

ARNOLD, G., HARRING, I.: Zur Bestimmung der Elastizitätsgrenze von Bindegewebsstrukturen in vitro. Experientia (Basel) 30, 835 (1974).

ARNOLD, G., HARTUNG, C.: Histomechanische Eigenschaften der Chordae tendinae des menschlichen Herzens. Z. Biomed. Techn. 17, 169–173 (1972).

ARNOLD, G., HARTUNG, C.: Methoden und Ergebnisse rheologischer Untersuchungen am hyalinen Knorpel. Z. Orthop. 111, 153–159 (1973).

ARNOLD, G., VOGT, C.-H.: Untersuchungen zur Relaxation menschlicher Sehnen. Res. exp. Med. 159, 50–57 (1972).

ARNOLD, G., ZECH, M.: Biorheologie fast reiner Faserstrukturen im Vergleich mit Probestücken aus hyalinem Knorpel. In: Biomechanik von Bindegewebssystemen. Berlin-Heidelberg-New York: Springer 1974.

ASHLEY, F.L., STONE, R.S., ALONSO-ARTIEDA, MIGUEL, SYVERUD, J.M., EDWARDS, J.W., SLOAN, R.F., MOONEY, S.A.: Experimental and clinical studies on the application of monomolecular cellulose filter tubes to create artificial tendon sheaths in digits. Plast. reconstr. Surg. **23**, 526–534 (1959).

Axhausen, W.: Die Bedeutung der Individual- und Artspezifität der Gewebe für die freie Knochen-verpflanzung. Hefte Unfallheilkd. 72 (1962).

Bassett, C.A.L., Carroll, R.E.: Formation of tendon sheath by silicone-rod implants. In: Proceedings of the American Society for Surgery of the Hand. J. Bone Jt Surg. A **45**, 884–885 (1963).

Baumgart, R.: Ist die Cutislappenplastik nach E. Rehn dem Perlonnetz bei Eingeweidebrüchen überlegen? Zbl. Chir. **80**, 1705 (1955).

Benedict, J.V., Walker, L.B., Harris, E.H.: Stress-strain characteristics and tensile strength of unembalmed human tendons. J. Biomech. **1**, 53–63 (1968).

Bezouglis, C.P., Eliopoulos, C.S.: Die Anwendung von Hautstreifen in der Orthopädie. Z. Orthop. **111**, 617 (1973).

Biesalski, K.: Über Sehnenscheidenauswechslung. Dtsch. med. Wschr. **36**, 1615–1618 (1910).

Billingham, R.E.: Ciba Symposium. Boston: Little, Brown 1954.

Billingham, R.E., Brent, L., Medawar, P.B.: "Enhancement" in normal homograft with a note on its possible mechanism. Transplant. Bull. **3**, 84 (1956a).

Billingham, R.E., Brent, L., Medawar, P.B.: Antigenic stimulus in transplantation immunity. Nature (Lond.), **178**, 514 (1956b).

Billingham, R.E., Medawar, P.B.: The freezing, drying and storage of mammalian skin. J. exp. Biol. **29**, (1952) 454.

Blanton, P.L., Biggs, N.L.: Ultimate tensile strength of foetal and adult human tendons. J. Biomech. **3**, 181 (1970).

Blümer, G.: Quoted by Flemming (1965).

Böhm, A.A., Davidoff, M.V.: Histologie des Menschen. Wiesbaden: Bergmann 1898.

Bornemisza, G.: In: Kettler, L.H., Serfling, H.J., Gewebekonserven, Bd. 11. Berlin 1965.

Boyes, J.H.: Flexor tendon grafts in the fingers and thumb. An evaluation of end results. J. Bone Jt Surg. **32** A, 489–499 (1950).

Bowitz, R., Nemetschek, T.: Struktur und Dehnungsverhalten von Kollagen. In: Biopolymere und Biomechanik von Bindegewebssystemen. Berlin-Heidelberg-New York: Springer 1974.

Brocklin, J.D. van, Ellis, D.G.: A study of the mechanical behavior of toe extensor tendons under applied stress. Arch. phys. Med. 360–373 (1965).

Brüchle, H.: Experimentelle Untersuchungen an konservierten Sehnen. Chir. plast. **6**, 62 (1969).

Bucsina, D., Ritter, L., B'alint, J.: Konservierte Faszie bei Operationen von Bauchwandbrüchen. Zbl. Chir. **97**, 1863 (1972).

Bunnell, S.: Repair of tendons in the fingers and description of two new instruments. Surg. Gynec. Obstet. **26**, 103 (1918).

Butler, H.C.: Teflon as a prosthetic ligament in repair of ruptured cruciate ligaments. Amer. J. vet. Res. **25**, 55 (1964).

Campbell, J.B., Bassett, C.A.L., Robertson, J.W.: Quoted by Seiffert (1967).

Crasselt, C.: Band- und Sehnenplastiken mit lyophilisiertem homologen Gewebe. Beitr. Orthop. Traum. **14**, 666 (1967).

Crawford, E.S., Dunn, J.R., Heard, J.B.: Quoted by Flemming (1965).

Cronkite, A.E.: The tensile strength of human tendons. Anat. Rec. **64**, (1936).

Dethloff, E.: Faszientransplantate. Beitr. Orthop. Traum. **14**, 672 (1967).

Diamant, J., Keller, A., Baer, E., Litt, N., Arridge, R.G.C.: Collagen: ultrastructure and its relation to mechanical properties as a function of ageing. Proc. roy. Soc. B **180**, 293 (1972).

Dick, J.C.: The tension and resistance to stretching of human skin and other membranes, with results from a series of normal and oedematous cases. J. Physiol. (Lond.) **112**, 102 (1951).

Diehl, E.: Beitrag zur plastischen Deckung von größeren Bauchbrüchen mit Cutislappen. Chirurg **30**, 322 (1959).

Eitner, E.: Über die Unterpolsterung der Gesichtshaut. Med. Klin. **16**, 93 (1920).

Elliot, D.H.: Structure and function of mammalian tendon. Biol. Rev. **40**, 392–421 (1965).

Elliot, D.H.: The biomechanical properties of tendon in relation to muscular strength. Ann. phys. Med. **9**, 1 (1967).

Ellis, D.G.: Cross-sectional area measurements for tendon specimens: A comparison of several methods. J. Biomech. **2**, 175 (1969).

Elo, J.O.: The effect of subperiosteally implanted autogenous wholethickness skin graft on growing bone. Acta orthop. scand. **30**, Suppl. 43 (1960).

FLEMMING, F.: In: KETTLER, L.H., SERFLING, H.J., Gewebekonserven. Berlin 1961.

FLEMMING, F.: Plastische Versorgung von Bauchnarbenbrüchen mit homologer Dura. Bruns' Beitr. klin. Chir. **206**, 357 (1963).

FLEMMING, F.: In: KETTLER, L.H., SERFLING, H.J., Gewebekonserven II. Berlin 1965.

FLEMMING, F., UNGER, R.: Zur Anwendung lyophilisierten Gewebes in der Chirurgie. Zbl. Chir. **86**, 375 (1961).

FRANCILLON, M.R.: Myokinesigraphie. In: HOHMANN, G., HACKENBROCH, M., LINDEMANN, K.: Handbuch der Orthopädie, Bd. I, S. 878. Stuttgart: Georg-Thieme 1957.

FRANCILLON, M.R.: Traitement des entorses récidivantes du cou-de-piepar rétraction du ligament latéral externe par greffe dermique. Acta orthop. belg. **25**, 559 (1959).

FRANCILLON, M.R.: Myokinetische und operative Befunde bei der Distorsio pedis. Bandersatz durch Kutisriemen. Verh. Dtsch. Orthop. Ges. 48 Kongr. 1960. Beih. Z. Orthop. **94**, 398 (1961).

FRANCILLON, M.R.: Distorsio pedis. Schweiz. med. Wschr. **91**, 117 (1961).

FRANCILLON, M.R.: Distorsio pedis with an isolated lesion of the ligamentum calcaneo-fibulare. Acta orthop. scand. **32**, 473 (1962).

FRANCILLON, M.R.: Utilizacion de la dermatodesis en el tratamiento de las paralisis del serrato mayor. Libro-Homenaje Prof. SANCHES OLMOS Hospital Provincial de Madrid 1965.

FRANCILLON, M.R.: Zur Analyse des Gehens. In: Aktuelle Diagnostik, Festschr. 75 Jahre Hommel. Zürich: Bühler 1965.

FRANCILLON, M.R.: Osteotomien und Gelenkplastiken in der Behandlung der primär chronischen Polyarthritis. Med. Welt **1965**, 2523–2525.

GIESE, R.: Quoted by FLEMMING (1965).

GLUCK, T.: Quoted by SEIFFERT (1967).

GLUCK, T.: Zur Behandlung der Ankylose des Kiefergelenkes. Verh. dtsch. Ges. Chir. **1**, 167 (1902).

GONZALEZ, R.I.: Experimental tendon repair within the flexor tunnels. Use of polyethylene tubes for improvement of functional results in the dog. Surgery **26**, 181–198 (1949).

GRASSMANN, W.: Unsere heutige Kenntnis des Kollagens. Das Leder **10**, 241 (1955).

GRASSMANN, W.: Kollagenforschungen. Das Leder **12**, 165 (1961).

GRASSMANN, W., ENGEL, J., HANNIG, K., HÖRMANN, H., KUHN, K., NORDWIG, A.: Kollagen. In: Fortschritte der Chemie organischer Nährstoffe (ed. L. ZECHMEISTER). Wien: Springer 1965.

GRATZ, C.M.: Tensile strength and elasticity tests on human fascia lata. J. Bone Jt Surg. A **13**, 334 (1931).

GRISCHIN, I.G.: II. Orthopädische Probleme bei der Behandlung der chronischen Polyarthritis. Arthroplastik der Ellbogen- und Handgelenke mit homoplastischer Faszie bei Patienten mit rheumatoider Arthritis. Beitr. Orthop. Traum. **17**, 745 (1970).

GRÜTER, H.: Desinfektionsversuche mit einem neuen Quecksilberpräparat „Cialit". Dissertation, Münster 1933.

GSCHWEND, N.: Die fibularen Bandläsionen. Eine häufig verkannte Folge der Fußverstauchungen. Praxis **47**, 809 (1958).

GSCHWEND, N.: Zur Häufigkeit und Aetiologie der lateralen Form der Osteochondrosis dissecans tali. Arch. orthop. Unfall-Chir. **51**, 491 (1960).

GSCHWEND, N.: Die operative Behandlung der progressiv chronischen Polyarthritis. Stuttgart: Thieme 1968.

GUEUKDJIAN, S.A.: A new method of canalization of tendon sutures with vein grafts. Arch. Surg. **73**, 1018–1021 (1956).

GUSTAVSON, K.H.: The Chemistry and Reactivity of Collagen. New York: Acad. Press 1956.

HAAS, S.L.: Quoted by PEER (1959).

HACKENSELLNER, H.A.: Gefriergetrocknete Dura — ein wertvolles Transplantationsmaterial. Klin. Med. **10**, 599 (1962).

HACKENSELLNER, H.A.: Quoted by METZ (1965).

HELFERICH, H.: Ein neues Operationsverfahren zur Heilung der knöchernen Kiefergelenkankylose. Langenbecks Arch. klin. Chir. **48**, 864 (1894).

HEMPEL, E.: Quoted by FLEMMING (1965).

HENNEBERT, P.N., MAKULU, A., NZEZA, L.: Quoted by SEIFFERT (1967).

HERZOG, K.H.: Sehnenkonservierung und -transplantation. Jena: Fischer 1965.

HERZOG, K.H.: Sehnenhomoplastik in Experiment und Klinik. Beitr. Orthop. Traum. **14**, 557 (1967).

HIRSCH, G.: Tensile properties during tendon healing. Acta orthop. scand., Suppl. 153 (1974).

HÖRMANN, H.: Zur Frage der Quervernetzung von Kollagen. Das Leder 13, 79 (1962).

HÖRMANN, H.: Bausteine des Stütz- und Bindegewebes (biochem. Referat). Binde- und Stützgewebe, Morphologische und biochemische Information (eds. H. BARTELHEIMER, N. DETTMER). Darmstadt: Steinkopff 1966.

HUESTON, J.T., HUBBLE, B., RIGG, B.R.: Homografts of the digital flexor tendon system. Aust. N. Z. J. Surg. 36, 269–274 (1967).

HUMPHREY, J.N., WHITE, R.G.: Kurzes Lehrbuch der Immunologie. Stuttgart: Thieme 1971.

HUNTER, J.: Artificial tendons. Early development and application. Amer. J. Surg. 109, 325–338 (1965).

HUNTER, J.M.: Tendon reconstruction using a gliding tendon prosthesis prior to flexor tendon grafting. In: Orthopaedic surgery and traumatology. Amsterdam: Excerpta medica 1973.

HUNTER, J.M., SALEM, A.W., STEINDEL, C.R., SALISBURY, R.E.: The use of gliding artificial tendon implants to form new tendon beds. Presented at the Annual Meeting of the American Society for Surgery of the Hand. New York, Jan. 17, 1969.

HUNTER, J.M., SALISBURY, R.E.: Flexor tendon reconstruction in severely damaged hands. A two-stage procedure using a silicone-dacron reinforced gliding prosthesis prior to tendon grafting. J. Bone Jt Surg. A 53, 829–858 (1971).

HYATT, G.W., TURNER, T.C., BASSETT, A.L., PATE, J.W., SAWEYER, P.N.: New methods for preserving bone, skin and blood vessels. Postgrad. Med. 12, 238 (1952).

HYOFF, H., HACKENSELLNER, H.A.: Das histologische Bild des Einbaus und Umbaus von gefriergetrockneten Duratransplantaten beim Menschen. In: Gewebekonserven, Herstellung und Anwendung. 2nd Symposium, 8. edn. (240) (eds. KETTLER, L.H., SERFLING, H.J.). Berlin: Volk & Gesundheit 1965.

IDELBERGER, K.: Palavit in der operativen Orthopädie. Z. Orthop. 86, Beilageheft (1955).

ISELIN, M.R., DE LA PLAZA, R., FLORES, A.: Surgical use of homologous tendon grafts preserved in Cialit. Plast. reconstr. Surg. 32, 4 (1963).

JÄGER, M.: Bindegewebstransplantationen in der orthopädischen Chirurgie. Fortschr. Med. 87, 1014 (1969a).

JÄGER, M.: Experimentelle Untersuchungen und erste klinische Anwendung der lyophilisierten Dura in der Orthopädie. Melsunger med. Mitt. 112, 157 (1969b).

JÄGER, M.: Homologe Bindegewebstransplantation. Biomechanische Untersuchungen zur Frage der Transplantateignung verschieden strukturierter und konservierter Bindegewebstexturen in der orthopädischen Chirurgie. Aktuelle Orthopädie, H. 2. Stuttgart: Thieme 1970.

JÄGER, M.: Experimentelle Untersuchungen und klinische Anwendung homologer Bindegewebstransplantate. Verh. Dtsch. Ges. Orthop. Traum. Stuttgart: Enke 1971a.

JÄGER, M.: Experimentelle Untersuchungen zur Verwendung der lyophilisierten Dura im Bereich der Wiederherstellungschirurgie. Chirurg 42, 266–269 (1971b).

JÄGER, M.: Indikation und Anwendungsmöglichkeiten verschieden konservierter homologer Transplantate. Acta traum. 3, 91 (1973).

JÄGER, M.: Biomechanical examinations for the usefulness of grafts with different structural and conservational connective tissue properties in orthopedic surgery. In: Biopolymere und Biomechanik von Bindegewebssystemen. Berlin-Heidelberg-New York: Springer 1974.

JÄGER, M.: Dura – ihre Verwendungsmöglichkeit bei Bandverletzungen des Kniegelenkes. Vortrag, geh. auf d. 3. Reisensburger Workshop, Februar 1975.

JÄGER, M., ANDERS, K.: Dehnungs- und Entdehnungsverhalten verschieden konservierter und strukturierter Bindegewebstexturen. Arch. orthop. Unfall-Chir. 66, 95 (1969).

JALIFIER: Quoted by SEIFFERT (1967).

JOHNSON, F.L.: Prosthetic anterior cruciate ligament of the dog. J. Amer. vet. med. Ass. 137, 646 (1960).

JOKINEN, T.: Tensile strength of the whole-thickness skin graft used for the replacement of tendon and ligament defects. Acta orthop. scand. 28, Suppl. 36 (1958).

JUDET, J., GUIGNARD, J.: Transplantation du tiers externe du tendon d'Achille à la face externe du calcaneum. Rev. Chir. orthop. 46, 634 (1960).

JUDET, J., JUDET, R., CLERIN, J.T.: Ligamentoplastie du genou à la peau conservée. J. Chir. (Paris) 82, 302 (1961).

JUDET, R., JUDET, J.: Arthroplastie avec interposition cutanée. Rev. Chir. orthop. 46, 663 (1960).

JUDET, R., LORD, G.: L'emploi de la peau conservée en chirurgie osseuse. Acta orthop. belg. **25**, 561 (1959).

JUDET, R., ROY-CAMILLE, R., LETOURNEL, E.: Le banque de peau en chirurgie orthopédique. Ann. Chir. **14**, 1367 (1960).

JUNGHANNS, H., JUZBASIC, D.M.: Quoted by FLEMMING (1965).

KALLIO, E.: Skin arthroplasty of the hip joint and corresponding alloplastic methods in the light of a clinical study. Acta orthop. scand., Suppl. **30**, (1958).

KALLIO, K.E.: Arthroplastie cutanée de la hanche; autogreffe fraiche de peau totale avec du tissu adipeux. Mém. Acad. Chir. **81**, 458 (1955).

KALLIO, K.E.: Skin cap arthroplasty. XX. Anniversary. International College of Surgeons, Geneva, 23–26 May 1955, p. 577.

KALLIO, K.E.: Skin arthroplasty of the hip joint. Ann. Chir. Gynaec. Fenn. **45**, 181 (1956).

KALLIO, K.E.: Arthroplastia Cutanea Coxae. Acta orthop. scand. **4**, 327 (1957).

KALLIO, K.E.: Traitement chirurgical de l'arthrite rheumatoïde de l'articulation du genou. Congres S.I.C.O.T. Vienne 1963, Impr. des Sciences, Bruxelles, p. 180 (1964).

KEL AMI, A.: Lyophilized human dura as a bladder wall substitute: Experimental and clinical results. Sc. J. Urol. **105**, 518–522 (1971).

KEL AMI, A., KORB, G., LUDTKE-HANDJERY, A., ROLLE, J., SCHNELL, J., LEHNHARDT, F.H.: Alloplastic replacement of the partially resected urethra in dogs. Invest. Urol. 55–58 (1971).

KETTLER, L.H., SERFLING, H.J.: Berlin: Volk & Gesundheit 1965.

KETTUNEN, K.O.: Skin arthroplasty in the light of animal experiments with special reference to functional metaplasia of connective tissue. Acta orthop. scand. Suppl. **29**, (1958).

KIRSCHNER, M.: Über freie Sehnen- und Faszientransplantation. Bruns' Beitr. klin. Chir. **65**, 472 (1909).

KIRSCHNER, M.: Der gegenwärtige Stand und die nächsten Aussichten der autoplastischen freien Faszienübertragung. Bruns' Beitr. klin. Chir. **86**, 1 (1913).

KIVILAAKSO, R.: Changes in the whole-thickness skin graft buried in tissue. Acta orthop. scand. **25**, Suppl. 18 (1955).

KLEINSCHMIDT, O.: Die freie autoplastische Faszientransplantation. Ergebn. Chir. Orthop. **8**, 206 (1914a).

KLEINSCHMIDT, O.: Experimentelle Untersuchungen über den histologischen Umbau der frei transplantierten Faszie und Beweis für die Lebensfähigkeit derselben unter Heranziehung der vitalen Färbung. Langenbecks Arch. klin. Chir. **104**, 933 (1914b).

KOCH, S.L.: Division of the flexor tendons within the digital sheath. Surg. Gynec. Obstet. **78**, 9 (1944).

KOONTZ, A.R.: Quoted by PEER (1959).

KORB, G., RUNGE, D., ARKENAU, C.: Histologische Untersuchungen von lyophilisierten, mit Gammastrahlen sterilisierten kollagenen Geweben. Melsunger med. Mitt. **41**, H. 108, 11, 38 (1967).

KREUZ, F.P., HYATT, G.W., TURNER, T.C., BASSETT, C.A.L.: The preservation and clinical use of freeze-dried bone. J. Bone Jt Surg. A **33**, 863 (1951).

LANGE, M.: Orthopädisch-Chirurgische Operationslehre, 2nd edn. München: Bergmann 1962.

LANGE, M.: Orthopädisch-Chirurgische Operationslehre. Ergänzungsband: Neueste Operationsverfahren. München: Bergmann 1968.

LANGER, K.: Quoted by PUNKUS, F.: Normale Anatomie der Haut. In: Handbuch der Haut- und Geschlechtskrankheiten, ed. J. JADASSOHN. Berlin: Springer 1927.

LEXER, E.: Die freien Transplantationen. Neue dtsch. Chir. **26a** (1919); Neue dtsch. Chir. **26b** (1924).

LOEFFLER, K.: Kreuzbandverletzungen im Kniegelenk des Hundes. Anatomie, Klinik und experimentelle Untersuchungen. Hannover: M. u. H. Scharper Verlag 1964.

LOEWE, O.: Über Hautimplantation an Stelle der freien Faszienplastik. Münch. med. Wschr. **24**, 1320 (1913).

LONGMIRE, W.P., JR., CANNON, J.A., WEBER, R.A.: General surgical problems of tissue transplantation. In: Preservation and transplantation of normal tissue (p. 23). Ciba Foundation General Symposia. London: Churchill 1954.

MAIR, G.B.: The use of whole skin graft in the treatment of hernia. Brit. J. Surg. **32**, 381 (1945).

MARCHAND, F.: Der Process der Wundheilung mit Einschluß der Transplantation. Dtsch. Chir. **16**, (1901).

Marquardt, P., Hedler, L.: Quoted by Seiffert (1967).
Marrangoni, A.G., Cecchini, L.P.: Homotransplantation of arterial segments preserved by the freeze-drying method. Ann. Surg. **134**, 977 (1951).
Mason, M.S., Raaf, J.: Quoted by Seiffert (1967).
Mason, M.L., Shearon, C.G.: The process of tendon repair. Arch. Surg. **25**, 615 (1932).
Masshoff, W.: Handbuch d. Allg. Pathol., Bd. VI/I. Berlin-Göttingen-Heidelberg: Springer 1955.
Matis, U., Schäffer, E.: Zur Frage des Kreuzbandersatzes mit lyophilisierter menschlicher Dura beim Hund — experimentelle Untersuchungen. Berl. Münch. tierärztl. Wschr. **86**, 245 (1973).
Mayer, Leo, Ransohoff, Nicholas: Reconstruction of the digital tendon sheath. A contribution to the physiological method of repair of damaged finger tendons. J. Bone Jt Surg. **18**, 607-616 (1936).
Medawar, P.B.: General problems of immunity. In: Preservation and transplantation of normal tissues (p. 1). Ciba Foundation General Symposia. London: Churchill 1954a.
Medawar, P.B.: Diskussionsbemerkung zum Vortrag von J.E. Lovelock. In: Preservation and transplantation of normal tissue. Ciba Foundation General Symposia. London: Churchill 1954b.
Medawar, P.B.: The immunology of transplantation. Harvey Lect. **52** (1958).
Metz, R.: Durakonservierung. Wehrmed. Mschr. **9**, 159 (1965).
Metz, R.: Erfahrungsbericht über Gewebskonservierung und -verpflanzung an der Gewebebank des Bundeswehr-Lazarettes Gießen, Wehrmed. Wschr. **11**, 66 (1967).
Metze, H.: Diskussionsbemerkung. In: Gewebekonserven, Herstellung und Anwendung. 2. Symposion, 8th edn (p. 196) (eds. L.H. Kettler, H.J. Serfling), Berlin: Volk & Gesundheit 1965.
Minns, R.J., Soden, P.D., Jackson, D.S.: The role of the fibrous components and ground substance in the mechanical properties of biological tissues: a preliminary investigation. J. Biomech. **6**, 153 (1973).
Müller, J., Willenegger, H., Schuster, K.: Autologe Cutisplastik bei Spätschäden von seiten der Bänder (Seitenband, Kreuzband). Z. Unfallmed. Berufskr. **63**, 23 (1970).
Nageotte, J.: Réfléxion sur quelques causes d'erreur dans l'examen histologique des greffes osseuses experimentales. C.R. Soc. Biol. (Paris) **84**, 828 (1921).
Nageotte, J.: L'organisation de la matière dans ses rapports avec la vie. Paris: Alean 1922.
Nageotte, J.: Über die Verpflanzung von abgetöteten Bindegewebsstücken. Virchows Arch. path. Anat. **263**, 69 (1927).
Nageotte, J., Sencert, L.: Quoted by Seiffert (1967).
Nasteff, D.: In: Kettler, L.H., Serfling, H.J., Gewebekonserven II. Berlin 1965.
Neumann, K.H.: Grundriß der Gefriertrocknung. Göttingen: Musterschmidt 1955.
Nicolle, F.V.: A silastic tendon prosthesis as an adjunct to flexor tendon grafting: An experimental and clinical evaluation. Brit. J. plast. Surg. **22**, 224 (1969).
Omrod, A.N.: Restabilisation of the femoro-tibial joint in the dog following rupture of the anterior cruciate ligament. Vet. Rec. **75**, 375 (1963).
Pahlke, G.: Elektronenmikroskopische Untersuchungen an der Interzellularsubstanz des menschlichen Bindegewebes. Z. Zellforsch. **39**, 421 (1954).
Pate, J.W.: Transplantation of preserved non-viable tissues. In: Preservation and transplantation of normal tissue. Ciba Foundation General Symposia. London: Churchill 1954.
Peacock, E.E., Jr.: The vascular basis for tendon repair. Surg. Forum **8**, 65 (1957).
Peacock, E.E., Jr.: A study of the circulation in normal tendons and healing grafts. Ann. Surg. **149**, 415 (1959).
Peacock, E.E., Jr.: Some aspects of fibrogenesis during the healing of primary and secondary wounds. Surg. Gynec. Obstet. **115**, 408 (1962).
Peacock, E.E., Jr.: Fundamental aspects of wound healing relating to the restoration of gliding function after tendon repair. Surg. Gynec. Obstet. **119**, 241 (1964).
Peacock, E.E., Jr.: Biological principles in the healing of long tendons. Surg. Clin. N. Amer. **45**, 461 (1965).
Peacock, E.E., Jr.: Biology of tendon repair. New Engl. J. Med. **276**, 680–683 (1967).
Peacock, E.E., Jr., Madden, J.N.: Human composite flexor tendon allografts. Ann. Surg. **166**, 624–629 (1967).
Peer, L., Paddock, R.: Histologic studies on the fate of deeply implanted dermal grafts. Arch. Surg. **34**, 268 (1937).
Peer, L.A.: Transplantation of tissues. I. Baltimore: 1955.
Peer, L.A.: Transplantation of tissues. II. Baltimore: 1959.

POTENZA, A.D.: The healing of autogenous tendon grafts within the flexor digital sheath in dogs. J. Bone Jt Surg. A **46**, 1462–1484 (1964).

PULVERTAFT, R.G.: Repair of tendon injuries in the hand. Ann. roy. Coll. Surg. Engl. **3**, 3 (1948).

PULVERTAFT, R.G.: Tendon grafts for flexor tendon injuries in the fingers and thumb. J. Bone Jt Surg. B **38**, 175 (1956).

RANK, B.K., WAKEFIELD, A.R.: Flexor tendon repair in the hand. Austr. N. Z. J. Surg. **19**, 232–238 (1950).

RANK, B.K., WAKEFIELD, A.R.: In: Surgery of repair as applied to hand injuries. Ed. 2. Edinburgh-London: Livingstone 1960.

REHN, E.: Das Verhalten der Faszie bei homoioplastischer Transplantation. Verh. dtsch. Ges. Chir. **40**, 1. Teil, 87 (1911 a).

REHN, E.: Experimentelle Erfahrungen über freie Gewebstransplantationen. Verh. dtsch. Ges. Chir. **40**, 1. Teil, 86 (1911 b).

REHN, E.: Versuche über Duraersatz. Verh. dtsch. Ges. Chir. **1**, 99 (1912).

REHN, E.: Zur Frage des Ersatzes großer Sehnendefekte. Langenbecks Arch. klin. Chir. **114**, 253 (1920).

REHN, E., MIYAUCHI, M.: Das kutane und subkutane Bindegewebe in veränderter Funktion. Langenbecks Arch. klin. Chir. **105**, 1 (1914).

RIGBY, B.J.: Effect of cyclic extension on the physical protperties of tendon collagen and its possible relation to biological ageing of collagen. Nature (Lond.) **202**, 1072 (1964).

ROESCH, H.: Die Kutisplastik bei Seitenbandschaden des Kniegelenkes und bei veraltetem Quadrizepssehnenriß. Z. Orthop. **111**, 383 (1973).

ROLLHÄUSER, H.: Konstitutions- und Altersunterschiede in Festigkeit kollagener Fibrillen. Gegenbaurs morph. Jb. **90**, 157 (1950 a).

ROLLHÄUSER, H.: Die Festigkeit menschlicher Sehnen nach Quellung und Trocknung in Abhängigkeit vom Lebensalter. Gegenbaurs morph. Jb. **90**, 180 (1950 b).

ROLLHÄUSER, H.: Die Zugfestigkeit der menschlichen Haut. Gegenbaurs morph. Jb. **90**, 249 (1950 c).

ROLLHÄUSER, H.: Untersuchungen über den mikroskopischen Bau kollagener Fasern. Morph. Jb. **51**, 1 (1951).

ROLLHÄUSER, H.: Der Einfluß der funktionellen Beanspruchung auf die Feinstruktur der Sehne. Morph. Jb. **93**, 153 (1953).

ROLLHÄUSER, H.: Funktionelle Anpassung der Sehnenfasern im submikroskopischen Bereich. Verh. anat. Ges. (Jena) **51**, 318 (1954).

ROLLHÄUSER, H., WENDT, G.: Zur inneren Mechanik des hypertrophierten Muskels. Morph. Jb. **95**, 151 (1955).

SAKELLARIDES, H.T.: Divided flexor tendons in the "no man's land" in the fingers and thumb and treatment by tendon grafting. In: Orthopaedic Surg. and Traum. Amsterdam: Excerpta medica 1973.

SALAMON, A., MAYER, F., TEMES, G.: Der experimentelle Ersatz des vorderen Kreuzbandes im Kniegelenk durch Transplantate verschiedenen Typs. Bruns' Beitr. klin. Chir. **218**, 182 (1970).

SALOMON, A.: Untersuchungen über die Transplantation verschiedenartiger Gewebe im Sehnendefekt. Langenbecks Arch. klin. Chir. **114**, 523 (1920).

SALOMON, A.: Über Sehnenersatz ohne Muskel; ein Beitrag zur Lehre von den funktionellen Reizen. Langenbecks Arch. klin. Chir. **119**, 608 (1922).

SANCHIS-OLMOS, V.: L'emploi de la peau conservée dans le Merthiolate en chirurgie orthopédique. Congrès Berne: SICOT 1954.

SARKIN, T.L.: A fifteen-year follow-up of the nylon replacement of cut flexor tendons of the fingers. In: Orthop. Surg. Traum. Amsterdam: Excerpta medica 1973.

SCHAFFER, J.: Vorlesungen über Histologie und Histogenese. Leipzig: Engelmann 1920.

SCHEIBE, G.: Freie Cutisplastik bei sakraler Narbenhernie. Zbl. Chir. **81**, 1066 (1956).

SCHMELZLE, R., SCHMIDT, U.: Results of animal experiments on the transplantability of Cialite-preserved human dura. J. max.-fac. Surg. **2**, 49 (1974).

SCHMIDT, A., SEIFFERT, K.E.: Zur Beeinflussung der Verwachsungen von Beugesehnentransplantaten. Handchirurgie, 85–87 (1973).

SCHNELL, J., PLENTO, H.G., PAULI, W., BRAUN, B., KORB, G.: The influence of ionizing radiation on various collagen-containing medical bioproducts **92**, 145 (1967).

SCHREIBER, A.: Die Verwendung von Hautimplantaten in der Orthopädie. Ergebn. Chir. Orthop. **50**, 1 (1967).

SCHREIBER, A.: Pers. comm. (1968).

SCHWARTZ, E.: Über die anatomischen Vorgänge bei der Sehnenregeneration und dem plastischen Ersatz von Sehnendefekten durch Sehne, Faszie und Bindegewebe. Dtsch. Z. Chir. **173**, 301 (1922).

SCHWARZ, W.: Elektronenmikroskopische Untersuchungen über die Differenzierung der Cornea- und Sklerafibrillen des Menschen. Z. Zellforsch. **38**, 78 (1953).

SCHWARZ, W.: Über Bindegewebsfibrillen im Interstitium der Lunge. Beitr. zur Silikose-Forsch. Sonderband II/**23**, 605 (1957).

SCHWARZ, W.: Bausteine des Stütz- und Bindegewebes. In: Binde- und Stützgewebe, hrsg. von BARTELHEIMER, H., DETTMER, N. Darmstadt: Steinkopff 1966.

SCHWARZ, W., PAHLKE, G.: Elektronenmikroskopische Untersuchungen an der Interzellularsubstanz des menschlichen Knochengewebes. Z. Zellforsch. **38**, 75 (1953).

SEIFFERT, K.E.: Biologische Grundlagen der homologen Transplantation konservierter Bindegewebe. Mschr. Unfallheilk. **93**, (1967).

SEIFFERT, K.E.: Biological aspects of collagenous homografts. Acta oto-rhino-laryng. belg. **24**, 27–33 (1970).

SEIFFERT, K.E., FILIPOVI, C.B.: Peritonealersatz mit konservierter Dura. Med. Mschr. **24**, 161–164 (1970).

SEIFFERT, K.E., HARTLEIB, J., SCHMIT, K.P.: Über den biologischen Umbau von frischem und in Cialit konserviertem Sehnengewebe in funktionstüchtige Sehnen. Bruns' Beitr. klin. Chir. **209**, 444 (1964).

SIEBER, E.: Biochemische Untersuchungen an konserviertem Knochengewebe. Zbl. Chir. **81**, 538 (1956).

SINGLETON, W.B.: Stifle joint surgery in the dog. Canad. vet. J. **4**, 142 (1963).

SPIRIG, B.: Vorläufige Mitteilung über die Anwendungsmöglichkeit von Cialit-Hautstreifen. Schweiz. med. Wschr. **91**, 60 (1961).

STEFFEN, C.: Allgemeine und experimentelle Immunologie und Immunpathologie. Stuttgart: Thieme 1967.

STEFFEN, C.: Pers. vomm. 1968.

STEFFEN, C., TIMPL, R.: Quoted by STEFFEN (1967).

STEFFEN, C., TIMPL, R., WOLFF, J., FURTHMAYR, H., WICK, G.: Immunbiologie und Immunpathologie des Kollagens. Melsunger med. Mitt. **41**, 27 (1967).

STERNEMANN, H.O., VOORHOEVE, A.: Die Kreuzbandplastiken des Kniegelenkes. Arch. orthop. Unfall-Chir. **74**, 329 (1973).

STÖHR, PH.: Lehrbuch der Histologie, 17. edn., ed. O. SCHULTZE. Jena: Fischer 1918.

STUCKE, K.: Über das elastische Verhalten der Achillessehne im Belastungsversuch. Langenbecks Arch. klin. Chir. **265**, 579 (1950).

SWENSON, S.A.: Cutis grafts. Arch. Surg. **61**, 881 (1950).

TRIEPEL, H.: Einführung in die physikalische Anatomie. Wiesbaden: Bergmann 1902.

TRIEPEL, H.: Die trajektorellen Strukturen. Wiesbaden: Bergmann 1908.

TURNER, T.C.: Symposium on treatment of trauma in the armed forces. Washington, D.C.: Army Medical Service Graduate School, 1952.

UNGER, R.R.: In: KETTLER, L.H., SERFLING, H.J., Gewebekonserven. Berlin 1961.

UNGER, R.R.: In: KETTLER, L.H., SERFLING, H.J., Gewebekonserven II. Berlin 1965.

URBANIAK, J.R., BRIGHT, D.S., GILL, L.H., GOLDNER, J.L.: Vascularisation and the gliding mechanism of free flexor tendon grafts inserted by the silicone-rod method. J. Bone Jt Surg. A **56**, 473 (1974).

VALENTIN, B.: Histologische Untersuchungen zur freien Fascientransplantation. Ztschr. f. Chir. **113**, 398 (1912).

VALENTIN, B.: Experimentelle Untersuchungen zur homoioplastischen Fascien-Transplantation. Bruns Beitr. klin. Chir. **85**, 574 (1913).

VALENTIN, G.G.: Lehrbuch der Physiologie des Menschen. Bd. I. Braunschweig: 1847.

VAUGHAN, L.C.: A study of the replacement of the anterior cruciate ligament in the dog by fascia, skin and nylon. Vet. Rec. **75**, 537 (1963).

VERDAN, C.E.: Primary repair of flexor tendons. J. Bone Jt Surg. A **42**, 647–656 (1960).

VERZAR, F.: The ageing of connective tissue. 4th Congr. Int. Assoc. Geront. Merano 1957.

VERZAR, F.: Molekulare Veränderungen des Kollagens beim Altern und bei Erkrankungen. Schweiz. med. Wschr. **33**, 1036 (1963).

VERZAR, F., HUBER, K.: Thermic-contraction of single tendon fibres from animals of different age after treatment with formaldehyde, urethane, glycerol, acetic acid and other substances. Gerontologia **2**, 81 (1958).

VERZAR, F., WILLENEGGER, H.: Das Altern des Kollagens in der Haut und in Narben. Schweiz. med. Wschr. **41**, 1234 (1961).

VIIDIK, A.: Biomechanics and functional adaptation of tendons and joint ligaments. In: EVANS, F.G., Studies on the anatomy and function of bone and joints. Berlin-Göttingen-Heidelberg: Springer 1966.

VIIDIK, A.: The effect of training on the tensile strength of isolated rabbit tendons. Scand. J. plast. reconstr. Surg. **1**, 141–147 (1967).

VIIDIK, A.: A rheological model for uncalcified parallel-fibred collagenous tissue. J. Biomech. **1**, 3–11 (1968a).

VIIDIK, A.: Function and structure of collagenous tissue. Göteborg: Elanders 1968b.

VIIDIK, A.: Tensile strength properties of Achilles tendon systems in trained and untrained rabbits. Acta orthop. scand. **40**, 261–272 (1969).

VIIDIK, A., LEWIN, T.: Changes in ligaments by postmortal storage. Acta orthop. scand. **37**, 141 (1966).

VIIDIK, A., SANDQUIST, L., MÄGI, M.: Influence of postmortal storage on tensile strength characteristics and histology of rabbit ligaments. Acta orthop. scand. **35**, Suppl. 79 (1965).

VOORHOEVE, A.: Verpflanzung konservierter homologer Sehnen. Z. Orthop. **110**, 986 (1972).

VOORHOEVE, A., STERNEMANN, H.O.: Ergebnisse freier Transplantationen konservierter homologer und heterologer Sehnen. Hefte Unfallheilk. **114**, 294 (1973).

WALKER, L.B., HARRIS, E.H., BENEDICT, J.V.: Stress-strain relationship in human cadaveric plantaris tendon: A preliminary study. Med. biol. Engng **2**, 31 (1964).

WALLRAFF, J.: Leitfaden der Histologie des Menschen. München: Urban & Schwarzenberg 1954.

WEICKMANN, F.: In: KETTLER, L.H., SERFLING, H.J., Gewebekonserven. Berlin 1961.

WEIDENREICH, F.: Über Transplantation konservierter Sehnen. Virchows Arch. path. Anat. **250**, 178 (1924).

WELSH, R.B., MACNAB, L., RILEY, V.: Biomechanical studies of rabbit rendon. Clin. Orthop. **81**, 171 (1971).

WERTHEIM, M.G.: Memoir sur l'elasticité et la cohésion des principaux tissus du corps humain. Ann. Chim. Phys. **21**, 385 (1847).

WESSELHÖFT, R.: Cutisplastik nach REHN und Infektion. Langenbecks Arch. klin. Chir. **291**, 162 (1959).

WHEELDON, THOMAS: The use of Cellophane as a permanent tendon sheath. J. Bone Jt Surg. **21**, 393–396 (1939).

WILHELM, K.: Die subcutane traumatische Achillessehnenruptur. Münch. med. Wschr. **7**, 386 (1969).

WILHELM, K.: Die statische und dynamische Belastbarkeit der Achillessehne. Res. exp. Med. **157**, 221 (1972a).

WILHELM, K.: Die maximale statische und dynamische Belastbarkeit der Achillessehne beim Menschen im Experiment. Habil.-Schrift, München 1972b.

WILHELM, K.: Die statische und dynamische Belastbarkeit der Achillessehne. Res. exp. med. **157**, 221 (1972).

WILHELM, K., BEDACHT, R., RUEFF, F.L.: Die Behandlung der Achillessehnenruptur. Ärztl. Prax. **83**, 3809 (1968).

WITT, A.N.: Skiverletzung der Fußaußenbänder. Med. Klin. **42**, 3 (1947).

WITT, A.N.: Die Sehnenverletzungen und Sehnenmuskeltransplantationen. München: Bergmann 1953.

WITT, A.N.: Traumatische Schäden des Bewegungssystems. In: Handbuch der Orthopädie, Bd. I. Eds. HOHMANN, G., HACKENBROCH, M., LINDEMANN, K., Stuttgart: Thieme 1957.

WITT, A.N.: Orthopädische Chirurgie der Hand. Medizinische **22**, 819 (1957).

WITT, A.N., COTTA, H., JÄGER, M.: Die angeborenen Fehlbildungen der Hand und ihre operative Behandlung. Stuttgart: Thieme 1966.

WITT, A.N., MITTELMEIER, H.: Unterschenkel und Fuß. In: Handbuch der Orthopädie, Bd. 4, 2. Teil, eds. HOHMANN, G., HACKENBROCH, M., LINDEMANN, K. Stuttgart: Thieme 1961.

WÖHLISCH, E., MESNIL DE ROCHEMONT, R., GERSCHLER, H.: Untersuchungen über die elastischen Eigenschaften tierischer Gewebe I, II. Z. Biol. **85**, 325 (1927).

ZIMCHES, J.L.: The fate of surface epithelium transplanted into deep tissues and its relations to epithelial cysts. Frankfurt. Z. Path. **42**, 203 (1931).

Transplantation of the Cornea in Man and Animal

E.N. Hinzpeter and G.O.H. Naumann

With 11 Figures and 9 Tables

I. Introduction and Historical Background

Although superficial excision of corneal opacities—keratectomy—has been practised for centuries, actual transplantation of corneal tissue began only approximately 150 years ago (Table 1). The most active pioneering work took place during the first 30 years of this century. It was, however, only after the second world war that keratoplasty became a routine procedure for the ophthalmic surgeon (Table 1). The most important factors responsible for this development are the improvement in surgical technique under the operating microscope with ultrafine suture material and instruments; the advent of antibiotics for the prophylaxis and treatment of postoperative infection; the use of corticosteroids in the prophylaxis and treatment of immunologic graft rejection and the increasing knowledge concerning the fate of the donor tissue with recognition of the importance of the

Table 1. Milestones in the historical background of keratoplasty

1789	Pellier de Quengsy	Describes operation for substituting cornea with convex glass mounted in silver ring
1813	Himly	Develops idea of corneal transplantation
1824	Reisinger	Performs series of homologous keratoplasties in animals
1837	Bigger	First successful homologous keratoplasty in gazelle
1838	Kissam	Unsuccessful heterologous penetrating keratoplasty (pig→man)
1840	v. Walther and Mühlbauer	Series of heterologous lamellar keratoplasties
1853	Nussbaum	Because of disappointing results from keratoplasty return to glass keratoprosthesis
1872	Power	Discovers importance but not reason for successful *homologous* penetrating keratoplasties in animals
1878	Sellerbeck	First attempt to use human donor corneas
1888	v. Hippel	First successful lamellar heterologous (rabbit→man) keratoplasty; mechanical trephine developed
1901	Fuchs	Large series homologous mostly lamellar keratoplasties (mainly tectonic)
1905	Zirm	*First successful penetrating homologous keratoplasty in man*

endothelium for the ultimate transparency and optical success of the graft. The introduction of alloplastic corneal tissue substitutes or keratoprostheses, in cases where a keratoplasty might have a poor prognosis, should also be mentioned (CARDONA et al., 1972).

Among the ophthalmic surgeons who are particularly responsible for recent development of keratoplasty, the following should be especially mentioned: ELSCHNIG (Prague); FILATOV (Odessa); ARRUGA, both father and son BARRAQUER (Spain); MAGITOT, SOURDILLE, OFFRET, PAUFIQUE (France); FRANCESCHETTI (Switzerland); FRIEDE (Austria); GÜNTHER, LÖHLEIN, HALLERMANN, H.K. MÜLLER, HARMS, MACKENSEN, SAUTTER (Germany); CASEY, TUDOR-THOMAS, RYCROFT, LEIGH (England); PATON, BURKE, CASTROVIEJO (USA). Excellent historical reviews have been written by CASTROVIEJO (1968), RINTELEN (1974), TOWNLEY-PATON (1970), and TREVOR-ROPER (1972).

II. Basic Principles of Keratoplasty

A. Terminology

The term *Keratoplasty* for corneal transplantation has been in use since 1824 (Table 1). Several additional terms exist relating to the various aspects of type of donor material used, shape of graft, thickness and circumference of host tissue to be replaced, and exact localization of the transplant in the host cornea (Table 2). Further definitions pertaining to the indications for surgery will be discussed later (Section II B). Most grafting is done with *homologous* material from fresh or eyebank stored enucleated or cadaver eyes. *Autologous* transplants are rarely used, e.g., for keratomileusis (see Section II D), and where the clear cornea of a blind eye is transplanted to replace the cloudy cornea of the fellow eye (BORUCHOFF and DOHLMAN, 1967), or in ring autokeratoplasty described by STRAMPELLI (1969). Full thickness *heterologous* transplants have no common use due to their poor prognosis regarding immune rejection when compared with homologous grafts. They have been advocated however as *lamellar* grafts, e.g., canine or fish cornea for metaherpetic keratitis (PAYRAU, 1965). In *lamellar* keratoplasty various depths of corneal stroma are replaced but the endothelium with Descemet's membrane remains. The donor tissue usually consits of superficial corneal stroma alone, although sometimes stroma complete with Descemet's membrane and endothelium are placed into the lamellar bed. *Penetrating* keratoplasty involves *all* the layers of the cornea so that the eye is opened during operation. *Mushroom* or stem grafts are a combination of a lamellar and penetrating transplant, with the latter comprising the central section of the graft (Fig. 1).

Table 2. Terminology used in corneal transplantation (keratoplasty)

Term used depending on		Diameter of host tissue excised	Shape of transplant	Locali- sation
donor material	depth of host tissue excised			
autogenous	lamellar	partial (usually trepan size up to 9 mm)	circular (most common)	central
homogenous (allograft)	penetrating		square	eccentric
heterogenous (xenograft)	mushroom or stem	total	triangular	marginal
alloplastic (keratoprosthesis)			sector-shaped rectangular annular	

Types of keratoplastik

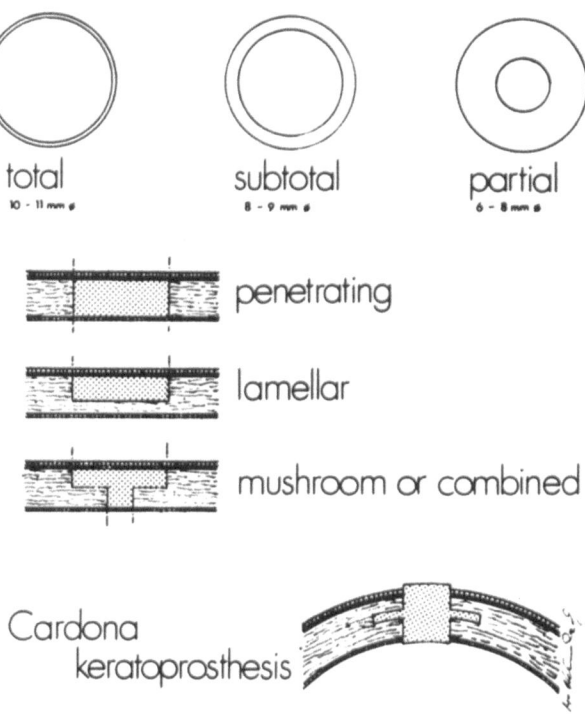

total
10 - 11 mm ∅

subtotal
8 - 9 mm ∅

partial
6 - 8 mm ∅

penetrating

lamellar

mushroom or combined

Cardona
keratoprosthesis

Fig. 1. Terminology of various types of keratoplasty

Most keratoplasties are *partial* and *circular* with a size varying from 6 mm to 8 mm diameter (rarely up to 9 mm). Grafts larger than this are considered *total* (normal corneal diameters being 11 × 12 mm) and some of these are even transplanted with a fringe of conjunctiva and sclera attached. The relation of prognosis to size of graft will be discussed in Section II E.

B. Indications for Keratoplasty

There are several reasons for performing keratoplasty (Table 3). The most common indication is an *optical* one, whereby opaque corneal tissue due to one of the numerous familial corneal dystrophies or due to scarring after inflammation, wounds, or chemical burns, is partially replaced by transparent donor cornea to improve visual acuity in an otherwise intact eye. Depending on the degree of the opacity, or on the depth of the corneal layer primarily involved in a particular dystrophy, a lamellar or a penetrating keratoplasty is necessary. Often a combination of the indications listed in Table 3 exists, as for instance in the case of a corneal scar with persisting herpetic inflammation where a keratoplasty is often performed not only for optical reasons, but to preserve the eye itself, i.e. curative reasons.

Refractive keratoplasty, first conceived by JOSÉ I. BARRAQUER (1969), will be described in Section II D. Keratomileusis is indicated in high myopia when the difference in refractive error of the two eyes is large (anisometropia). Keratophakia is performed for hypermetropic anisometropia e.g. monocular aphakia when a contact lens is not tolerated.

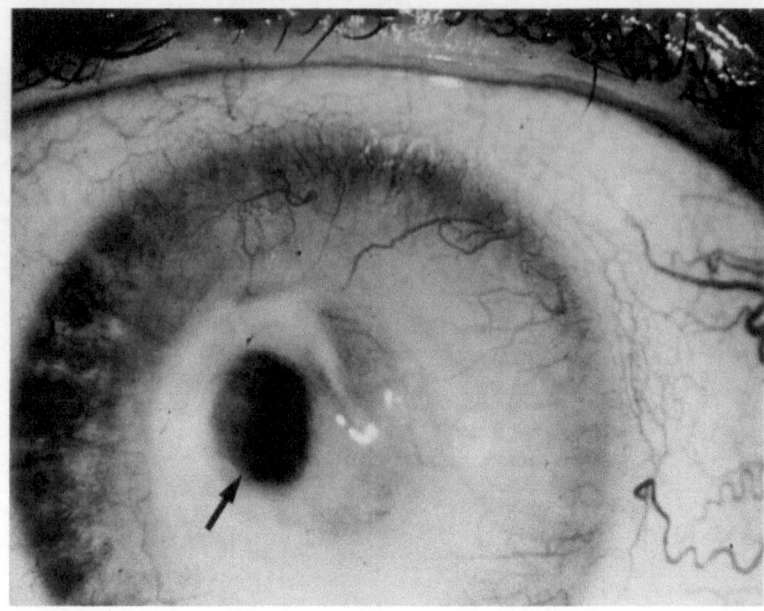

(a)

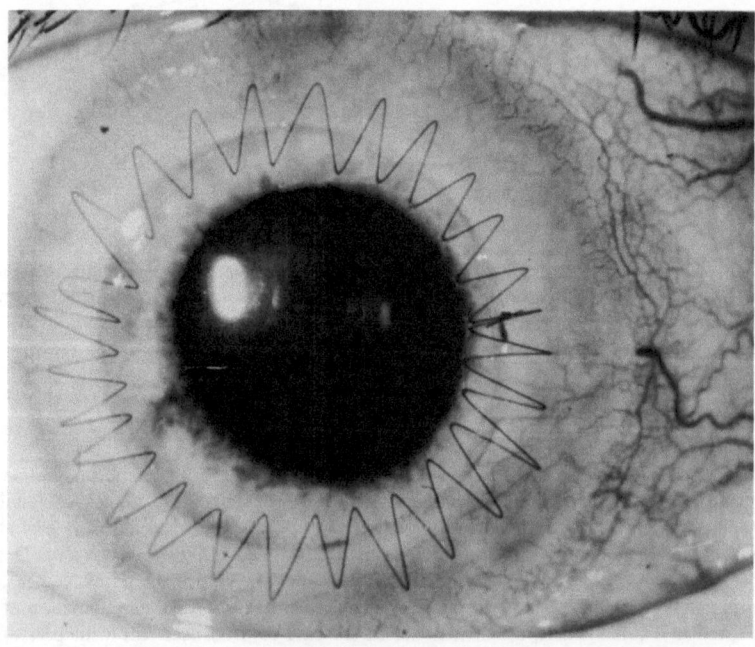

(b)

Fig. 2. (a) Perforated corneal ulcer (arrow) due to herpes simplex: Dense vascularized scar occupies entire cornea adjacent to ulcer. (b) 3 months after keratoplasty crystal-clear corneal graft of 7.5 mm diameter with running 10-0-(25 µ) nylon suture in situ. Removal of suture is performed 6 months after surgery (Univ. Eye Clinic, Hamburg)

Table 3. General indications for keratoplasty

Optical

to achieve transparence (mostly penetrating keratoplasties)

to alter refractive error (keratophakia, keratomileusis, cylindrical sectioning)

Therapeutic

tectonic-mostly preparatory (lamellar or mushroom keratoplasties)

curative-(keratoplasty "à chaud")

prophylactic

Among the *therapeutic* indications, lamellar keratoplasty has a special place as *preparatory* surgery (FILATOW's "meliorisation"; ASCHER's "tectonic" keratoplasty), prior to a final penetrating keratoplasty for optical reasons (see LEIGH, 1955). It is done to reduce vascularization and increase the thickness of the recipient cornea, as well as to provide a new Bowman's membrane which is important for fixation of subsequent sutures (EIMER, 1972). *Lamellar* keratoplasty more difficult to perform, but not having the dangers of an "open eye", is also indicated where possible in the very young or aged where postoperative restlessness would be expected, or when adequate anesthesia during keratoplasty is not possible. Lamellar keratoplasty to prevent recurrence of a pterygium is an example of a prophylactic indication.

Curative keratoplasty whether lamellar or penetrating, is primarily done to excise a therapy-resistant corneal disease or chronic infection. As transparence is often not achieved in addition to the elimination of the corneal process, this too is a tectonic keratoplasty. When performed in an acute stage to forestall or treat corneal perforation (TRAGAKIS *et al.*, 1974), i.e., to preserve the eye itself (Fig. 2) it is known as keratoplasty "à chaud" (FRANCESCHETTI and DORET, 1950).

When the disease process involves the deeper layers of the cornea, e.g. metaherpetic keratitis (granulomatous reaction against Descemet's membrane); or fungal keratitis, a lamellar keratoplasty is contraindicated even as a tectonic measure.

Tectonic keratoplasty is also used to replace scleral defects after excision of epibulbar (e.g. dermoids) or intraocular (e.g. ciliary melanoma) tumors. A further form of tectonic keratoplasty is the "Minikeratoplasty" to cover unwanted limbal fistula after filtrating surgery for glaucoma (SAUTTER *et al.*, 1972b).

In advanced corneal edema (bullous keratopathy) of varying etiology, relief of pain and sometimes slight improvement of vision can be obtained by a mushroom transplant; or a preliminary operation like a full thickness graft in a lamellar bed is undertaken before final optical penetrating keratoplasty.

Total keratoplasty is rarely indicated for instance after eye-burns when the anterior segment is severely damaged (TICHO and BEN-SIRA, 1973). Thus the indications for the *type* of keratoplasty to be performed are as important as the general indications for corneal transplantation.

C. Criteria for Donor Material and Storage

1. General

It is essential to have viable donor tissue—endothelium in particular, for penetrating but not for lamellar keratoplasty.

If fresh material is available, the cadaver eyes must be enucleated within the first 8 hours post mortem, at the very latest within 24 hours. Whole eyes, or just the corneas are placed in moist sterile chambers after inspection and refrigerated at +4° C. The donor cornea must be used within 24 hours postmortem for penetrating keratoplasty and within 48 hours postmortem for lamellar keratoplasty.

With fresh material, the *age* of the donor has no consequence on the subsequent success of the graft (FORSTER and FINE, 1971), although the corneas of donors over 60 years of age must be more carefully evaluated for potential endothelial deficiency. Corneas of infants are avoided unless the recipient is of similar age, because of the different diameters, thickness, and curvature involved. For long-term storage, corneas from donors under 50 years are preferable.

Donors with *systemic infection* such as syphilis, infective hepatitis, meningitis, and septicaemia of varying etiology at the time of death should not be used. It has been suggested that leukemia and metastatic carcinoma are also contraindications (KING, 1970). One case of probable transmission of Creutzfeldt-Jakobs disease via keratoplasty has been reported (DUFFY et al., 1974; DE VOE, 1975).

Donor *intraocular disease* is no contraindication provided the corneas are healthy. Many surgeons make use of the corneas of eyes enucleated because of malignant melanoma of the choroid. So far there has been no report of seeding of melanoma cells to the host. HATA (1939), however, described such transplantation of retinoblastoma tumor cells by keratoplasty.

Immune Selection of Donor. There is a diversity of opinion regarding the role of AB0-blood group incompatibility in graft rejection. Clinical studies which found AB0 mismatches to be harmful to the transplanted cornea either immediately or much later were published by NELKEN et al. (1957), HAVENER et al. (1958), RICHTER (1965). Others again are of the opinion that there is *no* certain relationship between AB0 donor-recipient incompatibility and graft failure (MEHRI et al., 1959; MEYER, 1971; ALLANSMITH et al., 1975; VOTOCKOVA and KAREL, 1975).

Since 1964 the major histocompatibility locus- the HL-A system has been used to test donors and recipients in renal and other major organ transplantations.

EHLERS and AHRONS found HL-A antigens present in the cornea (1971). GIBBS et al. found no certain correlation between HL-A matching of donors with recipients and graft failure (1973).

ALLANSMITH et al. (1974) came to similar results although they emphasised that so far the data are too few for definitive conclusions. All donor-recipient pairs were mismatched for two to four antigens but the degree of mismatch did *not* correlate to the fate of the graft.

WATSON and JOYSEY describe the difficulties and methods of prospective tissue typing of donors and potential corneal recipients for HL-A antigens and AB0 groups (1973). Matching donor to recipient according to AB0-Groups and HL-A system compatibility has not found general practice in corneal transplantation. It is probably advisable in cases of multiple rekeratoplasty or when the recipient's cornea is heavily vascularized, in other words where the cornea has lost its immunologic privileges and the risk of immune graft reaction is especially high (see also Section III B).

Reduction of the immune reaction is probably achieved by scraping off the epithelium of the donor cornea before grafting and thus reducing the amount of antigen. STOCKER (1965) believes that placing the donor cornea 48 hours in the recipient's serum before grafting reduces the immune response.

2. Donor-Cornea Evaluation (Laboratory and Clinical)

Means of evaluating the donor cornea are divided into laboratory methods and clinical staining methods (Table 4). The techniques are described in detail elsewhere.[1] Most of these methods are not used routinely prior to keratoplasty, but rather in experimental work for improving storage and banking methods.

The surgeon always inspects the donor cornea in the whole eye with the slit lamp microscope, paying special attention to the mosaic of endothelial cells and to Descemet's membrane. When fresh corneas are used this inspection is carried out immediately after enucleation because the rapidly developing stromal edema and folding of Descemet's membrane soon obscures the view of the endothelium. Although this method gives an indication of the number of cells showing gross morphologic changes it does not reveal the functional efficiency of the endothelium BROWN and TREVOR-ROPER (1968) found opacities on the posterior corneal surface in all of 400 eyebank eyes 24 hours post mortem on examination with the slit lamp microscope. These dots corresponded to endothelial degeneration areas when tested with the *PNT stain* (Para nitroblue tetrazolium). This stain has the disadvantage that it requires fixation of tissue so that the cornea cannot be used for keratoplasty afterwards. However as KAUFMANN et al. (1966) have shown that the endothelial pattern is similar in partner eyes in 98% of cases, the partner eye could then be used for keratoplasty if the donor was a cadaver.

---

[1] Corneal Preservation: Clinical and Laboratory Evaluation of Current Methods. CAPELLA, J.A., EDELHAUSER, H.F., VAN HORN, D.L. (eds.). Springfields, Illinois: Charles C. Thomas, 1973.

Table 4. Evaluation of Donor cornea Methods (mainly concerned with endothelial viability)

Vital staining
  Trypan Blue (STOCKER, 1970)
  Lissamine Green (JANS and HASSARD, 1967)
  (KUMING and RYCROFT, 1969)

Histochemical staining
  PNT (P-nitroblue tetrazolium) (KAUFMANN, 1964)
  NBT and MTT (COOPER and MCTIGUE, 1968)

Microscopy
  Examination with the slitlamp
  Transmission electron microscopy (SCHAEFFER, 1963)
  Specular microscopy (MAURICE, 1968), (HOEFLE *et al.*, 1970)

Corneal thickness measurements with Haag-Streit pachometer (MAURICE and GIARDINI, 1951)

Radioactive sulphate uptake (AURELL *et al.*, 1956)

Temperature reversal phenomenon measurements (DAVSON, 1955; SHENNAND, 1973)

Oxygen consumption (AURELL *et al.*, 1956)

Tissue culture (STOCKER *et al.*, 1959)

Permeability to nonelectrolytes (MISHIMA and KUDO, 1967; HOEFLE, 1969)

RNA Production: (HANNA *et al.*, 1969)

The advantage of the relatively simple *Trypan blue vital* stain test (STOCKER, 1971), is that the graft can be used afterwards. Only dead or diseased cells take up the stain. However there is no knowledge concerning the maximal number of nonviable endothelial cells that still permit a clear graft. Moreover, absence of staining does not indicate the degree of viability, nor staining the degree of reversibility of damage possible.

Direct information on what is probably endothelial function, is obtained by observing the *temperature reversal phenomenon*. On freezing an enucleated eye, the active fluid-transport mechanisms of the endothelium stop and the stroma swells with inflowing aqueous. On rewarming before use to body temperature, reactivation of the metabolic pump causes the stroma to dehydrate to normal thickness if the tissue is still viable (SHERRARD, 1974).

3. Storage

When fresh donor material is not available, or, as in some countries, impossible to obtain due to religious or legal prejudices, preserved human corneas from eyebanks elsewhere are used.

The first Eyebank was founded before World War II in the U.S.A. by PATON.

There are several recognized ways of preserving and banking corneas. They can roughly be divided into those for lamellar and those for penetrating keratoplasty, as well as into those for short-term storage and those for long-term preservation (Table 5).

a) The Fate of Corneal Donor Cells in Storage. Many investigations on human as well as on animal corneas show the rate of endothelial degeneration in stored eyes regarding both the rate and degree of damage to each individual cell as well as the increasing numbers of cells involved. None of the techniques listed in Table 4 are entirely satisfactory measurements of endothelial viability. Moreover, in most cases the age of the donor and the time and temperature of the interval between death and storage have not been taken into account. Still certain differences in the various methods of storage as regards the fate of especially the endothelial cells during the period of storage have been found (MCCAREY and KAUFMAN, 1974).

b) Fresh Donor Eyes Stored in a Moist Chamber at + 4° C Before Keratoplasty. In flat preparations of the corneal endothelium STOCKER (1971) has shown that after 24 hours the cell outline was still visible, and although small vacuoles were present within the protoplasm, the nuclei were not disintegrated. However in an eye 48 hours after such storage, there was a loss of continuity

Table 5. Methods of storage and preservation of donor cornea prior to keratoplasty

	Short-term storage (4–12 weeks)	Long-term preservation
Lamellar keratoplasty	cornea or eyeball in liquid paraffin at +4° C (Bürki, 1947)	lyophilization in glycerine with molecular sieve (King, 1961)
	freezing cornea −40° C to −80° C	spontaneous dessication (Urrets-Zavalia, 1964)
	cornea in glycerine	lyophilization with colloidal alumina-silicates (Payrau and Pouliquen, 1959)
Penetrating keratoplasty	(7–10 days)	Pretreatment with sucrose and DMSO (dimethylsulphoxide), step-freezing to −80° C, and storing in liquid nitrogen at −196° C (Mueller et al., 1964; Capella et al., 1965)
	cornea or eyeball in moist chamber at +4° C (up to 24 hours)	
	cornea or eyeball in liquid paraffin at +4° C (Bürki, 1947)	
	cornea in recipients serum at +4° C (Stocker, 1971)	
	cornea in artificial aqueous humour (Kuwahara, 1965) at +4° C	
	cornea in modified culture medium (M–K) at +4° C (McCarey and Kaufmann, 1974)	

of the endothelium with disintegration of nuclei. After 4 days, large parts of Descemet's membrane were also disrupted. Electronmicroscopically, Schaeffer (1963) found irreversible changes in the epithelium as early as 24 hours after enucleation, in the stroma at 24–36 hours, and in the endothelium "degeneration bodies" only after 96 hours. On the other hand Van Horn and Schultz (1973) stress severe endothelial damage can occur as early as 12 hours. Examining this type of short-term cold storage, Polack et al. (1968) concluded that in human donor corneas 30% of the endothelium could be damaged and still result in a clear penetrating graft.

Hanna et al. (1969) maintained that failure of clear penetrating grafts using corneas stored thus for 1–3 weeks was due to impaired protein and RNA synthesis of the cornea as a whole, rather than to the decreased viability of the endothelial cells alone.

A more recent investigation by Sherrard (1974) using a combination of specular microscopy and "temperature reversal" indicated that some of the damaged endothelial cells can recover or be replaced by protrusions from neighbouring cells, and that they are then functionally competent as shown by the temperature reversal effect.

c) Fresh Corneas Stored in Liquid Paraffin at +4° C. Successful grafts have been reported when donor corneas were used as long as 3 weeks after such storage (Rycroft, 1954).

The morphologic appearance of human corneas after 4 weeks storage is comparable to that after 48 hours storage in a moist chamber at +4° C.

d) Storage of Isolated Cornea in Autologous Serum. Stocker (1971) found 50% viability in these endothelial cells (Trypan Blue staining) after 2 weeks compared with 20–30% viability of endothelial cells when whole eyes were stored in a moist chamber at +4° C for the same period of time.

e) Long-Term Cryopreservation. The critical step for the viability of cells in cryopreservation is the thawing before use (Polack, 1971). The problems of cell survival after freezing and thawing have been discussed by Ashwood-Smith (1973).

Polack and McEntyre (1969) and Galun et al. (1971) believe that stromal cells do not survive after thawing.

HOEFLE (1969) testing corneal endothelial permeability to small electrolytes, found that the metabolic dehydrating pump could survive this storage. But GENOSKI and EDELHAUSER (1974) found that the freeze-thaw induced injury reduced overall energy yielding metabolism of cryo-preserved corneal tissue 13% when compared to that of fresh tissue.

VAN HORN *et al.* (1970) in light and electronmicroscopic studies found approximately 78% of endothelial cells intact (i.e. plasma membrane intact) although there was a great variability in appearance. However, only 50% of the endothelial cells could be regarded as actually viable (ability to incorporate tritium uridine into RNA). An exact correlation of this test for viability and cellular ultrastructure was not possible.

Several authors, however, claim that cryopreserved corneas show no significant difference compared to fresh material as regards the ultimate fate of the graft; (see Section II E). On the contrary the chances of immune rejection appear less in cryopreserved material (SCHULTZ and GALLUN, 1973).

D. Surgical Techniques in Keratoplasty

The basic facts influencing the different surgical techniques of lamellar and penetrating keratoplasty, are that in the former the eye remains intact — it is in this respect the safer procedure — and that in the latter the transparence of the graft depends on the integrity of the donor endothelium.

For both, microsurgery under a $\times 6$ to $\times 40$ magnification is the method of choice. General anesthesia, alternatively local anesthesia with complete akinesia of the globe is necessary. Except in the cases where a combined perforating keratoplasty and cataract extraction is to be performed the pupil is medically constricted preoperatively.

Preoperative osmotherapy renders the globe hypotonic and prevents vitreous loss during penetrating keratoplasty.

Choice of size of graft depends on the area of opaque and vascularized recipient cornea. Very small grafts (under 6 mm) are rarely indicated, having their place as optical penetrating keratoplasties after preparatory lamellar keratoplasty in a heavily vascularized cornea (AINSLIE, 1974). Grafts of 6–7 mm diameter are the ones most commonly used in penetrating keratoplasty. Larger grafts are accompanied by a poorer prognosis due to an increase in immune rejection as well as the technical difficulties of obtaining exact apposition of wound edges and the proximity of the wound to the chamberangle and drainage area of the eye with the resulting complications of raised intraocular pressure. In excisions exceeding 7 mm diameter, most ophthalmic surgeons prefer to use a 0.1 mm larger diameter donor disc to compensate for the shrinkage of the graft after excision from the donor eye.

The host corneal tissue to be removed, is excised usually with a circular trephine, a similar one being used on the donor cornea. The donor cornea epithelium is usually scraped off to reduce the antigenic material transplanted. However, when the host cornea is expected to be incapable of rapid epithelialization of the graft (severe alkali burns, Sjörgen's syndrome, Stevens-Johnson syndrome) it is important to graft an intact donor epithelium (BROWN *et al.*, 1974).

In lamellar keratoplasty a flat dissector or a keratome is preferred for excision of host tissue as well as for obtaining donor material (Barraquer's microkeratome; Castroviejo's electrokeratome).

Silk or nylon (Perlon, Ethilon) sutures are used. The advantages of the ultrafine monofilamentous synthetic sutures are their tensile strength and their ability to remain intact and inert for long periods of time in living tissue causing minimal foreign-body reaction. Formerly, (nowadays only for lamellar or very small penetrating keratoplasties) indirect crossover suturing or even splint-fixation of the graft was carried out. Direct continuous starshaped, or for very large grafts, interrupted sutures are the method of choice for penetrating keratoplasty. These sutures must be laid deep within the tissue (at least $^2/_3$ depth).

During trephining and suturing an air bubble inserted into the anterior chamber protects the deeper structures and allows accurate apposition of wound edges.

Iridectomies or iridotomies are performed with large grafts, or elsewhere when postoperative synechias are expected.

Postoperatively intraocular tension is kept low and antibiotics or corticosteroids are given topically and sometimes systemically according to each individual case. The monofilamentous nylon sutures are usually left in situ for several months before being removed under the operating microscope.

In *refractive keratoplasty* basic preparations for surgery are similar to those already mentioned. In *keratomileusis* an anterior lamellar resection is made with an electromicrokeratome. The resected disc is frozen with CO_2 and chiseled to the desired optical correction before being thawed and resutured into the same eye. In *keratophakia* a lens is carved from donor corneal stroma and inserted into a pocket incised into the recipient cornea. Cylindrical sectioning whereby freezing and thus a certain amount of damage to the tissue is avoided is still in an experimental stage (Katzin and Kaplan, 1969).

The various techniques of inserting keratoprosthesis have been dealt with by Choyce (1969), Cardona *et al.* (1972), Strampelli and Marchi (1972), Dohlman *et al.* (1974).[2]

E. Factors Determining Prognosis of Keratoplasty

The cornea was historically the first solid tissue to be sucessfully grafted from one individual to another. Keratoplasty with its mainly good prognosis has a special place in organ transplantation, because the cornea being normally avascular and free from lymphatic channels is regarded as an immunologically privileged site (Billingham and Boswell, 1953). Added to this, is the fact that the actual mass of antigenic material involved in corneal transplantation is small.

In the absence of a aesthetic or purely tectonic indications, successful keratoplasty can be defined as a healed graft, transparent enough, and with a curvature regular enough to improve on preoperative visual acuity. A minimum of 6 months must elapse before declaring a graft successful, although clouding occuring much later remains a possibility (Stansbury, 1949).

Factors which influence the prognosis of keratoplasty are the quality of the donor material, the state of the recipient cornea, other ocular disease, and the quality of surgical technique (Table 6).

1. Quality of the Donor-Cornea

The selection of *high quality donor material* has been discussed in Section II C. The age of the donor or the cause of his death have been regarded as factors not directly influencing the ultimate prognosis of the graft (Forster and Fine, 1971; Meyer and Arnecke, 1972); neither does ABO and HL-A system incompatibility between donor and recipient; though here opinions vary (see Sections II C and III B).

As regards use of deep-frozen tissue or fresh material, several clinical studies have revealed no difference in the outcome of the grafts (Kaufmann *et al.*, 1966; Irvine *et al.;* 1969; Mathieu, 1969. Clifton and Hanna (1974), actually suggest that cryopreserved corneas are superior to fresh material because antigenic material is lost. This could not be verified in xenograft animal experiments (Bourne, 1975).

---

[2] For further details in the surgical techniques of keratoplasty see Troutman (1970), Moore and Aronson (1971), Castroviejo (1972), Fine, M. (1972), Sautter *et al.* (1972a, b, 1973).

Table 6. Factors influencing the prognosis of keratoplasty

---

1. *Quality of donor cornea* (endothelium viability for penetrating grafts)

2. *State of recipient cornea* (presence of Bowman's membrane; degree of vascularization; circumference to be excised; etiology of corneal opacity; rekeratoplasty)

3. *Presence of other eye diseases* (malformations of eyelids, conjunctiva, lacrimal apparatus; glaucoma; anterior synechiae from iris)

4. *Quality of surgical technique* (avoidance of trauma to endothelium, accurate and watertight wound closure)

---

2. State of the Recipient Cornea

The state of the recipient cornea is also important in the prognosis of keratoplasty. Here several factors must be taken into account. *Compactness of the anterior layers of the recipient cornea* is necessary for the sutures to hold and the graft to heal without an inner or outer ridge. The presence of Bowman's membrane appears especially important for suture fixation (EIMER, 1972).

The diameter and circumference of the tissue to be excised and replaced is of great prognostic significance for the future clarity of the graft. The larger the graft, the nearer the antigenic mass to the corneal limbus blood vessels and therefore the higher the incidence of immune rejection. Also, very large or total grafts may interfere with the anterior drainage system of the eye, causing secondary glaucoma. The size of graft with the best visual prognosis is 6 mm (HALLERMANN, 1965).

Size is also important for the prognosis of keratoprosthesis. An impermeable endothelial prosthesis would be expected to starve the cornea (glucose from the aqueous humour), if its circumference is more than 4 mm (MAURICE, 1969).

Vascularization of the recipient cornea offers a poor prognosis for a clear graft because of the higher incidence of immune rejection (BASU and ORMSBY, 1957; POLACK, 1962). Attempts have been made to pretreat the cornea with Argon Laser, or β-radiation to diminish corneal vascularization prior to keratoplasty and thereby increase the chances of the graft remaining transparent.

Probably avascularity is important for both the prevention of initial sensitisation of the host as well as prevention of rejection once sensitisation has been achieved.

The underlying corneal disease in the recipient is important. Thus CASTROVIEJO (1968) divided patients into 5 prognostic groups based on the diagnosis of the corneal disease alone. Among Group I (with a 90% chance of the graft healing with improvement of vision), are keratoconus and a few of the familiar corneal dystrophies. The worst prognostic groups are those with heavily vascularized scars and glaucoma.

However, one must emphasize that in recent years with more experience in clinical keratoplasty, knowledge acquired from experimental work, and better surgical techniques, many corneal diseases have a better prognosis regarding keratoplasty. Thus in 1948 PAUFIQUE warned against penetrating keratoplasty for FUCHS' corneal dystrophy and other forms of bullous keratopathy (endothelial decompensation) because of the poor prognosis, but since 1972 patients with this disease have a 70–80% chance of success with the same operation (Brown, 1970; Fine and West, 1971; Rice, 1974; Sautter et al., 1972a). Also congenital endothelial defects can be treated successfully by penetrating kerato-plasty (Hinzpeter and Naumann, 1972). By preliminary tectonic surgery par-tial or total lamellar keratoplasty, or fullthickness grafts in a lamellar bed), corneal structure and function can be improved so that the final optical penetrat-ing keratoplasty has a better chance of survival in even very poor prognostic groups (Castroviejo, 1972). Those corneas with severe chemical (alkali) burns, and reduced tear secretion with cicatrizing disease of the conjunctiva, so that sufficient protection of the graft is not achieved have the worst prognosis.

The type of disease in the recipient cornea is also important prognostically, because certain corneal diseases tend to recur on the graft (Section III A), and others are actually predisposed in an unknown way to immune rejection (Sec-tion III B).

Rekeratoplasty which compared with other organ transplantation is carried out frequently (10–20% of all keratoplasties) has also improved its prognosis in recent years.

3. Other Ocular Disease

The presence of other ocular disease is naturally of great prognostic significance for the corneal graft.

a) Age alone plays no important role. Very young children (Brown, 1974), as well as the very old have been operated on successfully (Leigh, 1966).

b) Additional External Ocular Disease. Deformities of the lids, conjunctiva, and lacrimal apparatus which lead to insufficient mechanical protection of the cornea must be corrected as far as possible *before* keratoplasty. Any deficiency in the quantity or quality of the tear film decreases the chance for a successful corneal graft due to exposure.

c) Intraocular Disease. High intraocular pressure (*glaucoma*) must be ad-equately controlled medically or surgically before keratoplasty is attempted. The eye should also be free of external or endogenous inflammation. In chronic uveitis, a quiet interval should be selected for performing the keratoplasty. Keratoplasty performed during active herpetic keratitis suffers from a high rate of reinfection of the graft as well as other complications.

A *cataract* is no contraindication and can be extracted at the same time as keratoplasty is performed through the central-trephine-opening.

Conversely *aphakia* is also no contraindication to keratoplasty, but requires a modified surgical technique to prevent undue vitreous loss and collapse of the globe during surgery (Fine, 1972b; Sautter et al., 1973). Bronson suggests ultrasonic diagnostic examination prior to grafting in corneas so opaque that visualization of deeper structures is not possible. Thus anterior chamber organ-isation, cataract, vitreous hemorrhage and retinal detachment could be foreseen and treated before or during keratoplasty. Infrared photography permits visua-lization of anterior chamber structures through a dense corneal opacity (Huer-kamp, 1955).

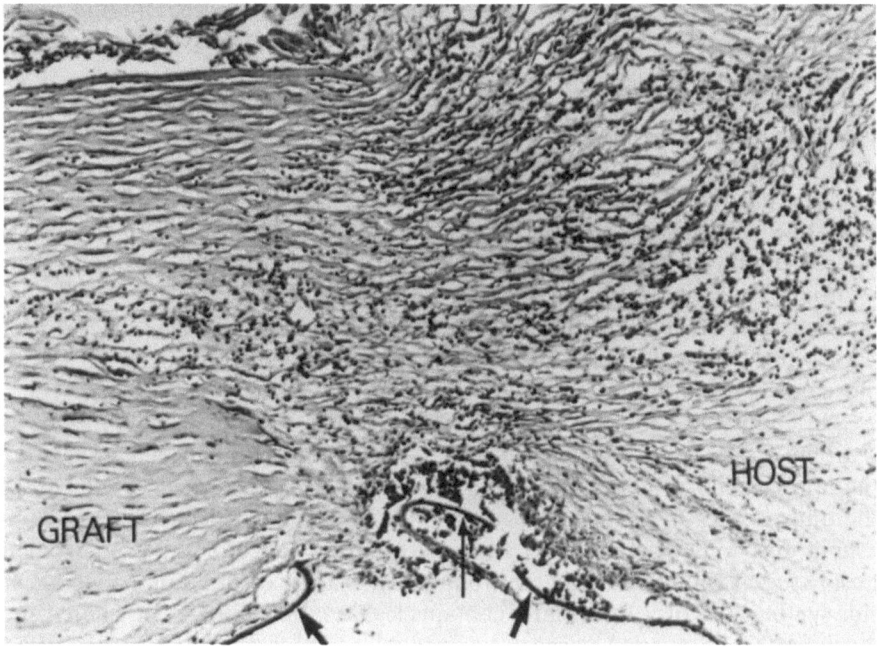

Fig. 3. Massive inflammatory infiltrate with granulomatous reaction to Descemet's membrane (typical of herpes simplex) extending from host into corneal graft. (No. 185/63 Histologic Laboratory, Univ. Eye Clinic, Hamburg)

4. Quality of Surgery

The *quality of surgical technique* during keratoplasty and the *adequacy of postoperative* care have great prognostic significance in keratoplasty. Important is the avoidance of trauma to the endothelium of donor and host cornea in penetrating keratoplasty, and accurate wound closure (see Section II D). Postoperative treatment of high intraocular pressure, and prompt application of antibiotics or corticosteroids where necessary is indicated. Improper selection of surgical technique, e.g. lamellar keratoplasty for herpes cornea with chronic granulomatous reaction against Descemet's membrane, maylead to failure from the start (VOGEL and NAUMANN, 1972) (Fig. 3).

F. Healing of the Corneal Wound in Keratoplasty

The healing process uniting the edges of the corneal graft to the cornea of the host is initially similar to that of a penetrating corneal wound. Swelling of the wound edges (due to inhibition of aqueous humour and tear fluid), and the formation of a fibrin plug occurs within hours after grafting. Polymorphonuclear leukocytes escaping from the limbal capillaries, are carried across the cornea within the tear film by the blinking reflex and enter the wound area within hours after grafting (ROBB and KUWABARA, 1962).

It has been estimated that approximately 35% of the cells in the healing area originate from corneal stroma (keratocytes), the rest deriving from invading monocytes (Weimar, 1958).

The epithelium of the donor cornea which has either been removed by the surgeon prior to grafting (Section II D) or which disappears within a few days is replaced by migration of epithelium from the adjacent host cornea. The first positive repair activity however occurs in the keratocytes immediately beneath the epithelium at the wound edges around the 5th day. In the absence of epithelium this healing process is delayed. Dohlman and Gasset also found retardation in gain of tensile strength of a corneal wound in such cases, suggesting some metabolic interaction between the epithelium and the adjacent fibroblasts, in the area of repair (1969). They also found peripheral wounds healed more quickly than more centrally placed corneal injuries.

On about the 15th day the gap in the stroma is bridged by fibrils having a variety of diameters mostly thicker than those of normal collagen, and without the normal regular horizontal pattern and equal spacing which contributes to the transparency of normal corneal stroma (Jakus, 1962). Thus there is always a nontransparent scar, however fine, marking the edges of the graft from the host tissue. Although initially the wound area is a site of rapid mucopolysaccharide synthesis, a corneal scar later contains less keratin sulphate and chondroitin-4-sulphate than normal corneal stroma. Also dermatan sulphate not usually found in the cornea has been isolated in nontransparent scars (Anseth, 1972). Internally, a wound in good apposition is bridged by mitosis of adjacent endothelial cells mainly derived from the host. The cut edges of Descemet's membrane are united by thin new basement membranes formed by these new bridging endothelial cells. In poor internal wound apposition, proliferating fibroblasts converting from adjacent keratocytes form a mass of connective tissue bulging into the anterior chamber (Inomata et al., 1970). This becomes covered with endothelium only after weeks to months. Alternatively overproliferation of the endothelium leads to reduplication or an extra thick Descemet's membrane in the wound area. It has been suggested that endothelial cells convert to fibroblasts and after several months back to their original form (Smelser and Ozanics, 1972).

G. Fate of the Donor Cells in Keratoplasty

Knowledge regarding the *ultimate fate of donor tissue in a successful graft,* has of necessity been largely derived from experimental work on animals. Chi *et al.* warns against too close a correlation with keratoplasty in human beings, also because the recipient corneas in the experimental animals used were free of disease (1965).

There is little doubt that *within days after grafting the donor epithelium is completely replaced* by that of the host (Castroviejo, 1937; Alberth, 1961) (Table 7). Experimentally, Khodadoust and Silverstein have shown however, that with careful handling fresh donor epithelium can survive (1969). Normal turnover rate of corneal epithelium is 1 week (Friedenwald and Buschke, 1944; Hanna and O'Brien, 1960).

Table 7. Fate of donor tissue in "successful" keratoplasty

Survival of	Replaced by host
Bowman's membrane	Epithelium
Stromal keratocytes and collagen	Nerves (often incomplete)
Descemet's membrane	
Endothelium	

On the other hand there is ample evidence that the *donor stomal and endothelial cells survive* in the host tissue as true chimeras for long periods of time in clear grafts. Thus BASU and ORMSBY (1960) using sex chromatin to identify stromal cells in penetrating keratoplasty of cats, found survival periods of 4–7 months. Using similar methods this was also verified for the endothelium by ESPIRITU et al., 1961.

POLACK et al. (1964) marking stromal and endothelial cells with H[3] Thymidine incorporated into the nuclear DNA showed survival of donor cells up to 12–13 months after keratoplasty in rabbits. CHI et al. (1965) found survival rates for the endothelium in rabbit keratoplasties up to 21 months, again using sex chromatin as a marker. The fact that an immune graft rejection can occur 10–15 years after keratoplasty is indirect evidence that at least the endothelium can survive that long (MAUMANEE et al., 1970). The fact that stromal and endothelial donor cells survive, means that foreign antigenic material remains for some time within the host, which is important regarding late immune rejection of the graft (Section III B).

(Normally the adult human endothelium never grows and stromal cells have a very slow turnover.)

Bowman's and Descemet's membrane are also *not replaced* by host tissue and the collagen fibers also remain.

Corneal nerves usually begin to proliferate into the graft from the host stroma after the 45th day, the palpebral reflex being recovered by the 12th month. However full corneal sensitivity is often not recovered even after 5 years (H.K. MÜLLER et al., 1961). ESCAPINI (1955) found that restoration of sensitivity started at the same time in clear as well as in opaque grafts and initial sensitivity was due to sprouting neurites from the nerves of the host. The new nerves in the transplant were present in the stroma as well as in the epithelium and were mostly sheathed with Schwann cells. Innervation progressed faster in an opaque vascularized transplant, the nerves following the pathway of the blood vessels.

III. Unsuccessful Keratoplasty

A failed or unsuccessful corneal graft is one which dislocates, or becomes opaque, the latter criterion applying especially to penetrating keratoplasty (GÜNTHER, 1961; H.K. MÜLLER et al., 1961; HALLERMANN, 1972).

Histopathologic examination of 36 failed human corneal transplants showed: epithelial thinning or hypertrophy in 90%, damage to Bowman's membrane in 57%, subepithelial fibrosis (anterior graft membrane) in 80%, stromal vascularization in 86%, retrocorneal membrane in 90%, and an abnormal endothelium in all cases (Winter, 1969).

Experimentally Zauberman and Sachs (1971), have shown that the cell population density of the endothelium decreased gradually in progressively more edematous grafts.

The presence of vascularization and inflammatory cell infiltration in 90% of cases (Winter) suggests that immune rejection of the graft played a role in the final opacification of the failed penetrating corneal transplant. However, there was evidence that a primary surgical defect was at least the initiating cause of graft failure in almost half these cases.

Surgical error as well as unsuitable donor material will cause *early* edema and opacification of the graft i.e. (within the first three weeks postoperatively). In failures occurring *three weeks to five years* after keratoplasty *the immunologic allograft reaction* is the commonest cause. *Very late graft opacification* is again more likely to be due to *deterioration* of the hitherto surviving *donor endothelium* (Stocker and Irish, 1969; Maumenee, 1973).

A. Nonimmunologic Factors for Graft Failure

Immunologic rejection of a corneal graft has probably been overemphasised in the past as the *primary* reason for failure (Hales and Spencer, 1963). It is more likely that other factors cause initial clouding which progresses to irreversible opacification directly or via immune rejection (Table 8).

The suitability of the donor cornea has been discussed already (Section II). The endothelium of the prospective graft is particularly difficult to evaluate and its viability is particularly important for the transparence of a penetrating

Table 8. Nonimmunologic reasons for graft failure

---

1. Unsuitable donor material (diseased or traumatized endothelium; cornea guttata)

2. Recurrence of disease in graft (herpetic keratitis; granular hereditary dystrophy, hydroquinone keratopathy)

3. Incomplete excision of inflammatory process in the host (keratomycosis)

4. Surgical errors
   anterior wound dehiscence (absence of Bowman's membrane in the host; epithelialization of the anterior chamber)
   posterior wound dehiscence (retrocorneal membrane)

5. Glaucoma
   primary
   secondary (flat anterior chamber, anterior synechia, steroid-provoked)

6. Incomplete postoperative protection of graft (defective lid closure; diminished tear secretion; mucus-deficiency syndrome)

7. Postoperative infection

---

keratoplasty. Decompensated endothelium with a consequently thickened Descemet's membrane (cornea guttata) may be overlooked and grafted into the host cornea (WINTER, 1969; STOCKER, 1971; EIMER, 1972). Such a graft will remain edematous, as will one where the initially healthy endothelium has been damaged during storage or at surgery. Edema of a corneal graft which does not clear, predisposes to vascularization from vessels in the scarred host cornea or from the limbus (COGAN, 1962; MAURICE, 1969).

The presence of these vessels will then lead to a donor-specific immune reaction (MAUMENEE, 1962). Even if this does not take place, vascularization of the graft in itself will result in irreversible opacification.

Recurrence of the original disease of the host cornea in the graft has long been suspected clinically for various hereditary corneal dystrophies and has been verified histologically for the commonest of these, namely granular dystrophy or GROENOUW's Type I (BROWNSTEIN et al., 1974). It is also known to occur in keratomykoses (NAUMANN et al., 1967) and hydroquinone damage to the cornea (NAUMANN and ROSSMANN, 1969).

Recurrence of herpetic keratitis is common. It cannot be regarded as true recurrence but rather as a continuation of the infection by the Herpes simplex virus due to the impossibility of complete excision of infected host cornea (HALLERMANN, 1965). Viral particles within the deep stromal keratocytes are responsible for the continued infection or rather reactivation, commonly occurring one or two years after keratoplasty (RICE and JONES, 1973; PFISTER et al., 1972). An additional factor for graft failure in the metaherpetic form of this disease is the fact that Descemet's membrane is destroyed due to a granulomatous reaction, so that only a penetrating keratoplasty has a chance of success (Fig. 3). The importance of surgical technique in producing perfect apposition of wound edges has also been emphasised (Section II). Faulty surgery is at least as frequent a primary cause of graft failure as immune rejection, to which it can also lead secundarily.

The surgeon must achieve a *water-tight closure of the wound*, taking care to centrate the graft, to keep the excision regular with a uniform bevel of the edges and to equalize suture tension. But most important of all is the *avoidance of trauma to the endothelium* in penetrating keratoplasty (MOORE and ARONSON, 1973). Anterior wound dehiscence is frequently associated with the absence of Bowman's membrane in the host cornea (so that the sutures are not anchored firmly, EIMER, 1972). In such cases the value of a preparatory tectonic lamellar keratoplasty to improve the host tissue structure cannot be overemphasised.

Epithelial growth inward is a serious but rare complication of penetrating keratoplasty, although a well-recognised cause of failure in prosthokeratoplasty (FERRY and GORDON, 1974).

Histopathologically a retrocorneal membrane is the commonest finding in a failed penetrating corneal transplant (Fig. 4). First described by FUCHS in 1901, it has been the subject of intense observation and investigation (HALES and SPENCER, 1963; TSUTSUI, 1966; BROWN and KITANO, 1966; SHERRARD and RYCROFT, 1967a, b; KURZ and D'AMICO, 1968; SHERRARD, 1969; SMITH, 1970; WERB, 1972).

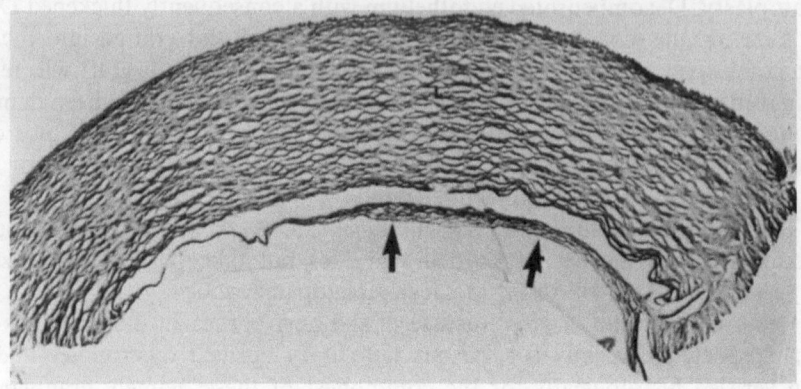

Fig. 4. Retrocorneal membrane (arrows) with corneal button obtained at rekeratoplasty. (No. 41/66 Univ. Eye Clinic, Histologic Laboratory, Hamburg)

Retrocorneal membranes are usually composed of connective tissue elements, with endothelium and sometimes a new Descemet's membrane. Kanai *et al.* (1972) found different endothelium cell types, including those whose cytoplasm resembled that of fibroblasts and which produced basement membrane-like strands.

The earliest occurrence of this membrane is within the third postoperative week. The source is the proliferating keratocytes (modified endothelial cells) at the internal wound site (Fig. 5). The membrane always develops centrally across the graft and not peripherally across host cornea. This is important as regards rekeratoplasty.

Any factor which causes insufficient apposition of the graft to the host tissue internally will predispose to retrocorneal membrane formation—(devitalized, or missing endothelium; retraction of the graft causing a gap internally; faulty suturing causing an internal ridge or step). It has also been claimed that iris stromal cells when adherent to the transplant (anterior synechia) can proliferate to form a retrocorneal membrane.

Most of the investigators in this field believe that only the integrity of the graft's endothelium prevents a retrocorneal membrane. Moreover, it is likely that it is a late manifestation of the immune response which leads to loss of the endothelial cells at the start (Maumenee, 1973).

Once formed the retrocorneal membrane will interfere with nutrition of the graft resulting in stromal edema with the ensuing chain of damage involving vascularization, scarring, and immune rejection.

Glaucoma either as a primary disease before keratoplasty or occurring secondarily after grafting (due to flat anterior chambers and the formation of anterior synechias, or provoked by the long-term administration of corticosteroids) will embarrass donor endothelial function, and therefore also predispose to graft edema and opacification. Thus it will hasten decompensation of the endothelium of marginal vitality.

Incomplete protection of the graft by defective lid closure or diminished or deficient tear production will predispose to scarring by causing ulceration

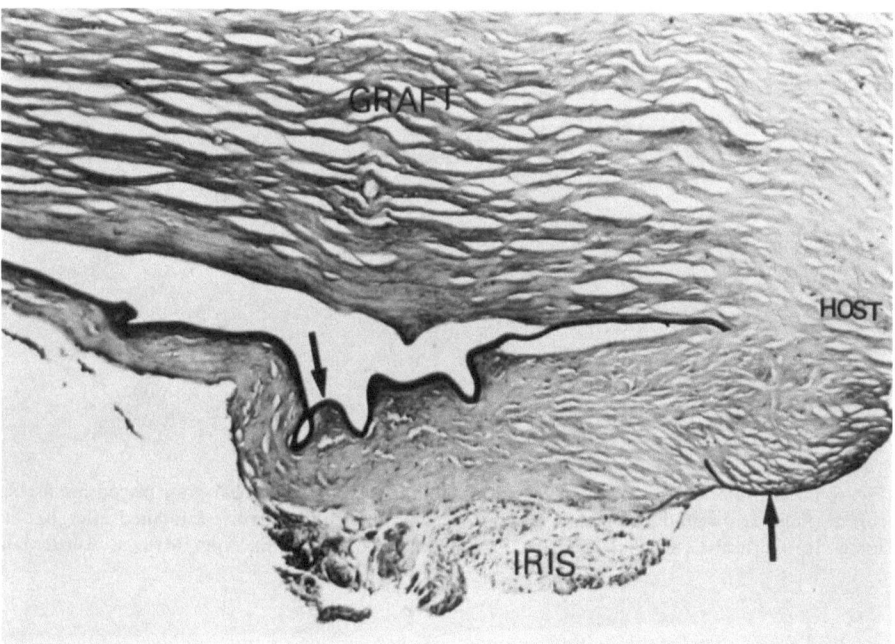

Fig. 5. Iris adherent to corneal host-graft-junction leading to massive retrocorneal membrane, causing infolding of the graft-Descemet's membrane (arrows). (No. 259/66 Hist. Lab. Univ. Eye Clinic, Hamburg)

of the epithelium and eventually the stroma of the corneal transplant. It is believed that certain serum proteins in normal tear fluid inhibit collagenases which are responsible for stromal destruction once the epithelium of a cornea is damaged.

Postoperative infection or inflammatory reactions to suture material are only very rarely involved in graft failure nowadays.

B. Immunologic Reasons for Graft Failure

Transplantation immunity is defined as an active immunologic process against histocompatibility antigens present in the donor tissue but absent in the host (ELLIOTT, 1971). It has been proved experimentally, that it is the *location* (Fig. 6) and not any specific property of corneal tissue that renders this organ an "immune-priviledged site" for transplantation (BILLINGHAM and BOSWELL, 1953). The in vitro models of BASU (1969) using corneal grafts in diffusion chambers provide evidence that host corneal cells in vivo do *not* play significant roles in the immune reaction, whereas host lymphoid cells do.

If cornea is transplanted as an allograft to an extracorneal site (Fig. 7) it will excite and result in a typical graft rejection (Fig. 8). When an allograft (or xenograft) is transplanted into corneal host tissue, usually the host T-lymphocytes cannot come into contact with the foreign antigens to become sensitized,

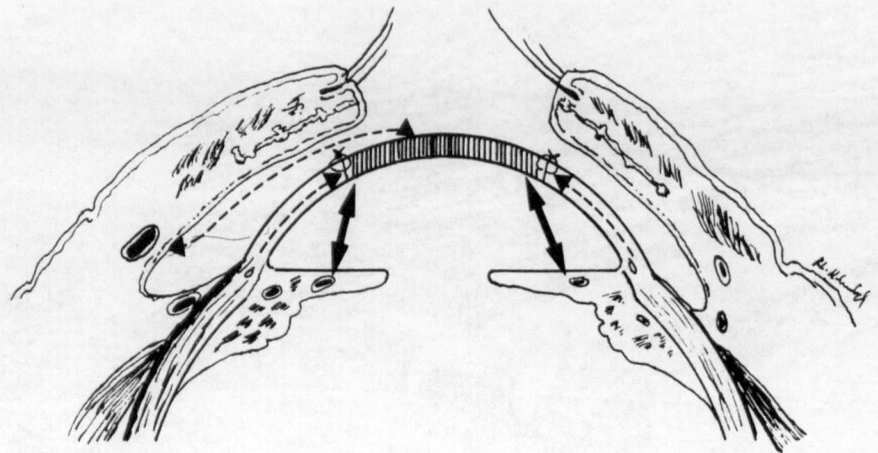

Fig. 6. Local routes of immunologic sensitization and response to corneal graft placed in vascular cornea (Solid arrows indicate higher significance than interrupted arrow) (modified after BARRIE, JONES. In: Corneal Graft Failure CIBA Foundation Symposium, Excerpta Medica, Amsterdam, 1973)

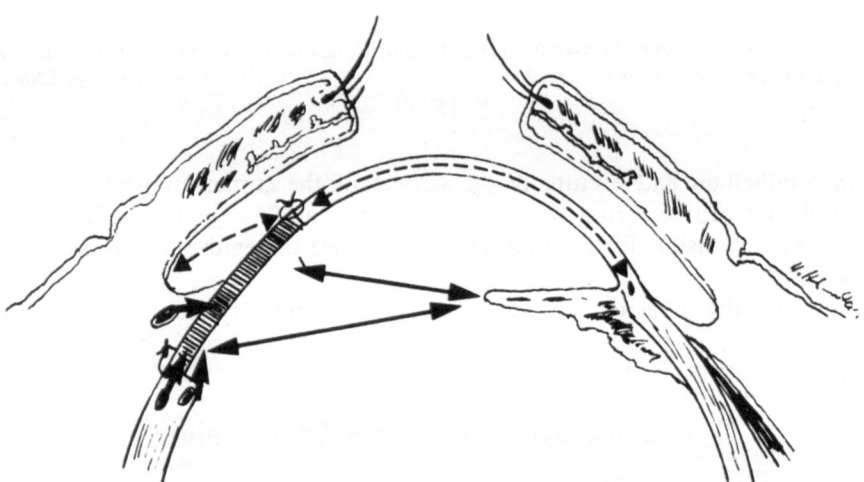

Fig. 7. Excentrically placed corneal graft exposed to close immunologic contact with vascularized tissues, conjunctiva, uvea, and sclera in addition to the transcameral route: Unprivileged site

because of the avascularity of the site. Also, even in a previously sensitized host (rekeratoplasty, blood transfusions, pregnancy) the sensitized lymphocytes usually cannot react with the graft in the absence of host corneal vascularization. Sensitization of the recipients T-lymphocytes (a prerequisite for graft immune rejection) can however also occur via diffusion of solid donor antigens leaving the graft through edematous corneal tissue or via aqueous humour (in penetrating keratoplasty); as well as by lymphocytes entering the graft in a vascularized

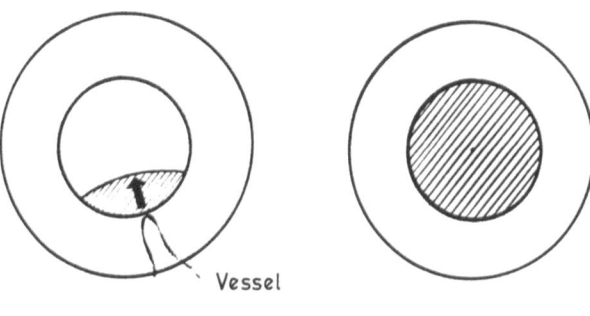

Focal - Progressive   Diffuse - Acute

Corneal Immune- Rejection

Fig. 8. Scheme of two principle clinical immune reactions

host, or when the graft is so large or eccentrically placed to be near the limbal vessels of the host.

Aqueous humour is usually free of cells, but it is conceivable that lymphocytes from the host uvea may reach the donor antigenic material via this route, which explains graft rejection in penetrating keratoplasty occurring in the absence of host vascularization (FRENCH, 1972), as well as the fact that lamellar keratoplasties are less liable to undergo rejection than penetrating ones (KORN-BLUETH and NELKEN, 1958). An electronmicroscopic study by INOMATA et al. (1970) showed the presence of lymphocytes from the aqueous humour pushing in between the endothelial cells of the corneal graft. The various biologic factors of transplantation which are unique to the corneal tissue were recently summed up by SILVERSTEIN and KHODADOUST (1973).

Cells having features common to both monocytes and lymphocytes have been described as "graft rejection cells", though their exact function and identity in the immune rejection is unknown (WIENER et al., 1964). The cornea contains soluble proteins having transplantation antigen activity also capable of stimulating an antibody response, the epithelium being especially strong in antigens (D'ERMO and SECCHIO, 1972). The role of these cornea specific antigens in graft rejection is still unclear (LEIBOWITZ and LUZZIO, 1970), although anticorneal antibody titers have been shown to rise after transplant surgery (ALBERTH, 1974). The antigens important for graft rejection in corneal transplantation are probably the HL-A (and perhaps less significant those of AB0 system) antigen. The former exist on cell membranes and over twenty antigenic specificities are known. They are released without cell death as soon as the graft is transplanted, and can produce delayed hypersensitivity and circulating antibodies.

Clinical retrospective studies on the significance of HL-A and AB0-system matching host to donor, on the ultimate fate of the graft are conflicting in their results: (see Section IIC). However, a recent publication by GIBBS et al. showed that the sharing of HL-A system antigens between host and donor affects mainly the reversibility of rejection reactions, and that cases at high risk (because of extreme vascularization of the host cornea) which share even only two HL-A system antigens have significantly better prognostic chances, than those where no sharing of these strong antigens was present (1974).

That some cases of corneal graft failure are due to immunologic graft rejection is a recognized fact. In 1948 Paufique *et al.* named unexpected unexplained graft clouding "maladie du greffon" which must now be considered a very general term including all reasons for graft failure. The clinical diagnosis remains empirical, and there are as yet no specific laboratory tests to confirm a diagnosis of immunologic graft rejection.

Criteria for the clinical diagnosis of an immunologic corneal graft-reaction are:

1. Clouding of a graft which has been initially clear and well healed for at least 2–3 weeks postoperatively

2. Absence of any other obvious cause of graft clouding (e.g. severe secondary glaucoma, trauma, woundseparation)

3. Localized bulbar conjunctival hyperemia with keratic precipitates on the endothelium of the transplant associated with localized graft stromal edema, as well as commonly—but not always—the presence of blood vessels at the graft margins where the clouding has begun (Elliott, 1972; Chandler and Kaufman, 1974).

Typical symptoms of onset are a red eye, vague ocular discomfort, photophobia, and blurring of vision. Nine to twelve percent of "good prognosis" penetrating grafts are unsuccessful because of immune graft reaction (Polack, 1973). In "poor prognosis" cases, up to 70% can fail because of graft immune rejection. The prompt recognition of these graft reactions is especially important since they are reversible at an early stage with corticosteroid therapy (Chandler and Kaufman, 1974).

The severity of the reaction is inversely proportional to the length of time in which the transplant has remained clear. Typical reactions have even been seen as late as 10, 12, and 15 years after keratoplasty, which is indirect proof of the length of donor tissue survival in the host (Maumenee, 1970).

Polack (1966 and 1973) has defined two different clinical forms of graft rejection, as seen by slitlamp microscopy:

1. The first begins insidiously in the periphery with precipitates on the donor endothelium beginning at the wound margins where there is vascularization of host cornea, and forming a line which slowly wanders across the transplant leaving behind edematous cloudy tissue ("Khodadoust line").

2. The second form is an acute diffuse edema of the entire corneal graft with a scattering of endothelial precipitates. Polack believes that circulating antibodies may play an important role in the second form of reaction, which is commoner among the poor prognostic groups (heavily vascularized host cornea, rekeratoplasty etc.) and is more resistant to treatment with corticosteroids.

In 1969 Khodadoust and Silverstein described the pattern of rejection of the individual layers of corneal allografts, when rabbit corneal grafts were sensitized by induced vascularization (1969b).

Epithelial rejection is characterized by a fine linear defect marking local destruction of donor cells followed practically immediately by regeneration from recipient epithelium. The corneal *stroma* shows a broad band of leukocytic infiltration also moving across the transplant and leaving behind dead kerato-cytes replaced by the host much later than epithelial cells. Within the *endothelium*, the "rejection line" contains plasma cells and lymphocytes. The stroma imme-diately above the line is nearly always edematous, and becomes clear only when endothelium from the recipient replaces that of the donor. The whole process takes several months. We like to call the first process *"chronic cir-cumscribed immune-reaction"*, the second *"acute diffuse immune reaction"* (Fig. 8).

Factors predisposing a graft to immune rejection are listed in Table 9. The most important single factor is the *proximity to blood vessels* either due to a vascularized host cornea or due to a very large or eccentrically placed graft which is near to the host limbal vessels. That avascularity of the corneal host bed is important for both the afferent as well as the efferent limb of the host allograft reaction has been proved experimentally (KHODADOUST and SILVER-STEIN, 1972). Deep vessels although structurally similar to superficial vessels especially aid an immune rejection.

The *original disease* in the recipient cornea is also important. Herpetic kerati-tis for instance appears to increase the susceptibility to immune response proba-bly due to the chronic inflammation in the deeper layers perhaps also due to hyperemia of the iris. In fact 60% of penetrating keratoplasties for this disease undergo a typical allograft reaction (RICE and JONES, 1973).

Any factor like *poor wound apposition,* or mechanical irritation of the graft postoperatively due to sutures or poor lid closure, will predispose to an antigen-antibody reaction, as will any *inflammatory process* of the anterior eye segments. POLACK (1965) was able to demonstrate experimentally, that these "immunomi-metic" reactions were not true transplant immune rejections. ELLIOTT (1972) calls them adventitious antigen-antibody reactions. That is to say, they are not initiated by direct combination or interaction of specific antigens with anti-bodies or by interaction of specific antigens with immunologically activated cells (ELLIOTT, 1971). They can however lead *secondarily* to a true immune graft tissue rejection. Silk sutures expecially cause this, due to their affinity for gamma globulins (MOORE and ARONSON, 1971). Evidence also exists, that bacterial endotoxins can cause such a reaction or even initiate a true graft immune rejection.

In short, any prolonged alteration of vascular permeability in the donor and host cornea when unsuppressed will inevitably lead to immunologic rejection of the graft resulting in edema and opaque scarring (ELLIOTT, 1971, 1972).

The histologic appearance of a corneal homograft rejection was first de-scribed by MAUMENEE in 1951.

Most clinical material can only be examined histologically in the *late* stages of the immune graft rejection (Fig. 9), so that studies on the early pathologic changes have been mainly confined to experimental work, usually on rabbits (MAUMENEE, 1951; POLACK, 1962; INOMATA et al., 1970; KANAI and POLACK, 1971; POLACK, 1972, 1973). Histologic examination of rejected human corneal transplants are described by LEVENSON and BRIGHTBILL (1973), POLACK (1975).

Electron microscopic studies of *epithelial* rejection shows lymphocytes and plasma cells infiltrating at the base from the superficial stroma as well as from

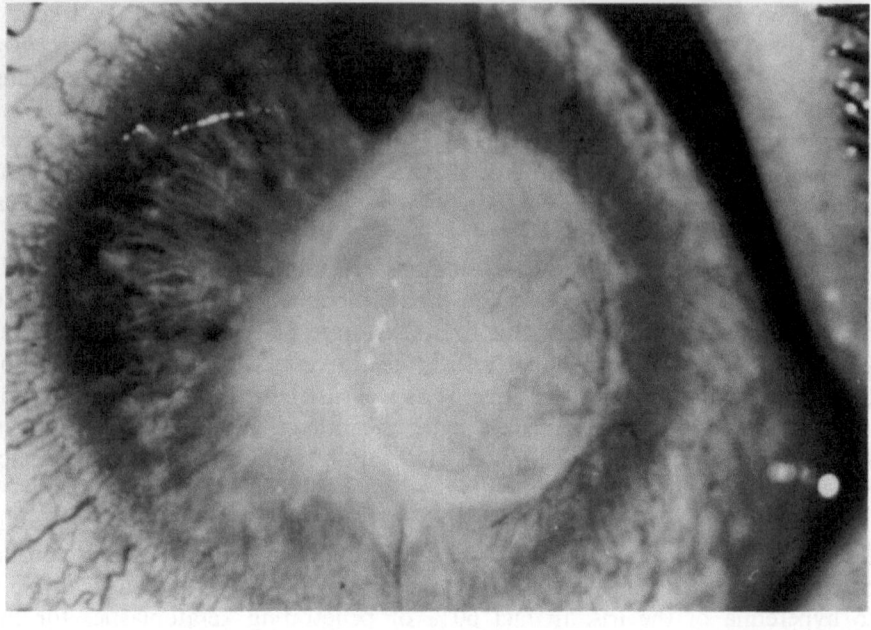

(a)

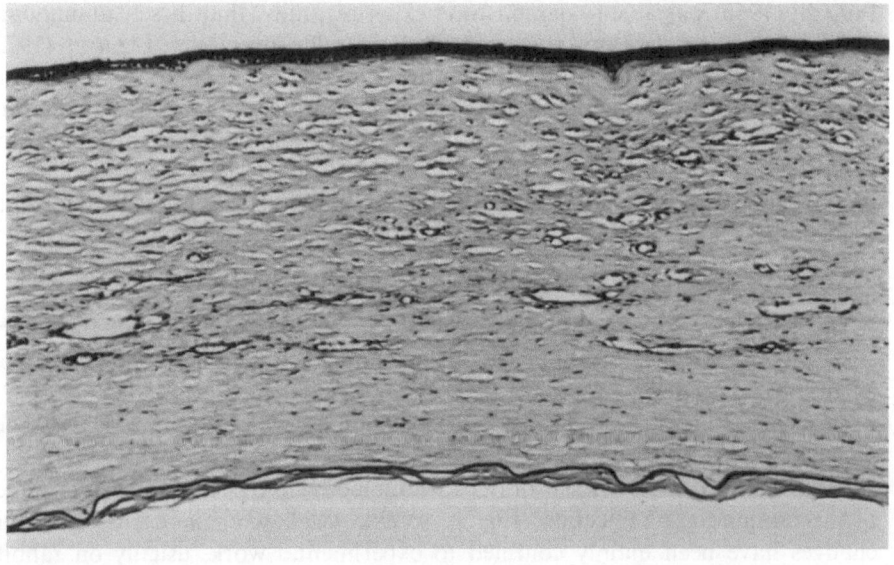

(b)

Fig. 9a and b. Final stage of irreversible focal or diffuse immune reaction: (a) vascularized scar replaced donor cornea. (b) histology shows thin epithelium, richly vascularized stroma with chronic inflammatory infiltrate and the endothelium replaced by retrocorneal membrane. Only Bowman's and Descemet's membrane remain. (No. 36/68 Univ. Eye-Clinic, Hist. Laboratory, Hamburg)

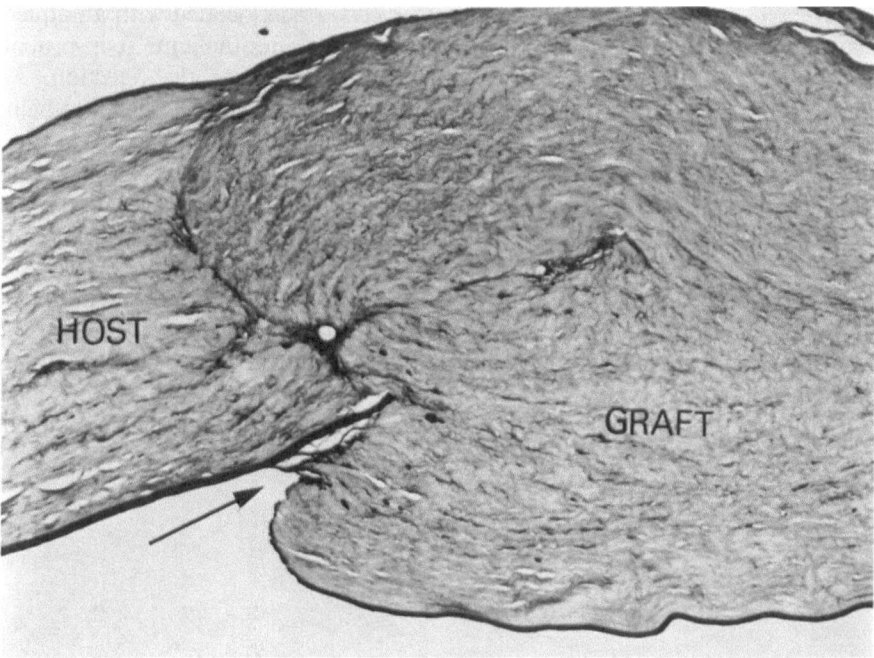

Fig. 10. Edematous corneal graft protruding beyond level of host cornea into anterior chamber exposing one edge to access (arrow) of aqueous humour (No. 144/68 Univ. Eye Clinic, Hist. Laboratory, Hamburg)

the vessels at the wound edge. POLACK believes that some anterior corneal membranes or pannus formation in human rejected grafts could represent the endstage of epithelial rejection.

Stromal rejection is characterized by infiltration of the stromal wound with lymphocytes usually with blood vessels which reach the endothelium via the space between Descemet's membranes of the host and the donor before this gap has bridged over (POLACK, 1962; INOMATA *et al.,* 1970). The lymphocytes *preceed* the endothelial capillary proliferation into the donor stroma. The gap between the donor- and host-Descemet's membranes where scar tissue is formed is the weak point whereby inflammatory cells can reach the stroma from the aqueous (Fig. 10). Normally it is bridged between 6–9 months, but if the inner wound edges are in poor apposition or Descemet's membrane and the endothelium traumatized, proliferation of fibroblasts (probably also of modified endothelial cells) of the host will cause a retrocorneal graft membrane.

The peripheral *endothelial "line rejection"* type of immune graft sickness is especially seen in experimental animals (POLACK, 1973) and is accompanied by deep stromal vascular invasion of the scar. The anterior chamber is usually free of inflammatory cells, but leukocytes are present, interspersed with the endothelial cells, POLACK, 1972; KHODADOUST and SILVERSTEIN, 1969b). This "Khodadoust-Line" is pathognomonic for endothelial rejection (Fig. 11).

The second type of diffuse *acute graft rejection* is associated with an aqueous flare and diffuse keratic precipitates on the graft endothelium. It is probable that sensitized lymphocytes from the host uvea initiates the rejection. Also active circulating antibodies may cause the acute reaction once the endothelium is damaged (POLACK, 1973).

The *prevention* of the corneal graft immune rejection lies firstly in the avoidance of the factors listed in Table 9. Careful surgery and protection of the graft postoperatively with the avoidance of inflammation are of paramount importance.

Many surgeons prefer to remove the epithelium of the donor tissue thereby reducing the antigenic mass introduced. However in poor lid closure, dry eye syndromes, and where reepithelialization from the host is expected to be delayed this should be avoided.

STOCKER recommends soaking the donor cornea in the prospective recipient's serum for 24 hours preoperatively (1968).

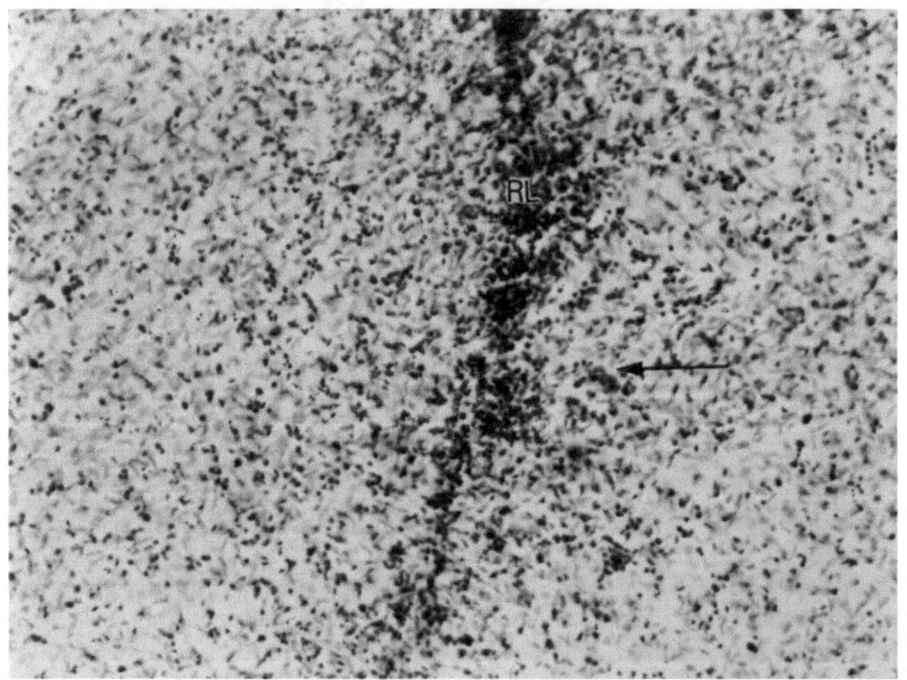

Fig. 11a–c. Reproduced (with kind permission of FRANK M. POLACK, M.D. from Investigative Ophthalmology, Vol. 11, 1–14, 1972)
(a) Flat endothelium preparation showing rejection line (*RL*) formed by lymphocytes and direction of endothelial reaction (arrow). Many lymphocytes are located in subendothelial layer (b) Scanning electron micrograph shows the lymphocytes from rejection line (c) Clump of lymphocytes (*Ly*) in area of active rejection showing cytoplasmic junction by pseudopodial extension and attachments to damaged endothelial cells (*En*). Degenerated cells show thick bodies (stars)

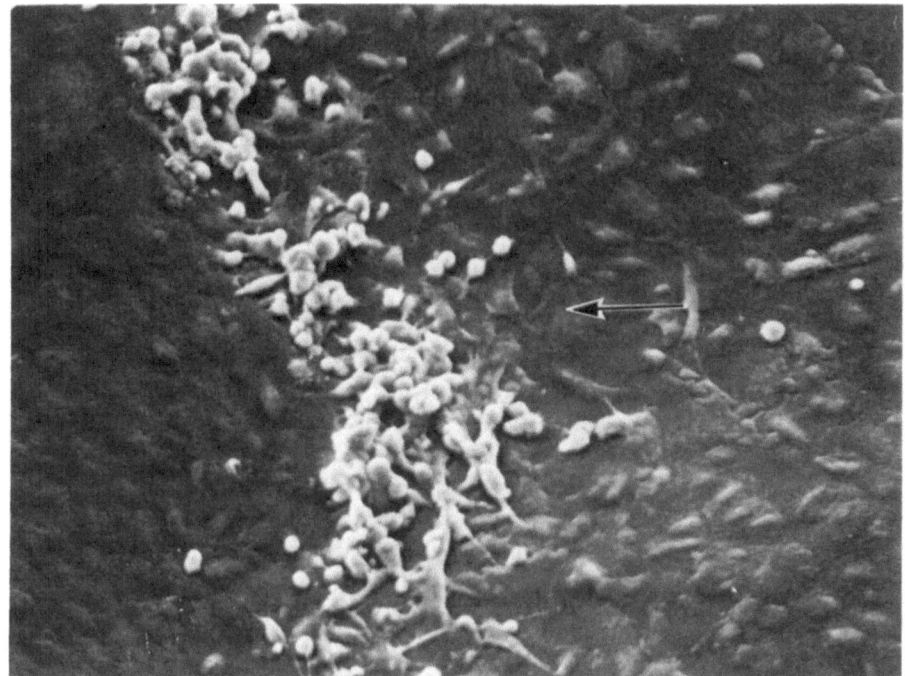

Fig. 11b

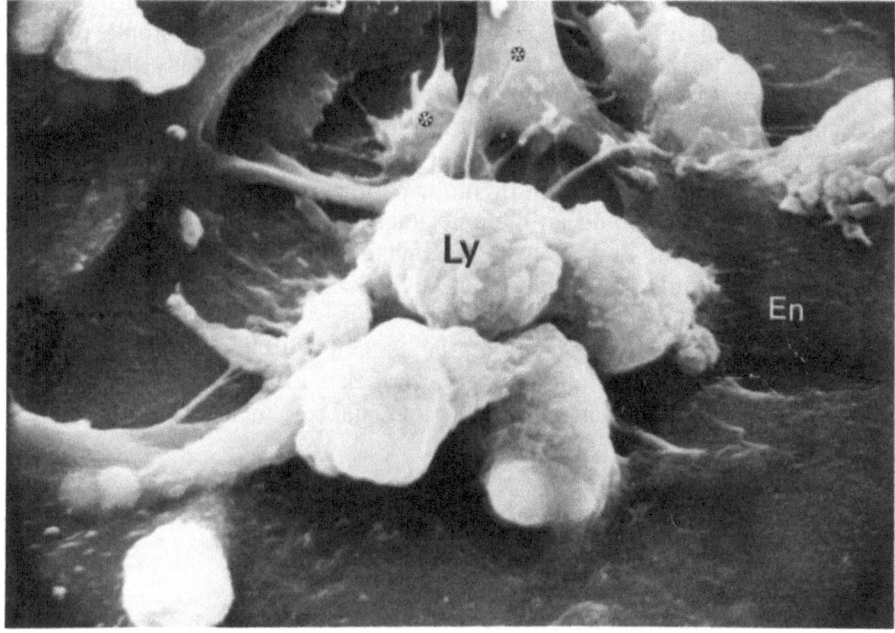

Fig. 11c

Table 9. Factors influencing immunologic graft failure

1. Size and location of graft
2. State of recipient cornea: *vascularization*, scarring, inflammation
3. Original disease of recipient cornea: increased susceptibility to immune response, e.g., herpetic keratitis
4. Surgical errors: poor wound apposition, mechanical irritation by sutures
5. Glaucoma
6. Poor protection of graft (lagophthalmos, "dry eye syndrome")

Preoperative reduction of the vascularization in the host cornea has been attempted with cauterization, Argon laser, beta radiation, thio-TEPA, cryocoagulation, and subconjunctival injections of methyl prednisolone (EY *et al.,* 1968). All measures proved unreliable.

The use of cryopreserved corneas instead of fresh donor material apparently also decreases the chances of immune rejection (SCHULTZ and GALLUN, 1973).

The future lies in tissue-typing donor with prospective recipient for the "strong" antigens of the HL-A (and AB0) systems. This of course involves a large organization for selection of donor material in an eyebank, and also a large group of prospective patients awaiting keratoplasty. Crossmatching for circulating antibodies is also recommended (i.e., incubation of lymphocytes of the prospective donor with the serum of the prospective recipient plus complement, whereby a negative result indicating absent circulating antibodies does not necessarily mean the host is not sensitized) (FRENCH, 1972).

Treatment of the corneal graft immune rejection rests mainly on the prompt local and usually also systemic application of glucocorticosteroids. [POLACK has been able to show in a scanning electron-microscopic study that topically applied dexamethasone in rabbit eyes with rejecting corneal grafts decreased the numbers of leukocytic endothelial infiltration (1973)].

Azathioprine (IMUREL) given together with these has also been recommended for the poor prognostic cases. In the experimental stage are treatment with antilymphocytic serum and antilymphocyticglobulin (SMOLIN, 1968; WALTMAN *et al.,* 1969). KROGH and WEEKE (1972) have described a case treated with extracorporeal irradiation of blood or "ECIB".

EVANS (1973) has summarized the main dangers of immunosuppressive treatment, which can be so severe that the patient with the eventually perhaps successfully clear corneal allograft is nevertheless crippled by such iatrogenic complications as bone marrow depression, diabetes mellitus, or osteoporosis to name but a few.

IV. Experimental Keratoplasty and Heterografting

In the history of corneal transplantation, keratoplasty in animals including heterografting to man, has played an important role (see Section I).

Heterografting in humans is rarely indicated nowadays although PAYRAU advocates the use of canine lamellar grafts for herpetic keratitis in humans (dogs do not suffer from this disease) (1965).

Other indications for heterografting corneas in man are:

1. To save the eye in an emergency (e.g. perforating ulcer or wound) when human donor material is not available.

2. For lamellar keratoplasties in countries where legal or religious prejudice forbids the use of human cadaver corneas.

Heterologous corneal grafting is successful in lamellar keratoplasty, especially when the donor tissue has been lyophilized or desiccated, so that antigenic material is minimized.

The immunologic aspects of heterografting have been reviewed by ROCHA and GALVÃO (1966). Species specific antigens are added to individual specific and organ specific antigens so that an immune rejection is all the more likely. Interestingly enough, there is considerable variation in the success of heterografting depending on the combination of species involved. Thus PAYRAU found an 80% success rate when cattle corneas were implanted to dogs, but only a 20% success rate when pig corneas were used in rabbits. The exact relationship between the zoologic class of the donor and recipient and the ultimate fate of the xenograft remains open to speculation.

Experimental keratoplasty has been responsible for the immense progress in all fields of keratoplasty. It is probably the most frequent surgical procedure performed in experimental animals, and is still important for:

1. Practising and improving the techniques of keratoplasty.

2. Investigating corneal healing.

3. Examining the effects of different suture materials.

4. Lightmicroscopic, electronmicroscopic, and biochemical aspects of the fate of individual cell layers of the donor tissue.

5. All aspects of immune graft rejection and the effect of different immuno-suppressive treatment.

6. Improving methods in storage and transportation of donor material for eyebanks and investigating techniques for measuring corneal viability.

It was an animal experiment in 1888 by WAGENMANN which led to the important recognition of the role of the corneal endothelium in maintaining transparence of the stroma.

The rabbit has been used for most experimental models of keratoplasty. The corneal anatomy resembles that of man except for the fact that a Bowman's membrane is missing, and the endothelium appears hardier than human corneal endothelium (STOCKER, 1965).

The price of rabbits as experimental animals is low and they are easy to handle and readily available. Techniques for experimental keratoplasty in rabbits have been discussed and reviewed by KHODADOUST (1968) and MUELLER (1963, 1964), MUELLER et al., 1964).

The only disadvantage in using rabbits is the weakness and variability of the corneal homograft rejection reaction so that methods have been developed to potentiate this reaction (e.g. with Freund's adjuvant) when studying aspects of the immune response (SMOLIN, 1972).

Acknowledgements

Thanks are due to Miss E. PORTWICH for preparing the histologic slides; Miss I. HADLOK for preparing the clinical photos; and Mr. H. HELMDACH for the diagrams.

References

AINSLIE, D.: Recent advances in keratoplasty. Brit. J. Ophthal. **58**, 335–343 (1974)

ALBERTH, B.: Keratoplastik. Bücherei des Augenarztes. No. 37, S. 126–130. Stuttgart: Enke 1961

ALBERTH, B.: Anticorneal antibody examination in human keratoplasty. v. Graefes Arch. klin. exp. Ophthal. **190**, 341–346 (1974)

ALLANSMITH, M.R., FINE, M., PAYNE, R.: Histocompatibility typing and corneal transplantation. Trans. Amer. Acad. Ophthal. Otolaryng. **78**, 445–460 (1974)

ALLANSMITH, M.R., DRELL, D.W., KAJIYAMA, G.: AB0 Blood groups and corneal transplantation. Amer. J. Ophthal. **79**, 493–501 (1975)

ANSETH, A.: Wound healing in corneal grafting. In: Corneal Grafting. CASEY, T.A. (ed.), p. 59–62. London: Butterworths 1972

ASCHER cited by LÖHLEIN, W.: Fortschritte auf dem Gebiet der Hornhauttransplantation. Dtsch. Ophthal. Ges. Heidelberg **52**, 72–80 (1938)

ASHWOOD-SMITH, M.J.: Problems of cell survival after freezing and thawing with special reference to the cornea. In: Corneal Graft Failure. Ciba Foundation No. 15, p. 57–77. North Holland: Elsevier 1973

AURELL, G., DOHLMAN, C.H., RODÉN, L.: The viability of the stored cornea. Acta Ophthal. **34**, 281–292 (1956)

BARRAQUER, J.I.: Keratomileusis and keratophakia. In: Corneoplastic Surgery. RYCROFT (ed.), p. 409–443. London: Pergamon 1969

BASU, P.K., ORMSBY, H.L.: Corneal Heterografts in Rabbits. Amer. J. Ophthal. **44**, 477–598 (1957)

BASU, P.K., ORMSBY, H.L.: Sex chromatin as a biologic cell marker in the study of the fate of the corneal transplant. Amer. J. Ophthal. **49**, 513–515 (1960)

BASU, P.K.: Studies on the mechanisms of corneal graft reaction using simplified systems. In: Corneo-plastic Surgery. RYCROFT (ed.), p. 163–172. London: Pergamon 1969

BILLINGHAM, R.E., BOSWELL, T.: Studies on the problem of corneal homografts. Proc. roy. Soc. London (Biol.) **141**, 392–406 (1953)

BORUCHOFF, S.A., DOHLMAN, C.H.: Corneal autografts. Amer. J. Ophthal. **63**, 1677–1681 (1967)

BOURNE, W.M.: Antigenicity of cryopreserved corneas. Arch. Ophthal. **93**, 215–218 (1975)

BRONSON, N.R.: Ultrasonic examinations in keratoplasty. Int. Ophthalmol. Clin. **10**, 253–259 (1970)

BROWN, R.M., TREVOR-ROPER, P.D.: A clinical method for assessment of endothelial viability in donor corneas. Brit. J. Ophthal. **52**, 882–886 (1968)

BROWN, S.I., KITANO, S.: Pathogenesis of the retrocorneal membrane. Arch Ophthal. **75**, 518–525 (1966)

BROWN, S.I.: Results of corneal transplantation in diffuse corneal oedema. Amer. J. Ophthal. **70**, 20–23 (1970)

BROWN, S.I.: Corneal transplantation of the infant cornea. Trans. Amer. Acad. Ophthal. Otolaryng. **78**, 461–466 (1974a)

BROWN, S.I., BLOOMFIELD, S.E., PEARCE, D.B.: A followup report on transplantation of the alkali burned cornea. Amer. J. Ophthal. **77**, 538–542 (1974b)

BROWNSTEIN, S., FINE, B.S., SHERMAN, M.E., ZIMMERMAN, L.E.: Granular dystrophy of the cornea. Light and electron microscopic confirmation of recurrence in the graft. Amer. J. Ophthal. **77**, 701–710 (1974)

BÜRKI, E.: Über ein neues Verfahren zur Konservierung von Hornhautgewebe. Ophthalmologica **114**, 288–293 (1947)

CAPELLA, J.A., EDELHAUSER, H.F., VAN HORN, D.L.: Corneal Prevervation. Clinical and laboratory evaluation of current methods. Illinois: Charles C. Thomas 1973

CAPELLA, J.A., KAUFMAN, H.E., ROBBINS, J.E.: Preservation of viable corneal tissue. Arch. Ophthal. **74**, 669–673 (1965)

CARDONA, H., CASTROVIEJO, R., DE VOE, A.G.: Advanced in prosthokeratoplasty. In: Corneal Grafting. CASEY, T.A. (ed.), p. 313–329. London: Butterworths 1972

CASTROVIEJO, R.: Keratoplasty: microscopic study of corneal grafts. Trans. Amer. Ophthal. Soc. **35**, 355–384 (1937)

CASTROVIEJO, R.: Keratoplastik. S. 17, S. 400–402. Stuttgart: Thieme 1968

CASTROVIEJO, R.: Keratoplasty and cataractextraction as separate or combined operations. In: Symposium on the cornea. Trans. New Orleans Acad. Ophthal., p. 152–162. Saint Louis: C.V. Mosby 1972a

CASTROVIEJO, R.: Report on unusual cases with special reference to those requiring multiple operations. In: Symposium on the cornea. Trans. New Orleans Acad. Ophthal., p. 163–187. Saint Louis: C.V. Mosby 1972b

CHANDLER, J.W., KAUFMAN, H.E.: Graft reactions after keratoplasty for keratoconus. Amer. J. Ophthal. **77**, 543–547 (1974)

CHI, H.H., TENG, C.C., KATZIN, H.M.: The fate of endothelial cells in corneal homografts. Amer. J. Ophthal. **59**, 186–191 (1965)

CHOYCE, P.: The treatment of bullous keratoplasty with acrylic inlays. In: Corneo-plastic Surgery, p. 399–403. London: Pergamon 1969

CLIFTON, E.C., HANNA, C.: Corneal cryopreservation and the fate of corneal cells in keratoplasty. Amer. J. Ophthal. **78**, 239–250 (1974)

COGAN, D.G.: Corneal vascularisation. Invest. Ophthal. **1**, 253–261 (1962)

COOPER, T.D., McTIGUE, J.W.: NBT-MTT Tetrazolium stains for the study of corneal endothelial cells. Invest. Ophthal. **7**, 227 (Abstract) (1968)

DAVSON, H.: The hydration of the cornea. Biochem. J. **59**, 24–28 (1955)

D'ERMO, F., SECCHI, A.G.: Immunität und allergische Erscheinungen bei Homo und Heterotransplantation der Hornhaut. Zbl. ges. Ophthal. **105**, 272 (1971/72)

DOHLMAN, C.H.: Artificial corneal endothelium—a new principle in penetrating keratoplasty. In: Corneo-plastic Surgery. RYCROFT (ed.), p. 229–240. London: Pergamon 1969

DOHLMAN, C.H., GASSET, A.R.: Studies on the healing of the corneal stroma. In: Corneo-plastic Surgery. RYCROFT (ed.), p. 179–183. London: Pergamon 1969

DOHLMAN, C.H., SCHNEIDER, H.A., DOANE, M.G.: Prosthokeratoplasty. Amer. J. Ophthal. **77**, 694–700 (1974)

DUFFY, P., WOLF, J., COLLINS, G., DE VOE, A.G., STREETEN, B., COWEN, D.: Letter to the Editor. New Eng. J. Med. **290**, 692–693 (1974)

DUKE-ELDER, S.: Corneal Grafts. In: Diseases of the outer eye. Vol. VIII, Part 2, p. 648–661. London: Kimpton 1965

EHLERS, N., AHRONS, S.: Corneal transplantation and histocompatibility. Acta Ophthalmol. **49**, 513–527 (1971)

EIMER, H.H.: Zur Klinik und Histopathologie von Re-Keratoplastiken. Unang. Diss. Hamburg 1972

ELLIOT, J.H.: Immune factors in corneal graft rejection. Invest. Ophthal. **10**, 216–234 (1971)

ELLIOT, J.H.: Immunologic factors in penetrating keratoplasty failures. In: Symposium on the Cornea. Trans New Orleans Acad. Ophthal., p. 64–77. Saint Louis: C.V. Mosby 1972a

ELLIOT, J.H., LEIBOWITZ, H.M.: Immunosuppression of corneal graft rejection. In: Symposium on the Cornea. Trans. New Orleans Acad. Ophthal., p. 53–63. Saint Louis: C.V. Mosby 1972b

ESCAPINI, H.: Nerve changes in the human corneal graft. Arch. Ophthal. **53**, 229–235 (1955)

ESPIRITU, R.B., KORA, G.B., TABOWITZ, D.: Studies on the healing of corneal grafts. The fate of endothelial cells of the graft as determined by sex chromatin. Amer. J. Ophthal. **52**, 91–95 (1961)

EVANS, D.B.: Some clinical problems of immunosuppression. In: Corneal Graft Failure. Ciba Foundation No. 15, p. 279–291. North Holland: Elsevier 1973

EY, R.C., HUGHES, W.F., BLOOME, M.A., TALLMAN, C.B.: Prevention of corneal vascularisation. Amer. J. Ophthal. **66**, 1118–1131 (1968)

FERRY, A.P., GORDON, B.L.: Epithelialisation of the anterior chamber, a complication of prosthokeratoplasty. Arch. Ophthal. **91**, 281–284 (1974)

FILATOW cited by NIŽETIC, Z.: Erweiterte Indikationen für Hornhauttransplantation. Dtsch. Ophthal. Ges. Heidelberg **52**, 72–80 (1938)

FINE, M., WEST, C.E.: Late results of keratoplasty for Fuch's dystrophy. Amer. J. Ophthal. **72**,
109–114 (1971)

FINE, M.: Techniques of penetrating keratoplasty. In: Symposium on the cornea. Trans. New
Orleans Acad. Ophthal., p. 132–142. Saint Louis: C.V. Mosby 1972a

FINE, M.: Problems of keratoplasty in aphakic eyes. In: Symposium of the cornea. Trans. New
Orleans Acad. Ophthal., p. 143–151. Saint Louis: C.V. Mosby 1972b

FORSTER, R.K., FINE, M.: Relation of donor age to success in penetrating keratoplasty. Arch.
Ophthal. **85**, 42–47 (1971)

FRANCESCHETTI, A., DORET, M.: Hornhauttransplantation „a chaud". Klin. Mbl. Augenheilk. **117**,
449–458 (1950)

FRENCH, M.E.: Immunological aspects of corneal graft rejection. In: Corneal Grafting. CASEY
(ed.), p. 63–80. London: Butterworths 1972

FRIEDENWALD, J.S., BUSCHKE, W.: Mitotic and corneal healing activities of the corneal epithelium.
Arch. Ophthal. **32**, 410–413 (1944)

FUCHS, E.: Zur Keratoplastik. Z. Augenheilk. **5**, 1–5 (1901)

GALUN, A.B., EDELHAUSER, H.F., SCHULTZ, R.O.: Experimental surgical evaluation of frozen corneal
tissue. Ann. Ophthalmol. **3**, 748–755 (1971)

GENOSKI, D.H., EDELHAUSER, H.F.: Metabolic evaluation of cryopreserved corneal tissue. Arch.
Ophthal. **91**, 130–133 (1974)

GIBBS, D.C., BATCHELOR, J.R., CASEY, T.A.: The influence of HL-A compatibility on the fate
of corneal grafts. In: Corneal graft failure. Ciba Foundation Symposium No. 15, p. 293–304.
North Holland: Elsevier 1973

GIBBS, D.C., BATCHELOR, J.R., WERB, A., SCHLESINGER, W., CASEY, T.A.: The influence of tissue-type
compatibility on the fate of full thickness corneal grafts. Trans. ophthal. Soc. U.K. **94**, 95–101
(1974)

GÜNTHER, G.: Spätergebnisse der Keratoplastik an 100 erfolgreichen Transplantationen. Ber. Dtsch.
ophthal. Ges. **64**, 159–164 (1961)

HALES, R.H., SPENCER, W.H.: Unsuccessful penetrating keratoplasties. Arch. Ophthal. **70**, 805–810
(1963)

HALLERMANN, W.: Ergebnisse der Keratoplastik bei Herpes. Klin. Mbl. Augenheilk. **146**, 161–171
(1965)

HALLERMANN, W.: Vorderkammertransplantationen bei der Keratoplastik. Klin. Mbl. Augenheilk.
146, 161–171 (1965)

HALLERMANN, W.: Probleme der Keratoplastik. Ber. Dtsch. ophthal. Ges. **71**, 279–289 (1972)

HANNA, C., O'BRIEN, J.E.: Cell production and migration in the epithelial layer of the cornea.
Arch. Ophthal. **64**, 536–539 (1960)

HANNA, C., BLOCKER, D., ALLEN, J.H.: RNA and protein synthesis by cells of human eye bank
corneas. Amer. J. Ophthal. **68**, 53–64 (1969)

HARMS, H., MACKENSEN, G.: Augenoperationen unter dem Mikroskop. Stuttgart: Thieme 1966

HATA, B.: The uses of corneae from gliomatous eyes in corneal transplantation. Acta Soc. Ophthal.
Jap. **43**, 1763–1767 (1939)

HAVENER, W.H., STINE, G.T., WEISS, L.L.: Corneal donor selection by blood type. Arch. Ophthal.
60, 443–447 (1958)

HINZPETER, E.N., NAUMANN, G.: Kongenitale hereditäre Hornhaut-Endothel-Dystrophie. Ber.
Dtsch. ophthal. Ges. **71**, 585–591 (1972)

HOEFLE, F.B.: Human corneal donor material in vitro studies. Arch. Ophthal. **82**, 361–367 (1969)

HOEFLE, F.B., MAURICE, D.M., SIBLEY, R.C.: Human corneal donor material. A method of examination before keratoplasty. Arch. Ophthal. **84**, 741–744 (1970)

HORN, D.L. VAN, HANNA, C., SCHULTZ, R.O.: Corneal cryopreservation ultrastructural and viability
changes. Arch. Ophthal. **84**, 655–667 (1970)

HORN, D.L. VAN, SCHULTZ, R.O.: Ultrastructural changes in the endothelium of human cornea
stored under eyebank conditions. In: Corneal preservation. CAPELLA, EDELHAUSER, VAN HORN
(eds.). Illinois: Charles C. Thomas 1973

Huerkamp, B.: Die Infrarot-Photographie in der Differentialdiagnostik von Pigmentveränderungen des vorderen Augenabschnittes. Ber. Dtsch. ophthal. Ges. **56**, 322 (1955)

Inomata, H., Smelser, G.K., Polack, F.M.: Fine structure of regenerating endothelium and Descemet's membrane in normal and rejecting corneal grafts. Amer. J. Ophthal. **70**, 48–64 (1970a)

Inomata, H., Smelser, G.K., Polack, F.M.: The fine structural changes in the corneal endothelium during graft rejection. Invest. Ophthal. **9**, 263–271 (1970b)

Irvine, A.R., Capella, J.A., Kaufman, H.E.: Corneal thickness, postoperative changes in refrigerated and cryopreserved corneal grafts. Arch. Ophthal. **82**, 232–238 (1969)

Jakus, M.A.: Further observations on the fine structure of the cornea. Invest. Ophthal. **1**, 202–225 (1962)

Jans, R.G., Hassard, D.T.R.: Lissamine green, a supravital stain for determination of corneal endothelial viability. Canad. J. Ophthal. **2**, 297–309 (1967)

Kanai, A., Mustakallio, A.H., Kaufman, H.E.: E.M. Studies of corneal endothelium: the abnormal endothelium associated with retrocorneal membrane. Ann. Ophthal. **4**, 564–567 (1972)

Kanai, A., Polack, F.M.: Ultramicroscopic changes in the corneal graft stroma during early rejection. Invest. Ophthal. **10**, 415–423 (1971a)

Kanai, A., Polack, F.M.: Ultramicroscopic alterations in corneal epithelium in corneal grafts. Amer. J. Ophthal. **72**, 119–126 (1971b)

Katzin, H.E., Kaplan, M.M.: Refractive keratoplasty-cylindrical sectioning. In: Corneo-plastic Surgery. Rycroft (ed.), p. 445–460. London: Pergamon 1969

Kaufman, H.E., Capella, J.A., Robbins, J.E.: A study of enzyme activity in corneal repair. Invest. Ophthal. **3**, 34–46 (1964)

Kaufman, H.E., Capella, J.A., Robbins, J.E.: The human corneal endothelium. Amer. J. Ophthal. **61**, 835–841 (1966a)

Kaufman, H.E., Escapini, H., Capella, J.A., Robbins, J.E., Kaplan, M.: Corneal endothelium and preservation of living corneal tissue. Excerpta Medica Int. Congress Series. **146**, 869–878 (1966b)

Khodadoust, A.A.: Penetrating keratoplasty in the rabbit. Amer. J. Ophthal. **66**, 892–905 (1968a)

Khodadoust, A.A.: Lamellar corneal transplantation in the rabbit. Amer. J. Ophthal. **66**, 1111–1117 (1968b)

Khodadoust, A.A., Silverstein, A.M.: The survival and rejection of epithelium in experimental corneal transplants. Invest. Ophthal. **8**, 169–179 (1969a)

Khodadoust, A.A., Silverstein, A.M.: Transplantation and rejection of the individual cell layers of the cornea. Invest. Ophthal. **8**, 180–195 (1969b)

Khodadoust, A.A., Silverstein, A.M.: Studies on the nature of the privilege enjoyed by corneal allografts. Invest. Ophthal. **11**, 137–148 (1972)

King, J.H., McTigue, J.W., Meryman, H.T.: Preservation of corneas for lamellar keratoplasty. A simple method of chemical glycerine-dehydration. Trans. Amer. ophthal. Soc. **59**, 194–199 (1961)

King, J.H.: Donor eyes and eyebanks. Int. ophthal. Clin. **10**, 313–328 (1970)

Kornblueth, W., Nelken, E.: A study on donor-recipient sensitisation. Amer. J. Ophthal. **45**, 843–847 (1958)

Krogh, E., Weeke, E.: Extracorporeal irradiation of the blood and corneal transplantation. Acta ophthal. **50**, 102–110 (1972)

Kuming, B.S., Rycroft, P.V.: A study of postmortem viability of corneal endothelial cells. In: Corneo-plastic Surgery, p. 507–510. London: Pergamon 1969

Kurz, G.H., D'Amico, R.A.: Histopathology of corneal graft failures. Amer. J. Ophthal. **66**, 184–199 (1968)

Kuwahara, Y. et al., cited by Stocker, F.W.: The endothelium of the cornea, p. 168. Illinois: Charles C. Thomas 1971

Leibowitz, H.M., Luzzio, A.J.: Transplantation antigens in keratoplasty. Arch. Ophthal. **83**, 215–222 (1970)

Leigh, A.G.: Corneal Transplantation, p. 78–79. Oxford: Blackwell 1966

Levenson, J.E., Brightbill, F.S.: Endothelial rejection in human transplants. Arch. Ophthal. **89**, 489–492 (1973)

Mathieu, M.: Results obtained in perforating keratoplasty with preserved corneas using liquid nitrogen. Trans. Amer. Acad. Ophthal. Otolaryng. **73**, 796 (1969)

MAUMENEE, A.E.: The influence of the donor-recipient sensitisation on corneal grafts. Amer. J. Ophthal. **34**, 142–152 (1951)

MAUMENEE, A.E.: Clinical aspects of the corneal homograft reaction. Invest. Ophthal. **1**, 244–252 (1962)

MAUMENEE, A.E.: Discussion in Int. Ophthal. Clinics **10**, 406 (1970)

MAUMENEE, A.E.: Clinical patterns of corneal graft failure. In: Corneal graft failure. Ciba Foundation Symposium No. 15, p. 5–15. North Holland: Elsevier 1973

MAURICE, D.M., GIARDINI, A.A.: A simple optical apparatus for measuring the corneal thickness and the average thickness of the human cornea. Brit. J. Ophthal. **35**, 169–177 (1951)

MAURICE, D.M.: Cellular membrane activity in the corneal endothelium of the intact eye. Experimentia **24**, 1094–1095 (1968)

MAURICE, D.M.: Nutritional aspects of corneal grafts. In: Corneoplastic Surgery. RYCROFT (ed.), p. 197–207. London: Pergamon 1969

McCAREY, B.E., KAUFMAN, H.E.: Improved corneal storage. Invest. Ophthal. **13**, 165–173 (1974)

MEHRI, P., BECKER, B., OGLESBY, R.: Corneal transplants and blood types. Amer. J. Ophthal. **47**, 48–53 (1959)

MEYER, H.J.: Zur Bedeutung von Blutfaktoren bei der Keratoplastik. Klin. Mbl. Augenheilk. **158**, 780–785 (1971)

MEYER, H.J., ARNECKE, H.: Der Einfluß verschiedener Faktoren des Hornhaut-Spendermaterials auf den Erfolg der Keratoplastik. Klin. Mbl. Augenheilk. **160**, 540–550 (1972)

MISHIMA, S., KUDO, T.: In vitro incubation of rabbit cornea. Invest. Ophthal. **6**, 329–339 (1967)

MOORE, T.E., ARONSON, S.B.: The corneal graft. A multiple variable analysis of the penetrating keratoplasty. Amer. J. Ophthal. **72**, 202–296 (1971)

MOORE, T.E., ARONSON, S.B.: Role of surgical factors in corneal graft failure. In: Corneal graft failure. Ciba Foundation Symposium No. 15, p. 209–217. North Holland: Elsevier 1973

MUELLER, F.O.: Techniques for full thickness keratoplasty in rabbits using fresh and frozen tissue. Brit. J. Ophthal. **48**, 377–393 (1964)

MUELLER, F.O., CASEY, T.A., TREVOR-ROPER, P.D.: Use of deep frozen human cornea in full thickness grafts. Brit. med. J. **2**, 473–475 (1964)

MUELLER, F.O., SMITH, A.U.: Some experiments on grafting frozen corneal tissue in rabbits. Exp. Eye Res. **2**, 237–246 (1963)

MÜLLER, H., MAUMENEE, E.A.: Eintrübung klarer Hornhaut-Transplantate durch individualspezifische Sensibilisierung des Empfängers. Graefes Arch. Ophthal. **152**, 1 (1951)

MÜLLER, H.K., SÖLLNER, F., VUCICEVIC, Z.: Spätergebnisse der Keratoplastik. Ber. dtsch. ophthal. Ges. **64**, 142–159 (1961)

NAUMANN, G., GREEN, W.R., ZIMMERMANN, L.E.: Mycotic keratitis: A histopathologic study of 73 cases. Amer. J. Ophthal. **64**, 668–682 (1967)

NAUMANN, G., ROSSMANN, H.: Hornhautschäden bei Hydrochinon. Arb. Ophthalmologica addit. ad **158**, 371–375 (1969)

NELKEN, E., MICHAELSEN, I.C., NELKEN, D., GUREVITCH, J.: Studies on antigens in the human cornea and their relationship to corneal grafting in man. J. Lab. clin. Med. **49**, 745–752 (1957)

PAUFIQUE, L., SOURDILLE, G.P., OFFRET, G.: Les greffes de la cornée, p. 258. Paris: Masson et Cie 1948

PAYRAU, P.: Heterografting of the cornea. In: Cornea World Congress. KING and McTIGUE (eds.), p. 639–653. London: Butterworths 1965

PAYRAU, P., POULIQUEN, Y.: A practical procedure for preserving corneas and sclera. Bull. Soc. Ophthal. France **3**, 209–301 (1959)

PFISTER, R.R., RICHARDS, J.S.F., DOHLMAN, C.H.: Recurrence of herpetic keratitis in corneal grafts. Amer. J. Ophthal. **73**, 192–196 (1972)

POLACK, F.M.: Histopathologic and histochemical alterations in the early stages of corneal graft rejection. J. exp. Med. **116**, 709–718 (1962)

POLACK, F.M.: The effect of ocular inflammation on corneal grafts. Amer. J. Ophthal. **60**, 259–269 (1965)

POLACK, F.M.: The pathologic anatomy of corneal graft rejection. Survey of Ophthal. **11**, 391–404 (1966)

POLACK, F.M.: Cryopreservation of corneas for penetrating keratoplasty. Amer. J. Ophthal. **71**, 505–515 (1971)

POLACK, F.M.: Scanning electron microscopy of corneal graft rejection: epithelial rejection, endothelial rejection and formation of posterior graft membranes. Invest. Ophthal. **11**, 1–14 (1972)

POLACK, F.M.: Scanning electron microscopy of the host-graft endothelial junction in corneal graft reaction. Amer. J. Ophthal. **73**, 704–710 (1972a)

POLACK, F.M.: Lymphocytic destruction during corneal homograft reaction. Arch. Ophthal. **89**, 413–416 (1973)

POLACK, F.M.: Clinical and pathologic aspects of the corneal graft reaction. Trans. Amer. Acad. Ophthal. Otolaryng. **77**, 418–430 (1973a)

POLACK, F.M.: Corneal graft rejection: Clinico-pathological correlation. In: Corneal graft failure. Ciba Foundation Symposium No. 15, p. 127–138. North Holland: Elsevier 1973b

POLACK, F.M.: The endothelium of failed corneal grafts. Amer. J. Ophthal. **79**, 251–261 (1975)

POLACK, F.M., KANAI, A.: Electronmicroscopic studies of graft endothelium in corneal graft rejection. Amer. J. Ophthal. **73**, 711–717 (1972b)

POLACK, F.M., KUDO, T., TAKAHASHI, G.H.: Viability of human eyebank corneas. Arch. Ophthal. **79**, 205–210 (1968)

POLACK, F.M., McENTYRE, J.M.: Incorporation of S^{35} by cryopreserved corneal grafts in vivo. Arch. Ophthal. **81**, 577–582 (1969)

POLACK, F.M., SMELSER, G.K., ROSE, J.: Longterm survival of isotopically labelled stromal and endothelial cells in corneal homografts. Amer. J. Ophthal. **57**, 67–77 (1964)

RICE, N.S.C.: The prognosis for penetrating keratoplasty. Trans. Ophthal. Soc. U.K. **94**, 94–100 (1974)

RICE, N.S.C., JONES, B.R.: Problems of corneal grafting in herpetic keratitis. In: Corneal graft failure. Ciba Foundation Symposium No. 15, p. 221–239. North Holland: Elsevier 1973

RICHTER, S.: Untersuchungen über Isoantikörper bei Keratoplastie. v. Graefes Arch. klin. exp. Ophthal. **168**, 131–135 (1965)

RINTELEN, F.: Zur Geschichte der Keratoplastik. Klin. Mbl. Augenheilk. **165**, 214–222 (1974)

ROBB, R.M., KUWABARA, T.: Corneal wound healing. The movement of poly morphonuclear leucocytes into corneal wounds. Arch. Ophthal. **68**, 636–642 (1962)

ROCHA, H., GALVÃO, P.G.: Immunological aspects of corneal heterografts. Int. ophthal. Clinics **6**, 19–52 (1966)

RYCROFT, B.W.: The scope of corneal grafting. Brit. J. Ophthal. **38**, 1–9 (1954)

SAUTTER, H., HINZPETER, E.N., NAUMANN, G.: Über Indikation, Technik und Ergebnisse bei Fuchs' Hornhaut-Dystrophie. Klin. Mbl. Augenheilk. **160**, 129–141 (1972a)

SAUTTER, H., NAUMANN, G., DEMELER, M.: Tektonische Minikeratoplastik bei persistierendem Hypotonie-Syndrom nach ELLIOT' Trepanation. Klin. Mbl. Augenheilk. **161**, 629–634 (1972b)

SAUTTER, H., NAUMANN, G., DEMELER, B.: Erfahrungen mit gleichzeitiger perforierender Keratoplastik und Katarakt-Extraktion. Klin. Mbl. Augenheilk. **163**, 290–298 (1973)

SCHAEFFER, E.M.: Ultrastructural changes in moist chamber corneas. Invest. Ophthal. **2**, 272–282 (1963)

SCHULTZ, R.O., GALLUN, A.B.: The effects of cryopreservation on the corneal heterograft reaction. In: Corneal preservation. CAPELLA, EDELHAUSER, VAN HORN (eds.), p. 300–307. Illinois: Charles C. Thomas 1973

SHERRARD, E.S.: Further studies on the retrocorneal membrane-endothelium relationship. Brit. J. Ophthal. **53**, 808–818 (1969)

SHERRARD, E.S.: The corneal endothelium in vitro, its survival during banking at 4° C. Trans. Ophthal. Soc. U.K. **94**, 80–93 (1974)

SHERRARD, E.S., RYCROFT, P.V.: Retrocorneal membranes. 1. Their origin and structure. Brit. J. Ophthal. **51**, 379–386 (1967a)

SHERRARD, E.S., RYCROFT, P.V.: 2. Factors influencing their growth. Brit. J. Ophthal. **51**, 387–393 (1967b)

SILVERSTEIN, A.M., KHODADOUST, A.A.: Transplantation immunobiology of the cornea. In: Corneal graft failure. Ciba Foundation Symposium, p. 105–125. North Holland: Elsevier 1973

SMELSER, G.K., OZANICS, V.: Reaction of the cornea to injury and wound healing. In: Symposium on the cornea. Trans. New Orleans Acad. Ophthal., p. 121–131. Saint Louis: C.V. Mosby 1972

SMITH, E.L.: A review of retrograft membranes. Canad. J. Ophthal. **5**, 127–135 (1970)

Smolin, G.: Suppression of corneal graft reaction by antilymphocytic serum. Arch. Ophthal. **79**, 603–610 (1968)

Smolin, G.: Potentiation of the corneal graft reaction. Arch. Ophthal. **87**, 60–66 (1972)

Stansbury, F.C.: Corneal transplantation. Visual and cosmetic results. Arch. Ophthal. **42**, 813–844 (1949)

Stocker, F.W.: Preservation of donor corneas in autologous serum prior to penetrating grafts. Amer. J. Ophthal. **60**, 21–24 (1965)

Stocker, F.W.: Storage of donor corneas in recipients serum prior to grafting. Pac. Med. Surg. **76**, 31–34 (1968)

Stocker, F.W.: The endothelium of the cornea and its clinical implication, p. 141–193. Illinois: Charles C. Thomas 1971

Stocker, F.W., Eiring, A., Georgiade, R., Georgiade, N.: Evaluation of viability of preserved rabbit corneas by tissue culture procedures. Amer. J. Ophthal. **47**, 772–782 (1959)

Stocker, F.W., Irish, A.: Ultimate fate of successful corneal grafts done for endothelial dystrophy. Trans. Amer. Ophthal. Soc. **67**, 196–206 (1969)

Stocker, F.W., King, E.H., Lucas, D.O., Georgiade, N.: Clinical test for evaluating donor corneas. Arch. Ophthal. **84**, 2–7 (1970)

Strampelli, B.: Ring autokeratoplasty. In: Corneo-plastic Surgery. Rycroft (ed.), p. 253–275. London: Pergamon 1969

Strampelli, B., Marchi, V.: Osteo-odonto-keratoprosthesis. In: Corneal grafting. Casey (ed.), p. 291–312. London: Butterworths 1972

Ticho, U., Ben-Sira, I.: Total keratoplasty. Arch. Ophthal. **90**, 104–106 (1973)

Townley Paton, R.: History of corneal transplantation. Int. Ophthal. Clinics **10**, 181–186 (1970)

Tragakis, M.P., Rosen, J., Brown, S.I.: Transplantation of the perforated cornea. Amer. J. Ophthal. **78**, 518–522 (1974)

Trevor-Roper, P.D.: The history of corneal grafting. In: Corneal grafting. Casey (ed.), p. 1–10. London: Butterworths 1972

Troutman, R.C.: Microsurgery for keratoplasty. Int. Ophthal. Clinics **10**, 297–311 (1970)

Tsutsui, J.: Clinicohistopathological classification of the graft illness in keratoplasty. Jap. J. Ophthal. **10**, 1–9 (1966)

Urrets-Zavalia, A., Jr.: Spontaneous dessication of corneal donor material. Amer. J. Ophthal. **57**, 247–255 (1964)

Voe, de A.G.: Complication of keratoplasty. Amer. J. Ophthal. **79**, 907–912 (1975)

Vogel, M., Naumann, G.: Die granulomatöse Reaktion gegen die Descemet'sche Membran. Ber. dtsch. ophthal. Ges. **71**, 35–42 (1972)

Votockova, J., Karel, I.: Cited by Allansmith et al., Amer. J. Ophthal. **79**, 493–501 (1975)

Wagenmann, A.: Experimentelle Untersuchungen zur Frage der Keratoplastik. Graefes Arch. klin. exp. Ophthal. **1**, 211–269 (1888)

Waltman, S.R., Faulkner, H.W., Burde, R.M.: Modification of the ocular immune response. Use of antilymphocytic serum to prevent rejection of penetrating corneal homografts. Invest. Ophthal. **8**, 196–200 (1969)

Watson, P.G., Joysey, V.C.: Difficulties in the use of tissue-typing for corneal grafting. In: Corneal graft failure. Ciba Foundation Symposium, No. 15, p. 323–335. North Holland: Elsevier 1973

Weimar, V.: The sources of fibroslasts in corneal wound repair. Arch. Ophthal. **60**, 93–109 (1958)

Werb, A.: Complications of full thickness keratoplasty. In: Corneal grafting. Casey (ed.), p. 110–120. London: Butterworths 1972

Wiener, J., Spiro, D., Russell, P.S.: An electron microscopic study of the homograft reaction. Amer. J. Path. **44**, 319–347 (1964)

Winter, F.C.: The histopathology of unsuccessful penetrating keratoplasty in man. In: Corneo-plastic Surgery. Rycroft (ed.), p. 557–569. London: Pergamon 1969

Zauberman, H., Sachs, U.: The endothelium in clear and progressively oedematous transplants. Amer. J. Ophthal. **71**, 495–499 (1971)

General Pathology
of the Transplantation Reaction
in Experimental and Clinical Organ Grafts

CHRISTOPH R. JERUSALEM and PAUL H.K. JAP

With 61 Figures

A. The Many Facets
of the Transplantation Reaction

I. Introduction

From the clinician's point of view, the wider use of transplantation as a remedy for disease is being restrained by a number of factors. Despite the considerable degree of success achieved in its most extensive clinical application – kidney transplantation – transplantation of organs must still be regarded as an experimental procedure (HUME, 1971). The central stumbling block is the rejection, since due to an apparently immutable law of immunity the transplantation of tissues to a genetically, i.e. antigenically dissimilar host inevitably mobilizes defense mechanisms against the foreign antigens. It has been suggested that this law may have a crucial loophole. The canine and, particularly, the porcine liver appear to be immunologically favored, since in unmodified hosts identifiable allograft rejection did not occur or reversed spontaneously, whereas in the same animals skin and kidney were regularly rejected (CALNE et al., 1969; GARNIER et al., 1970). In human liver transplantation it has become the usual practice to ignore the result of HL-A typing (STARZL, 1971; CALNE, 1974). Since other experimenters found that canine, porcine, and rat liver allografts were rejected in the usual way (PORTER, 1969; JERUSALEM et al., 1971b; JAP, 1971), the above findings may represent a particular modification of the immunologic network of responses, rather than an exception to the principle of the transplantation reaction.

There is clear evidence that in all organs so far studied, both the induction and the intensity of the transplantation reaction depend upon the extent of antigenic divergence between donor and recipient (VRIESENDORP, 1973; WEIL and REEMTSMA, 1974; DE LANGEN et al., 1975). The so-called autograft is obviously the most likely to be successful. This also applies to transplants between monozygotic twins, since their genetic make-up is in fact identical. A good match between siblings and littermates provides a favorable prognosis for both graft acceptance and efficacy of immunosuppression (TERASAKI et al., 1968;

STARZL, 1971). At the other extreme, i.e. transplantation between species of phylogenetic disparity, either the graft is rejected despite massive immunosuppression, or the recipient dies of complications resulting from the immunosuppressive therapy. For these reasons, clinical application of heterotransplantation has recently been abandoned (STARZL, 1974a), although kidneys of chimpanzees were found to function for several months in human recipients (REEMTSMA et al., 1964). The area between the two extremes is the domain of experimental and clinical allotransplantation. Unfortunately, the typing of nonrelated individuals seems to be incapable of providing consistently accurate predictions of the extent of the possible antigenic confrontation in individual instances (STARZL, 1971). It is beyond the scope of this review to discuss whether an occasional poor correlation between the results of histocompatibility determination and the final outcome of kidney, liver, or lung transplantation (VEITH and BLUMENSTOCK, 1971; HALGRIMSON et al., 1971; TERASAKI, 1974) might be due to the absence of organ-specific antigens on lymphocytes (MARTIN and LUNDAK, 1971), serologically silent genes linked to the H-2, HL-A, and probably DL-A antigens, which appear to specify the antigens that stimulate the transplantation reaction (EDIDIN and HENNEY, 1973), or to the problem of anomalous antigens (JONES and MOORE, 1970). However, hitherto unexplored mechanisms related to the recognition of foreign antigenic determinants by recipient cells, the transport of information to the lymphoid centers, the central lymphoid tissue response, and the efferent branch of this reaction may be responsible for the kaleidoscopic picture of the transplantation reaction. Although numerous workers have accumulated an impressive amount of basic data on the manifestations and temporal sequences of host reactions against transplanted organs, not only are the exact mechanisms by which they operate poorly understood, but opinions about this are even controversial in several features. Probably conventional descriptive methods are unsuited to appreciation of the mechanisms involved in graft rejection as modulations of the functional network of the immune system. This review attempts to interpret the transplantation reaction as the final common result of the activity of the highly diversified cellular system that is entrusted with self and nonself control. These considerations may hint at potentially valuable concepts to be refined by further studies of lymphoid cell kinetics, dynamics, and cellular co-operation.

II. Terminology

1. Donor-Recipient Relationship

Since there is no doubt that the outcome of each kind of transplantation depends ultimately on the extent of divergence of the genetically determined histocompatibility and differentiation antigens that may exist between the donor and the recipient, it is usual to indicate the degree of donor-recipient disparity by special terms. Several years ago it was proposed that the original terms, i.e. *autologous, isologous, homologous* and *heterologous* be replaced by the terms *autoplastic, syngenic* (or *isogenic*), *allogenic* and *xenogenic*, for linguistic reasons[1]. Many studies using donors and recipients of wide genetic disparity made the need for further division on the basis of genetic diversity apparent. PERPER and NAJARIAN (1966a) demonstrated that the rejection pattern in experimental hetero-(xeno-)transplantation was different according to whether widely divergent species, species of intermediate phylogenetic disparity (PERPER, 1971), or closely related species were involved (PERPER and NAJARIAN, 1966b). REEMTSMA (1969) suggested retention of the term *"heterologous"*, for use only if donors and recipients were relatively closely placed on the phylogeneic scale (e.g. baboon to man), and the word *"xenogenic"*, for use in the case of very distant relationships (e.g. pig to man, pig to dog). From other studies it also appeared advisable to distinguish between the terms *"homologous"* and *"allogenic"* (JAP, 1971; v.D. WERF, 1972), since reactions of an unmodified host to liver and kidney grafts from donors which should be designated *"homologous"* (or *"allogenic"*) can vary widely, and range between reactions typical of isografts and those seen with heterografts.

In summary, the following indicative terms have been used by various authors: *Autograft* (from the same individual), *isograft, syngenic graft* (from the same inbred, genetically homogeneous strain, or from an identical twin), *homograft* (from an individual of the same, but noninbred, genetically inhomogeneous strain, or from a "closed breeding colony"), *allograft* (from an individual of another, inbred or noninbred, strain of the same species), *heterograft* (from another species relatively closely placed on the phylogenetic scale, e.g. sheep and goat, chimpanzee and man), *xenograft (heterograft)* either between species of intermediate phylogenetic disparity (e.g. pig and goat, or baboon and man) or between widely divergent species (e.g. pig and dog, pig and man). However, all attempts to classify genetic disparities by simple terms appear unsatisfactory; it has been demonstrated that the relative speed of rejection can vary significantly when donor and recipient are interchanged: pig-to-dog kidney xenografts were rejected about ten times more rapidly than dog-to-pig xenografts; and whereas the unmodified Wistar rat rejects a PVG/C liver allograft constantly after 14 to 21 days (JAP, 1971) the untreated PVG/C rat survives a Wistar liver and/or kidney allotransplantation for more than 6 months (HESS and JERUSALEM, 1975). Therefore, in this review the donor-recipient disparity will be indicated in more detail, e.g. "baboon-to-man xenotransplantation", if this appears necessary to the interpretation of the course of events.

2. Chronologies of Rejection

Immune reactions to transplanted organs are generally categorized under four headings. These courses of events differ not only in the time of occurrence,

---

[1] The prefix "allo-" (Greek: allos—ἄλλος) meaning "other" or "differing", appears to be more appropriate for indicating the genetic disparity in largely mongrelized species like man and dog than the combining form "homo-" (Greek: homos—ὅμοιος) meaning the "same" or "alike". For the same reason the prefix "xeno-" (Greek: xenos—ξένος) meaning "strange" or denoting relation to "foreign" is preferred to the term "hetero" (Greek: heteros—ἕτερος) meaning "other" or "different" for indicating transplantation between species of wide genetic disparity (e.g., pig to dog).

but also in the mechanisms that appear to be preferentially involved (HUME, 1971). This classification is based mainly on changes occurring in kidneys transplanted into both modified and unmodified host. Identical patterns have been observed in the transplanted heart, liver, lung, and pancreas, although several organ-specific reactions have also been observed. There are, however, no fundamental differences between different species. Structural changes encountered in the pig-to-man liver xenograft were indistinguishable from those observed in pig livers transplanted to dogs (JERUSALEM et al., 1974). In baboon-to-man renal xenotransplants the cellular infiltrates were more marked than in human allografts, but not dissimilar to those in rejecting canine allografts. Usually, immunosuppressive therapy inhibits or delays the incidence of the transplantation reaction, but the rejection process can occasionally proceed regardless of the method of immunosuppression (Fig. 26, 28, 32). A chimpanzee-to-man liver xenograft (treated with azathioprine and prednisone) exhibited histologic changes (PORTER, 1969) closely resembling those commonly seen in light microscope preparations of PVG/C rat liver allografts in Wistar rat recipients.

The four commonly observed patterns can be summarized as follows:

a) *Hyperacute rejection* occurs within minutes or a few hours after the organ has been revascularized. It is triggered by naturally occurring and/or allo- or heterospecific antibodies (NOHA) present in the recipient prior to transplantation surgery.

b) *Delayed hyperacute or accelerated rejection* can be of the "hyperacute" type, developing slowly during the first 3 days after transplantation, or an acute rejection pattern mediated exclusively by antibody sensitized *de novo*.

c) *Acute or intermediate rejection* is regarded as the classic primary response of cellular immunity, mediated predominantly by the T-lymphocyte population. The roles both of cellular mechanisms that are independent of the thymus, including various types of macrophages, and of the primary humoral response are usually underestimated. The great majority of rejection episodes of this type occur after about 3 to 5 days and within 2 to 4 months. With cadaveric transplants the danger period may extend up to 2 years (HUME, 1971).

d) Changes characteristic of *chronic or late rejection* may be present after 2 months, but the rejection process can progress very slowly and insidiously over a period of years. This type is usually seen in recipients submitted to immunosuppressive therapy for prolonged periods. Circulating antibody appears to be involved in triggering vascular lesions in which proliferative changes predominate over destructive ones. However, the immunologic nature of this type of injury is not consistently demonstrable.

III. Elements of the Transplantation Reaction

1. Dichotomy of the Immune Response (see Figs. 1 and 2)

The transplantation reaction, particularly the acute reaction to solid organ grafts, is regarded as one of the classic, primary responses of cellular immunity, classified as cell-mediated or cellular immunity, immune lymphoid cell cytotoxicity, cell-mediated reaction, and cell-mediated cytotoxicity, including delayed hypersensitivity (Fig. 1).

Before entering on an analysis of details of this type of immune response it appears appropriate to describe some features of the total immune response in more general terms to provide a frame of reference for this discussion, which is necessary for the interpretation of the various and seemingly contradictory morphologic features of the transplantation reaction.

In recent years, we have become increasingly familiar with the two major lymphocyte classes and the divergent mechanisms of lymphocyte stimulation responsible for the dichotomy of the immune response: the *humoral reaction* and the *cell-mediated reaction* (Fig. 2). To some extent these definitions are inadequate, since even humoral immunity depends ultimately on cells (OWEN, 1974), and at least in certain instances, the true cell-mediated reaction is initiated by, or dependent on, humoral antibodies (HASEK *et al.*, 1969; MÖLLER, 1971).

Nevertheless, the concept of two types of immune response has proved useful, and indicates whether circulating antibody or direct participation of mononuclear effector cells is the predominant element in a given immune response. Whereas humoral immunity is usually defined as a response transferable by serum antibody alone, a cell-mediated reaction is implied when the typical response can be transferred by cells (CHASE, 1945; WESSLEN, 1952; JAFFER *et al.*, 1973), even to a tolerant host (BILLINGHAM *et al.*, 1962), and not by serum. It has been widely accepted that only cells from sensitized donors can transfer passively delayed hypersensitivity, including transplant immunity, from one individual to another (BLOOM *et al.*, 1964).

At the same time, two groups obtained and presented clear evidence that the thymus is essential for the development of certain immune reactions in mice (ARCHER and PIERCE, 1961; MILLER, 1961), and that deficiency of both cellular and humoral immunity is produced in rats, mice, rabbits, and chickens when the thymus is extirpated very early in life (JANKOVIC *et al.*, 1962; MILLER, 1964). Around the same time it was shown that the bursa of Fabricius was essential for full immunologic competence in chickens (GLICK *et al.*, 1956; GLICK, 1964), and that these two central lymphoepithelial organs exercise entirely different functions (COOPER *et al.*, 1965, 1966). Much controversy surrounds the question of the existence of an anatomic bursal equivalent in mammals, where B-lymphocytes in the peripheral lymphoid tissue have a remote origin in the bone marrow (MITCHEL and MILLER, 1968), an analogous situation to that in birds (OWEN, 1972). Whether B-cells only colonize the lymph nodes and spleen after they have undergone an intermediate stage of development in the gut-associated lymphoid tissue (GOWANS and KNIGHT, 1964; PEREY *et al.*, 1970; HENRY *et al.*, 1970; HOWARD *et al.*, 1972) cannot be decided without further experiments (GOWANS, 1974).

This problem is of particular interest with respect to the frequent occurrence of graft-*vs*-host reactions in recipients of extensive allografts of intestine (LILLEHEI *et al.*, 1959b; RUIZ *et al.*, 1972). However, it has become clear that the marrow-derived precursor of the B-lymphocyte acquires immunologic competence only after a period of residence in the lymph node or spleen (BASTEN *et al.*, 1971; ITO *et al.*, 1973; MOND and THORBECKE, 1973). The realization

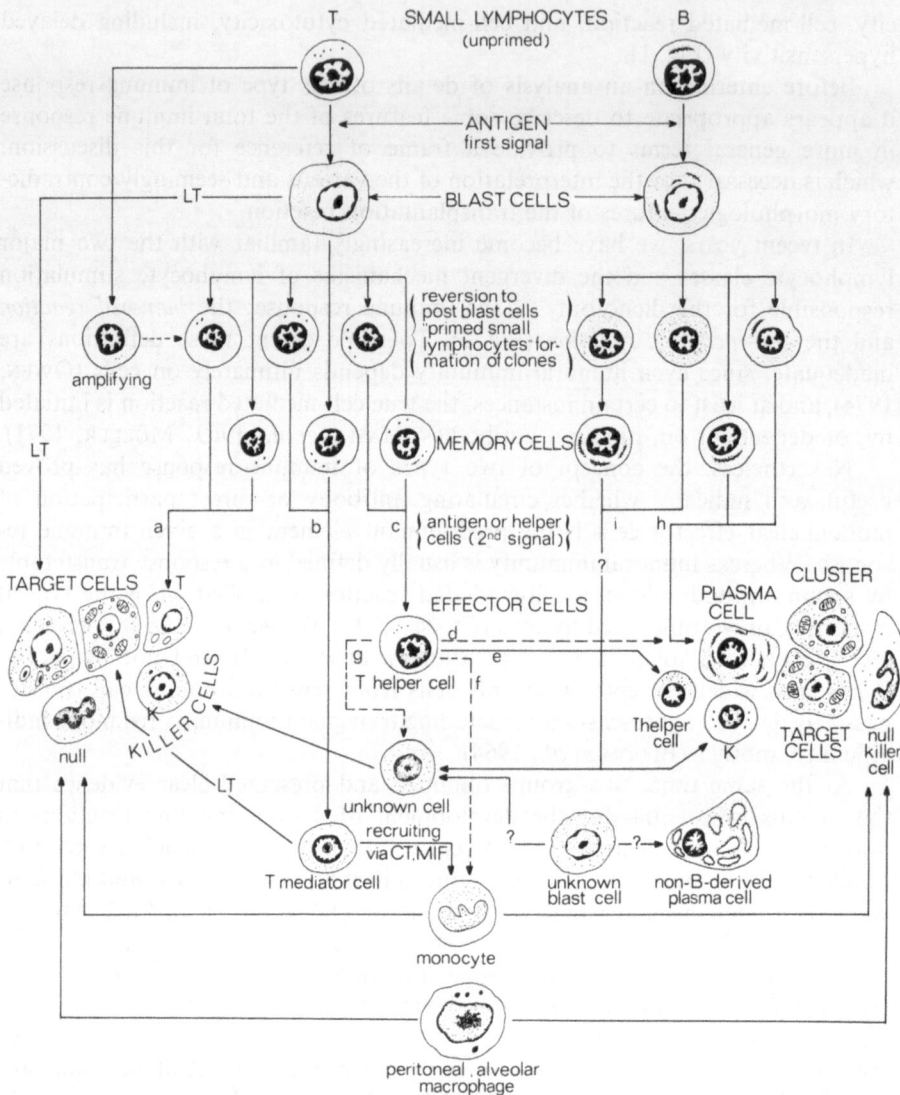

Fig. 1a–i. Elements of the transplantation reaction. T-cell response: Unprimed small T-lymphocytes transform into blast cells upon antigenic stimulation (first signal). After vigorous stimulation (by PHA, and possibly by immune complexes) transforming T-cells appear to secrete lymphotoxin (*LT*). Blast cell-derived lymphocytes are small, do not react with PHA, and form selected clones. It is uncertain whether potential effector cells and memory cells belong to different populations. Upon a second signal (by antigen or macrophages as possible "helper cells"), primed cells differentiate into cells capable of (a) autonomous T-cell cytotoxicity (T-killer cell, probably amplified by unprimed T-cells); (b) recruitment of monocytes and macrophages through secretion of CT and MIF, and killing through production of lymphotoxin; (c) exertion of helper cell functions; (d) stimulation of plasma cell activity (IgG); (e) participation in formation of peripheral "clusters" for antibody-dependent cytotoxicity; (f) sensitization of various macrophages for antibody-independent cytotoxicity; (g) a helper cell function in recruitment and sensitization of "unknown" cells for differentiation into K (killer) cells is uncertain.

(Fig. 1 continued see opposite page)

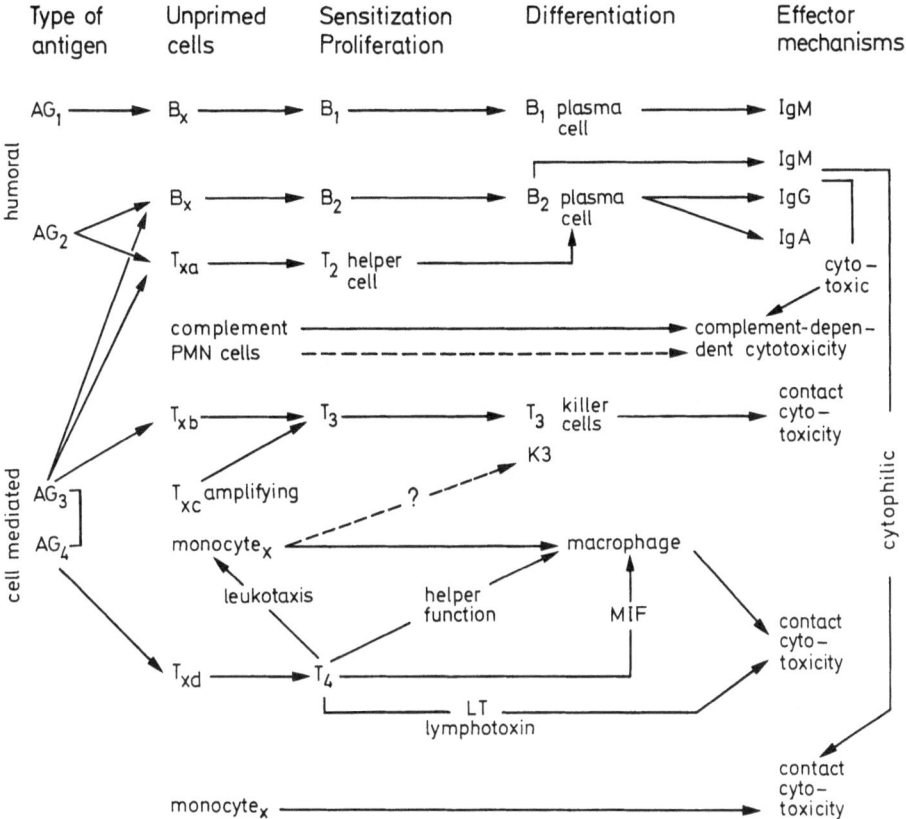

Fig. 2. Immunologic reaction patterns. AG_1: Antigens independent of thymus (e.g. lipopolysaccharides from *E. coli*, pneumococcal polysaccharide, flagellin, levan from *Corynebacterium levaniformis*, polyvinyl pyrrolidone, dextran) stimulate unprimed B-cells to proliferate (selected clones) and to produce IgM antibodies in absence of T-cells.

AG_2: Most other antigens (except for AG_3, AG_4) predominantly stimulate both unprimed B- and T-helper cells. Production of IgG, and particularly of IgA, is result of B-T-cell co-operation. In absence of T-helper cells the immunoglobulin released by B_2-cell-derived antibody-producing cells is almost exclusively of macromolecular class.

$AG_{3,4}$: Histocompatibility, differentiation, and/or tissue-specific antigens predominantly trigger either autonomous T-cell cytotoxicity (AG_3) or cell-mediated effector mechanisms independent of thyms (AG_4). In these reactions, T-T-cell ("amplifying") and T-cell-macrophage collaboration (mediator and "helper" function) appear to be important. In addition, most antigens of this group are able to evoke humoral responses, as do antigens of AG_2 group (e.g. xeno- and alloantibodies to H-2 and HL-A antigens). Thus, cytotoxic mechanisms or those independent of thymus initiate immunologic injury. T-cells involved in the various mechanisms may belong to different subpopulations (T_{xa-d}), and killer cells (K_3) may exhibit different characteristics than differentiated T-lymphocytes (T_3)

◁ B-cell response: The blast cell response and formation of selected clones is comparable to early T-cell response upon a first signal. (h) Primed B-cells usually differentiate into IgG secreting plasma cells through helper cell activity. Without second signal B-cell-derived plasma cells appear to produce predominantly IgM; (i) transformation of B-cells into killer cells has been suggested, but not confirmed. Occurrence of clusters consisting of plasma cells, small lymphocytes, and either macrophages or nonadherent monocytes is suggestive of antibody-dependent cytotoxicity independent of thymus. Proliferation of plasma cells from non-B-cells should be taken into consideration that the bursa functions in the development of antibody production, while the thymus controls development of allograft immunity (WARNER and SZENBERG, 1964) led to formulation of the two-component scheme of immunologic development (COOPER et al., 1968a, b). It was also concluded that the immune reaction is not an "either–or" situation of T-cells as against B-cells, since antibody responses to a variety of antigens, e.g. sheep red blood cells, simple soluble protein antigens, certain bacteriophage antigens, and *Salmonella* H antigens, were defective in neonatally thymectomized mice, whereas the antibody response to antigens of *Brucella* organisms, *Salmonella* organisms, and to pneumococcal polysaccharide seemed to develop normally (JANKOVIC et al., 1962; FAHEY et al., 1965; MOSSER et al., 1970). This paradox was first clarified by CLAMAN et al. (1966, 1969) and by MITCHEL and MILLER (1968) MILLER and MITCHEL (1969), DAVIES (1969), MOSIER (1969) and TAYLOR (1969), who showed that at least in mice the T-cell immune system often acts in co-operation with cells now referred to as bone marrow-derived, or B-lymphocytes (Fig. 2). Carrier-specific T-helper cells were more important for the induction of the synthesis of IgG than of IgM antibody (CHEERS and MILLER, 1972; GRUMET, 1972; KISHIMOTO and ISHIZAKA, 1973a, 1973b). It is largely unknown whether tissue and/or organ-specific antigens can trigger an immune reaction to solid organ grafts with no dependence on thymus. Cyclophosphamide, a compound known to deplete a host preferentially of B-lymphocytes (TURK and POULTER, 1972), has been shown to suppress kidney allograft rejection as competently as azathioprine (STARZL et al., 1972; LEVIN and MERRILL, 1972; KAWABE et al., 1972), although under cyclophosphamide treatment a proportional increase in theta-carrying lymphocytes was observed (POULTER and TURK, 1972), from which both helper cells and/or effector (killer) cells might be recruited.

2. T-Helper Cell Mechanisms

Although there is clear evidence that the T-helper cell is not identical with the T-lymphocytes involved in the cell-mediated immune reaction as killer cells (K-cell, cytotoxic effector cells) (DENNERT and LENNOX, 1972; GOLSTEIN et al., 1973; NOSSAL, 1974), T-helper cell activity may also be essential in the transplant reaction. Since the killer cell itself is frequently a cytotoxic cell independent of the thymus, the central role of T-cells in the cell-mediated immune response may be essentially the same as their role in humoral immunity, i.e. co-operation with the B-cell or with macrophages (SIEGEL, 1970; FELDMAN et al., 1972). It is possible that several quite different mechanisms of helper cell activity are involved in the immune response (DUTTON and HUNTER, 1974).

a) T-cells *specific for carrier determinants* might collect antigen and present the haptenic determinations to the B-cell surface in a concentrated form (FELD-MANN and BASTEN, 1971; TAYLOR et al., 1971; MITCHISON, 1971). In other systems, the T-cell dependence of stimulation of *haptenspecific* B-cells independently of carriers has been demonstrated (DOUGHTY and KLINMAN, 1973), and the macrophage implicated as a mediator (FELDMANN and NOSSAL, 1972).

b) A two-signal concept has been proposed for self-nonself discrimination (BRETSCHER and COHN, 1970) and for helper cell activity (DUTTON et al., 1971).

A soluble T-cell product (GORCZYNSKI *et al.*, 1972; WATSON, 1973), can replace intact T-cells as a source of helper activity and provide a secondary signal for B-cell responsiveness. The first signal is provided by the antigen (Fig. 1 pathway d).

c) *A third model* proposes restrictive requirements for effective T- and B-cell or macrophage interaction. In this concept the helper effect can only take place between partners sharing a common histocompatibility haplotype (KATZ *et al.*, 1973a, b); this also applies to effective macrophage T-cell co-operation (ROSENTHAL and SHEVACH, 1973; SHEVACH and ROSENTHAL, 1973) (Fig. 1 pathway f).

d) Studies on the allogenic effect strongly support the concept that T-cells have an important function in B-cell activation, quite apart from any antigen-focusing role (ELFENBEIN *et al.*, 1973). The infusion of allogenic lymphocytes, particularly T-cells from *nonimmune* donors, to *antigen-primed* guinea pigs and mice leads to the spontaneous production of *specific* antibodies directed at the antigens to which the recipient has been primed (HIRST and DUTTON, 1970; KATZ *et al.*, 1971; EKPAHA-MENSAH and KENNEDY, 1971; OSBORNE and KATZ, 1972). The allogenic effect may play a role in instances of delayed hyperacute rejection (Chapter E), in which neither naturally occurring nor heterospecific antibodies are detectable before transplantation.

e) When peripheral T-cells that were too few to yield good cytotoxicity responses were mixed with thymocytes, and the cell mixture was immunized *in vitro* against cell-bound antigens, cytotoxicity exceeding about 10–20 times that attributable to a purely additive effect was generated. The synoptic interpretation of these findings suggested strongly that peripheral T-cells provide the major source for precursor cells of cytotoxic lymphocytes, thymocytes acting mainly as helper (amplifier) cells (WAGNER, 1973a, b).

f) A T-cell-macrophage helper cell mechanism has been proposed (ZEMBALA *et al.*, 1973). Mouse lymphocyte cultures became specifically immunized in the presence of allogenic fibroblasts or syngenic polyoma virus-induced tumor cells, but were noncytotoxic by themselves. Target cell killing was only observed when normal macrophages were added to this system (Fig. 1, "null" killer cells).

3. Effector Mechanisms of Cell-Mediated Cytotoxicity

Since its classic description by KOCH (1890) the tuberculin reaction has become the prototype of delayed hypersensitivity and has long served as a model for investigations on the mechanism of cell-mediated immunity. As a consequence of the increased interest in this type of response, a broad spectrum of *in vitro* and *in vivo* methods using various natural, synthetic and frequently chemically standardized antigens has been developed in recent years (PERLMANN and HOLM, 1969; GREAVES *et al.*, 1973; REVILLARD, 1971). Because it is widely accepted that immune reactions directly mediated by cells (thus including the response against transplanted cells, tissues, and solid organs) are manifestations of delayed hypersensitivity, we feel justified in discussing whether the mechanisms found to cause the various types of delayed hypersensitivity might also be involved in the transplant reaction. One problem is encountered in consideration of this possibility. Most *in vitro* studies deal with well-characterized single cell lines and with defined antigens. In contrast, in the reaction to transplanted tissue and solid organs, one is generally unaware of the amount of transplantation and differentiation antigens, their antigenic properties, and the antigenic strength recognized by the host's immunocompetent system, although nowadays the donor-recipient relationship is determined by means of histocompatibility typing in clinical and frequently in experimental transplantation.

a) Autonomy of T-Lymphocyte Cytotoxicity
(Fig. 1 pathway a)

Evidence for T-cell implication particularly in the cell-mediated reaction has been obtained in experiments with neonatally thymectomized animals (Miller and Osoba, 1967; for review see Good, 1973) and, recently, with athymic nude (nu/nu) mice (Stutman, 1974; for review see Rygaard and Povlsen, 1974). Although the biological phenomenon of delayed type hypersensitivity consists of a variety of divergent events (Dumonde *et al.*, 1969), it has generally been agreed that the central reaction, i.e. the cytopathic or cytotoxic effect on target cell populations whose surfaces bear the specific antigen (Perlmann and Holm, 1968), is also mediated by sensitized T-lymphocytes (Cerottini *et al.*, 1970a, b; Halpern *et al.*, 1973). Generally, autonomous T-cell cytotoxicity is assumed, in particular when added antitheta serum inhibits the cytotoxic effect and the cytotoxic activity of supernatants from effector cell-target cell incubates is less than 1 percent above background (Canty and Wunderlich, 1970). The inhibition of the cytotoxic effect by incubation with isoantibody against target cell antigens may be a further indication, since sensitized lymphocytes appear to act directly and specifically on target cells bearing the specific antigen (Golstein *et al.*, 1972; Freedman *et al.*, 1972). However, the specificity of this reaction is disputable, since Feldman *et al.* (1972) suggested that the effector phase is composed of at least two stages, immunospecific activation by the sensitizing antigen and the mediation of the injury to target cells, which is not immunospecific but which appears to depend on close contact between activated lymphocytes and target cells. According to the above criteria, the autonomous killing potency of T-lymphocytes has been demonstrated with lymphoid tumor cells (Canty and Wunderlich, 1970), mastocytoma P 815 (Golstein *et al.*, 1972, 1973), and xenogenic fibroblasts (Feldman *et al.*, 1972) as target cells.

The proliferative response of allogenic lymphocytes cultured together has been widely used as an *in vitro* correlate of the antigenic recognition phase of the allograft response (Bach and Amos, 1967). Mixed lymphocyte culture responses can be initiated neither with cell populations depleted of T-cells by means of antitheta serum (Mosier and Cantor, 1971; Tyan and Ness, 1972), nor with B-cells alone (Andersson *et al.*, 1973). Since blast cells from one-way mixed lymphocyte cultures revert to lymphocytes *in vivo* and *in vitro*, and these in turn promptly react to the original H-2 stimulator cells and convert to strongly cytotoxic effector cells, it has been suggested that this phenomenon represents a T-cell response (Andersson and Häyry, 1973). Harrison (1973) proposed restrictive requirements for the mixed-lymphocyte reaction. In this model, T-cells were not the mandatory stimulators, although the ability to respond appeared to require the presence of T-lymphocytes. This mechanism resembles the two-signal concept of B-cell triggering mentioned above (BRETSCHER and COHN, 1970), and requires the presence of monocytes (GORDON, 1968). Rapid target cell lysis resulting from incubation with PHA-stimulated lymphocytes in the absence of other cell types (BIBERFELD et al., 1968) may also be an instance of autonomous T-cell killer function, since only T-lymphocytes respond to this mitogen (GREAVES et al., 1973). However, so-called killer lymphocytes appear to be remarkably inefficient in the destruction of target cells in vitro, since ratios of several hundred lymphocytes per target cell were often necessary (KELLER, 1973). In contrast, in most instances of cell-mediated organ-graft rejection, typical lymphocytes and lymphocyte-derived blast cells appear to be in the minority, compared with the number of target cells. An alternative hypothesis was offered by WAGNER (1973a, b). In this study T-T-cell co-operation was demonstrated, increasing the cytotoxicity of sensitized peripheral T-cells by 10 to 20 times (see Chapter A III 2). In vivo, the amplifying T-T-cell co-operation appears to be restricted to the autochthonous lymphatic organs (see Chapter C II). Other mechanisms proved to be effective in cell-mediated cytotoxicity are discussed in later chapters.

b) Mediators of the Cellular Immune Reaction

In studies on passive transfer of the delayed hypersensitivity reaction it was demonstrated that leukocyte extracts were as effective as viable cells (LAWRENCE, 1955), even in skin-graft rejection (LAWRENCE et al., 1960). Subsequently, a group of soluble and biologically active factors generated by antigen-activated lymphocytes was detected (for review see BLOOM and CHASE, 1967; DUMONDE et al., 1969; LAWRENCE and VALENTINE, 1970). The active mediators are quite different from classic antibodies; they are non-antigen-specific (GREAVES et al., 1973) and independent of complement, and cannot therefore be neutralized with antibodies to any immunoglobulin class or subclass. Since they are soluble, they sometimes deploy their activity at some distance from the locality where they are released (KELLEY et al., 1972; HAY et al., 1973).

α) *Transfer factor.* Among other properties, this substance produces intradermal inflammation when injected into normal skin (LAWRENCE and VALENTINE, 1970). The reaction is revealed as increased vascular permeability to protein, with subsequent cellular infiltration with mononuclear and polymorphonuclear cells at skin test sites. In contrast to the late onset of other phenomena of the delayed reaction, much of the protein was shown to accumulate even during the first hour after administration (MORLEY and DUMONDE, 1969). Thus, this factor appears to act as do certain mediators of the anaphylactic reaction.

β) *Lymphotoxin* (LT in Figs. 1 and 2). Upon specific membrane interaction between effector cell and target cell (GRANGER and KOLB, 1968), a toxic, cell-free factor termed lymphotoxin (LT) or lymphocyte cytotoxin factor (LCF) is released (RUDDLE and WAKSMAN, 1968; KOLB and GRANGER, 1968). Once it has been released, further cellular contact is not required (WALKER and LUCAS,

1972). This factor is nonspecifically toxic to cells and causes target cell damage that is morphologically similar to lymphocyte-directed cytolysis (Kolb and Granger, 1968). From the rapidity with which lymphotoxin associates with target cells it was concluded that lymphotoxin binds at the external surface of target cells, probably to a cell membrane glycoprotein (Hessinger et al., 1973). Since human lymphotoxin is soluble and nondialyzable, when released in grafts it can cause cellular damage that is histotopographically distant from sites of mononuclear infiltrations (Hay et al., 1973).

γ) *Inhibition of macrophage migration* (MIF in Figs. 1 and 2). The capillary migration technique (David et al., 1964) has been used not only for the study of mediators of cellular immunity in general (Amos et al., 1967), but also for detailed investigations such as the diagnosis of cell-mediated kidney graft rejection (Melnick and Friedman, 1971). It was discovered that (macrophage) migration inhibition is mediated by a factor (Bloom and Bennet, 1966; David, 1966) identified as a protein with a molecular weight of 30,000–80,000 (Dumonde et al., 1969). Only a few sensitive lymphocytes (about 2,5%) are able to produce enough active substance to inhibit migration of the whole population (David et al., 1964). The reaction is independent of any circulating antibody directed against the triggering antigen that may have been produced, and the specificity of the *in vitro* reaction is identical to the specificity of the dermal reaction (David, 1968).

δ) *Leukotactic factor* (leukotaxis in Fig. 2). The majority of cells present in the passively induced skin lesion are nonsensitized cells of host origin (Najarian and Feldman, 1961; McCluskey et al., 1963) and are attracted by a soluble factor chemotactic *in vitro* (Ward et al., 1969) for mononuclear macrophages and lymphocytes, but not for neutrophils (Cohen et al., 1973).

ε) *Mitogenic and potentiating factors* (amplifying in Fig. 1). The occurrence of large pyroninophilic cells of the blast cell type (immunoblasts) in numerous acutely rejected grafts suggests a peripheral proliferation of effector cells. Small numbers of sensitized leukocytes can recruit nonsensitive cells for clonal proliferation (Valentine and Lawrence, 1969) through secretion of the mitogenic factor (Dumonde et al., 1969). This factor is not identical with transplantation antigens (Spitler and Fudenberg, 1970); it appears to be released by stimulated T-lymphocytes (Greaves et al., 1973) and by macrophages (Gery and Waksman, 1972). It has potentiating effects and acts synergistically with PHA, exlusively on T-cells (Gery et al., 1972).

ζ) *Proliferation-inhibiting factor(s)*. According to Jerne's (1974) network theory, the essence of the immune system is the repression of its lymphocytes. The morphologic diversity of the transplantation reaction may therefore also be due to the blocking of suppressor mechanisms. Whereas the suppression of B-lymphocytes by anti-allotypic antibody is maintained by T-lymphocytes (Jacobson et al., 1972), B-cells remain functional or even enhanced to antigens independent of thymus in antithymocyte serum-treated animals (Baker et al., 1970; Kerbel and Eidinger, 1971). Soluble factors obtained from T-cells (Green et al., 1970) inhibited both DNA synthesis (Smith et al., 1971) and development of clones (Lebowitz and Lawrence, 1971).

c) Cell-Mediated Cytotoxicity Independent of Thymus
(compare Figs. 1 and 2)

Results of earlier experiments suggested that in several models of cell-mediated cytotoxicity either T-cells might not be involved or non-T-cells were implicated (McLennan, 1972; Podleski and Podleski, 1973; Golstein et al., 1973). Most of these experiments were carried out in systems known to be dependent on antibody bound to target cell antigens, particularly to xenogeneic erythrocytes, liver, and tumor cell lines. Since these antibodies fix little or no complement, they were believed to be incomplete (Lobuglio et al., 1967) or cytophilic (Boyden, 1964). Addition of either blood leukocytes or peritoneal macrophages from unsensitized donors to these systems gave rise to the formation of rosettes (Jandl and Tomlinson, 1958), erythrophagocytosis (Berken and Benacerraf, 1966), and target cell damage (Perlmann and Holm, 1969). The role of the antibody-dependent cell-mediated response within the scope of the transplantation reaction was shown by Hasek et al. (1969). They achieved skin graft rejection by passive administration of antibody, but demonstrated that host cells also participated in the reaction. Thus, when the animals were treated with ALS or total-body irradiation, the humoral antibody was insufficient to cause graft rejection. The most likely explanation is that in these instances the humoral antibody initiated the reaction, while it was executed by host cells (Möller, 1971). In other studies a dichotomy of cell-mediated cytotoxicity was suggested. In, irradiated golden hamsters with reconstituted bone marrow, the rejection of an allogenic lymphoma transplant was accomplished by direct action of immune cells, whereas a simultaneously occurring skin lesion of the delayed hypersensitivity type was due to an indirect effect mediated by normal macrophages (Nomoto et al., 1970).

α) Monocytes and Macrophages

Monocytes and macrophages were identified as effector cells for both cytolytic and rosette-forming cells (Archer, 1965; Bennett, 1965; Lobuglio et al., 1967). Using a system consisting of defined soluble antigens covalently bound to xenogenic target cells, Schirrmacher et al. (1974) confirmed that the lytic effector cell is neither an antigen-specific T-cell (as tested by helper cell function) nor an antigen-specific B-cell (as judged by antibody-forming precursor function), and that it has distinct adherent properties. Furthermore, the lysis of human erythrocytes treated with anti-A serum by blood monocytes of the red cell donor was supressed when the monocytes were loaded with heat killed *Candida albicans* or carbonyl iron particles. Isolated "immune" peritoneal macrophages were able specifically to suppress tumor growth (Bennett, 1965) or to transfer passively resistance to a subsequent melanoma graft in mice (Burger et al., 1973). *In vitro* macrophage-mediated contact cytotoxicity to allogenic target cells (Lohmann-Matthes et al., 1972) may be caused by membrane-associated antibodies on macrophages (Granger and Weiser, 1966) rather than by antibody coating of target cells. However, in the serum of patients carrying transitional carcinomas of the urinary tract a factor is present which induces Fc-receptor-bearing mononuclear cells from healthy donors to become cytotoxic against cultured tumor cells (HAKALA and LANGE, 1974). The type and source of the various mononuclear cells termed macrophages were morphologically determined only in some of the studies. Cells "adhering" to cotton-wool and nylon-wool columns are believed to be macrophages; thus the effluent of these columns is considered to be free of macrophages, not taking into account the presence of nonphagocytic monocytes (GREENBERG et al., 1973b). Adherent cells from various lymphoid organs display divergent functional properties (FOLCH et al., 1973). The assumption of an alternating action of divergent macrophage types might be strengthened by recent findings from our laboratory. Whereas in unmodified liver allografts the most prominent of the effector cells is the monocyte, large numbers of peritoneal macrophages were found to accumulate in the graft when the host was treated with cyclophosphamide. In T-cell-deprived dogs, lung allografts exhibited an abundant increase in alveolar macrophages (Fig. F9) (WILDEVUUR et al., 1973a).

The origin of the "bulk" phagocytosing macrophage frequently remains obscure, although there is clear evidence that circulating blood monocytes are at least one type of precursor cells of macrophages (VOLKMAN and GOWANS, 1965a) and that their progenitors derive from the bone marrow (VOLKMAN and GOWANS, 1965b). Some authors have suggested that small lymphocytes may differentiate into macrophages (REBUCK et al., 1958; BJÖRKLUND et al., 1972), but this has been denied by others (RABINOWITZ and SCHREK, 1962; BRÜCHER et al., 1969). However, on electron micrographs, cells containing phagocytosed sensitized erythrocytes are undoubtedly lymphocytes (BIBERFELD and PERLMANN, 1970). Cytoplasmic inclusions such as fat droplets are frequently seen both in transforming normal lymphocytes (TANAKA and LIDDY, 1966) and in leukemic lymphocytes (TANAKA and GOODMAN, 1972). In individual instances, inclusions might also result from antigen-mediated internalization of surface membrane immunoglobulin (M-IgG) (ROSENTHAL et al., 1973). Wistar rat liver allografts were infiltrated by cells closely resembling lymphocytes on electron micrographs, however, they exhibited numerous lysosomes.

In recent studies, HIBBS et al. (1972a, b, c) have established evidence for in vitro nonimmunologic destruction of cells with abnormal growth characteristics by activated peritoneal macrophages. Similar cytotoxicity to allogenic lymphoma cells was observed when macrophages were treated with fungal virus RNA, synthetic double-stranded polynucleotides, and Shigella endotoxin (ALEXANDER and EVANS, 1971). Phagocytosis was not involved, and only after 24 hours, when disintegration of the lymphoma cells became evident, did the macrophages show any degree of phagocytosis (ALEXANDER and EVANS, 1971). After stimulation with endotoxin and RNA, polymorphonuclear leukocytes exerted a general injurious effect on target cells similar to that of macrophages, although to a quantitatively lesser degree (KELLER, 1973). These results suggest that both macrophage and polymorphonuclear leukocyte activation can be effected by nonimmunologic means, as well as result from a specific immunologic event. Although the models mentioned above are restricted to tumor cells which appear to exhibit changes in membrane stability, favoring focal and temporary membrane fusions (LUCY, 1970; POSTE and ALLISON, 1971; HIBBS, 1974), they appear to parallel results obtained with liver homotransplantation in rats (ZELDER et al.,

1973). Unmodified Wistar rats of a closed-colony breeding reject liver homografts in a maximum of 4 percent of cases, when animals are kept under specific germ-free conditions. When the rats were transferred to a conventional environment, and transplanted 14 days after they had become "uncontrolled" gnotobionts, all liver grafts were rejected acutely. In these instances, the effector cells were initially nonphagocytosing monocytes, and the number of polymorphonuclear cells was distinctly increased.

β) B-lymphocytes

With respect to this type of effector cell the problem has become much more complex and controversial since antibody-dependent cytotoxicity that was independent of thymus was observed after depletion of active macrophages (MÖLLER, 1965; HOLM and PERLMANN, 1967; MCLENNAN and LOEWI, 1968; KEDAR et al., 1974). Several authors (BIBERFELD and PERLMANN, 1970; MÖLLER and SHEVAG, 1972) have suggested that the killer cells belong to a currently unrecognized subpopulation of lymphocytes resembling small lymphocytes ("unknown" cells, ALLISON, 1972). In studies on the lysis of target cells bearing Moloney sarcoma virus-determined antigen (LAMON et al., 1972), and in patients with a transitional cell carcinoma of the urinary bladder (O'TOOLE et al., 1973), there was some evidence in favor of a B-cell as at least one type of killer cell. Prior treatment of the effector population with antibody to kappa chains diminished cell-mediated cytotoxicity, suggesting the implication of B-lymphocytes (VAN BOXEL et al., 1972). A class of specific cytotoxic cells detected in a lymphoid population depleted of both T-cells and IgG-bearing cells was termed "null" cells (GREENBERG et al., 1973a; GREENBERG and SHEN, 1973) and subsequently identified as nonphagocytic monocytes (GREENBERG et al., 1973b). Thus GREAVES et al. (1973) argued that non-thymus-derived cytotoxic cells can be attributed to any type of non-T-cells bearing membrane-bound Fc receptors, (LAMON et al., 1972), e.g. macrophages (EVANS and ALEXANDER, 1970; LOHMANN-MATTHES et al., 1972), monocytes (HUBER and FUDENBERG, 1968; HOLM and HAMMARSTRÖM, 1973), and "unknown" cells (ALLISON, 1972; WISLÖFF and FRÖLAND, 1973). However, B-cells reveal a marked predilection for IgG_1, whereas mononuclear phagocytes bind preferentially IgG_{2a} (BASTEN et al., 1972).

γ) Plasma cells and clusters (right lower quadrant of Fig. 1)

It can be claimed that morphologic demonstration of plasma cells as part of an effector system would convincingly point to the participation of B-cells in cell-mediated cytotoxicity. During progressive destruction of cultured allogenic fibroblasts by specifically sensitized lymphoid cells, large IgG-containing cells, probably plasma cells, increased in number, as revealed by immunofluorescence (CLARK and WEISS, 1969) and electron microscopy (WEISS, 1968). Ultrastructural examination of hemolytic cell clusters responding in vitro to xenogenic erythrocytes revealed the existence of three cell types: plasma cells, large undifferentiated lymphoid (blast) cells, and macrophages (MCINTYRE et al., 1973). The composition of the cluster changed with time: small lymphocytes decreased in number and plasma cells increased, while the numbers of lymphoid blast cells and macrophages remained constant. Passive administration of the specific opsonizing antibody relieves the reactive system of the need to synthesize it, even when antibody-forming precursor cells are present. If the specific antibody is absent, but both the triggering antigen and the essential precursor cells are present, the *in vivo* reaction can be initiated *in vitro*, displaying the triad of cellular elements, as demonstrated by McINTYRE *et al.* (1973).

These results suggest a "peripheralization", i.e. "extranodular autonomous" histogenesis of the antibody-dependent cell-mediated immune response as one of the possible manifestations of the transplantation reaction in instances in which the cellular components of a plaque-forming cluster are present within the graft, i.e. lymphocytes, plasma cells and mononuclear macrophages (Figs. 20, 22, 23, 36, 52). Numerous plasma cells were seen invading implants of sub-maximillary glands (DARCY, 1952), canine kidney allografts (KOUNTZ *et al.*, 1963; PORTER, 1969), skin xenografts (BILSKI and JERUSALEM, 1969), and lung allografts (FUJIMURA *et al.*, 1970; SUZUKI *et al.*, 1973; NOIRCLERC *et al.*, 1973). A close arrangement of lymphocytes and alveolar macrophages in the presence of maturing plasma cells was clearly depicted on electron micrographs by GON-DOS *et al.* (1973). Recent investigations from our laboratory showed an increase in the number of plasma cells when liver allografted rats were treated with cyclophosphamide, a drug known to deplete a host preferentially of the B-cell population (TURK and POULTER, 1972; POULTER and TURK, 1972). These findings may cast some doubt on the recent reading of a single cytogenetic origin of plasma cells. Lymphatic origin of plasma cells is the classic and currently most widely accepted concept. A second major hypothesis includes their derivation from mesenchymal elements (KOLOUCH *et al.*, 1947; REBUCK and LOGRIPPO 1961; for references see McMILLAN and ENGELBERT, 1963; TANAKA and GOOD-MAN, 1972). Most of these studies were concerned with the blast cell problem. Since morphologically, "plasmablasts" appear to be indistinguishable from "lymphoblasts" ("immunoblasts" DAMESHEK, 1963), undifferentiated mesen-chymal elements known as germinocytes, hemocytoblasts and lymphoid reticular cells (LENNERT, 1961), isomorphism was held to be synonymous with isogenesis. However, immunohistochemical methods made it possible to distinguish two types of plasma cells (POTWOROWSKI and NAIRN, 1968). One type reacted nega-tively with an antiserum prepared against a common lymphoid cell antigen but positively with fluorescein-conjugated anti-rat globulin, while the other could be stained with the lymphoid-specific antiserum.

The various cell types that progressively accumulate in tissue and organ grafts may not be exclusively of host-nodular origin. They can apparently prolif-erate and mature within the graft, suggesting a certain autonomy of the peripher-al clusters and the developing lymphoid cell accumulation (DEMPSTER and WIL-LIAMS, 1963). The "cuffing" of lymphoid cells around the vasculature of primari-ly revascularized organ grafts is regarded as a classic feature of the cell-mediated transplantation reaction. These cuffs and the interstitial mononuclear infiltrates are frequently composed of lymphocytes, occasional plasma cells, monocytes and macrophages. The cells of these lines can exhibit various stages of maturation and mitotic figures, and label heavily with ^{3}H-thymidine.

δ) *Cell interaction in cell-mediated cytotoxicity*

The formation of peripheral clusters composed of cells with known helper and/or effector cell activity suggests cell interactions in cell-mediated cytotoxicity, and in particular of immune lymphocytes with macrophages (EVANS and ALEXANDER, 1970). In this system, lymphocyte products appear to affect macrophages by "activation" (increase in killing potentials), "arming" (induction of specific reactivity to antigen), and "firing" (dissemination of toxic factors) (ARIYAN and GERSHON, 1973). For an adoptively transferred delayed hypersensitivity reaction the co-operation of bone marrow and thymus cells was found to be essential to induce the most vigorous skin lesion (TUBERGEN and FELDMAN, 1971). Although there is clear morphologic evidence for the presence of B-cells (plasma cells) in numerous instances of tissue and organ graft rejection, the role of the B-cell system in this response remains uncertain, since there is an apparently normal expression of cell-mediated immunity in the absence of both B-cells and conventional antibody, e.g. in bursectomized chickens and patients with congenital agammaglobulinemia (GREAVES *et al.*, 1973; see also Section A III/1). Thus, normally undetectable cytophilic serum antibodies (BOYDEN and SORKIN, 1961), high-affinity antibodies of low concentration (KARUSH and EISEN, 1962), and/or local synthesis of antibody (SCHLOSSMAN *et al.*, 1966; HALL, 1969) do not seem to play a crucial role in the transplantation reaction. Because thymus-processed cells can be toxic by themselves, co-operation with non-T-cells may result in an intensification (amplification) of the cell-mediated reaction (EVANS and ALEXANDER, 1970). However, due to recent findings, the possibility of antibody involvement in cell-mediated immunity is being discussed again. Mouse T-cells can apparently synthesize and release an antibody-like molecule of the 7S IgM class (HÄMMERLING and RAJEWSKI, 1971), and the binding of antigen by human T-cells is inhibited by "capping" of the antigen receptors with anti-immunoglobulin (ROELANTS *et al.*, 1973). Furthermore, the T-cell-derived 7S IgM molecule exhibits an intense cytophilia for the macrophage surface (CONE *et al.*, 1974; for further references see NOSSAL, 1974). After assaying T-lymphocytes both for their capacity to co-operate *in vitro* with B-cells in the induction of plaque-forming cells and for their capacity to cause *in vitro* lysis of target cells independently of complement, DENNERT and LENNOX (1972) suggested that the role of the T-cell was the same both in the humoral and in the cell-mediated response, i.e. to co-operate with the B-cell: specific antibody, released by B-effector cells triggered by T-cells (plasma cells) opsonized the target cell which is subsequently attacked by a macrophage.

ε) *Polymorphonuclear (PMN) cells*

The vast amount of data concerning lymphocytes and macrophages in immune responses has tended to overshadow the importance of other cell types, particularly that of PMN cells (OWEN, 1974). Neutrophilic granulocytes are not only important effector cells in hyperacute graft rejection (HUME, 1971; MEJIA-LAGUNA *et al.*, 1972; see also Figures 4, 5, 6, 7b, 9, 12a, 13a, 16 and Chapter D II 1 b α), but are also able to kill target cells, apparently by a mechanism similar to that of activated macrophages. KELLER (1973) argued that PMN cells could participate in the elimination of tumor cells, particularly under circumstances where the number of conventional effector cells is limited. This may also be true of recipients of organ grafts who have been depleted of lymphocytes mainly by surgical procedures, either via a thoracic duct fistula (Irvin and Carbone, 1967; Murray et al., 1968) or by adult thymectomy and subsequent ATS treatment (Wildevuur et al., 1973a). Under the latter condition, lung allografts exhibited remarkable proliferative changes associated with the occurrence of numerous PMN cells. Since the observation of Lay and Nussenzweig (1968), it has been appreciated that peripheral blood leukocytes contain receptors for IgG which are discrete from the complement receptors present on the same cell. Furthermore, Henson (1971) and Weissmann et al. (1972) showed that endocytosis of immune complexes and the subsequent release of lysosomal hydrolases from PMN cells could be readily induced by aggregates containing IgG_1 and IgG_3. It therefore appears reasonable to suppose that PMN cells participate in organ graft rejection only in instances where conventional antibody and complement are important mediators of the reaction. However, except for hyperacute graft rejection, in each particular instance it remains to be proved whether PMN cells can be regarded as cells amplifying the transplant reaction or are a manifestation of a mild infection.

IV. Humoral Factors Involved in Graft Rejection

Although a large body of data has established the importance of cellular immunity in the processes of graft rejection (Wilson and Billingham, 1967), the role of humoral antibodies has also become firmly established (Stastny, 1970). Humoral-mediated tissue injury occurring subsequent to organ transplantation can be attributed to three distinct pathogenic mechanisms. The first is mediated by preformed circulating antibodies present in the recipient prior to transplantation. Such antibodies may react nonspecifically with antigens of the transplanted organ and unleash a course of events finally resulting in hyperacute graft rejection (see Section D). The second mechanism invokes the concept that antigens which trigger predominantly cell-mediated immune reactions also initiate a primary humoral response (Fig. 2). These antibodies are directed not only against donor-specific but also against species-specific antigens (Van Breda-Vriesman, 1972). The production of both species-specific antilymphocyte serum for immunosuppressive therapy and the various antisera for tissue-typing purposes is a practical application of the ability of histocompatibility and differentiation antigens to trigger humoral immune responses. Although immune reactions to transplanted organs can have either a cellular or a humoral pattern, it is not an either-or situation of cell versus antibody. The majority of clinical rejections present with more mixed characteristics (Carpenter and Merrill, 1969), and the predominance of one type may change during the post-transplantation course, particularly as the result of immunosuppressive therapy. Donor-specific antibodies have been demonstrated after the transplantation of skin (Woodruff and Forman, 1950), and high titers of circulating cytotoxic antibodies were still observed when the cytotoxic effect expressed by the sensitized lymphocytes had disappeared (DEGIOVANNI and LEJEUNE, 1973). Humoral antibodies were assumed to contribute to acute kidney graft rejection (LINDQUIST *et al.*, 1968a; BOHLE, 1970; BUSCH *et al.*, 1971; PILLAY *et al.*, 1973), and measurement of IgG was recommended as a guide to immunosuppression and cytotoxicity in renal allograft patients (KU *et al.*, 1973). Several patients who underwent a classic cell-mediated homograft rejection developed complement-dependent humoral antibody activity against cultured cells from the transplanted kidney (WOLF *et al.*, 1971). Subsequently evidence was obtained on the role of humoral factors in human cardiac graft rejection (DALLOCHIO *et al.*, 1970; ELLIS *et al.*, 1970a, b). However, in several instances, circulating antibodies were not demonstrable, although the deposition of IgG and β 1 C in various cardiac tissues was almost associated with severe degeneration of both vascular media and myocardial fibers (BIEBER *et al.*, 1970). It appears, therefore, that the present tests for detecting such antibodies are relatively insensitive (CARPENTER and MERRILL, 1969), that low- and high-affinity antibody titers may alternate and oscillate (MACARIO and DE MACARIO, 1971), or that antibody is synthesized locally in the graft by proliferating plasma cells, as assumed for lung allografts (FUJIMURA *et al.*, 1970; SUZUKI *et al.*, 1973). Whereas in mixed rejection patterns it appears difficult to distinguish lesions induced by humoral mechanisms from those mediated by cells, experimental studies have provided evidence that antibody alone could produce changes identical to those seen in accelerated kidney allograft rejection (NAJARIAN and PERPER, 1967; COCHRUM *et al.*, 1969). There was a positive correlation between the severity of the lesion and the titer of the passively transferred donor-specific antibody (DUBERNARD *et al.*, 1968). After successful transplantation to immunosuppressed recipients, skin allografts were rejected in an accelerated manner when antidonor allo-antiserum was administered either alone (OLUWASANMI, 1973) or together with complement (GERLAG *et al.*, 1973). Thirdly, in contrast to mechanisms involving antibodies which upon fixing of complement are directly cytotoxic to cells (see Chapter B III 1), non-complement-fixing immunoglobulins can trigger cell-mediated cytotoxicity that is independent of the thymus. The occurrence of characteristic "hemolytic" clusters consisting of plasma cells, macrophages and small lymphocytes in various organ grafts suggests the peripheral synthesis of cytophilic antibody (see Chapter A III 3c).

B. Effector Cells and the Target Cell Injury

I. Morphology of Infiltrating "Lymphoid Cells"

The terms "lymphoid", "mononuclear" and "round" cells are frequently used to characterize a collective of cells having only one, more or less round, nucleus. Unfortunately, various cells of different lines involved in the transplantation reaction (Chapter A III 3) exhibit these features. Of course, under the light microscope the typical small lymphocyte, the mature plasma cell, and the large macrophage are fairly distinctive. However, a large majority of cells appear

to be intermediate stages between mature and immature, e.g. in blast cell transformation; immature and mature, e.g. during reversal to blast cell derived clonal
cells, or between precursor and effector cells, e.g. during differentiation to plasma
cells and to supposed lymphocyte-derived killer cells. Although the differences
in the ultrastructural characteristics of these cell types are too slight to allow
clear categorization of the various cell lines, the main ultrastructural features
are outlined in this chapter.

1. Small Lymphocytes (Figs. 18, 22, 23, 29)

The average size of small lymphocytes is about 8 μm. The nucleus is round,
electron-opaque with relatively condensed chromatin, and exhibits a small indentation. Several short microvilli are usually present at the surface of the
cytoplasm, which is only a narrow rim. Adjacent to the small Golgi area,
there are centrioles and a small number of spherical mitochondria. Compound
vacuoles, multivesicular and, occasionally, osmiophilic bodies (lysosomes) may
represent the small "azurophilic" granules. Small bundles of filaments and
glycogen are sometimes present. The basophilia of the cytoplasm is due to
a relatively large number of free ribosomes (monosomes) rather than to the
few profiles of RER. Although only these cells have the ability to form rosettes,
not all of them are thymus-derived, since the same cell type is frequently present
in the follicular corona. Furthermore, it is impossible to distinguish between
"unprimed" cells, which are sensitive to PHA and pokeweed mitogens, and
specifically sensitized blast cell-derived lymphocytes.

2. Medium-Sized Lymphocytes

Medium-sized lymphocytes (Figs. 14, 20, 39) measure up to 10 μm, and are
round or slightly oval. Compared with the small lymphocyte, the ratio of the
cytoplasmic to the nuclear diameter is larger, as is the nucleus itself. The chromatin is either somewhat denser, or distinctly less dense. Occasionally the nucleus
is slightly indented and exhibits 1 or 2 nucleoli. Whereas microvilli appear
to be less frequent in these cells than in the small lymphocytes, single pinocytotic
vesicles may be increased in number. Frequently the cells exhibit a distinct
perinuclear space. A Golgi complex is present, with well-developed saccules
and vesicles. There are usually 1 or 2 centrioles in same cytoplasmic areal.
Mitochondria are more numerous and tend to accumulate in one hemisphere.
In most instances the ribosomes are less densely packed, and single narrow
cisternae of the RER can be detected. Occasionally these cells exhibit Gall
bodies. However, the degree of cytoplasmic differentiation varies considerably,
even in the same individual. Although these cells are most prominent in the
bursa of Fabricius (Clawson et al., 1967) and in bone marrow-dependent areas,
it is uncertain whether they represent B-cells in every instance.

3. Atypical Lymphocytes

Occasionally cells resembling medium-sized lymphocytes exhibit an increased
number of cisternae of RER which are sometimes irregularly shaped, either

closed or open, but have a tendency to circular arrangements. These cells are unlike mature plasma cells because of their small size and the comparatively underdeveloped RER profiles, but are also unlike maturing plasma cells in that the degree of nuclear differentiation is too high.

4. Large Lymphocytes

Large lymphocytes are round or slightly oval, with an average size of 12–18 µm. The large nucleus is electron-light and is usually round but sometimes exhibits deep surface indentations. The heterochromatin is reduced to small and finely granulated patches randomly distributed throughout the nucleus and concentrated in a thin rim adjacent to the nuclear envelope. The nucleoli are large, prominent, and coarsely granular. The central nucleolar portion is enlarged and frequently electron-light. Usually one part of the nucleolus is connected with the peripheral nuclear heterochromatin. The cell surface exhibits several microvilli. A Golgi complex is generally absent, but if present, its lamellae surround the centrioles. The spherical mitochondria tend to be grouped at one pole of the cell. The presence of large numbers both of free ribosomes and of randomly distributed clusters of polysomes is striking. Whereas short profiles of RER are only occasionally seen, several membranous channels are usually present. Furthermore, the cytoplasm exhibits bundles of filaments, microtubules, and some glycogen. One or two lysosomes, and one lipid-containing Gall body measuring 0.3–0.7 µm can also be present. The large lymphocytes have numerous features in common with cells of stimulated lymph nodes, but differ from lymphoblasts, e.g. in the increased number of microtubules (BESSIS, 1973). Since among other characteristics the nuclear shape, the chromatin patterns, and particularly the content and distribution of monosomes and polysomes can vary considerably, there are probably at least two different classes of large lymphocytes (JOHNSON et al., 1966). Occasionally cells resembling large lymphocytes develop an increased number of somewhat longer strands of RER adjacent to the nuclear envelope. Others exhibit parallel profiles of RER in a circumscript region. The resemblance of these cells to proplasmacytes becomes closer with increasing amounts of RER and, correspondingly, decreasing numbers of free ribosomes, (ISHII et al., 1973).

5. Transformed Lymphocytes (Figs. 21, 41)

Cells of this type derive from small lymphocytes upon stimulation by PHA and pokeweed mitogens, specific antigens, mixed lymphocyte cultures etc., and are commonly termed blast cells. The diameter of individual cells can increase up to 20 to 30 µm, i.e. three to four times the diameter of small lymphocytes. The nucleus enlarges considerably, its shape becomes variable, and it frequently develops more than one indentation. Usually the finely granulated chromatin is regularly dispersed within the electron-light nucleoplasm, and a thin, patchy layer of heterochromatin is sometimes condensed adjacent to the nuclear envelope. The nucleoli are prominent, frequently elongated, ramified, and occasionally hyperplastic. The periphery of the cytoplasm, which is greatly increased in volume, is irregular; it exhibits cytoplasmic projections and distinct pinocytotic activity. Usually, the cytoplasmic organelles appear to be increased in both number and size. A well-developed Golgi complex, centrioles, and numerous microtubules are found in the same area. The mitochondria are large, voluminous, oval or cylindrical, and have characteristic rows of densely packed parallel cristae. The number of ribosomes increases. They are arranged in rosettes and/or chain-like organizations (polysomes). The appearance of the RER is variable, ranging from a few small vesicles to an increased number of flattened cisternae. The degree of differentiation of the RER appears to depend upon the kind of stimulating agent. The development of profiles of RER is more pronounced after incubation with pokeweed mitogens than after incubation with PHA, although both mitogens stimulate exclusively T-cells. Transformed lymphocytes usually exhibit a variety of cytoplasmic inclusions. Lamellated structures that have a positive reaction for acid phosphatase and large electron-dense bodies of round, oval, or occasionally stellate appearance are present in considerable numbers. Multivesiculated bodies are less frequent. It has been suggested that these membrane-bound bodies are lysosomal in nature. They correspond in size and shape to the clear vacuoles frequently seen in Giemsa-stained smears. Electron-opaque spheres which probably contain protein are less common. Sporadically a spherule consisting of neutral fat and a substantial quantity of filaments can be detected.

6. Lymphoid Killer Cells (Fig. 19)

Although the general consensus of opinion is that cells infiltrating an organ graft are involved in the transplantation reaction, it is impossible to attribute functions suggestive of cell-mediated target cell destruction to a morphologically well-defined lymphocyte-derived "killer cell". As revealed by the vast amount of morphologic studies presently available, all the cell types mentioned above can be present, occasionally in overwhelming numbers but frequently in various combinations. Even taking into account that ancestors and successors of different lymphocyte families have different functions but appear morphologically identical, the problem of the lymphocyte-derived effector cell in the transplantation reaction remains unsolved.

7. Monocytes (Figs. 25, 38)

The size of mature cells ranges from 10 to 15 μm. The horseshoe- or kidney-shaped nucleus is eccentrically localized and exhibits only lightly staining aggregates of heterochromatin. Occasionally one or two nucleoli are present. The surface of the cytoplasm is either smooth or rough. Numerous vacuoles near the cytoplasmic membrane suggest active pinocytosis. Microvilli, philopodia, and pseudopodia are usually present. The Golgi complex is small but exhibits well-developed vesicles and vacuoles; in most cases its location is perinuclear. A topographic association with centrioles and occasionally with large pinocytotic vesicles is evident. Mitochondria tend to localize at the periphery of the cytoplasm. They are small, slim, and oval with closely packed cristae in a dense matrix almost devoid of granules. The number of mitochondria varies from 2 to over 20. Monosomes are sparsely distributed, and the presence of polysomes is abnormal in mature cells. Profiles of RER are present in modest numbers. They are short and flattened. In instances where they are more numerous the RER is arranged in circular arrays adjacent to the nucleus, but more randomly in the periphery. Occasionally some SER is present. The ("azurophilic") membrane-bound, dense granules are a characteristic feature. They measure 100 to 200 nm, are uniformly dense, and are regularly distributed throughout the cytoplasm. These granules are smaller but more numerous than those found in lymphocytes, and obviously represent primary lysosomes because of their hydrolytic and peroxidatic activity. Small arrays of filaments (3–7 nm) are present in the perinuclear region, and after appropriate fixation microtubules (15 nm) are demonstrable in the periphery of the cytoplasm, particularly in the base of uropods.

8. Macrophages

It has been claimed that monocytes are not the only cells capable of phagocytosis that can be involved in the transplantation reaction (Chapter A III 3c, α). All these cells presumably derive from a common ancestor, the bone marrow-dependent promonocyte:

Promonocyte — Monocyte	histiocyte (macrophage of connective tissue)
	peritoneal macrophages (serous cavity)
	Kupffer cell (liver)
	alveolar phagocyte (lung)
	free and fixed macrophages, sinusoidal lining cells (spleen, lymph node, bone marrow)
	osteoclast (bone)
	microglia (nervous system)

Although there are several species-dependent differences, the ultrastructural and cytochemical characteristics are of surprising uniformity, except for the osteoclasts. We therefore summarize the minute differences that exist between the fixed macrophage (e.g. the resident peritoneal macrophage) and the exudate macrophage (e.g. the monocyte-derived exudate peritoneal macrophage), or the peripheral monocyte, in tabular form.

General features of macrophages (compare Figs. 20, 23, 30, 31, 32, 37, 40, 41, 43, 45, 49).

Although most "fixed" macrophages are spindle-shaped or multiangular, in contrast to "free" macrophages which are round or oval, the following description applies to all macrophages with few exceptions.

The trilaminar cell membrane (8 nm) exhibits a ruthenium red-positive fuzzy (mucoid) coat (7–16 nm) for adhesion and phagocytosis. Characteristic differentiations of the cell surface are fingerlike processes (philopodia-like projections), flap-like ruffles, and microvilli. Large, irregularly shaped electron-lucent vacuoles (400–800 nm) beneath the surface represent cross-sectioned convoluted superficial surface invaginations with ill-defined filamentous substructures. During phagocytosis pseudopodia develop a distinct hyaloplasm and long membranous channels, microspikes, organelles (bundles of microtubules), and small micropinocytotic vacuoles (50–100 nm). Furthermore, bristle-coated micropinocytotic vesicles, "wormlike structures" (pinocytosis vermiformis, with a patchy distribution of the cell coat) are conspicious for phagocytosis. The eccentrically localized nucleus measures about 8–11 μm and varies in shape from oval kidney-shaped to highly irregular. Deep infoldings of the nuclear membrane are evident. Nuclear pores can vary considerably in number. Some macrophages exhibit one, others several nucleoli. A rim of dense peripheral heterochromatin is always distinct.

On appropriate sections 1 to 2 nuclear bodies may be detected. These spherical structures consist of fine filamentous material of moderate density. Two types of these bodies can be distinguished:

1. The simple form (occurring singly or in multiples) is a hollow spherical or ovoid structure and consists of filaments (250 nm) of a moderate density in a concentric arrangement. They are surrounded by a variable electron-lucent zone.

2. Complex bodies: a) Single structures (500–1500 nm) composed of a central part of osmiophilic granules and hollow granules (25–30 nm) in addition to larger dense aggregates. b) A larger and more complex type than type 2a. Simple hollowed nuclear bodies are arranged in chainlike formation or solid agglomerates of similar material around a core of dense granules or aggregates. Several microcylindric elements are present. The electron-light cytoplasm is abundant. The amount of rough endoplasmatic reticulum is somewhat species-dependent, e.g., in macrophages of mice and rats there is a moderate amount of RER, whereas human macrophages mostly exhibit only few RER profiles. The RER is preferentially localized at one side near the nucleus but opposite the Golgi complex and/or at the cell periphery. It consists of a varying number of parallel lamellae with communicating cisternae. Ribosomes attached to the trilaminar membrane (6 nm) of the cisternae have a polysomal configuration. A low to moderate amount of free ribosomes is present, but free polysomes are rarely observed. Continuous with the rough endoplasmatic reticulum is the tubular smooth endoplasmatic reticulum (SER). In macrophages of most species the SER is poorly developed, except for macrophages of cats, where the SER is prominent. In the space between the nuclear indentation (an area of the cytoplasm which is referred to as the "hof" of the nucleus), two centrioles and a well-developed Golgi apparatus are localized. The Golgi areas vary in size and number. In general the Golgi apparatus is well developed, and is composed of several stacks of parallel, smooth lamellae. Frequently smooth membrane-bound vesicles and small bristle-coated vesicles can be detected adjacent to the lamellar system. Around the centrioles and their pericentriolar satellites, microtubules (20 nm) are radially arranged. Vacuoles of varying size and number exhibiting an electron-lucent matrix, and several lysosomes are located in the same area.

The few mitochondria with a trilaminar membrane of 6 nm thickness vary in shape and size. They are round-oval to elongated in shape, measure between 200–1000 nm, and are moderately rich in cristae. They are randomly distributed but frequently to be found at that side of the nucleus where RER lamellae are localized. The Golgi area is the preferred site of localization of radially

Fixed macrophage	*Monocyte-derived exudate macrophage*
Cell diameter 10–50 μm	Cell diameter 10–50 μm
Close membrane interrelationship	Close membrane interrelationship
("loops")	("loops")
Abundant microvilli, labyrinth formation	Fewer microvilli, no labyrinth formation
Folded or deeply indented nucleus	Kidney-shaped nucleus
Endoplasmic reticulum well represented	Less well-developed endoplasmic reticulum
Golgi complex well developed	Golgi complex less developed
More mitochondria	Fewer mitochondria
Abundant vesicles and vacuoles	Few vesicles and vacuoles
Few polysomes	More polysomes
Peroxidatic activity in nuclear envelope, R.E.R. and Golgi complex	Peroxidatic activity in cytoplasmatic granules
Bundles of filaments	Few filaments
Abundant lysosomes	Fewer lysosomes
No lysosomal peroxidatic activity	Heterogeneous peroxidatic activity
No peroxidatic activity in phagocytic vacuoles	Phagocytic vacuoles show peroxidatic activity (by release of the peroxidase-positive granules)
Lysozyme not present	Lysozyme present as an antibacterial agent
High acid phosphatase activity	Low acid phosphatase activity
No NaF-sensitive esterase	NaF-sensitive esterase
High NaF-resistant esterase	Low NaF-resistant esterase
Bactericidal activity differs from granulocytes	Bactericidal activity same as granulocytes

orientated microtubules which extend from the centrioles to the peripheral cytoplasm. A limited number of filaments (8–10 nm) frequently accompanies the microtubules. Bundles of thinner filaments (5–6 nm) can be found near the nucleus, in the "hof", and in the outer periphery of the cell, but also scattered throughout the cytoplasm. Some lipid droplets and either dispersed or aggregated glycogen particles may be detected, too, in the cytoplasm. Crystalloid and fibrillar structures exhibiting periodicity are occasionally seen. The cytoplasm is filled with a number of lysosomal structures varying in size from 200–800 nm. They include primary (H granula) and secondary lysosomes, which are bounded by a single trilaminar membrane and separated from the matrix by a clear halo. Further characteristic features are residual bodies containing lipid droplets, degradation products rich in iron, ingested erythrocytes, fragments of granulocytes, as well as multivesicular bodies. Autophagous vacuoles with myelin figures, fragments of organelles, e.g., mitochondria or banded rodlike structures can also be observed.

II. Morphology of the Cell-Mediated Target-Cell Destruction *in vitro*

In vitro systems of cell-mediated cytotoxicity were found to be appropriate models for morphologic studies on target cell lysis, because they deal with both well-characterized single cell lines as target cells and identifiable effector cells. Although varying models were investigated, several features of the chain of destructive events were surprising uniform.

1. Membrane Contact

It is unequivocally accepted that the essential and crucial step in the initiation of the final effector phase is the close contact which has to be established between the effector and the target cell (Rosenau, 1963; Möller, 1965; Hellstrom and Hellstrom, 1966; Kolb and Granger, 1968; Feldman et al., 1972). Inhibition of this membrane contact preserves the target cell from damage (Rosenau, 1963; Wilson, 1965; Wolberg et al., 1973; Hibbs, 1974). Membrane stabilizers such as hydrocortisone have an inhibitory effect (Weissmann and Dingle, 1961; De Duve et al., 1962). However, the absence of initial membrane interaction is occasionally reported (Holm, 1967). Establishment of membrane contact is promoted by active movement of effector cells including both lymphocytes and macrophages. No difference was observed in the overall rate of translational movement of normal and stimulated macrophages (Carr and Carr, 1970). Sensitized and PHA-stimulated lymphocytes, however, appear to contact their isogenic target cells more frequently than do unsensitized controls (Biberfeld et al., 1968; Ax et al., 1968). There was no evidence of chemotaxis (Able et al., 1970); sensitized lymphocytes were seen crawling across the fibroblast layer and colliding at random with target cells. Results of Biberfeld et al.

(1968) suggest that lymphocytes which have established contact with allogenic target cells *in vitro* move around on their surface (ROBINEAUX *et al.*, 1962) in a fashion reminiscent of an interaction of macrophages and lymphocytes that is observed only after skin homografting and is termed "peripolesis" by SHARP and BURWELL (1960). Occasionally, the lymphocytes developed more elongated and tapered foot processes and penetrated between the cells of the monolayer, reaching its bottom side and raising the peripheral portions of the target cells (BIBERFELD *et al.*, 1968). These pictures resemble those observed in acute cell-mediated organ graft rejection, when mononuclear cells penetrate the vascular intima (Fig. 25). By means of electron microscopy three features of membrane approximation were observed (LOBUGLIO *et al.*, 1967; ABLE *et al.*, 1970; McIN-TYRE *et al.*, 1973): an attachment extended over a considerable area of the cell surface; the cell membranes showed points or plaques of intimate contact, frequently regularly spaced; and there were spike-like interdigitating junctions between effector and target cells. Coated vesicles and accumulations of cell organelles were frequently prominent adjacent to plaques of intimate contact, suggesting a certain destabilization of cytoplasmic membranes (HIBBS, 1974).

However, in WEISS's (1968) model of homograft rejection, lymphocytes adherent to the fibroblastic target cells displayed no specialized junctional complexes, and in virtually all instances the membrane of each cell remained intact and separate. In solid organ grafts the types of membrane association mentioned above were detected more frequently 2 to 6 hours after revascularization, i.e. during the phase of recognition (PORTER, 1965; FELDMAN and LEE, 1967; KOUNTZ *et al.*, 1963), than during the acute effector phase of cell-mediated rejection (Figs. 14, 21, 30).

2. Morphology of Cell-Mediated Target Cell Lysis

The cardinal features of lymphocyte-mediated cytotoxicity suggest that primarily osmoregulatory mechanisms of the target cells are impaired (ROSENAU, 1963). These changes closely resemble alterations observed after both specific inhibition of the plasma membrane-associated adenosine triphosphatase (Na^+/K^+-ATPase) with ouabain (GINN *et al.*, 1968; TRUMP and BULGER, 1971) and the decrease in nonspecific ATPase activity in the donor liver perfused over a long period (JAP, 1971), particularly when procaine is added to the perfusate (CREMERS-VAN DIJCK, 1973). The first indication of lymphocyte-mediated target-cell lysis is a loss of electron density of cytoplasmic organelles and occasionally of the cytoplasm at sites of close contact with the effector cell. Subsequently, edema of the whole cell develops, numerous membrane-bound vacuoles may appear, and finally the plasma membrane ruptures (ABLE *et al.*, 1970). Almost the same changes are characteristic for the "ballooning" type of cytolysis induced by purified human lymphotoxin (RUSSEL *et al.*, 1972). Lymphocytotoxin can cause a second type of target cell damage characterized by a sudden shrinkage of the cell body followed by a violent agitation of the residuum (RUSSEL *et al.*, 1972). Again, development of both large cytoplasmic vesicles and cellular edema with subsequent damage to cytoplasmic organelles is obvious when plasma cells act as effector cells (WEISS, 1968).

Similar cytoplasmic changes were also observed in the aggressor cell, which subsequently died (Granger and Weiser, 1966; Granger and Kolb, 1968; Able *et al.*, 1970). In other systems this reaction was not found to be suicidal (Wilson, 1963; Perlmann *et al.*, 1968; Biberfeld *et al.*, 1968). Weiss (1968) and Russel *et al.* (1972), both working with fibroblasts, described small, dark-stalked protrusions from the cytoplasm, which were morphologically consistent with virus particles and which increased in number as degenerative changes in the target cells became more severe (compare Fig. 50). Immediate cytolysis is not the inevitable result of contact with aggressor lymphocytes. Target cells to which lymphocytes had been attached can still divide mitotically (Ax *et al.*, 1968). Numerous mitotic figures of parenchymal cells are also a characteristic feature of the acutely rejected PVG/C rat-liver allograft (Jap, 1971). However, in this instance proliferation of hepatocytes was explained as "internal compensatory growth" of the remaining cells, due to their functional overload (Fig. 42).

The period necessary for lymphoid cell-mediated cytotoxicity *in vitro* is the subject of some controversy. When sensitized lymphocytes were added to target cell monolayers, the first signs of target cell lysis were observed after 24 to 30 hours, and almost all cells were damaged after 2 days (Weiss, 1968; Able *et al.*, 1970). Under conditions which exclude orthodox immune phenomena (Möller, 1965; Holm *et al.*, 1964), e.g. mixed culture of unsensitized lymphocytes with allogenic fibroblasts, the monolayer was also destroyed after 2 days (Björklund *et al.*, 1972). Surprisingly, only about 17 hours were necessary to destroy target cells when normal lymphocytes were added to a Chang cell line monolayer and simultaneously stimulated with PHA (Biberfeld *et al.*, 1968). The time was reduced to 4 hours when suspension cultures were used (Ax *et al.*, 1968), and to 2 hours when the incubation mixture was gently rocked (Canty and Wunderlich, 1970). These values are the same as those observed with lymphotoxin-mediated target cell lysis (Russel *et al.*, 1972).

Of particular interest is the early cytotoxic activity of normal lymphocytes stimulated not only nonspecifically by PHA but also by anti-immunoglobulin antibodies (Sell and Gell, 1965; Sell, 1970). It remains an open question whether strong, nonspecific stimulation plays a role in those instances of organ transplantation in which changes characteristic for rejection become manifest before a specific transplantation reaction can be expected to occur (Busch *et al.*, 1969; see also Chapters D II 1b, F I 2).

3. Morphology of Antibody-Dependent Cell-Mediated Cytotoxicity

When IgG and Rh (anti-D) antibody-coated erythrocytes were attached to normal blood monocytes, the red cells rapidly transformed from their normal shape to spherocytes and became very sensitive to hypotonic lysis. On adhering, the monocytes gripped the cells with long, delicate, finger-like processes. Subsequently the red cell underwent puckering in the region of attachment, with the formation of numerous folds and tubular processes (Lobuglio *et al.*, 1967). Complete lysis after contact with monocytes was noted within 18 hours (Holm and Hammarström, 1973). In contrast, when spleen cells were explanted in the presence of antigen but in the absence of antibody, the essential microenvironment was established by the spontaneous increase in the number of both IgG antibody-forming cells and hemolytic clusters from very low levels to a peak on day 4 (McIntyre et al., 1973). In vitro studies suggest that monocytes were more effective than lymphocytes in cell-mediated cytotoxicity. Whereas in most studies ratios of 50 to several hundred so-called killer cells per target cell are often required, one monocyte was able to lyse 2 to 3 red blood cells (Holm and Hammarström, 1973), and tumor-cell proliferation was significantly inhibited at a macrophage-to-tumor cell ratio of 1:1 (Keller, 1973).

4. Other Mechanisms of Cell-Mediated Target Cell Destruction

An unusual mechanism of target cell destruction was described by Hibbs, (1974). When lysosomal markers identifiable under the light microscope were used, activated macrophages were seen to transfer the content of secondary lysosomes directly into the cytoplasm of susceptible target cells, which subsequently underwent heterolysis. Exocytosis of lysosomes of polymorphonuclear (PMN) cells into the intercellular space is occasionally depicted in instances of lung allograft rejection (Klika et al., 1973) (Fig. 14), and lysosomes derived from PMN cells within the cytoplasm of target cells were detected in advanced stages of alcoholic liver cirrhosis (Leevy and Jap, pers. comm., 1974). Furthermore, in several models of organ transplantation, neither lymphoid cells of the monocyte series nor those of the macrophage series appear to exert direct cytotoxicity on target cells. In rat liver allografts, infiltrating cells frequently encompass the hepatocytes, separating them from each other by large cytoplasmic extensions, thus interfering with local blood flow and competing with the liver cells for nutrients. Ultrastructural and histochemical changes appear to be a nonspecific form of hepatocellular damage, e.g. atrophy (Jap, 1971) (Fig. 40). A similar mechanism was suggested as the reason for parenchymal atrophy in several instances of canine pancreaticoduodenal allotransplantation (v. Hee, 1973).

III. Features of Antibody-Mediated Injury

The nature of the antibody-induced injury varies widely, since its character, localization, and severity are dependent on a variety of factors such as the type, the avidity, and the quantity of antibody involved, the immunologic specificity, and the site and structure of the antigen. For purposes of this chapter we are not only concerned with antigens that are tissue-fixed components of the transplanted organ, but also with the role of immune complexes and mechanisms mimicking autoimmune diseases. Most of these mechanisms are either dependent on, or amplified by, complement. It should be stressed that polymorphonuclear (PMN) leukocytes, but not, as would be expected, lymphocytes, are usually involved in reactions induced by complement-fixing antibodies (see Chapter D II 1 b and Fig. 6c).

1. Morphology of Complement-Dependent Immune Cytolysis

Transplantation of organs to a presensitized host results in an immediate contact of the vascular endothelium as the main target with a large amount of complement-fixing antibody (see Chapter D I). Under these circumstances the reaction can be explosive (DIXON, 1971a), as demonstrated *in vitro*: upon treatment with immune gamma globulin plus complement, virtually all Krebs ascites tumor cells displayed remarkable cytoplasmic swelling after less than 2 minutes (GOLDBERG and GREEN, 1959, 1960). After 15 to 20 minutes the normal cytoplasmic organization was disrupted, there was a moderate to marked degree of vacuolar change and swelling of membrane-bound structures. Ribosomes were liberated into the incubation medium by passage across an obviously continuous cell membrane. Fragmentation of swollen cells yielded large numbers of membrane-bound spheres derived from segments of the cell surface. The cytoplasmic membrane of cellular ghosts appeared to be coated by a small rim of an amorphous substance. Although coated membranes of erythrocytic ghosts were also observed upon treatment with hemolytic antibody, but not after hypotonic lysis (JERUSALEM and ELING, 1969), it remains to be shown whether the associated amorphous substance represents the attached antibody-complement complex. Cell lysis was not observed in the presence of inactivated complement (GOLDBERG and GREEN, 1959). Compared with the manifestations of cell-mediated cytotoxicity, changes resulting from complement-dependent immune cytolysis appear to be more dramatic, and vacuolar changes are more obvious. These results are consistent with endothelial changes observed in several instances of hyperacute graft rejection (see Chapter D II).

2. Relationship Between Immune Complexes and Clotting

Antigen-antibody reactions usually result in the formation of immune complexes, which either remain fixed to the antigen-bearing tissue component or circulate, if the antigen is a component of the circulating blood. In the presence of complement, very low concentrations of immune complexes can induce the aggregation of platelets. Subsequently a number of biologically active constituents are liberated from disintegrating thrombocytes, and the chain reaction of clotting events is initiated, ultimately resulting in the various features of intravascular coagulation (local and generalized Shwartzman reaction). The general consensus of opinion is that the hyperacute reaction (see Section D) and probably also the delayed hyperacute rejection of kidney grafts are an expression of this mechanism (see Section E).

Thus, although immunologic injury to the vascular endothelium promotes and enhances clotting mechanisms alternatively and/or additively (HUME, 1971), microthrombosis can on occasion be observed without detectable endothelial damage (SHARMA *et al.*, 1972, 1973) (Fig. 10). RATNOFF (1971) emphasized the influence of the RES on the sequence of clot-promoting events: the platelet-aggregating immune complexes may be handled by macrophages and removed from the circulation. This may explain the rare occurrence of microthrombosis in transplanted livers and lungs after hyperacute (and accelerated) rejection (see Chapter D II 3, 4, Fig. 5).

3. Pathogenesis of Tissue Injury Mediated
by Immune Complexes

When antibodies are evoked by a primary response against tissue-fixed antigens of the transplanted organs, these target structures appear to be the preferred site for an antigen-antibody interaction, e.g. the renal glomerulus and the wall of larger vessels. The tissue damage sometimes develops gradually, increasing as the amount of antibodies increases, though apparently dependent on the type of antibody. Non-complement-fixing IgG antibodies apparently produce relatively mild injury (DIXON, 1971a), and the reparative-proliferative reponse may be more the obvious (see Section G). Antibodies of the IgG class and/or complement have frequently been demonstrated by means of immunofluorescent techniques in rejected kidneys (LINDQUIST et al., 1968b; ROSENAU et al., 1969; BUSCH et al., 1969) heart (BIEBER et al., 1970; ROSSEN et al., 1971), and liver (PORTER, 1969), and IgM antibody in kidneys (MCKENZIE and WHITTINGHAM, 1968; VAN BREDA-VRIESMAN, 1972) and also in lungs (FUJIMARA et al., 1970; SUZUKI et al., 1973). Circulating lymphotoxins sedimenting exclusively at 19S were most abundant in sera from human cardiac allograft recipients who died of infection (ROSSEN et al., 1971). The nonspecific trapping of circulating complexes in structures that function as physiologic filters, in particular within the glomerulus (MARKHAM et al., 1973), appears to play a minor role in the pathogenesis of the post-transplantation injury. Diffuse glomerular changes observed after administration of ALS (THIEL et al., 1971; WILSON et al., 1971) appear to result from antibodies directed against common basement membrane antigens present in these preparations. True autoimmunity is involved if the antibody reacts against natural tissue- or organspecific antigens, e.g. in patients redeveloping ("recurrent") glomerulonephritis after transplantation of a kidney isograft from their identical twin (GLASSOCK et al., 1968) or secondarily in the transplant lung syndrome observed after kidney allograft rejection (SLAPAK et al., 1968; TISON and BARUZZI, 1969).

The involvement of pulmonary vessels by antiglomerular antibody was explained by the presence of antigenic determinants common to both glomerular and pulmonary basement membranes (SEEGAL et al., 1955; READ, 1958; MERCOLA and HAGADORN, 1973).

C. Pathways of Host Sensitization

I. Cellular Mechanisms (see Fig. 3)

1. Central Reactions

In lymph nodes draining the site of skin allografts and contact sensitivity reactions, an immunoblast reaction occurs preferentially in the thymus-dependent (PARROTT et al., 1966) paracortical areas (SCOTHORNE and MCGREGOR, 1955; TURK and STONE, 1963; DE SOUSA and PARROTT, 1969). In the spleen of rats bearing liver and kidney allografts, both the thymus-dependent periarteriolar

lymphatic sheath (PALS) and the marginal zone increase distinctly, while follicular structures appear to decrease in size. The immunoblast reaction in thymus-
dependent areas may represent the specific cellular reaction (Veldman, 1970;
Nieuwenhuis, 1971) of delayed-type hypersensitivity (De Petris et al., 1966).
Following subcutaneous or intravenous administration of antigens capable of
evoking humoral responses, the corticomedullary border of lymph nodes and
the marginal zone cells of splenic follicles appear to be the preferential site
for plasma cell proliferation (Oort and Turk, 1965; Nieuwenhuis, 1971). However, after rat liver and kidney allotransplantation, plasma cells can be shown
to differentiate in the medullary cords of mesenteric lymph nodes and to be
randomly distributed throughout the splenic red pulp. The germinal center
(follicular center) reaction appears to be coupled to the antibody response,
rather than to the cell-mediated reaction (reviewed by Veldman, 1970), although
normal antibody responses have been observed in the absence of germinal centers
(Keuning et al., 1963; Diener and Nossal, 1966). In rats splenic germinal
centers largely disappear by 3 to 5 days after liver and kidney allotransplantation,
but reappear when the graft ist resorbed. This may support the hypothesis
that germinal center cells are concerned in the production of secondary antibody-
forming ("memory") cell precursors (Thorbecke et al., 1964; Thorbecke, 1969;
Wakefield and Thorbecke, 1968a, b).

2. Recirculation of Immunocompetent Cells

Recirculating lymphocytes appear to play a particular role in organ transplantation. The majority of thoracic duct small lymphocytes are not newly formed
cells, but cells recirculating from the blood through the lymph nodes into the
efferent lymphatics and back via the thoracic duct to the blood (Gowans,
1959; Gowans and Knight, 1964). These recirculating cells have a long life
span (Little et al., 1962) and are immunologically competent (Gowans et al.,
1962; Miller, 1965), and there is some relationship between the thymus and
the pool of recirculating small (T) lymphocytes (Miller and Mitchell, 1969;
Miller, 1974). However, the immediate effect of adult thymectomy on modification of the immune response is poor in adult animals (McLean et al., 1957;
Miller, 1962; Claman et al., 1968), although thymectomy has led to a fall
in the lymphocyte population of the blood, thoracic duct lymph and lymphoid
tissues (Bierring, 1960; Metcalf, 1960). Essentially the same results were obtained with children beyond the neonatal stage, who were thymectomized on
the occasion of corrective heart surgery and simultaneously treated with a skin
allograft (Zollinger et al., 1964).

Thus, beyond the neonatal stage the thymus-dependent areas of peripheral
lymphatic organs and the pool of recirculating lymphocytes appear to represent
a system with a certain functional and proliferatory autonomy, in which the
thymus acts as a facultative stem cell source demonstrable in instances of rapid
loss of recirculating lymphocytes, e.g. after prolonged and continuous drainage
of the thoracic duct and after sublethal total-body irradiation with thymus
shielding (Mulder, 1972). Although the majority of recirculating lymphocytes
are cells competent for the transplantation reaction, and large proportions of

cells of the thymus-dependent areas belong to the recirculating pool (GOWANS and MCGREGOR, 1965; GREAVES et al., 1973; OWEN, 1974), repletion of lymphoid follicles has been observed following local irradiation of lymph nodes and subsequent infusion of the full complement of blood lymphocytes (BOS, 1967). Since this follicular reconstitution was specifically associated with the return of antibody responsiveness, it was concluded that the follicle-repleting (short-lived) B-lymphocytes are present in abundance in both the blood and the thoracic duct lymph (HOWARD, 1972; HOWARD et al., 1972). With recirculating B-cells, the occurrence of plasma cells and their precursors in various organ grafts can easily be explained (see also Chapter A III, c, β, γ).

The massive recirculation of lymphocytes appears to fulfill a dual function closely related to both the theory of peripheral sensitization to organ grafts (MEDAWAR, 1958) and the theory of central sensitization by passenger leukocytes (SNELL, 1957; STROBER and GOWANS, 1965). Recirculating lymphocytes seem to be an effective means of interaction with those antigens which do not enter immunocompetent tissues, e.g. those of organ grafts (ROWLEY et al., 1972; SPRENT et al., 1971). Then, by recirculating, sensitized lymphocytes may be disseminated to the various peripheral lymphatic organs. Surgicomechanical depletion of the host pool of recirculating lymphocytes via a thoracic duct fistula prevents both experimental skin allograft (MCGREGOR and GOWANS, 1964) and human renal allograft rejection for certain periods (IRVIN and CARBONE, 1967; MURRAY et al., 1968; SARLES et al., 1970). In various species, including man (SARLES et al., 1967, 1970) dog, and rat, prolonged diversion of thoracic duct lymph results in distinct depletion of the thymus-dependent paracortical areas and also of the follicular lymphocytic corona, leaving the germinal centers isolated. It is not known whether "resident" (noncirculating) T-lymphocytes are also decreased in number. These cells may have a helper function, since prolonged thoracic duct drainage does not inhibit secondary T-cell-dependent humoral responses (MCGREGOR and GOWANS, 1964). Under normal conditions, recirculating T-cells enter the paracortex of lymph nodes via the "epitheloid" postcapillary venules (GOWANS and KNIGHT, 1964; NIEUWENHUIS, 1971). After passing through the thymus-dependent areas they leave the lymph node via the efferent lymphatics and return to the blood via the thoracic duct (OWEN, 1974). Recirculating B-cells have the ability to home in on B-dependent follicular structures (BOS, 1967). In contrast, the majority of recirculating T-cells entering the lymph node via the efferent lymphatics (e.g. after tissue passages) were found to remain intrasinusal, even in those adjacent to follicles (PATTENGALE et al., 1972). Higher extra- to intrasinusal ratios were found with peripheral blood leukocytes (ELVES, 1970) and cells generated by a local intradermal immune response, which occasionally entered the follicular corona (KELLEY, 1970). It is important to be aware that antigens, too, are trapped, particularly in the outer follicular zone of the lymph node (NOSSAL et al., 1964, 1965). In the spleen both the antigen (NOSSAL et al., 1965, 1966) and recirculating T-cells appear to leave the circulating blood via the perifollicular capillaries, and are immediately trapped in the marginal zone (FORD, 1969). T-lymphocytes never enter follicular structures, but migrate within one to two days to the perifollicular sheaths (GOWANS and KNIGHT, 1964; NIEUWENHUIS, 1971). Whether these cells leave the spleen *via* periarteriolar lymphatics (MEDZIHRADSKY, 1958; KELLNER, 1963) or the sinuses of the red pulp is uncertain. Whereas the thymus was not the target of administered isologous thoracic duct lymphocytes (GOWANS and KNIGHT, 1964), lymphoid cells from lymph nodes draining a skin graft were present in small numbers, accumulating to some extent in the corticomedullary junctional region (GALTON and REED, 1966).

II. Pathways of Sensitization to Solid Organ Grafts (see Fig. 3)

It can be assumed that for the initiation of a transplantation reaction, the antigens of the graft have to be brought into intimate association with immunocompetent cells of the host. The pathways of sensitization to solid organ grafts appear to differ from those to cellular grafts and skin grafts. Intravenously administered cells are distributed *via* the general circulation and sensitize the host centrally. Tissue grafts are primarily not revascularized, but are in close contact with the lymphatic capillaries of the surrounding tissue. Extended wound areas stimulate lymphatic flow, suggesting an important role of the lymph nodes draining the sites of implantation. In contrast, solid organ grafts are primarily vascularized, but lack significant lymphatic drainage, at least during the first weeks after transplantation. In small bowel autografts new growth of lymphatics across the line of repair of resected mesentery was demonstrated after 2 weeks,

---

Fig. 3. Cellular pathways of host sensitization. *Skin graft.* Unprimed lymphocytes leave blood ▷ capillaries supplying wound area and become sensitized through contact with graft antigens. They enter the draining lymph node via afferent lymphatic capillaries (LC_1) and may migrate into both the cortical (B_1) and paracortical areas (T). However, the majority of sensitized cells apparently remains within the sinuses, and contact with sinusal (reticular) macrophages (M) appears to be a crucial step in induction of a proliferative response of effector cells in thymus-dependent paracortical area (T). This is also the pathway for soluble as well as macrophage-processed antigens, but not for recirculating sensitized lymphocytes and passenger cells, which enter lymph node via postcapillary venules (PV). Although recirculating sensitized lymphocytes home directly in thymus-dependent paracortical area (T), a host-*vs*-graft reaction is hardly triggered. Potential effector cells return via thoracic duct (TD) to general circulation, and transform into killer cells within the graft upon a second signal.

Organ graft. Unprimed lymphocytes become sensitized upon contacting endothelial surfaces or migrating through extracellular space. Emigrated host lymphocytes either leave the graft as passenger cells via general circulation after re-entering blood capillaries or remain in interstices, since their normal route of return—the organdraining lymphatics—has been sacrificed ($LC_{2\ x}$). Sensitized lymphocytes arrive in splenic lymphatic tissue via marginal capillaries (MC) between follicular corona (C) and marginal zone (MZ). This region is rich in fixed macrophages (M) and, in contrast to the lymph node, represents the joint entrance gate for sensitized and recirculating lymphocytes, and passenger cells, as well as for soluble and macrophage-processed antigens. The lymphatic sheath is the site of the proliferative response of potential effector cells which leave the spleen for the general circulation probably via the sinuses and transform into killer cells as the result of a second signal while entering the grafted organ. Sensitization of host via regional lymphatics (LC_3) and regional lymph nodes draining site of organ implantation (peritoneal and pleural cavity, mediastinum) is only an additional, secondary pathway. However, in case of prevention from regional lymphatic drainage, splenectomy delays or even inhibits graft rejection, although recirculating sensitized lymphocytes and passenger cells are allowed to enter thymus-dependent areas of distant lymph nodes (see above: skin grafts)

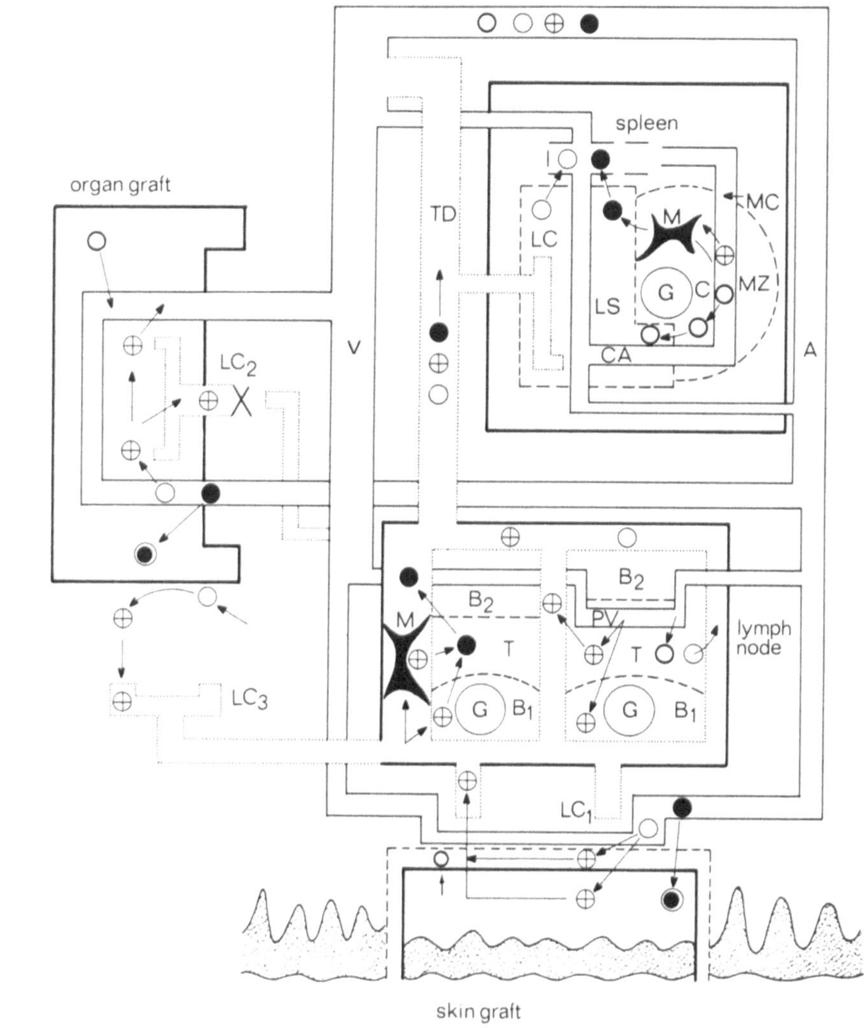

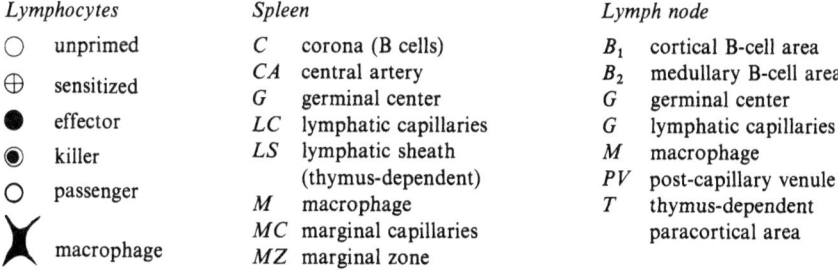

TD thoracic duct, *A* arterial system, *V* venous system

Lymphocytes		Spleen		Lymph node	
○	unprimed	*C*	corona (B cells)	*B₁*	cortical B-cell area
⊕	sensitized	*CA*	central artery	*B₂*	medullary B-cell area
●	effector	*G*	germinal center	*G*	germinal center
◉	killer	*LC*	lymphatic capillaries	*G*	lymphatic capillaries
○	passenger	*LS*	lymphatic sheath	*M*	macrophage
			(thymus-dependent)	*PV*	post-capillary venule
✶	macrophage	*M*	macrophage	*T*	thymus-dependent
		MC	marginal capillaries		paracortical area
		MZ	marginal zone		

and after 1 month spontaneous lymphatic anastomoses enabled fat absorption to proceed normally (LILLEHEI et al., 1959a; GOOTT et al., 1960; KOCANDRLE et al., 1966). Complete interstitial lymphatic regeneration from 5 months to one year postoperatively was demonstrated by ALICAN et al. (1971). After bilateral lung autotransplantation and lung hilar stripping, recanalization of lymphatics was found to occur after 2 to 4 weeks (HARDY et al., 1963; WAGENVOORT et al., 1973). Thus, the spleen may be considered to be the main draining lymphatic organ of transplanted organs, at least during the initial period of antigenic recognition. However, passenger leukocytes, i.e. mobile cells of donor origin accompanying the graft, may sensitize a host centrally, like cellular grafts. Although MEDAWAR (1958) voiced reservations against any attempt at regarding the reaction to skin grafts as norms for reactions to grafts in general, it appears advantageous to discuss the possible pathway of host sensitization to organ grafts as outlined for tissue homotransplantation and contact sensitivity (SNELL, 1957; DE SOUSA and PARROTT, 1969).

1. Soluble Antigens

It might be supposed that soluble isoantigens or tissue-specific or differentiation antigens pass in solution to lymph nodes or spleen. One factor that seems inconsistent with this supposition is the insolubility of the major transplantation antigens (KANDUTSCH and REINERT-WENK, 1957). However, antigens other than histocompatibility antigens appear to provoke immune responses (SELA, 1973). Most of the tissue-specific and differentiation antigens are also insoluble, and the soluble ones are accessible for immunological recognition only upon mild cytolysis or tissue damage. Furthermore, the type of antigen appears to influence the type of immune response. In human recipients of kidney transplants the macrophage inhibitory factor, but not the blast cell transformation factor, was stimulated by organ-specific antigens, whereas histocompatibility antigens provoke the elaboration of both (MELNICK and FRIEDMAN, 1971). Injection of heterologous serum albumin stimulated the production of antibody but no detectable delayed-type hypersensitivity. In contrast, serum albumin heavily conjugated with an immunologically indifferent lipid resulted in sustained delayed-type hypersensitivity but did not stimulate antibody formation (COON and HUNTER, 1973). This change in type of immune response was associated with a change in the area of antigen localization in the draining lymph node. Whereas native albumin was localized in the germinal centers, lipid-conjugated antigen accumulated predominantly in the T-cell areas and not in the germinal centers. Protein-lipid combinations may be possible in skin transplantation, since, unlike the cornea and most internal organs, the skin biosynthesizes and excretes unusual fat-soluble substances (NICOLAIDES, 1974). Type II alveolar cells were also considered to be the source of surfactant, a saturated phospholipid, in the lungs (MACKLIN, 1954; WANG et al., 1971; HARRISON and WEIBEL, 1968); Clara cells may be an alternative source of this substance (NIDEN, 1967). Antiserum to isolated, soluble pulmonary surface-active material revealed activity against three antigenic components, two of which were immunologically identical to serum proteins while the third appeared to be alveolar-specific (KLASS, 1973; SCARPELLI *et al.*, 1973). Surfactant can be transported from the surface to the circulation (DERMER, 1970), and lung allograft rejection is associated early with increased turnover of dipalmitol lecithin, a quantitative indicator for surfactant (DREWS *et al.*, 1974).

In addition to tissue-specific antigens of liver cells (SHEFFIELD and EMMELOT, 1972) and a hepatic lectin (STOCKERT *et al.*, 1974), hepatocytes normally contain actin, and occasionally they exhibit microfilaments resembling those of smooth muscle (GABBIANI *et al.*, 1973). Damage to liver cells can result in the production of antibody reacting particularly with smooth muscle actomyosin (JOHNSON *et al.*, 1965; FARROW *et al.*, 1970, 1971). The smooth muscle antibody reacts also with cells of the renal glomerulus (WHITTINGHAM *et al.*, 1966) and with thymus medullary cells, suggesting that lymphocytes greatly increase their layer of the antigen resembling smooth muscle actomyosin within the membrane during maturation (FAGRAEUS *et al.*, 1973). This may explain why smooth muscle antibody is present in a large majority of patients with a history of infectious mononucleosis (HOLBOROW *et al.*, 1973). It is not yet known whether smooth muscle antibodies can block T-lymphocytes, thus preserving liver grafts and successive kidney grafts from rejection under certain conditions (CALNE *et al.*, 1969), or whether they are responsible for the necrosis of the vascular media in several types of late rejections (BUSCH *et al.*, 1969).

The importance for skin grafts of the included serum proteins in the immune response has been emphasized (KRAKOWER and GREENSPAN, 1973), since tissue antigens such as protein-dermaten sulfate, heavy and light protein-mucopolysaccharides, and nonstructural glycoproteins were less effective in accelerated rejection. Remarkable concentrations of autologous serum albumin were detected in the lung interstitium, endothelial cells, and type I alveolar epithelial cells (BIGNON *et al.*, 1975). The processing of collagen for immunologic recognition may be facilitated by macrophages observed in tissue and organ grafts (BILSKI and JERUSALEM, 1969; JAP, 1971). Certain tissue-specific antigens appear to trigger humoral immune response to solid organ grafts. Three out of nine rat cardiac proteins were antigenic for rabbits (CHATURVEDI *et al.*, 1973). Circulating heart-reactive antibody was detected in patients who exhibited histologic evidence of cardiac rejection at the time of death (DALLOCCHIO *et al.*, 1970; ELLIS *et al.*, 1970a, b; BIEBER *et al.*, 1970).

2. Macrophage-Processed Antigen

A second mechanism involves macrophage-processed cell debris, and stresses the importance of draining lymphatic organs in peripheral sensitization. Since the afferent lymph of lymph nodes draining the site of skin homografts, or contact sensitivity reactions, contained very few lymphocytes but numerous macrophages (HALL, 1967), and the thymus-dependent areas exhibited a blast cell reaction (OORT and TURK, 1965), it was concluded that sensitization to skin grafts occurs within lymph nodes (BARKER and BILLINGHAM, 1967). In contrast, in neonatally thymectomized mice which failed to develop contact sensitivity, blast cell transformation was absent, although the marginal sinus was also stuffed with macrophages (DE SOUSA and PARROTT, 1969). Since surgically revascularized solid organ grafts initially have no significant lymphatic drainage, the host becomes sensitized *via* the general circulation. Renal homografts isolated from the regional lymphatics by a plastic bag were rejected in a manner indistinguishable from that observed in controls (Hume and Egdahl, 1955), and regional lymphadenectomy failed to prolong the survival time of kidney homotransplants (Knox *et al.*, 1964). Thus, the draining organ of the circulating blood, i.e. the spleen, appears to play the central role in host sensitization to renal allografts. Although there were indications in recipients receiving a related kidney that splenectomy resulted in a higher proportion of transplants functioning for longer periods than in control groups (Gleason and Murray, 1967; Pierce and Hume, 1968; Tinbergen, 1971), clinical splenectomy in association with renal transplantation has been abandoned because of harmful side effects such as increased risk of sepsis and reduced tolerance to drugs (Veith *et al.*, 1965).

In contrast, recent studies in our laboratory have revealed that in addition to the spleen, lymph nodes draining the area of operation (not the graft itself) occasionally also become sensitized. One day after rat liver allotransplantation, intermediate sinuses of mesenteric lymph nodes were stuffed with macrophages, and by 4 days a proliferative response of the paracortical areas was observed. Obviously "virgin" immunocompetent cells (among others peritoneal macrophages) migrated into the peritoneal cavity due to irritation of the peritoneal membrane by the operating procedure, and sensitized cells returned via the mesenteric lymphatics to the lymph nodes. In rats carrying liver isografts, accumulations of macrophages were seen in the mesenteric lymph nodes, but no proliferation response of T-cell areas. The proliferative response was more obvious in the liver allograft than in the kidney allograft model, suggesting that the size of the graft and exudation *via* the liver capsule have some influence. This may explain both the wide range of individual survival of rat kidney allografts in splenectomized recipients (although the mean survival time was increased by about 580 percent; Tinbergen, 1971) and also the significantly prolonged survival of skin allografts following the removal of regional lymph nodes (Stark *et al.*, 1960), which contrasts with the inability of splenectomy to preserve skin grafts from rejection (Veith *et al.*, 1965; Haller *et al.*, 1966).

3. Peripheral Sensitization

The concept of peripheral sensitization (as opposed to central) was first suggested by Medawar (1958) and has been largely confirmed by *in vitro* and *in vivo* perfusion experiments (Strober and Gowans, 1965) and by spontaneous transformation of lymphocytes collected from capsular lymphatic ducts of human kidney allografts (Hamburger *et al.*, 1971). Furthermore, a "minimal contact time" was postulated as necessary to initiate a transplantation reaction by repeated passages of lymphocytes through the vascular bed, rather than through the parenchyma of kidney allografts. With thoracic duct lymphocytes this period was found to be about one hour *in vitro*. *In vivo* the graft had to be linked to the circulation for 5–12 hours. Thus, the lymphocytes shown to contact endothelial surfaces of human kidney allografts soon after revascularization

(KOUNTZ *et al.*, 1963; PORTER, 1965; FELDMAN and LEE, 1967) may be cells of the afferent arc of the immune response. Systematic electron microscope studies in our laboratory on canine lung allografts revealed an increase in the number of small lymphocytes 30 to 60 minutes after revascularization within alveolar capillaries with increasing histoincompatibility, except in instances of impending hyperacute rejection, where polymorphonuclear cells were more numerous.

4. Passenger Leukocytes

SNELL (1957) suggested a fourth fundamental pathway of host sensitization: "passenger leukocytes", i.e. the various types of nucleated blood cells and mobile cellular elements from the soft connective tissue, particularly lymphocytes that accompany the graft from the donor, may pass directly to the lymph nodes *via* the lymphatic vessels and to the spleen *via* the general circulation. The effectiveness of lymphoid tissue in evoking immune responses to subsequent grafts has long been known (WOGLOM, 1929), and the antigenicity of kidney and liver was drastically reduced when the lymphoid elements of the donor were destroyed by lymphocytolytic agents (STOERK, 1953). Since lymphocytes appear to be relatively abundant in the skin (HAGERMAN, 1954; MCCREIGHT and ANDREW, 1956), serum of rats rejecting skin allografts displays donor-specific antilymphocyte activity (WOODRUFF and FORMAN, 1950). The majority of passenger leukocytes appear to be long-lived recirculating T-lymphocytes (see Chapter C I 2). In chickens, T-cells are found to be eight times more antigenic than the lymphocytes of the bursa (FORGET *et al.*, 1970). However, mouse lymphoid cell populations enriched for either B- or T-lymphocytes were equally immunogenic *in vitro*, but were about 20–40 times more immunogenic than fibroblasts (WAGNER and WYSS, 1973). About one million lymphocytes can both stimulate transplantation immunity by the intraperitoneal route (BILLINGHAM *et al.*, 1957, 1959) and raise an effective ALS (GOZZO *et al.*, 1971). These numbers are clearly available in grafts which are prepared for transplantation by simple flushing and cool storing; only a specially developed asanguineous perfusion washed out 98 percent of blood cells from heart grafts (O'CONNELL *et al.*, 1974). There have been various attempts to remove allogenic passenger leukocytes from grafts, e.g. by total-body irradiation of the donor and local irradiation of the kidney graft (HUME *et al.*, 1960; TINBERGEN, 1971), pretreatment of the donor rat for kidney and heart grafts with ATS/ALS and cytotoxic drugs such as cyclophosphamide (GUTTMANN *et al.*, 1967a; GUTTMANN and LINDQUIST, 1969; FREEMAN *et al.*, 1971), intensive perfusion of lung and heart grafts of dogs (IWAHASHI *et al.*, 1972; O'CONNELL *et al.*, 1974), and replacement of the hemopoietic system in radiation-chimeric donors with bone marrow of recipient specificity (STUART *et al.*, 1971). These experiments confirmed that removal and/or destruction of allogenic passenger leukocytes delayed the onset of rejection significantly but did not prevent it.

Furthermore, passenger leukocytes alone are sufficient to stimulate rejection, and the rejection process ensues when the hematopoietic system in chimeric donors of kidney transplants is genetically different from that of the recipient, even when the organ parenchyma is compatible (ELKINS and GUTTMANN, 1968). In these instances target cell destruction appears to be mediated by mechanisms that are nonspecific in their final effector phase, such as lymphotoxin (A III, 3b) or antibody-dependent cytotoxicity (B III, c). Thus, unexpected immune responses may be caused by antigenic changes of passenger leukocytes. On the occasion of a positive response between siblings displaying HL-A identity, the twin whose lymphocytes caused cytotoxicity in the mixed lymphocyte culture was found to be suffering from a heavy cold (BALFOUR et al., 1972).

In some sinstances, passenger lymphocytes accompanying cadaver donor kidneys with previously existing pathology appeared to undergo proliferation and produced a localized graft-vs-host (GVH) reaction (ENDE, 1974). Absence of the characteristic picture of rejection and death from a vigorous GVH reaction in the recipient was regularly seen when large segments of the small bowel were allografted to unmodified or modified hosts (LILLEHEI et al., 1959a, b; RUIZ et al., 1972). In contrast to the above findings, short (10–15 cm) segments of ileal allografts were normally rejected (LILLEHEI and MANAX, 1966). This suggests that the induction of a GVH reaction depends on the number of escaping passenger leukocytes. Atypical rejection patterns in small bowel allografts (20 cm), i.e. the accumulation of PMN cells in the absence of round-cell infiltrations (BARNETT et al., 1962), indicate complement-dependent antibody-mediated reactions, probably by host ALS production to passenger leukocytes (WOODRUFF and FORMAN, 1950; see also Chapter B II, 6). Although lungs exhibited substantial amounts of autochthonous lymphatic tissue, GVH reaction is not the logical consequence of pulmonary allotransplantation since the majority of pulmonary-associated lymphocytes appear to be of the B-type (KALTREIDER and SALMON, 1973). However, atypical rejection patterns are also frequently encountered in lung transplantation (VEITH et al., 1972a, b; HAGLIN et al., 1973).

D. Hyperacute Rejection

I. Pathogenesis

Hyperacute immunologic rejection ("violent immediate rejection", "accelerated graft rejection"), defined as the disastrous loss of a transplanted organ immediately after revascularization ("rejection on the operating table"), has been studied extensively, including rejection of xenotransplants, since xenograft and allograft rejection may be mediated by essentially the same mechanisms (WEIL and REEMTSMA, 1974). Particular attention was paid to renal transplants, because it was thought that the course of histopathologic events was similar to those occurring in other solid organ grafts, although functional consequences might be organ-specific to varying degrees (BIEBER et al., 1970). These generalizations are now known to be inaccurate.

The immediate loss of kidney grafts was first (although not invariably) seen when donor and recipient belonged to different ABO red cell groups

(STARZL, 1964; STARZL *et al.*, 1964a). A rational explanation was available, since it was possible to demonstrate the blood group antigen A and B on cells of human liver, lung, kidney and heart (HOGMAN, 1959; SZULMAN, 1960). Subsequently, it was generally accepted that the rules applicable to blood transfusion in man also apply to the transplantation of organs (JOYSEY *et al.*, 1973). In dogs, however, the A antigen cannot be demonstrated on erythrocytes, although dog sera exhibit both anti-A and anti-B activity and dogs secrete blood group substances in their sputum (SLEE *et al.*, 1972); Swisher blood groups appear to be present in beagles (FERREBEE *et al.*, 1970). However, hyperacute rejection of renal allografts has also been observed in the absence of "naturally occurring" (CALNE, 1963; CLARK *et al.*, 1964) red cell isoantibodies (TERASAKI *et al.*, 1965; WILLIAMS *et al.*, 1967). In these instances patients exhibited preformed heterospecific lymphocytotoxic antibodies (KISSMEYER–NIELSEN *et al.*, 1966; WILLIAMS *et al.*, 1968), or heterospecific cytotoxins (PERPER and NAJARIAN, 1966a; GILES *et al.*, 1970). Natural antibodies of surprising specificity occurring in most animal species including man were described as early as 1930 by GIBSON. Subsequently, various naturally occurring and heterospecific antibodies (abbreviated to "NOHA"; WILDEVUUR *et al.*, 1973b) were demonstrated in cytotoxicity cross-match techniques. However, not all recipients who have NOHA's to the donor's lymphocytes experience violent rejection (PATEL and TERASAKI, 1969); on the other hand several allografts were hyperacutely rejected although the recipient's serum was not cytotoxic to the donor's lymphocytes (STARZL *et al.*, 1968). This suggests that NOHA's may not only be directed against transplantation antigens, but can also react with differentiation antigens, e.g. the "natural (anti-Θ) thymocytic antibody" (PARKER *et al.*, 1974) and tissue antigens, e.g. pre-existing heart-reactive antibodies (ELLIS *et al.*, 1970b). Therefore, the ideal target cell for cross-match purposes might be the endothelial cell (DE PLANQUE *et al.*, 1971).

The most common causes of recipient sensitization are a blood transfusion administered during the weeks before transplantation (CARPENTER and WINN, 1969; SPECK, 1975), and the rejection of a previous graft. Multiple pregnancies can induce the production of antibodies to red cell antigens and to white cell isoantigens in about 25 percent of cases (ZMIJEWSKI *et al.*, 1967). In addition, placenta and kidney share common antigens (SEEGAL *et al.*, 1955), and at least enhancing (cytophilic) auto-antibodies against the trophoblast can be expected in pregnancy (V.D. WERF, 1972). Particular attention was focused on the reaction of antibody independent of ABO and Forssman with the vascular endothelium in chronic pulmonary tuberculosis and toxoplasmosis (KREISLER *et al.*, 1971; LINDQUIST and OSTERLAND, 1971), on heterospecific cytolysis of cells originating from Forssman-positive species, cytotoxic activity of infectious mononucleosis sera (KANO and MILGROM, 1971), and the cross-reaction between streptococcal proteins and human transplantation antigens (HIRATA and TERASAKI, 1970). THOMPSON *et al.* (1973) showed changes in the antigenic nature of lymphocytes caused by common viruses, such as influenza A2, herpes simplex type 1, and adenovirus type 2, which may account both for anomalous reactions in mixed lymphocyte cultures and for the unexpected hyperacute rejection after the transplantation of a kidney from an HL-A identical sibling suffering from a viral infection. The presence and specificity of NOHA's was confirmed in most cases by inference, since the actual quantities of immunoglobulins picked up by the new organ may be too small for antibody localization by immunofluorescent assay (Carpenter and Merrill, 1969; Giles *et al.*, 1970). Thus, in general the various antidonor antibodies were demonstrated by preoperative *in vitro* testing and their clearance by organs of this donor (and not of any other) subsequent to transplantation, or by prolonged survival of the last organ of a series of successively transplanted kidneys from the same donor, or by specific absorption through administration of donor-specific erythrocyte stroma (Linn *et al.*, 1968; Mozes *et al.*, 1971; Giles *et al.*, 1970). However, not only circulating autochthonous antibodies can cause hyperacute rejection. When rat renal autografts were perfused *ex vivo* with heterologous ALS, revascularization was followed by immediate thrombosis and cortical necrosis (Collste, 1971). We have also observed the violent rejection of canine renal autografts after perfusion with pooled dog serum. The speed of xeno- and allograft rejection appears to be a function of both previous sensitization and the degree of species or individual disparity (Weil and Reemtsma, 1974). When pig kidneys were transplanted to dogs rejection was ten times more rapid than when dog kidney grafts were revascularized in pigs (Perper and Najarian, 1966a). However, hyperacute rejection is not the inevitable consequence of xenotransplantation between closely related species, e.g. between sheep and goat (Perper and Najarian, 1966b). Furthermore, chimpanzee and baboon kidney heterografts functioned for one to nine months in human patients (Reemtsma *et al.*, 1964; Cortesini, 1967). Autopsy findings revealed either minimal changes (Cortesini, 1967) or pronounced cellular infiltration (Porter, 1964; Porter *et al.*, 1965). In most instances of hyperacute rejection complement was found to be essential for the final cytolytic event (Clark *et al.*, 1965; McDowall *et al.*, 1973). It is activated by the Fc fragment of the NOHA bound to the target. Prolongation of the survival of xenografts was achieved by inactivation of circulating complement by means of the administration of aggregated Ig and cobra venom (Clark *et al.*, 1966; Gewurz *et al.*, 1966; Snyder *et al.*, 1966). However, when dogs were sensitized by multiple skin grafts, the hyperacute rejection of kidney allografts could not be delayed by treatment with the anticomplementary factor Co F (Kobayashi *et al.*, 1971). Furthermore, all patients with a positive lymphocytotoxic test had a positive indirect fluorescent antibody reaction against arterial tissue. This antibody is distinct from the cytotoxic antibody and is not complement-dependent (Cerilli *et al.*, 1972).

II. Pathology of the Hyperacute Rejection

Although a large body of work has established the role of NOHA's in the pathogenesis of hyperacute rejection, it appears unwarranted in our present state of knowledge to relate the pattern of pathologic alteration to a particular causative factor, and to make a direct comparison of changes observed in hyperacutely rejected kidneys with those in other organ grafts lost on the operating table.

1. Kidney

a) Course of Events

CALNE (1963) gave a classic description. Immediately after revascularization the xenograft turned a normal color, but within a few minutes the cortex had a mottled appearance and became increasingly cyanotic, and the blood flow ceased almost completely. Microscopic examination revealed interstitial edema, disruption of cortical vessels, and numerous hemorrhages. This report includes the two main, and representative, features of hyperacute graft rejection: (i) the rapidly increasing vascular permeability with profuse extravasation of corpuscular and noncorpuscular blood constituents; (ii) the spontaneous devascularization. Subsequent to the first detailed analyses of this course of events (KISS-MEYER–NIELSEN et al., 1966; PORTER et al., 1967; KINCAID–SMITH, 1969) an increasing number of studies have dealt in particular with the mechanisms of intravascular coagulation pointing out the similarity of the renal lesion to those observed in the Arthus phenomenon and the Shwartzman reaction (STARZL et al., 1968; MYBURGH et al., 1969; MEJIA–LAGUNA et al., 1972). Four phases are distinguishable, which largely overlap and may differ with respect to the mechanisms involved, though the variations appear to be largely quantitative.

During the first phase (1 to 5 min) the vascular endothelium appears to be the preferred target of NOHA's (GEWURZ et al., 1966; WILLIAMS et al., 1968; DE PLANQUE et al., 1971). Immediately after revascularization the endothelial cells are swollen and may exhibit an increase of pinocytotic vesicles and a great number of vacuoles of various sizes. Subsequently, disruption of the cytoplasm and the cytoplasmic membrane, with lifting off the cell surface from the basement membrane ("arcading") becomes obvious. In a second phase (2–10 min), increasing numbers of platelets aggregate, first within arterioles and then mainly within peritubular capillaries. At places where endothelial damage has taken place the basement membrane can become disrupted and marked edema develops in the interstitial space, manifested by distinct separation of collagen fibrils. Platelet pseudopods have been seen touching and/or extending through the vascular endothelium, and platelets exhibit the first signs of degranulation. Although it is generally thought that microthrombosis results from adherence of platelets to created rough surfaces of damaged endothelial cells (HUME, 1971), in systematic studies aggregated thrombocytes were noted before any evidence of injury of the capillary endothelium was detectable. When graft survival was prolonged by treatment with azathioprine (LÖWENHAUPT et al., 1971) and with the platelet inhibitor sulfinpyrazone (SHARMA et al., 1972), the initial endothelial lesion in capillaries was minimal.

During the first and second phases there is an almost complete sequestration of platelets within the graft, and within a few minutes large quantities of white and red cells are also retained; ultimately complement and clotting factors fail to be discharged into the venous outflow (GEWURZ et al., 1966; GILES et al., 1970).

The third phase (10–30 min) is characterized by further degranulation of platelets, progressive fibrin deposits even in glomerular capillaries, and extravasation of red cells due to progressive vascular damage. Immunofluorescent studies also revealed fibrin deposits within the wall of the cortical arterioles, while faint traces of IgG and $\beta 1 C$ were interpreted as the result of protein "trapping" rather than a specific immunologic reaction (STARZL et al., 1968). With the propagation of intravascular coagulation the venous outflow gradually decreases.

The fourth phase (15 min to several hours) is the aggravation of the third one. There is a confluence of focal hemorrhages, finally resulting in total necrosis, particularly of the renal cortex. The organ is almost completely devascularized.

b) Cellular Mechanisms and Mediators Involved in Hyperacute Rejection

The previous paragraph may have made it clear that the final steps of hyperacute rejection of kidney grafts are not necessarily due to the toxic effects of the antibody alone, even though rejection is initiated by these effects. Apart from the immunologically triggered intravascular coagulation, cellular defense mechanisms of the recipient and vasoactive soluble mediators may contribute in varying degrees to the morphologic lesion (BUSCH et al., 1969).

α) It appears important to note that cells involved in hyperacute rejection are *polymorphonuclear neutrophilic leukocytes* (PMN), and not the lymphocytes that would be expected to be involved in primary immunologic reactions (HUME, 1971). Although the presence of PMN cells is not specific, their number is often increased at the time of hyperacute rejection of both xenografts (LINN et al., 1968; MEJIA–LAGUNA et al., 1971) and allografts in animals and man (PORTER et al., 1967; STARZL et al., 1968; LINDQUIST et al., 1968a, b; WEYMOUTH et al., 1970). Prognostic evidence concerning the clinical outcome of renal cadaver allografts was gained from histologic evaluation of the number of PMN cells in the one-hour biopsy (KINCAID–SMITH et al., 1968).

The occurrence of "pavement-like" formations, i.e. the margination of PMN cells in larger vessels is more characteristic than the absolute number (MARCEAU et al., 1965; WILLIAMS et al., 1968). It was suggested that PMN cells adhere to activated antibody(NOHA)-complement complexes at the target cell surfaces by bridge-like and finger-like cytoplasmic processes, and contribute only secondarily to the damage to the lining endothelium, by releasing certain cytotoxic substances (JANOFF, 1970; HUME, 1971). This feature appears to be a specific example of the more general phenomenon of PMN cell infiltration in complement-mediated inflammatory processes, such as the Arthus phenomenon (BIRO, 1966), where complement fixation subsequent to the interaction of antibody with antigen in the wall of blood vessels (COCHRANE, 1965) leads to the accumulation of PMN cells within the vascular wall and the perivascular compartment (LETTERER, 1959; MYBURGH et al., 1969). Thus, a marked decrease in this infiltration was observed upon depletion of C_3 by means of treatment with cobra venom factor (COCHRANE et al., 1970), while the increased survival time of dog-to-rabbit kidney xenografts in leukopenic recipients was related to a diminution of the PMN-to-glomeruli ratio (MEJIA–LAGUNA et al., 1972). However, antibody-induced neutropenia does not prevent the generalized Shwartzman

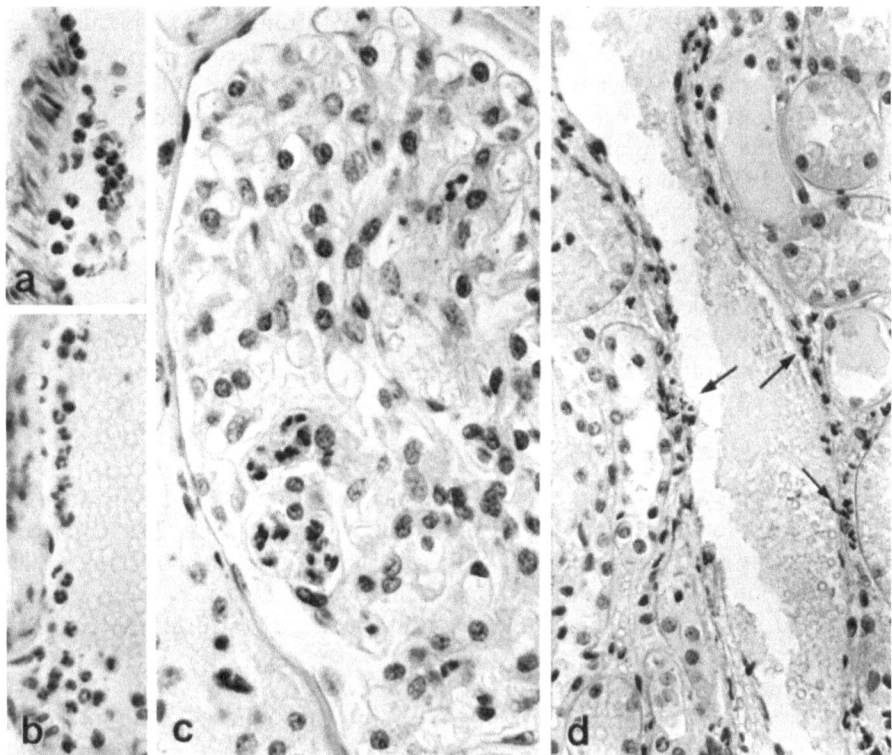

Fig. 4a–d. Canine renal allograft transplanted to sensitized host, 30 min after revascularization. PMN cells stick to damaged endothelial surfaces of cortical arteries (a, b), accumulate in several glomerular capillaries (c), and migrate through damaged wall of cortical veins (arrows, d). Graft was hyperacutely rejected after 2 h. (Hematoxylin and eosin: a, b ×350; PAS reaction: c ×500; d ×250)

reaction (MARGARETTEN and McKAY, 1969), another important component of kidney allograft rejection (Chapter D II a).

In severely damaged grafts it may be difficult to distinguish the pavementing of PMN cells induced by NOHA's from the adherence of white cells to vascular endothelium in instances of damage to the surrounding tissue (rather than to the vessels itself), and/or of stasis. Granulocytes initially adhering to endothelial surfaces were seen not only to pass through the endothelial junctions, but also to cause extensive separation and desquamation of the lining cells with subsequent exposure of subendothelial structures (STEWART et al., 1974). However, ischemic damage to kidney allografts before transplantation and vascular spasm affected neither the PMN cell count nor their pattern of distribution (PERLOFF et al., 1973).

β) *Soluble mediators possible involved in hyperacute graft destruction.* It has been speculated that NOHA's may not immediately destroy the graft because of low affinity for the binding sites, but that they may contribute to a variety of changes that finally lead to the loss of the transplant (KIRKPATRICK and WILSON, 1964). The involvement of additional mechanisms has been suggested, e.g. the production of vasoactive polypeptides by thrombin, plasmin, and Hageman factor, with resultant vasospasm and simple mechanical occlusion of blood vessels (Busch et al., 1969). Surprisingly few studies have called attention to the striking similarity between the circulatory disturbances seen in hyperacute rejection and those in anaphylactic shock, such as increased capillary fragility (Zander, 1937) and perivascular hemorrhage (Cannon et al., 1941), suggesting that mediators of anaphylaxis have an active role in the hyperacute destruction of grafts in presensitized hosts.

In addition, release of C 1 esterase following either antigen-antibody complexing or plasmin activation leads to increased vascular permeability. Increased vascular permeability and intravascular accumulation of PMN cells are also manifestations of the shock syndrome, and are particularly apparent in lungs.

2. Heart

There is practically no evidence that hyperacute rejection of a human cardiac allograft has occurred on the operating table. Webb (1969) has reported a case that may represent an example of this; the heart initially showed an excellent response, but after the heparin was neutralized with codamine, the graft failed and could not be resuscitated. Pathological studies revealed all the hallmarks of hyperacute rejection.

In numerous instances the initial lesion following transplantation to a presensitized host may be similar in both cardiac and renal allografts; the functional consequences appear to be organ-specific to varying degrees (Bieber et al., 1970). Morphologic sequelae of the primary NOHA-mediated injury may be absent when both the myocardial blood supply and the myocardial complicance are markedly impaired in instances of long-lasting ventricular fibrillation. Upon release of the aortic clamp, calf, sheep, goat, and pig hearts transplanted to dogs immediately became pink, and defibrillation has been possible only in the pig-to-dog experiments (Neville et al., 1969). Occlusion of capillaries by packed erythrocytes was the most striking histologic and ultrastructural finding, but platelet aggregates, fibrin deposits, and inflammatory cells were notably absent. Endothelial damage, distinct interstitial edema, and occasional extravasated erythrocytes at sites of occlusion were associated with nuclear margination and clumping of muscle fibers. In contrast, hearts of dogs sutured orthotopically into dog, calf, sheep, or goat functioned for the duration of the experiment and showed few histologic and ultrastructural changes even 2 hours after perfusion. Goat cardiac xenografts survived in unmodified calves for more than 4 days (Donawick et al., 1971). Although these results are consistent with those observed in the xenologous kidney implants (Perper and Najarian, 1966a), an alternative hypothesis for NOHA-mediated injury was offered: the larger size of dog erythrocytes may have been responsible for the occlusion of the correspondingly smaller myocardial capillaries of the species-divergent animals (Neville et al., 1969). Canine cardiac allografts placed heterotopically into hosts presensitized by multiple skin grafts were rejected hyperacutely within several minutes (Sharma et al., 1973). The histologic lesions, such as platelet aggregation, vascular injury, fibrin deposits, and occasional leukocytes, were essentially the same as observed in the comparable kidney allograft model. Differences in the course of events were related either to variations in the level of cytotoxic antibody or to the divergent capacity of AG-AB complexes to cause platelet aggregation (SHARMA *et al.*, 1972).

3. Liver

Except for two cases, there are as yet no fully documented examples of hyper-acute rejection of a human orthotopic liver allograft (STARZL and PUTNAM, 1969; STARZL, 1974a). It has been pointed out that in all species so far studied, including man, liver allografts are less aggressively rejected than allografts of kidney and heart (CALNE, 1974), and a good surgical technique appeared to be more important than either HL-A typing or determination of NOHA's (TERA-SAKI, 1974). However, liver xenotransplantation between widely divergent species (pig-to-dog, pig-to-man) results in hyperacute rejection as rapid as that observed with kidney xenografts (Figs. 5, 6). Hepatic xenotransplantation has been studied with especial reference to temporary liver replacement in acute hepatic failure (WEGMANN *et al.*, 1969; HÄRING, 1974), heterotopic auxiliary transplantation being used as the preferred model (KUSTER, 1974; JERUSALEM *et al.*, 1974), while extracorporal perfusion (ABOUNA *et al.*, 1972; HELL *et al.*, 1974) and occasionally orthotopic xenotransplantation (LIE *et al.*, 1974; THEMANN *et al.*, 1974) were used in other studies.

Although the pathogenic factors triggering the rejection are apparently the same, the course of events in hyperacutely rejected liver grafts differs from that observed in renal xenografts in many features (ROESSNER *et al.*, 1972). The ultimate extent of xenograft destruction depends largely on mechanical, particularly hemodynamic, factors (JERUSALEM *et al.*, 1974). In heterotopic liver xenografts (pig-to-dog, rabbit-to-rat) provided with venous blood only and occa-sionally in incompatible canine liver allografts the lining endothelium was inten-sely swollen, showed bulk endocytosis, and was either partly damaged or stripped off about 5 minutes after revascularization. Numerous exfoliated endothelial and phagocytozing Kupffer cells, trapped white blood cells, and cell debris subsequently accumulated within the central veins and the adjacent sinuses. The remaining space of Disse was hemorrhagically infiltrated. Between 10 and 40 minutes after revascularization the blood flow through the liver graft gradual-ly decreased and finally ceased, because of an intrasinusoidal outflow block due to settling of sludge (Fig. 7) rather than to microthrombosis. In xenografts provided with arterial blood the initial occlusion of the central sinusoids resulted in a sudden enlargement of the liver lobule caused by trapping of large numbers of erythrocytes. After a central or midzonal hemorrhagic necrosis, hepatocytes were separated from their trabecular connections, and isolated liver cells and fragments of the liver lobule were pressed into the collecting veins and embolized into the general circulation (Fig. 8). Platelets appeared to accumulate only secon-darily to the mechanically induced outflowblock, and then mainly in vessels supplying the lobular periphery, but were more frequent in orthotopic liver xenografts (LIE *et al.*, 1974; THEMANN *et al.*, 1974). The same disastrous course of events was observed after the connection of a pig liver with the circulation

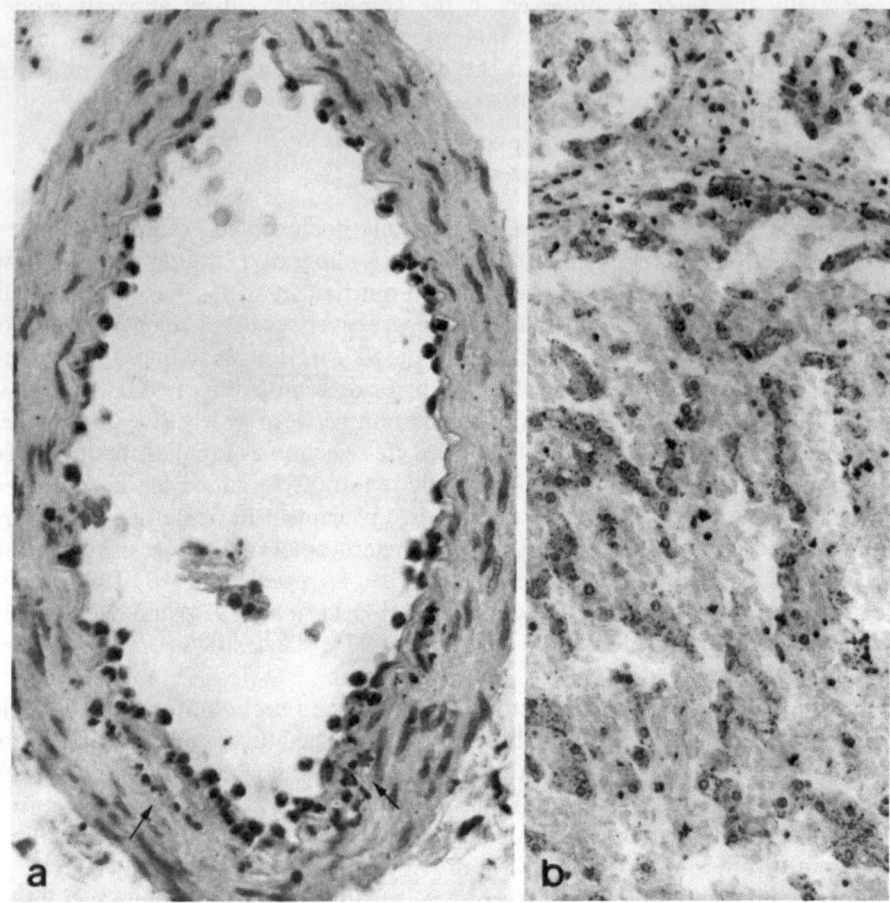

Fig. 5a and b. Porcine liver extracorporally connected to patient suffering from hepatic coma. After 8 h numerous PMN cells were found to be attached to damaged endothelial surface of branches of hepatic artery and to have invaded arterial wall locally (arrows, a). Hepatocytes are atrophic (by pressure) and loaded with pigment. Note disruption of trabecular architecture and severe congestion of hepatic parenchyma (b). (Hematoxylin and eosin: a ×350; b ×250)

of a patient suffering from hepatic coma. In addition to extended hemorrhagic necrosis and loss of hepatic parenchyma, changes histologically resembling the Arthus reaction were obvious (Figs. 5, 6).

There is some experimental evidence for an active role of the liver RES in xenograft rejection (Zimmermann and Rehfeld, 1971). Sinusoidal macrophages are apparently able not only to recognize worn-out components but also to distinguish between "self" and "nonself". Foreign serum globulin and peroxidase could be detected in immunohistochemical and submicroscopic cytochemical preparations 1–30 minutes after intravenous administration (Jerusalem et al., 1974), and up to 95 percent of virus inocula were cleared by the liver within a few minutes (Mims, 1959). In the case of xenotransplantation, macrophages may find all passing compounds worthy of phagocytosis. In addition,

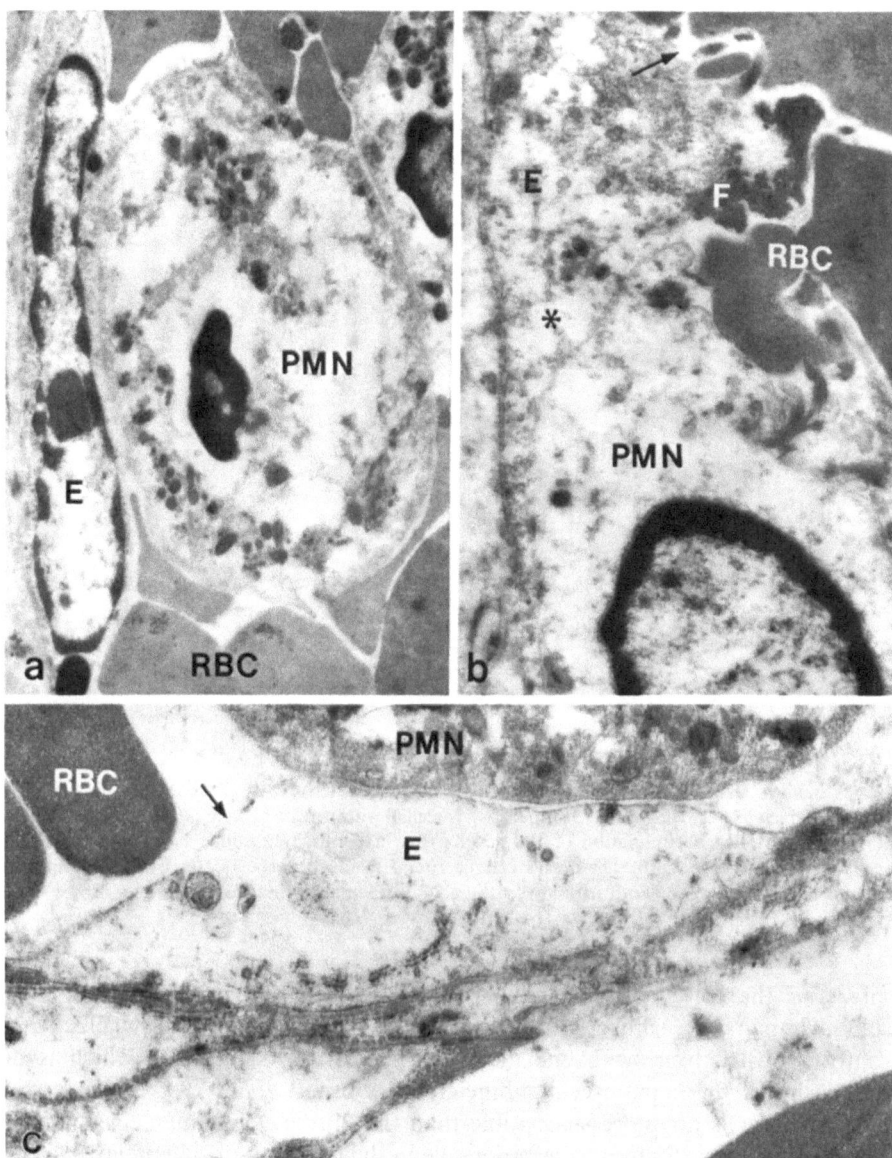

Fig. 6a -c. Porcine liver extracorporally connected to patient suffering from hepatic coma. After 8 h. *PMN* cells stick to endothelium (*E*) of small interlobular vein. Next to close cellular contact endothelial surface is either damaged (arrows, b, c) or endothelial cytoplasm is locally swollen (asterisk, b). Note disintegration of cytoplasmic organelles of endothelial cells (*E*), deposits of fibrin (*F* in b), and absence of thrombocytes in all preparations. RBC: red blood cells. (Fixation: formaldehyde, a, b, c × 15,000)

Kupffer cells also appear to phagocytose the clot-promoting immune complexes, which may explain the invariable occurrence of microthrombi (see Chapter B III 2). Overcrowded macrophages, however, tend either to rupture or to exfoli-

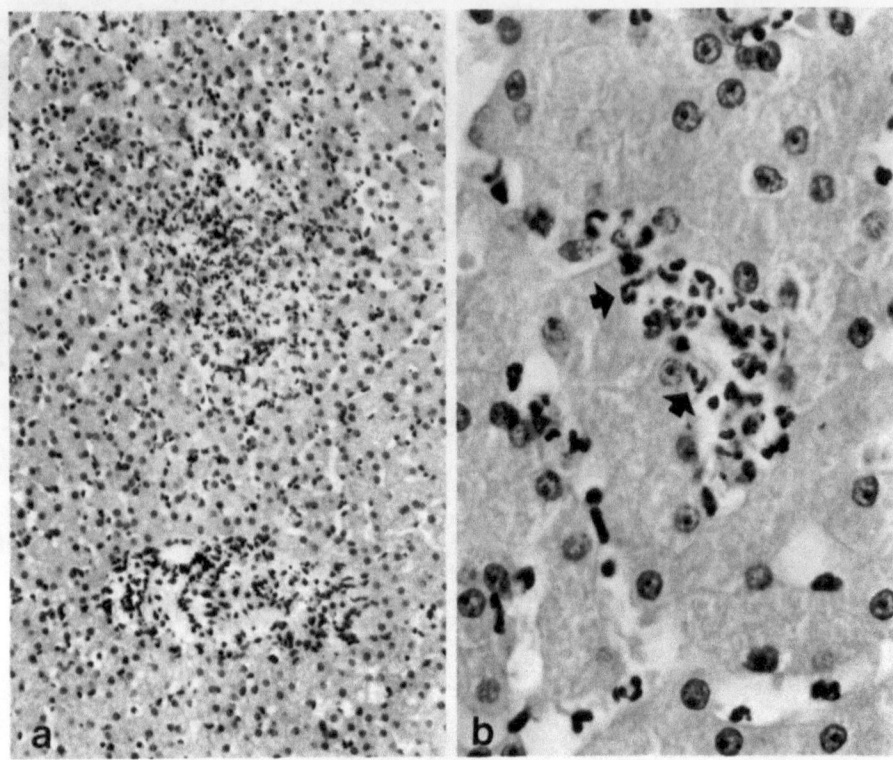

Fig. 7a and b. Canine orthotopic hepatic allograft 30 min after revascularization. Settling of sludge (exfoliated endothelial cells and trapped PMN cells) within central vein and adjacent sinusoids (a), and sinusoidal accumulation of PMN cells (b). In contrast to shock liver, numerous PMN cells have entered space of Disse and can be found inside hepatocytes (arrows, emperipolesis). Hemorrhagic necrosis of graft at autopsy after 24 h. (Hematoxylin and eosin: a ×250; b ×600)

ate, and the cell debris together with trapped cells and compounds of the blood impairs the sinusoidal microcirculation (sinusoidal outflow block). An outflow obstruction syndrome including hemorrhagic diathesis, which is due to spasms of the hepatic vein sphincters (GOODRICH et al., 1956) and to which the dog liver is far more susceptible than the porcine or human liver (STARZL et al., 1960), appears to play a minor role in the rejection of a hepatic xenograft. The damage to hepatocytes appears to be of a secondary nature, e.g. as a result of hypoxemia (THEMANN et al., 1974). Not unexpectedly, during the hyper-acute phase of rejection the activity of numerous hepatocytic enzymes decreased, particularly that of the ATPases and dehydrogenases, whereas the activity of glucose-6-phosphatase, which is low during cold perfusion, recovered quickly after 1 to 30 minutes, even in severely damaged grafts. Heterotopically inserted auxiliary liver grafts can be damaged rapidly and exclusively by unfavorable hemodynamic conditions, in particular high venous outflow pressure. The pressure in the systemic venous circulation also increases with increasing distance from the right atrium. Therefore, liver grafts being inserted distant from the

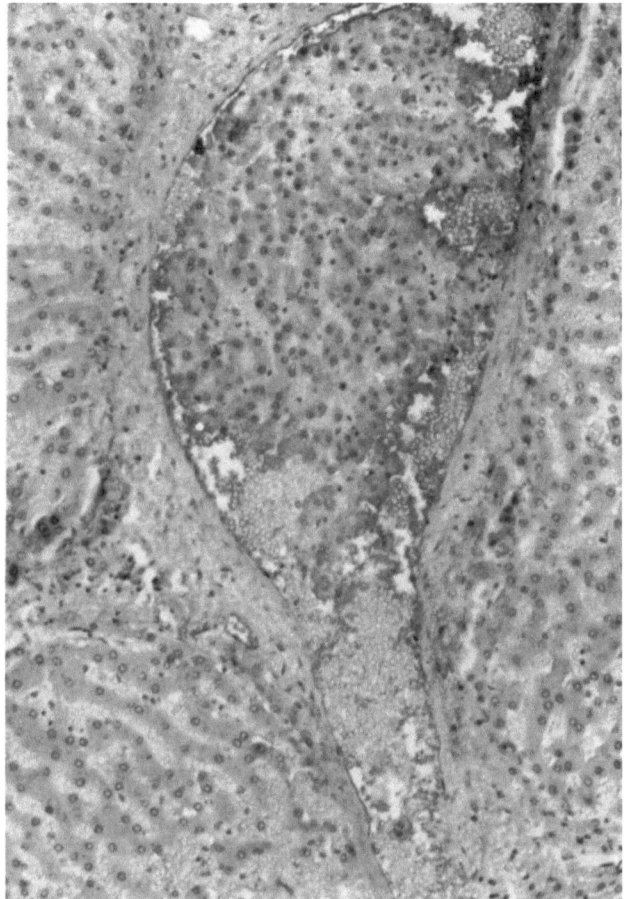

Fig. 8. Porcine to canine heterotopic liver xenograft 30 min after revascularization. Fragment of liver lobule within hepatic vein. Distinct congestion of all sinusoids and massive hemorrhagic infiltration. Complete graft destruction due to hemorrhagic necrosis after 2 h. (Goldner's trichrome: × 350)

orthotopic position have to overcome an outflow pressure that is above average (HESS *et al.*, 1972). In fact, almost all auxiliary livers have been inserted far distant from the recipient's liver (GOODRICH *et al.*, 1956; STARZL *et al.*, 1964b; MARCHIORO *et al.*, 1965a; ABSOLON *et al.*, 1965; HALGRIMSON *et al.*, 1966; SHEIL *et al.*, 1969). A rapid increase in outflow pressure due either to distal insertion of the graft or to experimental narrowing and accidental kinking of the outflow anastomosis can result in a disastrous course of events even in autografts (V.D. HEYDE *et al.*, 1970; JERUSALEM *et al.*, 1971a). The initial feature of rapid congestion of central veins and adjacent sinusoids, centrilobular hemorrhagic necrosis, and formation of congestive bridges histologically resembles changes seen in the acute Budd-Chiari syndrome and in veno-occlusive desease. A sinusoidal outflow block with subsequent total hemorrhagic necrosis of the liver lobules and thrombosis of the supplying vessels can develop from settling of the sludge of cell debris. Except for the absence of changes reminiscent of the Arthus phenomenon, the final picture is indistinguishable from that of hyperacutely rejected xenografts. In contrast, in heterotopic liver grafts inserted as proximally as possible, parenchymal damage due to unfavorable hemodynamic conditions was absent (Hess et al., 1972).

4. Lungs

No systematic studies are available on the rejection of orthotopic pulmonary xenografts nor are there any indications that a human allograft has ever been hyperacutely rejected. In dogs a characteristic course of histopathologic changes pointed to hyperacute rejection of several simultaneous bilateral and unilateral lung allografts (Fig. 9). Margination of PMN cells to endothelial surfaces of medium-sized vessels was most obvious in biopsies taken 30 minutes after revascularization. Endothelial cells showed arcading and detachment. In some small veins and arteries, exfoliated endothelial cells, trapped white cells, and cell debris appeared to occlude the vascular lumen (Wildevuur et al., 1973b). However, platelet aggregation was notably absent. Damage to, or loss of, the endothelium of alveolar capillaries was almost ubiquitous (Jap et al., 1973), rather than restricted to sites of contact with disrupting PMN cells (Klika et al., 1973). After an initial slight alveolar transudate containing scattered pneumocytes, macrophages and/or blood cells, the alveoli filled up with a richly proteinous substance and with increasingly more fibrin and/or red blood cells. Extended hemorrhagic or fibrinoid necrosis, including disruption of interstitial structures, was present in several grafts 5 to 12 hours after transplantation. Although this course of events suggests a NOHA-mediated lesion, it appears extremely difficult to demonstrate the active role of pre-existing antibodies in the deterioration of pulmonary structures. Specializations peculiar to the lung appear to mitigate a certain type of immunologic injury, but may promote others.

In connection with self-cleansing mechanisms that deal expeditiously with the inadvertent breath of contaminated air (Fishman and Pietra, 1974) the lungs function as an important antigenic trap (Roberts and Haurowitz, 1962; Patterson et al., 1962). High concentrations of antigens were demonstrated within the fixed lung macrophages (Roberts, 1963). It is unknown to what extent the local Shwartzman reaction is delayed or even prevented by the phagocytosis of clot-promoting immune complexes by the capillary endothelium. The cleaning-up of immunologically active substances may be facilitated by a "dilution effect", since the lungs are unique in that they receive the entire cardiac output, and the blood is spread over the largest capillary bed in the body (see also Chapters B III 2, C II 1, D II 3). In dogs the type of early endothelial lesions was virtually correlated to the extent of histoincompatibility (Langen et al., 1975): cellular changes were absent when the MCL test was negative. The endothelium was swollen and highly active in the MLC-positive group, and frequently damaged in instances of a double positive reaction (MLC + +). On the other hand, antigen trapping in lungs may partially explain the rapid release

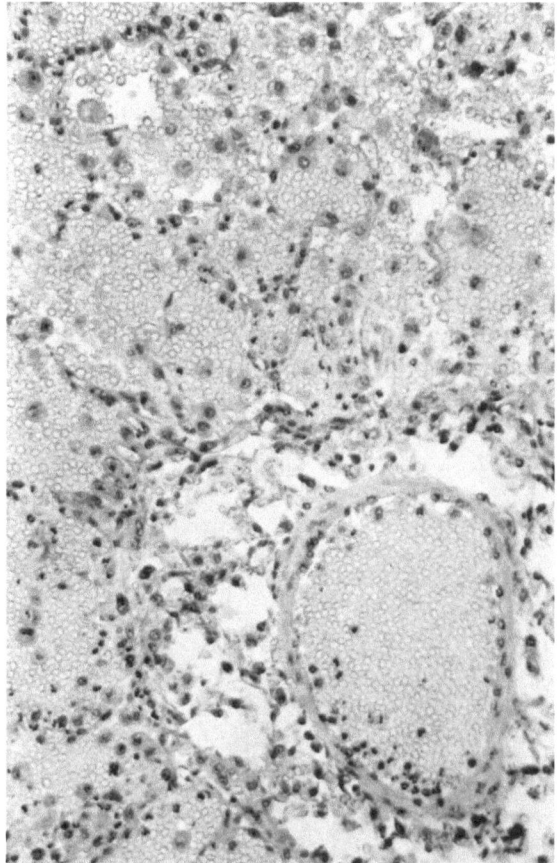

Fig. 9. Canine orthotopic pulmonary allograft 6 h after transplantation. Extended hemorrhagic necrosis. Note almost complete loss of endothelium of pulmonary vein with PMN cells sticking to wall, dilatation of perivascular lymphatic spaces, disruption of alveolar septa, and presence of PMN cells and alveolar macrophages in alveolar space. (Goldner's trichrome: × 350)

of chemical mediators of anaphylaxis from sensitized lungs (KALINER and AUSTEN, 1973; BRODER, 1974), which results in increased capillary fragility and permeability (see Chapter D II 1 b). Furthermore, in hyperacutely destroyed grafts, the breakdown of the blood-air barrier presents features that are histologically similar to those observed in Goodpasture's syndrome (BENOIT et al., 1964) and lesions induced by the application of heterologous pulmonary antibody (HAGADORN et al., 1969; HAGADORN and MERCOLA, 1971). In the latter model the antibody-induced acute immunologic injury was complement-dependent (MERCOLA and HAGADORN, 1973). However, shortly after simultaneous denervation and resection of the bronchial circulation of both lungs numerous dogs died of acute pulmonary edema and alveolar hemorrhage (REVENTOS et al., 1973). Although this complication was not observed in other studies (IRIE et al., 1975), it stresses the importance of the water-drainage machinery that normally prevents excess water from flooding the gas-exchanging surfaces (FISHMAN and

PIETRA, 1974). Numerous factors are known to be capable of a deleterious effect on this mechanism, including disregulation and abolition of baroreceptor reflexes (CAMERON, 1948; WIDDICOMBE, 1964), hypervolemia caused by a shift in blood volume from the systemic capillary circulation to the capillary bed of the lung, and chronic ischemic damage to the capillary endothelium (DRINKER, 1945). In contrast, cold ischemia prior to transplantation for up to two hours, and in exceptional cases for as long as 11 hours (HAGLIN *et al.*, 1973) appears to be tolerated readily. Some of the reported changes are of a transient nature per se, but may persist and even increase in combination with additional pathogenic events, e.g. NOHA's (WILDEVUUR *et al.*, 1973b). The influence of the sacrifice of the lymph flow on early graft failure has not yet been clearly demonstrated. Pulmonary lymphatics are normally able to drain more than three times their

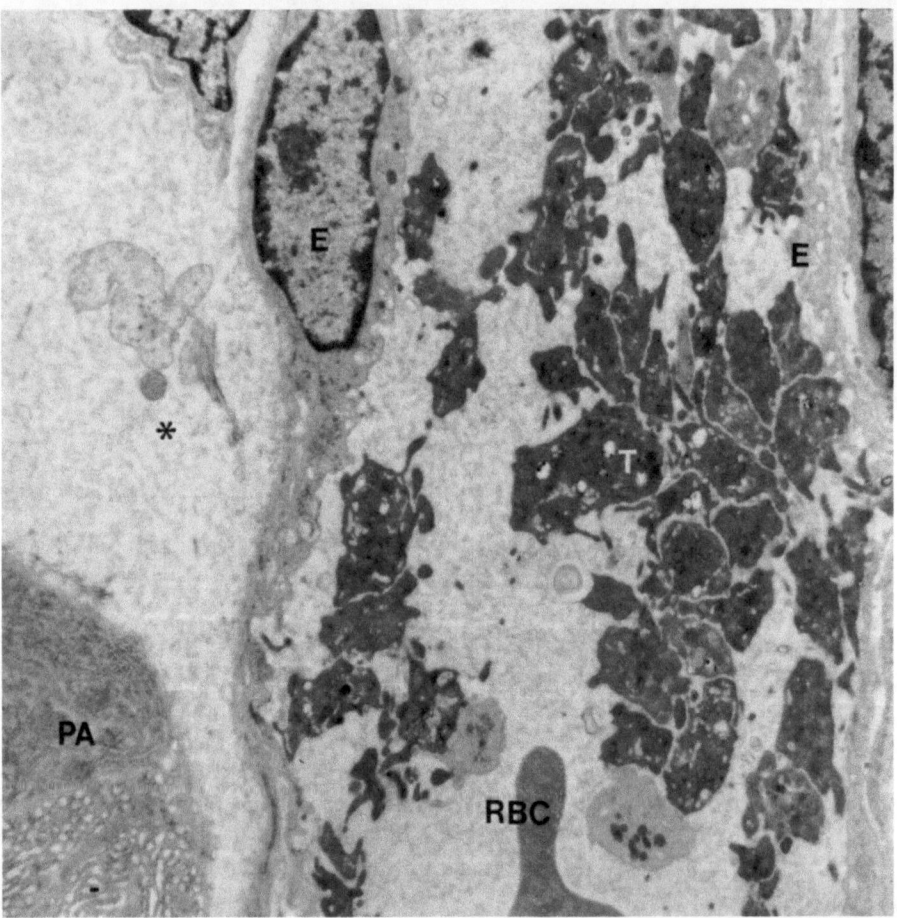

Fig. 10. Canine pancreatic allograft 30 min after revascularization. On right: wide lumen of capillary containing numerous thrombocytes (*T*) that tend to stick to endothelial cells (*E*). Note still intact endothelium. *RBC:* profile of red blood cell. On left: extensive interstitial edema (asterisk) and (portions of) 2 pancreatic acinar cells (*PA*). Graft hyperacutely rejected. (Fixation: glutaraldehyde × 5,000)

normal flow (SPENCER, 1968), but escaped protein-rich fluid, which would ordinarily be expected to be removed from the interstices *via* the lymphatic vessels (COURTICE, 1963), is only slowly resorbed from the alveolar spaces (COURTICE and SIMMONDS, 1949). The interruption of this draining mechanism may contribute to the establishment of a vicious circle.

5. Pancreas

Systematic studies on allotransplantation of the pancreas in dogs (v. HEE, 1973) revealed that early hemorrhagic necrosis of the graft and/or thrombosis of larger vessels followed margination of neutrophils to the damaged endothelium of medium sized arteries and veins quite closely, as seen in biopsies taken 30–60 minutes after revascularization. Damage to the capillary endothelium was less obvious. Subsequent infiltration of the vascular wall by PMN cells, platelet aggregates (Fig. 10), and fibrin thrombi in small veins and capillaries were the primary event resonsible for the final necrosis of the graft (ACOSTA *et al.*, 1973).

III. Nonimmunologically Caused Primary Graft Failure and Damage

1. Pretransplantation Anoxemic Lesions

In the previous chapters consideration has been occasionally given to a variety of structural changes caused by nonimmunologic events which may contribute to or accelerate the early destruction of organ grafts. Ischemic damage to the donor organ prior to transplantation is considered of particular importance by those interested in cadaveric organ transplantation and has probably been responsible for many primary failures (CALNE, 1967). In instances of successful transplantation of cadaveric kidney allografts (HALL *et al.*, 1974), the kidney can either function early and sufficiently enough after transplantation to obviate the need for further dialysis (immediate function), or the onset of secretion of urine is delayed (delayed function) and dialysis is required on one or more occasions until the life-supporting function is established (BAXBY et al., 1974a). A primary failure is a transplant that fails to maintain the recipient's life without the need for continuing dialysis, because secretion of urine is never resumed. It is obvious that this classification can only be applied to kidney transplantation. In orthotopic transplantation of the liver, and particularly of lung and heart, the recipient's life depends on the immediate function of the graft (see also Chapter H I, III). Morphologists are well acquainted with the rapid disintegration of histologic structures, particularly at the ultrastructural level, when an ischemic organ is kept at body temperature. Thus the cardinal rule for organ transplantation is that the shorter the warm ischemic period, the better the organ (TURNER, 1971). Unfortunately in those cases, where kidneys were imported to transplantation centers, often only limited information was available on ante-mortem hypotension, the anoxic interval, or the treatment of donors with vasoactive drugs, anticoagulants, or plasma expanders before nephrectomy (HALL *et al.*, 1974). Since there is no doubt that cooling the tissues decreases structural damage (PALADE, 1952) and preserves the viability of an organ for longer periods than under normothermic conditions (BOGARDUS and SCHLOSSER, 1956; STUEBER *et al.*, 1958; SCHLOERB *et al.*, 1957, 1959), cold perfusion and/or storage of the graft at 2–4° C to induce a metabolic break has become a common method of organ preservation (BELZER, 1974). Oxygen consumption virtually decreases exponentially with falling temperature (SEMB *et al.*, 1960), reaching less than 5 percent of normal at 5° C (LEVY, 1959). At this temperature, active tubular transport of water becomes immeasurable (HARVEY, 1959).

However, cold superimposed on anoxia also largely inhibits cellular functions necessary to maintain physiologic ion gradients between intra- and extracellular fluids. As a result of decreased Na^+-K^+ ATPase activity (JAP, 1971; MARTIN *et al.*, 1972) sodium ions, normally actively extruded by this cation pump into the intercellular space, accumulate within the cell. Simultaneously, the net influx of potassium ions is interrupted and the normally high intracellular K^+ concentration decreases (STATES *et al.*, 1972). Long lasting changes in ion gradients are fatal to the cell, and cold inhibition of the Na^+-K^+ ATPase enzyme system was considered a primary cause of unsuccessful preservation of liver and heart (MARTIN *et al.*, 1972). This process may be accentuated by procaine which is frequently added to perfusion media at a concentration of 1 percent to avoid an increase in vascular resistance during cold perfusion. Although to a somewhat lesser degree than the specific inhibitor ouabain, procaine inhibits the activity of the Na^+-K^+ ATPase activity in both the dog and rat kidney (CREMERS-VAN DIJCK, 1973), thus possibly contributing to the major loss of K^+ and Mg^{++} observed in rat kidneys after 1 to 3 hours of continuous hypothermic perfusion (KEELER *et al.*, 1966). In attempt to prevent this ion flux COLLINS *et al.* (1969) employed a solution rich in K^+ and Mg^{++} for kidney perfusion. Whereas several authors confirmed the advantages of solutions with an intracellular electrolyte composition (WATKINS et al., 1971; JOHNSON *et al.*, 1972), WELCH and FLANIGAN (1973) questioned the role excess Mg^{++} in COLLINS's C4 and SACKS's II (SACKS *et al.*, 1973) flush solution. They suggest two ways in which Mg^{++} may be potentially harmful: spontaneous precipitation of $MgHPO_4$. $3H_2O$ within the stored kidney; and a possibly toxic effect of magnesium at the concentration used (60 mEq./L). In contrast, ROSS and WERTHER (1974) reported a dramatic improvement in the renal function of autotransplanted kidneys upon 24 hours storage of the grafts after initial flushing with a solution containing 60 mEq./L of magnesium sulphate.

It is quite possible that variations in the survival time between imported and domestic cadaveric renal allografts, compared with laboratory studies on kidney preservation, are due to the (insufficiently documented) ante-mortem events and variations in the agonal hypoxemic interval (SELLS and MCLOUGHLIN, 1974), rather than to the advantages or disadvantages of a certain flushing solution. The concept of the "resting cell" as a desirable result of simple hypothermic storage must be re-examined (CALNE, 1967; BELZER, 1974). In hypothermically stored cells the two main energy sources are turned off: proteins or fats cannot be used as substrates for energy production due to a lack of oxygen;

and the pathway of anaerobic glycolysis is not available, because of the inhibition of the activity of glycolytic enzymes at low temperatures. A period of warm ischemia, prolonged shock, and anuric states before preservation (BELZER, 1974), and possibly the action of drugs administered ante mortem may accentuate the need for an energy-consuming metabolic demand for renewal processes by which the slow but gradual degradation may be delayed. FRANCAVILLA *et al.* (1973) suggested a possible diametrical effect of rapid cooling, resulting in a "thermal shock" characterized by a significant loss in activity of the glycolytic enzyme system. The change was greater in the liver than in the kidney and could be prevented by more gradual cooling. On the other hand, enzyme activity was found to return quickly to almost normal levels even in morphologically severely damaged livers immediately after revascularization (JAP, 1971). Furthermore, a slow reduction of glycolytic activity may rapidly diminish the amount of stored energy precursors which may be essential for the immediate function of the graft during the early post-transplantation period (SCHALM, 1972).

From the above it may have become clear that there is an urgent need for reliable viability tests of stored organs since the histology at the end of the preservation period may give misleading results (CALNE, 1967). Immediately before transplantation, preserved grafts may exhibit only minimal morphologic changes, and the maximum damage may not become apparent until some hours after restoration of the blood supply. In other instances the regenerative capacity of dogs' kidneys subjected to continuous pulsatile perfusion for 96 hours is impressive. According to studies in our laboratory some grafts exhibited an extended tubular necrosis at the end of the preservation time and were oliguric during the first 2 days after re-implantation. However, 4 to 5 days after auto-transplantation the life-supporting functions were resumed and there was an almost complete regeneration of the initially deteriorated tubular epithelium. This suggests that not the lesion per se, but the inability to restore the morphologic or metabolic defect is the main cause of primary graft failure. There are various attempts to correlate, on the one hand, the metabolic activity and the morphologic picture with the functional state of the graft after implantation, or on the other hand, using different histochemical, cytochemical, and biochemical techniques (ŠIŠKA *et al.*, 1970a, b; JAP, 1971). Generally either little relationship existed between early cellular structural and metabolic changes and the eventual functional capacity of the preserved organ, or the methods were too complicated and time-consuming. However, promising results in quick prediction of organ viability were recently obtained with the determination of the ability of preserved kidneys to maintain total adenine nucleotide levels (CALMAN and BELL, 1973) and through incorporation of p-aminohippuric acid (ROGERS and SLAPAK, 1974). Furthermore, the lactate level in the perfusate effluent at 1 hour was found to give an accurate indication (93% accuracy) of whether or not the kidney would function immediately (BAXBY *et al.*, 1974b).

2. Mechanical Traumatization

In view of the fact that a "no-touch nephrectomy" technique appears to be important even for a firm organ such as the kidney, SCHALM (1972) determined that the liver which has a partially low pressure circulation, might be extremely sensitive to external pressure. Local circulation disturbances, in the dog even outflow block and cellular necrosis, are the consequences of mechanical trauma to the liver. The same holds true for the lung and pancreas. Perfusion under unphysiologically high pressure (in compensation for the increase in vascular resistance) and, in instances of lung preservation, extracorporal inflation are further sources of mechanical traumatization.

3. Morphology of the Pretransplantation Ischemic and Mechanical Damage

After an extended cold ischemic storage period the organ may exhibit a variety of histologic and ultrastructural changes. However, with few exceptions the viability of the organ cannot be judged with certainty, neither from the type of lesion nor from its extent. Many changes may also be the result of rapid processing techniques (cryostat sectioning), and only occasionally can the post-transplantation course be retrospectively correlated with pretransplantation lesion through the evaluation of optimally fixed, embedded, and sectioned material. Furthermore, in instances of lung and liver transplantation the histologic diagnosis is rendered more difficult because of the relatively small size of the biopsy compared to the size of the whole graft. The biopsies are mostly taken from the wedges, thus from the outer periphery of these organs where histopathologic changes may differ widely from those in the central portions (Fig. 11 a). Of necessity, pretransplantation biopsies of preserved cardiac transplants are hardly available, and morphologic descriptions of clinical material are almost exclusively limited to post-mortem specimens. Nevertheless, with respect to the assessment of the post-transplantation course it appears essential to distinguish between immunologically triggered hyperacute rejection and a primary graft failure, particularly because the initial morphologic changes resulting from an extended hypoxemic interval may be minimal and the maximum damage may not become apparent until several hours after transplantation.

Some changes induced by anoxemia are similar in all preserved organs. They consist of a disturbance of the cell volume homeostasis (McLoughlin, 1973) and an increased capillary permeability resulting in interstitial edema (Jap et al., 1973; Van Hee, 1973). Characteristic features are vacuolar changes of parenchymal cells, swelling of mitochondria and nuclei (Šiška et al., 1970b), dissociation of cellular organelles combined with a loss of matrical density, an increase in pinocytotic vesicles, and occasional large vacuoles within the endothelial cytoplasm (Benjamin et al., 1974). Dissociation of parenchymal cells due to a marked interstitial edema and exfoliation of endothelial cells appear to indicate a more severe but still reversible injury. From the practical point of view it appears important that the degree of disturbance of the cell and tissue volume homeostasis apparently parallels the increase in organ weight. In lung allografts with immediate function after transplantation only a slight increase in organ weight was noticed after 6 to 21 hours of preservation (Modry et al., 1973). By better tissue oxygenation, maintainance of the perfusate at an osmolarity close to that of normal plasma, and the oncotic effect of proteins in the perfusate, SUROS and WOODS (1974) were able to keep the increase of weight of preserved hearts to only 20 percent. This compared favorably with weight increases of 40–60 percent reported by other authors (PROCTOR *et al.*, 1969; ŠIŠKA *et al.*, 1970a; COPELAND *et al.*, 1972). One should be aware that structural changes in kidneys and livers removed under optimal experimental conditions from beating-heart donors (initial warm ischemic period = 0, no pre-treatment, and no preceding shock) are not necessarily related in a causal manner to the constituents of perfusates and the type of short-term preservation. Results of a study on simple hypothermic storage of canine and porcine livers showed that postoperative life-sustaining function was obtained in 100 percent of cases, with histologic, biochemical, and clinical insignificant differences between the experimental groups, indicating the minor importance of the composition of the four preservation fluids examined (supplemented Ringer-lactate, TISSOL, and 2 modifications of Collins' C2 solution), cold ischemia up to 6 hours, and the species used for the experiments (SCHALM *et al.*, 1975). Thus, occasionally reported damage to histologic structures, e.g., rupture of the glomerular capillary-mesangial connections in kidneys preserved with pulsatile flow (JERUSALEM and VAN DE WERF, 1969) may be caused rather by a marked and uncontrolled increase in the perfusion pressure, since electron microscopy of biopsies taken 60 minutes post-transplantation of 24 hours hypothermically preserved kidneys of dogs revealed no significant differences between surviving kidneys preserved with pulsatile or nonpulsatile flow, or between organs perfused with plasma or an albumin solution (JESKE and ABOUNA, 1973). A potential danger may rise from the use of homologous (allogeneic) cryoprecipitated plasma added to perfusates in order to produce oncotic pressure, and to supply the perfused organ with trace substances, such as fatty acids, probably advantageous for the metabolic maintenance of the hypothermic organ. Cryoprecipitation of plasma was recommended to eliminate lipoproteins (BELZER *et al.*, 1968) which tend to aggregate spontaneously and may subsequently block the vessels during perfusion and after revascularization (BELZER *et al.*, 1967). However, neither by cryoprecipitation nor by silica gel precipitation (to remove fibrinogen, TOLEDO–PEREYRA *et al.*, 1974a) are naturally occurring and possibly cross-reacting heterospecific antibodies (NOHA's) cleared from the plasma. These antibodies may bind to the endothelium during the perfusion period and initiate a course of events similar to that described in Chapter D II 1. JESKE and ABOUNA (1973) demonstrated that unsuccessful preservation of canine kidneys by perfusion with solutions containing cryoprecipitated plasma was caused by the occlusion of peritubular capillaries with PMN cells. Since this phenomenon was not observed in any of the grafts perfused with albumin, it may be related to NOHA's and the differential diagnosis of hyperacute or accelerated rejection as a result of presensitization of the host may become extremely difficult. Furthermore, in instances where low molecular weight dextran was used as a perfusate, glomerular lesions were seen in biopsies taken 30 minutes after restoration of the blood flow. These consisted of local hyaline deposits within the capillary lumina of the glomerular tufts. In later biopsies some glomeruli were sclerotic, probably as a result of thrombosis (CALNE, 1967). However, in only a small number of cases did a latent ischemic lesion become manifest immediately after revascularization. According to our experience, there is a latent period of several hours to about 1 day, but once started the course of events may be dramatic. Surprisingly, it is capillary alteration and its sequels rather than the parenchymal lesion that are prominent, as indicated by a marked interstitial edema and massive interstitial hemorrhage. In contrast to antibody-mediated hyperacute rejection (Chapter E II 1a) and acute cell-mediated rejection characterized by capillary alteration (Chapter F I2b), lesion of the endothelium of medium-sized vessels,

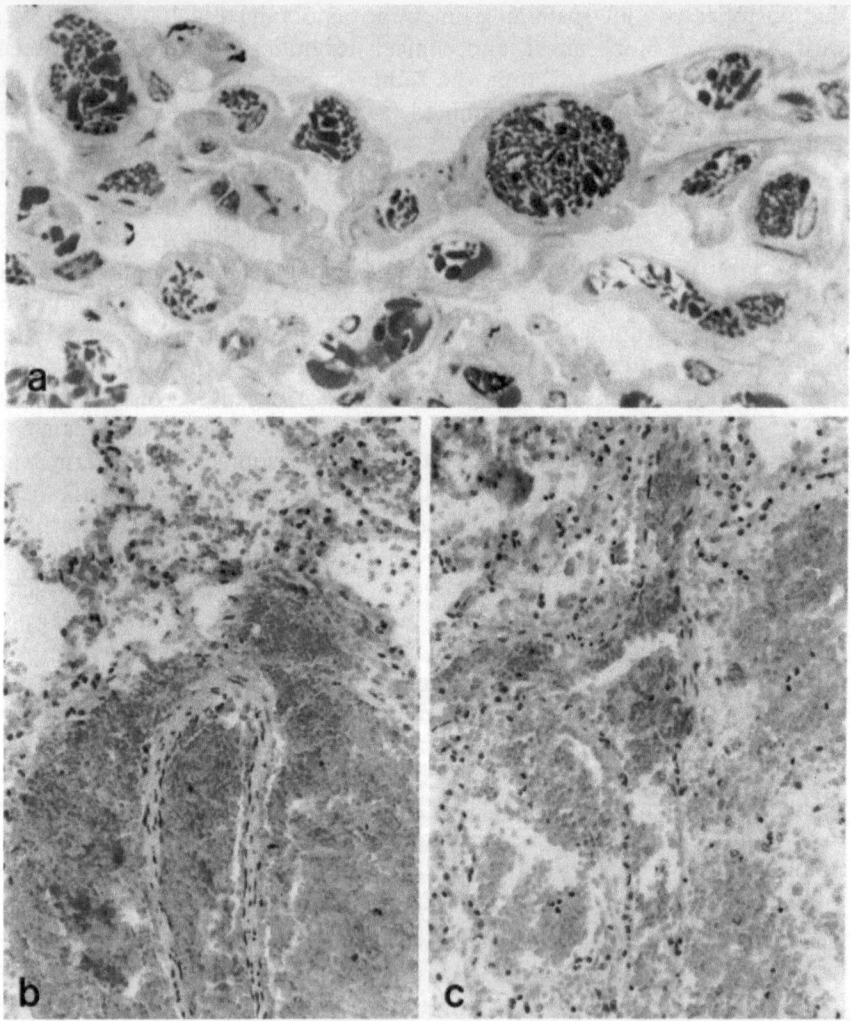

Fig. 11. (a) Canine pulmonary allograft before revascularization. Accumulation of thrombocytes in capillaries and blood vessels of lobar periphery probably resulting from insufficient cold flushing of small segment. Upon transplantation graft was not rejected (Toluidine blue stained semi-thin section: × 900). (b) and (c). Autopsy specimen (24h after reimplantation) of canine pulmonary autografts. These grafts were stored hypothermically for 24 h prior to transplantation. Note extended perivascular (b) and alveolar hemorrhage (c), and in both preparations absence of PMN cells in contrast to Fig. 9. (Hematoxylin and eosin: × 250)

sticking of PMN cells, the escape of fibrin, and thrombosis are almost absent (Fig. 11 b, c). In the ensuing paragraph several changes peculiar to various organs which may point to ischemic damage are summarized.

a) Kidney

Swelling, vacuolar degeneration, and even necrosis of the epithelium of the proximal convolutions indicate severe ischemic damage. Our own studies revealed that slight to moderate deterioration of the tubular epithelium occurred only when kidneys preserved hypothermically under optimal experimental conditions (warm ischemic period = 0) were stored for at least 36 hours or longer. This suggests that major damage to the parenchyma is likely to occur prior to donor nephrectomy in clinical cadaveric transplantation (CALNE, 1967). It is extremely difficult to determine whether the graft will recover from the ischemic injury after transplantation or not. Immediately after revascularization of ischemically damaged renal grafts capillaries may be dilated but do not contain erythrocytes (JESKE and ABOUNA, 1973), and the interstitial edema may become more prominent. In contrast to immunologically triggered hyperacute rejection the preferred site of focal hemorrhagic necrosis was the outer zone of the medulla rather than the cortical area.

b) Heart

Recently, we studied a series of 33 orthotopic simian allografts; however, neither mitochondrial changes (COPELAND et al., 1968), behavior of birefringence (BROWN et al., 1973), degree of interstitial edema, nor the loss of glycogen (ŠIŠKA et al., 1970b) could be used as a standard in predicting the mechanical performance of the myocardium after resuscitation. In instances of pulsatile flow preservation a final perfusion pressure greater than 60% of the initial pressure was indicative of unsatisfactory preservation (SUROS and WOODS, 1974). In post-mortem specimens, after fruitless attempts to resuscitate the cardiac graft, areas of myocardial necrosis may be due to electrical burning as a result of defibrillation with direct current shocks (LEANDRI, 1967).

c) Liver

The gradual loss of glycogen is an outstanding feature of the hypothermically preserved liver. The porcine liver appears more susceptible to the dissimilation of glycogen during cold storage (6 hours) than the rat or canine liver (12–24 hours). Although orthotopically transplanted porcine livers with largely reduced glycogen contents survive in 100% of the cases (SCHALM et al., 1975), the loss of energy precursors appeared to be disadvantageous (SCHALM, 1972). Swelling or arcading and desquamation of the sinusoidal endothelium are other changes observed after simple hypothermic storage. Upon revascularization exfoliated endothelial cells and trapped white cells may settle in the centrilobular area and block the outflow through the central vein (Fig. 12). After preservation with continuous flow for 19 hours (pulsatile or nonpulsatile) the sinusoidal lining endothelium was almost absent. Surprisingly, in these instances hyperacute rejection of the porcine to canine liver xenograft was largely delayed and mitigated (Jerusalem *et al.*, 1974).

d) Lung

Ischemic damage to the lung can be assumed in instances of swelling, fragmentation, and desquamation of alveolar lining cells, and pyknosis of bronchiolar epithelial cells. These changes may be prominent already after 3 to 4 hours of cold storage (Sekiguchi *et al.*, 1973). Isolated lungs, kept at ambient temperatures (18°–23° C) in a ventilation-perfusion circuit, deteriorated functionally (regression of the percentage of venous-arterial oxygen saturation) simultaneous with a retraction of both membranous pneumocytes and capillary endothelial cells after about 150 minutes (Rioux *et al.*, 1973). However, whereas even after 24 hours of simple cold storage, and 30 minutes after revascularization of the preserved pulmonary transplant the histologic changes may be minimal, the same graft may be found to be completely hemorrhagically necrotic at autopsy 1 day later (Fig. 11 b, c).

e) Pancreas

The most impressive change resulting from simple hypothermic storage was marked interstitial edema which increased in proportion to the preservation time. Surprisingly, the longer the preservation time, the longer the dogs survived. On the other hand, perfusion preservation using a commercial pulsatile flow apparatus yielded by far poorer results (Van Hee, 1973). In his series of 44 pancreatic allotransplantations incidences of early hemorrhagic necrosis were not related to the duration of the preservation time.

E. Accelerated (Delayed Hyperacute) Rejection

Changes characteristic for hyperacute rejection may be only slight or even absent for the first 1 or 2 days after transplantation, but then manifest themselves rapidly and earlier than a specific transplantation reaction could be expected to occur. Special attention is called to instances where patients had negative cross-matches before and after the rejection, indicating that a delayed form of hyperacute rejection can occur in the absence of detectable donor-specific antibody (Busch *et al.*, 1969). Since accelerated rejection of human kidney allografts is associated with more profound endothelial damage and vascular lesions, microthrombosis, abundant fibrin deposits, and a fall in complement titers in the absence of mononuclear infiltration, it is reminiscent of events observed in experimental xenograft rejection (Gewurz, 1971). On the basis of experiments in our laboratory, accelerated rejection was assumed to occur in canine and porcine auxiliary liver allotransplantation, but could not be fully documented, since the immunopathologic injury was largely superposed by other changes, e.g. those resulting from extrahepatic thrombosis of the portal vein and of the hepatic artery, and an outflow block due to kinking of the outflow anastomo-

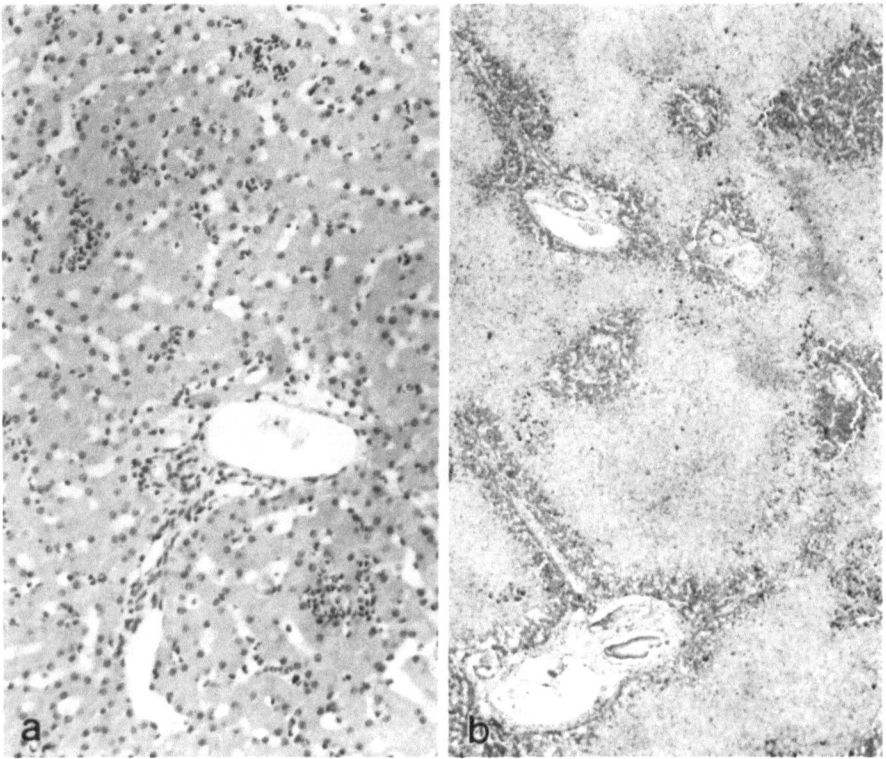

Fig. 12a and b. Canine orthotopic liver allograft. Treated with immunosuppressive drugs. (a) focal increase in sinusoidal PMN cells 30 min after revascularization. (Hematoxylin and eosin: ×250), (b) extended central and midzonal ischemic necrosis due to thrombosis of hepatoarterial anastomosis, 2 days after transplantation. (Hematoxylin and eosin: ×40)

sis. In typed beagles and pigs submitted to orthotopic liver transplantation a coincidence was observed between the occurrence of an increase in sinusoidal PMN cells early after revascularization and thrombosis of the hepatic arterial anastomosis 2 to 4 days later (Fig. 12). However, when instead of an end-to-end technique being used the hepatic artery was anastomosed directly to the aorta by means of a Carrel patch and isoproterenol administered via the portal vein, both PMN-cell sticking and thrombosis failed to appear (SCHALM et al., 1975).

It is highly speculative to suggest that there is a relationship between vascular compliance and binding capacity, e.g. of low avidity antibody. In unmodified dogs the occurrence of accelerated lung allograft rejection appeared to depend on differences in the major histocompatibility complexes (LANGEN et al., 1975). Whereas, in donor-recipient combinations in which lymphocytes reacted negatively when cultured together, accelerated rejection occurred only incidentally, about 40 percent of the lung allografts were lost by this type of rejection when the lymphocytes of both the donor and the recipient were stimulated in the MLC test. Thirty minutes after revascularization there was a margination of PMN cells in the larger vessels, local endothelial damage, severe perivascular

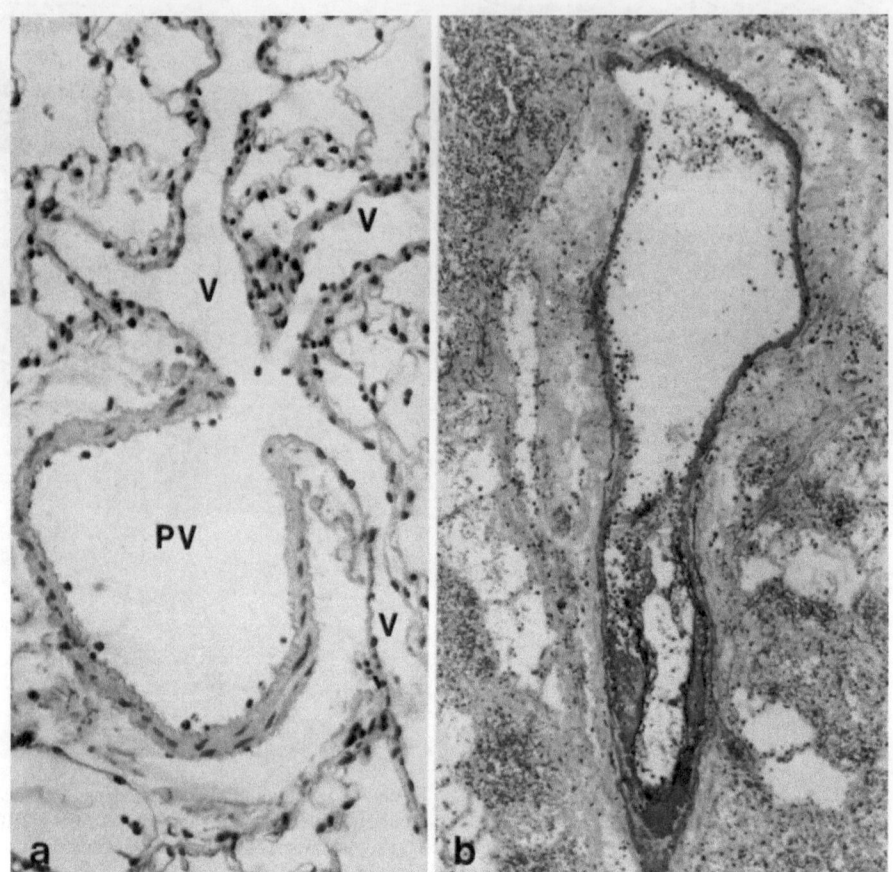

Fig. 13a and b. Incompatible (MLC test double positive) canine pulmonary allograft. No administration of immunosuppressive drugs. (a) 30 min after revascularization. Small pulmonary vein (*PV*) completely lacks endothelial cells but only few PMN cells are attached to damaged surface. Note perivascular edema. In contrast, in adjoining venules (*V*) endothelium is not injured. (Goldner's trichrome: × 350), (b) 4 days after transplantation. Mural thrombus in medium-sized vein and alveolar hemorrhagic necrosis. Note severe perivascular proteinaceous edema and absence of MN cells. The number of PMN cells slightly increased. On X-rays graft exhibited gradual increase in opacity between 1st and 3rd day after transplantation. (Goldner's trichrome: × 100)

edema, and occasional peribronchial and perivascular hemorrhage. However, platelet aggregates, fibrin deposits, and alveolar exudate were absent initially (Fig. 13). Even after one day, radiodiagnosis revealed densifications which became increasingly as time went on. When the animals died 4 and 5 days later, both Shwartzman-like and Arthus-like reactions were found to have contributed to complete fibrinoid and hemorrhagic necrosis of the graft, whereas mononuclear cell infiltration was minimal or even absent (Fig. 14).

Since individual profiles of NOHA's are maintained for long periods (Landy and Weidanz, 1964), and the induction of a primary response has been attributed

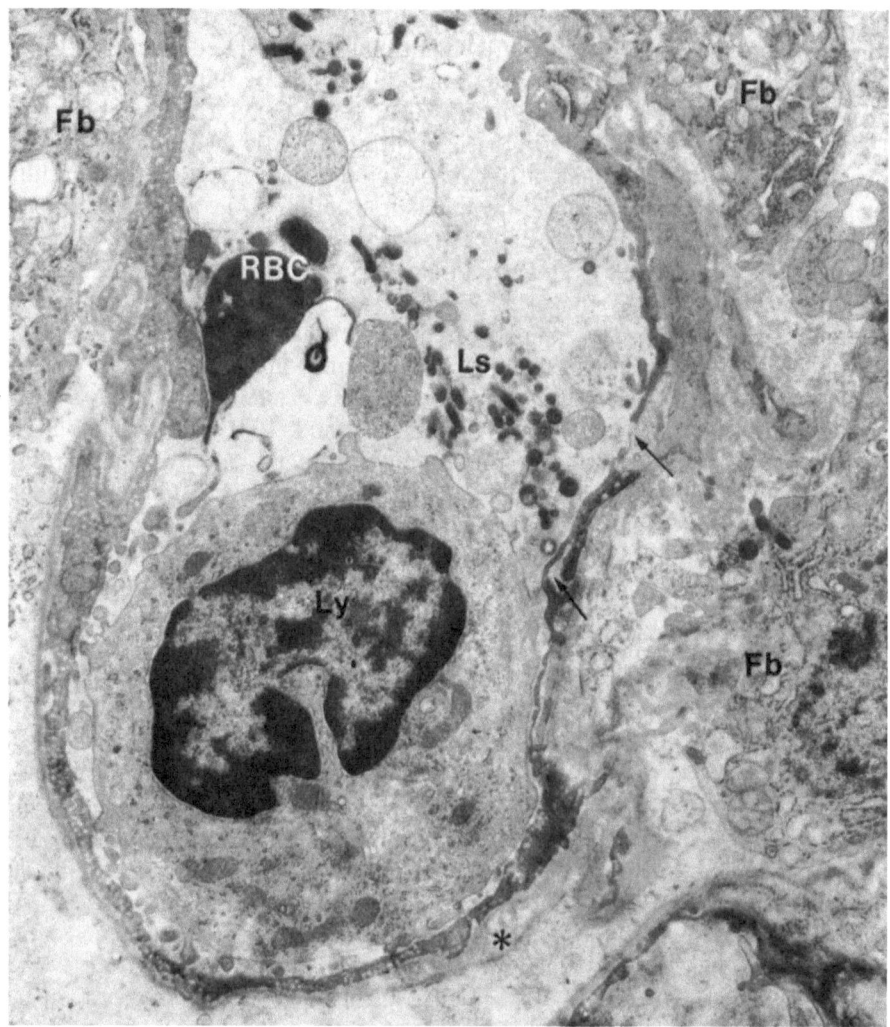

Fig. 14. Incompatible (MLC positive) canine pulmonary allograft 5 days after transplantation. No immunosuppressive treatment. Occasionally a medium-sized lymphocyte (*Ly*) can be detected within alveolar capillaries. However, no endothelial damage at sites of cytoplasmic contact. At other places, endothelium is locally either lifted off or discontinuous (arrows). Note free lysosomes (*Ls*) derived from disrupted PMN cells, splitting of basement membrane (asterisk), and increased number of fibroblasts (*Fb*). *RBC*: profile of red blood cell. (Fixation: glutaraldehyde × 12,000)

to the depletion of the specific natural antibody (MURRAY, 1968), it seems that classic feedback mechanisms may play a role in accelerated graft rejection. A homeostatic role for antibody in the immune response was first suggested by UHR and BAUMANN (1961), and was later demonstrated by BYSTRYN *et al.* (1971): Whereas passive elevation of the serum level of a given antibody resulted in a decreased synthesis of that antibody, depletion of a given antibody by means of exchange blood transfusion resulted in increased synthesis that not only repleted the amount of withdrawn antibody, but resulted in levels considerably in excess of the control levels. Since donor-specific antibodies are cleared by organs of this donor (CLARK et al., 1964, 1965; GEWURZ et al., 1966; LINN et al., 1968), and antibody, resynthesized through classic feedback mechanisms, may be trapped again by the graft, a vicious circle might be established, resulting in gradually advancing, humoral-mediated destruction of the graft. The allogenic effect may serve as an alternative hypothesis (see Chapter A III 2d). The infusion of allogenic lymphocytes from nonimmune donors antigen-primed animals leads to spontaneous production of the antigen-specific antibody and, upon challenge, to a secondary response of distinctly greater intensity than observed in a normal secondary response (KATZ et al., 1971). This phenomenon has been observed in mice and guinea pigs in vivo (OSBORNE and KATZ, 1972) and in vitro (HIRST and DUTTON, 1970; EKPAHA–MENSAH and KENNEDY, 1971). A principal characteristic of this allogenic effect is the elimination of the specific carrier-primed helper cells (Chapter A III 2) that are usually necessary to obtain a hapten-specific secondary antibody response (ELFENBEIN et al., 1973), and it appears to be mediated by a massive activation of the infused donor T-cells by means of a slight and transient GVH reaction, which in turn stimulates the response of host B-cells (KRETH and WILLIAMSON, 1971). In organ transplantation, an allogenic effect involving cross-reacting NOHA's might be triggered by passenger leukocytes (Chapter C II 4) and accentuated by the cross-reacting antigen released from the graft.

The major problem that has to be solved is the differentiation of nonspecific changes and rejection events during the early posttransplantation phase. Whereas changes resulting from denervation, abolition of the lymphatic flow, and surgical intervention per se in either sham operated or reimplanted kidneys and hearts are minimal, more than 60 percent of the dogs died several hours to 7 days after simultaneous denervation of both lungs (REVENTOS et al., 1973). After one and two days, pathologic changes in the necropsy specimens ranged from interstitial edema, focal atelectasis and alveolar exudation (NOIRCLERC et al., 1969; DOUGHERTY et al., 1971; VEITH et al., 1973) to pulmonary edema and hemorrhage (REVENTOS et al., 1973). However, fibrin deposits were an unusual finding (BECKER et al., 1972; BLÜMCKE et al., 1973), and pavementing of PMN cells was almost absent. Acute pneumonia was the cause of death in animals which succumbed three to seven days after hilar stripping.

Occasionally, a renal lesion histologically resembling hyperacute rejection (delayed form of hyperacute rejection; PILLAY et al., 1973) occurs several days (BOHLE, 1970), weeks, or even months after transplantation (BUSCH et al., 1971) (Fig. 15). Obviously, this pattern of rejection is seen after the type of transplantation which is mediated exclusively by de novo synthesized antibodies rather than by pre-existing ones. It may come about predominantly by way of an immunosuppressive regimen which inhibits T- but not B-lymphocyte activity (Fig. 2). Thus the determination of IgG as a guide to immunosuppression and cytotoxicity was recommended (KU et al., 1973). Mononuclear cells were notably absent in small bowel grafts undergoing accelerated rejection, but the grafts were heavily infiltrated with PMN cells (BARNETT et al., 1962), and a human

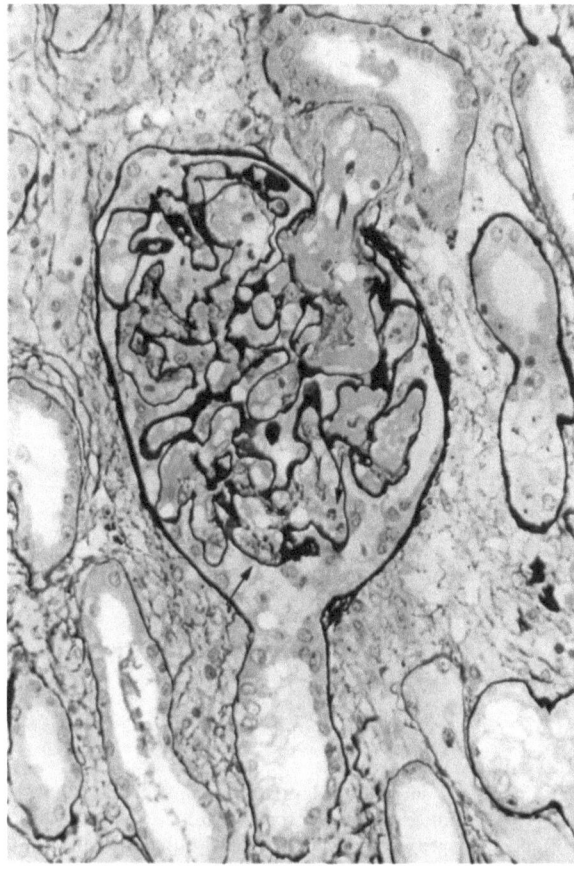

Fig. 15. Human renal allograft 4 weeks after transplantation (44 years, female). Treated with immu-nosuppressive drugs. Afferent arteriole and glomerular tufts are filled with amorphous substance (local Shwartzman reaction). Several PMN cells are trapped within casts (arrows). Infiltrating MN cells are notably absent. Note irregular thickening of basement membranes (Jones' silver-methenamine: ×350). By courtesy of Prof. Dr. P.H.M. SCHILLINGS, Dept. of Pathology, and Prof. Dr. P.G.A. WIJDEVELD, Dept. of Nephrology, University of Nijmegen, The Netherlands

cardiac allograft was rejected in a manner resembling hyperacute rejection after 10 days (BIEBER et al., 1970).

Other data from our laboratory may suitably demonstrate the complex etiolo-gy of the delayed hyperacute rejection. Poor renal function was observed after re-implantation of several canine kidneys subsequent to a period of 24 hours continuous perfusion with a solution containing pooled allogeneic serum. At autopsy 2 to 4 days later accumulations of PMN cells in large vessels, peritubular, and glomerular capillaries, and large foci of hemorrhagic necrosis were an outstanding feature (Fig. 16). Remarkably enough, these kidneys exhibited no changes in biopsies taken 30 minutes after restoration of the blood flow. The possible etiology of this alteration was discussed in the previous Chapter D III 3.

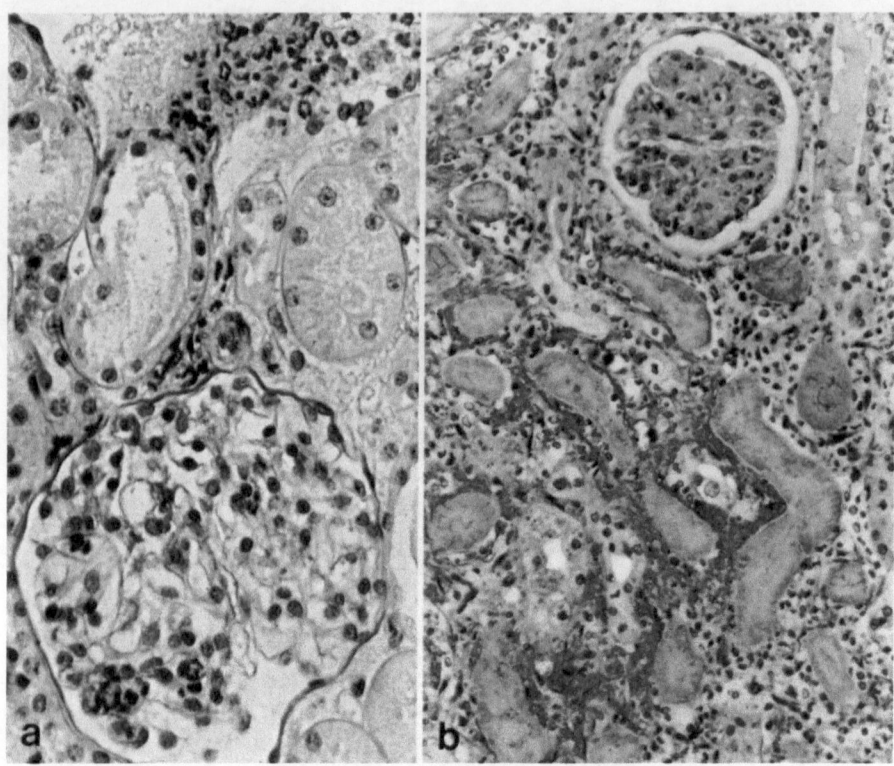

Fig. 16a and b. Canine renal autograft 4 days after reimplantation. Graft was cold perfused with solution containing pooled allogeneic serum for 24 h prior to reimplantation (a) accumulation of PMN cells at (partially damaged) wall of vein, within peritubular capillaries, and in some glomerular tufts. (PAS reaction: ×350) (b) area of focal interstitial hemorrhage and early ischemic necrosis of epithelial cells of proximal convolutes. Note interstitial infiltration with MN cells. (Hematoxylin and eosin: ×250)

F. Acute (Intermediate) Rejection

I. Pathogenesis

The acute rejection of tissue and organ grafts is regarded as the classic manifestation of cell-mediated immunity. Medawar (1944) was the first to regard the infiltrating lymphoid cells as a contributory factor in the death of skin allografts. He also stressed the importance of the humoral response, particularly in the "second-set" phenomenon (Medawar, 1945). About ten years later the role of accumulating mononuclear cells in the actual destruction of renal allografts was emphasized (Simonsen et al., 1952; Dempster, 1953). In addition, plasma cells were recognized (Dempster, 1955), but interpreted as a defense of the kidney against host antibody (Simonsen et al., 1952). With the demonstration of a dichotomy of immune responses (Chapter A III 1) it was widely accepted

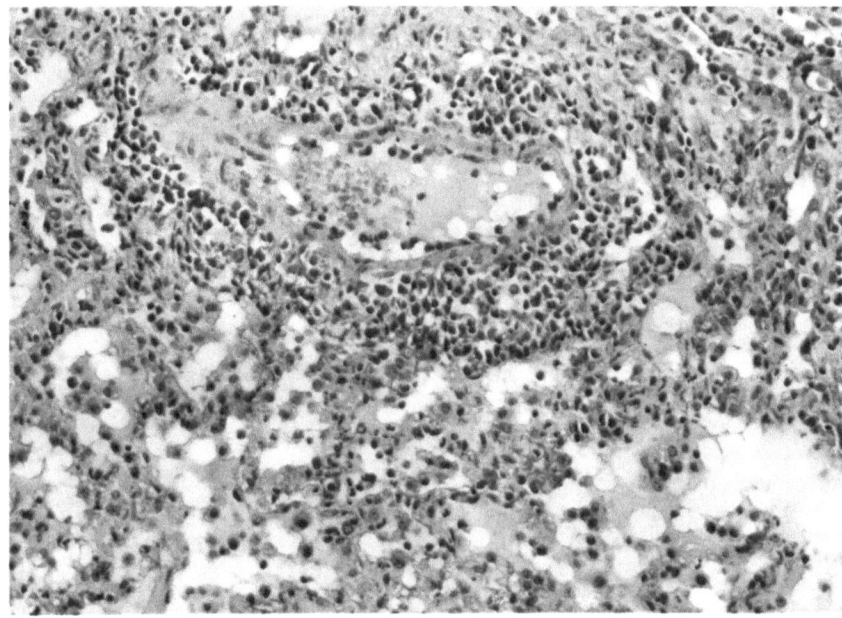

Fig. 17. Canine pulmonary allograft 12 days after transplantation. No immunosuppressive treatment. Accumulation of various types of MN cells around small vein (cuffing) and in adjacent interstices. Note thickening of alveolar septa and severe proteinaceous and cellular alveolar exudate. (Hematoxylin and eosin: ×250)

that the effector phase of the transplantation reaction, i.e. the cytotoxic effect on target cell populations, is almost exclusively mediated by T-lymphocytes (Chapter A III 3a). However, as outlined in Chapters A III 3b, c and A IV, cell-mediated mechanisms independent of T-cells, secondary mediators, and complement-dependent humoral factors may all be involved in graft rejection. The majority of clinical renal allograft rejection reactions were found in fact to occur with mixed characteristics (CARPENTER and MERRILL, 1969). Undoubtedly, the type, the degree, and the speed of rejection of organ grafts are fundamentally dependent upon the extent of histo-incompatibility, the type of antigen, the antigenic strength, and both the procedure and the intensity of immunosuppression. The data summarized above may explain the extreme variability in the course of events of rejection episodes and in the number and type of infiltrating cells. However, although an impressive amount of basic knowledge of lymphoid cell kinetics has been accumulated, the exact mechanism by which it goes into effect is not yet fully understood (LEVEY, 1974). The extant literature on this topic is so massive that it is beyond the scope of the handbook to review it adequately. Therefore, this chapter attempts to outline a common denominator of the cell-mediated reaction, to draw attention to some paradoxical phenomena of cellular infiltrations, to deal with divergent patterns of allograft destruction and with the modification of the transplantation reaction through immunosuppressive therapy, and to consider several nonimmunologic factors that interfere with the host response to transplanted organs.

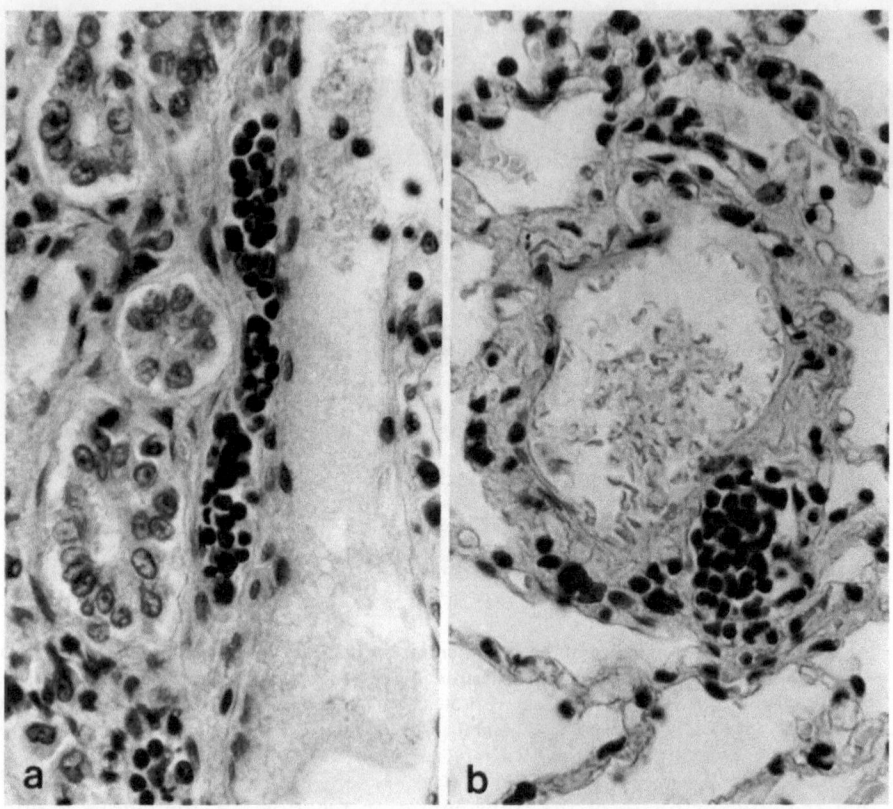

Fig. 18a and b. Accumulation of small lymphocytes within perivascular lymphatics in rat liver allograft (a) and in canine pulmonary allograft (b) 6 and 4 days after transplantation, respectively. No administration of immunosuppressive drugs. Note in (a) proliferating bile ductuli. (Goldner's trichrome: a and b × 600)

1. Cellular Infiltration and Vascular Lesions

Microscopically the outstanding feature of acute rejection is the observation of cellular infiltration. The sequence of events was first analyzed in kidney allografts (Simonsen et al., 1952; Dempster, 1953; Dempster et al., 1964; Porter, 1965), but basically identical patterns have been observed in the transplanted heart (Saunders and Bieber, 1968; Kosek et al., 1968; Ellis et al., 1971), liver (Porter, 1969; Beaudoin et al., 1970; Jerusalem et al., 1971 b), lung (Fujimura et al., 1970; Dougherty et al., 1971; Veith et al., 1972 b), and pancreas (Idezuki et al., 1968; Mori, 1968; Acosta et al., 1973; v. Hee, 1973). The time of inception, the tempo of manifestation, the density of cellular infiltration, and the extent of subsequent lesions are independent of species, but are largely related to the genetics of histocompatibility, the balance between humoral and cell-mediated responses, and, of course, to immunosuppression. However, the cell-mediated reaction can occasionally proceed regardless of the method of immunosuppression. Thus, morphologic manifestations of the acute cell-mediated reaction may be present as early as 24 hours after the circulation is re-established (FELDMAN and LEE, 1967), and in cadaver transplants the danger period extends up to two years (HUME, 1971).

a) *Perivascular and interstitial infiltration* is characterized by the progressive accumulation of mononuclear (MN) cells in connective tissue septa carrying medium-sized vessels and their branches. The early aggregates are adjacent to, or contiguous with, thin-walled vessels. Subsequently, MN cells mostly accumulate in a characteristic "cuff" around both small and medium-sized arteries and veins (LINDQUIST *et al.*, 1968b). As time goes on, the spread of the infiltrates

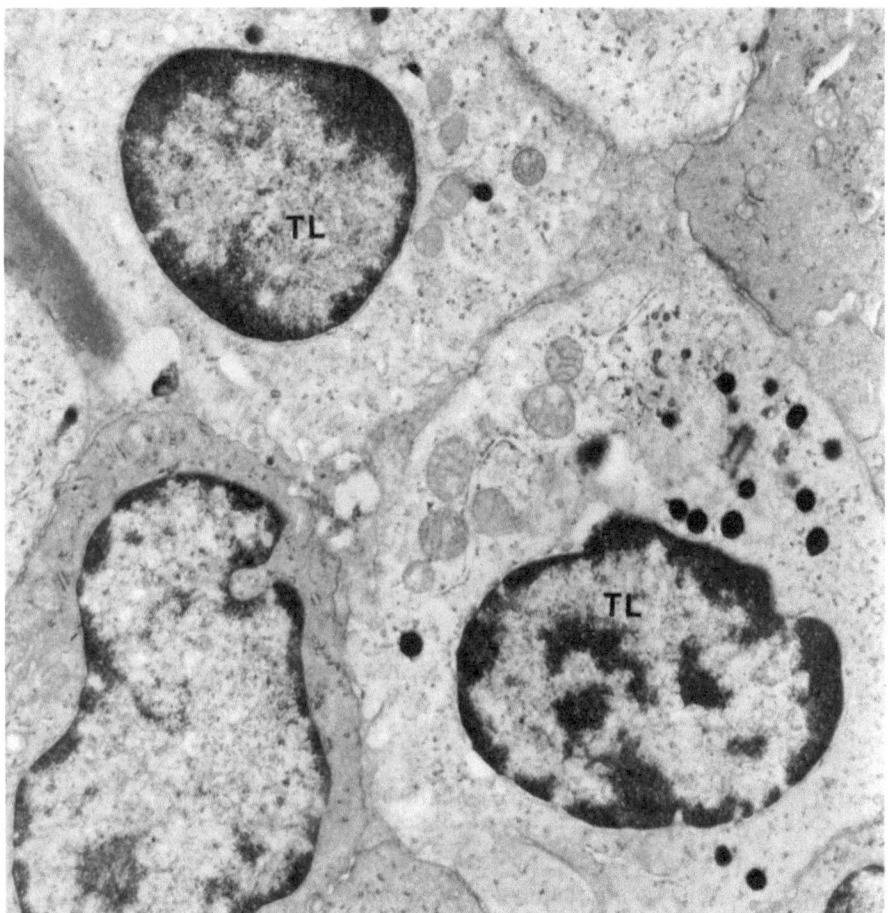

Fig. 19. Simian cardiac allograft, treated with Imuran and cortisone, 6 weeks after transplantation. These light cells (*TL*) may be postblast cell-derived T-lymphocytes transforming upon a second immunologic signal. Their nuclei still exhibit features of the mature lymphocyte. The cytoplasm is electron-light and contains several profiles of R.E.R., but only few clusters of polysomes and free ribosomes. Several mitochondria are concentrated in 1 portion of cytoplasm. Characteristic are electron-dark structures, probably of lysosomal nature, which surround the centriole. (Fixation: glutaraldehyde ×8,500)

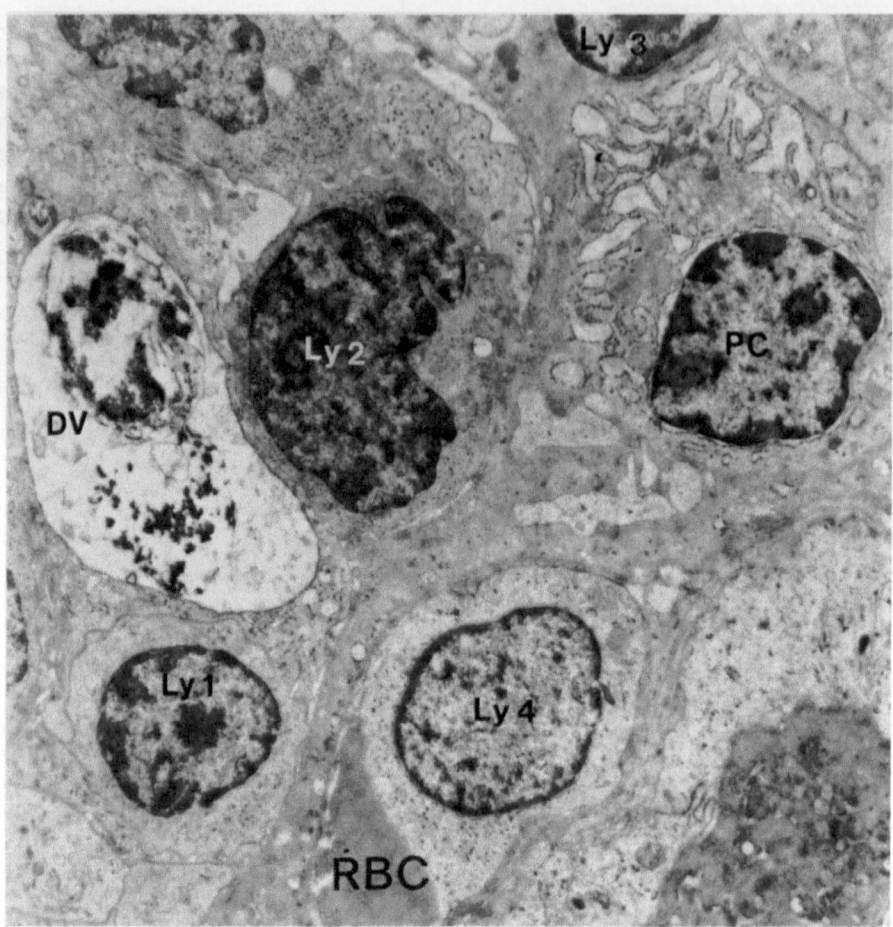

Fig. 20. Canine pulmonary allograft 12 days after transplantation. No immunosuppressive treatment. Perivascular cellular infiltrate is composed of lymphocytes (*Ly 1*) of varying degrees of maturity. Dark cell in centre of electron micrograph may be a lymphocyte (*Ly 2*) in early prophasic organization. Large digestive vacuole (*DV*) belongs to a bulk phagocytosing macrophage. Note plasma cell (*PC*) within capillary in close association with a mature lymphocyte (*Ly 3*) and immature lymphocyte (*Ly 4*). *RBC*: red blood cell. (Fixation: glutaraldehyde × 7,500)

appears to be centrifugal, and a gradually increasing number of cells become dispersed within the supporting tissue and interstitial spaces (Fig. 17). The actual cellular infiltrate is obviously governed by divergent cellular kinetics. Cells contacting the capillary endothelium during the first few hours (KOUNTZ *et al.*, 1963) (see also Chapter B II 1) either return to the spleen or migrate through the capillary wall (peripheral sensitization, Chapter C II 3). Since the lymphatic flow is sacrificed (Fig. 3), lymphocytes of the afferent branch of the immune response, which are almost exclusively of the small nonpyroninophilic type, accumulate preferentially within the distal lymphatic capillaries located in the surroundings of medium-sized vessels (Fig. 18). Similar infiltrates have occasionally been seen in autografts (LUND and JENSEN, 1970). The second generation of infiltrating cells comprises the various types of effector cells, e.g. transformed lymphocytes (Fig. 19), monocytes, macrophages capable of contact cytotoxicity, and plasma cells (Figs. 1, 2, 20).

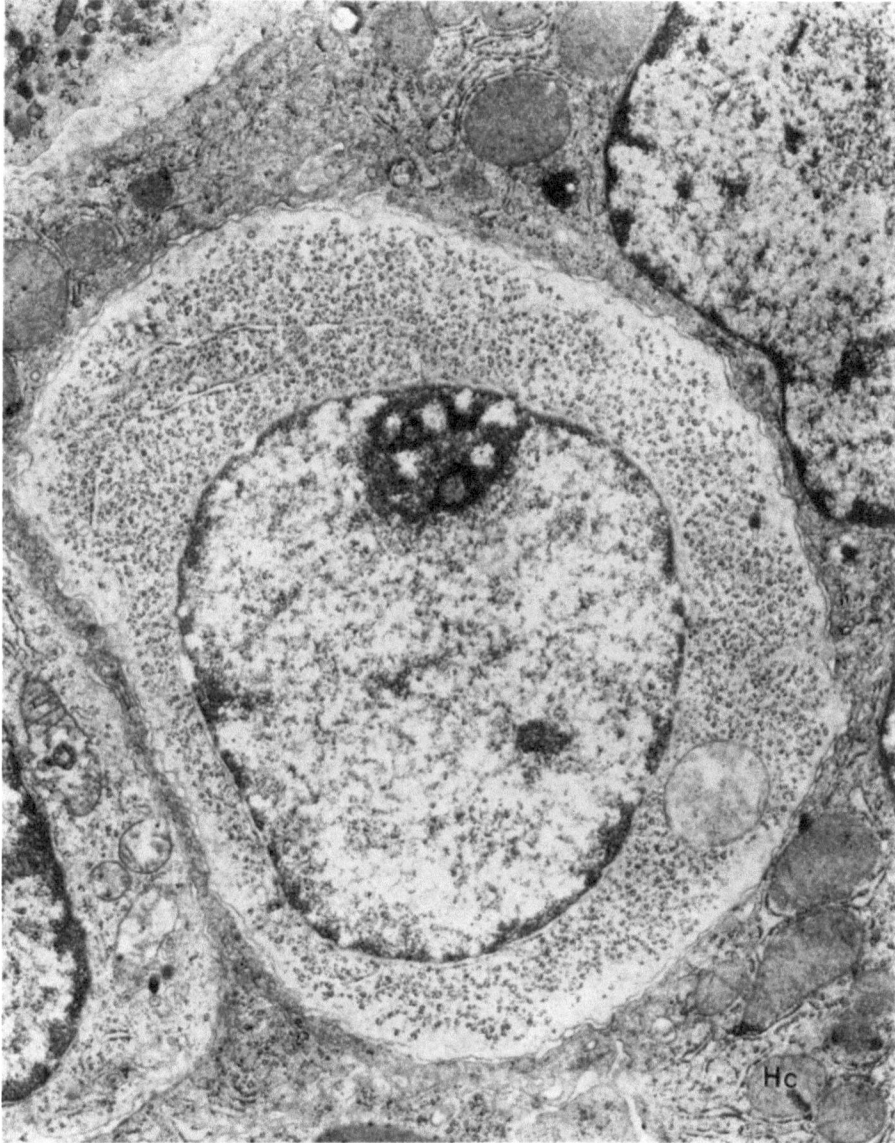

Fig. 21. Untreated canine orthotopic hepatic allograft 4 days after transplantation. Cell lying within cytoplasm of hepatocyte (*Hc*) exhibits all features of a blast cell. Heterochromatin is reduced to a small rim and nucleolus is connected with peripheral heterochromatin. Cytoplasm exhibits only few, short profiles of RER but abundant clusters of polysomes. Although close cytoplasmic contact is established between infiltrating immunoblast and the parenchymal cell, there are no indications for direct contact cytotoxicity (Fixation: glutaraldehyde, original enlargement × 16,500). By courtesy of Prof. Dr. H. THEMAN, Dept. of Medical Cytology, University of Münster, German Federal Republic

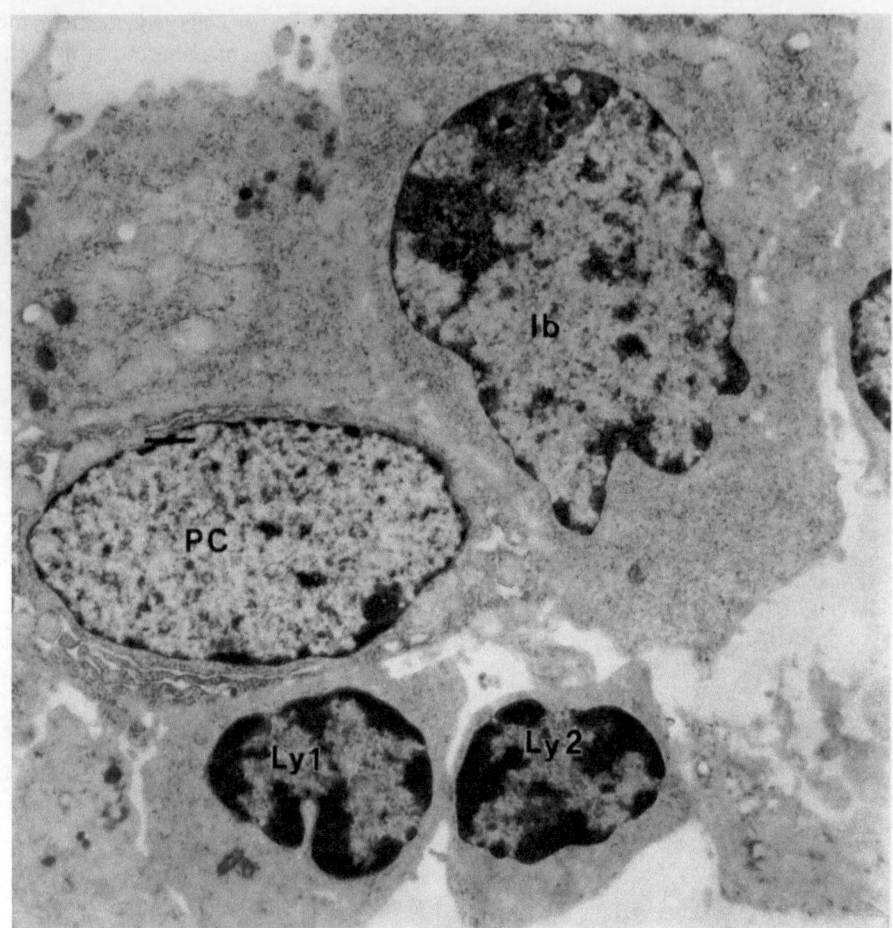

Fig. 22. Rat renal allograft, 7 days after transplantation. No immunosuppressive treatment. Cluster composed of immunoblast (*Ib*) with 2 nucleoli attached to small rim of peripheral nuclear heterochromatin and abundant polysomes, an immature plasma cell (*PC*; note thin rim of nuclear heterochromatin and developing profiles of RER), and 2 small lymphocytes (*Ly 1* and *2*). Close cytoplasmic contact between 1 lymphocyte (*Ly 1*) and developing plasma cell (*PC*). (Fixation: glutaraldehyde × 7,500)

A third group is represented by cells of the self-perpetuating machinery. Ultrastructurally they exhibit characteristics of blast cells (Fig. 21), transitional forms between lymphocytes and blasts, and of immature and mature plasma cells (KOUNTZ *et al.*, 1963; VANWIJCK *et al.*, 1968) (Figs. 22, 23). Immature cells incorporate tritiated thymidine (HÄYRY *et al.*, 1972; PASTERNACK *et al.*, 1973). In addition, various organ grafts exhibit cell clusters composed of "stimulated" lymphocytes, maturing and mature plasma cells which are in close contact with various types of macrophages (Fig. 23). They closely resemble autonomous hemolytic clusters suggestive of both peripheral helper cell activity and antibody synthesis (Chapter A III 3c γ; Fig. 1). In most instances cellular infiltration is associated with widespread moderate to severe interstitial edema.

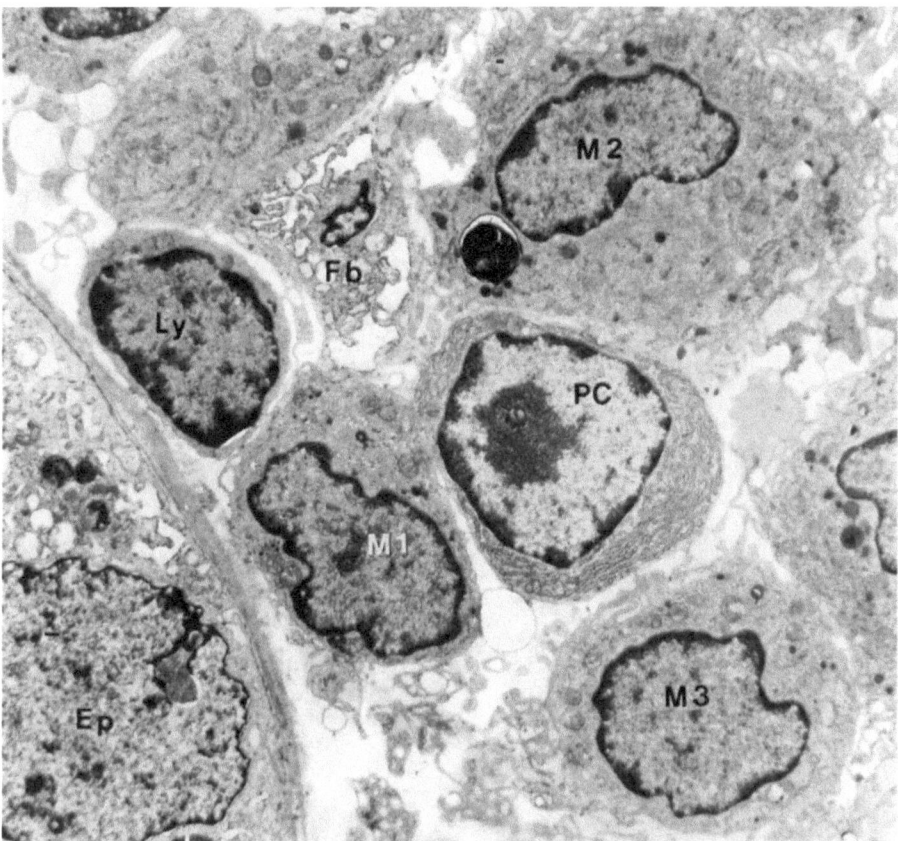

Fig. 23. Rat renal allograft, 7 days after transplantation. No immunosuppressive treatment. Peritubular interstitial accumulation of infiltrating cells arranged in cluster composed of mature plasma cell (*PC*), small lymphocyte (*Ly*), and several mononuclear macrophages (*M 1, 2* and *3*) with irregular loop-forming filopodia. Note close association between plasma cell and macrophage *M 1*.
Ep: tubular epithelial cell, *Fb*: fibroblast. (Fixation: glutaraldehyde × 5,000)

b) *Infiltrative and proliferative vascular lesions.* The infiltration of the subendothelial connective tissue (in heart graft also of the endocardium (Fig. 24) is somewhat less frequent, but pathognomonically more important (HUME et al., 1955; DEMPSTER et al., 1964). Since various cell types were observed to squeeze through lining endothelial surfaces (Fig. 25) among other mature plasma cells (PORTER, 1969), the cellular composition of the subendothelial infiltrates resembles that of the interstitial aggregates (Fig. 26). The most affected are medium-sized and small veins, and arterioles. Frequently, the endothelial cells are separated from the underlying tissue. Subsequent disruption of the endothelium favors the formation of both platelet thrombi, which appear to be rapidly replaced by fibrin (BOHLE, 1968; KINCAID–SMITH, 1970), (Fig. 27) and either mural or occlusive arterial and venous thrombosis (ROSENAU et al., 1969; PAZ, 1970). There are indications of early fibrous repair of the acute injury to the intima.

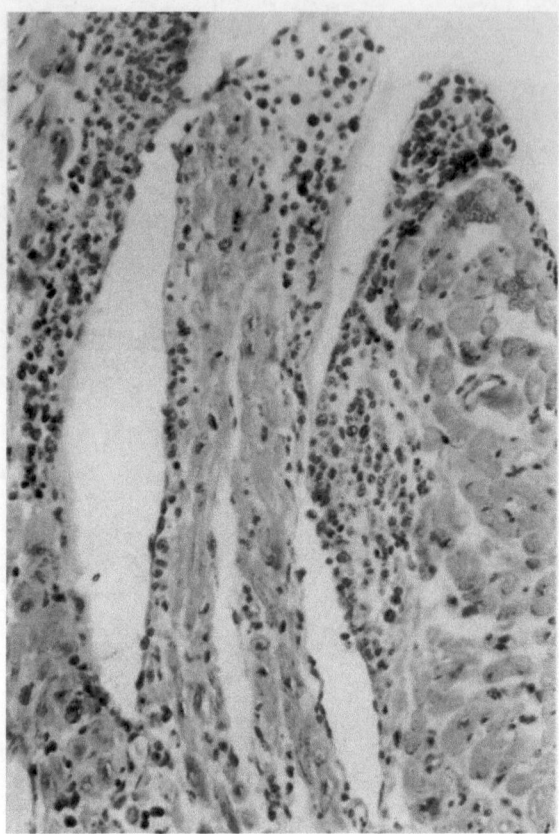

Fig. 24. Simian cardiac allograft, treated with Imuran and cortisone, 9 weeks after transplantation. Infiltration of endocardium of left ventricle predominantly consisting of small and medium-sized lymphocytes, several plasma cells, and a few lymphoblasts. Note intact lining endothelium. (Hematoxylin and eosin: ×250)

Frequently endothelial cells proliferate and form bridges across the lumen. Progressive thickening of the intima by infiltrating cells and edema, and the occlusion of smaller vessels by various MN cells (Kountz, et al., 1963; Guttmann et al., 1967b) are regarded as one of the reasons for the gradual decrease in the total blood flow through the graft.

c) *Necrotizing vascular lesion.* Focal fibrinoid necrosis of the media of arterioles and of small and medium-sized arteries is also seen in acute cell-mediated rejection (Dempster et al., 1964; Kincaid–Smith, 1964; Stinson et al., 1969; Paz, 1970) (Fig. 28). The necrotic process is often accompanied by rupture of the internal elastic lamina. Deposits of fibrin and platelets occur on the intima adjacent to damaged parts of the vessel wall. The IgG and $\beta 1$ C semidiscretely precipitated in the wall of altered vessels (Horowitz et al., 1965) suggests deposition of antibody or immune complexes as a pathogenic mechanism in the induction of necrosis of smooth muscle cells (Lindquist et al., 1968b).

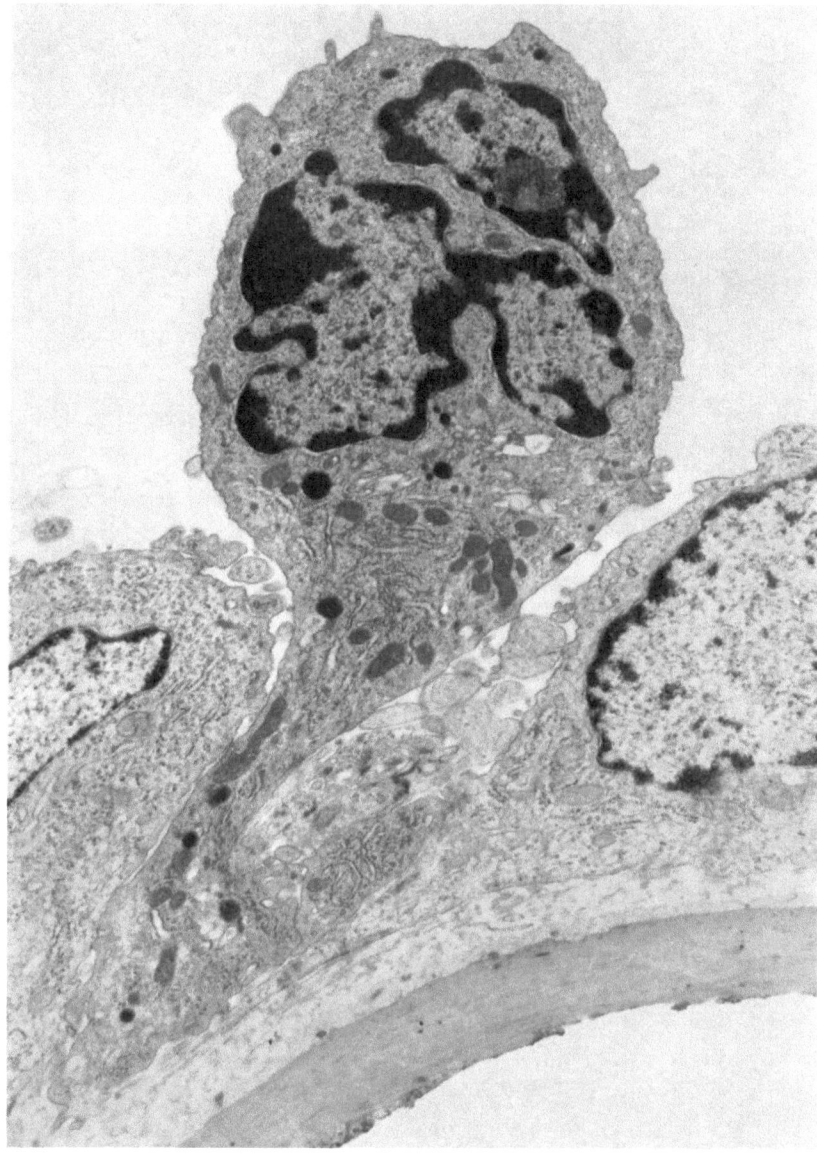

Fig. 25. Rat aortic allograft 5 days after transplantation. No administration of immunosuppressive drugs. Typical monocyte in diapedesis insinuates a cytoplasmic extension between 2 adjacent endothelial cells (Fixation: glutaraldehyde ×10,000). By courtesy of Dr. A.M. TER HAAR, Municipal Hospital Arnhem, The Netherlands

Since during the rejection of a second canine renal allograft the recipient's gastric and pancreatic arterioles were also damaged (SHEIL and MURRAY, 1968), smooth-muscle antibody may be involved (Chapter C II). Damage to the vasa vasorum may also result in areas of segmental medial necrosis (LOWER et al., 1969).

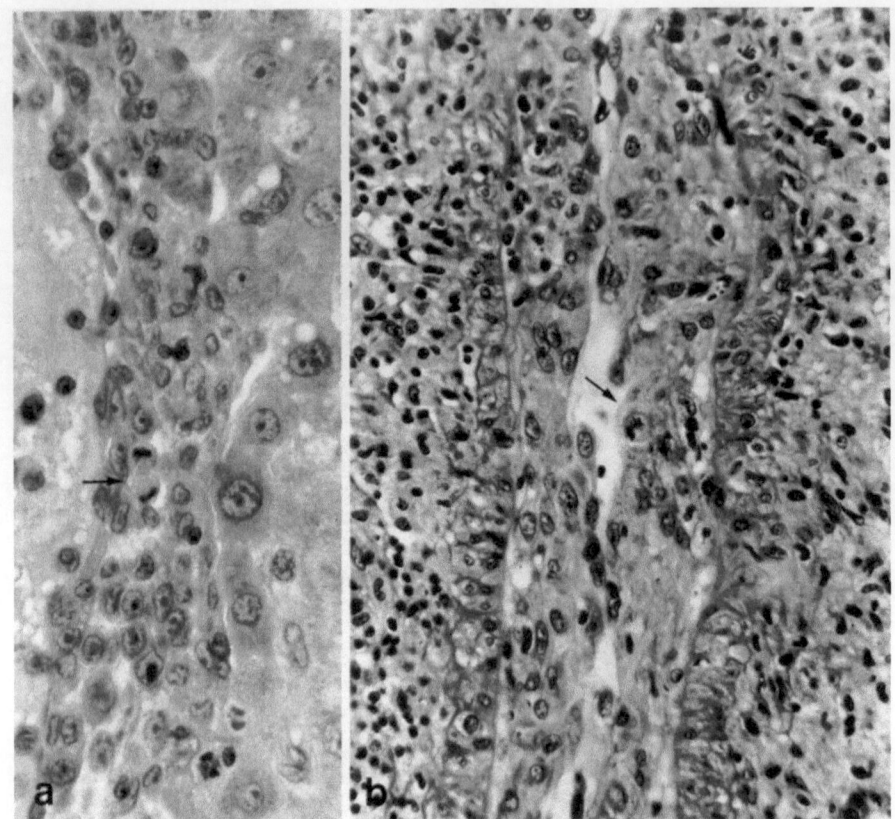

Fig. 26

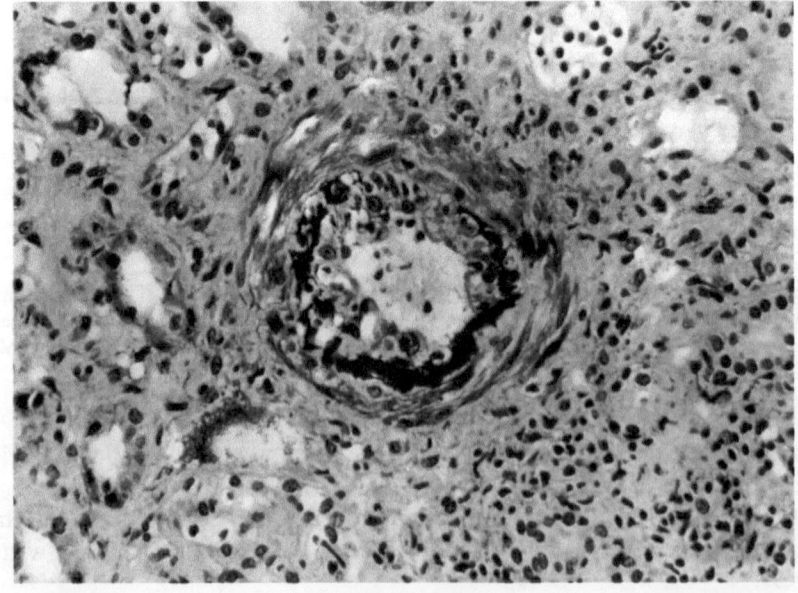

Fig. 27

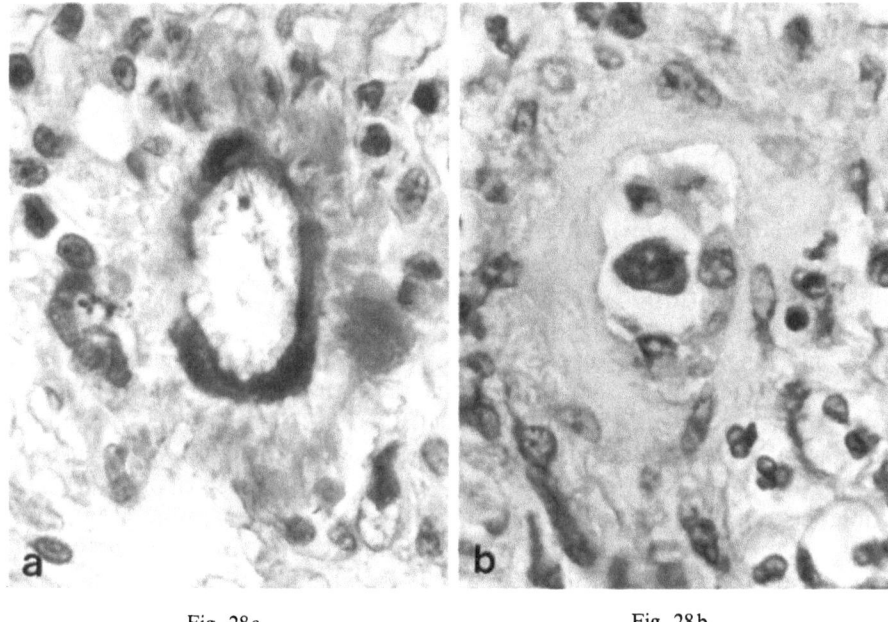

Fig. 28 a   Fig. 28 b

Fig. 28a. Canine pulmonary allograft, untreated, 7 days after transplantation. Fibrinoid necrosis of wall of small artery. (Goldner's trichrome: × 1,000)

Fig. 28b. Canine orthotopic hepatic allograft, treated with Imuran and cortisone, 7 days after transplantation. Hyalinization of media of small artery. Note damage to endothelium in both preparations and plasma cell in lumen of artery in b

◁ Fig. 26a and b. Infiltrative vascular lesion in rat heterotopic hepatic allograft, untreated, 4 days after transplantation (a), and in human renal allograft treated with immunosuppressive drugs, 4 weeks after transplantation (b). Note similarity of cellular infiltrate and occurrence of mitotic figures (arrows), although preparations are derived from different species and organs, from untreated or treated recipients respectively, and from different periods after transplantation. (Goldner's trichrome: × 500; hematoxylin and eosin: × 350). (b) By courtesy of Prof. Dr. P.H.M. SCHILLINGS, Dept. of Pathology and Prof. Dr. P.G.A. WIJDEVELD, Dept. of Nephrology, University of Nijmegen, The Netherlands

Fig. 27. Human kidney allograft, treated with immunosuppressive drugs, 4 weeks after transplantation. Mural fibrin deposits have replaced damaged endothelial surface of small artery. Lumen is narrowed by lipophages and infiltrating MN cells (Hematoxylin and eosin: × 350). By courtesy of Prof. Dr. P.H.M. SCHILLINGS, Dept. of Pathology and Prof. Dr. P.G.A. WIJDEVELD, Dept. of Nephrology, University of Nijmegen, The Netherlands

2. Mechanisms of Acute Cell-Mediated Graft Rejection

In necropsies, or biopsies taken during an acute rejection crisis, most grafts exhibit various combinations of histopathologic changes. Occasionally, however, one type of lesion predominates over the others, and the resulting changes can be used for a detailed analysis of histopathologic events contributing to graft destruction.

a) *Characterized by interstitial cellular infiltration.* The issue is very complex and rather controversial, involving consideration of the role of infiltrating cells in target cell destruction. Although renal tubular cells, cardiac myocytes, hepatocytes, and pancreatic acinar cells frequently exhibit changes like those triggered by contact cytotoxicity (Chapter B II 2, 3), these injuries can occur in the absence of intimate membrane contact between the infiltrating and the parenchymal cells (LINDQUIST et al., 1968b) (Chapter B II 1). In other instances, though close contact was established, parenchymal cells exhibited minimal lesions (ROSENAU et al., 1969; v. HEE, 1973; Figs. 14, 21). Furthermore, the degree of graft destruction does not seem to be related in any simple way to the number of infiltrating cells. In many instances of severe tissue injury they are suprisingly sparse, whereas in other cases accumulating cells are abundant, but destructive events may be minimal or, exceptionally, even absent. In one series of canine lung allotransplantation studied in our laboratory a graft exhibited diffuse interstitial and local perivascular infiltration between 14 and 40 days after transplantation (Fig. 29). After 80 days the cellular infiltrates were substantially reduced, and they were almost absent when the dog was sacrificed after 500 days. At no time was any indication of rejection present. The recipient had been submitted to adult thymectomy and subsequent treatment with ALS for 10 days four months before transplantation. No immunosuppressive drugs were administered during the posttransplantation period. Similarly, although human kidney allografts exhibited a distinctly increased number of lymphocytes within tubular epithelial cells (emperipolesis), their number was correlated neither to the type of rejection (acute or chronic) nor to the severity of the tubular and glomerular lesion (VOGT et al., 1970). Since a complete reversal of the cellular infiltrate was noticed after retransplantation of the unaccepted renal allograft back into the original recipient (MURRAY et al., 1962) it was suggested that in certain instances mononuclear cells and lymphocytes may cause target cell destruction only secondarily to a preceding humoral response (VAN BOXEL et al., 1972). After passive transfer of allospecific antibody, dogs rejected their own kidneys acutely. Simultaneously observed classic morphology of perivascular mononuclear cell infiltration indicated that the cellular response may occur as the result of antibody-induced damage, and does not necessarily represent a cellular response to transplantation antigens (DUBERNARD et al., 1968). Taking into account that both target cells and infiltrating cells were of host origin, these results are comparable to those observed after administration of allogenic anti-lung antibody (BURRELL et al., 1974; CATE and BURRELL, 1974).

However, it is easy to supplement these data with numerous examples where maximal tissue injury was observed at sites of maximal cell infiltration (BIEBER et al., 1970) or where aggressor cells were shown to attack their target cells

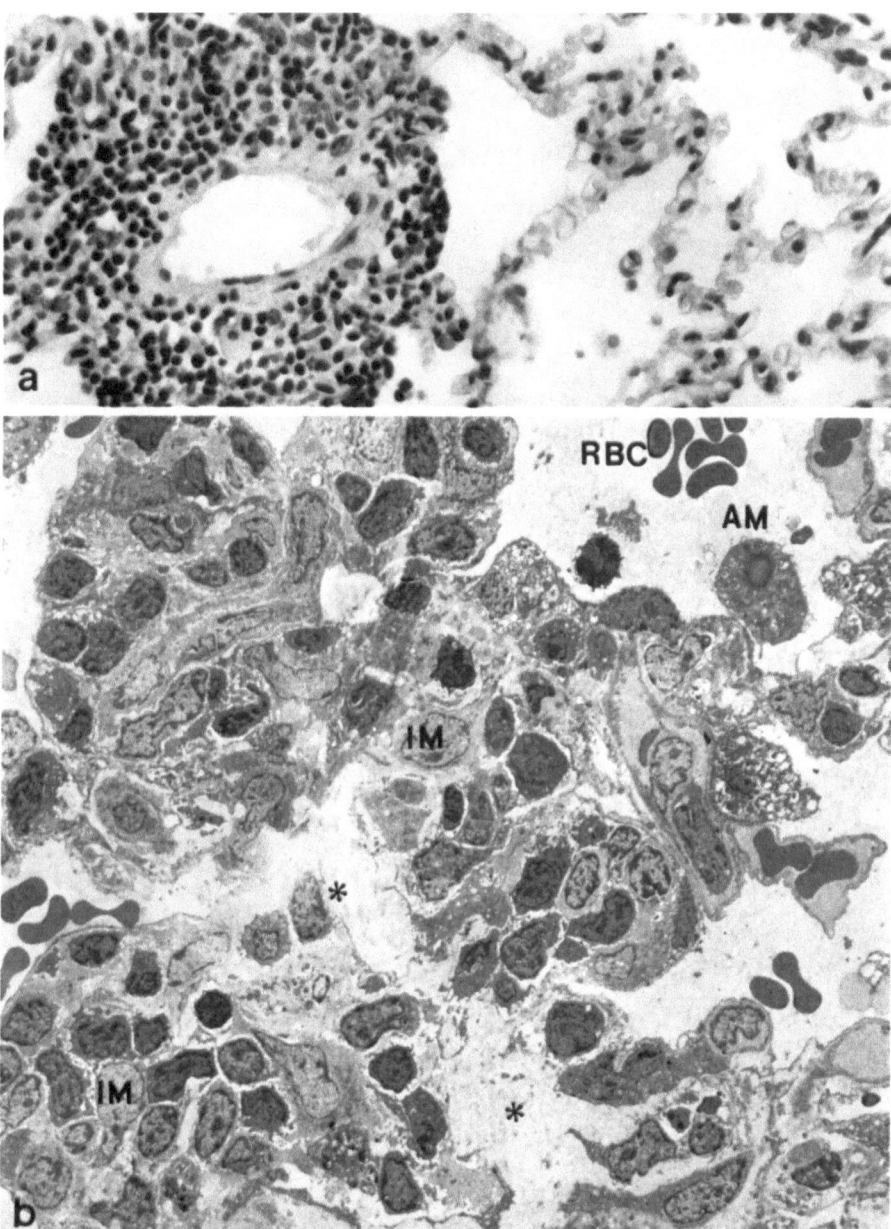

Fig. 29a and b. Canine pulmonary allograft 80 days after transplantation. The recipient was T-cell depleted through thymectomy and subsequent treatment with ATS for 10 days, 5 months prior to transplantation. No immunosuppressive treatment during post-transplantation course. Distinct perivascular cuffing (a) which on electron micrographs (b) is composed of dark and light staining small lymphocytes. Frequently lymphocytes are arranged around interstitial macrophages (*IM*). Note several alveolar macrophages (*AM*) within alveolar space. Presence of red blood cells (*RBC*) in alveolar space is probably a preparation artifact. Note slight interstitial edema and interstitial fibrosis (asterisks). (Goldner's trichrome: a × 350; Fixation: glutaraldehyde, b × 1,700)

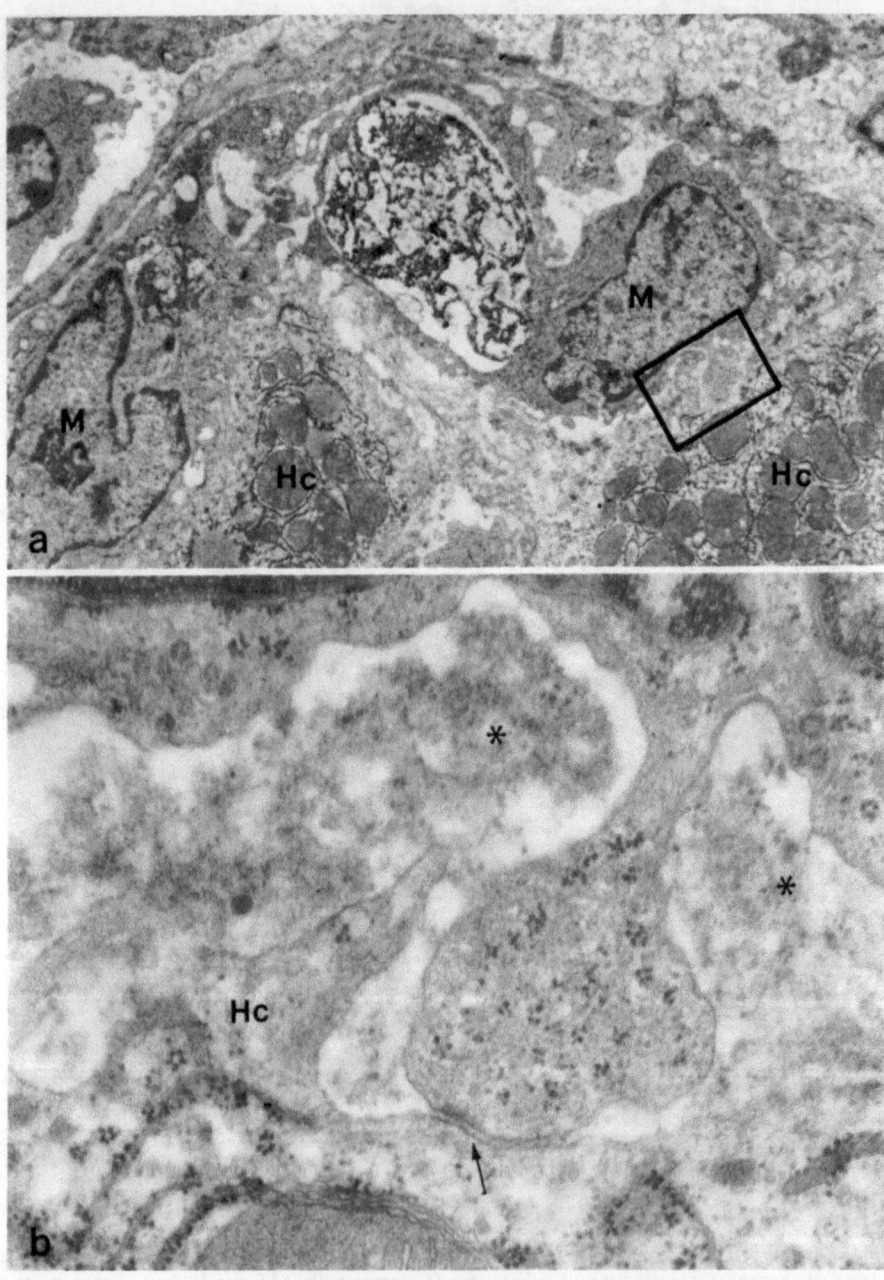

Fig. 30a and b. Rat heterotopic, auxiliary liver allograft 6 days after transplantation. No immunosuppressive treatment. Bulk phagocytosing macrophages (*M*) have infiltrated space of Disse (a). A pseudopodlike cytoplasmic extension of 1 macrophage (frame and b) appears to invaginate the cytoplasm of adjacent hepatocyte (*Hc*). Note "contact plate" between both cells (arrow). Space of Disse exhibits moderately dense fluffy basement membrane-like substance (asterisks, b). (Fixation: glutaraldehyde, a ×3,400; b ×21,000)

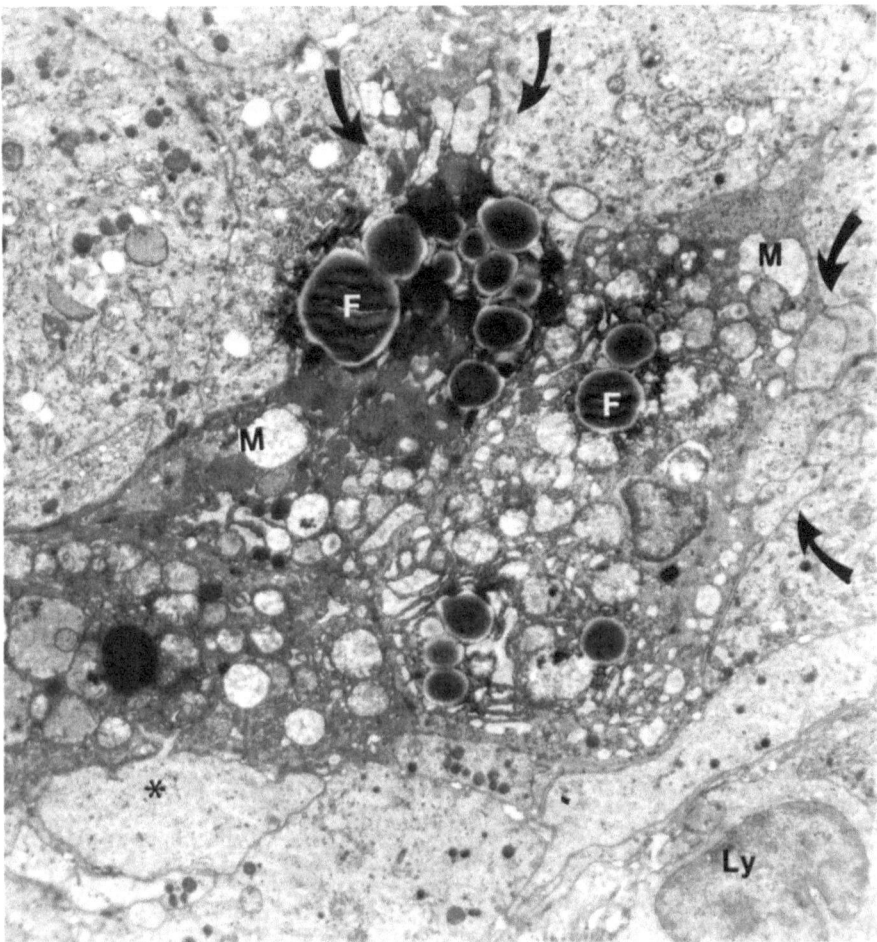

Fig. 31. Rat heterotopic, auxiliary liver allograft 10 days after transplantation. No immunosuppressive treatment. Large labyrinthine and electron-light cytoplasmic processes of numerous macrophages clinging closely to 3 hepatocytes and appearing to abrade portions of hepatocytic cytoplasm (arrows). Small finger-like projection is seen to penetrate 1 hepatocyte (asterisk). Remaining cytoplasm of hepatocytes exhibits swollen mitochondria (M) and large quantities of fat droplets (F). A lymphocyte (Ly) can be seen at some distance from scene of action. (Fixation: glutaraldehyde × 5,000)

(Kosek *et al.*, 1968) (Figs. 30, 31). The reader is therefore referred again to Chapter A III, in which the various mechanisms of transplantation reactions are summarized, and in particular to the importance of T-helper cell activities for the differentiation of effector cells, and to the role of lymphotoxin as a soluble mediator. What we do *not* know is the diversity of modes of sensitization to histocompatibility, differentiation or tissue-specific antigens (Chapter C II 1). The second signal for firing the soluble mediator may be specific, triggered by contact with the corresponding antigen, e.g. during migration through the capillary wall, or mediated by specialized cells; the resulting cytotoxicity, however, is nonspecific (Chapter A III 3b β).

Little attention has been paid to differences in the latent period in *in vitro* models and the *in vivo* manifestation of the cell-mediated reaction. Mouse peripheral lymphocytes stimulated with PHA exhibit maximum DNA synthesis on day 3. When they were stimulated by *in vitro* culturing with allogenic lymphocytes, the peak for incorporation of tritiated thymidine was found to fall between days 5 to 7 (HÄYRY and DEFENDI, 1970; ANDERSSON and HÄYRY, 1973). Lymphocytes collected from cannulated lymphatics of a human kidney exhibited both maximal incorporation of tritiated thymidine and blast cell transformation on days 5 and 6 after transplantation. Supposing that maximum DNA synthesis represents the peak transformation of unprimed small lymphocytes (see Fig. 1 and T_x, B_x, Fig. 2) into blast cells and their differentiation to postblast effector cells ($B_{1,2}$, T_3, Fig. 2), the times observed are coincident both with the IgG and IgM log phase after sensitization, e.g. with flagellin (v.D. BROEK, 1971), and with the first of the six stages postulated by MEDAWAR (1958) to establish the immunologic character of the skin homograft reaction, i.e. the latent period before its inception. However, they are, in part, not coincident with changes occasionally seen early after transplantation of solid organ grafts. Within 3 to 6 hours after revascularization of rat renal allografts, mononuclear cells traversed thin-walled vessels and accumulated in the perivascular space. Dense agglomerations present as little as 24 hours after surgery (FELDMAN and LEE, 1967) were associated with endothelial changes, slight focal injury of tubules, and increased vascular permeability. The extent of pathologic lesions increased gradually rather than occurring suddenly after a latent period. This sequence of events suggests a possible involvement of the transfer factor (Chapter A III 3b) and the early cytotoxic activity of strongly stimulated normal lymphocytes (Chapter B II b, Fig. 1).

Whatever mechanism of the cell-mediated reaction has caused the tissue injury, there are early attempts at gradual replacement of necrotic areas with fibrous connective tissue. First the number of classic bulk phagocytes increases (Fig. 32), then pyroninophilic fibroblasts progressively infiltrate the damaged area, and both collagenous fibers and, occasionally, outgrowing capillaries become visible. Finally, the lymphoid cells disappear. In grafts with longer survival, the size of the resulting fibrotic area is usually related to the magnitude of the primary lesion. Afunctional, non-life supporting auxiliary transplants are finally entirely replaced by fibrous tissue.

b) *Characterized by capillary alteration.* Interstitial cellular infiltration is generally associated with marked interstitial edema (PORTER, 1965, 1969; NORA et al., 1969; v. HEE, 1973), but severe edema may be an outstanding feature, even in the absence of significant numbers of MN cells (LINDQUIST et al., 1968b). In several instances it appears simply to result from both the absence of the (sacrificed) lymph flow and vascular denervation and it is only slightly progressive. Since diminution of lung functions (pO_2 and dynamic lung compliance) after bilateral hilar stripping was directly correlated to the severity of the postoperative interstitial edema in this organ (IRIE et al., 1975), a permanent increase in interstitial fluid may also impair the functions of parenchymal cells in other organs. Histochemically, decreased activity of various dehydrogenases, including those of the Krebs citric acid cycle, was detected in canine renal allografts

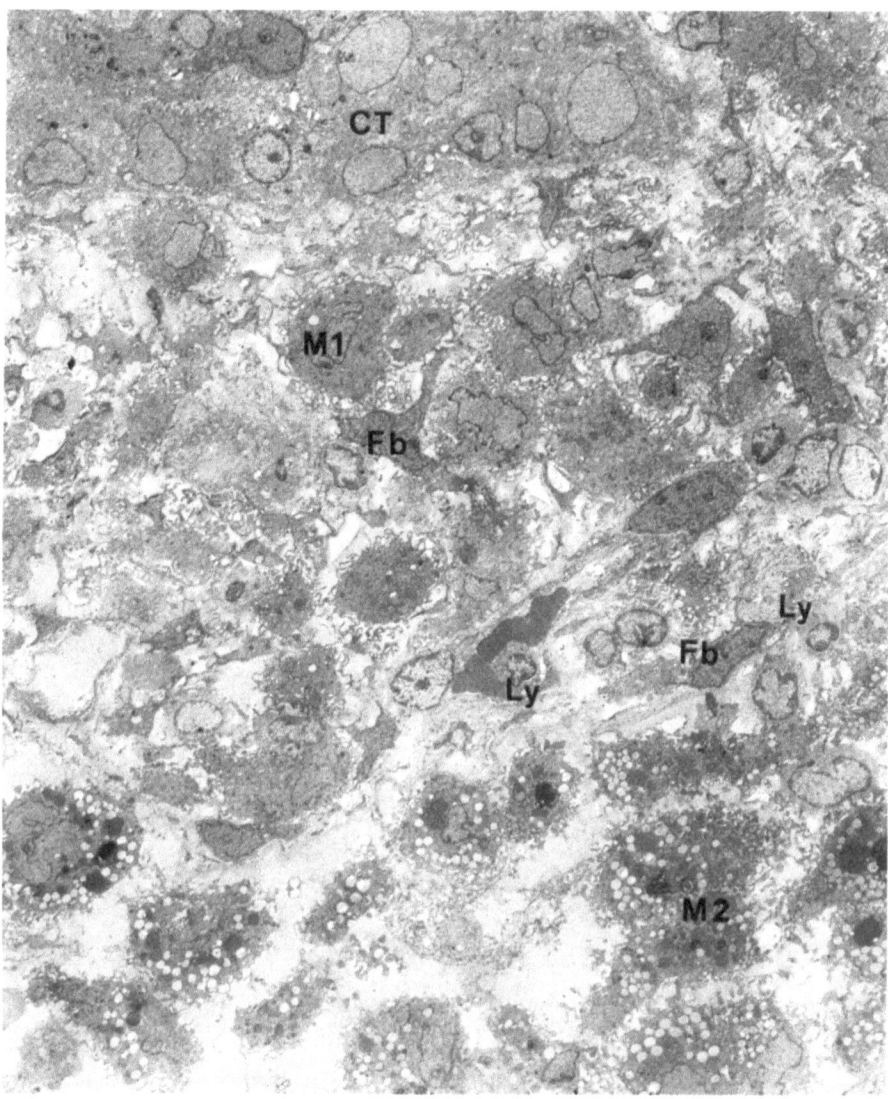

Fig. 32. Rat kidney allograft 10 days after transplantation. No immunosuppressive treatment. A collapsed collecting tubule (*CT*) is surrounded by large number of macrophages (*M 1*) which exhibit numerous long labyrinthine filopodia, but only few lipid droplets. Venule in lower part of picture is occupied by bulk phagocytosing macrophages (*M 2*) characterized by short and plump cytoplasmic extensions and numerous lipid droplets. Few small lymphocytes (*Ly*) and fibroblasts (*Fb*) are interspersed. Delicate collagenous fibrils are deposited in interstices between macrophages. (Fixation: glutaraldehyde ×2,000)

on the second day and before morphologic changes were perceived (LINDQUIST and HAGER, 1964). Abnormal increases in permeability of morphologically only slightly altered capillaries lead to nonspecific accumulation of serum proteins, but with a low fibrin content in the interstices. Renal tubuli, myocardial fibers and pancreatic acini are separated from each other and from the capillaries

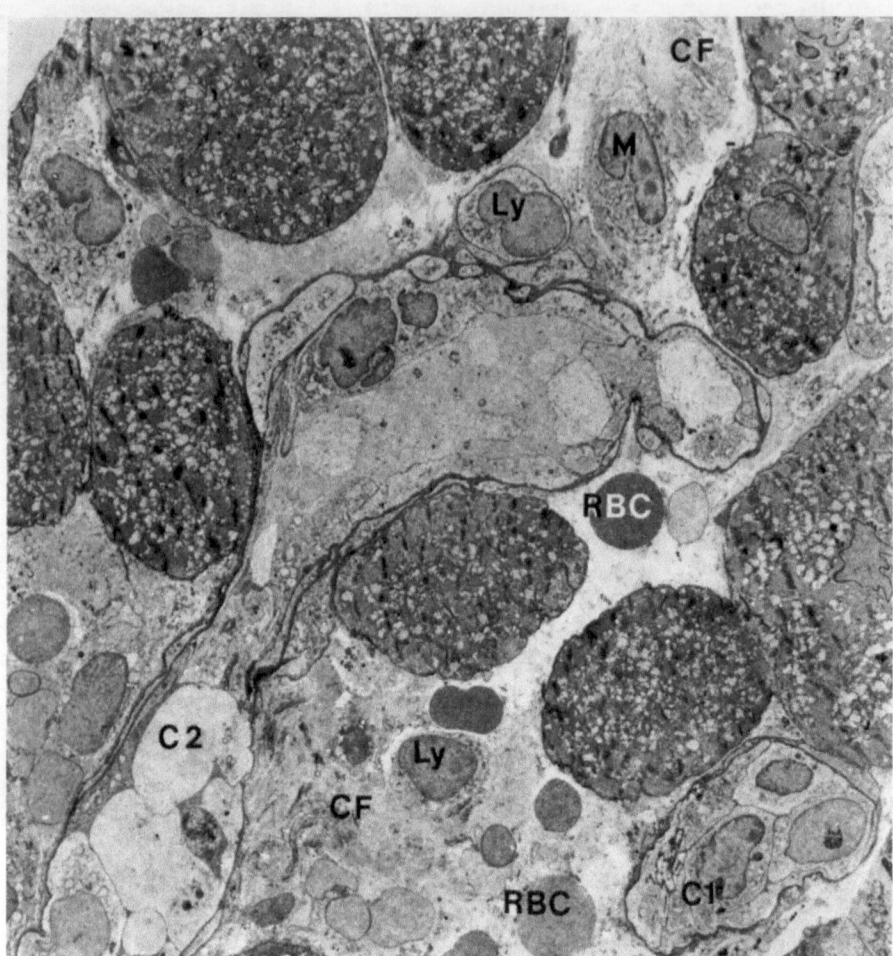

Fig. 33. Simian cardiac allograft, treated with Imuran and cortisone, 9 weeks after transplantation. Ventricular muscle cells are separated from each other and from capillaries by severe interstitial proteinaceous edema in which several strands of collagenous fibrils (*CF*) are embedded. Interstices are infiltrated by macrophages (*M*) and few lymphocytes (*Ly*). Increase in capillary permeability is further indicated by diapedesis of (occasionally degenerating) red blood cells (*RBC*). Capillaries are partly occluded either by hyperplastic and hypertrophic endothelium (*C 1*) or by cytoplasmic extensions of endothelial cells and/or white blood cells or their swollen remains (*C 2*). Whereas cardiac muscle cells exhibit swollen mitochondria, their contractile elements are still intact. (Fixation: osmic acid ×2,000)

by abundant edema; hypoxemic injury and atrophy of parenchymal cells may result from this change (v. HEE, 1973).

   The escape of larger quantities of fibrin and/or cells others than lymphocytes is linked to both progressive changes of capillaries and severe tissue injury (Fig. 33). Focal and total fibrinoid necrosis of a graft can occur in the absence of discernible damage to the larger vessels (ELLIS *et al.*, 1971; WILDEVUUR *et al.*, 1973b), but is frequently associated with deposition of fibrin in small arteries and veins. It has been suggested that both humoral mechanisms (LINDQUIST *et al.*, 1968a, b) and direct contact cytotoxicity (KOUNTZ *et al.*, 1963; PORTER, 1965; KOSEK *et al.*, 1969) contribute to the capillary damage in these instances. Specifically sensitized thoracic duct lymphocytes had the capacity to induce acute and severe interstitial hemorrhage in goats (JANSEN *et al.*, 1970).

However, interstitial hemorrhage rarely occurs as an isolated syndrome. The frequent association with venous thrombosis suggests a possible involvement of increased venous pressure in the chain of reactions: interstitial edema — fibrinoid necrosis — interstitial hemorrhage. Ischemia may operate as an additional pathogenic mechanism in capillary endothelial damage (DRINKER, 1945; JAP *et al.*, 1973). Recently we studied a series of lung autografts revascularized after 24 hours in cool storage. All transplants developed severe interstitial and alveolar hemorrhage 6 to 24 hours after reimplantation. Changes in small and medium-sized vessels were notably absent (Fig. 11 b, c).

c) *Characterized by vaso-occlusive changes.* The fate of numerous grafts undergoing acute rejection is largely determined by the extent of developing vascular injuries. Some lesions occur very rapidly, in particular when rejection commences within a few days of transplantation, while others become manifest only after some weeks or even months. Whatever type of vascular lesion and subsequent change is predominant, whether thrombotic or proliferative, it can cause marked narrowing or occlusion of almost every vessel. Progressive ischemic atrophy and necrosis of the parenchyma, local infarction (Fig. 34a) distal to narrowed arteries, and hemorrhagic necrosis (Fig. 34b) proximal to occluded veins are the almost inevitable subsequent histopathologic changes. In kidneys, the lesions in arterial branches of all sizes from the main renal artery down to the arterioles are histologically similar (KINCAID–SMITH, 1970). According to experience in our laboratory, the same holds true for the vasculature of hepatic and pancreatic grafts. However, immunologically triggered lesions of the main pulmonary artery were distinctly less frequent, suggesting an influence of the flow velocity. A solitary smooth stenosis of the renal artery just distal to the anastomosis was observed in instances where an end-to-side anastomosis to the iliac artery was the technique most often used (MORRIS *et al.*, 1971). Less efficient renal blood flow (MIMS, 1961) and replacement of laminar flow by turbulent flow in the vicinity of an unphysiological angle of take-off, or kinking of the artery, were considered to be mechanical factors that predispose to platelet deposition.

d) *Characterized by minimal lymphoid cell infiltration.* Sometimes grafts are rejected acutely even though infiltration with lymphoid cells is minimal or even absent (Fig. 35). There is unanimity about the role of *preformed* antibody as a consequence of pre-existing antigenic exposure, e.g. through a previous transplant, in triggering both microvascular diseases and hyperacute rejection (Chapters A III 2, 3, D I). However, the involvement of primary humoral immune reactions to the acute rejection of first-set organs is controversial. A positive correlation was suggested by studies where deposits of immunoglobulin, particularly of IgM, complement, and fibrin in various vessels were significantly associated with the rejection of kidney allografts two days to two years after transplantation (McKENZIE and WHITTINGHAM, 1968). Antibody of the IgM class

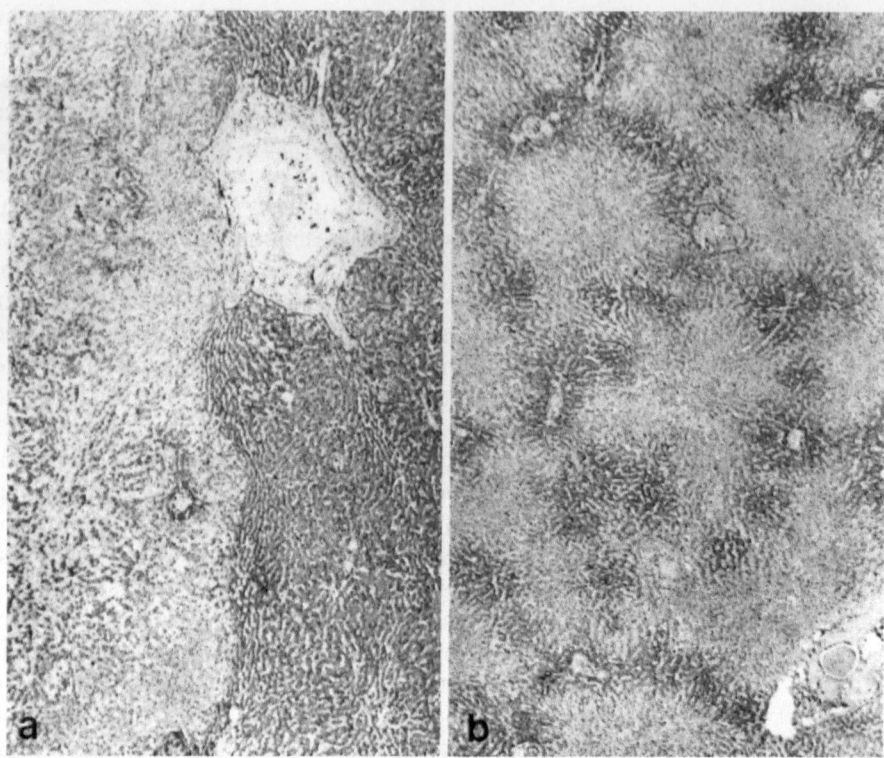

Fig. 34a and b. Canine orthotopic liver allografts exhibiting either segmental necrosis 5 days after transplantation (a) or extended central and midzonal hemorrhagic necrosis 9 days after transplantation (b). Both recipients underwent immunosuppressive treatment. (Hematoxylin and eosin: a and b × 40)

from rats rejecting kidney allografts fixed promptly to endothelia of capillaries and of medium-sized arteries (v. Breda–Vriesman and Feldman, 1972). Elevated serum IgM levels suddenly fell in patients during episodes of kidney allograft rejection, and IgM was deposited within the wall of small arteries (Zühlke, 1968). In contrast, immunoglobulin deposits were also noted in kidneys where rejection was *not* observed (Williams *et al.*, 1967), or were absent during the early phase of cardiac allograft rejection (Kosek *et al.*, 1969; Bieber *et al.*, 1970). Since characteristic staining patterns of immunoglobulin and complement in arterial walls were also present in rat renal isografts, and because the arterial wall is permeated by various plasma constituents even under normal conditions (Bleyl, 1969), the nonimmunologic fixation of these proteins to ischemically damaged tissue was suggested (Lubbe *et al.*, 1973). Fixation may be favored by changes in the transcapillary gradient, since the lymph drainage, which seems to be important for the maintenance of the fluid balance, is sacrificed (Hauck, 1973). Although in cardiac allografts deposition of IgG within myocardial fibers was always associated with severe necrosis, ischemia secondary to vascular lesions may account for this injury, since myocardial necrosis is predominantly

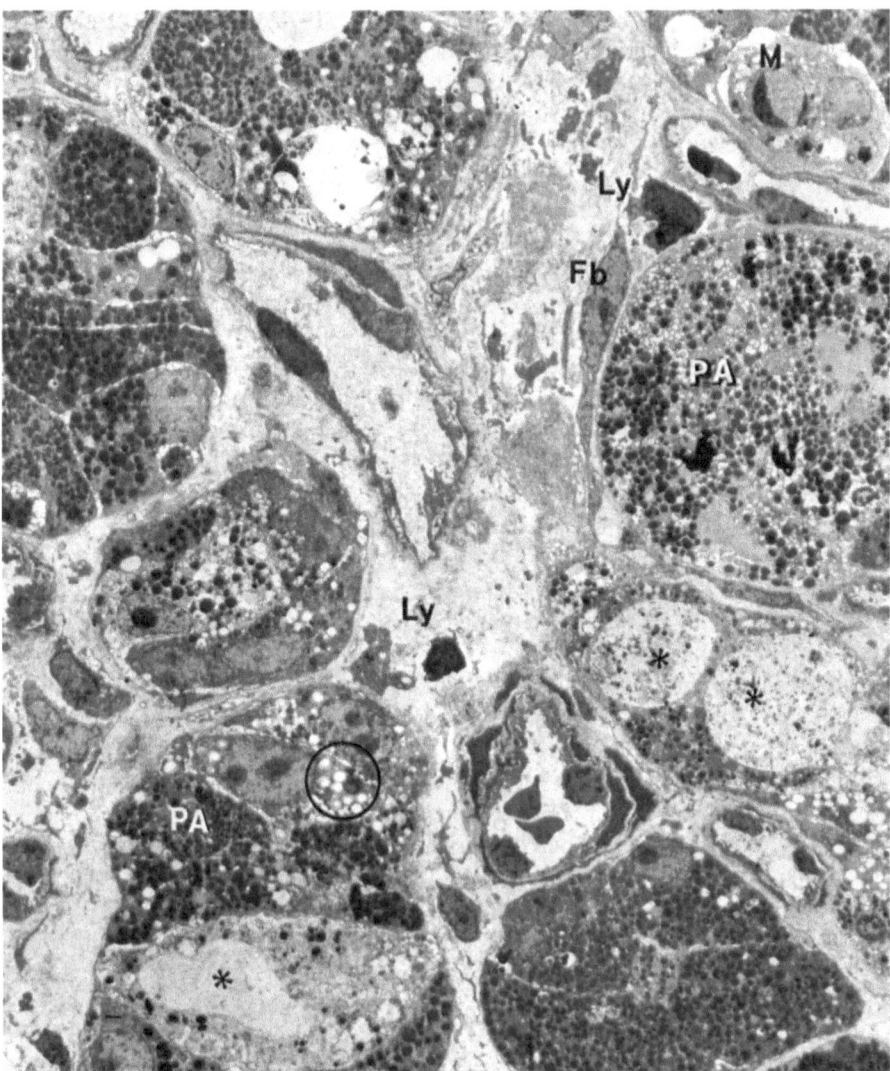

Fig. 35. Canine pancreatic allograft, treated with Imuran and cortisone, 17 days after transplantation. This surgical biopsy exhibits dilated blood vessels, distinct interstitial edema, and slight interstitial fibrosis (*Fb*: fibroblasts), but only occasionally small and obviously unstimulated lymphocytes (*Ly*), and a macrophage (*M*). Despite satisfactory function of exocrine part of graft at this time, the pancreatic acini (*PA*) exhibit ultrastructural abnormalities. In addition to abnormal acinar microarchitecture, zymogen granules are markedly polymorphic, and incipient necrosis is indicated by both lipid infiltration of most of acinar cells (circle) and focal cytoplasmic necrosis (asterisks). (Fixation: glutaraldehyde × 1,700)

localized in the subendocardial regions and the papillary muscles (BIEBER *et al.*, 1970). However, immunofluorescent antibody tests either demonstrate antibodies distinct from the cytotoxic ones (CERILLI *et al.*, 1972) or do not detect the small quantities of highly cytotoxic antibodies attached to target structures

(CARPENTER and MERRILL, 1969; GILES *et al.*, 1970). Thus the triggering of acute rejection by primary humoral responses is mostly supported by inference, strengthened by experimental studies in which the characteristic lesion of endothelial proliferation, i.e. fibrinoid necrosis of the arterial wall with subsequent cellular infiltration, was induced by a 5- to 7-day course of administration of specific antibody (DUBERNARD *et al.*, 1968).

II. Particular Patterns of Acute Rejection

1. Kidney

The pathologic changes described above (Chapter F I 2) are well exemplified by those seen in kidney allograft rejection. Most affected are the cortical arteries, arterioles and peritubular capillaries. The tubular alterations are varied and range from hyaline droplet formation, extreme vacuolation, isolated necrosis of tubular cells, and changes commonly observed in extensive acute tubular necrosis. Final tubular necrosis appears to be secondary to the primary immunological injury to the blood vessels (KOUNTZ *et al.*, 1963). Of particular interest, of course, are the glomerular changes. In acutely rejected renal allografts these may be slight, although swelling of the glomerular endothelial and mesangial cells is frequently seen. A major glomerular lesion is interpreted as an acute phenomenon (LINDQUIST *et al.*, 1968b), histologically paralleling the picture of acute proliferative and/or thrombotic glomerulopathy (GUTTMANN *et al.*, 1967b; GEWURZ, 1971; DIXON 1971a). There is little evidence for the participation of any delayed hypersensitivity mechanism. The alterations are frequently focal and local, involving only a portion of some glomerular tufts. Initially they are characterized by hypercellularity. Endothelial and mesangial cells exhibit mitotic figures, and the swelling of endothelial cells compromises the patency of glomerular capillaries. The mesangial matrix is often somewhat increased (ROSENAU *et al.*, 1969) and the basement membrane slightly thickened. Subsequently, the number of intracapillary PMN cells distinctly increases (GUTTMANN *et al.*, 1967b; PAZ, 1970), the capillary loops are thickened and focally occluded by eosinophilic, fibrillar, PAS-positive material which was shown on the electron micrograph close-up to be composed predominantly of platelets and fibrin. A local "chew up" (DIXON, 1971b) of the basement membrane is occasionally seen. Ensuing necrosis of both endothelial and mesangial cells causes diminution of the previously observed glomerular hypercellularity, while crescent proliferation may still be present in others. Finally, large portions of the glomerular tufts become bloodless and occluded by amorphous material (Fig. 27). KINCAID SMITH (1970) emphasized the striking similarity between the glomerular lesion during early allograft rejection and that in a variety of other diseases affecting the renal glomerulus primarily and secondarily. Although in developing proliferative glomerulopathy IgG and complement are frequently not demonstrable (LINDQUIST *et al.*, 1968b), mechanisms similar to those known to trigger both antibasement nephritis and the injury resulting from circulating nonglomerular antigen-antibody complexes were considered to be involved (MILGROM *et al.*, 1971). Neither the interaction between antibody and fixed glomerular antigens nor the deposition of immune complexes is injurious by itself. Damage to the basement membrane and the capillary endothelium results rather from subsequent fixation and activation of complement, and from attracted PMN cells (Chapter D I). However, non-complement-mediated glomerular injury may be present, at least in the initial phase of the Masugi nephritis model (KOBAYASHI *et al.*, 1973) (see also Chapter G III).

2. Heart

Histologic examination of rejected human cardiac allografts and of sequential canine cardiac allografts revealed a sequence of events and morphologic lesions

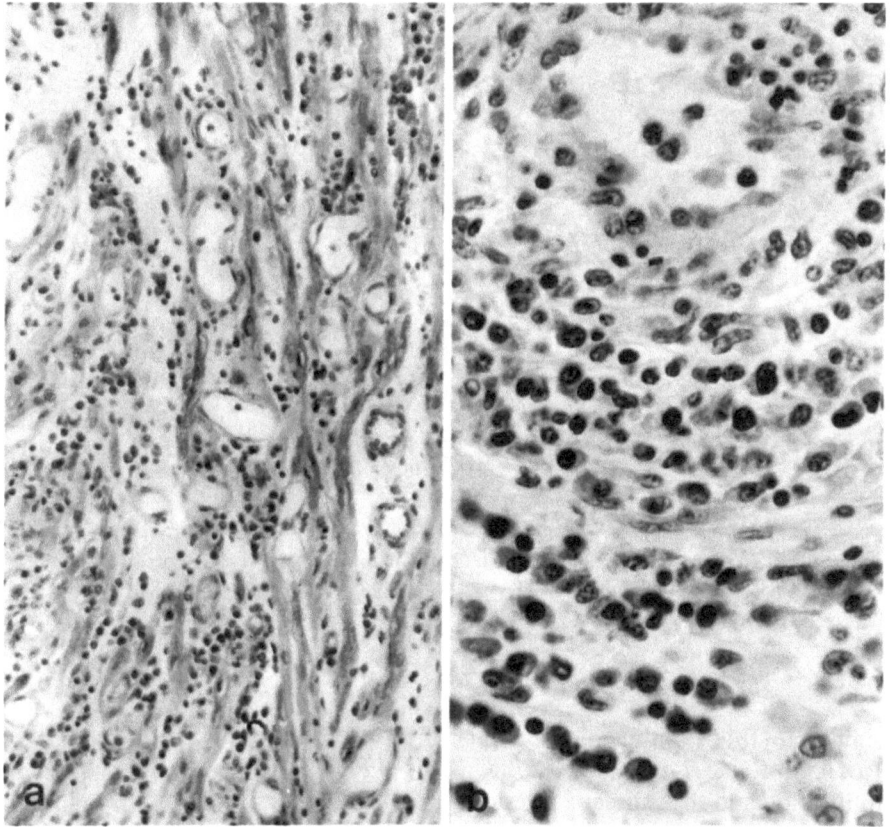

Fig. 36a and b. Simian cardiac allograft, treated with Imuran and cortisone, 9 weeks after transplantation. (a) Marked interstitial edema, infiltration by cells of lymphocytic and plasma-cellular series, and atrophy of ventricular muscle cells. Note dilated and patent blood vessels. (b) Although wall of interventricular branch of coronary artery is densely infiltrated by plasma cells and small lymphocytes, lumen is not markedly narrowed by infiltrative and/or proliferative changes of intima. (Hematoxylin and eosin: a ×250; b ×500). Remarkably enough, there were no distinct electrocardiographic abnormalities 2 days before the animal was sacrificed because of sudden deterioration of cardiac functions

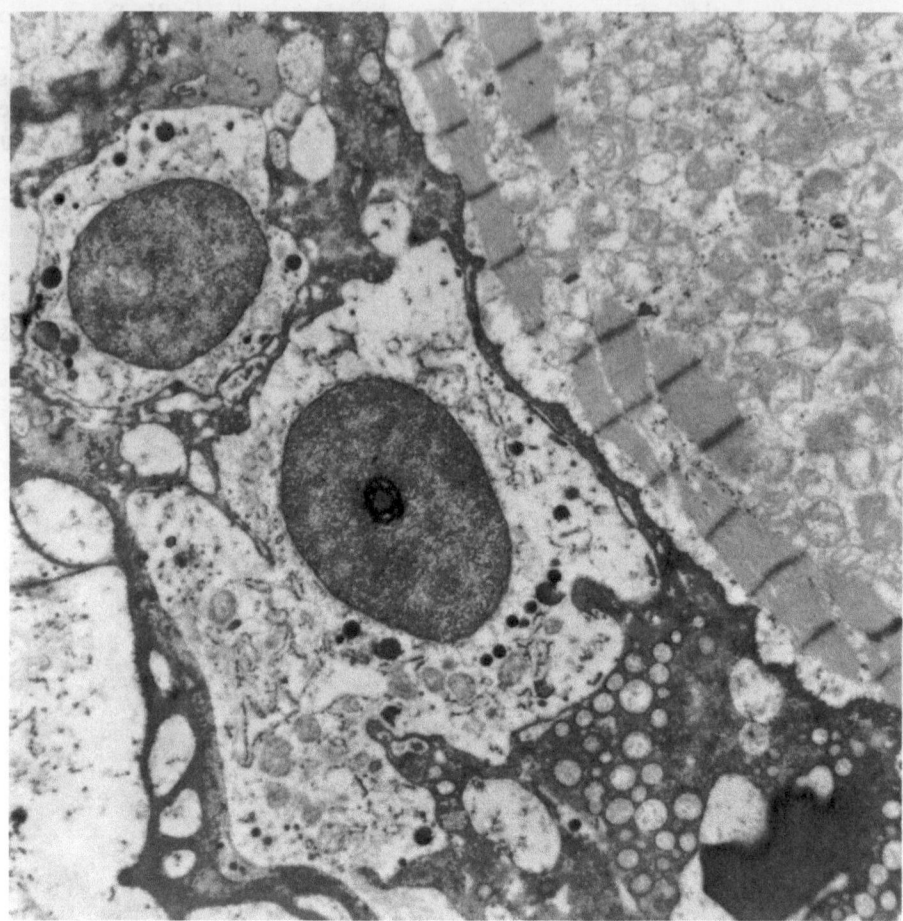

Fig. 37. Same cardiac allograft as in Fig. 36. Two electron-light infiltrating cells have penetrated endothelium of ventricular capillary. Irregular cytoplasmic extensions, an increased number of profiles of RER, and randomly distributed lysosomal structures suggest these cells belong to the group of macrophages. In the cardiac muscle cell disintegration of contractile elements evident. (Fixation: osmic acid ×8,000)

similar to those outlined in Chapter F I 1, 2 (SAUNDERS and BIEBER, 1968; ROWLANDS JR. et al., 1968; KOSEK et al., 1968). Perivascular and interstitial infiltration and the subsequent lesions are of surprising uniformity. In damaged areas the myocardial fibers exhibit collections of lipochrome pigment, mitochondrial swelling, focal vacuolation and fragmentation of myofibrils. The predominance of localization of myocardial damage to the subendocardial regions and papillary muscles suggests that ischemia secondary to vascular lesions may be a predominant mechanism in injury (BIEBER et al., 1970). Several large foci of myocardial necrosis, observed also in autotransplanted hearts, are undoubtedly due to electrical burning (defibrillation) (LEANDRI, 1967). Whereas the absence of consistent electrocardiographic abnormalities in acutely rejected canine and/or simian cardiac allografts was frequently in contrast with the severity of the myocardial lesion (Figs. 36, 37), incidences of arrhythmia closely paralleled the severity of the rejection injury to the conduction system (BIEBER et al., 1969).

3. Liver

Several studies have suggested that the liver of dogs and particularly of pigs may enjoy a better fate than other transplants, since occasionally identifiable allograft rejection did not occur, or reversed spontaneously in unmodified hosts, whereas the same animals regularly rejected skin and kidneys (CALNE et al., 1969; GARNIER et al., 1970). The human liver also seemed to be an immunologically favored organ (STARZL, 1971; CALNE, 1974). However, in other experiments it was clearly shown that the liver of various species, including man, was rejected in the usual way (PORTER, 1969; JERUSALEM et al., 1971 b; JAP, 1971). There are various events that are characteristic of acute rejection. MN cells accumulate in the portal spaces, particularly around small portal veins, and occasionally in the proximal portion of central veins exhibiting some adventitial connective tissue (PORTER, 1969). Infiltrating mononuclear cells also accumulate in the space of Disse. In the massive form of acute rejection perivascular infiltration may be minimal while the hepatic parenchyma is teeming with MN cells. The histologic feature of the sinusoidal type of acute rejection closely parallels the process of peripolesis (Chapter B II 2). The sinusoidal endothelium is disrupted, focally stripped off, or even absent. The space of Disse is sometimes dilated by fluid even at sites where cellular infiltrates are absent, and occasionally contains cell fragments and fibrin (PORTER, 1969; ANDRES et al., 1972). It has not been proved whether parenchymal injury can result from alterations in the sinusoidal microarchitecture, since rat auxiliary liver grafts survived for months in the conspicuous absence of sinusoidal endothelium (JAP et al., 1972; WARNIER et al., 1974). Proliferative vascular lesions, patchy media degeneration, and deposits of immunoglobulins are present (PORTER, 1969; CALNE et al., 1969; GARNIER et al., 1970; ANDRES et al., 1972). With respect to the cellular infiltrate the liver allograft appears to be a collecting center for all possible mechanisms of the cell-mediated reaction, as summarized in Chapter A III. Some liver grafts exhibit the basic infiltration patterns as outlined in Chapter F Ia (Figs. 17–22, 30). In other hepatic allografts monocyte derived macrophages are the main infiltrating cells (Fig. 38). Monocytes were found to be replaced by peritoneal macrophages in cyclophosphamide-treated rats (Fig. 39), and in numerous canine hepatic allografts the interlobular veins were completely occluded by monoculture-like accumulations of peritoneal macrophages. Several types of peculiar effector cells were detected in the canine and rat hepatic allograft (JAP, 1971; ROESSNER et al., 1971). They either resemble stimulated large lymphocytes but exhibit membrane-bound electron-dense granules, or are nearly as large as the remaining hepatocytes, by virtue of their abundant cytoplasm, and develop complex projections and foldings of a restricted portion of their surface (Figs. 40, 41). The origin of these cells remains obscure. The final pathway of cell-mediated destruction of hepatocytes is not fully understood. Both the "balloon-

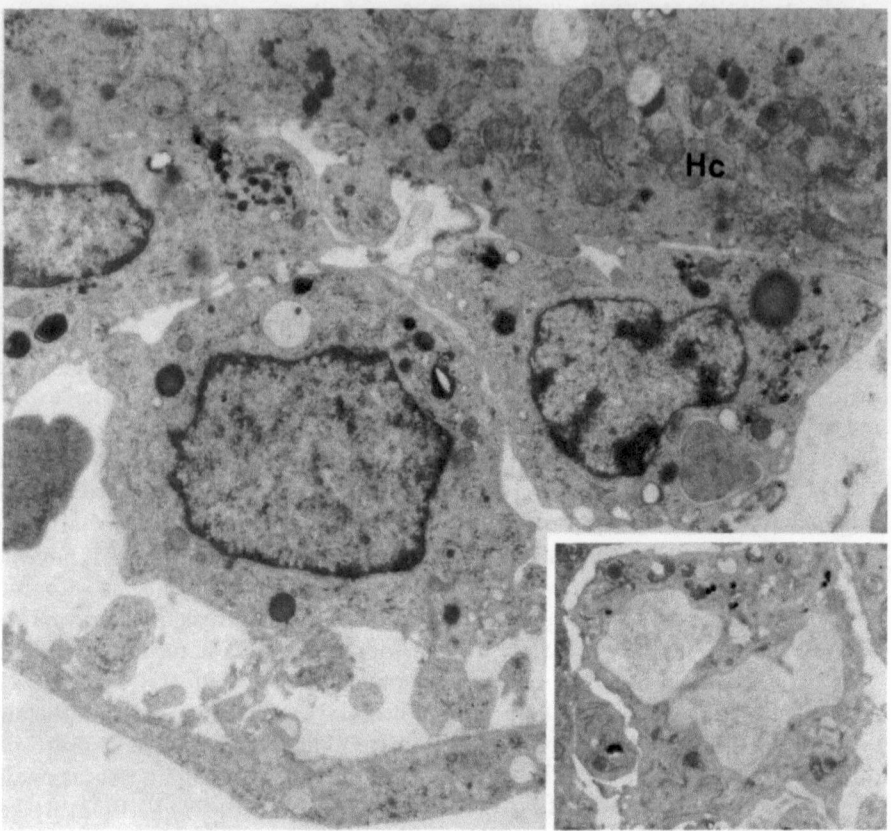

Fig. 38. Rat heterotopic auxiliary liver allograft, untreated, 7 days after transplantation. Cells infiltrating space of Disse are mainly of monocytic series. In cytochemical preparations (inset) they exhibit endogenous peroxidase activity of several (not of all) granular structures. *Hc*: hepatocyte.
(Fixation: glutaraldehyde × 8,000. Inset × 6,000)

ing type" and the sudden shrinkage of the cell body characteristic of lymphotoxin activity (Chapter B II 2) are found (Figs. 42, 43) not only in hepatocytes adjacent to cells infiltrating the space of Disse but also at sites where MN cells are absent (Porter, 1969; Roessner et al., 1971, 1974). However, the hepatic parenchyma may be well preserved quite close to dense lymphoid cell accumulations in the portal space. In rat hepatic allografts the hepatocytes frequently atrophy after being encompassed by obviously noncytotoxic MN cells which appear to interfere with the local blood flow and probably impair blood- hepatocyte exchange (Jap, 1971) (Chapter B II 3). Furthermore, in these grafts the number of hepatocytes exhibiting mitotic figures is suprisingly high (Fig. 42 b). Apparently the rapid loss of viable liver cells causes a maximal functional overload in the remaining hepatocytes, stimulating frequent mitotic division. These findings suggest that in many instances the acute rejection of liver allografts is the result of competitive metabolic activity of individual cells, rather than a

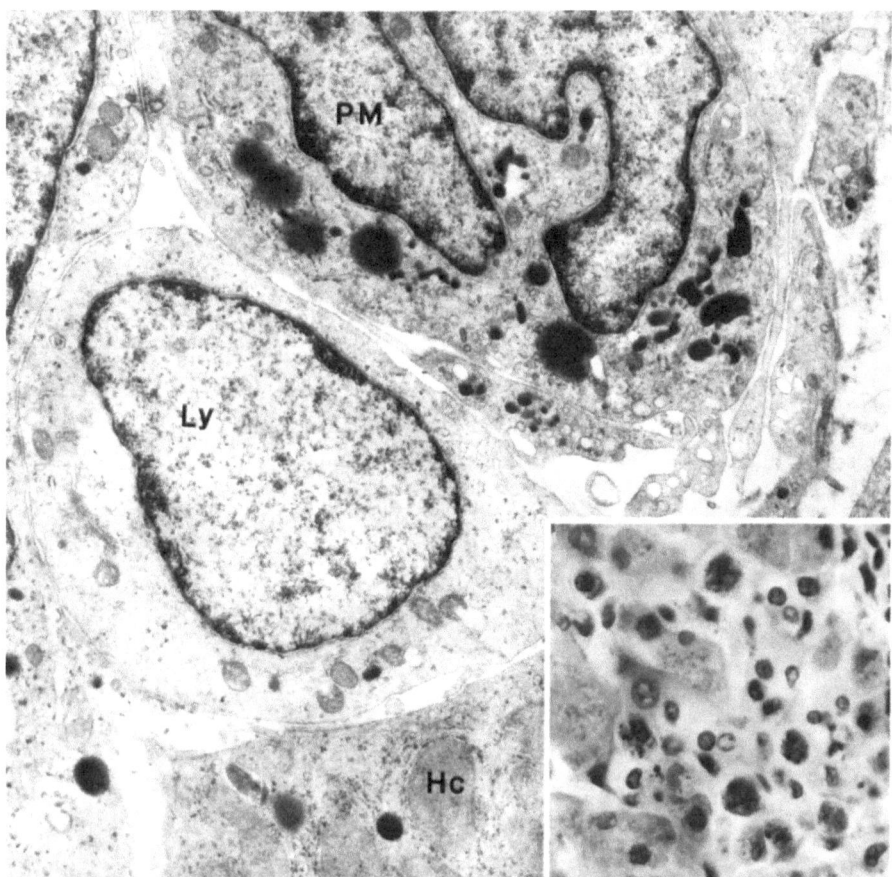

Fig. 39. Rat heterotopic auxiliary liver allograft treated with cyclophosphamide. Numerous macrophages have infiltrated sinusoids (inset). Ultrastructurally they exhibit characteristic features of peritoneal macrophages (*PM*), such as a horseshoe-shaped nucleus, numerous lysosomal structures, and several fat droplets. Medium-sized lymphocyte (*Ly*) is sandwiched between macrophage and hepatocyte (*Hc*). (Fixation: glutaraldehyde ×10,000. Inset: hematoxylin and eosin ×500)

general hepatocytotoxic event. However, general intoxication cannot be excluded, as indicated by the ultrastructural and histochemical changes involving almost all allogenic hepatocytes in untreated hosts. These changes are uncommon in nonrejecting isograft models. Functional lesions may contribute in part to the severe centrilobular and midzonal dense cholestasis and the deposits of lipofuscin and bile pigments in hepatocytes of human, canine, and rat liver allografts undergoing acute rejection (PORTER, 1969; JAP, 1971). Since foci of biliary acid necrosis and the proliferation of pseudo-bile ducts and cholangioles only indicated a disturbance in bile flow, these changes are not specific for allograft rejection. Large macrophages exhibiting cell fragments, erythrocytes, bile pigments, hemosiderin, and lipofuscin increase progressively in number, the increase obviously being secondary to parenchymal damage. Centrilobular

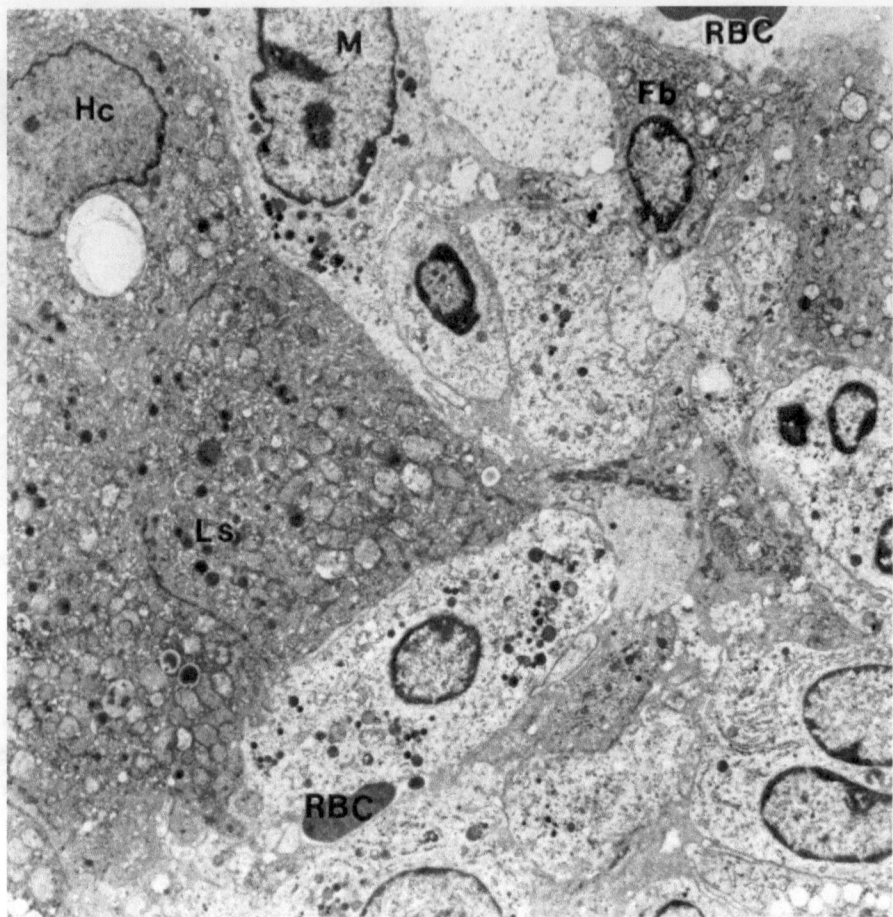

Fig. 40. Rat heterotopic auxiliary liver allograft 9 days after transplantation. No immunosuppressive treatment. Main infiltrating cells are large electron-light macrophages (*M*), occasionally as large as hepatocytes (*Hc*). Complete loss of sinusoidal microarchitecture. Although infiltrating cells impinge directly upon remaining hepatocytes, hepatocytic cytoplasm exhibits only swollen mitochondria, increase in lysosomal structures (*Ls*), and occasional fat droplets. This picture is suggestive of "asphyxia" of hepatocytes due to impaired exchange of metabolites between blood (*RBC*) and hepatocytes rather than to direct cytotoxicity. *Fb*: fibroblast. (Fixation: glutaraldehyde × 3,500)

and midzonal atrophy and necrosis with subsequent collapse of reticulin results mainly from intra- and extrahepatic vascular changes. Occasionally only a small rim of hepatocytes remains viable at the lobular periphery. It should be emphasized that bile ducts are frequently not affected. In completely resorbed afunctional grafts they are the only remaining recognizable hepatic structures.

The reactions in the liver may be representative of a particular type of nonimmunologic change that possibly interferes with the transplantation reaction. It has been claimed that the transplantation of a second liver or portions of a second liver would be technically less difficult than an orthotopic liver

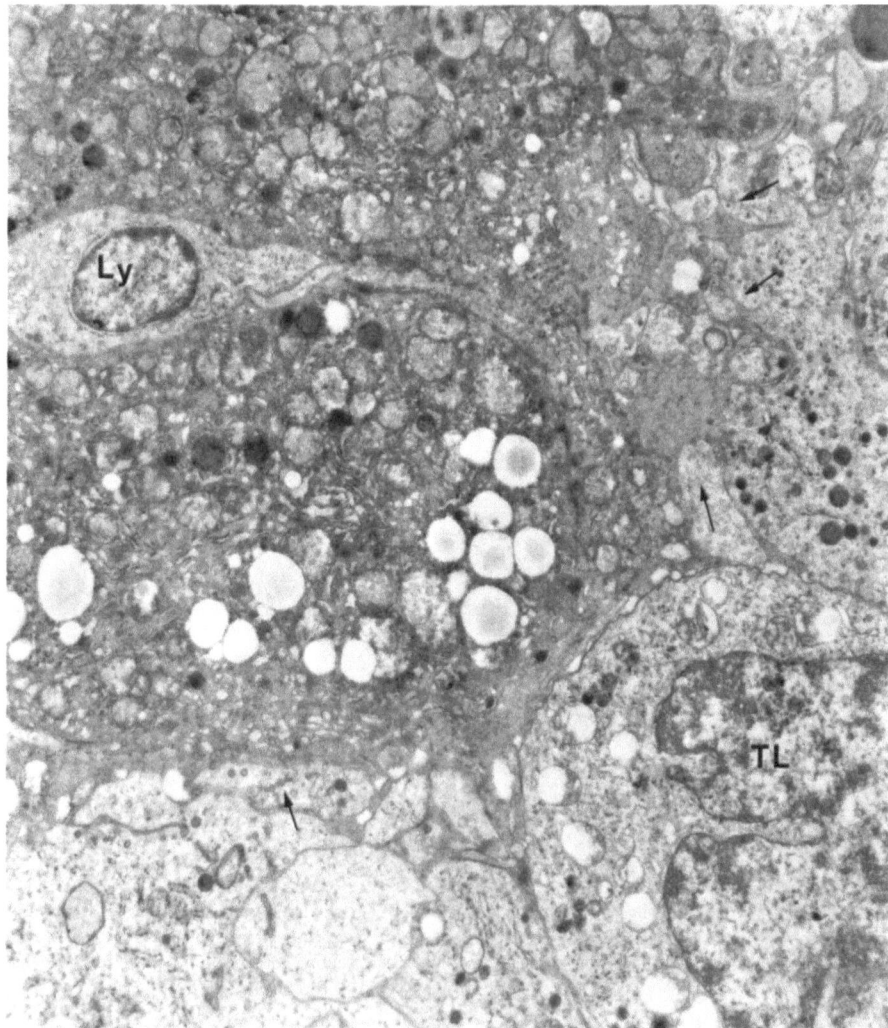

Fig. 41. Rat heterotopic auxiliary liver allograft 9 days after transplantation. No immunosuppressive treatment. Frequently light infiltrating macrophages develop complex folding of their cytoplasmic surface (arrows) which appear to interdigitate with protruding portions of hepatocytic cytoplasm. In contrast, contacting cell membranes of both hepatocyte and transformed lymphocyte (*TL*) are smooth. In addition an emperipolized and slightly stimulated electron-light lymphoid cell is shown (*Ly*). Since liver cells exhibit numerous fat droplets and swollen disintegrating mitochondria, it may be suggested that phagocytic activity is stimulated by deterioration in target cell. (Fixation: glutaraldehyde ×6,000)

transplantation. However, results of clinical heterotopic auxiliary liver transplantation have been rather dissappointing, only a few patients surviving for as long as several months (FORTNER *et al.*, 1970, 1973). In the early studies, experimentors were faced with the problem of rapid graft atrophy (STARZL *et al.*, 1964b; FARIS *et al.*, 1966), which was ascribed to the inevitable changes

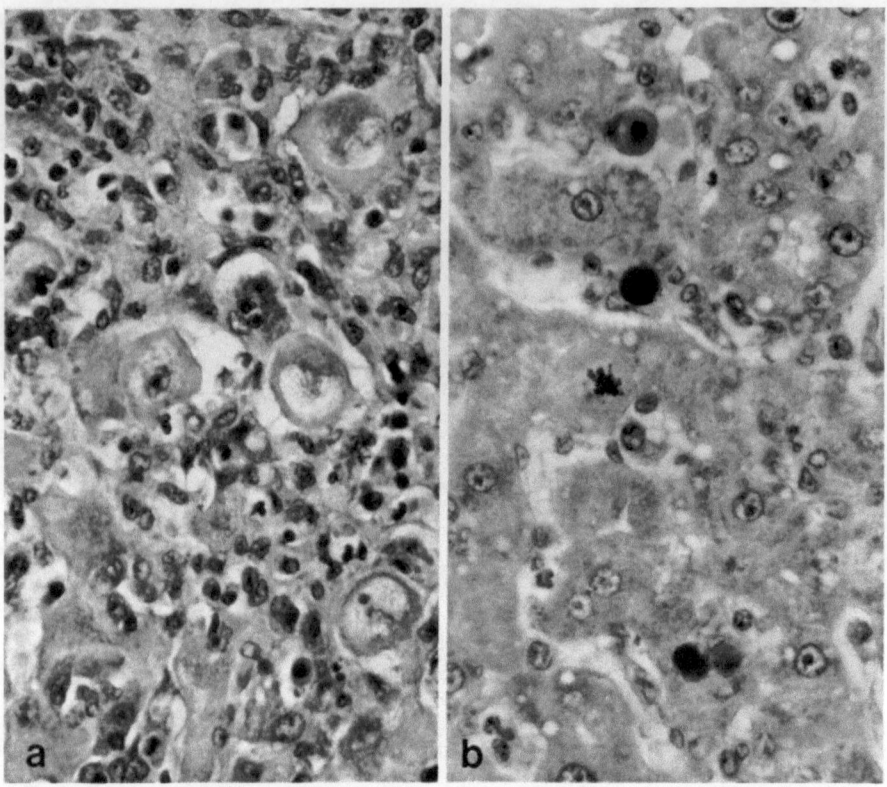

Fig. 42a. Porcine orthotopic liver allograft 6 days after transplantation. Treated with immunosuppressive drugs. "Ballooning" of several hepatocytes evident. (Goldner's trichrome: × 500)

Fig. 42b. Rat heterotopic auxiliary liver allograft 4 days after transplantation. No administration of immunosuppressive drugs. Coagulation necrosis of single liver cells resulting in Councilman bodies (eosinophilic globules, acidophilic bodies) is another but infrequent feature of target cell destruction. Note mitotic figure in hepatocyte beneath second eosinophilic globule. (Goldner's trichrome: × 500)

in the quality of the blood supply (MARCHIORO *et al.*, 1965a, b). Nevertheless, it was possible to induce moderate hypertrophy of the canine auxiliary liver allograft, although it was supplied with arterial blood only (V.D. HEYDE and SCHALM, 1968; V. D. HEYDE *et al.*, 1971); and dogs carrying a heterotopic autograft without portal inflow were able to complete a pregnancy to term (V.D. HEYDE *et al.*, 1974). Furthermore rat auxiliary liver grafts supplied only with portal blood had increased in size by about 4 times one year after transplantation (HESS *et al.*, 1972). Previous studies had made it clear that the atrophy of auxiliary liver grafts results predominantly from functional competition between two coexisting livers (SCHALM *et al.*, 1956; SCHALM, 1966), since changes in the intensity of the appropriate functional stimulus beyond that required in basic conditions (JERUSALEM, 1963a, b; JATROPULOS, 1965) cause complementory

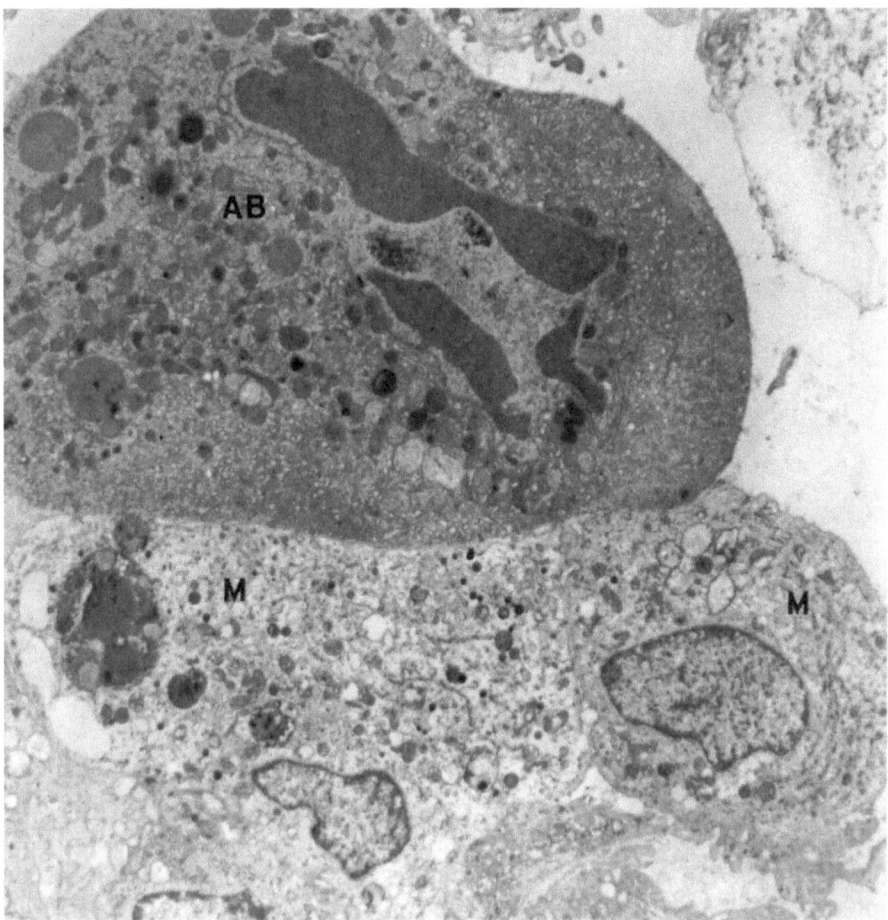

Fig. 43. Rat heterotopic auxiliary liver allograft 4 days after transplantation. Untreated. Occasional isolated hepatocyte undergoing coagulation necrosis (transformation to acidophilic bodies: *AB*) found in close contact with infiltrating light macrophages (*M*), rather than with lymphocytes. Note unusual variety of cellular organelles in deteriorating hepatocyte, polymorphism of mitochondria, and pyknosis. (Fixation: glutaraldehyde × 4,500)

or compensatory functional atrophy or hypertrophy, respectively. The insertion of an additional liver without functional handicapping of the recipient's own liver results in a surplus of liver parenchyma and subsequent atrophy of the graft, because it is exposed to unfavorable hemodynamic (outflow) conditions. In livers atrophying in compensation, a centrilobular numeric atrophy (in the absence of congestion) with slight collapse of the central reticulin and subsequent shrinkage of the whole lobule with slight prominence of reticulin in the lobular periphery has usually been noted. Metallactic changes were almost absent. In contrast, the atrophy occurring after the establishment of various types of portacaval shunts was characterized by a simple atrophy of hepatocytes throughout

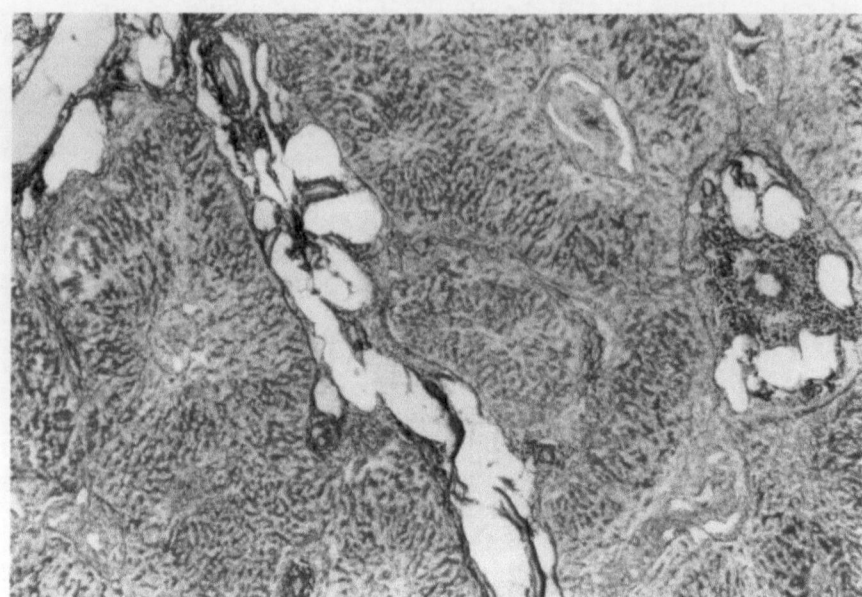

Fig. 44. Canine heterotopic auxiliary hepatic autograft 6 weeks after transplantation. Severe cirrhosis of mixed portal and cardiac type. Note extremely dilated lymphatics. (Bielschowsky: × 40)

all lobular zones. However, after resection of the donor liver by 30 to 50 percent prior to transplantation, and an additional handicap to the recipient's liver, e.g. ligation of its common bile duct, the functional stimulus is in favor of the graft (Schalm and Schalm, 1974); it hypertrophies and can sustain life for prolonged periods (Jap et al., 1972; Warnier et al., 1974). In clinical liver transplantation to the heterotopic (auxiliary) position, these interventions are unnecessary in instances where the recipient's liver is fatally damaged (Fortner et al., 1973). The functional balance resulting from the optimal body weight/liver weight ratio also appears to be important in orthotopic liver transplantation. The transplantation of a rather small liver to a large recipient was found to be relatively safe, while it was quite dangerous to transplant a large liver graft to a small recipient (Starzl, 1974b). In addition, the blood circulation to and from the graft may become choked off upon closure of the abdomen by oversized livers or the presence of a second (auxiliary) liver. The chronically increased outflow pressure to which most heterotopic livergrafts are exposed (Hess et al., 1972) cirrhosis of the mixed cardial and portal type, metallaxis of the lobular architecture, and congestive bridges were more frequent in the canine heterotopic auto- and allografts than in the recipient's own liver, or in orthotopic liver grafts (Jerusalem et al., 1972) (Fig. 44). Since these changes partly interfere with those resulting from rejection episodes, heterotopic liver allografts appear to be rejected more violently than orthotopically implanted livers (Calne et al., 1969).

4. Lungs

The histopathologic changes in pulmonary allografts appropriately illustrate the multiplicity of transplantation reactions. Although there are numerous grafts exhibiting the classic features of cellular infiltration and vascular lesions (Chapter F I 1 and Fig. 17). (BARNES *et al.*, 1963; RIBET *et al.*, 1969; LEBROS *et al.*, 1969), others are seemingly destroyed through atypical patterns (VEITH *et al.*, 1971). The importance of pulmonary osmoregulation has been outlined in Chapter D II 4. Whereas interstitial edema resulting from increased capillary fragility may be tolerated by the kidney, and even better by the liver, in the lungs it can lead to pulmonary edema (COTTRELL *et al.*, 1967), with subsequent impairment of the ventilation-perfusion balance. Actually, one of the early difficulties

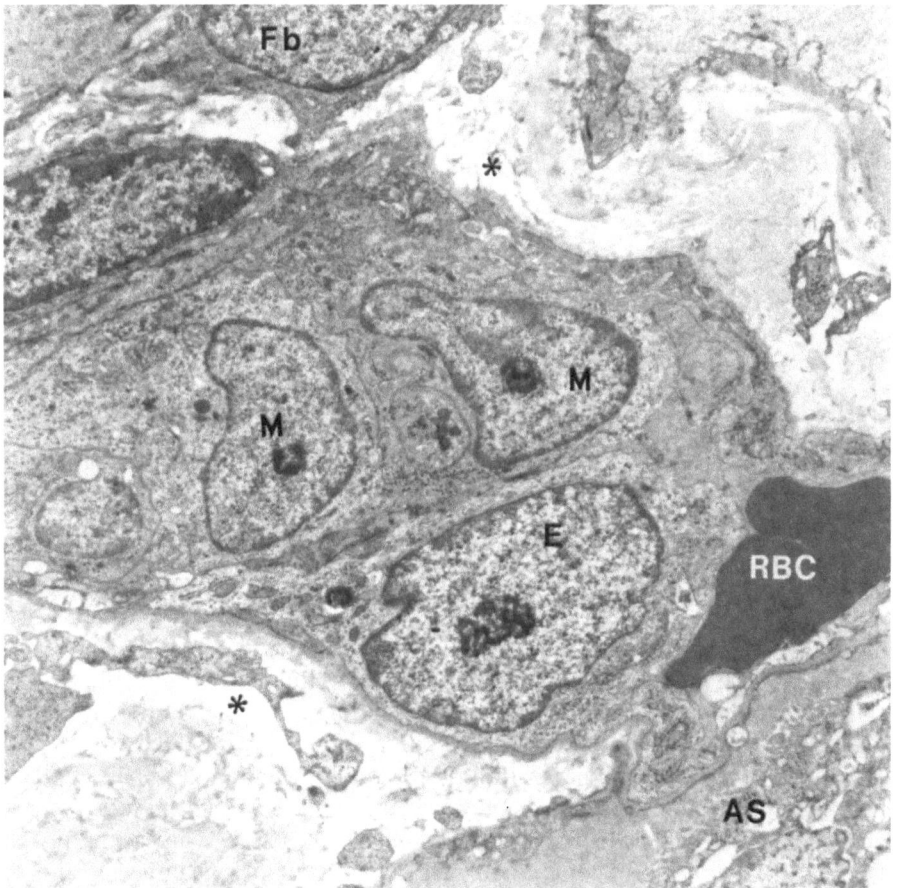

Fig. 45. Canine pulmonary allograft 5 days after transplantation into recipient depleted of T-cells (adult thymectomy and subsequent treatment with ATS for 10 days, 5 months prior to transplantation). Capillary is almost completely occluded by undifferentiated (blood-borne) macrophages (*M*). Note distinct interstitial edema (asterisks). *RBC*: red blood cell, *AS*: alveolar space, *Fb*: fibroblast, *E*: endothelial cell. (Fixation: Karnovsky ×6,000)

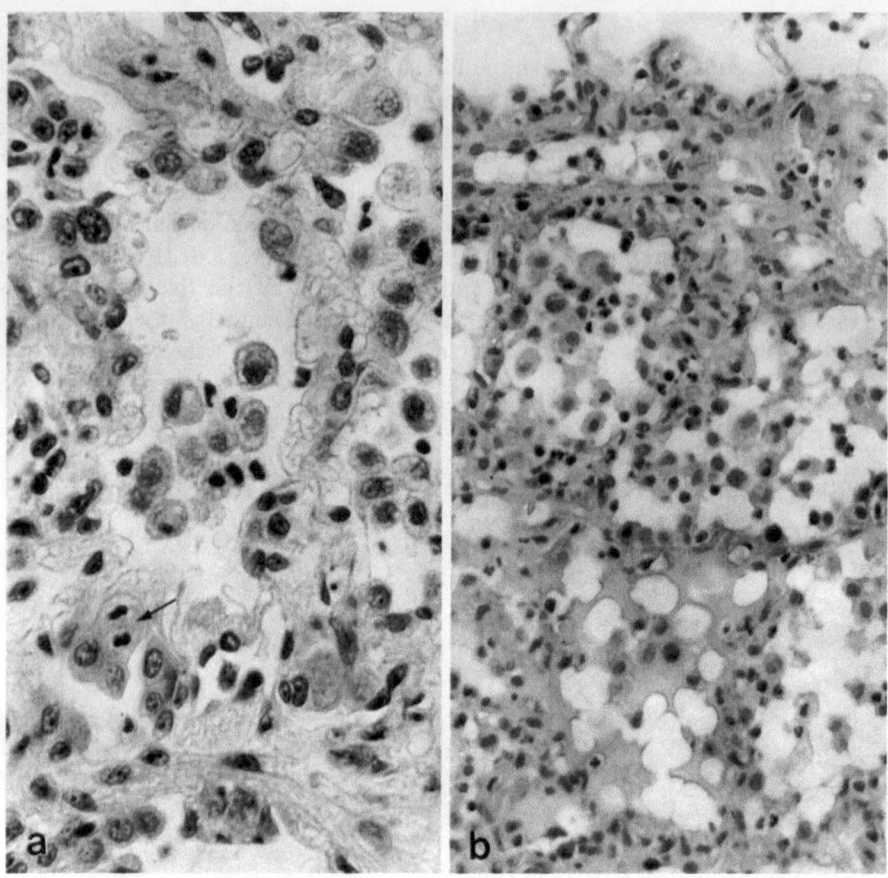

Fig. 46a and b. Canine pulmonary allograft 5 days after transplantation. Treated with ATS and Imuran. Hyperplasia and hypertrophy particularly of granular pneumocytes with subsequent break-down of blood-air barrier in absence of obvious infiltration by lymphocytes is suggestive of the alveolar pattern of rejection. Note mitotic figure in pneumocyte (a, arrow), cellular and proteinaceous alveolar exudate, and absence of cuffing pattern of lymphocytes (b). (Goldner's trichrome: a × 500; b × 350)

associated with lung allotransplantation is the development of interstitial edema (DE BONO, 1966) (Fig. 45). In contrast to autografts, where early interstitial edema is transient, it is progressive in the allograft. Two to three days after allotransplantation a disorganization of both endothelial and alveolar epithelial cells becomes evident, and increasingly more proteinaceous and fibrinoid exudate accumulates within the alveolar spaces (BECKER et al., 1972). Whereas this process is associated with a moderately intense sloughing off of pneumocytes and the occurrence of free alveolar macrophages, the escape of larger numbers of red blood cells appears to be due to the invariably occurring disruption of the septal architecture due to obstruction of alveolar capillaries with sludge (WARREN and DE BONO, 1969). These alveolar changes generally precede vascular lesions and are obviously independent of vascular pathology or MN cell infiltration,

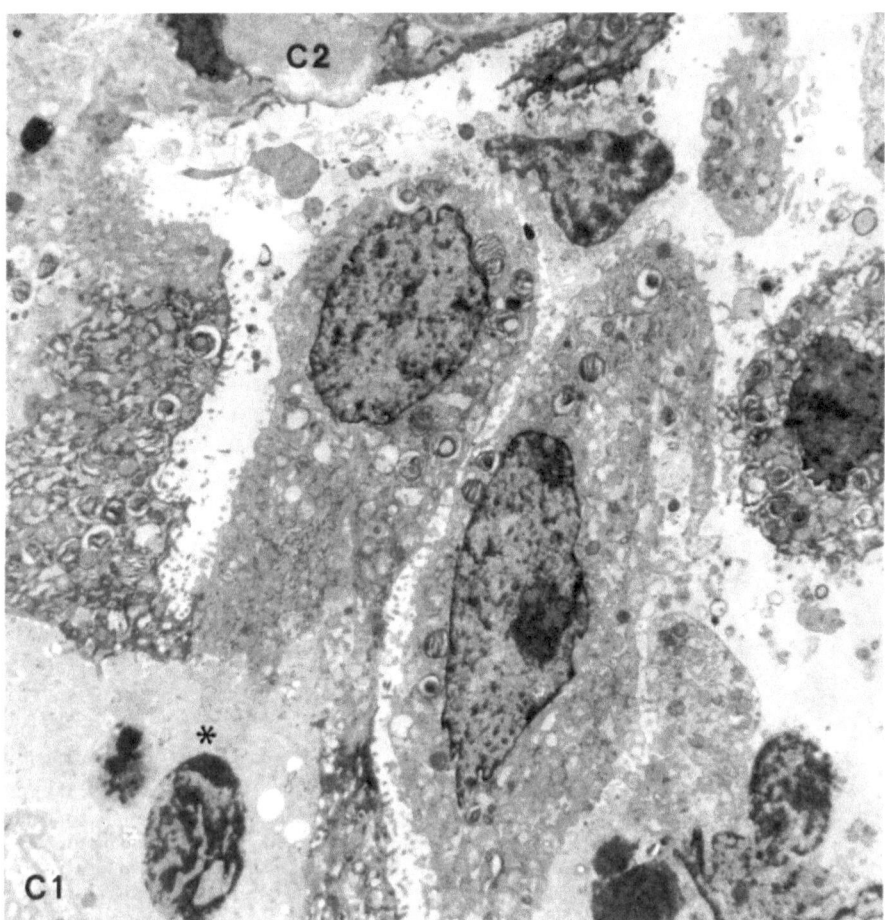

Fig. 47. Canine pulmonary allograft 5 days after transplantation. No administration of immunosuppressive drugs because of negative MLC test. During early phase of alveolar pattern of pulmonary allograft rejection granular pneumocytes frequently proliferate in a shape resembling columnar epithelium. On left, granular pneumocytes appear to be lifted off by homogeneous substance (asterisk) which is in contact with a remnant of an alveolar capillary (*C 1*). Note nuclear debris within this homogeneous substance, and cell debris and macrophages within alveolar space. Another damaged capillary is seen at upper border (*C 2*). (Fixation: Karnovsky × 5,000)

since it is possible to repress the appearance of round cells, but neither the extent nor the severity of the alveolar manifestation of rejection by immunosuppression (VEITH *et al.*, 1971). This phenomenon has been observed in the dog (STAUDACHER *et al.*, 1973) and the baboon (ANDERSON *et al.*, 1973), and was considered to be an important cause of the poor results obtained in human pulmonary transplantation (VEITH *et al.*, 1972a).

The "alveolar pattern" can be either the manifestation of a general rejection mechanism (Chapter F I 2 d) being promoted by the particular microarchitecture of the alveolar wall, or an alveolar-specific component of the pulmonary allograft rejection (BECKER *et al.*, 1972) (see alveolar antigens, Chapter C II 1). The strik-

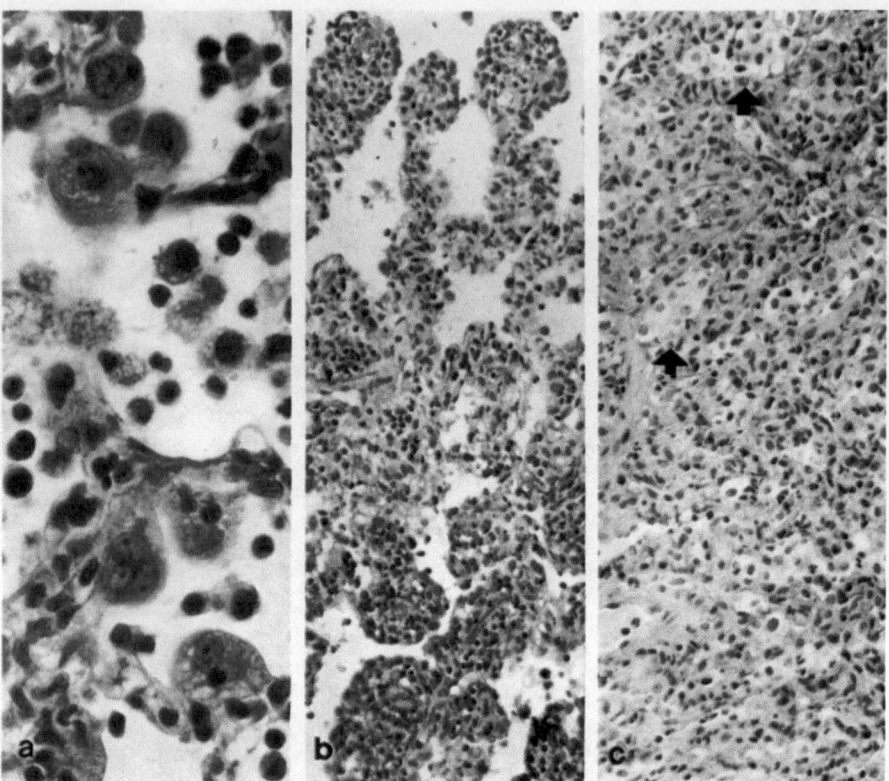

Fig. 48a–c. Canine pulmonary allografts in T-cell depleted recipient (adult thymectomy and subsequent treatment with ATS for 10 days, 5 months prior to transplantation). No immunosuppressive treatment during post-transplantation course. (a) 5 days after transplantation changes resembling giant cell pneumonia are obvious. (b) After 7 days distinct interstitial proliferative reaction. (c) After about 2-3 weeks several grafts revealed a complete "carnification" of pulmonary parenchyma. Note scattered clusters of epitheloid light cells (arrows). (Goldner's trichrome: a ×500; b ×150; c ×250)

ing similarity of this lesion with changes observed in Goodpasture's syndrome (Staudacher *et al.*, 1973) and the transplant lung syndrome (Slapak *et al.*, 1968; Tison and Baruzzi, 1969), as well as the occasional involvement of the recipient's own lung in instances of unilateral transplantation (Gondos *et al.*, 1971) suggest the implication of circulating antibody as a triggering factor. Circulating lung-binding antibody was demonstrable immediately before rejection episodes (Cullum *et al.*, 1972). In contrast to accelerated rejection of pulmonary allografts, cuboidal metaplasia of the alveolar lining epithelium and proliferation of type-II pneumocytes were common when the rejection was of the alveolar pattern (Veith *et al.*, 1972a; Haglin *et al.*, 1973) (Figs. 46, 47). In addition, intense hyperplasia of the capillary endothelium and lamellation of the basement membrane were observed (Staudacher *et al.*, 1973). Whereas impressive proliferation of granular pneumocytes may occur secondary to a primary, nonimmunologic injury, e.g. in instances of chronic pulmonary edema

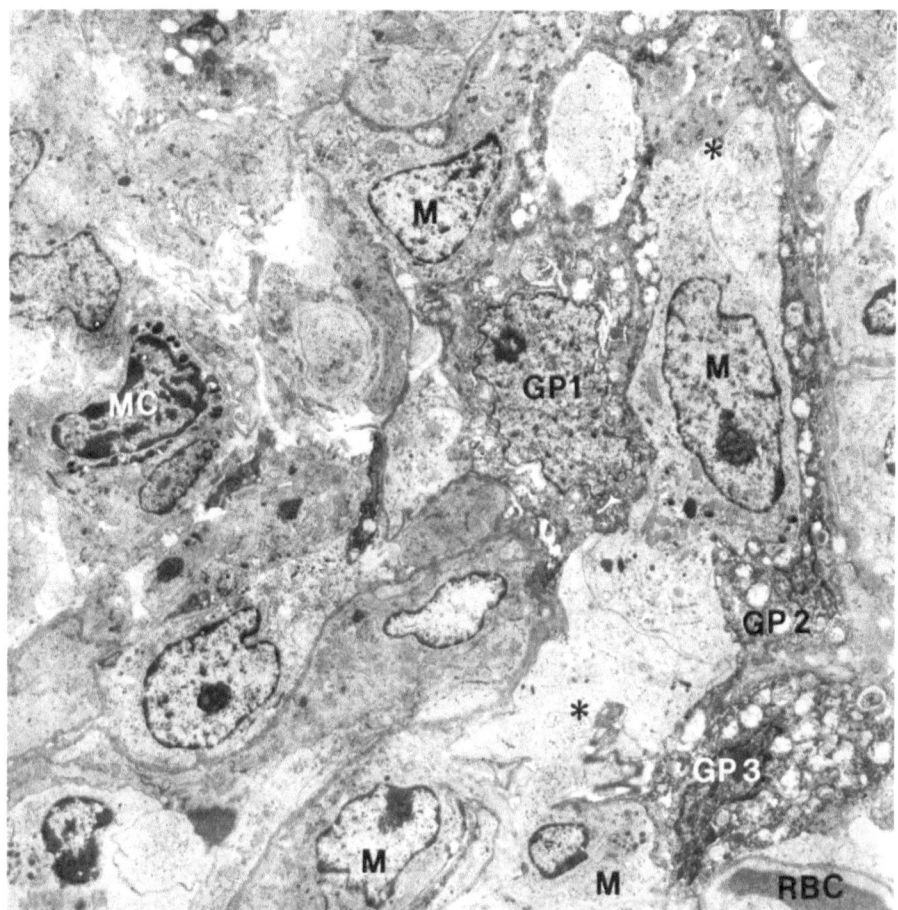

Fig. 49. Detail of graft in Fig. 48c. Even by means of electron microscopy, original pulmonary architecture is hardly recognizable. Erythrocytes (*RBC*) mark capillaries, almost occluded by undifferentiated macrophages (compare Fig. 45); and flattened granular pneumocytes (*GP 1, 2,* and *3*) indicate border of narrowed alveolar spaces. Most infiltrating cells belong to group of macrophages (*M*). Several macrophages appear to migrate into remaining free spaces (asterisks). Single mast cell (*MC*) is shown. Note absence of lymphocytes. (Fixation: Karnovsky ×3,500)

(ORTEGA *et al.*, 1970), the triad of endothelial and epithelial hyperplasia associated with alteration of the basement membrane appears to parallel changes characteristic of early proliferative glomerulopathy (Chapter F II 1).

In canine pulmonary allografts transplanted either to T-cell-deprived recipients or to compatible littermates, another atypical reaction was noted (WILDE-VUUR *et al.*, 1973a; DE LANGEN *et al.*, 1975). After an initial phase resembling either the alveolar pattern or a transient attack of viral interstitial or giant cell pneumonia (Fig. 48), not only alveolar epithelial cells but also various types of macrophages proliferated intensely (Fig. 49). The alveolar spaces were rapidly filled with densely packed alveolar macrophages, and the interstices enlarged. Various lymphoid cells and plasma cells were found throughout, fre-

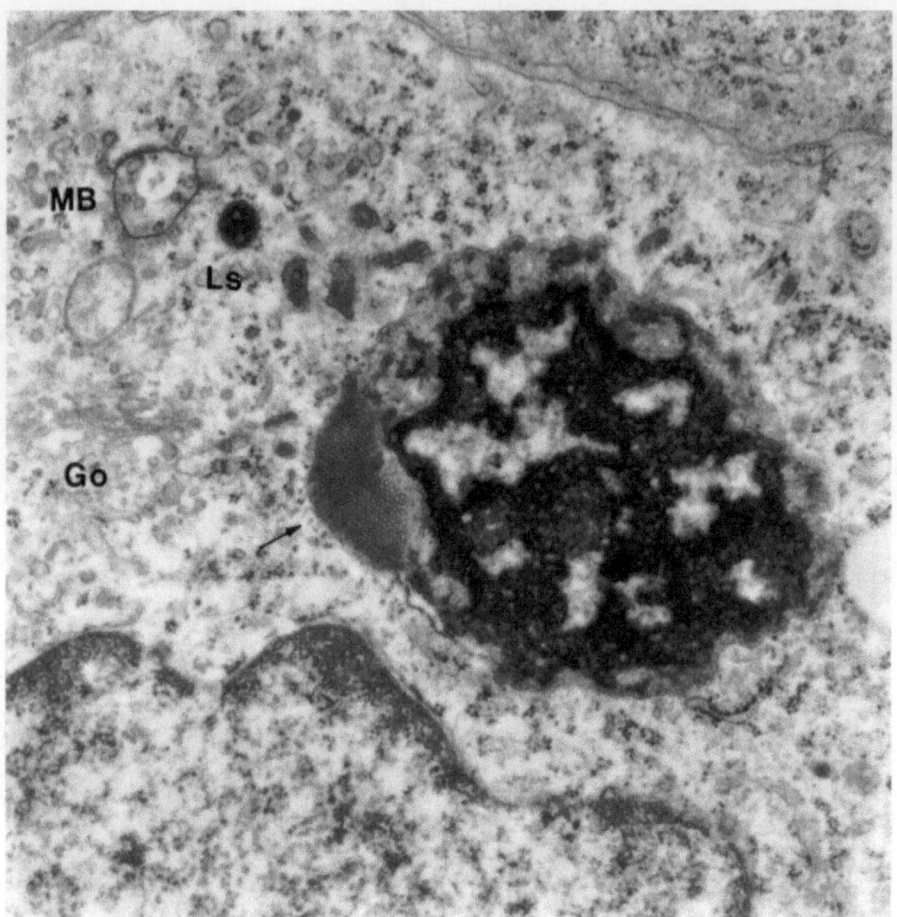

Fig. 50. Untreated canine pulmonary allograft 13 days after transplantation. Phagocytosis of lymphocytes occasionally seen in lung transplants in dogs. This lymphocyte was phagocytosed by an intracapillary macrophage during acute rejection of incompatible graft. Nucleus of lymphocyte is pyknotic, cytoplasm exhibits clustered polysomes and, most obvious, extensive paracrystalline inclusion, strongly suggestive of viral material (arrow). Note electron-light cytoplasm of macrophages containing a Golgi area (*Go*), a multivesicular body (*MB*), and small polymorphic lysosomal structures (*Ls*). (Fixation: Karnovsky ×25,000)

quently arranged in clusters. Ten to 21 days after transplantation, histologic preparations revealed carnification of these grafts and the absence of vascular lesions and necrosis (Fig. 48c). This peculiar proliferative response in pulmonary allografts suggests, but does not prove, either a reaction of immunologically competent alveolar cells, or a concurrence of viral infection and rejection. The immunologic activities of alveolar cells have rarely been studied. Isolated, perfused lungs of immunized animals are competent to synthesize and to secrete specific antibody (Askonas and Humphrey, 1958). When rabbits were sensitized via the intravenous or intratracheal route, cells obtained by washing the lungs exhibited a plaque-forming response specific to the immunizing antigen (Ford and KUHN, 1973a, b). Plaque formation required complement. The lung is provided with autochthonous cell lines competent of plaque formation (Chapter C II 4), and in allotransplantation these cells can react to the host's antigens. Immunologic clusters are easily detected in pulmonary allografts (STAUDACHER et al., 1973) (Fig. 20).

If we accept a viral etiology (Fig. 50), the reason why the allograft is preferentially involved, rather than the autograft and/or the recipient's own lung, requires some explanation. Murine leukemia viruses, for instance, apparently do not induce leukemia by a direct action on host cells, but rather leukemia results when a host's immune response produces secondary damage to virus-infected cells (METCALF, 1966). Whereas small lymphocytes are incapable of replicating various viruses, an increase of virus plaque-forming cells was observed when cells obtained from donors with delayed type hypersensitivity were stimulated with specific antigen (KANO et al., 1973). The budding of virus particles from fibroblasts attacked by sensitized effector lymphocytes was mentioned in Chapter B II 2. Furthermore, neuroretinal cells transformed by Roux's sarcoma virus proliferated for up to 12 generations, whereas uninfected cells did not grow in vitro (PESSAC and CALOTHY, 1974). An increased susceptibility of pulmonary grafts to viral infections may result from a lesion of the "first and second lines of mucosal defence" (BRANDTZAEG, 1973). The major quantity of IgA in the external secretions derives from plasma cells in the submucosa. It is a 7 S globulin which combines with the secretory component from epithelial cells to form dimers with 11 S characteristics. The interruption of the bronchial circulation apparently impedes the strongly T-helper cell-dependent synthesis of mucosal antibody. HAGLIN et al. (1973) emphasized the need to restore the bronchial arterial circulation to avoid fatal bronchial complications.

5. Pancreas

The rejection patterns of pancreatic allografts do not vary fundamentally from those described in Chapter F I 1, 2 (GRENIER et al., 1967; MORI et al., 1968). The intense interstitial proteinaceous edema which developed in almost all grafts during the first 10 minutes after revascularization was striking (v. HEE, 1973) (Fig. 10). The edematous fluid was insufficiently resorbed, and it either condensed to a hyaline substance or was only poorly organized in prednisolone-treated recipients (ZIMMERMANN and HELL, 1971), whereas the exudate was rapidly replaced by fibrous connective tissue when corticosteroids were not administered (ACOSTA et al., 1973). Pancreatic fibrosis rather than cell-mediated rejection appeared to be the major cause of atrophy of the acinar cells (v. HEE, 1973). In such instances the pancreatic islets were remarkably well preserved. Surprisingly, in several transplantations of the pancreaticoduodenal block in modified dogs studied in our laboratory only the pancreas and not the duodenal segment was rejected by classic cell-mediated mechanisms (Fig. 51); while in most instances both organs were attacked simultaneously, a preferential rejection of the duodenal portion of the transplant was never observed.

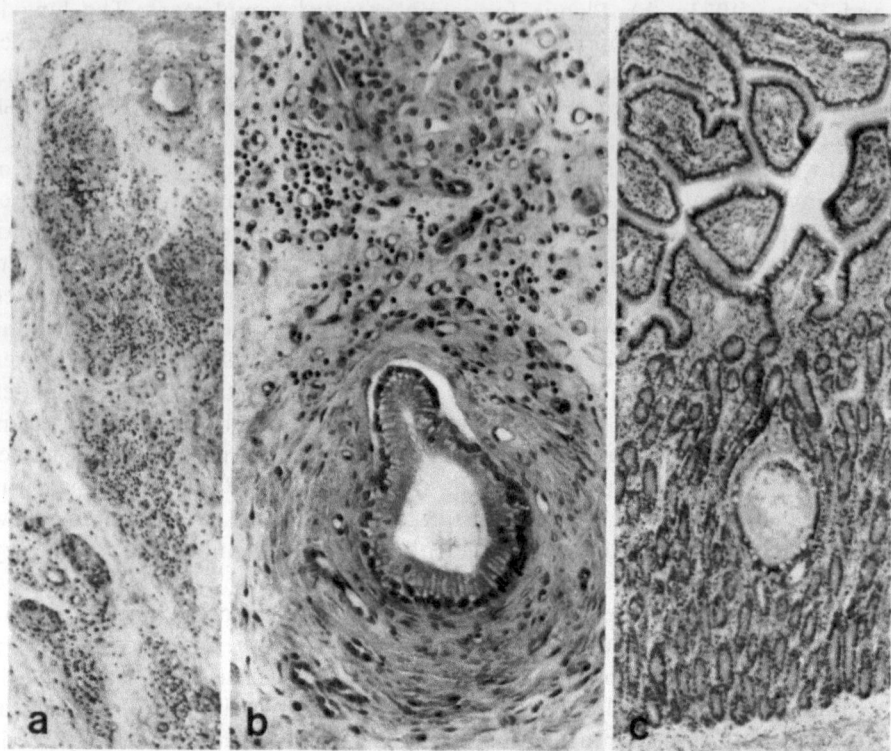

Fig. 51a–c. Canine pancreaticoduodenal allograft, treated with Imuran, 56 days after transplantation. Whereas exocrine part of graft is completely rejected (a, note lymphocytes infiltrating remnants of acini) pancreatic islands and, particularly, pancreatic excretory ducts are well preserved. Note periductular fibrosis (b). Simultaneously transplanted duodenum exhibits no signs of rejection (c). (Hematoxylin and eosin: a × 100; b × 250; c × 100)

6. Small Bowel

Short segments of about 10–15 cm of canine ileal allografts were normally rejected (Lillehei and Manax, 1966). However, the accumulation of numerous PMN cells in the absence of round-cell infiltration (Barnett et al., 1962) indicated complement-dependent antibody-mediated immune reactions when rather longer segments of the small bowel were used as an allograft. In contrast, when large segments of the small bowel were allografted into unmodified or modified dogs, rejection reactions failed to develop, and the recipients died of a vigorous graft-vs-host reaction (Lillehei et al., 1959a, b; Ruiz et al., 1972). The use of different parental and F_1 hybrid donor and recipient combinations in experiments with rats has made the isolation of unidirectional GVH and recipient reactions possible (Monchik and Russell, 1971). Allografts between strains differing at the Ag-B locus have been shown to sensitize the host, causing allograft rejection. Parental-to-F_1 transplant resulted in a GVH reaction, which could be prevented by donor x-irradiation. These findings emphasize the importance of passenger lymphocytes (Chapter C II 4).

Using Wistar rats as both donors and recipients full length small bowel grafts were not rejected although the lamina propria and submucosa were densely infiltrated with plasma cells of various degrees of maturity, and with small lymphocytes (Fig. 52).

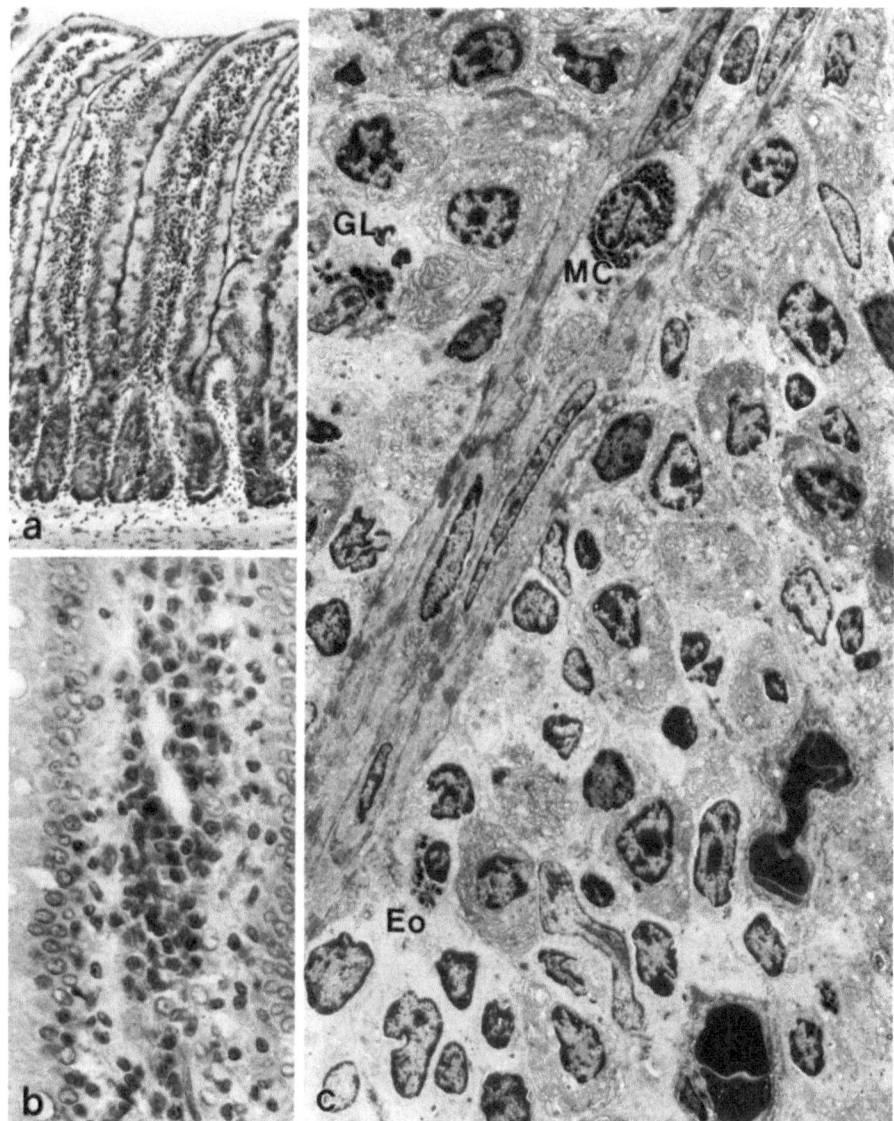

Fig. 52a–c. Rat (Wistar-to-Wistar) small bowel graft 5 months after transplantation. No administration of immunosuppressive drugs. (a) Epithelium is well preserved and exhibits functioning goblet cells. (PAS reaction: ×70). (b) Both lamina propria and submucosa densely infiltrated by large pyroninophilic cells. (Methylgreen and pyronin: ×400). (c) On electron-micrograph infiltrate consists predominantly of plasma cells of various degrees of maturity and of lymphocytes. Mast cells (*MC*), globular leukocytes (*GL*), and eosinophilic granulocytes (*Eo*) usually interspersed. (Fixation: glutaraldehyde ×2,000)

G. Chronic or Late Rejection

With the improvement of surgical techniques, organ storage, histocompatibility typing, international registration of data, patient management, and immunosuppressive therapy, increasingly more transplanted organs are having a long survival. However, a large number of these grafts exhibit changes which appear to be the expression of chronic rejection events. This fourth major pattern of rejection usually progresses slowly and insidiously, sometimes over a period of years (Hume, 1971), but occasionally it is manifest even several weeks after transplantation (Porter, 1965, 1969; Bieber et al., 1970). Although the pathogenesis of certain lesions remains obscure, it is agreed that most represent some form of immunologic injury mediated by circulating antibody. The suggestion that this course of events involves primarily the endothelium of blood vessels seems too simple to explain the preferred site of the vascular lesion, i.e. medium-sized and small arteries in which a progressive and intensive thickening of the intima is produced. Irreversible, ischemic parenchymal damage may result after progressive vascular stenosis. In kidney allografts, chronic glomerulopathy is another frequent finding, and the multiplicity of the glomerular lesion suggests the involvement of several pathogenic mechanisms (Lindquist et al., 1968b; Porter et al., 1968; Milgrom et al., 1971). The importance of cellular infiltrates of various kinds in late rejection of organ grafts is, however, questionable. The main, distinctive morphologic features of chronic rejection can be summarized as follows:

I. Arterial Obliterative Lesion

As the average survival of human allografts lengthened, this type of lesion was found more frequently first in the transplanted kidney (Dempster et al., 1964; Porter, 1965; Lindquist et al., 1968b), then in the heart (Kosek et al., 1969; Bieber et al., 1970), and in the liver (Porter, 1969). The lesion commonly consists of circumferential intimal thickening with luminal narrowing in medium-sized and small arteries, and occasionally in arterioles. In heart allografts the coronary arteries and the first portions of the intramyocardial branches are preferentially affected. The obliterative intimal thickening is due to an increase of intimal fibrous tissue and myointimal cells. Frequently foam cells (lipophages) are interspersed or predominant (Porter, 1969). The disruption of elastic lamellae that is occasionally seen in these vessels (Porter, 1965; Lindquist et al., 1968b) suggests a prior episode of acute arteritis (Chapter F I 1c), although healed vasculitis appears not to contribute significantly to an overall narrowing of vessels (Bieber et al., 1970). The close similarity of the arterial change in malignant hypertension, periarteritis nodosa, and thrombotic microangiopathy suggests that thrombosis and subsequent organization of mural thrombi may cause the vascular lesion in organ allografts. The occasional presence of fibrin and the morphologic similarity of the intimal thickening and the organizing thrombus appear to support this assumption (Fig. 27). Layered concentric bands may indicate that recurrent vascular deposition of fibrin is secondary to immunologic damage to the endothelium. The use of antithrombotic drugs and anticoagulant therapy was advocated to interrupt the chain of events consisting of aggregation of platelets resulting from antibody-mediated damage to endothelial cells, activation of the clotting system, and mobilization of cells that remove the clots (KINCAID–SMITH, 1969). However, the patchy and focal involvement, especially of arteries, and the rare presence of endothelial slough give rise to doubts of the concept that the endothelium is the only primary target of serum antibody.

HOLLENBERG et al. (1968) suggested a period of arterial vasocontriction occasioned by the release of vasoactive mediators resulting from antigen-antibody interaction prior to the manifestation of the obliterative lesion. In fact, the association of deposits of both immunoglobulin and complement together with the chronic manifestation of the proliferative lesion in renal (MCKENZIE and WHITTINGHAM, 1968; ROSENAU et al., 1969), cardiac (DALLOCHIO et al., 1970; ROSSEN et al., 1971), and hepatic allografts (PORTER, 1969) is much more common than the acute infiltrative and proliferative vascular lesion (Chapter F I 1 b). As in chronic glomerulopathy (Chapter G III), several authors emphasized the presence or even the preponderance of IgM antibody in the vascular wall (MCKENZIE and WHITTINGHAM, 1968; ZÜHLKE, 1968; ROSSEN et al., 1971). Antibodies of the IgM class can fix complement, are often more potent than antibodies of other classes in producing glomerular injuries (UNANUE and DIXON, 1965), and may have a specific reactivity for denatured IgG, as is known for the rheumatoid factor. Since rheumatoid factors were frequently present in patients bearing renal allografts (BRAVO et al., 1967), IgM antibody may be produced secondarily to preceding combinations of IgG with fixed tissue antigens (PORTER et al., 1968). In human cardiac allografts the striking similarity of the intimal lesion of the coronary arteries to changes commonly seen in active rheumatic carditis has been emphasized (BIEBER et al., 1970). Another explanation is that increased synthesis of IgM antibody is a direct result of immunosuppression, since in the antibody reaction against thymus-dependent antigens, switching from early IgM antibody production to the synthesis of immunoglobulin G needs T-helper cell activity (Chapter A III 1, 2, Fig. 2). For instance, treatment of rabbits with large doses of the purine analogue azathioprine during the immunization period caused the animals to develop highly effective antilymphocyte antibody of the IgM class (JAKOBSEN and FLATMARK, 1973). Thus, the arterial obliterative lesion appears to be the expression of an almost successful regimen of immunosuppression (HUME, 1971).

Occasionally, the intimal lesions have features in common with atherosclerosis (BIEBER et al., 1970). In one particular case, the recipient's high blood cholesterol was regarded as the main etiologic factor in the development of severe atheroma of the coronary arteries and of that portion of the aorta grafted with the heart (THOMSON, 1969). The role of antiheparin immunoglobulins in the pathogenesis of chronic obliterative arteriopathy has not yet been adequately investigated. These antibodies may cause hyperlipemia due to the blockage of heparin lipases, and thrombosis due to a blocking of physiologic anticoagulant activity (BEAUMONT and LEMORT, 1974). However, proliferation of myointimal cells is also a nonspecific reaction to a variety of mechanical and metabolic

injuries to the arterial wall, and spontaneous atheromatosis is occasionally stimulated through disruption of altered smooth muscle cells and subsequent infiltration with lipophages (BIEBER et al., 1970). The contribution of host cells to
the intimal hyperplasia has been suggested by TRENTIN (1966). Since deposits
of both endothelium and subendothelial tissue at Dacron arterial prostheses
(STUMP et al., 1963; TYSON et al., 1971), and exposed arterial surfaces following
extensive endothelial injury (CHRISTENSEN, 1973) can derive from blood-borne
cells, the arterial intimal hyperplasia appears to represent recipient rather than
graft tissue (WILLIAMS and ALVAREZ, 1969; BOHLE, 1968; BOHLE and HINRICH-
SEN, 1966). Host endothelial cells may provide a buffer zone between fixed
arterial antigens and humoral antibodies (TRENTIN, 1966), but on the other
hand, the various types of subendothelial infiltrating cells may perpetuate an
insidious host-*vs*-graft reaction.

II. Interstitial Fibrosis, Parenchymal Atrophy and Chronic Cellular Infiltration

In several long-surviving grafts a slowly progressing deterioration of function
was attributed to advancing interstitial fibrosis and atrophy of the parenchymal
portion of the organ graft. Some interstitial fibrosis or fibro-edema was found
in almost all human kidney allografts several months to one year after transplantation (HAMBURGER et al., 1965; LINDQUIST et al., 1968b; KHASTAGIR et al.,
1969). The interstitial fibrosis is usually moderate, focal and irregular, and
is associated with various degrees of tubular atrophy. Postmortem examination
of canine and human cardiac allografts one to several months after transplantation revealed the presence of areas of recent myocardial infarction, large areas
of infarct scars reminiscent of fibrosis, and, frequently, multiple residual scars
in the subendocardial region and papillary muscles (KOSEK et al., 1969; BIEBER
et al., 1970). In the mildest form, the interstitial fibrotic changes of liver allografts
consist of a collapse of the central part of the reticulin framework (Fig. 53a).
In more severe cases there is an appreciable lattice-work of fibrosis (GARNIER
et al., 1970). Later, distinct fibrosis, both periportal and around collecting and
hepatic veins becomes obvious, with early septum formation between the central
areas, subdividing the lobules (PORTER, 1969; WILLIAMS et al., 1969) (Fig. 53b).
However, nodule formation is uncommon. These events are ass ociated with
atrophy of hepatocytes incorporated within the fibrous lattice, dense centrilobular
cholestasis and loading of Kupffer cells with hemosiderin, lipofuscin and bile
pigment. Severe interstitial fibrosis is a common feature in the longer-surviving
pulmonary (GONDOS et al., 1973) (Fig. 54a) and pancreatic allograft (v. HEE,
1973) (Fig. 54b).

Most of these changes appear to reflect fibrous repair of a variety of previous
injuries, such as direct parenchymal damage caused by (reserved) intermittent
rejection episodes, and ischemia secondary to vascular lesions (KOSEK et al.,
1969; SHEIL, 1969). Although lymphoid cells are frequently distributed
throughout fibrotic areas (BOHLE, 1970), it is uncertain whether these infiltrates
are the manifestation of a mitigated rejection process. Most infiltrating cells

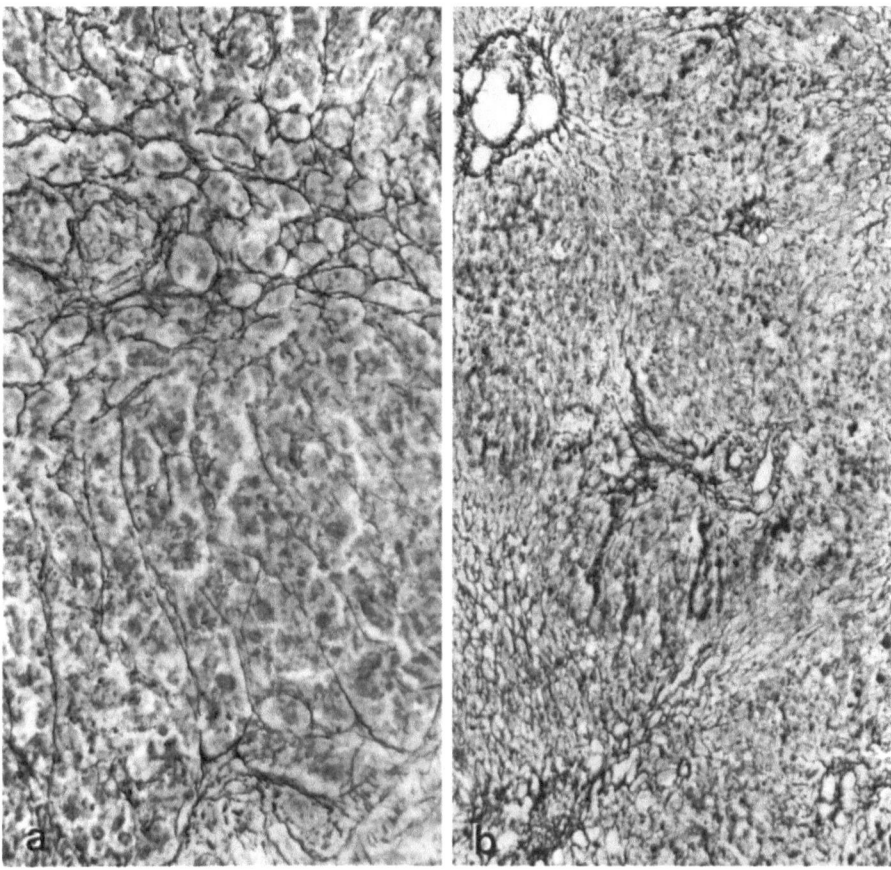

Fig. 53a and b. Canine heterotopic auxiliary liver allografts treated with Imuran. (a) Collapse of reticulin fibers adjacent to central vein 6 weeks after transplantation. (b) Distinct cirrhosis of mixed portal and cardiac type 8 weeks after transplantation. Note distorted reticulin pattern. (Bielschowsky: a ×250; b ×60)

are mature lymphocytes (LINDQUIST *et al.*, 1968b; BIEBER *et al.*, 1970) accompanied by a few plasma cells and a variable number of large macrophages. Since similar cellular compositions were demonstrated in infiltrates in renal autografts, after pulmonary bilateral hilar stripping, particularly in dogs (JERUSALEM and V.D. WERF, 1969; IRIE *et al.*, 1975) and in the indigenous liver of rats bearing auxiliary liver grafts (JAP, 1971), they may reflect chronic (interstitial) infection, bearing in mind that patients treated with immunosuppressive drugs become particularly vulnerable hosts (LIE, 1970; LAGRANGE, 1972). In numerous individual instances it may therefore be difficult to distinguish between the immunologically produced lesion and structural changes resulting from unphysiologic conditions to which an organ graft is exposed, e.g. denervation with a subsequent increase in hypersensitivity to vasoconstrictive agents (OHNISHI, 1969), impairment of lymphatic flow and/or bile flow, unfavorable hemodynamic conditions, and functional competition (Chapter F II 3). Indeed,

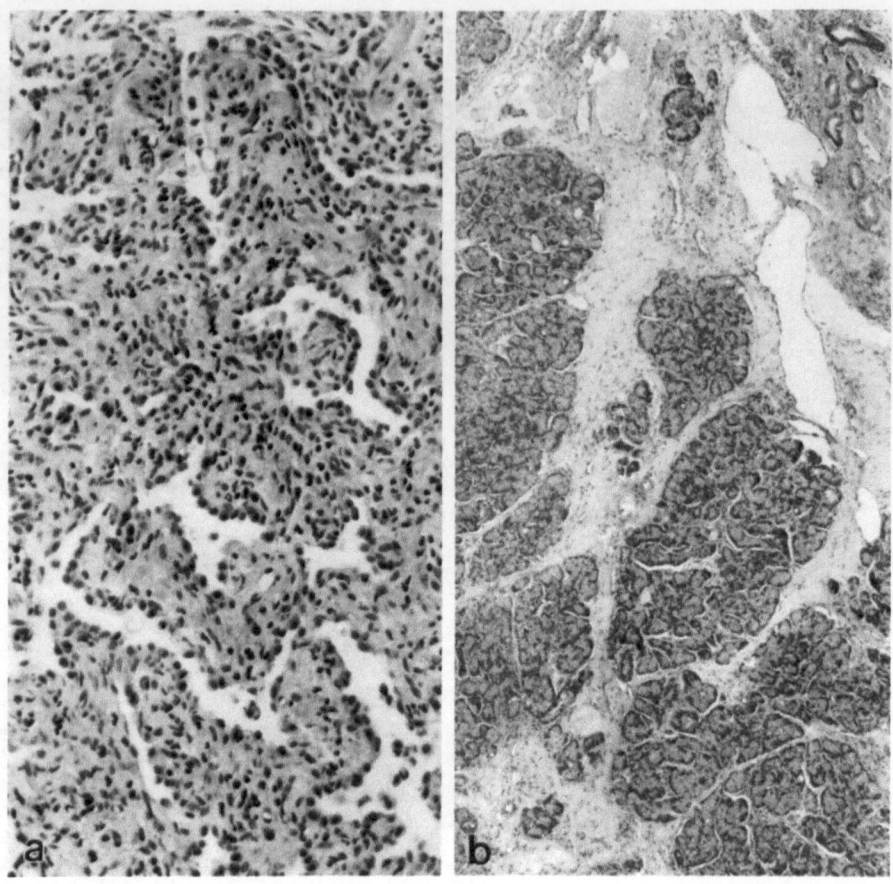

Fig. 54a. Canine pulmonary allograft 15 months after transplantation to a T-cell depleted recipient. (Adult thymectomy and subsequent treatment with ATS for 10 days, 5 months prior to transplantation.) Severe interstitial fibrosis of several portions of graft. Local distribution suggests infection, rather than rejection as causative event. (Hematoxylin and eosin: × 250)

Fig. 54b. Canine pancreatic allograft, treated with Imuran and cortisone, 31 days after transplantation. Distinct interstitial fibrosis. Note dilated lymphatics and proliferating pancreatic ductules in right upper quadrant, and irregular shape of pancreatic acini. (Hematoxylin and eosin: × 60)

the terminal aspect of some hepatic and pulmonary autografts is indistinguishable from that of allografts rejected late (Jerusalem et al., 1972; Wagenvoort et al., 1973).

III. Chronic Glomerulopathy

As the frequency of recourse to kidney transplantation to with the goal of prolonging and improving the quality of life increased, the grafts were found increasingly often to exhibit glomerular alterations similar to the well-known lesions of chronic glomerulopathy (Hamburger et al., 1965; Porter, 1965; Dix-

ON, 1971 b; HUME, 1971). Moreover, as in glomerulonephritis in man, the multiplicity of morphologic and immunofluorescent features suggests the implication of several pathogenic mechanisms (PORTER et al., 1967, 1968; ANDRES et al., 1970). The simplest pathogenic event offered as an explanation for the chronic glomerulopathy is the recurrence of the original renal disease of the recipient in the graft. In identical twin cases about 75 percent of the patients suffering from glomerulonephritis prior to nephrectomy and transplantation developed a similar disease in their renal isografts (GLASSOCK, et al., 1968). Although the immunologic nature of this lesion is indisputable, it is not a rejection, since it results from autoantibodies (or antigen-antibody complexes) against the glomerular basement membrane (GBM) of the original kidney. These antibodies can persist after transplantation and attack the glomerular filtering structures of the graft (DIXON, 1971 b). In contrast, after transplantation of kidneys from nonrelated donors the renal allograft exhibited a much lower rate of recurrence (HUME, 1968; ENDE, 1974) probably because these patients were treated with immunosuppressants which might have modified the course of the original disease, whereas in recipients of isografts being left without immunosuppression the formation of GBM antibodies remained undisturbed (HUME, 1971; MILGROM et al., 1971). Since there is clear evidence that this type of glomerular lesion also developed in grafts transplanted to recipients whose original renal disease was not of an immunologic nature (PORTER et al., 1967, 1968; ANDRES et al., 1970; HUME et al., 1968), mechanisms other than pre-existing GBM antibodies were considered as possibly responsible for the frequent deposits of amorphous material on the subendothelial aspects of the glomerular capillary basement membrane. In these instances a de novo immunologic process induced by the response to antigens shared by graft and recipient has been suggested (MILGROM et al., 1971). Rats submitted to several successive auxiliary renal allotransplantations developed granular deposits of IgG along the glomerular capillary walls and proliferation of both endothelial and mesangial cells in their own kidneys (KLASSEN and MILGROM, 1969). This type of glomerular lesion is apparently produced by the deposition of complexes composed of a tubular cell-derived antigen and its corresponding antibody (GRUPE and KAPLAN, 1969; CREMERS–V. DIJCK, 1973). Preceding rejection episodes and/or ischemic damage to the renal parenchyma may trigger or enhance this mechanism by way of the liberation of abundant tubular antigens. However, this type of glomerular injury is also obviously not due to rejection, since it corresponds to the postulated second pathogenic mechanism of spontaneous glomerulonephritis in man, i.e. the formation of circulating complexes in the vasculature, which reach and lodge in the glomeruli (DIXON, 1971 b). Although the responsibility of other antigens in the formation of immune complexes in recipients of renal allografts has not yet been demonstrated, consideration should be given to transplantation antigens (LINDQUIST et al., 1968 b). Several observations seem to indicate that a renal allograft may also stimulate the formation of antibodies to alloantigens of the tubular basement membrane (MILGROM et al., 1971) and to "anomalous" glomerular antigens, since it has been suggested that an individual can only express four antigens on the HL-A system, whereas the glomeruli of three individuals examined appeared to carry five antigens and those of another patient carried six (JONES and MOORE, 1970). Several authors emphasized the preponderance of deposits of IgM antibody in the glomerulopathy of chronic rejection. Deposits of exclusively IgG were only incidentally demonstrated. In almost all instances where the staining pattern was positive for IgG, IgM antibody was also fixed to the glomerular capillary wall, but in the majority of cases only IgM antibody was present (MCKENZIE and WHITTINGHAM, 1968; PORTER et al., 1968; HULME et al., 1972). As outlined in the previous Chapter (G II), IgM antibodies may be produced secondarily to preceding combinations of IgG with fixed tissue antigens (rheumatoid factor). However, increased synthesis of IgM also results from inhibition of T-helper cell activity in immunosuppressed recipients. In addition, deficiency in T-effector cell activity may allow the proliferation of "forbidden" clones, which are considered to be a possible source of autoantibodies (FUDENBERG, 1971). In mice, at least, the number and activity of immunologically competent cells was found to decline as the animals grew older, and the localization of mouse IgM immune complexes in the renal glomerulus increased with age (MARKHAM et al., 1973). Although the stimulation for this aberrant response may be exogenous, it results in the production of IgM antibody, which is often more potent than antibodies of other classes in the production of glomerular injuries in mice (UNANUE and DIXON, 1965).

It should be noted again that neither the interaction between antibody and fixed glomerular antigens nor the deposition of immune complexes along the glomerular capillary wall are in themselves injurious to the basement membrane, but these precipitates may fix complement as a secondary mediator and become activated, though not in every case. Fibrinogen is rarely demonstrable in the common type of late glomerular lesion (HULME et al., 1972) but has been found in a focal mesangial pattern in instances characterized by subepithelial humps as well as subendothelial deposits of IgG and IgM (PORTER et al., 1968).

In necropsies or biopsies of chronically rejected kidneys the glomeruli mostly exhibit various combinations of histopathologic changes (Figs. 55, 56). Occasionally, however, one type of lesion is dominant, and together with considerations of the nature of the original disease and the clinical post-transplantation course, it can be used as a criterion for the analysis of the pathogenic mechanism of the late glomerular lesion.

1. *Recurrent nephritis of the GBM type* in unmodified isogenic grafts (this type accounts for only 5 percent of all "spontaneous" adult cases of glomerulonephritis (DIXON, 1971b): linear arrays of IgG deposits and less pronounced endothelial proliferation are the characteristic features.

2. *Recurrent nephritis of the immune complex type* in unmodified isogenic grafts (this type accounts for the majority of the "spontaneous" cases of adult glomerulonephritis): coarsely granulated deposits of IgG, frequently irregularly distributed. More pronounced reaction of both epithelial and mesangial cells are typical.

3. *De novo glomerulopathy of the rejecting type,* induced by antibodies against histocompatibility antigens (experimental in unmodified hosts) (MILGROM et al., 1971): regular linear staining pattern for IgG. General hypercellularity is noted.

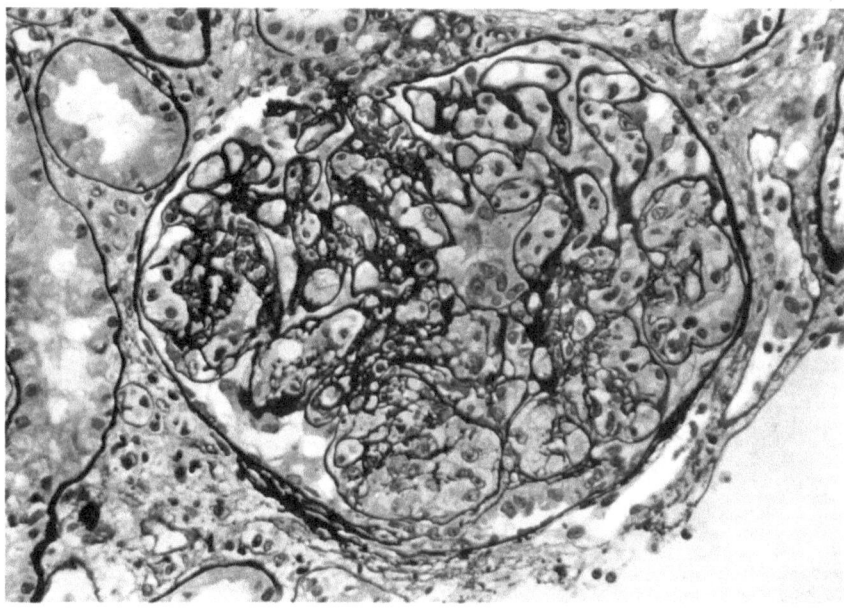

Fig. 55. Human kidney allograft, 24 weeks after transplantation to 32-years-old male (standard immunosuppressive treatment). Severity of mesangial and capillary changes lacks uniformity in glomerular tufts of same glomerulus. Several loops are occluded by swollen and proliferated endothelial cells and occasionally by lipophages, indicating preceding microthrombotic events. Furthermore, proliferation of both mesangial and epithelial cells is evident. Glomerular loops are irregular, and several tufts exhibit thickened and occasionally split basement membrane. Note irregularly thickened and split capsular membrane (Jones' silver-methenamine: × 500). By courtesy of Prof. Dr. P.H.M. SCHILLINGS, Dept. of Pathology and Prof. Dr. P.G.A. WIJDEVELD, Dept. of Nephrology, University of Nijmegen, The Netherlands

4. *De novo glomerulopathy of the nonrejecting complex type,* triggered by defined tubular antigens (experimental in unmodified hosts) (KLASSEN and MILGROM, 1969): regular deposits of coarsely granulated IgG along the glomerular capillary walls and along the tubular basement membranes are the typical features.

5. *De novo glomerulopathy of the nonrejection complex type,* triggered by hitherto undefined antigens in modified recipients: Finely granulated deposits of IgM, frequently irregularly distributed. Pronounced reaction of the capillary endothelium is characteristic of this type.

However, none of these criteria proved to be absolute in distinction between the various types of the chronic glomerulopathy in renal transplants. Since the commonly used immunosuppressive agents (ALS, ATG, purine antimetabolites and various C_{21}-Δ^4-3-keto—corticosteroids) are known to depress primary rather than secondary immune responses, in instances of type-1 or type-2 nephritis IgG fixation to the glomerular capillary walls can also be expected in modified recipients. The same is true of those instances of type-3 or type-4 nephritis where in the absence of T-helper cell activity IgG is compensatorily produced by B-lymphocytes through an increased turnover of membrane-bound immunoglobulin.

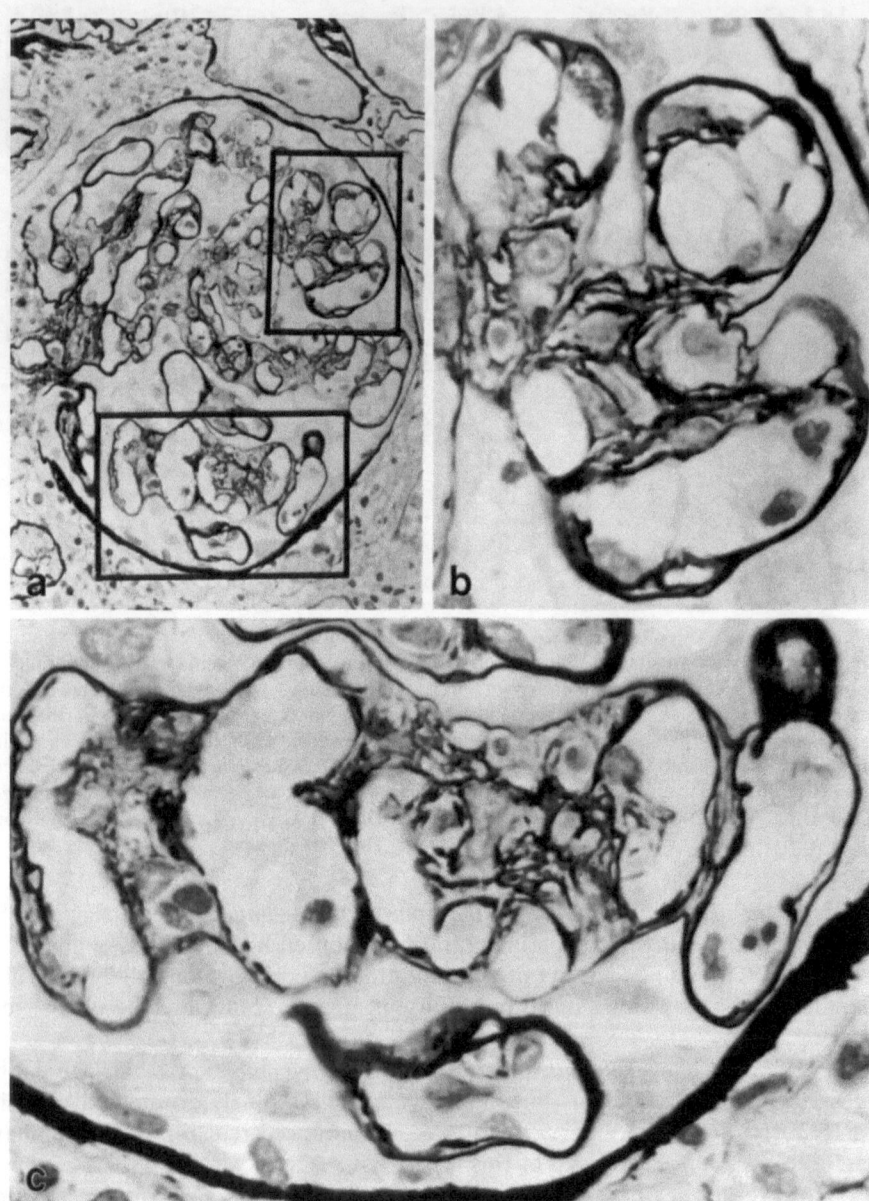

Fig. 56a–c. In other glomeruli of human renal allograft depicted in Fig. 55, changes of glomerular basement membranes dominate over proliferative ones (a). In addition to irregular increase in mesangial structures, basement membranes are locally thickened and almost split apparently due to deposits particularly on endothelial side (b). Note irregular thickening of capsular basement membrane (c) (Jones' silver-methenamine: a ×350; b and c ×1,200). By courtesy of Prof. Dr. P.H.M. SCHILLINGS, Dept. of Pathology and Prof. Dr. P.G.A. WIJDEVELD, Dept. of Nephrology, University of Nijmegen, The Netherlands

Clearly, the problem of the chronic glomerulopathy of transplants is a field in which many problems have still to be solved, particularly at the molecular level of the immune response, before we can understand the pathogenesis of changes which result ultimately in the functional deterioration of grafts.

H. Future Prospects of Organ Transplantation

I. Current Experience in Organ Transplantation

In the previous chapters we found ourself compelled to analyze predominantly the various events possibly contributing to the destruction of transplanted organs, and to disregard the promising results obtained in clinical and experimental organ transplantation. In view of the short history of organ transplantation, and the initial lack of basic data, most of the clinical work so far has been empirical (CALNE, 1967). At least renal transplantation, however, has reached a point where it is generally accepted as a treatment of choice for most patients with terminal renal disease. Through recent advances in research directed at clinical application, and the collaboration of workers of widely different training and skills we have a wide approach to the actual goal of clinical organ transplantation: to prolong and to improve the quality of life (HUME, 1971). Whereas 79% of the recipients and 52% of transplanted cadaveric kidneys survived for 1 year during the years 1968 to 1972, the 1-year survival rates were 93% and 64% respectively for 1972 and 1973. Still surviving related recipient and graft survival was 86% and 73% in the earlier group, but 100% and 88% in the current group (SALVATIERRA JR. et al., 1974). After the establishment of an interdisciplinary kidney center in 1971, the 3-year transplant mortality decreased from 38% (1963–1970) to 9% (1971–1974), despite the inclusion of more high-risk patients during the latter period (STENZEL et al., 1974). These results show good promise that the percentages of long-term survivors, too, (longer than 10 years) will further increase. Actually, 34% of those recipients of unrelated renal transplants and 52% of patients carrying a related kidney transplanted 8 to 12 years ago are alive (THOMAS et al., 1974). Moreover, RIFLE and TRAEGER (1974) counted 106 pregnancies in 92 women with renal allografts: 79 viable infants were born, 7 spontaneous abortions occurred, and 20 therapeutic abortions were performed, but only 3 for nephrologic reasons.

Results reported on long-term survivors of heart transplantation cannot be directly compared with those of kidney transplantation. Recipients of cardiac allografts are patients in whom all drug and nonoperative treatment had proved inadequate for continued survival. Mostly, they are in very bad condition, or even in shock from terminal cardiac disease. Their life expectancy may be hours, or, at best, a week or two. Of course, a related donor is not at the surgeons disposal, and an acceptable unrelated donor is available only by chance immediately when an acute emergency or impending death threatens. In spite of intensive efforts at medical centers throughout the world the developed

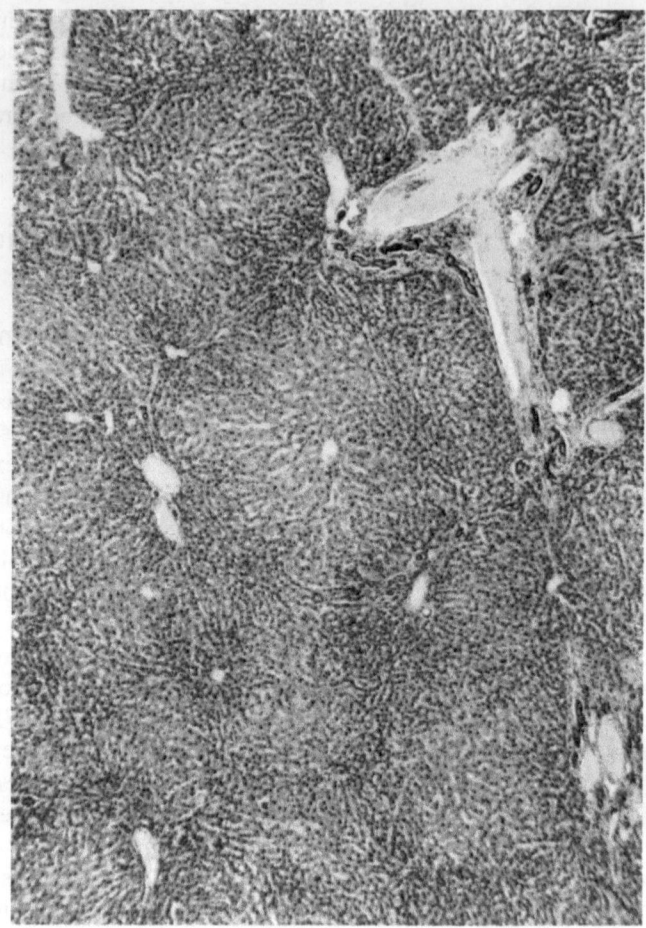

Fig. 57. Untreated Wistar-to-Wistar rat heterotopic liver graft 34 months after transplantation. Except for slight increase in portal connective tissue and prominent bile ductules, graft exhibits no distinct histopathologic changes. Animal died of uremia due to extended glomerular sclerosis. (Hematoxylin and eosin: × 40)

artificial hearts of various designs (bypass-type and series-type assist devices, total artificial hearts) are only suitable for acute experiments (AKUTSU, 1971). However, two efforts to bridge the time between cardiac arrest and cardiac transplantation by two-stage surgery were successful (COOLEY et al., 1969; DE-BAKEY et al., 1969). Furthermore, the cardiac graft has to function immediately in contrast to a kidney transplant which may eventually recover from pretransplantation ischemic damage; meanwhile the recipient's life is supported by repeated hemodialysis (see Section D III 1). The more remarkable are the results achieved by SHUMWAY (reported by GRIEPP et al., 1974) where 38 of the 66 patients who received heart grafts at Stanford have survived longer than 3 months. In this group 1, 2, and 3-year survival is 75%, 67%, and 40%. The careful management of long-term survivors of heart transplantation results in successful physical and social rehabilitation. Similar problems as in cardiac transplantation are encountered with extracorporal support and replacement of the terminal diseased lung and liver. So far, the artificial lung has not been developed to a point where long-term clinical use is successful (HARDY and ALICAN, 1971). Proposals (KIMOTO, 1959) to use membrane dialysis of the comatose patient's blood against a liver mash are still in an early experimental stage. Parabiotic attachment of patients in hepatic coma with a healthy volunteer of the same blood type (BURNELL et al., 1965) are less recommendable. This brief review cannot give appropriate recognition to the large number of investigations in the field of extracorporal hepatic support and auxiliary liver transplantation. The possible future role of these techniques has been summarized by EISEMAN and VELASQUES (1971). Extended studies in our laboratory suggest certain limitations of the extra- and intracorporal support of diseased livers, although we regularly obtain rats surviving 24 to 36 months with a heterotopic nonauxiliary hepatic graft (Fig. 57).

Despite the above mentioned difficulties, 26% of the first 42 patients receiving an orthotopic liver graft at the University of Colorado and the Veterans Adminis-

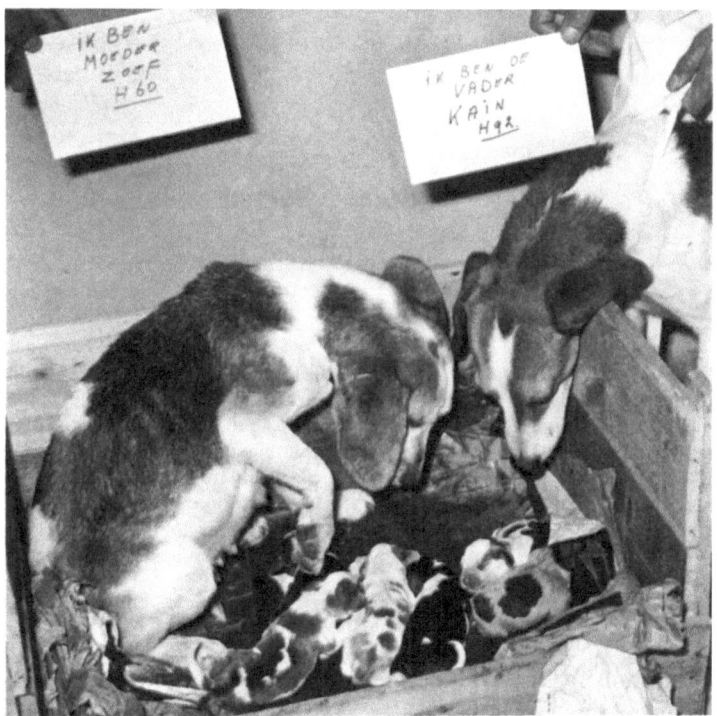

Fig. 58. "I am mother ZOEF" (H60) and "I am the father KAIN" (H92). Mother received an orthotopic liver allograft on October 24, 1972 and Father on Februar 21, 1973, at the University of Leiden, The Netherlands. Both dogs had several slight rejection crises which were treated with Imuran. On March 14, 1975 mother delivered 6 puppies. A surgical biopsy of liver of this dog (H60) was taken on August 4, 1975 (see Fig. 59). By courtesy of Dr. H.J. STOL, Dr. S.W. SCHALM and Prof. Dr. J.L. TERPSTRA, University of Leiden, The Netherlands

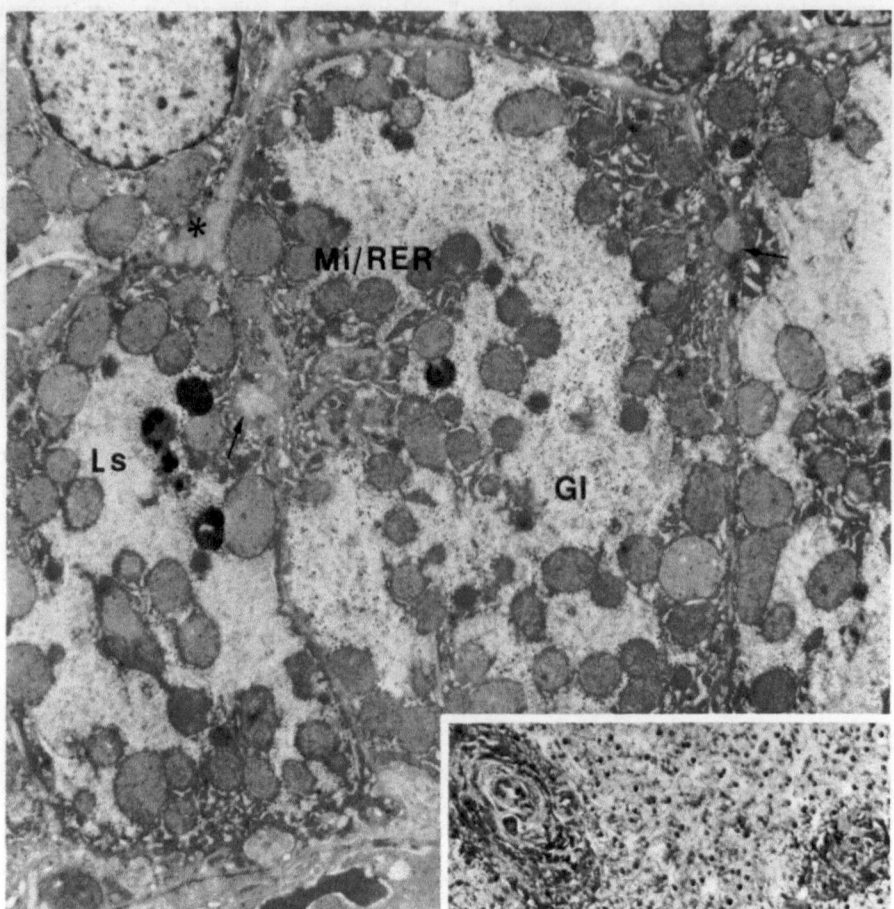

Fig. 59. Canine orthotopic liver allograft, treated with Imuran and cortisone, 30 months after transplantation. Surgical biopsy of dog H60, depicted in Fig. 58. Light microscopy reveals moderate increase in connective tissue (moderate fibrosis) and slight disarray of trabecular architecture. Ultrastructurally, borders of hepatocytes are prominent, due to unusual presence of delicate collagenous fibrils, indicating slight fibrosis (asterisk). Bile canaliculi are not dilated (arrows). Hepatocytes exhibit extended glycogen areas (*Gl*) and peripheral localization of mitochondrial/RER complexes (*Mi/RER*). In depicted area, number of lysosomal structures (*Ls*) is not increased. (Fixation: glutaraldehyde × 4,500. Inset: hematoxylin and eosin: × 100)

tration Hospital in Denver survived for 1 year or longer (PENN *et al.*, 1974), and a survival time of longer than 5 years has been reported from King's College Hospital Cambridge, although there were 4 major points of mismatch between the recipient and the donor (CALNE, 1974). Since the rate of long-term survivors is higher in experimental animals, and a significant number of clinical and experimental hepatic allografts were lost due to causes other than rejection, we would suppose that avoidance of technical pitfalls, control of viral and bacterial infection (SCHALM *et al.*, 1975), and restriction of liver transplantation almost exclusively to patients with benign hepatic disease (PENN *et al.*, 1974) will result in better long-term survival figures. There is no doubt that hepatic allotransplantation can result in successful physical rehabilitation, since both pigs (CALNE, 1974) and dogs carrying an orthotopic allograft were able to complete a pregnancy to term (Fig. 58), despite slight histopathologic changes of the graft (Fig. 59). Up to present, the success of vascularized pancreatic graft appears to have been relatively ignored, although allotransplantation of pancreatic segments has been proved to be an effective and simple method of aborting the pathophysiologic effects in juvenile onset diabetics. Four of seven recipients, some of them in addition provided with a renal allograft, survived for longer than 1 year (GLIEDMAN *et al.*, 1974). Canine pancreatic allografts exhibited a largely normal appearance 15 months after transplantation (Fig. 60), and Wistar rat to Wistar rat full-length small bowel grafts survived for longer than 20 months (Fig. 61).

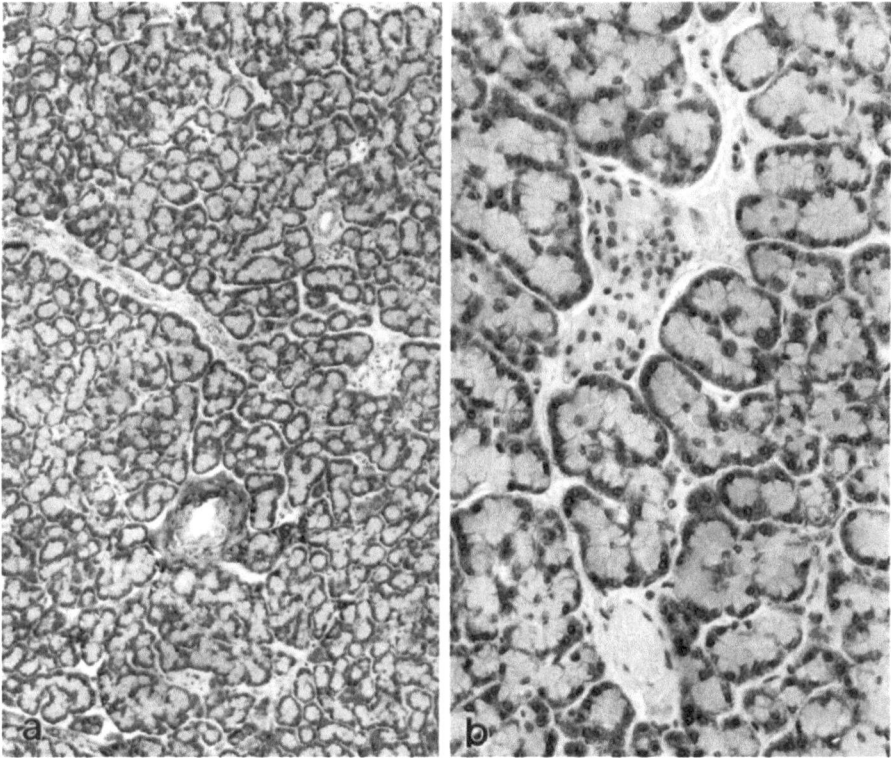

Fig. 60a and b. Canine pancreatic allograft, treated with Imuran and cortisone, 15 months after transplantation. Except for slight interstitial fibrosis no histopathologic changes of pancreatic acini and islands. Note scarcity of centroacinar cells in canine pancreas. (Hematoxylin and eosin: a × 100; b × 250)

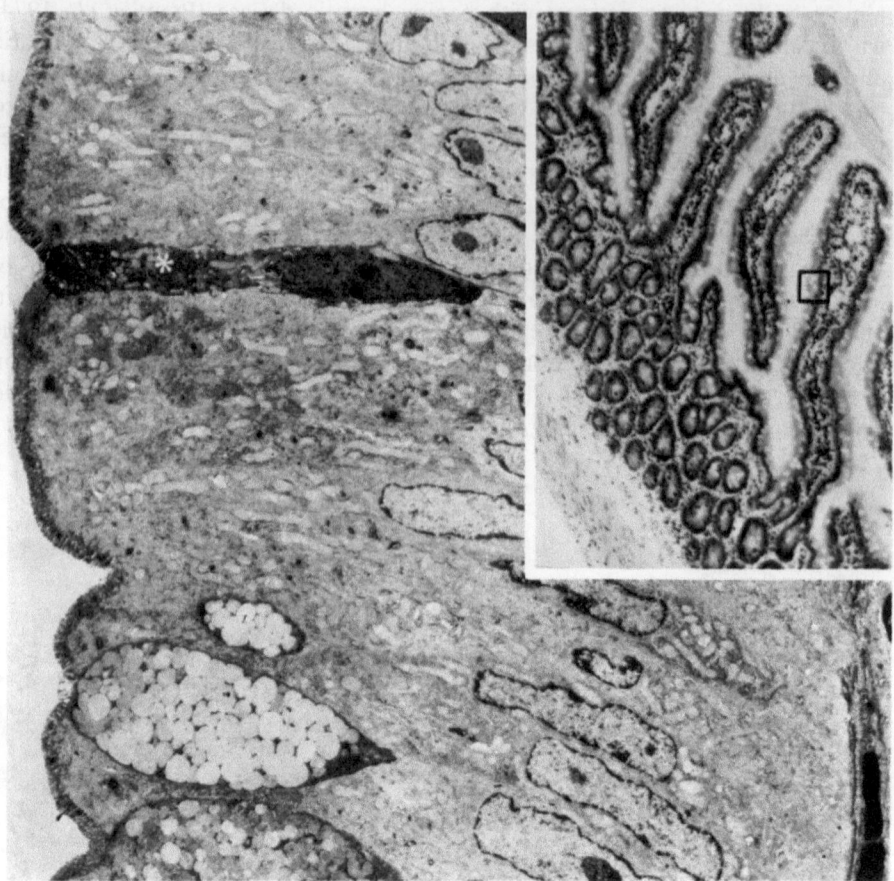

Fig. 61. Rat (Wistar-to-Wistar) full length small bowel graft 20 months after transplantation. No administration of immunosuppressive drugs. Regular columnar lining cells with interspersed goblet cells. Neither increase in apical lysosomal structures nor in number of cells undergoing pyknosis within the scope of physiologic regeneration (asterisk). As shown in inset, submucosa is slightly infiltrated with mononuclear cells. (Fixation: glutaraldehyde ×2,000. Inset: hematoxylin and eosin: ×70)

II. Histocompatibility Typing

Since it has become generally accepted that the rules applicable to blood transfusion in man also apply to the transplantation of organs (JOYSEY et al., 1973), compatibility tests between donor and recipient (donor selection) would seem to be indicated for solid organ transplantation also (VRIESENDORP, 1973). In practice, selection of donors on the basis of their transplantation antigens is restricted to the field of kidney transplantation. It is beyond the scope of this review and out of the competence of the authors to discuss the reasons for the occasional poor correlation between the results of histocompatibility determination and the final outcome of, particularly, the transplantation of lung and liver (VEITH and BLUMENSTOCK, 1971; HALGRIMSON *et al.*, 1971; CALNE, 1974; TERASAKI, 1974). However, there is clear evidence that in general in all organs so far studied both the induction and the intensity of the transplantation reaction depend upon the extent of antigenic difference between donor and recipient (WEIL and REEMTSMA, 1974; VRIESENDORP, 1973; DE LANGEN *et al.*, 1975). We have every reason to expect that the prognosis of each transplanted organ will improve further, due to further improvements in serologic typing techniques (for review see DAUSSET and COLOMBANI, 1972), the general application of recently introduced techniques of cellular testing of histocompatibility (see below), and computer analysis of results (VAN ROOD, 1962) for the establishment of the optimal donor-recipient relationship (REEMTSMA, 1971). Several investigators have claimed better correlation between serologic typing and graft survival of unrelated donors when the mixed lymphocyte culture (MLC) reactivity was also taken into account. It could be shown that in the mouse (BACH *et al.*, 1972), man (EIJSVOOGEL *et al.*, 1972), rhesus monkey (BALNER *et al.*, 1973), and the dog (VRIESENDORP, 1973) the MLC reactivity is not governed by serologically defined (SD) antigens, but by at least one other genetic system, closely linked to the system recognizing SD antigens, i.e., the lymphocyte defined (LD) locus. In this way major histocompatibility structures (H-2, HL-A, RhL-A, DL-A) can be divided into those which are serologically defined (SD) and those which control lymphocyte reactivity in mixed cultures. It has been supposed that in the transplantation reaction, LD and SD structures have different functions (EIJSVOOGEL *et al.*, 1973). During the sensitization phase the recipient would recognize, and be sensitized to, the allogeneic material through the difference between the LD characteristics, whereas the antigens controlled by the SD loci appear to serve as targets during the effector phase. In addition, most of the so-called immune response (Ir) genes, which control the ability of an individual to react by antibody formation to applied simple antigens, are linked to the major histocompatibility complex. This leads to the hypothesis that Ir structures probably play an additional role in the recognition phase of the immune response (BENACERRAF and McDEVITT, 1972), and may explain why in patients nonreactive to presensitization (blood transfusion, preceding graft) a long survival rate can be observed, despite serologically bad matches (TERASAKI, 1974). Since combined methods of donor-recipient matching are time consuming, their routine clinical application in instances of cadaveric organ transplantation depends on methods which will not preclude the storage of organs for 2 to 3 weeks (BELZER, 1974).

III. Organ Preservation and Storage

1. Simple Hypothermic Storage

The gradual acceptance of prospective tissue typing in organ transplantation has meant that the transportation of organs to centers where recipients with the best tissue match are available has become a routine procedure (VAN ROOD, 1969). The elaboration of simple and efficient methods of organ preservation during transportation was closely related to this development. If the donor can be tissue-typed before death, an average preservation time of 6 to 10 hours is considered to be sufficient for kidney and liver transplantation for the removal of the organ, its transportation over a distance of at least 120 to 300 miles, and for implantation (Schalm et al., 1975). Simple hypothermic storage has proved to be an excellent method for this purpose. Either before or after it is removed from the donor, the organ is usually flushed with a chilled solution for rapid core cooling and is then stored at temperatures between 2 and 4 °C to induce a metabolic break. Many flush-out solutions in conjunction with hypothermia have been recommended, but the important constituents of each, and their optimal concentrations, have not been clearly defined (see also Chapter D III 3). Four solutions have been widely used in various modifications 1) supplemented Ringer-lactate, 2) Collins' C2 solution (Collins et al., 1969), 3) Gelin's three-stage perfusates (Brunius et al., 1968; Sells and Pena, 1970) and 4) Sack's solution (Sacks et al., 1973). Whereas with ideal donors (experimental animals) the preservation time of kidneys may be extended up to 48 and even 72 hours (Sacks et al., 1974) and that of lungs up to 24 hours (Grosjean et al., 1972) it appears inadvisable to preserve livers longer than 8 hours (Otte et al., 1973). In cadaveric kidney transplantation an average preservation time of only 5 hours (Belzer, 1974) to $7^1/_2$ hours (Hall et al., 1974) is recommended to avoid a high percentage of primary graft failures. However, kidneys derived from well-prepared donors and subjected to a minimal anoxic interval (initial warm ischemic period, see also Chapter D III 1) can tolerate much longer periods of storage on ice (Baxby et al., 1974a), at least for 24 to 30 hours (Kreis and Barbanel, 1973). Since Manax et al. (1964) demonstrated the superiority of a combination of hyperbaric oxygen with hypothermia over hypothermic storage alone in canine kidneys, this method has undergone extensive laboratory as well as clinical testing. Oxygen enters organs by direct diffusion and reaches their core over a period of time also in the absence of circulation. As the temperature is lowered, oxygen actually diffuses more rapidly and is bound at higher concentrations to tissues; however, a considerable period of decompression is required before transplantation. The results of hyperbaric oxygenation are not uniform in the hands of different investigators (Turner, 1971). High oxygen pressures may even be harmful to preserved lungs as indicated by the induction of acute edema (Grosjean et al., 1972). Several transplantation units combine simple hypothermic storage (transportation of imported kidneys) with pulsatile flow perfusion (conservation of imported kidneys during preparation of the recipient, and preservation of domestic cadaveric grafts). Continuous flow perfusion permits assessment of suspect kidneys (increase in perfusion pressure and lactate levels) and discarding of those unfit for use (Baxby et al., 1974a).

2. Short-Term Preservation

The preservation of organs up to about three days would allow intercontinental transport of organs to the most suitable recipient, extension of histocompatibility tests (except for the MLC reaction), the handling of a sudden influx of a larger number of cadaveric organs to a transplantation center by a small team, and the actual transplantation at a time most advantageous to both the patient and the surgical team (BELZER, 1974). The basic principles of short-term preservation are continuous, mostly pulsatile perfusion, hypothermia, membrane oxygenation, and addition of albumin or (cryoprecipitated, silica gel precipitated) plasma to induce oncotic pressure. Theoretically, chemical inhibitors of specific metabolic reactions should be advantageous as supplements. Oxamic acid, e.g., completely inhibits the lactic dehydrogenase conversion of pyruvate to lactate (NOVOA et al., 1959). However, only phenoxybenzamine (CALMAN and BELL, 1972) and chlorpromazine are routinely used in several transplantation centers. These drugs apparently have the ability both to protect the membranes of cells and subcellular particles (lysosomes and mitochondria) against a number of noxious influences, and to reduce oxygen requirements (EYAL et al., 1965a, b; LILLEHEI and MANAX, 1966).

A short review may indicate that the relevant clinical problem of a 100% survival of short-term preserved organs has not yet been solved, not even in dogs used as experimental animals:

Kidney. Survival less than 100% after a preservation period of 24 hours (JESKE and ABOUNA, 1973); 90% after 48 hours; and 25% after 120 hours (TOLEDO–PEREYRA et al., 1974a).

Heart. After a preservation period of 24–28 hours 60% of the grafts functioned immediately, and 23% survived for longer than 30 hours (COPELAND et al., 1973); 79% survival of cardiac grafts after 24 hours preservation was obtained by SUROS and WOODS (1974).

Liver. Preserved for 24 hours, 63% of the grafts were able to support life, (PETRIE and WOODS, 1973) but only 26% functioned for longer than 3 days after a preservation period of 48 hours (SUNG and WOODS, 1974).

Small intestine. Graft survival did not exceed 24 hours after a preservation period of 3 days (TOLEDO–PEREYRA et al., 1974b).

3. Intermediate-Term Storage and Long-Term Preservation

There is a general consensus that the development of methods allowing preservation of organs for 2 to 3 weeks would provide an important breakthrough in clinical organ transplantation (BELZER, 1974). Only then will the more time-consuming methods of donor-recipient matching, e.g., mixed lymphocyte culture, be practical. However, there are few indications that this goal may soon be achieved using hypothermic storage. Since at low temperatures (2–4° C) cellular functions are largely delayed, but not entirely blocked, substrates and oxygen must be delivered to the organ, and metabolic end products removed. The implication of simultaneous inactivation of enzyme systems responsible for the maintenance of intercellular/extracellular ion gradients in hypothermically preserved tissues is insufficiently investigated (see Chapter D III 1). Sometimes we have the feeling that in the concept of hyperthermic preservation of organs one important factor of cellular homostasis is disregarded. In Chapter F II 3 we focused attention on the problem of functional competition between coexisting organs in auxiliary liver transplantation. Only an organ which labors under a functional stimulus, survives, while the functionally relieved organ inevitably atrophies. Functional, compensatory, and complementary atrophy or hypertrophy, respectively, are the immutable results of a distinct functional under- or overload of tissues. Perhaps, the organ to be stored for longer periods should be connected to an artificial host which would not only supply the graft with essential nutrients but also with precursors of the organspecific function, e.g., urea and sodium bicarbonate to the kidney, bilirubin, glucose, and (intermittent) glucagon to the liver, and carbon dioxide to the lungs. The preservation of lungs by perfusion with blood in a simple recirculation system at 29° C (MODRY et al., 1973) does not appear to be disadvantageous compared with simple hypothermic storage, and the functional *ex vivo* preservation of self-perfusing heart-lung preparations at 37° C was demonstrated by RIEDESEL et al. (1973). Although in the latter study the mean survival time of blood perfused preparations was only about 8 hours, these results certainly suggest lines for further research.

Intermediate-term storage of allografts may offer another important advantage. Canine pancreatic allografts preserved for 24 hours by hypothermic perfusion were shown to be more resistant to rejection (mean survival time [MST] 11.7 days) than allografts implanted immediately (MST 6.1 days). When hypothermic preservation was preceded by a warm ischemic period of 30 minutes, the MST was extended to 15.7 days (DE GRUYL et al., 1973). In another experimental series the mean survival times of canine pancreatic allografts after 2, 4, and 6 hours preservation time were 8.1, 15.3, and 43.6 days, respectively (VAN HEE, 1973). However, the prolongation of the MST with increasing preservation time appeared to be related to the progressive development of technical skill rather than to a favorable factor induced by storage, since the experiments were not randomized but carried out in the sequence of increasing preservation times. Nevertheless, in a randomized experimental set-up for studies on simple hypothermic storage of both canine and porcine liver allografts the survival was shortest in the 1 hour ischemic group compared with an ischemic time of 3 and 6 hours (SCHALM et al., 1975). Although several authors questioned the significance of their observations, the results could be analogous to those obtained by SUMMERLIN et al. (1970, 1973) who found that certain types of animal and human tissues lose their ability to provoke an immune response in a new host, if the tissues have been grown in a culture medium for a critical period of time prior to transplantation. Human skin, e.g., could be transplanted after 4 to 6 weeks in culture into individuals whose histocompatibility antigens were grossly different from those of the donor. SUMMERLIN's findings have sparked off a great deal of scepticism among immunologists, because they appear to contradict the conventional wisdom of the field (MAUGH, 1973). Culturing of viruses and occasionally of malaria parasites (WEISS and DIGIUSTI, 1966) does not appear to parallel this phenomenon, since the produced attenuated strains predominantly loose their infectivity rather than their antigenicity. With respect to clinical importance, the reduction or even the loss of antigenic strength of cultured cells awaits confirmation on a larger scale.

Most workers in the field of organ conservation pin large hopes on the freezing of organs (LILLEHEI and MANAX, 1966; TURNER, 1971; BELZER, 1974). The discovery of the cryoprotective agents glycerol (POLGE et al., 1949) and dimethylsulfoxide (DMSO) (LOVELOCK and BISHOP, 1959) stimulated the development of methods for freeze preservation of cell suspensions. In subsequent studies on freezing of solid organs a variety of problems was encountered, such as the control of the rate of freezing and subsequent warming throughout the tissue mass, intracellular crystallization of water, shift of electrolytes, and the disproportion in concentration of cryoprotective agents, necessary on the one hand to prevent damages by freezing and rewarming, and tolerated by the tissue, on the other (TURNER, 1971). Actually there are only few published reports on long-term functional success following freezing of organs and subsequent implantation. Two of 14 canine renal autografts (14%) survived after freezing to −6° C (MUNDTH et al., 1965), and life-supporting function was observed in two instances of 9 reimplanted surviving kidneys of dogs after freezing to −22° C (DIETZMAN et al., 1973). HAMILTON et al. (1973) used a chilled (5° C) cryoprotective solution containing DMSO, low-molecular-weight dextran, and glucose for initial perfusion of small segments of the small bowel. After freezing to −70° C in a dry ice chamber, the grafts were transferred to a liquid nitrogen refrigator at −196° C. One week later, the bowel segments were prewarmed on dry ice, thawed rapidly in warm physiologic saline, and heterotopically reimplanted. Five of 14 grafts (35,7%) were considered survivors, as judged by the microscopic identification of all layers of the bowel, including a regenerated mucosa, 14 days after transplantation. Four grafts were found to produce mucus and to absorb glucose, and 3 had peristaltic activity. These results appear more promising than those obtained with continuous hypothermic perfusion for 3 days (survival time shorter than 24 hours, see Chapter H III 2). However, it should be taken into account that HAMILTON et al. (1973) worked with non-life-supporting heterotopic autografts, whereas TOLEDO–PEREYRA et al. (1974 b) transplanted allografts orthotopically. In conclusion, freezing of organs may become the procedure of choice in the future. Storage at the temperature of liquid nitrogen appears to be essential. In our laboratory this method is used for the preservation of various cultures' cell lines, e.g., rat hepatocytes, rat hepatoma cells, and calf ocular lens epithelium, which can be kept viable after transfer into a liquid nitrogen refrigator (at about −190° C) as long as for more than 12 months. Kept on dry ice (at about −70° C) the survival time of cell culture suspensions is distinctly shorter. Further development will probably depend on the detection of nontoxic cryoprotective agents that remain liquid at much lower temperatures than is possible now (BELZER, 1974). Referring again to our tissue culture experiments, most of the damage to DMSO incubated cells appears to occur during the freezing period (about 30%) rather than during storage at −196° C for between 1 week and 1 year (about 15%). Since freezing of organs requires not only expensive equipment, but also experienced cryobiologists, the long-term preservation of grafts (banking of organs) will probably become the method of choice for large transplantation centers only.

IV. Artificial Organs

Artificial organ support and replacement have a long history, extending back for about a century, and remains an actively investigated field today. Organ transplantation and artificial organ support are not in conflict, on the contrary, they supplement and complement each other, and both modalities will retain an autonomous field of application (HARDY, 1971). In Chapter H I we emphasized the need for suitable devices to assist also the failing lung and heart as long as necessary to bridge the period between impending death and transplantation, since there is no doubt that the recent success in clinical renal transplantation is largely due to routine application of the life-sustaining artificial kidney.

The heart-lung machine has become a common tool in the armamentarium for open heart or great vessel surgery, and for the short-term support of, e.g., acute congestive heart failure, pulmonary embolism, or severely impaired pulmonary functions in candidates for surgery (RATLIFF, 1971). Whereas the heart-lung machine can be regarded as a result of combined research on both gas exchangers ("oxygenators") and pump systems, current experimental trends attempt to develop separate units for differential support of impaired lung or heart function. Advantages and disadvantages of supplanting lung functions by blood-biological membrane-gas interface exchangers (temporary lung transplants), blood-gas interface gas exchangers (direct exposure of blood to various gaseous mixtures) and blood-synthetic membrane-gas interface gas exchangers (exchange through hydrophobic synthetic membranes) have been summarized by RATLIFF (1971). Although rapid progress is apparent, mechanical gas exchange systems are not yet perfected to such an extent of efficiency that they could compete with lung transplants for chronic support. For the construction of artificial hearts technical problems presented by materials are fundamental (AKUTSU, 1971). For devices to be permanently implanted the demands on materials are extremely severe, concerning particularly their durability and compatibility. Polyurethane implanted in dogs in the form of strips (MIRKOVITCH et al., 1962) or mitral valves (SEIDEL et al., 1962) had become stiff and brittle with loss of much of its tensile strength after 8 months, and was completely demolished after 16 months. Compatibility with blood is another important requirement, since a certain amount of damage to corpuscular elements of circulating blood by conventional heart-lung machines is unavoidable, although their action is restricted to a relatively short period of time (SCHMIDT et al., 1974). Theoretically, all problems concerning the artificial heart could be solved: materials, design, energy sources including nuclear energy and protection from radioactivity, energy conversion systems, and automatic (computer) control of driving systems (AKUTSU, 1971). However, such a device would become too expensive for permanent implantation. Furthermore, the artificial heart cannot grow in proportions with a growing body when implanted in a newborn child, or in an infant, as do biologic cardiac grafts.

Finally, the awareness that their life depends on the continuous function of a machine may be unbearable for a number of patients carrying an artificial organ. Higher incidences of suicidal attempts are registered among patients submitted to chronic renal dialysis. Therefore, we have every reason to believe that the artificial lung and heart will be most suitable for temporary support, rather than permanent implantation.

V. Modification of the Immune Response

Among the many advances in immunology the development of modalities to depress immune reactivity has contributed to successful application of clinical organ transplantation. Depression of immune reactivity, brought about by a variety of agents, is the result of a nonspecific reaction, and is mainly produced by the destruction, or at least the inactivation, of immunocompetent cells. Recently used immunosuppressive agents cannot select between, e.g., the undesirable transplantation reactions and immune responses necessary for the defense against various infectious agents. However, the progress to date has led immunologists into lines of investigation that appear to converge on what must be regarded as the ultimate goal of transplantation immunology—the ability to suppress the response to a single antigen, or constellation of antigens, while leaving all other immune responses intact (SCHWARTZ, 1971). In studies dealing with selectivity two agents are involved in which specifity is inherent: antibody and antigen. It is not the purpose of this chapter to review the entire subject, but to summarize, albeit very briefly, the immunochemical approaches to immunosuppression as based on recent information on the nature of interactions between either antigen or antibody and immunocompetent cells, and of possible cellular interactions. As in any new field, transplantation terminology continues to change from year to year, becoming more precise with increasing understanding of the factors involved. Since it appears important to know specifically what is meant by a given term, particularly if the term is new but actually refers to a subject which the reader previously knew by another name (HARDY, 1971) we range the following discussion according to terms actually used in connection with attempts to modify the immune response.

1. Immunosuppression

This means the artificial suppression of immune responses by a variety of modalities, such as a) physical agents (e.g., x-irradiation), b) surgical ablation of lymphatic tissues and cells (e.g., thymectomy, splenectomy, thoracic duct fistula), c) chemical agents (e.g., antimetabolites), d) biological agents (e.g., antilymphocyte serum), and e) physiologic agents (e.g., cortisone). Attempts to mitigate the transplantation reaction by means of irradiation of the whole body, the graft, and (extracorporally) the circulating blood were soon abandoned after the introduction of immunosuppressive drugs in experimental and clinical transplantation. KAPLAN and CALABRESI (1973) focused attention on the common misconception concerning the specific effector mechanism of cytotoxic chemicals, which may cause damage to rapidly proliferating tissues (NEIDHARDT, 1972), and therefore, due to myelosuppressive toxicity (BACH and DARDENNE, 1971), patients treated with these drugs become "particularly vulnerable hosts", resulting in infection as a frequent complication after clinical and experimental transplantation (Lie, 1970; Lagrange, 1972; Hess *et al.*, 1973). Thus, suppression of the immune response may be considered to be a side effect of the depression of various enzymes involved, e.g., in purine biosynthesis, in addition to other cytotoxic effects. Alkylating agents (nitrogen mustard, cyclophosphamide) known as inhibitors of nucleic acid synthesis, cause interphase death of marginal zone cells, follicular small lymphocytes, and induce characteristic lesions in plasmablasts and immature plasma cells (Van de Broek, 1971). Lymphocytes of the B-type are apparently the main target of alkylating agents (Turk and Poulter, 1972; Poulter and Turk, 1972). In terms of current clinical practice, the most effective cytotoxic chemical is azathioprine (Imuran), a derivate of the classical purine antagonist 6-mercaptopurine. The purine analogues were found to exert a relatively selective effect on suppression of both the primary response to new tissue antigens (Meeker *et al.*, 1960), and the primary antibody formation (Schwartz *et al.*, 1959), in particular IgG antibody formation (Sahiar and Schwartz, 1966). Since secondary antibody responses and established delayed hypersensitivity reactions are usually not suppressed, azathioprine appears to affect predominantly dividing T-cells including those of the helper cell population. It is unlikely that the full potential of folic acid antagonists (e.g., amethopterin, methotrexate) has been completely exploited. Since the kidney provides the major route of elimination of methotrexate, its use in patients with any degree of renal impairment (rejection) is contraindicated. Although in man the mode of action of cortisone in immunosuppression has not been clarified, in clinical practice corticosteroids have been proven to facilitate allograft acceptance (Schwartz, 1971). In rodents, cortisone preferentially damages TL-antigen carrying thymocytes of the outer cortex and subsequently depletes the total thymic cortex. Furthermore it causes interphase death of cells of the follicular corona, inactivates germinal center cells (Van de Broek, 1971), and the short-lived lymphocytes rather than the long-lived category disappear from the peripheral blood (Everett and Tyler, 1967); in man greater depletion of T- than of B-lymphocytes occurred (Yu *et al.*, 1974). In addition, corticosteroids can impair the bactericidal and fungicidal activity of human monocytes and induces monocytopenia (Rinehart *et al.*, 1975). In this way, thymus-independent effector mechanisms of the cell-mediated immune response may become impaired (see Chapter A III 3c).

With the realization of the important role of lymphocytes in the transplantation reaction interest in antilymphocytic serum (ALS) was renewed. Xenogenic ALS was first produced in 1899 by Metchnikoff, but the current interest in ALS undoubtedly dates from 1963 when the ability of this agent to significantly prolong the survival of skin allografts in rats was demonstrated (Woodruff and Anderson, 1963). The rationale of ALS appeared to be simple: a direct immunologic attack on cells involved in delayed hypersensitivity reactions, seemingly without other cytotoxic side effects, except for side effects resulting from a response to the foreign protein (Schwartz, 1971). For this reason antisera against T-cells (antithymocyte serum, ATS) are frequently preferred to preparations directed against all lymphocyte classes (ALS); and purified immunoglobulin fractions (ALG, ATG) are superior to total serum. The high hopes placed on the clinical use of ALG and ATG in clinical organ transplantation, however, have not been realized. Unavoidable hematologic side effects and the potential risk of renal damage (immune complex disease) have prompted caution in the clinical application of this agent (COLLSTE, 1971). In spite of numerous investigations, which cannot be adequately reviewed and appreciated within the scope of this chapter, the action of ALS and ATS are incompletely understood. The general view is that these agents inactivate recirculating T-lymphocytes while actually circulating (TRAEGER et al., 1969; MITCHISON, 1970; COLLSTE, 1971). In the presence of complement both complexing and cell disruption can occur which renders the attacked cells vulnerable to phagocytosis (LANGE and MEDAVAR, 1971). Depletion of paracortical areas but sparing of lymph follicles in the lymph node of guinea pigs treated for 6 days with ATS may result from the lack of recirculating lymphocytes (TURK, 1967). However, the degree of immunosuppression brought about by ALS does not seem to be related in any simple way to the degree of lymphopenia that it produces (GOWANS, 1971). Furthermore, ALS too, can neither select between the undesirable cell-mediated transplantation reaction and cellular immune responses necessary for the defense against viruses and neoplasm, nor between various T-helper cell activities involved in the production of cytotoxic graft-binding antibodies on the one hand, and neutralizing antibodies necessary for the protection from bacterial infectious agents, on the other.

2. Immunologic Enhancement

Originally the term was introduced to indicate the increased rate of growth of subsequent tumors in animals previously actively immunized against the same tumor (CASEY and SCOTT, 1932). The delayed rejection of skin allograft in presensitized hosts (HALASZ and ORLOFF, 1965) and accelerated multiplication of malaria parasites in actively and passively immunized mice (JERUSALEM et al., 1971 c) were also considered to be a manifestation of the enhancement phenomenon. Immunologic enhancement is attributed to the presence of specific antibody to cellular antigens which may either be evoked through active immunization or passively administered antibody. Incubation of isolated tumor cells with specific antibody for about 30 minutes prior to inoculation into an unsensitized host also enhances the growth of the tumor. The enhancing antibody may act in different ways. The hypothesis for a peripheral mechanism suggests a noncytotoxic antibody that combines with the isoantigen determinant on the surface of the target cell. This combination could either wall off soluble antigens originating from the target cell (SNELL et al., 1960), or impair the contact between surfaces antigens and cells responsible for recognition. On the other hand, the combination of noncytotoxic antibody with a cellular antigen could shield the target cell against destruction by the host's effector cells (MÖLLER and MÖLLER, 1965). An alternative hypothesis was proposed by authors working with lymphocytes from animals bearing enhanced tumor grafts (MITCHISON and DUBE, 1955; HELLSTRÖM and MÖLLER, 1965; WRIGHT, 1968). These cells were found to be selectively unresponsive to H-2 antigens, but fully competent against the H-2^k antigen of unrelated third strains. The H-2:AB combination appears to be a more important factor than the enhancing antibody in the induction of selective cellular nonreactivity at the host level (central site). In studies on abrogation of cell-mediated immunity by hyperimmune alloantiserum Cohen et al. (1974) isolated a fraction from a mixture of alloantiserum and ascitic fluid containing alloantibody against lymphoma cells, which dissociated into IgG and a small molecular species with some antigenic properties analogous to H-2 fragments. Successful blocking of effector cells was possible with the AG:AB complex-containing fraction, but not with alloantibody alone. It was supposed that cells with antibody alone bound to their antigens would lose these complexes either by simple shedding, or by capping and phagocytosis. In instances where cells rapidly generate new antigens, preliminary treatment with antiserum would alter only the kinetics of the response by delaying the immune response (Frelinger et al., 1975). Prolonging the survival time of skin grafts by means of methods suitable to induce tumor grafts is easily achieved in models where donor and recipient are closely related, but difficult in fully mismatched "hard" models (Van De Werf, 1972). Studies in our laboratory revealed an increase in survival time of rabbit to rat skin xenografts from 5 to 14 days when tissues of low antigenicity (cornea) from the same donor were grafted simultaneously. Surprisingly, hypothermic perfusion of canine small intestinal allografts with human plasmanate for 24 hours resulted in significant prolongation of graft survival (Toledo–Pereyra et al., 1974c). The authors suggest that human plasmanate contains (cytophilic) cross-reacting antibodies which bind at hypothermic temperatures, thereby interfering with the perception of allogeneic receptors on the graft by unrelated recipients.

3. Immunosuppressive Antibodies

Primary interest in the immunosuppressive activity of antibodies rose from observations on the inhibition of antigen-induced antibody production in infants with high circulating titers of maternal antibody (Murray, 1968). The most striking example of clinical application of immunosuppressive activity of specific antibody can be seen in the prevention of erythroblastosis fetalis by anti-Rh antiserum (Freda et al., 1966; Woodrow, 1970). The phenomenon of specific suppression of immune responses by antibody directed against either antigen or receptors of antigens may be caused by a feedback type mechanism (see also Chapter E, page 503), by prevention of selective recruitment of recirculating lymphocytes, or by activation of nonspecific physiologic control mechanisms. Suppression of the antibody response by passive immunization has been studied most extensively. Relatively small amounts of antibody against sheep red blood cells (SRBC) given to normal animals specifically suppress their primary IgM and IgG antibody response (Haughton et al., 1969, 1970; Rowley et al., 1973). Since depletion of natural antibody against either SRBC or a metabolizable antigen was shown to be the cause of the induction of the primary immune response (Murray, 1968), the addition of specific antibody may result in suppression of antibody synthesis through a similar feedback regulation (Graf and Uhr, 1969). A similar conclusion was drawn for the regulation of the antibody response against *Escherichia coli* endotoxin (BRITTON and MÖLLER, 1968). Although the most straightforward form of feedback regulation is the inhibitory effect of antibody operating by direct competition with B-cell receptors, it is clear that antibody can also interfere with the antigen processing function of macrophages and with helper cells. HAUGHTON (1974) achieved reversal of immunosuppression caused by passively administered anti-SRBC through transfer of stimulated macrophages harvested from mice immunized against SRBC. A relation between immunosuppressive antibodies and a normally circulating immunosuppressant factor present among the class of alpha globulins (KAMRIN, 1959; COOPERBAND et al., 1968) that appears to bind to larger molecules and to interfere with antigen recognition (KARPAS and SEGRE, 1973) remains uncertain. There are only a few reports on the inhibition of cell-mediated responses induced by passive administration of antireceptor antibody (MCKEARN, 1974). Since antigen-antibody complexes were found to block the function of activated T-cells more effectively (BALDWIN et al., 1972), and to induce a longer survival of rat renal allografts (STUART et al., 1968; ROWLEY et al., 1973), the active mechanism may be more closely related to the phenomenon of immunologic tolerance than to suppressor activity of the antibody.

4. Immunologic Tolerance

This term refers to the state of specific nonreactivity (formely: immunologic paralysis) of immunocompetent cells to a given antigen as a result of previous exposure to the same antigen. The term "acquired tolerance" is preferred when immunologic tolerance is induced by application of either very small or very large doses of antigen. This state of "immunologic unresponsiveness" apparently persists only as long as the antigen is present (HOPE, 1971). The possibility of rendering an antigen nonmetabolizable is largely unexplored (LYLE and PARKER, 1974). Nonmetabolizable antigens apparently keep cells in a chronic state of antigen excess without the necessity of maintaining high concentration of circulating antigen to induce immunologic tolerance. Poly-D-amino acids are poorly immunogenic presumably because they are poorly metabolized (GILL et al., 1963). Recent investigations failed to support the concept that tolerance may be induced at two separate dosage thresholds of antigen, i.e., the "low zone (dose) tolerance" and "high zone (dose) tolerance" (BELL and SHAND, 1973). In recent attempts to achieve "low dose tolerance" in the adult, immunosuppressive agents (see Chapter H V 1) and antigen were administered simultaneously (BRENT et al., 1974). A state of immunologic tolerance induced by passive transfer of lymphoid cells obtained from a tolerant donor into an unprimed (usually irradiated) recipient (UPHOFF, 1969; MCCULLAGH, 1973) is termed "adoptive tolerance". A "tolerogen" is an antigen capable of including immunologic tolerance.

New approaches to specific immunosuppression turned to the use of antigens as pharmacologic agents in the above mentioned sense. Injection of very small amounts of antigens during the neonatal period classically tends to result in the induction of immunologic tolerance. In the adult animal either repeated subimmunogenic doses of antigen or a single but excessively high dose of antigen are necessary to induce a long-lasting state of immunologic unresponsiveness (Batshon et al., 1963; Sercarz and Coons, 1963; Mitchison, 1964). The mechanisms which lead to acquired tolerance are not known. They may include the specific destruction of a line of cells (Bell, 1973) in combination with complement (Azar et al., 1968), the modified ability to recognize "self" and "nonself" (Uphoff, 1969), the activation of "repressor" cells (McCullach, 1973), and the reversible inhibition of cellular functions (Katz et al., 1972) particularly the production of high affinity antibody, whereas passive antibody (see Chapter HV 3) predominantly suppresses the synthesis of low affinity antibody (Siskind, 1974). Like immunosuppressive antibodies, antigens are most effective in the suppression of humoral antibody responses, rather than cell-mediated reactions. The reported effect of administering alloantigen extracts to recipients of tumor-, kidney-, and skin allografts are contradictory, ranging from accelerated rejection (Graff and Nathenson, 1971) to prolonged survival (Koene et al., 1971; Von Haefen et al., 1973). Bonavida and Zighelboim (1974) emphasized that the alloantigen must be soluble to induce suppression of cell-mediated immunity, and evidence was presented that serum factors from tolerant animals that block lymphocyte-mediated immunity in vitro are soluble antigen-antibody complexes (Wright et al., 1973). Salfner et al. (1974) focused attention on the possibility of isolating, of characterizing and of solubilizing human histocompatibility antigens from platelets to avoid concomitant extraction of nucleic acids, which makes further preparation of transplantation antigens from nucleated cells difficult. The greatest difficulty appears to be the necessity for pretreatment of the recipient with donor-specific tissue extract—a procedure that cannot be applied to human recipients of cadaveric kidneys, unless a "cocktail" of the most common HL-A antigens proves to be efficacious (Brent et al., 1974).

5. Specific Immunologic Unresponsiveness

Whereas a nonspecific unresponsiveness to many antigens is a generalized immunologic unresponsiveness, e.g., as a result of therapy with an immunosuppressive agent, or as encountered in immunologic deficiency states, in new approaches to immunosuppression the eradication of a particular group of specific antigen-sensitive cells is attempted. The antigen "suicide" technique (Basten et al., 1971) is an attractive approach to the production of specific immunologic unresponsiveness. The principle of this idea is to render the antigen cytotoxic which would damage the specific antigen-sensitive cell upon attachment to the cell membrane, thus preventing the proliferation of potential immunoreactive clones. Two largely unexplored techniques merit careful attention. The first profits from the ability of antigens to incorporate a radiolabel of high specific activity. Radioactive H antigen (flagellin) was shown to kill selectively antigen-sensitive cells in vitro (Ada and Byrt, 1969) and T- and B-cells were specifically inactivated by incorporation of ^{125}I-labeled fowl gamma globulin (Basten et al., 1971). Lyle and Parker (1974) questioned whether immunologic unresponsiveness could be obtained by administering highly radioactive antigens in vivo, since the information available indicates that sensitized T-cells are relatively radioresistant and high levels of radioactivity are needed to kill antigen-sensitive cells *in vitro*. Furthermore, nonspecific immunosuppression may result in addition (WEBBER, 1967). In the second technical approach the antigen is combined with toxins, e.g., diphtheria toxin (MOOLTEN and COOPERBAND, 1970), or chlorambucil (GHOSE *et al.*, 1972). Since this method requires an extremely toxic molecule, the use of antigens conjugated with an enzyme with a high turnover number and the capacity to generate a potent toxic product was advocated (PARKER, 1973). LYLE and PARKER (1974) concluded from their experiments with glucose oxidase and galactose oxidase protein-antigen conjugates that the concept of "affinity cytotoxicity" may be applicable for the induction of immunologic unresponsiveness *in vivo*. However, it remains an open question whether or not the eradicated group of specific antigen-sensitive cells may regenerate from undifferentiated bone marrow cells through processing by the thymus.

6. Attempts to Render the Graft Nonantigenic

Approaches to the modification of the immune response by reducing the immunogenicity of the graft partly parallels the procedures for the induction of immunologic enhancement. Recently, in place of specific antibody a variety of substances was investigated which may be able to mask the histocompatibility antigens upon either specific or unspecific binding. Acid mucopolysaccharides (LIPPMANN, 1968) and ribonucleic acid (LEMPERLE, 1968) were found to reduce the immunogenicity of grafts, and histocompatibility antigens on suspended lymphoid cells, while kidney allografts could be masked by phytomitogens (RAY and SIMMONS, 1973; SIMMONS and TOLEDO-PEREYRA, 1974). Protection from hyperacute rejection and prolonged survival of renal allografts resulted from pretreatment with the Fab fragments of antibodies directed against the histocompatibility antigens (STUART *et al.*, 1968; SUTHERLAND *et al.*, 1973). TOLEDO–PEREYRA *et al.* (1974c) explained a distinct increase in survival time of canine orthotopic small-intestinal allografts preserved for 24 hours by hypothermic perfusion with human plasmanate with the unspecific masking of the canine tissue antigens by heterospecific binding (noncytotoxic) NOHA's. So far, these attempts to reduce the antigenicity of grafts have not led to indefinite survival, probably because cells shed the masking substance during the normal physiologic turnover of their histocompatibility antigens. CALNE (1967) focused attention on the considerable literature, reviewed by MAY (1959), testifying that fetal tissues are often less antigenic. Puppy kidneys grafted into adult dogs survived longer than transplants from mature animals (CALMAN *et al.*, 1963), and pancreatic islands derived from rat embryos appear to be particularly suitable for transplantation (BROWN *et al.*, 1974). Perhaps, the culturing of organs may become a method of reducing the antigenicity of a graft. Some immunologists have suggested that cultured cells differentiate into an immunologically more primitive, embryonic state in which they are unable to produce those proteins, sugars, or other substances (histocompatibility antigens?) that might be recognized as foreign by the future host (MAUGH, 1973). In this context, we refer again to findings according to which certain types of animals and human tissues permanently lose their ability to provoke an immune response in a new host after growth in tissue culture for a critical period of time prior to transplantation (SUMMERLIN *et al.*, 1970, 1973) (see also Chapter H III 3).

VI. Xenotransplantation

In summary, the transplantation of organs has led to the prolongation of useful life in many cases. We are convinced that by further advances in basic research directed at clinical application the replacement of organs will be facilitated convincingly. First, advantages in organ preservation and storage will allow the application of refined techniques of histocompatibility typing, and the modification of the antigenicity of the graft as well as the ability of the host to respond to possibly remaining antigenic structures of the transplants. Artificial organs will be available to bridge the time between an acute emergency and the transplantation of the heart, lung, and liver. The transplantation of the pancreas may be replaced by the inoculation of nonimmunogenic pancreatic islands. Although the realization of approaches to render a graft completely nonimmunogenic, or to highly selectively suppress the host's immune response remain problems for the future, the time does not seem to lie too far ahead, when the transplantation of xenogeneic organs could become a routine procedure, if it can be shown that the life expectancy of those organs is comparable to human organs. Among other advantages, e.g., availability of organs of best quality at every time, xenotransplantation evades an important implication of organ transplantation: the ethical problem (GRÜNDEL, 1969), although it introduces another one: will anybody be disposed to live with a heart of a pig or a chimpanzee?

VII. Abbreviations and Definitions

AG-AB complex
   Antigen-antibody complex (*see* antibody).

Ag-B locus
   Part of the histocompatibility system in the rat.

ALS
   Antilymphocyte serum.

Antibody
   Immunoambocepter, originally defined a body or substance evoked by an antigen; but it is now generally accepted that antibodies may also exist naturally without being the result of an antigenic stimulus (naturally occurring antibody). Antibody reacts specifically with the antigen, but cross reactions (allo-, heterospecific) are possible. Antibodies belong to one or other of the classes of globulins (immunoglobulins, Ig) and consist of at least two pairs of polypeptide chains. The two heavy chains (H) are linked to each other and to the light chains

(L), by disulfide bonds. The different classes, e.g., IgG or γG (7S), IgM or γM (19S), IgA or γA, are recognized on the basis of particular structural and antigenic characteristics of their heavy chains. Subclasses of IgG have been well defined on the basis of differences in their heavy chains and are referred as to IgG 1, IgG 2, IgG 3, IgG 4. A similar nomenclature is used for IgG subclasses in other species, e.g., in the mouse IgG 1, IgG 2a, and IgG 2b. When antibody is treated with papain, it splits into three parts. One fragment has two halves of heavy chains still linked by disulfide bonds and is crystallizable. This crystallizable fragment (Fc) is immunologically inactive but can be bound to receptors at the surface of various cells. The other two parts each contain half of a heavy chain (Fd fragment), and a complete light chain and include the combining site of the antibody (Fab fragment). The bivalence of the intact antibody permits the formation of a framework (aggregate, complex) with antibody and antigen alternating in the structure. These aggregates also activate the complement system.

anti-A
Antibody against the A antigen of the blood group system.

anti-B
Antibody against the B antigen of the blood group system.

anti-D
Antibody against the D antigen of the Rhesus blood group system.

ATG
Antithymocyte globulin.

ATPase
Adenosine triphosphatase.

ATS
Antithymocyte serum.

B-cells, B-lymphocytes, B-type
Bone marrow-derived (bursa-dependent) lymphocytes which are not processed by the thymus.

β 1 C
Serum globulin with activity of the C 3 component of the complement system.

C 1
The first of the complement components which reacts directly with the antigen-modified antibody. It is made up of three subunits (C 1g, C 1r, and C 1s). After activation through binding at AG:AB complexes an active esterase (C'1 esterase, C $\overline{1}$ esterase) is released. This esterase activates the complement components C 2 and C 4.

C 3
The third component is quantitatively dominant in the complement group. One of the fragments which is cleared by the tryptic convertase activity of the C 4, 2, 3 complex may be active in the hemolytic sequence, another fragment

(C 3a) has anaphylotoxin activity and is probably also a neutrophil cytotoxin. C 3 is also known as β 1 C globulin.

C 5–9
Further components of the complement system.

Cobra venom
Two macromolecular factors of the venom of the Indian cobra *Naja naja* have anticomplementary activity.

Co F
Substance of known anticomplementary activity. Several antisera and antigens initiate the complement cascade reaction, i.e., fix complement, in the absence of any specific union of antibody with antigen.

DMSO
Dimethylsulphoxide.

DNA
Desoxyribonucleic acid.

DL-A
see histocompatibility antigens.

Fc receptor
Receptors at the surface of cells (B-cells, macrophages) able to bind the electrophoretically mobile anodal immunoglobulin fragment Fc (*see* antibody).

GBM
Glomerular basement membrane.

GVH
Graft-versus-host reaction. Reaction of immunologically competent cells accompanying a graft against the tissues of a genetically nonidentical recipient. A GVH reaction is particularly stimulated when the number of accompanying T-cells is large and the recipient's defense system is deficient.

H antigens
Antigens of the flagella of mobile gram-negative enterobacteria, such as the *Salmonella* group.

H-2 histocompatibility antigens
Isoantigens at the surface of cells of mice (*see* histocompatibility antigens).

Histocompatibility antigens (major histocompatibility locus)
A group of isoantigens (transplantation antigens) at the surface of cells of mammalian species termed H-2 (murine), DL-A (dog), HL-A (human), RhL-A (Rhesus monkey). The histocompatibility antigens are genetically controlled. All species appear to have at least two SD loci and one LD locus, and in those species in which Ir genes have been defined, at least some of the Ir systems appear to be linked with the major histocompatibility locus.

HL-A

see histocompatibility antigens.

IgA

Immunoglobulin of the external secretions. A dimer (11S) consisting of a 7S molecule and a secretory (transport) piece (*see* antibody).

IgG

The major circulating immunoglobulin in most species. Sedimentation coefficient of about 7S (*see* antibody).

IgM

High molecular weight immunoglobulin (sedimentation coefficient of about 19S). Phylogenetically the most primitive antibody. Cyclic pentamer of 5 basic units of heavy and light chains (*see* antibody). The monomeric form has a sedimentation coefficient of 7-8S.

Ir (immune response) genes

A group of genes controlling the ability of an individual to react by antibody formation.

LCF

Lymphocyte cytotoxin factor. Term occasionally used for lymphotoxin (LT).

LD

Lymphocyte-defined.

LT

Lymphotoxin (*see* LCF).

MIF

Migration inhibition factor derived from primed lymphocytes. The factor inhibits the migration of macrophages out of capillary tubes *in vitro*.

M-IgG

Immunoglobulin G bound to the cell membrane particularly of B-lymphocytes.

MLC

Mixed lymphocyte culture. In the MLC test small T-cells transform into blast cells when equal numbers of lymphocytes from genetically different donors are cultured together for about 5 days.

MLR

Mixed lymphocyte reaction.

MN cells

Mononuclear cells. Collective name for mobile circulating cells, their ancestors, and successors exhibiting but one, mostly round shaped nucleus. This term excludes polymorphonuclear cells.

MST

Mean survival time.

NaF
   Sodium fluoride.

Na⁺/K⁺

Na^+/K^+
   Related to sodium and potassium. Used in combination with ATPase. The Na^+/K^+-ATPase is the major enzyme responsible for the maintenance of the intra- and extracellular ion gradient.

NOHA
   Abbreviation for naturally occurring hetero- or allospecific antibody, respectively. Naturally occurring antibody (anti A, anti B) reacts with the isoantigens B and A of the blood group system. Hetero- and allospecific (preformed) antibodies produced by previous sensitization against antigens, having the specifity for a different species (probably also for germs) and which can cross react with histocompatibility and tissue-specific antigens (*see* antibody).

nu/nu mice
   Inbred strain of congenitally athymic, and hairless (nude) mice. These mice largely lack immunocompetent T-cells.

PAS
   Periodic acid Schiff reagent. For the demonstration of polysaccharides and their conjugates, e.g., glycogen, glycoproteins, and mucopolysaccharides.

PHA
   Phytohemagglutinin. Lectin extracted from *Phaseolus vulgaris* or *P. communis* (beans). PHA unspecifically stimulates the transformation of T-lymphocytes into blast cells, The term derives from the ability to agglutinate certain red blood cells.

PMN cells
   Polymorphonuclear cells, neutrophilic granulocytes.

PVG/C
   An inbred strain of rats originally deriving from the Glaxo laboratories (USA). In 1947 they were imported to Compten, Berks. (UK), and from there (1955) to the central animal laboratory of the University of Nijmegen.

RER
   Rough endoplasmic reticulum.

RES
   Reticuloendothelial system.

Rh
   Rhesus, *see* anti D.

RhL-A
   see histocompatibility antigens.

RNA
   Ribonucleic acid.

SD
Serologically defined.

SER
Smooth endoplasmic reticulum.

7 S IgM
see IgM.

SRBC
Sheep red blood cells.

T-cells, T-lymphocytes, T-type
Thymus-derived lymphocytes. Characterized by specific antigens at the cell surface.

TL antigen
Thymus and leukemia antigen. A particular antigen of thymocytes of the outer thymic cortex and also of circulating cells of several murine leukemias. TL antigen carrying cells are cortisone-sensitive.

Wistar rats
A strain of rats, originating from the Glaxo laboratories (USA). Originally inbred, recently mostly kept in "closed colonies" in various laboratories. Rats from the TNO Laboratory Zeist (The Netherlands) can reject skin from donors of the same strain, but only occasionally the liver and kidney.

Acknowledgements

The authors would like to acknowledge the financial support of the ICRP/MII program of the Netherlands and of the World Health Organization for supplemental studies on elements of the cell-mediated immune reaction. We are also indepted to Prof. Dr. S. BENGMARK (Lund), Dr. R. BILSKI (Nijmegen), Dr. R. V. HEE (Nijmegen), F. HESS (Nijmegen), Dr. M.N. V. D. HEYDE (Arnhem), Dr. S.W. SCHALM (Leiden), Prof. Dr. L. TERPSTRA (Leiden), Dr. M. THERMAN (Marburg), Dr. CH. WILDEVUUR (Groningen), and Dr. O. ZELDER (Marburg) who entrusted us with all of the biopsy and autopsy specimens of their experimental series.

We would also like to express our sincere gratitude to Dr. M. WEISS-OPPÉ for her assistance in preparing the English version of the manuscript, and to the collaborators of the laboratory of Cytology and Histology for technical aid, checking of references, and last but not least the onerous chore of typing.

References

ABLE, M.E., LEE, J.C., ROSENAU, W.: Lymphocyte-target cell interaction in vitro. Am. J. Pathol. **60**, 421–434 (1970).

ABOUNA, G.M., ANEMIYA, H., FISHER, L.M., ANDRES, G., PORTER, K.A.: Experience in hepatic support by intermittent multi-species liver perfusion. Eur. Surg. Res. **4**, 241–242 (1972).

ABSOLON, K.B., HAGIHARA, P.E., GRIFFEN JR., W.O., LILLEHEI, R.C.: Experimental and clinical heterotopic liver homotransplantation. Rev. Int. Hépat. **15**, 1481 -1490 (1965).

582   CHR.R. JERUSALEM and P.H.K. JAP: General Pathology of the Transplantation Reaction

ACOSTA, J.M., NARDI, G.L., REEVES, G., PINN, V., BUCETA, J.C., SOLOAGA, J.C.: Histopathologic changes in the allografted canine pancreas. Arch. Surg. **106**, 844–847 (1973).
ADA, G.I., BYRT, P.: Specific inactivation of antigen-reactive cells with ^{125}I-labelled antigen. Nature **222**, 1291–1292 (1969).
AKUTSU, T.: Artificial heart: Partial support and total replacement. In: Human organ support and replacement, HARDY, J.D. (ed.) pp. 384–414. Springfield: C.C. Thomas 1971.
ALEXANDER, P., EVANS, R.: Endotoxin and double stranded RNA render macrophages cytotoxic. Nature (New Biol.) **232**, 76–78 (1971).
ALICAN, F., HARDY, J.D., CAYIRLI, M., VARNER, J.E., MOYNIHAN, P.C., TURNER, M.D., ANAS, P.: Intestinal transplantation: Laboratory experience and report of a clinical case. Am. J. Surg. **121**, 150–159 (1971).
ALLISON, A.C.: Immunity and immunopathology in virus infections. Ann. Inst. Pasteur (Paris) **123**, 585–608 (1972).
AMOS, H.E., GURNER, B.W., OLDS, R.J., COOMBS, R.R.A.: Passive sensitization of tissue cells. II. Ability of cytophilic antibody to render the migration of guinea pig peritoneal exudate cells inhibitable by antigen. Int. Arch. Allergy Appl. Immunol. **32**, 496–505 (1967).
ANDERSON, W.R., CROSSON, J.T., HAGLIN, J.J.: Light microscopic and ultrastructural characteristics of rejected baboon lung allografts. In: Morphology in lung transplantation, WILDEVUUR, CH.R.H., JERUSALEM, C.R., LAUWERIJNS, J.M., WILDEVUUR-VAN HAMERSVELD, C. (eds.) pp. 27–36. Basel: Karger 1973.
ANDERSSON, L.C., HÄYRY, P.: Specific priming of mouse thymus-dependent lymphocytes to allogeneic cells in vitro. Eur. J. Immunol. **3**, 595–599 (1973).
ANDERSSON, L.C., NORDLING, S., HÄYRY, P.: Allograft immunity in vitro. IV. Autonomy of T-lymphocytes in target cell destruction. Scand. J. Immunol. **2**, 107–113 (1973).
ANDRES, G.A., ACCINNI, L., HSU, K.C., PENN, I., PORTER, K.A., RENDALL, J.M., SEEGAL, B.C., STARZL, T.E.: Human renal transplants. III. Immunopathologic studies. Lab. Invest. **22**, 588–604 (1970).
ANDRES, G.A., ANSELL, I.D., HALGRIMSON, C.G., HSU, K.C., PORTER, K.A., STARZL, T.E., ACCINNI, L., CALNE, R.Y., HERBERTSON, B.M., PENN, I., RENDALL, J.M., WILLIAMS, R.: Immunopathological studies of orthotopic human liver allografts. Lancet **1**, 275–280 (1972).
ARCHER, G.T.: Phagocytosis by human monocytes in red cells coated with Rh antibodies. Vox Sang. **10**, 590–598 (1965).
ARCHER, O.K., PIERCE, J.C.: Role of thymus in the development of the immune response. Fed. Proc. **20**, 26 (1961).
ARIYAN, S., GERSHON, R.K.: Augmentation of the adoptive transfer of specific tumor immunity by non-specifically immunized macrophages. J. Natl. Cancer Inst. **51**, 1145–1148 (1973).
ASKONAS, B.A., HUMPHREY, J.H.: Formation of antibody by isolated perfused lungs of immunized rabbits. The use of ^{14}C amino acids to study the dynamics of antibody secretion. Biochem. J. **70**, 212–222 (1958).
AX, W., MALCHOW, H., ZEISS, I., FISHER, H.: The behaviour of lymphocytes in the process of target cell destruction in vitro. Exp. Cell. Res. **53**, 108–116 (1968).
AZAR, M.M., YUNIS, E.J., PICKERING, P.J., GOOD, R.A.: On nature of immunological tolerance. Lancet **1**, 1279–1281 (1968).
BACH, J.F., AMOS, D.B.: Hu-1: Major histocompatibility locus in man. Science **156**, 1506–1508 (1967).
BACH, J.F., DARDENNE, M.: The metabolism of azathioprine in renal failure. Transplantation **12**, 253–259 (1971).
BACH, F.H., BACH, M.L., KLEIN, J.: Genetic and immunological complexity of major histocompatibility regions. Science **176**, 1024–1027 (1972).
BAKER, P.J., BARTH, R.F., STASHAK, P.W., AMBAUGH, D.F.: Enhancement of the antibody response of type III pneumococcal polysaccharide in mice treated with antilymphocyte serum. J. Immunol. **104**, 1313–1315 (1970).
BALDWIN, R.W., PRICE, M.R., ROBINS, R.A.: Blocking of lymphocyte-mediated cytotoxicity for rat hepatoma cells by tumor-specific antigen-antibody complexes. Nature **238**, 185–187 (1972).
BALFOUR, I.C., EVANS, C.A., MIDDLETON, V.I., PEGRUM, G.D.: Observations on the cytotoxicity of lymphocytes to a target cell system. Clin. exp. Immunol. **10**, 67–75 (1972).

BALNER, H., D'AMARO, J., TOTH, E.K., DERSJANT, H., VREESWIJK VAN, W.: The histocompatibility complex of rhesus monkeys. Relation between RhL and the main locus controlling reactivity in mixed lymphocyte cultures. Transpl. Proc. **5**, 323–329 (1973).

BARKER, C.F., BILLINGHAM, R.E.: The role of regional lymphatics in the skin homograft response. Transplantation **5**, 962–966 (1967).

BARNES, B.A., FLAX, M.H., BURKS, J.F., BARR, G.: Experimental pulmonary homografts in the dog. I. Morphologic studies. Transplantation **1**, 351–364 (1963).

BARNETT, W.O., TRUETT, G., STONE, J.: Experimental small bowel homografts. Am. J. Dig. Dis. **7**, 833–838 (1962).

BASTEN, A., MILLER, J.F.A.P., WARNER, N.L., PYE, J.: Specific inactivation of thymus-derived (T) and non-thymus-derived (B) lymphocytes by ^{125}I-labelled antigen. Nature (New Biol.) **231**, 104–106 (1971).

BASTEN, A., WARNER, N.L., MANDEL, T.: A receptor for antibody on B-lymphocytes. II. Immuno-chemical and electronmicroscopic characteristics. J. Exp. Med. **135**, 627–642 (1972).

BATSHON, B.A., BAER, H., SHAFFER, M.F.: Immunologic paralysis produced in mice by *Klebsiella pneumoniae* type 2 polysaccharide. J. Immunol. **90**, 121–126 (1963).

BAXBY, K., TAYLOR, R.M.R., SWINNEY, J.: Ischaemic-times and kidney transplants. Lancet **1**, 984 (1974a).

BAXBY, K., ANDERSON, H., TAYLOR, R.M.R., JOHNSON, R.W.G., SWINNEY, J.: Assessment of cadaver kidneys by perfusion. In: Abstracts of the 5th International Congress of the Transplantation Society, Jerusalem, 1974, pp. 172.

BEAUDOIN, J.G., SLAPAK, M., PHILLIPS, M.J., CHANDRASEKARAN, A.K., McLEAN, L.D.: Function of auxiliary liver allografts. Surg. Gynecol. Obstet. **130**, 622–635 (1970).

BEAUMONT, J.L., LEMORT, N.: Les immunoglobulines anti-héparine; un facteur de thromboses, d'hyperlipidémies et d'athérosclerose. Path.Biol. **22**, 67–76 (1974).

BECKER, N.H., SINHA, S.B.P., HAGSTROM, J.W.C., BLÜMCKE, S., VEITH, F.J.: Fine structure alterations in canine lung transplantation. J. Thorac. Cardiovasc. Surg. **63**, 81–93 (1972).

BELL, E.B.: Cellular events in protein tolerant inbred rats: II. Antibody activity maturation during induction and loss of tolerance. Eur. J. Immunol. **3**, 267–272 (1973).

BELL, E.B., SHAND, F.L.: Cellular events in protein tolerant inbred rats. I. The fate of thoracic duct lymphocytes and memory cells during tolerance induction to human serum albumin. Eur. J. Immunol. **3**, 259–267 (1973).

BELZER, F.O.: Renal preservation. N. Engl. J. Med. **291**, 402–404 (1974).

BELZER, F.O., ASHBY, B.S., DUNPHY, J.E.: Twenty-four and 72 hour preservation of canine kidneys. Lancet **2**, 536–568 (1967).

BELZER, F.O., ASHBY, B.S., HUANG, J.S., DUNPHY, J.E.: Etiology of rising perfusion pressure in isolated organ perfusion. Ann. Surg. **168**, 382–391 (1968).

BENACERRAF, B., McDEVITT, H.O.: Histocompatibility-linked immune response genes. Science **175**, 273–279 (1972).

BENJAMIN, J.L., DICKSON, L.G., SELL, K.W.: Ultrastructural degeneration and hypothermic function of in vitro perfused kidneys. In: Abstracts of the 5th International Congress of the Transplantation Society, Jerusalem, 1974, pp. 172.

BENNETT, B.: Specific suppression of tumor growths by isolated peritoneal macrophages from immunized mice. J. Immunol. **95**, 656–664 (1965).

BENOIT, F.L., RULON, D.B., THEIL, G.B., DOOLAN, P.D., WATTAN, R.H.: Goodpasture's syndrome. A clinicopathologic entity. Am. J. Med. **37**, 424–444 (1964).

BERKEN, A., BENACERRAF, B.: Properties of antibodies cytophilic for macrophages. J. Exp. Med. **123**, 119–144 (1966).

BESSIS, M.: Living blood cells and their ultrastructure. Berlin-Heidelberg-New York: Springer 1973.

BIBERFELD, P., PERLMANN, P.: Morphologic observations on the cytotoxicity of human lymphocytes for antibody—coated chicken erythrocytes. Exp. Cell. Res. **62**, 433–440 (1970).

BIBERFELD, P., HOLM, G., PERLMANN, P.: Morphological observations on lymphocyte peripolesis and cytotoxic action in vitro. Exp. Cell. Res. **52**, 672–677 (1968).

BIEBER, CH.P., STINSON, E.B., SHUMWAY, N.E.: Pathology of the conduction system in cardiac rejection. Circulation **39**, 567–575 (1969).

BIEBER, CH.P., STINSON, E.B., SHUMWAY, N.E., ROSE, R., KOSEK, J.: Cardiac transplantation in man. VII. Cardiac allograft pathology. Circulation **41**, 753–772 (1970).

Bierring, F.: Quantitative investigations on the lymphomyeloid system in thymectomized rats. In: Ciba Foundation Symposium on Haemopoiesis: Cell production and its regulation, Wolsten-holme, G.E., O'Conner, M. (eds.) pp. 185–203. London: Churchill 1960.

Bignon, J., Chahinian, P., Feldmann, G., Sapin, C.: Ultrastructural immunoperoxidase demonstrating of autologous albumin in the alveolar capillary membrane and the alveolar lining material in normal rats. J. Cell. Biol. 64, 503–509 (1975).

Billingham, R.E., Brent, L., Mitchinson, A.: The route of immunization immunity. Br. J. Exp. Path. 38, 467–472 (1957).

Billingham, R.E., Brent, L., Brown, J.B., Medawar, P.B.: Time of onset and duration of transplantation immunity. Transpl. Bull. 6, 410–414 (1959).

Billingham, R.E., Silvers, W.K., Wilson, D.B.: Adoptive transfer of transplantation immunity by means of blood-borne cells. Lancet 1, 512–515 (1962).

Bilski, R., Jerusalem, C.: Histochemische und elektronenmikroskopische Untersuchungen an Hauttransplantaten. In: Organtransplantation. Immunologie und Klinik, Heymer, A., Ricken, D. (eds.) pp. 103–112. Stuttgart-New York: Schattauer 1969.

Biro, C.E.: The role of the sixth component of complement in some types of hypersensitivity. Immunology 10, 563–565 (1966).

Björklund, B., Björklund, V., Lindström, R., Eklund, G., Nilsson, L., Grönneberg, R.: Cytokinetics of the destruction of HEp-2 in vitro by lymphoid cells from subjects immunized with HeLa antigen and demonstration of a mechanism for biologic amplification of certain lymphoid cells by phase contrast, time-lapse cinemicrography, and scanning electron microscopy. J. Reticuloendothel. Soc. 11, 29–59 (1972).

Bleyl, U.: Arteriosklerose und Fibrininkorporation. Untersuchungen zur Pathogenese der Aortensklerose. Berlin-Heidelberg-New York: Springer 1969.

Bloom, B.R., Bennet, B.: Mechanism of a reaction in vitro associated with delayed-type hypersensitivity. Science 153, 80–82 (1966).

Bloom, B.R., Chase, M.W.: Transfer of delayed-type hypersensitivity. A critical review and experimental study in the guinea pig. Prog. Allergy 10, 151–245 (1967).

Bloom, B.R., Hamilton, L.D., Chase, M.W.: Effects of mitomycin C on the cellular transfer of delayed-type hypersensitivity in the guinea pig. Nature 201, 689–691 (1964).

Blümcke, S., Becker, N.H., Sinha, S., Veith, F.J.: Electron microscopic studies of canine lung transplants. In: Morphology in lung transplantation, Wildevuur, Ch.R.H., Jerusalem, C.R., Lauwerijns, J.M., Wildevuur-Van Hamsersveld, C. (eds.) pp. 64–71. Basel: Karger 1973.

Bogardus, G.M., Schlosser, R.J.: The influence of temperature upon ischemic renal damage. Surgery 39, 970–974 (1956).

Bohle, A.: Über die pathologische Anatomie der Nierentransplantation. Langenbecks Arch. Chir. 322, 87–93 (1968).

Bohle, A.: Zur Pathomorphologie der akuten, perakuten und chronischen Abstoßung von Nierentransplantaten. Verh. Dtsch. Ges. Pathol. 54, 136–145 (1970).

Bohle, A., Hinrichsen, K.: Morphologischer Beitrag zur sog. Transplantatadaption. Klin. Wochenschr. 47, 74–77 (1966).

Bonavida, B., Zighelboim, J.: Modulation of the immune response toward allografts in vivo. I. Selective suppression of the development of cell-mediated immunity by soluble alloantigens. Cell. Immunol. 13, 52–65 (1974).

Bono de, A.H.B.: Problems of lung transplantation. Br. J. Surg. 53, 993 (1966).

Bos, W.H.: Recirculatie en transformatie van lymphocyten. Thesis. Groningen, The Netherlands 1967.

Boyden, S.V.: Cytophilic antibody in guinea-pigs with delayed-type hypersensitivity. Immunology 8, 474–483 (1964).

Boyden, S.V., Sorkin, E.: The absorption of antibody and antigen by spleen cells in vitro–some further experiments. Immunology 4, 244–252 (1961).

Boxel van, J.A., Stobo, J.D., Paul, W.E., Green, I.: Antibody-dependent lymphoid cell-mediated cytotoxicity no requirement for thymus-derived lymphocytes. Science 175, 194–196 (1972).

Brandtzaeg, P.: Structure, synthesis and external transfer of mucosal immunoglobulins. Ann. Immunol. (Paris) 124, 417–438 (1973).

Bravo, J.F., Herman, J.H., Smyth, C.J.: Musculoskeletal disorders after renal homotransplantation. A clinical and laboratory analysis of 60 cases. Ann. Intern. Med. 66, 87–104 (1967).

BREDA VAN-VRIESMAN, P.J.C., FELDMAN, J.D.: γM alloantibody elicited by first set renal allografts in vivo and in vitro studies. J. Immunol. **108**, 1188–1198 (1972).

BRENT, L., KILSHAW, P.L., PINTO, M.: Induction of specific unresponsiveness with tissue extracts and antilymphocytic serum. In: Liver transplantation, LIE, T.S., GÜTGEMANN, A. (eds.), pp. 241–247. Baden-Baden: Witzstrock 1974.

BRETSCHER, P.A., COHN, M.: A theory of self-nonself discrimination. Science **169**, 1042–1049 (1970).

BRITTON, S., MÖLLER, G.: Regulation of antibody synthesis against Escherichia coli endotoxin. I. Suppressive effect of endogenously produced and passively transferred antibodies. J. Immunol. **100**, 1326–1334 (1968).

BRODER, I.: Mechanism of histamine release from guinea-pig lung by soluble immune complexes. II. Role of anaphylatoxin. Immunology **26**, 125–135 (1974).

BROEK VAN DEN, A.A.: Immune suppression and histophysiology of the immune response. Thesis, Groningen, The Netherlands 1971.

BROWN, A.H., NILES, N.R., BRAIMBRIDGE, M.V., AUSTEN, W.G.: Preservation of the myocardium by means of cold physiological solutions, as assessed by ventricular function, histochemistry and birefringence. J. Surg. Res. **14**, 46–57 (1973).

BROWN, J., MOLNAR, J.G., CLARL, W., MULLEN, Y.: Control of experimental diabetes mellitus in rats by transplantation of fetal pancreases. Science **184**, 1377–1379 (1974).

BRÜCHER, H., GRÄBER, M., KIETZMANN, E.: Kurze wissenschaftliche Mitteilungen. Klin. Wochenschr. **3**, 161–162 (1969).

BRUNIUS, V., BERGETZ, B.E., EKMAN, H., GELIN, L.E., WESTBERG, G.: The cadaveric kidney in clinical transplantations. Scand. J. Urol. Nephrol. **2**, 15–23 (1968).

BURGER, D.R., HU, F., PASZTOR, L.M., MALLEY, A.: A model for immunity to melanomas in mice. Proc. Soc. Exp. Biol. Med. **144**, 426–430 (1973).

BURNELL, J.M., THOMAS, E.D., ANSELL, J.S., CROSS, H.E., DILLARD, D.H., EPSTEIN, R.B., ESHBACK, J.W., HOGAN, R., HUTCHINGS, R.H., MOTULSKY, A., ORMSBY, J.W., POTTENBARGER, P., SCHRIBNER, B.H., VOLWEILER, W.: Hepatic coma observations on cross-circulation in man. Am. J. Med. **38**, 832–841 (1965).

BURRELL, R., FLAHERTY, D.K., DENEE, P.B., ABRAHAM, J.L., GELDERMAN, A.H.: The effect of lung antibody on normal lung structure and function. Am. Rev. Resp. Dis. **109**, 106–113 (1974).

BUSCH, G.J., BRAUN, W.E., CARPENTER, C.B., CORSON, J.M., GALVANEK, E.R., REYNOLDS, E.S., MERRILL, J.P., DAMMIN, G.J.: Intravascular coagulation (IVC) in human renal allograft rejection. Transplant. Proc. **1**, 267–270 (1969).

BUSCH, G.J., REYNOLDS, E.S., GALVANEK, E.G., BRAUN, W.E., DAMMIN, G.J.: Human renal allograft. The role of vascular injury in early graft failure. Medicine (Baltimore) **50**, 29–81 (1971).

BYSTRYN, J.-C., SCHENKEIN, I., UHR, J.W.: A model for the regulation of antibody synthesis by serum antibody. In: Progress in immunology, AMOS, B. (ed.) pp. 627–636. New York: Academic Press 1971.

CALMAN, K.C., BELL, P.R.F.: Experimental organ preservation. Br. J. Surg. **59**, 758–764 (1972).

CALMAN, K.C., BELL, P.R.F.: The prediction of organ viability. Br. J. Surg. **60**, 322 (1973).

CALMAN, M., BALFOUR, J., FORBES, D.: Survival of homologous transplants of neonatal kidneys in dogs. Surg. Gynecol. Obstet. **116**, 227–231 (1963).

CALNE, R.Y.: Renal transplantation. Baltimore: The Williams and Wilkins Co. 1963.

CALNE, R.Y.: Renal transplantation, 2nd ed. London: Edward Arnold 1967.

CALNE, R.Y.: Observations on liver transplantation. In: Liver transplantation, LIE, T.S., GÜTGEMANN, A. (eds.) pp. 39–46. Baden-Baden: Witzstrock 1974.

CALNE, R.Y., SELLS, R.A., PENA, J.R., DAVIS, D.R., MILLARD, P.R., HERBERTSON, B.M., BINNS, R.M., DAVIES, D.A.L.: Induction of immunological tolerance by porcine liver allografts. Nature **223**, 472–476 (1969).

CAMERON, G.R.: Pulmonary oedema. Br. Med. J. **1**, 965–972 (1948).

CANNON, P.R., WALSH, T.E., MARSHALL, C.E.: Acute local anaphylactic inflammation of the lungs. Am. J. Pathol. **17**, 777–784 (1941).

CANTY, T.G., WUNDERLICH, J.R.: Quantitative in vitro assay of cytotoxic cellular immunity. J. Natl. Cancer Inst. **45**, 761–771 (1970).

CARPENTER, C.B., MERRILL, J.P.: Modification of renal allograft rejection in man. Arch. Intern. Med. **123**, 501–513 (1969).

CARPENTER, C.B., WINN, H.J.: Hyperacute rejection. N. Engl. J. Med. **280**, 47–48 (1969).

CARR, K., CARR, I.: How cells settle on glass: A study by light and scanning electron microscopy of some properties of normal and stimulated macrophages. Z. Zellforsch. Mikrosk. Anat. **105**, 234–241 (1970).

CASEY, A., SCOTT, G.: Experimental enhancement of malignancy in Brown-Pearce rabbit tumor. Proc. Soc. Exp. Biol. Med. **29**, 816–818 (1932).

CATE, C.C., BURRELL, R.: Lung antigen induced cell-mediated immune injury in chronic respiratory diseases. Am. Rev. Resp. Dis. **109**, 114–123 (1974).

CERILLI, J., JESSEPH, J.E., MILLER, A.C.: The significance of antivascular endothelium antibody in renal transplantation. Surg. Gynecol. Obstet. **135**, 246–252 (1972).

CEROTTINI, J.C., NORDIN, A.A., BRUNNER, K.T.: In vitro cytotoxic activity of thymus cells sensitized to alloantigens. Nature **227**, 72–73 (1970a).

CEROTTINI, J.C., NORDIN, A.A., BRUNNER, K.T.: Specific in vitro cytotoxicity of thymus-derived lymphocytes sensitized to alloantigens. Nature **228**, 1308–1309 (1970b).

CHASE, M.W.: The cellular transfer of cutaneous hypersensitivity to tuberculin. Proc. Soc. Exp. Biol. Med. **59**, 134–135 (1945).

CHATURVEDI, V.C., DAVIES, J.W., FLEWETT, T.H.: Separation and characterization of cardiac antigen proteins. Clin. Exp. Immunol. **15**, 613–622 (1973).

CHEERS, C., MILLER, J.F.A.P.: Cell-to-cell interaction in the immune response. Regulation of hapten-specific antibody classes by carrier priming. J. Exp. Med. **136**, 1661–1665 (1972).

CHRISTENSEN, B.C.: Repair in arterial tissue. A scanning electron microscopic (SEM) and light microscopic study on the endothelium of rabbit thoracic aorta following a single dilatation injury. Virchows Arch. (Pathol. Anat.) **360**, 93–106 (1973).

CLAMAN, H.N., CHAPERON, E.A.: Immunologic complementation between thymus and marrow cells–a model for the two-cell theory of immunocompetence. Transpl. Rev. **1**, 92–113 (1969).

CLAMAN, H.N., CHAPERON, E.A., TRIPLETT, R.F.: Thymus-marrow cell combinations. Synergism in antibody production. Proc. Soc. Exp. Biol. Med. **122**, 1167–1171 (1966).

CLAMAN, H.N., CHAPERON, E.A., SELNER, J.C.: Thymus-marrow immunocompetence III. The requirement for living thymus cells. Proc. Soc. Exp. Biol. Med. **127**, 462–466 (1968).

CLARK, J.M., WEISS, L.: An immunofluorescence study of the in vitro interaction between lymphoid cells and target cells. J. Immunol. **103**, 1006–1013 (1969).

CLARK, D.S., GEWURZ, H., GOOD, R.A., VARCO, R.L.: Complement fixation during homograft rejection. Surg. Forum **15**, 144–146 (1964).

CLARK, D.S., GEWURZ, H., VARCO, R.L.: Serologic studies on accelerated graft rejection. Fed. Proc. **24**, 621 (1965).

CLARK, D.S., FOKER, J.E., PICKERING, R., GOOD, R.A., VARCO, R.L.: Evidence for two platelet populations in xenograft rejection. Surg. Forum **17**, 264 (1966).

CLAWSON, C.C., COOPER, M.D., GOOD, R.A.: Lymphocyte fine structure in the bursa of Fabricius, the thymus and the germinal centres. Lab. Invest. **16**, 407–421 (1967).

COCHRANE, C.G.: Arthus reaction. In: The inflammatory process, ZWEIFACH, B.N., GRANT, L., McCLUSKEY, R.T. (eds.) pp. 613–648. New York: Academic Press 1965.

COCHRANE, C.G., MÜLLER-EBERHARD, H.J., AIKIN, B.S.: Depletion of plasma complement in vivo by a protein of cobra venom: its effect on various immunologic reactions. J. Immunol. **105**, 55–59 (1970).

COCHRUM, K.C., DAVIS, W.C., KOUNTZ, S.L., FUDENBERG, H.H.: Renal autograft rejection initiated by passive transfer of immune plasma. Transplant. Proc. **1**, 301–304 (1969).

COHEN, S., WARD, P.A., YOSHIDA, T, BUREK, C.L.: Biologic activity of extracts of delayed hypersensitivity skin reaction sites. Cell. Immunol. **9**, 363–376 (1973).

COHEN, J.M., YANG, S.S., LAW, L.W.: Abrogation of cell-mediated immunity by hyperimmune alloantiserum: mechanisms and correlation with allograft enhancement. Int. J. Cancer **13**, 463–477 (1974).

COLLINS, C.M., BRAVO-SHUGMAN, M., TERASAKI, P.I.: Kidney preservation for transportation, initial perfusion and 30 hours storage. Lancet **2**, 1219–1222 (1969).

COLLSTE, L.G.: Antilymphocyte globulin in experimental and clinical transplantation. Thesis, Stockholm, Sweden 1971.

CONE, R.E., FELDMANN, M., MARCHALONIS, J.J., NOSSAL, G.J.V.: Cytophilic properties of surface immunoglobulin of thymus-derived lymphocytes. Immunology **26**, 49–60 (1974).

COOLEY, D.A., LIOTTA, D., HALLMAN, G.L., BLOODWELL, R.D., LEACHMAN, R.D., MILAM, J.D.: Discussion: First human implantation of cardiac prosthesis for staged total replacement of the heart. Trans. Am. Soc. Artif. Intern. Organs **15**, 252–263 (1969).

COON, J., HUNTER, R.: Selective induction of delayed hypersensitivity by a lipid conjugated protein antigen which is localized in thymus dependent lymphoid tissue. J. Immunol. **110**, 183–190 (1973).

COOPER, M.D., PETERSON, R.A.D., GOOD, R.A.: Delineation of the thymic and bursal lymphoid systems in the chicken. Nature **205**, 143–146 (1965).

COOPER, M.D., RAYMOND, D.A., PETERSON, R.A.D., SOUTH, M.A., GOOD, R.A.: The functions of the thymus system and the bursa system in the chicken. J. Exp. Med. **123**, 75–102 (1966).

COOPER, M.D., PEREY, D.Y., GABRIELSEN, A.E., SUTHERLAND, D.E.R., McKNEALLY, M.F., GOOD, R.A.: Production of an antibody deficiency syndrome in rabbits by neonatal removal of organized interstinal lymphoid tissues. Int. Arch. Allergy Appl. Immunol.**33**, 65–88 (1968a).

COOPER, M.D., PEREY, D.Y., PETERSON, R.A.D., GABRIELSEN, A.E., GOOD, R.A.: The two component concept of the lymphoid system. In: Immunologic deficiency diseases in man, BERGSMA, D., GOOD, R.A. (eds.) pp. 7–10. New York: National Foundation Press 1968b.

COOPERBAND, S.R., BONDEVIK, H., SCHMID, K., MANNICK, J.A.: Transformation of human lymphocytes: Inhibition of homologous alpha globulins. Science **159**, 1243–1244 (1968).

COPELAND, J., KOSEK, J.C., HURLEY, E.J.: Early functional and ultrastructural recovery of canine cadaver hearts. Circulation (Supplement II) *XXXVII* and *XXXVIII*, 188–199 (1968).

COPELAND, J., JONES, M., SPRAGG, R., STINSON, E.: A successful method for preservation of canine hearts for 24 to 28 hours. Abstracts 4th International Congress of the Transplantation Society, San Francisco, California, p. 54, 1972.

COPELAND, J.G., JONES, M., SPRAGG, R., STINSON, E.B.: In vitro preservation of canine hearts for 24 to 28 hours followed by successful orthotopic transplantation. Ann. Surg. **178**, 687–692 (1973).

CORTESINI, U.R.: Discussion of a paper by Reemtsma, K., on renal heterotransplantation. In: Transplantation von Organen und Geweben, SEIFFERT, K.E., GEISENDORFER, R. (eds.) pp. 153–155. Stuttgart: Thieme 1967.

COTTRELL, T.S., LEVINE, O.R., SENIOR, R.M., WIENER, J., SPIRO, D., FISHMAN, A.P.: Electron microscopic alterations at the alveolar level in pulmonary edema. Circ. Res. **21**, 783–797 (1967).

COURTICE, F.C.: Lymph flow in the lungs. Br. Med. Bull. **19**, 76–79 (1963).

COURTICE, F.C., SIMMONDS, W.J.: Absorption from the lungs. J. Physiol. (London) **109**, 103–115 (1949).

CREMERS–VAN DIJCK, M.J.E.S.: Phosphatases in the kidney of normal and experimental rodents. Thesis, Nijmegen, The Netherlands 1973.

CULLUM, P.A., BEWICK, M., SHILKIN, K., TEE, D.F.M., AYLIFFE, P., HUTCHINSON, D.C.S., LAWS, J.W., MASON, S.A., LYNNE REID, HUGH, J.P., McARTHUR, A.M.: Distinction between infections and rejection in lungtransplantation. Brit. Med. J. **2**, 71–74 (1972).

DALLOCHIO, M., BAUDET, F.E., BEZIAN, J., BRICAUD, H., PAUTRIZEL, R., BROUSTET, P.: Les lésions artérielles d'un coeur humain de sujet jeune transplanté sur un sujet jeune. Arch. Mal. Coeur **63**, 935–950 (1970).

DAMESHEK, W.: "Immunoblasts" and "immunocytes". An attempt at a functional nomenclature. Blood **21**, 243–245 (1963).

DARCY, D.A.: A study of the plasma cell and lymphocyte reaction in rabbit tussue. Philos. Trans. R. Soc. Lond. (Biol. Sci.) **236**, 463–503 (1952).

DAUSSET, J., COLOMBANI, J.: Histocompatibility testing. In: Histocompatibility testing, DAUSSET, J., COLOMBANI, J. (eds.) Copenhagen: J. Munksgaard 1973.

DAVID, J.R.: Delayed hypersensitivity in vitro: Its mediation by cell-free substances formed by lymphoid cell-antigen interaction. Proc. Natl. Acad. Sci. U.S.A. **56**, 72–77 (1966).

DAVID, J.R.: Macrophage migration. Fed. Proc. **27**, 6–13 (1968).

DAVID, J.R., AL-ASKARI, S., LAWRENCE, H.S., THOMAS, L.: Delayed hypersensitivity: I. The specificity of inhibition of cell migration by antigens. J. Immunol. **93**, 264–273 (1964).

DAVIES, A.J.S.: The thymus and the cellular basis of immunity. Transplant. Rev. **1**, 43–91 (1969).

DEBAKEY, M.E., HALL, C.W., HELLUMS, J.D., O'BANNON, W., BOURLAND, H., FELDMAN, L., WIETING, D., CALVIN, S., SMITH, P., ANDERSON, S.: Orthotopic cardiac prosthesis preliminary experiments in animals with biventricular artifical heart. Cardiovasc. Res. Center Bull. **7**, 127 142 (1969).

Degiovanni, G., Lejeune, G.: Antibody response, measured by a plaque assay, compared to cellular response after skin allograft in mice. Eur. J. Immunol. **3**, 653–654 (1973).

Dempster, W.J.: Kidney homotransplantation. Br. J. Surg. **40**, 447–465 (1953).

Dempster, W.J.: A consideration of the cause of functional arrest of homotransplanted kidneys. Br. J. Urol. **27**, 66–86 (1955).

Dempster, W.J., Williams, M.A.: Cellular infiltration in homotransplanted kidneys. Br. Med. J. **1**, 18–23 (1963).

Dempster, W.J., Harrison, C.V., Shackman, R.: Rejection processes in human homotransplanted kidneys. Br. Med. J. **2**, 969–976 (1964).

Dennert, G., Lennox, E.: Cell interactions in humoral and cell-mediated immunity. Nature (New Biol.) **238**, 114–116 (1972).

Dermer, G.B.: The fixation of pulmonary surfactant for electron microscopy II. Transplant of surfactant through the air-blood barrier. J. Ultrastruc. Res. **31**, 229–246 (1970).

Diener, E., Nossal, G.J.V.: Phylogenetic studies on the immune response I. Localization of antigens and immune response in the toad, Bufo marinus. Immunology **10**, 535–542 (1966).

Dietzman, R.H., Rebeld, A.E., Graham, E.F.: Long-term functional success following freezing of canine kidneys. Surgery **74**, 181–189 (1973).

Dixon, F.J.: Mechanisms of immunologic injury. In: Immunobiology, Good, R.A., Fisher, D.W. (eds.) pp. 161–166. Stamford: Sinauer Associates, Inc. 1971 a.

Dixon, F.J.: Glomerulonephritis and immunopathology. In: Immunobiology, Good, R.A., Fisher, D.W. (eds.) pp. 167–173 Stamford: Sinauer Associates, Inc. 1971 b.

Donawick, W.J., Shaffer, C.F., Dodd, D.D., Buchanan, J.W., Fregin, G.F.: Cardiac and skin heterograft rejection: Suppression with antilymphocyte serum. Transplant. Proc. **3**, 551–553 (1971).

Doughty, R.A., Klinman, N.R.: Carrier independent T-cell helper effects in antigenic stimulation. J. Immunol. **111**, 1140–1146 (1973).

Dougherty, J.C., Siegelman, S.S., Sinha, S., Boley, S.J., Veith, F.J.: Mechanisms of lung allograft rejection in untreated dogs. In: Current topics in surgical research, Skinner, D.B., Ebert, P.A. (eds.) Vol. III, pp. 301–311. New York: Academic Press 1971.

Drews, J.A., Tierney, D.F., Benfield, J.R.: Effect of immunosuppression and lung transplantation upon surfactant. Surgery **76**, 80–87 (1974).

Drinker, C.K.: Pulmonary oedema and inflammation. Cambridge: Harvard University Press 1945.

Dubernard, J.M., Carpenter, C.B., Busch, G.J., Diethelm, A.G., Murray, J.E.: Rejection of canine renal allograft by passive transfer of sensitized serum. Surgery **64**, 752–760 (1968).

Dumonde, D.C., Wolstengroft, R.A., Panay, G.S., Matthew, M., Morley, J., Howson, W.T.: "Lymphokines": non-antibody mediators of cellular immunity generated by lymphocyte activation. Nature **224**, 38–42 (1969).

Dutton, R.W., Hunter, P.: The effects of mitogen-stimulated T-cells on the response of B-cell to antigen and the mechanism of T-cell stimulation of the B-cell response. In: Cellular selection and regulation in the immune response, Edelman, E.M. (ed.) Vol. XXIX, pp. 199–215. New York: Raven Press 1974.

Dutton, R.W., Falkoff, R., Hirst, J.A., Hoffmann, M., Kappler, J.W., Kettman, J.R., Leslie, J.R., Vann, D.: Is there evidence for a non-antigen specific diffusable chemical mediator from the thymus-derived cell in the initiation of the immune response? In: Progress in immunology, Amos, B. (ed.) pp. 355–368. New York: Academic Press 1971.

Duve de, J.T., Wattiaux, R., Wibo, M.: Effects of fat-soluble compounds on lysosomes in vitro. Biochem. Pharmacol. **9**, 97 116 (1962).

Edidin, M., Henney, C.S.: The effect of capping H-2 antigens on the susceptibility of target cells to humoral and T-cell-mediated lysis. Nature (New Biol.) **246**, 47–49 (1973).

Eiseman, B., Velasques, A.: Extracorporeal and auxiliary liver support. In: Human organ support and replacement, Hardy, J.D. (ed.) pp. 100–110. Springfield: C.C. Thomas 1971.

Ekpaha-Mensah, J.A., Kennedy, J.C.: New indicator of histocompatibility differences in vitro. Nature (New Biol.) **233**, 174–176 (1971).

Elfenbein, G.J., Green, I., Paul, W.E.: The allogeneic effect: increased affinity of serum antibody produced during a secondary response. Eur. J. Immunol. **3**, 640–644 (1973).

Elkins, W.L., Guttmann, R.D.: Pathogenesis of a local graft versus host reaction immunogenicity of circulating host leukocytes. Science **159**, 1250–1251 (1968).

ELLIS, R.J., LILLEHEI, C.W., ZABRISKIE, J.B.: Immunofluorescent studies in cardiac rejection. Rev. Surg. **27**, 376–377 (1970a).

ELLIS, R.J., LILLEHEI, C.W., ZABRISKIE, J.B.: The significance of heartbinding antibody in human cardiac rejection. Ann. Thorac. Surg. **10**, 432–442 (1970b).

ELLIS, B., MADGE, G., KOLHOTHAR, M., STILL, W.: Clinical and pathological findings in human cardiac rejection. Arch. Pathol. **92**, 58–66 (1971).

ELVES, M.W.: Migration of small lymphocytes from the skin to the regional lymph nodes. Nature **227**, 725–727 (1970).

ENDE, N.: Course of transplanted cadaver donor kidneys with previously existing pathology. Am. J. Pathol. **75**, 543–572 (1974).

EVANS, R., ALEXANDER, P.: Cooperation of immune lymphoid cells with macrophages in tumor immunity. Nature **228**, 620–622 (1970).

EVERETT, N.B., TYLER, C.R.W.: Lymphopoiesis in the thymus and other tissues: functional implication. Int. Rev. Cytol. **22**, 205–237 (1967).

EYAL, Z., MANAX, W.G., BLOCH, J.H., LILLEHEI, R.C.: Successful in vitro preservation of the small bowel, including maintenance of mucosal integrity with chlorpromazine, hypothermia and hyperbaric oxygenation. Surgery **57**, 259–268 (1965a).

EYAL, Z., MANAX, W.G., BLOCH, J.H., LILLEHEI, R.C.: Utilization of chlorpromazine in heart storage and its combined use with hyperbaric oxygen and hypothermia. Surg. Gynecol. Obstet. **120**, 1237–1245 (1965b).

EIJSVOOGEL, V.P., DU BOIS, R., MELIEF, C.J.M., ZEYLENMAKER, Z., RAAT-KONING, L., GROOT DEKOOY, L.: Lymphocyte activation and destruction in vitro in relation to MLC and HL-A. Transplant. Proc. **5**, 415–420 (1973).

EIJSVOOGEL, V.P., ROOD, VAN J.J., DUTOIT, E.D., SCHELLEKENS, P.TH.A.: Position of a locus determining mixed lymphocyte reaction, distinct from the known HL-A loci. Eur. J. Immunol. **2**, 413–418 (1972).

FAGRAEUS, A., THE, H., BIBERFELD, G.: Reaction of human smooth muscle antibody with thymus medullary cells. Nature (New Biol.) **246**, 113–115 (1973).

FAHEY, J.L., BARTH, W.F., LAW, L.W.: Normal immunoglobulins and antibody response in neonatally thymectomized mice. J. Natl. Cancer Inst. **35**, 663–678 (1965).

FARIS, T.D., DICKHAUS, A.J., MARCHIORO, T.L., STARZL, T.E.: Liver radioisotope scanning in auxiliary hepatic homografts. Surg. Gynecol. Obstet. **123**, 1261–1266 (1966).

FARROW, L.J., HOLBOROW, E.J., JOHNSON, G.D., LAMB, S.G., STEARD, J.S., TAYLOR, P.E., ZUCKERMAN, A.J.: Autoantibodies and the hepatitis–associated antigen in acute infective hepatitis. Br. Med. J. **2**, 693–695 (1970).

FARROW, L.J., HOLBOROW, E.J., BRIGHTON, W.D.: Reaction of human smooth muscle antibody with liver cells. Nature (New Biol.) **232**, 186–187 (1971).

FELDMAN, J.D., LEE, S.: Renal homotransplantation in rats. I. Allogenic recipients. J. Exp. Med. **126**, 783–803 (1967).

FELDMAN, M., COHEN, J.R., WEKERLE, H.: T-cell mediated immunity in vitro; an analysis of antigen recognition and target cell lysis. Transplant. Rev. **12**, 57–90 (1972).

FELDMANN, M., BASTEN, A.: The relationship between antigenic structure and the requirement for thymus-derived cells in the immune response. J. Exp. Med. **134**, 103–119 (1971).

FELDMANN, M., NOSSAL, G.J.V.: Tolerance, enhancement and the regulation of interactions between T-cells, B-cells and macrophages. Transplant. Rev. **13**, 3–34 (1972).

FERREBEE, J.W., CANNON, F.D., MOLLEN, N., JOHN, D.S.: Beagles for studies of histocompatibility and organ transplantation. Transplantation **9**, 68–69 (1970).

FISHMAN, A.P., PIETRA, G.P.: Handling of bioactive materials by the lung. N. Engl. J. Med. **291**, 884–890 (1974).

FOLCH, H., YOSHINAGA, M., WAKSMAN, B.H.: Regulation of lymphocyte responses in vitro. III. Inhibition by adherent cells of the T-lymphocyte response to phytohemagglutinin. J. Immunol. **110**, 835–839 (1973).

FORD, W.L.: The kinetics of lymphocyte recirculation within the rat spleen. Cell Tissue Kinet. **2**, 171–191 (1969).

FORD, R.J., KUHN, C.: Immunologic competence of alveolar cells. I. The plaque-forming response to particulate and soluble antigens. Am. Rev. Resp. Dis. **107**, 763–770 (1973a).

FORD, R.J., KUHN, C.: Immunologic competence of alveolar cells. II. Modification of the plaque-forming response by inhibitors, tolerance and chronic stimulation. Am. Rev. Resp. Dis. **107**, 771–775 (1973 b).

FORGET, A., POTWOROWSKI, E.F., RICHER, G., BORDUAS, A.G.: Antigenic specifities of bursal and thymic lymphocytes in the chicken. Immunology **19**, 465–468 (1970).

FORTNER, J.G., BEATTIE, E.G., SHIU, M.H., KAWANO, N., HOWLANDS, W.S.: Orthotopic and heterotopic liver homograft in man. Ann. Surg. **172**, 23–32 (1970).

FORTNER, J.G., KINNE, D.W., SHIU, M.H., HOWLANDS, W.S., KIM, D.K., CASTRO, E.B., YEH, S.D.J., BENUA, R.S., KRUMINS, S.: Clinical liver heterotopic (auxiliary) transplantation. Surgery **74**, 739–751 (1973).

FRANCAVILLA, A., BROWN, T.H., FIORE, R., CASCARDO, S., TAYLOR, P., GROTH, C.G.: Preservation of organs for transplantation. Evidence of detrimental effect of rapid cooling. Eur. Surg. Res. **5**, 384–389 (1973).

FREDA, V.J., GORMAN, J.G., POLLACK, W.: Rh factor: prevention of isoimmunization and clinical trial on mothers. Science **151**, 828–830 (1966).

FREEDMAN, I.R., CEROTTINI, J.C., BRUNNER, K.T.: In vivo studies of the role of cytotoxic T-cells in tumor allograft immunity. J. Immunol. **109**, 1371–1378 (1972).

FREEMAN, J.S., CHAMBERLAIN, E.C., REEMTSMA, K., STEINMÜLLER, D.: Prolongation of rat heart allografts by donor pretreatment with immunosuppressive agent. Transplant. Proc. **3**, 580–582 (1971).

FRELINGER, J.A., NIEDERHUBER, J.E., SHREFFLER, D.C.: Inhibition of immune responses in vitro by specific antiserum to Ia antigens. Science **188**, 268–270 (1975).

FUDENBERG, H.M.: Are autoimmune diseases immunologic deficiency states? In: Immunobiology, GOOD, R.A., FISHER, D.W. (eds.) pp. 175–183. Stamford: Sinauer Associates, Inc. 1971.

FUJIMURA, S., NAKADA, T., KAWAKAMI, M., SUKENO, T., YONECH, M., OKANIWA, G., KAGAMI, Y., SUZUKI, C.: Detection of immunoglobulins (γM and γG) by fluorescent antibody method in canine lung allotransplantation. Tohoku J. Exp. Med. **101**, 183–198 (1970).

GABBIANI, G., RYAN, G.B., LAMELIN, J.P., VASSALLI, P., MAJNO, G., BOUVIER, C.A., CRUCHAUD, A., LÜSCHER, E.F.: Human smooth muscle autoantibody. Its identification as antiactin antibody and a study of its binding to "nonmuscular" cells. Am. J. Pathol. **72**, 473–488 (1973).

GALTON, M., REED, P.B.: Entry of lymph node cells into the normal thymus. Transplantation **4**, 168–177 (1966).

GARNIER, H., CLOT, J.P., CHOMETTE, G.: Orthotopic transplantation of the procine liver. Surg. Gynecol. Obstet. **130**, 105–111 (1970).

GERLAG, P.G.G., KOENE, R.A.P., HAGEMAN, J.F.H.M., HAELST, VAN U.J.G., WIJDEVELD, P.G.A.B.: Hyperacute rejectie van huidtransplantaten bij de muis door toediening van alloantiserum van konijne complement. Ned. Tijdschr. Geneeskd. **117**, 1719 (1973).

GERY, I., WAKSMAN, B.H.: Potentation of the T-lymphocyte response to mitogens. II. The cellular source of potentiating mediators. J. Exp. Med. **136**, 143–155 (1972).

GERY, I., GERSHON, R.K., WAKSMAN, B.H.: Potentiation of the T-lymphocyte response to mitogens. I. The responding cell. J. Exp. Med. **136**, 128–142 (1972).

GEWURZ, H.: The immunological role of complement. In: Immunobiology, GOOD, R.A., FISHER, D.W. (eds.) pp. 95–103. Stamford: Sinauer Associates, Inc. 1971.

GEWURZ, H., CLARK, D.S., FINSTAD, J., KELLY, W.D., VARCO, R.L., GOOD, R.A., GABRIELSEN, A.E.: Role of the complement system in graft rejections in experimental animals and man. Ann. N.Y. Acad. Sci. **129**, 673–713 (1966).

GHOSE, T., NORVELL, S.T., GUDU, A., CAMERON, D., BODURTHA, A., DONALS, A.S.: Immunochemotherapy of cancer with chlorambucil antibody. Br. Med. J. **3**, 495–499 (1972).

GIBSON, H.J.: Observations on occurrence characteristics and specificity of natural agglutinins. J. Hyg. **30**, 337–356 (1930).

GILES, G.R., BOEHMIG, H.J., LILLY, J., AMEMIYA, H., TAKAGI, H., COBURG, A.J., HATHAWAY, W.E., WILSON, C.B., DIXON, F.J., STARZL, T.E.: The mechanism and modification of rejection of heterografts between divergent species. Transplant. Proc. **2**, 522–538 (1970).

GILL, T.J., GOULD, H.J., DOTY, P.: Role of optimal isomers in determining the antigenicity of synthetic polypeptides. Nature **197**, 746–747 (1963).

GINN, F.L., SHELBURNE, J.D., TRUMP, B.F.: Disorders of cell volume regulation. I. Effects of inhibition of plasma membrane adenosine triphosphatase with ouabain. Am. J. Pathol. **53**, 1041–1071 (1968).

GLASSOCK, J.R., FELDMAN, D., REYNOLDS, E.S., DAMMIN, G.J., MERILL, J.P.: Recurrent glomerulonephritis in human renal isograft recipients. A clinical and pathological study. In: Advance in transplantation, DAUSSER, J., HAMBURGER, J., MATHÉ, G. (eds.) pp. 361–364. Copenhagen: Munksgaard 1968.

GLEASON, R.E., MURRAY, J.E.: Report from kidney transplant registry: analysis of the variables in the function of human kidney transplants. I. Blood group compatibility and splenectomy. Transplantation 5, 343–373 (1967).

GLICK, B.: The bursa of Fabricius and the development of immunologic competence. In: The thymus in immunobiology, GOOD, R.A., GABRIELSEN, A.E. (eds.) pp. 343–358. New York: Harper 1964.

GLICK, B., CHANG, T.S., JAAP, R.G.: The bursa of Fabricius and antibody production. Poult. Sci. 35, 224–225 (1956).

GLIEDMAN, M.L., VEITH, F.J., SOBERMAN, R., TELLIS, V., RIFKIN, H., FREED, S.: Segmental pancreatic transplantation. Abstracts of the 5th International Congress of the Transplantation Society, Jerusalem, p. 89, 1974.

GOLDBERG, B., GREEN, H.: The cytotoxic action of immune gamma globulin and complement on Krebs ascites tumor cells. I. Ultrastructural studies. J. Exp. Med. 109, 505–510 (1959).

GOLDBERG, B., GREEN, H.: Immune cytolysis. I. The release of ribonucleoprotein particles. II. Membrane-bounded structures arising during cell fragmentation. J. Biophys. Biochem. Cytol. 7, 645–650 (1960).

GOLSTEIN, P., WIGZELL, H., BLOMGREN, H., SVEDMYR, E.A.J.: Cell mediating specific in vitro cytotoxicity. II. Probable autonomy of thymus-processed lymphocytes (T-cells) for the killing of allogeneic target cells. J. Exp. Med. 135, 890–906 (1972).

GOLSTEIN, P., SCHIRRMACHER, V., RUBIN, B., WIGZELL, H.: Cytotoxic immune cells with specificity for defined soluble antigens. II. Chasing the killing cells. Cell. Immunol. 9, 211–225 (1973).

GONDOS, B., WHITE, P., BENFIELD, J.R.: Histologic changes associated with rejection of canine lung transplants. J. Thorac. Cardiovasc. Surg. 62, 183–187 (1971).

GONDOS, B., SHIMADA, K., PETER, M.E., BENFIELD, J.R.: Light and electron microscopic findings in canine lung transplants. In: Morphology in lung transplantation, WILDEVUUR, CH.R.H., JERUSALEM, C.R., LAUWERIJNS, J.M., WILDEVUUR-VAN HAMERSVELD, C. (eds.) pp. 72–84. Basel: Karger 1973.

GOOD, R.A.: Immunodeficiency in the developmental perspective. In: The Harvey lectures, AXELFORD, J., BENACERRAF, B., BERG, P., BOYSE, E.A., DOLE, V.P., GOOD, R.A., MERRIFIELD, B., OLD, L.J., SELA, M. (eds.) pp. 1–107. New York: Academic Press 1973.

GOODRICH, E.O., WELCH, H.F., NELSON, J.A., BEECHER, T.S., WELCH, C.S.: Homotransplantation of the canine liver. Surgery 39, 244–251 (1956).

GOOTT, B., LILLEHEI, R.C., MILLER, F.A.: Mesenteric lymphatic regeneration after autografts of small bowel in dogs. Surgery 48, 571–575 (1960).

GORCZYNSKI, R.M., MILLER, R.G., PHILIPS, R.A.: Initiation of antibody production to sheep erythrocytes in vitro: replacement of the requirements for T-cells with a cellfree factor isolated from cultures of lymphoid cells. J. Immunol. 108, 547–551 (1972).

GORDON, J.: Role of monocytes in the mixed leukocyte culture reaction. Proc. Soc. Exp. Biol. Med. 127, 30–33 (1968).

GOWANS, J.L.: The recirculation of lymphocytes from the blood to lymph in the rat. J. Physiol. 146, 54–69 (1959).

GOWANS, J.L.: Immunobiology of the small lymphocyte. In: Immunobiology, GOOD, R.A. and FISHER, D.W. (eds.) pp. 18–27. Stamford: Sinauer Associates, Inc. 1971.

GOWANS, J.L.: Differentiation of the cells which synthesize the immunoglobulins. Ann. Inst. Pasteur (Paris) 125, 201–211 (1974).

GOWANS, J.L., KNIGHT, E.J.: The route of re-circulation of lymphocytes in the rat. Proc. R. Soc. Lond. (Biol.) 159, 257–282 (1964).

GOWANS, J.L., MCGREGOR, D.D.: The immunological activities of lymphocytes. Prog. Allergy 9, 1–78 (1965).

GOWANS, J.L., MCGREGOR, D.D., COWEN, D.M., FORD, C.E.: Initiation of immune responses by small lymphocytes. Nature 196, 651–655 (1962).

GOZZO, J.J., WOOD, M.L., MONACO, A.P.: Use of minimal doses of lymphoid cells for production of heterologous antilymphocyte serum. Transplant. Proc. 111, 779–783 (1971).

GRAF, M.W., UHR, J.W.: Regulation of antibody formation by serum antibody. I. Removal of specific antibody by means of immunoadsorption. J. Exp. Med. **130**, 1175–1186 (1969).

GRAFF, R.S., NATHENSON, S.G.: Immunogenic proporties of papain-solubilized alloantigen. Transplant. Proc. **3**, 249–252 (1971).

GRANGER, G.A., KOLB, W.P.: Lymphocyte in vitro cytotoxicity: Mechanisms of immune and non-immune small lymphocyte mediated target L cell destruction J. Immunol. **101**, 111–120 (1968).

GRANGER, G.A., WEISER, R.S.: Homograft target cells: contact destruction in vitro by immune macrophages. Science **151**, 97–99 (1966).

GREAVES, M.F., OWEN, J.J.T., RAFF, M.C.: T- and B-lymphocytes: origins, properties and roles in immune responses. New York: American Elsevier Publishing Co. 1973.

GREEN, J.A., COOPERBAND, S.R., RUTSTEIN, J.A., KIBRICH, S.: A lymphocyte-produced factor which inhibits proliferation of other cells. Fed. Proc. **29**, 306 (1970).

GREENBERG, A.H., SHEN, L.: A class of specific cytotoxic cells demonstrated in vitro by arming with antigen-antibody complexes. Nature (New Biol.) **245**, 282–285 (1973).

GREENBERG, A.H., HUDSON, L., SHEN, L., ROITT, I.M.: Antibody-dependent cell-mediated cytotoxicity due to a "null" lymphoid cell. Nature (New Biol.) **242**, 111–113 (1973a).

GREENBERG, A.H., SHEN, L., ROITT, I.M.: Characterization of the antibody-dependent cytotoxic cell: a non-phagocytic monocyte? Clin. Exp. Immunol. **15**, 251–259 (1973b).

GRENIER, J.F., GILLET, M., SANTIXO LEPE, G., KLEIN, A., BARTH, A.M., WEISS, A.G.: Les greffes de pancréas chez le chien, étude de la survie et des potentialités fonctionelles du transplant. Ann. Chir. **21**, 1523–1537 (1967).

GRIEPP, R.B., STINSON, E.B., OYER, P.F., DONG, JR. E., SHUMWAY, N.E.: Management of long-term survivors of heart transplantation. In: Transplantation Today, vol. 3, SCHLESINGER, M., BILLINGHAM, R.E., RAPAPORT, F.T. (eds.), pp. 595–599. New York: Grune & Stratten 1975.

GROSJEAN, O., NOIRCLERC, M., DUVINAGE, J.F., SUDAN, N., TEDESCHI, J., COUTANT, P., LEJEUNE, G.: Mise au point d'un procédé simple de conservation du poumon assurant une reprise immédiate de fonction après vingt-quatre heures d'ischémie. Acta Chir. Belg. **71**, 321–333 (1972).

GRUMET, F.C.: Genetic control of the immune response. A selective defect in immunologic (IgG) memory in non responder mice. J. Exp. Med. **135**, 110–125 (1972).

GRÜNDEL, J.: Ethics of organ transplantation. In: Organ transplantation today, MITCHINSON, N.A., GREEP, J.M., HATTINGA-VERSCHURG, J.C.M. (eds.) pp. 333–344. Amsterdam: Excerpta Medica Foundation 1969.

GRUPE, W.E., KAPLAN, M.H.: Demonstration of an antibody to proximal tubular antigen in the pathogenesis of experimental autoimmune nephrosis in rat. J. Lab. Clin. Med. **74**, 400–409 (1969).

GRUYL DE, J., WESTBROEK, D.L., DIJKHUIS, C.M., VRIESENDORP, H.M., MacDICKEN, I., ELION-GERRITSEN, W., VERSCHOOR, L., HULSMANS, H.A.M., HÖRCHNER, P.: Influence of DL-A matching, ALS, and 24-hour preservation on isolated pancreas allograft survival. Transplant. Proc. **5**, 755–759 (1973).

GUTTMANN, R.D., LINDQUIST, R.R.: Renal transplantation in the inbred rat. XI. Reduction of allograft immunogenecity by cytotoxic drug pretreatment of donors. Transplantation **8**, 490–495 (1969).

GUTTMANN, R.D., CARPENTER, C.B., LINDQUIST, R.R., MERRILL, J.P.: Renal transplantation in the inbred rat. III. A study of heterologous antithymocyte sera. J. Exp. Med. **126**, 1099–1126 (1967a).

GUTTMANN, R.D., LINDQUIST, R.R., PARKER, R.M, CARPENTER, C.B., MERRILL, J.P.: Renal transplantation in the inbred rat. I. Morphologic, immunologic and functional alterations during acute rejection. Transplantation **5**, 668–681 (1967b).

HAEFEN VON, U., WREN, S.F.G., SHAIPANICH, T., MARTINS, A.C.P., BUSCH, G.J., WILSON, R.E.: Active enhancement of rat renal allografts with papain-released specific antigens. Transplantation **16**, 295–303 (1973).

HAGADORN, J.E., MERCOLA, K.E.: Immunologic and morphologic studies of the acute effect of anti-lung serum. Exp. Mol. Pathol. **15**, 97–107 (1971).

HAGADORN, J.E., VASQUEZ, J.J., KINNEY, T.R.: Immunopathological studies of an experimental model resembling Goodpasture's syndrome. Am. J. Pathol. **57**, 17–30 (1969).

HAGERMAN, G.: How is epidermal hypersensitivity transmitted through lymphocytes? Acta Derm. Venerol. **34**, 51–56 (1954).

HAGLIN, J.J., RUIZ, E., BAKER, R.C., ANDERSON, W.R.: Histologic studies of human lung allotransplantation. In: Morphology in lung transplantation, WILDEVUUR, CH.R.H., JERUSALEM, C.R., LAUWERIJNS, J.M., WILDEVUUR-HAMERSVELD, C. (eds.), pp. 13–22. Basel: Karger 1973.

HAKALA, T.R., LANGE, P.H.: Serum induced lymphoid cell mediated cytotoxicity to human transitional cell carcinomas of the genitourinary tract. Science 184, 795–797 (1974).

HALASZ, N., ORLOFF, M.: The passive transfer of enhancement as applied to skin homografts. J. Immunol. 94, 253–256 (1965).

HALGRIMSON, C.G., MARCHIORO, T.L., FARIS, T.D., PORTER, K.A., PETERS, C.N., STARZL, T.E.: Auxiliary liver homotransplantation: Effect of host portacaval shunt. Arch. Surg. 93, 107–118 (1966).

HALGRIMSON, C.C., RAPAPORT, F.T., TERASAKI, P.I., PORTER, K.A., ANDERS, G., PENN, I., PUTMAN, C.W., STARZL, T.E.: Net histocompatibility ratios (NHR) for clinical transplantation. Transplant. Proc. 3, 140–144 (1971).

HALL, J.G.: Studies of the cells in the afferent and efferent lymph nodes draining the site of skin homografts. J. Exp. Med. 125, 737–754 (1967).

HALL, J.G.: Effector mechanisms in immunity. Lancet 1, 25–28 (1969).

HALL, C.L., THOMSON, R.W., DAWSON-EDWARDS, P., BARNES, A.D., BLAINEY, J.D.: Importance of warm and cold ischaemia times in primary failure of human cadaver kidney transplants. Lancet 1, 532–534 (1974).

HALLER, J., SALM, T., RAVENHORST, J.: Effect of newborn splenectomy on homograft survival in inbred mice. Transplantation 4, 505–506 (1966).

HALPERN, B., FRAY, A., CREPIN, Y., PLASTICA, O., LORINET, A.M., RABOURDIN, A., SPARROS, L., ISAC, R.: Corynebacterium parvum, a potent immunostimulant in experimental infections and in malignancies. In: Ciba Foundation Symposium 18: Immunopotentiation, pp. 217–236. New York: Elsevier Publishing Co. 1973.

HAMBURGER, J., CROSNIER, J., DORMONT, J.: Experience with 45 renal homotransplantations in man. Lancet 1, 985–992 (1965).

HAMBURGER, J., DIMITRIU, A., BANKIR, L., DEBRAY-SACHS, M., AUVERT, J.: Collection of lymph from kidneys homotransplanted in man: Cell transformation in vivo. Nature 232, 633–634 (1971).

HÄMMERLING, U., RAJEWSKI, K.: Evidence for surface-associated immunoglobulin on T- and B-lymphocytes. Eur. J. Immunol. 1, 447–452 (1971).

HAMILTON, R., HOLST, H.I., LEHR, H.B., HAZEL, B., MERNDON, B.: Successful preservation of canine small intestine by freezing. J. Surg. Res. 14, 313–318 (1973).

HARDY, J.D.: Summation and concluding discussion. In: Human organ support and replacement, HARDY, J.D. (ed.), pp. 431–446. Springfield: C.C. Thomas 1971.

HARDY, J.D., ALICAN, F.: Transplantation of the lung. In: Human organ support and replacement, HARDY, J.D. (ed.), pp. 252–287. Springfield: C.C. Thomas 1971.

HARDY, J.D., ERASLAN, S., DALTON, M.L.: Autotransplantation and homotransplantation of the lung: Further studies. J. Thorac. Cardiovasc. Surg. 46, 606–615 (1963).

HÄRING, R.: Temporary and permanent liver replacement in acute hepatic failure. Indication and prognosis. In: Liver transplantation, LIE, T.S., GÜTGEMANN, A. (eds.), pp. 13–18. Baden-Baden: Witzstrock 1974.

HARRISON, G.A., WEIBEL, J.: The membranous component of alveolar exudate. J. Ultrastruct. Res. 24, 334–342 (1968).

HARRISON, M.R.: Thymus independent stimulator cells in the mixed lymphocyte reaction. J. Immunol. 111, 1270–1273 (1973).

HARVEY, R.B.: Effect of temperature on function of isolated dog kidney. Am. J. Physiol. 197, 181–186 (1959).

HASEK, M., KARAKOZ, I., SKAMENE, E., CHUTNA, J., NOUZA, K., BUBINEK, J., NEMES, M., SOVOVA, V.: Protective action of homologous serum component on graft rejection. Transpl. Proc. 1, 527–529 (1969).

HAUCK, G.: Physiological and pathophysiological aspects of the venous microvasculature. Basic Res. Cardiol. 68, 443–451 (1973).

HAUGHTON, G.: Specific immunosuppression by passive antibody. V. Participation of macrophages in reversal of suppression by peritoneal exudate cells from immune animals. Cell. Immunol. 13, 230–240 (1974).

HAUGHTON, G., ADAMS, D.O.: Specific immunosuppression by minute doses of passive antibody. II. The site of action. J. Reticuloendothel. Soc. 7, 500–517 (1970).

HAUGHTON, G., NASH, D.R.: Specific immunosuppression by minute doses of passive antibody. Transpl. Proc. 1, 616–618 (1969).

HAY, J.B., LACHMANN, P.J., TRNKA, Z.: The appearance of migration inhibition factor and a mitogen in lymph draining tuberculin reaction. Eur. J. Immunol. 3, 127–130 (1973).

HÄYRY, P., DEFENDI, V.: Mixed lymphocyte cultures produce effector cell model in vitro for allograft rejection. Science 168, 133–135 (1970).

HÄYRY, P., LINDSTRÖM, B.L., VIROLAINEN, M., PASTERNACK, A., LINDFORS, O.: Immunobiological diagnosis of rejection in dogs with renal allografts. Surgery 71, 494–506 (1972).

HEE VAN, R.H.G.G.: Pancreaticoduodenal preservation and transplantation. An experimental study. Thesis, Nijmegen, The Netherlands 1973.

HELL, E., BOEDEL, O., ZIMMERMANN, G., LETNANSKY, K.: Protein synthesis during extracorporeal perfusion of pig livers with human blood. In: Liver transplantation, LIE, T.S., GÜTGEMANN, A. (eds.), pp. 285–287. Baden-Baden: Witzstrock 1974.

HELLSTRÖM, I., HELLSTRÖM, K.E.: Recent studies of the mechanism of the allogeneic inhibition phenomenon. Ann. N.Y. Acad. Sci. 129, 724–733 (1966).

HELLSTRÖM, K.E., MÖLLER, G.: Immunological and immunogenetic aspects of tumor transplantation. Progr. Allergy 9, 158–245 (1965).

HENRY, C., FAULK, W.P., KUHN, L., YOFFEY, J.M., FUDENBERG, H.H.: Peyer's patches: immunologic studies. J. Exp. Med. 131, 1200–1210 (1970).

HENSON, P.M.: Interaction of cells with immune complexes: adherence release of constituents and tissue injury. J. Exp. Med. 134, 114 (1971).

HESS, F., JERUSALEM, C.: Self elimination of T and B lymphocytes in the spleen of the PVG/C rat after auxiliary liver allotransplantation. Eur. Surg. Res. in press 1975.

HESS, F., JERUSALEM, C., HEYDE VAN DE, M.N.: Advantages of auxiliary liver homotransplantation in rats. Arch. Surg. 184, 76–80 (1972).

HESS, F., POLAK, M., JERUSALEM, C.: Imuran in the treatment of heterotopic (auxiliary) rat liver allotransplantation. Eur. Surg. Res. 5, 133–134 (1973).

HESSINGER, D.A., DAYNES, R.A., GRANGER, G.A.: Binding of human lymphotoxin to target-cell membranes and its relation to cell-mediated cytodestruction. Proc. Natl. Acad. Sci. U.S.A. 70, 3082–3086 (1973).

HEYDE VAN DE, M.N., SCHALM, L.: Auxiliary livergraft without portal blood. Experimental autotransplantation of left liver lobes. Br. J. Surg. 53, 114–118 (1968).

HEYDE VAN DE, M.N., JERUSALEM, C., SCHMIDT, W.J., BILSKI, R., REINKING, J.W., TJEBBES, F.A., JAP, P.: The influence of hemodynamics on the microstructure of the heterotopic livergraft. Eur. Surg. Res. 2, 150 (1970).

HEYDE VAN DE, M.N., JERUSALEM, C., SCHMIDT, W.J., TJEBBES, F.A.: Heterotopic livertransplantation. I. Postoperative course and histological feature of the canine auxiliary homograft. Eur. Surg. Res. 3, 454–463 (1971).

HEYDE VAN DE, M.N., JERUSALEM, C., REINKING, J.W., SCHMIDT, W.J., JAP, P.: Heterotopic livertransplantation. In: Liver transplantation, LIE, T.S., GÜTGEMANN, A. (eds.), pp. 123–126. Baden-Baden: Witzstrock 1974.

HIBBS, J.B.: Heterocytolysis by macrophages activated by Bacillus Calmette-Guérin: Lysosome exocytosis into tumor cells. Science 184, 468–471 (1974).

HIBBS, J.B., LAMBERT, L.H., REMINGTON, J.S.: In vitro non-immunologic destruction of cells with abnormal growth characteristics by adjuvant activated macrophages. Proc. Soc. Exp. Biol. Med. 139, 1049–1052 (1972a).

HIBBS, J.B., LAMBERT, L.H., REMINGTON, J.S.: Control of carcinogenesis: a possible role for the activated macrophage. Science 177, 998–1000 (1972b).

HIBBS, J.B., LAMBERT, L.H., REMINGTON, J.S.: Possible role of macrophage mediated non-specific cytotoxicity in tumor resistance. Nature (New Biol.) 235, 48–50 (1972c).

HIRATA, A.A., TERASAKI, P.I.: Cross-reactions between streptococcal M. proteins and human transplantation antigens. Science 168, 1095–1096 (1970).

HIRST, J.A., DUTTON, R.W.: Cell components in the immune response III. Neonatal thymectomy: restoration in culture. Cell. Immunol. 1, 190–195 (1970).

HOGMAN, C.F.: Blood group antigens A and B determined by means of mixed agglutination on cultured cells of human fetal kidney, liver, spleen, lung, heart, and skin. Vox Sang. **4**, 319–332 (1959).

HOLBOROW, E.J., HEMSTED, E.M., MEAD, S.V.: Smooth muscle autoantibodies in infectious mononucleosis. Br. Med. J. **3**, 323–325 (1973).

HOLLENBERG, N.K., RETIC, A.B., ROSEN, S.M.: The role of vasoconstriction in the ischemia of renal allograft rejection. Transplantation **6**, 59–69 (1968).

HOLM, G.: The in vitro cytotoxicity of human lymphocytes. Comparison with other cells. Exp. Cell Res. **48**, 327–333 (1967).

HOLM, G., PERLMANN, P.: Cytotoxic potential of stimulated human lymphocytes. J. Exp. Med. **125**, 721–736 (1967).

HOLM, G., HAMMARSTRÖM, S.: Haemolytic activity of human blood monocytes. Lysis of human erythrocytes treated with anti-A serum. Clin. Exp. Immunol. **13**, 29–43 (1973).

HOLM, G., PERLMANN, P., WERNER, B.: Phytohaemagglutinin-induced cytotoxic action of normal lymphoid cells on cells in tissue culture. Nature **203**, 841–843 (1964).

HOMMA, Y., ONODERA, I., IRIE, T., HEESTRA, H., JERUSALEM, C., WILDEVUUR, CH.R.H.: Simultaneous bilateral hilar stripping (BHS) of the lungs: Alterations in lung function and corresponding lung morphology. Eur. Surg. Res. in press 1975.

HOPE, U.: Immunologische Toleranz. Klin. Wochenschr. **49**, 177-192 (1971).

HOROWITZ, R.E., BURROWS, L., PARONETTO, F., DREILING, D., KARK, A.F.: Immunologic observations on homografts. II. The canine kidney. Transplantation **3**, 318–325 (1965).

HOWARD, J.C.: The life-span and recirculation of marrow-derived small lymphocytes from the thoracic duct. J. Exp. Med. **135**, 185–199 (1972).

HOWARD, J.C., HUNT, S.V., GOWANS, J.L.: Identification of marrow-derived small lymphocytes in the lymphoid tissue and thoracic duct lymph of normal rats. J. Exp. Med. **135**, 200–219 (1972).

HUBER, H., FUDENBERG, H.H.: Receptor sites of human monocytes for IgG. Int. Arch. Allergy Appl. Immunol. **34**, 18–31 (1968).

HULME, B., ANDRES, G.A., PORTER, K.A., OGDEN, D.A.: Human renal transplants. IV. Glomerular ultrastructure, macromolecular permeability and hemodynamics. Lab. Invest. **26**, 2–10 (1972).

HUME, D.M.: Kidney transplantation. In: Human transplantation, RAPAPORT, F.T., DAUSSET, J. (eds.), pp. 110–130. New York: Grune & Stratton, Inc. 1968.

HUME, D.M.: Organ transplants and immunity. In: Immunobiology, GOOD, R.A., FISHER, D.W. (eds.), pp. 185–194. Stamford: Sinauer Associates, Inc. 1971.

HUME, D.M., EGDAHL, R.H.: Progressive destruction of renal homografts isolated from the regional lymphatics of the host. Surgery **38**, 194–214 (1955).

HUME, D.M., MERILL, J.P., MILLER, B.F., THORN, G.W.: Experience with renal homotransplantation in human. J. Clin. Invest. **34**, 327–382 (1955).

HUME, D.M., JACKSON, B.T., ZUKOSKI, C.F., LEE, H.M., KAUFFMAN, H.M., EGDAHL, R.H.: The homotransplantation of kidneys and of fetal liver and spleen after total body irradiation. Ann. Surg. **152**, 354–373 (1960).

IDEZUKI, Y., FEEMSTER, J.A., DIETZMAN, R.H., LILLEHEI, R.C.: Experimental pancreaticoduodenal preservation and transplantation. Surg. Gynecol. Obstet. **126**, 1002–1014 (1968).

IRIE, U., HOMMA, Y., HEEMSTRA, H., JERUSALEM, C., WILDEVUUR, CH.R.H.: Simultaneous bilateral hilar stripping (BHS) of the lungs: Alteration in lung function and corresponding lung morphology. Eur. Surg. Res. in press 1975.

IRVIN, G.L., CARBONE, P.P.: Immunosuppression with lymph depletion in man. Surg. Gynecol. Obstet. **124**, 1283–1287 (1967).

ISHII, Y., VENO, H., KIKUCHI, K.: Ultrastructure of lymphoid cells involved in local graft-versus-host reaction. Virchows Arch. (Zellpathol.) **14**, 105–115 (1973).

ITO, T., KINO, T., CUDKOWIZ, G.: B-cell differentiation in the splenic environment: acquired susceptibility to the helper function of irradiated T-cells. J. Immunol. **110**, 596–599 (1973).

IWAHASHI, H., NAGAYA, H., SEALY, W.C.: Effect of in situ perfusion of donor lung on the survival of canine lung allografts. Transplantation **13**, 183–186 (1972).

JACOBSON, E.B., HERZENBERG, L.A., RIBLET, R.: Active suppression of immunoglobulin allotype synthesis. II. Transfer of suppressing factor with spleen cells. J. Exp. Med. **135**, 1163–1176 (1972).

JAFFER, A.M., JONES, G., KASDON, E.J., SCHLOSSMAN, S.F.: Local transfer of delayed hypersensitivity by T-lymphocytes. J. Immunol. 111, 1268–1269 (1973).

JAKOBSEN, A., FLATMARK, A.: Immunosuppression mediated by IgM antibodies. Eur. Surg. Res. 5, 17 (1973).

JANDL, J.H., TOMLINSON, A.S.: The destruction of red cells by antibodies in man. II. Pyrogenic, leukocytic and dermal responses to immune hemolysis. J. Clin. Invest. 37, 1202–1228 (1958).

JANKOVIC, B.C., WAKSMAN, B.H., ARNASON, B.: Role of the thymus immune reactions in rats. I. The immunologic response to borne serum albumin (antibody formation, Arthus reactivity and delayed hypersensitivity) in rats thymectomized or splenectomized at various times after birth. J. Exp. Med. 116, 159–176 (1962).

JANOFF, A.: Mediators of tissue damage in human polymorphonuclear neutrophils. Ser. Haematol. 3, 96–130 (1970).

JANSEN, C.R., LOUBSER, J.S., JOOSTE, S.V.: Hyperacute renal rejection in goats. S. Afr. Med. J. 44, 1184–1186 (1970).

JAP, P.H.K.: Ultrastructural and histochemical investigations on auxiliary liver grafts in rats with some notes on the application to other species. Thesis, Nijmegen, The Netherlands 1971.

JAP, P., JERUSALEM, C., HESS, F., HEYDE VAN DE, M.N.: Ultrastructural and histochemical investigations on long surviving rat auxiliary liver homografts. Cytobiol. 5, 165–180 (1972).

JAP, P.H.K., WARNIER, B.H.M., WILDEVUUR, CH.R.H., JERUSALEM, C.R.: Ultrastructural studies on isolated and transplanted lungs of dogs. In: Morphology in lung transplantation, WILDEVUUR, CH.R.H., JERUSALEM, C.R., LAUWERIJNS, J.M., WILDEVUUR-HAMERSVELD, C. (eds.), pp. 159–179. Basel: Karger 1973.

JATROPULOS, M.J.: Form und Verlauf der kompensatorischen Leberhypertrophie bei der Ratte. Z. Anat. Entwicklungsgesch. 124, 455–470 (1965).

JERNE, N.K.: Towards a network theory of the immune system. Ann. Inst. Pasteur (Paris) 125, 373–389 (1974).

JERUSALEM, C.: Untersuchungen zur kompensatorischen Nierenhypertrophie. I. Gewichtszunahme und Wassergehalt verbleibender Nieren bei einseitig nephrektomierten Ratten. Anat. Anz. 114, 86–102 (1963a).

JERUSALEM, C.: Untersuchungen zur kompensatorischen Nierenhypertrophie. II. Der Einfluß des Alters auf die Gewichtszunahme hypertrophierender Rattennieren. Z. Anat. Entwicklungsgesch. 123, 549–556 (1963b).

JERUSALEM, C., ELING, W.: Active immunization against Plasmodium berghei malaria in mice, using different preparations of plasmodium antigen and different pathways of administration. Bull. WHO 40, 807–818 (1969).

JERUSALEM, C., WERF VAN DE, B.: Electronenmikroskopische Untersuchungen an unterkühlten autotransplantierten Nieren. In: Organtransplantation, Immunologie und Klinik, HEYMER, A., RICKEN, D., LETTERER, E. (eds.), pp. 315–324. Stuttgart-New York: Schattauer 1969.

JERUSALEM, C., HEYDE VAN DE, M.N., JAP, P., REINKING, J.W., SCHMIDT, W.J.H., BILSKI, R., TJEBBES, F.A.: Zum Problem der heterotopen Lebertransplantation. Anat. Anz. 124, 69–76 (1971a).

JERUSALEM, C., HEYDE VAN DE, M.N., JAP, P., REINKING, J.W., SCHMIDT, W.J.A., BILSKI, R., TJEBBES, F.A.: Rejection phenomena in heterotopic liver homo- and heterografts. Transplant. Proc. 3, 554–557 (1971b).

JERUSALEM, C., WEISS, M.L., POELS, L.: Immunologic enhancement in malaria infection (Plasmodium berghei). J. Immunol. 107, 260–267 (1971c).

JERUSALEM, C., HEYDE VAN DE, M.N., SCHMIDT, W.J., TJEBBES, F.A.: Heterotopic liver transplantation. II. Unfavorable outflow conditions as a possible cause for late graft failure. Eur. Surg. Res. 4, 186–197 (1972).

JERUSALEM, C., HEYDE VAN DE, M.N., JAP, P., REINKING, J.W., HEE VAN, R.H.G.G., WARNIER, B.: Pathogenesis of hyperacute liver xenograft rejection. In: Liver transplantation, LIE, T.S., GÜTGEMANN, A. (eds.), pp. 277–283. Baden-Baden: Witzstrock 1974.

JESKE, A.H., ABOUNA, M.: Ultrastructure of canine renal autografts following 24-hour hypothermic preservation. Eur. Surg. Res. 5, 424–435 (1973).

JOHNSON, G.D., HOLBOROW, E.J., GLYNN, L.E.: Antibody to smooth muscle in patients with liver disease. Lancet 2, 878–879 (1965).

JOHNSON, H.A., SCHNAPPAUF, H., CHANANA, A.D., CRONKITE, E.P.: Variability of ribosomal aggregation in lymphocytes. Nature 211, 420 (1966).

JOHNSON, R.W.G., ANDERSON, M., FLEAR, C.T.G., MURRAY, G.H., SWINNEY, J.: Evaluation of new perfusion solution for kidney preservation. Transplantation 13, 270–275 (1972).

JONES, J.V., MOORE, B.: Problems of anomalous glomerular antigens. Lancet 1, 1056–1058 (1970).

JOYSEY, V.C., ROGER, R.H., EVANS, D.B., HERBERTSON, B.M.: Kidney graft survival and matching for HL-A and ABO antigens. Nature 246, 163–165 (1973).

KALINER, M., AUSTEN, K.F.: A sequence of biochemical events in the antigen-induced release of chemical mediators from sensitized human lung tissue. J. Exp. Med. 138, 1077–1094 (1973).

KALTREIDER, H.B., SALMON, S.E.: Immunology of the lower respiratory tract. Functional properties of bronchoalveolar lymphocytes obtained from the normal canine lung. J. Clin. Invest. 52, 2211–2217 (1973).

KAMRIN, B.B.: Successful skin homografts in mature non-littermate rats treated with fractions containing alpha-globulins. Proc. Soc. Exp. Biol. Med. 100, 58–61 (1959).

KANDUTSCH, A.A., REINERT-WENK, U.: Studies on a substance that promotes tumor homograft survival (the enhancing substance) its distribution and some properties. J. Exp. Med. 105, 125–139 (1957).

KANO, J.T., MILGROM, F.: Antibody induced lysis of nucleated cells in agar gel. Int. Arch. Allergy Appl. Immunol. 41, 739–753 (1971).

KANO, S., BLOOM, B.R., HOWE, M.L.: Enumeration of activated thymus-derived lymphocytes by the virus plaque assay. Proc. Natl. Acad. Sci. U.S.A. 70, 2299–2303 (1973).

KAPLAN, S.R., CALABRESI, P.: Immunosuppressive agents. N. Engl. J. Med. 289, 1234–1236 (1973).

KARPAS, A.B., SEGRE, D.: A nonspecific immunosuppressive material derived from normal bovine serum. Proc. Soc. Exp. Biol. Med. 144, 141–147 (1973).

KARUSH, F., EISEN, H.N.: A theory of delayed hypersensitivity. Science 136, 1032–1039 (1962).

KATZ, D.H., PAUL, W.E., GOIDL, E.A., BENACERRAF, B.: Carrier function in anti-hapten antibody responses. III. Stimulation of antibody synthesis and facilitation of hapten-specific secondary antibody responses by graft-versus-host reactions. J. Exp. Med. 133, 169–186 (1971).

KATZ, D.H., HAMAOKA, T., BENACERRAF, B.: Immunological tolerance in bone marrow derived lymphocytes. I. Evidence for an intracellular mechanism of antibody-forming cells. J. Exp. Med. 136, 1404–1429 (1972).

KATZ, D.H., HAMAOKA, T., BENACERRAF, B.: Cell interactions between histoincompatible T- and B-lymphocytes. II. Failure of physiologic cooperative interaction between B- and T-lymphocytes from allogeneic donor strains in humoral response to hapten-protein conjugates. J. Exp. Med. 137, 1405–1418 (1973a).

KATZ, D.H., HAMAOKA, T., DORF, M.E., BENACERRAF, B.: Cell interactions between histoincompatible T- and B-lymphocytes. III. Demonstration that the H-Z gene complex determines successful physiologic lymphocyte interactions. Proc. Natl. Acad. Sci. U.S.A. 70, 2624–2628 (1973b).

KAWABE, K., GUTTMANN, R.D., LEVIN, B., MERRILL, J.P., WINDQUIST, R.R.: Renal transplantation in the inbred rat. XVIII. Effect of cyclophosphamide on acute rejection and long survival of recipients. Transplantation 13, 21–26 (1972).

KEDAR, E., ORTIZ DE LANDAZURI, M., FAHEY, J.L.: Comparative studies of immunoglobulin receptors and antibody-dependent cell cytotoxicity (ADCC) in rat lymphoid organs. J. Immunol. 112, 37–46 (1974).

KEELER, R., SWINNEY, D.J., TAYLOR, M.R., ULDALL, P.R.: The problem of renal preservation. Br. J. Urol. 38, 653–656 (1966).

KELLER, R.: Cytostatic elimination of syngeneic rat tumor cells in vitro by nonspecifically activated macrophages. J. Exp. Med. 138, 625–644 (1973).

KELLEY, R.H.: Localization of afferent lymph cells within the draining node during a primary response. Nature 227, 510–513 (1970).

KELLEY, R.H., WOLSENCROFT, R.A., DUMONDE, D., BALFOUR, B.M.: Role of lymphocyte activation products (LAP) in cell-mediated immunity. II. Effects of lymphocyte activation products on lymph node architecture and evidence for peripheral release of LAP following antigen stimulation. Clin. Exp. Immunol. 10, 49–65 (1972).

KELLNER, G.: Die Blut- und Lymphwege der menschlichen Milz. Wien. Klin. Wochenschr. 35, 610–620 (1963).

KERBEL, R.S., EIDINGER, D.: Variable effects of anti-lymphocyte serum on humoral antibody formation: role of thymus dependency of antigen. J. Immunol. 106, 917–926 (1971).

KEUNING, F.J., MEER VAN DER, J., NIEUWENHUIS, P., OUDENDIJK, P.: The histophysiology of the antibody response. II. Antibody responses and splenic plasma cell reactions in sublethally X-irradiated rabbits. Lab. Invest. **12**, 156–170 (1963).

KHASTAGIR, B., MONTANDON, A., NAKAMOTO, S., KOLFF, W.J.: Early and late failures of human cadaveric renal allografts. Arch. Intern. Med. **123**, 8–14 (1969).

KIMOTO, S.: The artificial liver. Experiments and clinical application. Trans. Am. Soc. Artif. Intern Organs **5**, 102–112 (1959).

KINCAID-SMITH, P.: Vascular changes in homotransplants. Br. Med. J. **1**, 178–179 (1964).

KINCAID-SMITH, P.: Modification of the vascular lesions of rejection in cadaveric renal allografts by dipyridamole and anticoagulants. Lancet **2**, 920–922 (1969).

KINCAID-SMITH, P.: The pathogenesis of the vascular and glomerular lesions of rejection in renal allografts and their modification by antithrombotic and anticoagulant drugs. Aust. Ann. Med. **3**, 201–214 (1970).

KINCAID-SMITH, P., MORRIS, P.J., SAKER, B.M., TING, A., MARSHALL, V.C.: Immediate renal-graft biopsy and subsequent rejection. Lancet **2**, 748–749 (1968).

KIRKPATRICK, C.H., WILSON, W.E.C.: Immunologic studies of baboon-to-man renal heterotransplantation. In: Experience in renal transplantation, STARZL, T.E. (ed.), pp. 284–298. Philadelphia: W.B. Saunders Company 1964.

KISHIMOTO, T., ISHIZAKA, K.: Regulation of antibody response in vitro. V. Effect of carrier-specific helper cells on generation of haptenspecific memory cells of different immunoglobulin classes. J. Immunol. **111**, 1–9 (1973a).

KISHIMOTO, T., ISHIZAKA, K.: Regulation of antibody response in vitro. VII. Enhancing soluble factors for IgG and IgE antibody response. J. Immunol. **111**, 1194–1205 (1973b).

KISSMEYER-NIELSEN, F., OLSEN, S., PETERSEN, V.P., FJELDBORG, O.: Hyperacute rejection of kidney allografts with pre-existing humoral antibodies against donor cells. Lancet **2**, 662–665 (1966).

KLASS, D.J.: Immunochemical studies of the protein fraction of pulmonary surface active material. Am. Rev. of Resp. Dis. **107**, 784–789 (1973).

KLASSEN, J., MILGROM, F.: Autoimmune concomitants of renal allografts. Transplant. Proc. **1**, 605–608 (1969).

KLIKA, E., KRÁKORA, P., POHUNKOVÁ, H.: Ultrastructure of allo and autografts in canine lungs. In: Morphology in lung transplantation, WILDEVUUR, CH.R.H., JERUSALEM, C.R., LAUWERIJNS, J.M., WILDEVUUR-VAN HAMERSVELD, C. (eds.), pp. 148–158. Basel: Karger 1973.

KNOX, W.G., McCABE, R.E., NAY, H.R., ZINTEL, H.A., STARK, R.B.: Effect of regional lymphatic ablation on kidney homograft survival. Am. J. Surg. **107**, 547–552 (1964).

KOBAYASHI, K., HRICKO, G.M., LUKL, JR. P., HUNSICKER, L., PATEL, R., REISNER, G.S., BIRTCH, A.G.: Hyperacute renal allograft rejection in presensitized monkeys. Surg. Forum **22**, 246–248 (1971).

KOBAYASHI, Y., SKIGEMATSU, H., TADE, T.: Nephritogenic properties of nephrotoxic guinea pig antibodies. I. Glomerulonephritis induced by guinea pig IgG_1 antibody in rats. Virchows Arch. (Zellpathol.) **14**, 259–271 (1973).

KOCANDRLE, V., HOUTTUIN, E., PROHASKA, J.V.: Regeneration of the lymphatics after autotransplantation and homotransplantation of the entire small intestine. Surg. Gynecol. Obstet. **122**, 587–592 (1966).

KOCH, R.: Weitere Mitteilung über ein Heilmittel gegen Tuberkulose. Dtsch. Med. Wochenschr. **16**, 1029 (1890).

KOENE, R., McKENZIE, I.C.F., PAINTER, E., SACHS, D.H., WINN, H.J., RUSSELL, P.S.: Soluble mouse histocompatibility antigens. Transpl. Proc. **3**, 231–233 (1971).

KOLD, W.P., GRANGER, G.A.: Lymphocyte in vitro cytotoxicity characterization of human lymphotoxin. Proc. Natl. Acad. Sci. **61**, 1250–1256 (1968).

KOLOUCH, F., GOOD, R.A., CAMPBELL, B.: The reticuloendothelial origin of the bone marrow plasma cells in hypersensitivity states. J. Lab. Clin. Med. **32**, 749–755 (1947).

KOSEK, J.C., HURLEY, E.J., LOWER, R.R.: Histopathology of orthotopic canine cardiac homografts. Lab. Invest. **19**, 97–112 (1968).

KOSEK, J.C., HURLEY, E.J., SEWELL, D.H.: Histopathology of orthotopic canine cardiac allografts and its clinic correlation. Transplant. Proc. **1**, 311–315 (1969).

KOUNTZ, S.L., WILLIAMS, M.A., WILLIAMS, P.L., KAPROS, C., DEMPSTER, W.J.: Mechanism of rejection in homotransplanted kidneys. Nature **199**, 257–260 (1963).

KRAKOWER, C.A., GREENSPAN, S.A.: The importance of the included serum proteins in the immune response in rabbits to a rat skin xenograft. Am. J. Pathol. **73**, 549–568 (1973).

KREIS, H., BARBANEL, C.: Preservation of cadaver kidneys. Lancet 2, 1445 (1973).

KREISLER, M., NAITO, S., TERASAKI, P.I.: Cytotoxins in disease. V. Various diseases. Transplant. Proc. 3, 112–114 (1971).

KRETH, H.W., WILLIAMSON, A.R.: Cell surveillance model for lymphocyte cooperation. Nature 234, 454–456 (1971).

KU, G., VARGHEX, Z., FERNANDO, O.N., BAILLOD, R., HOPEWELL, J.P., MOORHEAD, J.F.: Serum IgG and renal transplantation. Br. Med. J. 4, 702–707 (1973).

KUSTER, G.G.R.: Experimental auxiliary liver transplantation in acute liver failure. In: Liver transplantation, LIE, T.S., GÜTGEMANN, A. (eds.), pp. 121–122. Baden-Baden: Witzstrock 1974.

LAGRANGE, P.: Kidney transplantation. Infectious complications of active immunosuppression. Concours Med. 94, 5637–5642 (1972).

LAMON, E.W., SKURZAK, H.M., KLEIN, E., WIGZELL, H.: In vitro cytotoxicity by a nonthymus-processed lymphocyte population with specificity for a virally determined tumor cell surface antigen. J. Exp. Med. 136, 1072–1079 (1972).

LANDY, H., WEIDANZ, W.P.: In: Bacterial endotoxins, LANDY, H., BRAUN, W. (eds.). New Brunswick: Rutgers, the State University 1964.

LANGE, E.M., MEDAWAR, P.B.: Antilymphocytic serum: Its properties and potential. In: Immunobiology, GOOD, R.A., FISHER, D.W. (eds.), pp. 248–256. Stamford: Sinauer Associetes, Inc. 1971.

LANGEN DE, Z.J., JONG DE, B., EIJSINK-SMEETS, M., VRIESENDORP, H.M., JERUSALEM, C., WILDEVUUR, CH.R.H.: Unmodified lung allograft survival related to the major histocompatibility complex in the dog. Eur. Surg. Res. in press 1975.

LAWRENCE, H.S.: Transfer in humans of delayed skin sensitivity to streptococcal M substance and to tuberculin with disrupted leukocytes. J. Clin. Invest. 34, 219–230 (1955).

LAWRENCE, H.S., VALENTINE, F.T.: Transfer factor and other mediators of cellular immunity. Am. J. Pathol. 60, 437–451 (1970).

LAWRENCE, H.S., RAPAPORT, F.T., CONVERSE, J.M., TILLETT, W.S.: Transfer of delayed hypersensitivity to skin homografts with leukocyte extracts in man. J. Clin. Invest. 39, 185–198 (1960).

LAY, N.W., NUSSENZWEIG, V.: Receptor for complement on leukocytes. J. Exp. Med. 128, 991–1001 (1968).

LEANDRI, J.: Some histological features of canine cardiac transplants. Thorax 22, 397–403 (1967).

LEBOWITZ, A.S., LAWRENCE, H.S.: The technique of clonal inhibition: a quantitative assay for human lymphotoxin activity. In: In vitro methods in cell-mediated immunity, BLOOM, B.R., GLADE, P.R. (eds.), pp. 375–379. New York: Academic press 1971.

LEBROS, F., VUILLARD, P., GADOT, P., RADICE, P., LAMOTHE, P., FALCONNET, J., DESCOTES, J.: Étude microscopique du poumon transplanté chez le chien. Arch. Anat. Pathol. 17, 159–166 (1969).

LEMPERLE, G.: Prolonged survival of skin allografts after incubation with recipient DNA or RNA. J. Surg. Res. 8, 511–521 (1968).

LENNERT, K.: Cytologie des ruhenden, aktivierten und entzündeten Lymphknotens. In: Lymphknoten, Diagnostik und Cytologie. Handbuch der speziellen pathologischen Anatomie und Histologie, LENNERT, K. (ed.), Vol. III. Berlin: Springer 1961.

LETTERER, E.: Allgemeine Pathologie. Grundlagen und Probleme. Ein Lehrbuch. Stuttgart: Thieme 1959.

LEVEY, R.H.: Cellular aspects of transplantation immunity. In: Mechanisms of cell-mediated immunity, McCLUSKEY, R.T., COHEN, S. (eds.), pp. 257–287. New York: John Wiley & Sons 1974.

LEVIN, B., MERRILL, J.P.: Immunosuppressive effects of cyclophosphamide and L-asparaginase in the inbred rat renal transplant model. Transplantation 13, 160–163 (1972).

LEVY, M.N.: Oxygen consumption and blood flow in the hypothermic, perfused kidney. Am. J. Physiol. 197, 1111–1114 (1959).

LIE, T.S.: Beitrag zur immunosuppressiven Therapie bei der experimentellen und klinischen Lebertransplantation. Zentralbl. Chir. 95, 1001–1009 (1970).

LIE, T.S., KOLLOCH, R., FASSKE, E., ROESSNER, A.: Inhibition of hyperacute rejection in xenogenic liver transplantation from dog to pig. In: Liver transplantation, LIE, T.S., GÜTGEMANN, A. (eds.), pp. 289–295. Baden-Baden: Witzstrock 1974.

LILLEHEI, R.C., MANAX, W.G.: Organ transplantation: A review of past accomplishments, present problems and future hopes. Anesth. Analg. 45, 707–732 (1966).

LILLEHEI, R.C., GOOTT, B., MILLER, F.A.: The physiological response of the small bowel of the dog to ischemia including prolonged in vitro preservation of the bowel with successful replacement and survival. Ann. Surg. **150**, 543–560 (1959a).

LILLEHEI, R.C., GOOTT, B., MILLER, F.A.: Homografts of the small bowel. Surg. Forum **10**, 197–201 (1959b).

LINDQUIST, K.J., OSTERLAND, C.K.: Human antibodies to vascular endothelium. Clin. Exp. Immunol. **9**, 753–760 (1971).

LINDQUIST, R.R., HAGER, E.B.: Histochemical studies of renal grafts. Ann. N.Y. Acad. Sci. **120**, 52–80 (1964).

LINDQUIST, R.R., GUTTMANN, R.D., MERRILL, J.P.: Renal transplantation in the inbred rat. II. An immunohistochemical study of acute allograft rejection. Am. J. Pathol. **52**, 531–545 (1968a).

LINDQUIST, R.R., GUTTMANN, R.D., MERRILL, J.P., DAMMIN, G.J.: Human renal allograft interpretation of morphologic and immunohistochemical observations. Am. J. Pathol. **53**, 851–881 (1968b).

LINN, B.S., JENSEN, J.A., PORTAL, P., SNYDER, G.B.: Renal xenograft prolongation by suppression of natural antibody. J. Surg. Res. **8**, 211–213 (1968).

LIPPMANN, M.: Transplantation and cytotoxicity changes induced by acid mucopolysaccharides. Nature **219**, 33–36 (1968).

LITTLE, J.R., BRECHER, G., BRADLEY, T.R., ROSE, S.: Determination of lymphocyte turnover by continuous infusion of H3 thymidine. Blood **19**, 236–242 (1962).

LOBUGLIO, A.E., COTRAN, R.S., JANDL, J.H.: Red cells coated with immunoglobulin G: Binding and sphering by mononuclear cells in man. Science **158**, 1582–1585 (1967).

LOHMANN-MATTHES, M.L., SCHIPPER, H., FISCHER, H.: Macrophage-mediated cytotoxicity against allogeneic target cells in vitro. Eur. J. Immunol. **2**, 45–49 (1972).

LOVELOCK, J.E., BISHOP, M.W.H.: Prevention of freezing damage to living cells by dimethylsulfoxide. Nature **183**, 1394–1395 (1959).

LÖWENHAUPT, R.W., NATHAN, P., MENEFEE, M.G.: Correlation of platelet aggregation in canine renal allotransplants with serum cytotoxic antibody following treatment with azathioprine. Transplant. Proc. **3**, 453–456 (1971).

LOWER, R.R., KOSEK, J.C., KEMP, V.E., GRAHAM, W.H., SEWELL, D.H., LIM, F.: Rejection of the cardiac transplant. Am. J. Cardiol. **24**, 492–499 (1969).

LUBBE, F.H., EASTHAM, W.N., HERIC VAN DEN, A.: The significance of early immunoglobulin and β_{1c}-globulin deposition in the arterial walls of transplanted rat kidneys. Transplantation **14**, 649–652 (1973).

LUCY, J.A.: The fusion of biological membranes. Nature **227**, 815–817 (1970).

LUND, B., JENSEN, O.M.: Renal transplantation in rabbits. II. Morphologic alterations in autografts. Acta Path. Microbiol. Scand. **78**, 701–712 (1970).

LYLE, L.R., PARKER, C.W.: New approaches to immunosuppression. Fed. Proc. **33**, 1888–1893 (1974).

MACARIO, A.J.L., MACARIO DE, E.: Low and high affinity antibodies can alternate during the immune response. Nature **245**, 263–264 (1973).

MACKLIN, C.C.: The pulmonary alveolar mucoid film and the pneumonocytes. Lancet **1**, 1088–1099 (1954).

MANAX, W.G., BLOCH, J.H., LONGERBEAM, J.K., LILLEHEI, R.C.: Successful 24 hour in vitro preservation of canine kidney by combined use of hyperbaric oxygenation and hypothermia. Surgery **56**, 275–282 (1964).

MARCEAU, J.P., HALLENBECK, G.A., ZOLLMAN, P.E., BUTLER, H.C., SHORTER, R.G.: A comparison of autoplastic allogeneic and xenogeneic perfusion of isolated kidneys. J. Surg. Res. **5**, 492–502 (1965).

MARCHIORO, T.L., PORTER, A., DICKINSON, T.C., FARIS, T.D., STARZL, T.E.: Physiologic requirements for auxiliary liver homotransplantation. Surg. Gynecol. Obstet. **121**, 17–31 (1965a).

MARCHIORO, T.L., PORTER, K.A., ILLINGWORTH, B., FARIS, T.D., HERRMANN, T.J., SUDWEEKS, A., STARZL, T.E.: The specific influence of nonhepatic splanchnic venous blood flow upon the liver. Surg. Forum **16**, 280 (1965b).

MARGARETTEN, W., MCKAY, D.G.: The effect of leukocyte antiserum on the generalized Shwartzman reaction. Am. J. Pathol. **57**, 299–305 (1969).

MARKHAM, R.V., SUTHERLAND, J.C., MARDINEY, M.R.: The ubiquitous occurrence of immune complex localization in the renal glomeruli of normal mice. Lab. Invest. **29**, 111–120 (1973).

MARTIN, D.C., LUNDAK, R.L.: Histocompatibility testing of renal cells, fibroblasts and lymphocytes. In: Current topics in surgical research, SKINNER, D.R., EHERT, P.A. (eds.), Vol. III, pp. 327–339. New York: Academic Press 1971.

MARTIN, D.C., SCOTT, D.F., DOWNES, G.L., BELZER, F.O.: Primary cause of unsuccessful liver and heart preservation. Cold sensitivity of the ATPase system. Ann. Surg. 175, 111–117 (1972).

MAUGH, T.H.: Tissue cultures: transplantation without immunosuppression. Science 181, 929–931 (1973).

MAY, R.M.: Bibliography of brephoplastic transplantation; addendum No. 1. Transplant. Bull. 6, 458–461 (1959).

MCCLUSKEY, R.T., BENACERRAF, B., MCCLUSKEY, J.W.: Studies on the specificity of the cellular infiltrate in delayed hypersensitivity reactions. J. Immunol. 90, 466–477 (1963).

MCCREIGHT, C.E., ANDREW, W.: Diversity of cell types in epidermis of mouse under normal conditions and following renal application of estrogen. Anat. Rec. 125, 761–775 (1956).

MCCULLAGH, P.: The transfer of immunological tolerance with tolerant lymphocytes. Aust. J. Exp. Biol. Med. Sci. 51, 445–459 (1973).

MCDOWALL, R.A.W., BATCHELOR, J.R., FRENCH, M.E.: Hyperacute rejection and enhancement of rabbit kidney allografts. Lancet 1, 797–801 (1973).

MCGREGOR, D.D., GOWANS, J.L.: Survival of homografts of skin in rats depleted of lymphocytes by chronic drainage from the thoracic duct. Lancet 1, 629–632 (1964).

MCINTYRE, J.A., LAVIA, M.F., PRATER, T.F.K., NIBLACK, G.D.: Studies of the immune response in vitro. I. Ultrastructural examination of cell types and cluster formation and functional evaluation of clusters. Lab. Invest. 29, 703–713 (1973).

MCKEARN, T.L.: Antireceptor antiserum causes specific inhibition of reactivity to rat histocompatibility antigens. Science 183, 94–96 (1974).

MCKENZIE, I.F.C., WHITTINGHAM, S.: Deposits of immunoglobulin and fibrin in human allografted kidneys. Lancet 1, 1313–1316 (1968).

MCLEAN, L.D., ZAK, S.J., VARCO, R.L., GOOD, R.A.: The role of the thymus in antibody production; an experimental study of the immune response in thymectomized rabbits. Transpl. Bull. 4, 21–22 (1957).

MCLENNAN, I.C.M.: Antibody in the induction and inhibition of lymphocyte cytotoxicity. Transplant. Rev. 13, 67–90 (1972).

MCLENNAN, I.C.M., LOEWI, G.: Effect of specific antibody to target cells on their specific and non-specific interactions with lymphocytes. Nature 219, 1069–1070 (1968).

MCLOUGHLIN, G.A.: Proceedings: a method of evaluation of renal preservation techniques. Br. J. Surg. 60, 906 (1973).

MCMILLAN, D.B., ENGELBERT, V.E.: The developmental history of the plasmocyte. Am. J. Pathol. 42, 315–335 (1963).

MEDAWAR, P.B.: The behavior and fate of skin autografts and skin homografts in rabbits. J. Anat. 78, 176–199 (1944).

MEDAWAR, P.B.: A second study of the behavior and fate of skin homografts in rabbits. J. Anat. 79, 157–176 (1945).

MEDAWAR, P.B.: The homograft reaction. Proc. R. Soc. Lond. (Biol.) 140, 145–166 (1958).

MEDZIHRADSKY, J.: Über die lymphatische Drainage der Milzpulpa. Z. Zellforsch. Mikrosk. Anat. 64, 448–465 (1958).

MEEKER, W.R., CONDIE, R.M., GOOD, R.A.: Alteration of the homograft response by antimetabolites. Ann. N.Y. Acad. Sci. 87, 203–213 (1960).

MEJIA-LAGUNA, J.E., MARTINEZ-PALOMA, A., LOPEZ-SORIANO, F., GARCIA-CORNEJO, M., BIRO, C.E.: Prolonged survival of kidney xenografts in leukopenic rabbits. Immunology 21, 879–882 (1971).

MEJIA-LAGUNA, J.E., MARTINEZ-PALOMA, A., BIRO, C.E., CHAVEZ, B., LOPEZ-SORIANO, F., GARCIA-CORNEJO, M.: Morphologic study of the participation of the complement system in hyperacute rejection of renal xenotransplants. Am. J. Pathol. 69, 71–78 (1972).

MELNICK, H.D., FRIEDMAN, H.: Cellular immunity to a purified kidney antigen assessed by macrophage migratory inhibition and MIF release by human leukocytes. Transplant. Proc. 3, 465–469 (1971).

MERCOLA, K.E., HAGADORN, J.E.: Complement-dependent acute immunologic lung injury in an experimental model resembling Goodpasture's syndrome. Exp. Mol. Pathol. 19, 230–240 (1973).

METCALF, D.: The effect of thymectomy on the lymphoid tissues of the mouse. Br. J. Haematol. 6, 324–333 (1960).

METCALF, D.: The thymus: its role in immune response, leukemia development and carcinogenesis. Berlin: Springer 1966.

METCHNIKOFF, E.: Etudes sur la resorption des cellules. Ann. Inst. Pasteur (Paris) 13, 737–769 (1899).

MILGROM, F., KLASSEN, J., FUJI, H.: Immunologic injury of renal homografts. J. Exp. Med. 134, 193–207 (1971).

MILLER, J.F.A.P.: Immunological function of the thymus. Lancet 2, 748–749 (1961).

MILLER, J.F.A.P.: Role of the lymphoid system in homotransplantation reaction; Part 1. Role of the thymus in transplantation immunity. Ann. N.Y. Acad. Sci. 99, 340–354 (1962).

MILLER, J.F.A.P.: Effect of thymic ablation and replacement. In: The thymus in immunobiology, GOOD, R.A., GABRIELSEN, A.E. (eds.), pp. 436–460. New York: Harper 1964.

MILLER, J.F.A.P.: The thymus and transplantation immunology. Br. Med. Bull. 21, 111–117 (1965).

MILLER, J.F.A.P.: Role of the cells which originate from the thymus and bone marrow. Ann. Inst. Pasteur (Paris) 125, 213–229 (1974).

MILLER, J.F.A.P., OSOBA, D.: Current concepts of the immunological function of the thymus. Physiol. Rev. 47, 437–520 (1967).

MILLER, J.F.A.P., MITCHELL, G.F.: Thymus and antigen-reactive cells. Transplant. Rev. 1, 3–42 (1969).

MIMS, M.M.: Hemodynamics of renal transplantation. J. Urol. 86, 493–500 (1961).

MIMS, C.A.: The response of mice to large intravenous injections of ectromelia virus. I. The fate of injected virus. Br. J. Exp. Pathol. 40, 533–542 (1959).

MIRKOVITCH, V., AKUTSU, T., KOLFF, W.J.: Polyurethane aortas in dogs. Three-year results. Trans. Am. Soc. Artif. Intern. Organs 8, 79–84 (1962).

MITCHEL, G.F., MILLER, J.F.A.P.: Cell to cell interaction in the immune response. II. The source of hemolysin forming cells in irradiated mice given bone marrow and thymus or thoracic duct lymphocytes. J. Exp. Med. 128, 821–837 (1968).

MITCHISON, N.A.: Induction of immunological paralysis in two zones of dosage. Proc. R. Soc. London 161, 275–292 (1964).

MITCHISON, N.A.: Mechanism of action of antilymphocyte serum. Fed. Proc. 29, 222–223 (1970).

MITCHISON, N.A.: The carrier effect in the secondary response to haptoprotein conjugates. I. Measure of the effect with transferred cells and objections to the local environment hypothesis. Eur. J. Immunol. 1, 10–17 (1971).

MITCHISON, N.A., DUBE, O.L.: Studies on the immunological response to foreign tumor transplants in the mouse; relation between hemagglutinating antibody and graft resistance in the normal mouse and mice pretreated with tissue preparations. J. Exp. Med. 102, 179–197 (1955).

MODRY, D.L., JIRSCH, D.W., BOEHME, G., OVERTON, T., FISK, R.L., COUVES, C.M.: Hypothermic perfusion preservation of the isolated dog lung. Ann. Thorac. Surg. 16, 583–597 (1973).

MÖLLER, E.: Contact induced cytotoxicity by lymphoid cells containing foreign isoantigens. Science 147, 873–879 (1965).

MÖLLER, G.: Immunocompetent cells in graft rejection. Transplant. Proc. 3, 15–20 (1971).

MÖLLER, G., MÖLLER, E.: The cytotoxic effect of antigenic and/or structural incompatibility in vitro. In: Isoantigens and cell interactions, PALM, J. (ed.), pp. 65–70. Philadelphia: The Wistar Institute Press 1965.

MÖLLER, G., SHEVAG, S.E.: Specifity of lymphocyte-mediated cytotoxicity induced by in vitro antibody-coated target cells. Cell. Immunol. 4, 1–19 (1972).

MONCHIK, G.J., RUSSELL, P.S.: Transplantation of small bowel in the rat: Technical and immunological considerations. Surgery 70, 693–702 (1971).

MOND, J.J., THORBECKE, G.J.: Greater sensitivity to inhibition by anti-immunoglobulin of splenic than of bone marrow B-lymphocytes. J. Immunol. 110, 605–607 (1973).

MOOLTEN, F.L., COOPERBAND, S.R.: Selective destruction of target cells by diphteria toxin conjugated to antibody directed against antigens on the cells. Science 169, 68–70 (1970).

MORI, S., OTA, K., NOBORI, M., INOU, T.: Vascular changes in the pancreaticoduodenal allograft. Vasc. Surg. 2, 61–77 (1968).

MORLEY, J., DUMONDE, D.: Allergic inflammation. I. Simultaneous measurement of vascular permeability to isotope labelled cells and protein in immediate and delayed hypersensitivity. Bibliotheca Anatomica 10, 244–251 (1969).

MORRIS, P.J., YADAV, R.V.S., KINCAID-SMITH, P., ANDERTON, J., HARE, W.S.C., JOHNSON, N., JOHNSON, W., MARSHALL, V.C.: Renal artery stenosis in renal transplantation. Med. J. Aust. 1, 1255–1257 (1971).

MOSIER, D.E.: Cell interactions in the primary immune response in vitro: A requirement for specific cell clusters. J. Exp. Med. 129, 351-362 (1969).

MOSIER, D., CANTOR, H.: Functional maturation of mouse thymic lymphocytes. Eur. J. Immunol. 1, 459–461 (1971).

MOSSER, G., GOOD, R.A., COOPER, M.D.: The immune response and lymphoid tissues of neonatally thymectomized, X-irradiated mice. Int. Arch. Allergy Appl. Immunol. 39, 62–81 (1970).

MOZES, M.F., SHONS, A.R., HARRIS, N.S., MERINO, G.E., MOBERG, A.W., CAMPOS, R.A., NAJARIAN, J.S.: Specificity of the heteroantibody in xenograft rejection. Surg. Forum 22, 244–246 (1971).

MULDER, N.H.: Thymus afhankelijkheid van de humorale immuun-reactie. Thesis, Groningen, The Netherlands 1972.

MUNDTH, E.D., DE FALCO, A.J., JACOBSON, Y.G.: Functional survival of kidneys subjected to extracorporal freezing and reimplantation. Cryobiology 2, 62–67 (1965).

MURRAY, I.M.: Induction of the primary immune response. Nature 217, 430–432 (1968).

MURRAY, J.E., BALANKURA, O., GREENBURG, J.B., DAMMIN, G.J.: Reversibility of the kidney homograft reaction by retransplantation and drug therapy. Ann. N.Y. Acad. Sci. 99, 743–761 (1962).

MURRAY, J.E., WILSON, R.E., TILNEY, N.L.: Five years experience in renal transplantation with immunosuppressive drugs: Survival function, complications and the role of depletion by thoracic duct fistula. Ann. Surg. 168, 416–435 (1968).

MYBURGH, J.A., COHEN, I., GECELTER, L., MEYERS, A.M., ABRAHAMS, C., FURMAN, K.I., GOLDBERG, B., BLERK VAN, P.J.P.: Hyperacute rejection in human-kidney allografts — Shwartzman or Arthus reaction? N. Engl. J. Med. 281, 131–135 (1969).

NAJARIAN, J.S., FELDMAN, J.D.: Passive transfer of tuberculin sensitivity by tritiate thymidine-labeled lymphoid cells. J. Exp. Med. 114, 779–790 (1961).

NAJARIAN, J.S., PERPER, R.J.: Participation of humoral antibody in allogeneic organ transplantation rejection. Surgery 62, 213–220 (1967).

NEIDHARDT, M.: Nebenwirkungen der Immunsuppressiven Therapie. Monatsschr. Kinderheilkd. 120, 210–215 (1972).

NEVILLE, W.E., BALIS, J.U., PIFARRÉ, R., COX, W.D., DWAN, F., LUNCH, R.D., RAPPAPORT, E.S.: The microcirculation of the transplanted heart. J. Thorac. Cardiovasc. Surg. 58, 625–673 (1969).

NICOLAIDES, N.: Skin lipids: their biochemical uniqueness. Science 186, 19–26 (1974).

NIDEN, A.H.: Bronchiolar and large alveolar cell in pulmonary phospholipid metabolism. Science 158, 1323–1324 (1967).

NIEUWENHUIS, P.: On the origin and fate of immunologically competent cells. Thesis, Groningen, The Netherlands 1971.

NOIRCLERC, M., CHAUVIN, G., PONS, R., MALMEJAC, C., COURBIL, J.L., LEBREUIL, G., FIERE, M., DONNAREL, G.: Problèmes techniques et de surveillance dans les transplantation pulmonaires d'après 120 expérimentations. Ann. Chir. Thorac. Cardiovasc. 8, C 331–338 CT 215–222 (1969).

NOIRCLERC, M., SUDAN, N., GROSJEAN, O., PAYAN, H., LEBREUIL, G., OTTE, H., GAYRARD, P.: Ultrastructural study of rejection phenomena in the homografted dog lung. In: Morphology in lung transplantation, WILDEVUUR, CH.R.H., JERUSALEM, C.R., LAUWERIJNS, J.M., WILDEVUUR-VAN HAMERSVELD, C. (eds.), p. 37–45. Basel: Karger 1973.

NOMOTO, K., GERSHON, R.K., WAKSMAN, B.H.: Role of nonimmunized macrophages in rejection of an allotransplanted lymphoma. J. Natl. Cancer Inst. 44, 739–745 (1970).

NORA, J.J., COOLEY, D.A., FERNBACH, D.J., ROCHELLE, D.G., MILAM, J.D., MONTGOMERY, J.R., LEACHMAN, R.D., BUTLER, W.T., ROSSEN, R.D., BLOODWELL, R.D., HALLMAN, G.L., TRENTIN, J.J.: Rejection of the transplanted human heart. Indexes of recognition and problems in prevention. N. Engl. J. Med. 280, 1079–1086 (1969).

NOSSAL, G.J.V.: Various forms of specialization in cells which synthesize immunoglobulins. Ann. Inst. Pasteur (Paris) 125, 239 251 (1974).

NOSSAL, G.J.V., ADA, G.L., AUSTIN, C.M.: Antigens in immunity. IV. Cellular localization of ^{125}I-labelled and ^{131}I-labelled flagella in lymph nodes. Aust. J. Exp. Biol. Med. Sci. 42, 311–330 (1964).

NOSSAL, G.J.V., ADA, G.L., AUSTIN, C.M., PYE, J.: Antigens in immunity. VIII. Localization of ^{125}I-labelled antigens in the secondary response. Immunology 9, 349–357 (1965).

Nossal, G.J.V., Austin, C.M., Pye, J., Mitchell, J.: Antigens in immunity. XII. Antigen trapping in the spleen. Int. Arch. Allergy Appl. Immunol. **29**, 368–383 (1966).

Novoa, W.B., Winer, A.D., Glain, A.J., Schwert, G.W.: Lactic dehydrogenase. V. Inhibition by oxamate and by oxalate. J. Biol. Chem. **234**, 1143–1148 (1959).

O'Connell, T.X., Gonzalez-Lavin, L., Milton, J.D., Mowbray, J.F.: Improved survival in canine heterotopic cardiac transplants without immunosuppression. J. Thorac. Cardiovasc. Surg. **67**, 459–465 (1974).

Ohnishi, H.: Serial measurement of the cortical blood flow in the canine renal allografts during the rejeetion crisis. Arch. Jap. Chir. **38**, 372–393 (1969).

Oluwasanmi, J.O.: The role of hyperimmune alloantiserum in allograft survival. Immunology **25**, 881–889 (1973).

Oort, J., Turk, J.L.: A histological and autoradiographic study of lymph nodes during the development of contact sensitivity in guinea pig. Br. J. Exp. Pathol. **46**, 147–154 (1965).

Ortega, P., Uhley, H.N., Leeds, S.E., Freedman, M., Sampson, J.J.: Serial electron and light microscopic studies on the dog lung in chronic experimental pulmonary edema. Am. J. Pathol. **60**, 57–73 (1970).

Osborne, D.P., Katz, D.H.: The allogeneic effect in inbred mice. I. Experimental conditions for the enhancement of hapten-specific secondary antibody responses by the graft-versus-host reaction. J. Exp. Med. **136**, 439–454 (1972).

O'Toole, C., Perlmann, P., Wigzell, H., Unsgaard, B., Zetterland, C.G.: Lymphocyte cytotoxicity in bladder cancer. No requirement for thymus-derived effector cells. Lancet **1**, 1085–1089 (1973).

Otte, J.B., Lambotte, L., Squifflet, J.P., Moriau, M., Kestens, P.J.: Successful orthotopic transplantation of the canine liver after prolonged preservation by initial perfusion and cold storage. Eur. Surg. Res. **5**, 273–281 (1973).

Owen, J.J.T.: The origins and development of lymphocyte populations. In: Carbon-fluorinecompounds. Chemistry, Biochemistry and biologic activities, pp. 35. A Ciba Foundation Symposium. Amsterdam: North-Holland, 1972.

Owen, J.J.T.: Anatomy of the lymphoid system. In: Biochemistry series one, Kornberg, H.L., Philips, D.C. (eds.) (MTP internal review of science), Vol. X, pp. 35–64. London: Butterworths University Park Press 1974.

Palade, G.E.: Study of fixation for electron microscopy. J. Exp. Med. **95**, 285–298 (1952).

Parker, C.W.: The immunotherapy of cancer. Pharmacol. Rev. **25**, 325–342 (1973).

Parker, L.M., Chused, T.M., Steinberg, A.D.: Immunofluorescence studies on thymocytotoxic antibody from New Zealand black mice. J. Immunol. **112**, 285–292 (1974).

Parrott, D.M., De Sousa, M.A.B., East, J.: Thymus-dependent areas in the lymphoid organs of neonatally thymectomized mice. J. Exp. Med. **123**, 191–204 (1966).

Pasternack, A., Virolainen, M., Häyry, P.: Fine-needle aspiration biopsy in the diagnosis of human renal allograft rejection. J. Urol. **109**, 167–171 (1973).

Patel, R., Terasaki, P.I.: Significance of the positive crossmatch test in kidney transplantation. N. Engl. J. Med. **280**, 735–739 (1969).

Pattengale, P.K., Stahl, W.M., Thorbecke, G.J.: Fate of autogenous canine lymphocytes after injection into an afferent lymphatic of the popliteal lymph node. Am. J. Pathol. **67**, 527–540 (1972).

Patterson, R., Suszko, I.M., Pruzansky, J.J.: In vitro uptake of antigen-antibody complexes by phagocytic cells. J. Immunol. **89**, 471–482 (1962).

Paz, R.A.: Estudio precoz de las lesiones arterio esclerotical cronicas observadas en un homoinjerto renal humano. Medicina **30**, 360–366 (1970).

Penn, I., Corman, J., Gustafsson, A., Halgrimson, C.G., Putnam, W., Schroter, G., Groth, C.G., Starzl, T.E.: Experience in orthotopic liver transplantation. Indications. Result and future prospects. In: Liver transplantation, Lie, T.S., Gütgemann, A. (eds.), pp. 27–38. Baden-Baden: Witzstrock 1974.

Perey, D.Y.E., Frommel, D., Hong, R., Good, R.A.: The mammalian homologue of the avian bursa of Fabricius. Lab. Invest. **22**, 212–227 (1970).

Perlmann, P., Holm, G.: Studies on the mechanism of lymphocyte cytotoxicity. In: Immunopathology, 5th International Symposium, Miescher, P.A., Grabar, P. (eds.), pp. 325–341. Basel: Schwabe 1968.

PERLMANN, P., HOLM, G.: Cytotoxic effects of lymphoid cells in vitro. Adv. Immunol. **11**, 117–193 (1969).

PERLMANN, P., PERLMANN, H., HOLM, G.: Cytotoxic actions of stimulated lymphocytes on allogeneic and autologous erythrocytes. Science **160**, 306–309 (1968).

PERLOFF, L.J., GOODLOE, S., JENIS, E.H., LIGHT, J.A., SPEES, E.K.: Value of one-hour renal allograft biopsy. Lancet **2**, 1294–1295 (1973).

PERPER, R.J.: Renal heterotransplants rejection. A model for separation of humoral and cellular mechanisms. Transplantation **12**, 519–521 (1971).

PERPER, R.J., NAJARIAN, J.S.: Experimental renal heterotransplantation. I. In widely divergent species. Transplantation **4**, 377–388 (1966a).

PERPER, R.J., NAJARIAN, J.S.: Experimental renal heterotransplantation. II. Closely related species. Transplantation **4**, 700–712 (1966b).

PESSAC, B., CALOTHY, G.: Transformation of chick embryo neuroretinal cells by Rous sarcoma virus in vitro: induction of cell proliferation. Science **185**, 709–710 (1974).

PETRIE, C.R., WOODS, J.E.: Successful 24 hour preservation of the canine liver. Arch. Surg. **107**, 461–464 (1973).

PETRIS DE, S., KARLSBAD, G., PERNIS, B., TURK, J.L.: Ultrastructure of cells present in lymph nodes during the development of contact sensitivity. Int. Arch. Allergy Appl. Immunol. **29**, 112–130 (1966).

PIERCE, J.C., HUME, D.M.: The effect of splenectomy on survival of first and second renal homotransplants in man. Surg. Gynecol. Obstet. **127**, 1300–1306 (1968).

PILLAY, V.K.G., KURTZMAN, N.A., MANALIGAD, J.R., JONASSON, O.: Selective thrombocytopenia due to localised microangiopathy of renal allografts. Lancet **2**, 988–991 (1973).

PLANQUE DE, B.A., WILLIAMS, G.M., BORST-EILERS, E., HUME, D.: Antibodies and early human transplants rejection. Transplant. Proc. **3**, 376–379 (1971).

PODLESKI, W.K., PODLESKI, U.G.: Circulating cytotoxic lymphocytes in human tuberculosis. Am. Rev. Resp. Dis. **108**, 791–798 (1973).

POLGE, C., SMITH, A.V., PARKS, A.S.: Revival for spermatozoa after vitrification and dehydration at low temperatures. Nature **164**, 666 (1949).

PORTER, K.A.: Pathological changes in transplanted kidneys. In: Experience in renal transplantation, STARZL, T.E. (ed.). Philadelphia: W.B. Saunders 1964.

PORTER, K.A.: Morphological aspects of renal homograft rejection. Br. Med. Bull. **21**, 171–175 (1965).

PORTER, K.A.: Pathology of the orthotopic homograft and heterograft. In: Experience in hepatic transplantation, STARZL, T.E., PUTMAN, C.W. (eds.), pp. 422–471. Philadelphia: Saunders 1969.

PORTER, K.A., MARCHIORO, T.L., STARZL, T.E.: Pathological changes in six treated baboon to men renal heterotransplants. Br. J. Urol. **37**, 274–284 (1965).

PORTER, K.A., DOSSETOR, J.B., MARCHIORO, T.L., PEART, W.S., RENDALL, J.M., STARZL, T.E., TERASAKI, P.I.: Human renal transplants. I. Glomerular changes. Lab. Invest. **16**, 153–181 (1967).

PORTER, K.A., ANDRES, G.A., CALDER, M.W., DOSSETOR, J.B., HSU, K.C., RENDALL, J.M., SEEGAL, B.C., STARZL, T.E.: Human renal transplants. II. Immunofluorescent and immunoferritin studies. Lab. Invest. **18**, 159–171 (1968).

POSTE, G., ALLISON, A.C.: Membrane fusion reaction: A theory. J. Theor. Biol. **32**, 165–184 (1971).

POTWOROWSKI, E.F., NAIRN, R.C.: Lymphoid-specific antigen: distribution and behavior. Immunology **14**, 591–597 (1968).

POULTER, L.W., TURK, J.L.: Proportional increase in the θ carrying lymphocytes in peripheral lymphoid tissue following treatment with cyclophosphamide. Nature (New Biol.) **238**, 17–18 (1972).

PROCTOR, E., PARKER, R., TURNER, D.: Preservation of the isolated heart for 72 hours: a preliminary report on the development of a heart bank. Guys Hosp. Rep. **118**, 75–84 (1969).

RABINOWITZ, Y., SCHREK, R.: Studies of cell source of macrophages from human blood in slide chambers. Proc. Soc. Exp. Bio. Med. **110**, 429–431 (1962).

RATLIFF, J.L.: Extracorporal support of respiration. In: Human organ support and replacement, HARDY, J.D. (ed.), pp. 240–251. Springfield: C.C. Thomas 1971.

RATNOFF, O.D.: The interrelationship of clotting and immunologic mechanisms. In: Immunobiology, GOOD, R.A., FISHER, D.W. (eds.), pp. 135–144. Stamford: Sinauer Associetes, Inc. 1971.

RAY, P.K., SIMMONS, R.L.: Masking of cellular histocompatibility antigens with phytomitogens. J. Immunol. **110**, 1693–1698 (1973).

READ, J.: The pathological changes produced by anti-lung serum. J. Pathol. Bact. **76**, 403–417 (1958).

REBUCK, J.W., LOGRIPPO, G.A.: Characteristics and interrelationship of the various cells in the RE cell, macrophage, lymphocyte, and plasma cell series in man. Lab. Invest. **10**, 1068–1093 (1961).

REBUCK, J.W., MONTO, R.W., MONAGHAN, E.A., RIDDLE, J.M.: Potentialities of the lymphocyte, with an additional reference to its dysfunction in Hodgkin's disease. Ann. N.Y. Acad. Sci. **73**, 8–38 (1958).

REEMSTMA, K.: Heterotransplantation. Transplant. Proc. **1**, 251–255 (1969).

REEMSTMA, K.: Heterotransplantation: Theoretical considerations. Transplant. Proc. **3**, 49–52 (1971).

REEMSTMA, K., McCRACKEN, B.H., SCHLEGEL, J.V., PEARL, M.A., PEARCE, C.W., DE WITT, C.W., SMITH, P.E., HEWITT, R.L., FLINNER, R.L., CREECH JR., O.: Renal heterotransplantation in man. Ann. Surg. **160**, 384–410 (1964).

REVENTOS, J., VICENS, B., LEON, C., PALACIOS, C.: Early and late effects of pulmonary denervation in the dog. In: Morphology in lung transplantation, WILDEVUUR, CH.R.H., JERUSALEM, C.R., LAUWERIJNS, J.M., WILDEVUUR-VAN HAMERSVELD, C. (eds.), pp. 185–195. Basel: Karger 1973.

REVILLARD, J.P.: Cell-mediated immunity in vitro correlates. Basel: Karger 1971.

RIBET, M., QUANDALLE, P., FLORIN, M., BRENNER, A., HASSOUN, A., GUERIN, F., GROSSELIN, B., CAPRON, A.: Expériences de greffe pulmonaire chez le chien. I. Etude des conséquences de la section-suture bilatérale des troncs souches avec dénervation et dévascularisation bronchiques. II. Homotransplantation. Etude histologique de la réaction de rejet. Lille Med. **14**, 1133–1142 (1969).

RIEDESEL, W.M., ERDAMAR, I., DOS, S.J.: Functional preservation of canine heart-lung preparations by perfusion with pure haemoglobin solution. Nature **243**, 530–531 (1973).

RIFLE, G., TRAEGER, G.: Pregnancy after renal transplantation. An international survey. In: Transplantation Today, Vol. 3, SCHLESINGER, M., BILLINGHAM, R.E., RAPAPORT, F.T. (eds.), pp. 723–728. New York: Grune & Stratten 1975.

RINEHART, J.J., SAGONE, A.L., BALCERZAK, S.P., ACKERMAN, G.A., LE BUGLIO: Effects of corticosteroid therapy on human monocyte function. N. Engl. J. Med. **292**, 236–241 (1975).

RIOUX, C., LECA-CHETOCHINE, F., PARIENTE, R., LALANDE, J., RUFF, F., MAUREL, A., NEVEUX, J.Y., MATHEY, J.: Analysis of degeneration of the isolated dog lung by functional and ultrastructural study after reimplantation. In: Morphology in lung transplantation, WILDEVUUR, CH.H.R., JERUSALEM, C.R., LAUWERIJNS, J.M., WILDEVUUR-VAN HAMERSFELD, C. (eds.), pp. 137–147. Basel: Karger 1973.

ROBERTS, A.N.: Quantitative cellular distribution of tritiated antigen in immunized mice. Am. J. Pathol. **44**, 411–430 (1963).

ROBERTS, A.N., HAUROWITZ, F.: Intracellular localization and quantitation of tritiated antigens in reticuloendothelial tissue of mice during secondary and hyperimmune responses. J. Exp. Med. **116**, 407–422 (1962).

ROBINEAUX, R., PINET, J., KOURLILSKY, R.: Etude morphodynamique de l'îlot réticulaire lymphoplasmocytaire en culture sous membrane de dialyse. C.R. Soc. Biol. **156**, 1025–1032 (1962).

ROELANTS, G.E., FORNI, L., PERNIS, B.: Blocking and re-distribution ("capping") of antigen receptors on T- and B-lymphocytes by anti-immunoglobulin antibody. J. Exp. Med. **137**, 1060–1077 (1973).

ROESSNER, A., LIE, T.S., SCHULZ, D.V., BASSEWITZ, D.B., THEMANN, H.: Zur Feinstruktur der orthotop transplantierten allogenen Hundeleber. Virchows Arch. (Zellpathol.) **9**, 354–370 (1971).

ROESSNER, A, LIE, T.S., SCHULZ, D.V., BASSEWITZ, D.B., THEMANN, H.: The ultrastructure of the orthotopic transplanted allogeneic dog liver. In: Liver transplantation, LIE, T.S., GÜTGEMANN, A. (eds.), pp. 131–133. Baden-Baden: Witzstrock 1974.

ROESSNER, A., FASSKE, E., LIE, T.S., KOLLOCH, R., V. BASSEWITZ, D.B., THEMANN, H.: Zur Feinstruktur der hyperakuten Abstoßung xenogener Lebertransplantate. Beitr. Pathol. **147**, 119–132 (1972).

ROGERS, S., SLAPAK, M.: An evaluation of two predictive tests of eventual kidney function, p. 79. Abstracts of the 5th International Congress of the Transplantation. Society, Jerusalem 1974.

ROOD VAN, J.J.: Leucocyte grouping. A method and its application. Thesis, Leiden, The Netherlands 1962.

ROOD VAN, J.J.: Tissue typing and organ transplantation. Lancet **1**, 1142–1146 (1969).

ROSENAU, W.: Interaction of lymphoid cells with target cells in tissue culture. In: Cell bound antibodies, AMOS, B., KOPROWSKI, H. (eds.), pp. 75–80. Philadelphia: Wistar Institute Press 1963.

ROSENAU, W., LEE, J.C., NAJARIAN, J.S.: A light, fluorescence, and electron microscopic study of functioning human renal transplants. Surg. Gynecol. Obstet. **128**, 62–76 (1969).

ROSENAU, W., GOLDBERG, M.L., BURKE, G.C.: Early biochemical alterations induced by lymphotoxin in target cells. J. Immunol. **111**, 1128–1135 (1973).

ROSENTHAL, A.S., SHEVACH, E.M.: The function of macrophages in antigen recognition by guinea pig T-lymphocytes. I. Requirement for histocompatible macrophages and lymphocytes. J. Exp. Med. **138**, 1194–1212 (1973).

ROSENTHAL, A.S., DAIRE, J.M., ROSENSTREICH, D.L., CEHRS, K.U.: Antibody-mediated internalization of B-lymphocyte surface membrane immunoglobulin. Exp. Cell Res. **81**, 317–329 (1973).

ROSS, H., WERTHER, M.: Kidney preservation. Lancet **1**, 867 (1974).

ROSSEN, R.D., BUTTER, W.T., JOHNSON, A.H., MITAL, K.K.: Immunofluorescent and serologic studies of the humoral antibody response to cardiac allotransplantation in man. Transplant. Proc. **3**, 445–448 (1971).

ROWLANDS JR., D.T., VANDERBEEK, R.B., SEIGLER, H.F., EBERT, P.A.: Rejection of canine cardiac allografts. Am. J. Pathol. **53**, 617–629 (1968).

ROWLEY, D.A., GOWANS, J.L., ATKINS, R.C., FORD, W.L., SMITH, M.E.: The specific selection of recirculating lymphocytes by antigens in normal and preimmunized rats. J. Exp. Med. **136**, 499–513 (1972).

ROWLEY, D.A., FITCH, F.W., STUART, F.P., KÖHLER, H., COSENZA, H.: Specific suppression of immune responses. Science **181**, 1133–1141 (1973).

RUDDLE, N.H., WAKSMAN, B.H.: Cytotoxicity mediated by soluble antigen and lymphocytes in delayed hypersensitivity. J. Exp. Med. **128**, 1267–1279 (1968).

RUIZ, J.O., UCHIDA, H., SCHULTZ, L.S., LILLEHEI, R.C.: Problems in absorption and immunosuppression after entire intestinal allotransplantation. Am. J. Surg. **123**, 297–303 (1972).

RUSSEL, S.W., ROSENAU, W., LEE, J.C.: Cytolysis induced by human lymphotoxin cinemicrographic and electron microscopic observations. Am. J. Pathol. **69**, 103–111 (1972).

RYGAARD, J., POVLSEN, C.O.: Proceedings of the first international workshop on nude mice. Stuttgart: Gustav Fischer 1974.

SACKS, S.A., PETRISCH, P.H., KAUFMAN, J.J.: Canine kidney preservation using a new perfuse. Lancet **1**, 1024–1028 (1973).

SACKS, S.A., PETRISCH, P.H., LEONG, C.H., KAUFMAN, J.J.: Experiments in renal preservation: 48 and 72 hours canine kidney preservation by initial perfusion and hypothermic storage. J. Urol. **3**, 434–438 (1974).

SAHIAR, K., SCHWARTZ, R.S.: The immunoglobulin sequence. II. Histological effects of the suppression of gamma-M and gamma-G antibody synthesis. Int. Arch. Allergy Appl. Immunol. **28**, 52–68 (1966).

SALFNER, B., VOIGTMANN, R., UHLENBRUCK, G.: Isolation and characterization of transplant antigens with the purpose of induction of immune tolerance. In: Liver transplantation, LIE, T.S., GÜTGEMANN, A. (eds.), pp. 249–251. Baden-Baden: Witzstrock 1974.

SALVATIERRA, JR. O., COHRUM, K., BELZER, R.O.: Patient survival in renal transplantation, p. 192. Abstracts of the 5th International Congress of the Transplantation Society, Jerusalem 1974.

SARLES, H.E., RENMERS, A.R., FISH, J.C., CANALES, C.O., THOMAS, F.D., TYSON, K.R.T., BEATHARD, G.A., RITZMANN, S.E.: Depletion of lymphocytes for the protection of renal allografts. Arch. Intern. Med. **125**, 443–450 (1970).

SARLES, H.E., SMITH, G.H., ASCH, J.C.: Observations concerning human lymphocyte homeostasis during prolonged thoracic duct lymph diversion. Tex. Rep. Biol. Med. **25**, 573–583 (1967).

SAUNDERS, A.M., BIEBER, CH.: Pathologic findings in a case of cardiac transplantation. J.A.M.A. **206**, 815–820 (1968).

SCARPELLI, E.M., WOLFSON, D.R., COLACICCO, G.: Protein and lipid-protein fractions of lung washings: immunological characterization. J. Appl. Physiol. **34**, 750–753 (1973).

SCHALM, L.: Heterotopic auxiliary liver transplantation. I. A physiological concept of functional competition. Arch. Chir. Neerl. **18**, 283–284 (1966).

SCHALM, S.W.: Liver preservation without perfusion. Folia Med. Neerl. **15**, 198–206 (1972).

SCHALM, L., SCHALM, S.W.: The concept of functional competition in auxiliary liver grafting.

In: Liver transplantation, LIE, T.S., GÜTGEMANN, A. (eds.), pp. 117–122. Baden-Baden: Witzstrock 1974.

SCHALM, L., BAX, H.R., MANSENS, B.J.: Atrophy of the liver after occlusion of the bile ducts or portal vein and compensatory hypertrophy of the unoccluded portion and its clinical importance. Gastroenterology 31, 131–155 (1956).

SCHALM, S.W., V.D. WAAY, D., HENDRIKS, W.D.H., JERUSALEM, C., POPESCU, D.T., KROM, R.A.F., TERPSTRA, J.L.: Orthotopic liver transplantation. An experimental study on the prevention of infections with gram-negative organisms. Br. J. Surg. 62, 513–517 (1975).

SCHIRRMACHER, V., RUBIN, B., PROSS, H., WIGZELL, H.: Cytotoxic immune cells with specifity for defined soluble antigens. IV. Antibody as mediator of specific cytotoxicity. J. Exp. Med. 139, 93–107 (1974).

SCHLOERB, B.R., WALDORF, R.D., WELSH, J.S.: The protective effect of kidney hypothermia on total renal ischemia. Surg. Forum 8, 633–635 (1957).

SCHLOERB, B.R., WALDORF, R.D., WELSH, J.S.: The protective effect of kidney hypothermia on total renal ischemia. Surg. Gyn. Obstet. 109, 561–565 (1959).

SCHLOSSMAN, S.F., BEN-EFRAIM, S., YRRON, A.: Immunochemical studies on the antigenic determinants required to elicit delayed and immediate hypersensitivity reactions. J. Exp. Med. 123, 1083–1095 (1966).

SCHMIDT, K., STUNKAT, R., HELLER, W.: Bestimmung der Hämolyse nach einer neuen Mikromethode bei Operationen mit der Herz-Lungen-Maschine. Med. Welt. 25, 98–102 (1974).

SCHWARTZ, R.S.: Immunosuppression: the challenge of selectivity. In: Immunobiology, GOOD, R.A., FISHER, D.W. (eds.), pp. 240–256. Stamford: Sinauer Associates, Inc. 1971.

SCHWARTZ, R.S., EISNER, A., DAMESHEK, W.: The effect of 6-mercaptopurine on primary and secondary immune responses. J. Clin. Invest. 38, 1394–1403 (1959).

SCOTHORNE, R.J., McGREGOR, I.A.: Cellular changes in lymph nodes and spleen following skin homografts in the rabbit. J. Anat. 89, 283–292 (1955).

SEEGAL, B.C., HASSON, M.W., GAYNOR, E.C., ROTHENBERG, M.S.: Glomerulonephritis produced in dogs by specific antisera. I. The course of the disease resulting from injection of rabbit antidog-placenta serum or rabbit antidog-kidney serum. J. Exp. Med. 102, 789–805 (1955).

SEIDEL, W., AKUTSU, T., MIRKOVITCH, V., KOLFF, W.J.: A mitral valve prosthesis and a study of thrombosis on heart valves in dogs. J. Surg. Res. 2, 168–175 (1962).

SEKIGUCHI, N., HAYATA, Y., HAGIWARA, K., YOSHIOKA, T., KANEKO, H., KADOWAKI, O.: Histological studies on the isolated human lung. In: Morphology in lung transplantation, WILDEVUUR, CH.R.H., JERUSALEM, C.R., LAUWERIJNS, J.M., WILDEVUUR-VAN HAMERSVELD, C. (eds.), pp. 128–136. Basel: Karger 1973.

SELA, M.: Antigen design and immune response. In: The Harvey Lectures, AXELROD, J., BENACERRAF, B., BERG, P., BOYSE, E.A., DOLE, V.P., GOOD, R.A., MERRIFIELD, B., OLD, L.J., SELA, M. (eds.), pp. 213–246. New York: Academic Press 1973.

SELL, S.: Development of restrictions in the expression of immunoglobin specifities by lymphoid cells. Transplant. Rev. 5, 19–44 (1970).

SELL, S., GELL, P.G.H.: Studies on rabbit lymphocytes in vitro. I. Stimulation of blast transformation with anti-allotype serum. J. Exp. Med. 122, 423–440 (1965).

SELLS, R.A., PENA, J.R.: Preservation of cadaveric kidneys for transplantation. Lancet 2, 539–542 (1970).

SELLS, R.A., McLOUGHLIN, G.A.: Ischaemia times in renal transplants. Lancet 1, 801 (1974).

SEMB, G., KROG, J., JOHANSEN, K.: Renal metabolism and blood flow during local hypothermia studied by means of renal perfusion in situ. Acta Chir. Scand. 253, 196–202 (1960).

SERCARZ, E.E., COONS, A.H.: The absence of antibody-producing cells during unresponsiveness to BSA in the mouse. J. Immunol. 90, 478–491 (1963).

SHARMA, H.M., MOORE, S., MERRICK, H.W., SMITH, M.R.: Platelets in early hyperacute allograft rejection in kidneys and their modification by sulfinpyrazone (Anturan) therapy. Am. J. Pathol. 66, 445–460 (1972).

SHARMA, H.M., ROSENSWEIG, J., CHATTERJEE, S., MOORE, S., DE CHAMPLAIN, M.L.: Platelets in hyperacute rejection of heterotopic cardiac allografts in presensitized dogs. Am. J. Pathol. 70, 155–173 (1973).

SHARP, J.A., BURWELL, R.G.: Interaction (peripolesis) of macrophages and lymphocytes after skin homografting or challenge with soluble antigens. Nature 188, 474–475 (1960).

SHEFFIELD, J.B., EMMELOT, P.: Studies on plasma membranes. XVI. Tissue specific antigens in the liver cell surface. Exp. Cell Res. **71**, 97–105 (1972).

SHEIL, A.G.R.: Pathologic changes in canine renal allografts with prolonged function. Aust. J. Exp. Biol. Med. Sci. **47**, 55–62 (1969).

SHEIL, A.G.R., MURRAY, J.E.: Sensitized rejection of second renal allografts in dogs after long function of first renal allografts. Preliminary communication. Surgery **64**, 954–957 (1968).

SHEIL, A.G.R., ROGERS, J., MAY, J., STOREY, B., KURUVILA, J.T., GEORGE, C., BERRY, F.R., STEWART, J.H.: Simplified technique for human auxiliary liver transplantation. Am. J. Surg. **117**, 359–362 (1969).

SHEVACH, E.M., ROSENTHAL, A.S.: The function of macrophages in antigen recognition by guinea pig T-lymphocytes. II. Role of macrophages in the regulation of genetic control of the immune response. J. Exp. Med. **138**, 1213–1229 (1973).

SIEGEL, I.: Autologous macrophages-thymocyte interactions. J. Allerg. **46**, 190–194 (1970).

SIMONSEN, M., BUEMANN, J., GAMMELTOFT, A., JENSEN, F., JØRGENSEN, K.: Biological incompatibility in kidney transplantation in dogs. Acta Pathol. Microbiol. Scand. **32**, 1–108 (1952).

SIMMONS, R.L., TOLEDO-PEREYRA, L.H.: Masking kidney graft antigens with phytomitogens, p. 100. Abstracts of the 5th International Congress of the Transplantation Society, Jerusalem 1974.

ŠIŠKA, K., HOLEC, V., FEDELEŠOVÁ, M., ZIEGELHÖFFER, A., SLEZAK, J., STYK, J., PETRÁŠ, J., TRÉGEROVÁ, V.: Investigation of heterotopically transplanted dog hearts after preservation. Transplantation **9**, 93–109 (1970a).

ŠIŠKA, K., HOLEC, V., FEDELEŠOVÁ, M., ZIEGELHÖFFER, A., SLEZAK, J., STYK, J., PETRÁŠ, J., TRÉGEROVÁ, V.: Investigation of heterotopically transplanted dog hearts after preservation. Eur. Surg. Res. **2**, 203–212 (1970b).

SISKIND, G.W.: Selective immunosuppression using antigens and antibodies as pharmacologic agents. Fed. Proc. **33**, 1886–1888 (1974).

SLAPAK, M., LEE, H.M., HUME, D.M.: Transplant lung—a new syndrome. Br. Med. J. **1**, 80–84 (1968).

SLEE, G., HENNEVELD, L., VRIESENDORP, H.M., WESTBROEK, D.L.: ABO antigens and "natural occurring" antibodies against ABO antigens in the dog. Eur. Surg. Res. **4**, 350 (1972).

SMITH, R.T., ADLER, W.H., TAKIGUCHI, T., PEAVY, D., BAUSHER, J.: Studies of cellular recognition in vitro: Role of T-lymphocytes and some effects of a lymphoblast—derived inhibitor of cell proliferation. In: Cell interactions and receptor antibodies in immune responses, MAKELA, O., CROSS, A., KOSUNEN, T.U. (eds.), pp. 399 410. New York: Academic Press 1971.

SNELL, G.D.: The homograft reaction. Ann. Rev. Microbiol. **11**, 439–458 (1957).

SNELL, G.D., WINN, H.J., STIMPFLING, J.H., PARKER, S.J.: Depression by antibody of the immune response to homografts and its role in immunological enhancement. J. Exp. Med. **112**, 293–314 (1960).

SNYDER, G.B., BALLESTEROS, E., ZARCO, R.M., LINN, B.S.: Prolongation of renal xenografts by complement suppression. Surg. Forum. **17**, 478–480 (1966).

SOUSA DE, M.A.B., PARROTT, D.M.V.: Induction and recall in contact sensitivity, changes in skin and draining lymph nodes of intact and thymectomized mice. J. Exp. Med. **130**, 671–690 (1969).

SPECK, B.: Möglichkeiten und Probleme der klinischen Knochenmarktransplantation. Med. Welt. **26**, 39–42 (1975).

SPENCER, H. (ed.): Pathology of the lung. Oxford: Pergamon Press 1968.

SPITLER, L.E., FUDENBERG, H.H.: Products of interaction of antigensensitized leukocytes and antigen: Further characterization of the mitogenic factor. J. Immunol. **104**, 544–549 (1970).

SPRENT, J., MILLER, J.F.A.P., MITCHELL, G.F.: Antigen-induced recruitment of circulating lymphocytes. Cell. Immunol. **2**, 171–181 (1971).

STARK, R.B., DWYER, E.M., DEFOREST, M.: Effect of surgical ablation of regional lymph nodes on survival of skin homografts. Ann. N.Y. Acad. Sci. **87**, 140–148 (1960).

STARZL, T.E. (ed.): Experience in renal transplantation. Philadelphia: Saunders 1964.

STARZL, T.E.: The current status of liver transplantation. In: Immunobiology, GOOD, R.A., FISHER, D.W. (eds.), pp. 195–208. Stamford: Sinauer Associetes, Inc. 1971.

STARZL, T.E.: Discussion remarks. In: Liver transplantation, LIE, T.S., GÜTGEMANN, A. (eds.), pp. 301 304. Baden-Baden: Witzstrock 1974a.

STARZL, T.E.: Discussion remarks. In: Liver transplantation, LIE, T.S., GÜTGEMANN, A. (eds.), pp. 53–54. Baden-Baden: Witzstrock 1974b.

STARZL, T.E., PUTMAN, C.W.: Experience in hepatic transplantation. Philadelphia: Saunders 1969.

STARZL, T.E., KAUPP, JR. H.A., BROCK, D.R., LAZARUS, R.E., JOHNSON, R.V.: Reconstructive problems in canine liver homotransplantation with special reference to the postoperative role of hepatic venous flow. Surg. Gynecol. Obstet. 111, 733–743 (1960).

STARZL, T.E., MARCHIORO, T.L., HERMANN, G., BRITTAIN, R.S., WADDELL, W.R.: Renal homografts in patients major donor-recipient blood group incompatibilities. Surgery 55, 195–200 (1964a).

STARZL, T.E., MARCHIORO, T.L., HUNTLEY, R.T., RIFKIND, O., ROWLANDS, D.T., DICKINSON, T.C., WADDELL, W.R.: Experimental and clinical homotransplantation of the liver. Ann. N.Y. Acad. Sci. 120, 739–765 (1964b).

STARZL, T.E., LERNER, R.A., DIXON, F.J., GROTH, C.G., BRETTSCHNEIDER, L., TERASAKI, P.I.: Shwartzmann reaction after human renal homotransplantation. N. Engl. J. Med. 278, 642–648 (1968).

STARZL, T.E., PUTNAM, C.W., HALGGIMSON, C.G.: Renal transplantation under cyclophosphamide. Transplant. Proc. 4, 461–464 (1972).

STASTNY, P.: Bound immunoglobulin and complement in heart allografts undergoing rejection. Transplantation 10, 248–257 (1970).

STATES, B., HOLTZAPPLE, P., ROSENHAGEN, M., SEGAL, S.: Effect of hypothermic storage of kidney slices on membrane ATP-ase and electrolyte transport. Kidney int. 2, 17–21 (1972).

STAUDACHER, C., DI CARLO, V., BEVILACQUA, G., BRAGHERIO, G., SIBILLA, E., STAUDACHER, V.: Ultrastructural changes in canine lung allografts. In: Morphology in lung transplantation, WILDE-VUUR, CH.R.H., JERUSALEM, C.R., LAUWERIJNS, J.M., WILDEVUUR-VAN HAMERSVELD, C. (eds.), pp. 46–63. Basel: Karger 1973.

STENZEL, K.H., STUBENBORD, W.T., WHITSELL, J.C., CHEIGH, J.S., LEWY, J.E., SULLIVAN, J.F., RIGGIO, R.R., TAPIA, L.S., RUBIN, A.L.: Kidney transplantation: Results of a multidisciplinary, kidney center approach, p. 193. Abstracts of the 5th International Congress of the Transplantation Society, Jerusalem 1974.

STEWART, G.J., RITCHIE, W.G.M., LYNCH, P.R.: Venous endothelial damage produced by massive sticking and emigration of leukocytes. Am. J. Pathol. 74, 507–532 (1974).

STINSON, E.B., DONG, E., BIEBER, C.P., POPP, R.L., SHUMWAY, N.E.: Cardiac transplantation in man. II. Immunosuppressive therapy. J. Thorac. Cardiovasc. Surg. 58, 326–337 (1969).

STOCKERT, R.J., MORELL, A.G., SCHEINBERG, I.H.: Mammalian hepatic lectin. Science 186, 365–366 (1974).

STOERK, H.C.: Cortisone and immunity to homoiogeneous tissue loss of "individual differentials" from tissues of cortisone-treated rats. Ann. N.Y. Acad. Sci. 56, 742–747 (1953).

STROBER, S., GOWANS, J.L.: The role of lymphocytes in the sensitization of rats to renal homografts. J. Exp. Med. 122, 347–361 (1965).

STUART, F.P., SAITOM, T., FITCH, F.W.: Rejection of renal allografts: specific immunologic suppression. Science 160, 1463–1465 (1968).

STUART, F.P., BUSTEIN, E., HOLTER, A., FITCH, F.W., ELKINS, W.L.: Role of passenger leukocytes in the rejection of renal allografts. Transplant. Proc. 3, 461–464 (1971).

STUEBER, P., KOVACS, S., KOLETSKY, S., PERSKY, L.: Regional renal hypothermia. Surgery 44, 77–83 (1958).

STUMP, M.M., JORDAN, G.L., DEBAKEY, M.E., HALPERT, B.: Endothelium growth from circulating blood on isolated intravascular dacron hub. Am. J. Pathol. 43, 361–367 (1963).

STUTMAN, O.: Tumor development after 3-methylcholanthrene in immunological deficient athymic nude mice. Science 183, 534–536 (1974).

SUNG, D.T., WOODS, J.E.: Forty-eight-hour preservation of the canine liver. Ann. Surg. 179, 422–426 (1974).

SUMMERLIN, W.T., CHARLTON, E., KARASEK, M.J.: Transplantation of organ cultures of adult human skin. J. Invest. Dermatol. 55, 310–316 (1970).

SUMMERLIN, W.T., BROUTBAR, C., FOANES, R.B., PAYNE, R., STUTMAN, O., HAYFLICH, L., GOOD, R.A.: Acceptance of phenotypically differing cultured skin in man and mice. Transplant. Proc. 5, 707–710 (1973).

SUROS, J., WOODS, J.E.: Twenty-four hour preservation of the canine heart. J. Surg. Res. 16, 672–678 (1974).

SUTHERLAND, D.E.R., HOWARD, R.J., NAJARIAN, J.S.: Immunological enhancement of renal allografts in an outbred animal susceptible to hyperacute rejection. Fed. Proc. 32, 971 (1973).

SUZUKI, C., NAKADA, T., FUJIMURA, S.: Immunohistological assessment of mononuclear cells in canine lung allografts undergoing rejection. In: Morphology in lung transplantation, WILDEVUUR, CH.R.H., JERUSALEM, C.R., LAUWERIJNS, J.M., WILDEVUUR-VAN HAMERSVELD, C. (eds.), pp. 112–117. Basel: Karger 1973.

SZULMAN, A.E.: The histological distribution of blood group substances A and B in man. J. Exp. Med. 111, 785–800 (1960).

TANAKA, Y., LIDDY, T.J.: Lipids and acid phosphatase in cultured lymphocytes of peripheral blood. A histochemical and electron microscopic study. Lab. Invest. 15, 455–463 (1966).

TANAKA, Y., GOODMAN, J.R.: Electron microscopy of human blood cells. In: New York: Harper and Row 1972.

TAYLOR, R.B.: Cellular cooperation in the antibody response of mice to two serum albumins: specific function of thymus cells. Transplant. Rev. 1, 114–149 (1969).

TAYLOR, R.B., DUFFUS, P.H., RAFF, M.I., DE PETRIS, S.: Redistribution and pinocytosis of lymphocyte surface immunoglobulin molecules induced by immunoglobulin antibody. Nature (New Biol.) 233, 225–229 (1971).

TERASAKI, P.: Significance of HLA-typing in human organ transplantation. In: Liver transplantation, LIE, I.S., GÜTGEMANN, A. (eds.), pp. 191–193. Baden-Baden: Witzstrock 1974.

TERASAKI, P.I., MARCHIORO, T.L., STARZL, T.E.: Sero-typing of human lymphocyte antigens: preliminary trials on long-term kidney homograft survivors. In: Histocompatibility testing, TERASAKI, P.I. (ed.), pp. 83–96. Washington, O.C.: National Academy of Science 1965.

TERASAKI, P.I., MICKE, M.R., SINGAL, P.D., MITTAL, K.K., PATEL, R.: Serotyping for homotransplantation. XX. Selection of recipients for cadaver donor transplants. N. Engl. J. Med. 279, 1101–1103 (1968).

THEMANN, H., ROESSNER, A., FASSKE, E., LIE, T.S., KOLLOCH, R., V. BASSEWITZ, D.B.: On the ultrastructure of hyperacute rejection of xenogeneic liver grafts. In: Liver transplantation, LIE, T.S., GÜTGEMANN, A. (eds.), pp. 297–298. Baden-Baden: Witzstrock 1974.

THIEL, G., MOPPERT, J., MAHLICH, J., BUHLER, F., FISCHER, T., ENDERLIN, F., WEBER, H., ZOLLINGER, H.V.: Glomerular damage after intravenous administration of antilymphocyte globulin (ALG) in man and rhesus monkeys. Transpl. Proc. 3, 741–744 (1971).

THOMAS, F., LEE, H.M., WOLF, J., PIERCE, J.C., HUME, D.: Long term (8–12 year) prognosis in related and unrelated renal transplantation. In: Transplantation Today, vol. 3, SCHLESINGER, M., BILLINGHAM, R.E., RAPAPORT, F.T. (eds.), pp. 707–711. New York: Grune & Stratten 1975.

THOMSON, J.G.: Production of severe atheroma in a transplanted human heart. Lancet 2, 1088–1092 (1969).

THOMPSON, E., LEWIS, C.M., PEGRUM, G.D.: Changes in antigenic nature of lymphocytes caused by common viruses. Br. Med. J. 4, 709–711 (1973).

THORBECKE, G.J.: Germinal centers and immunological memory. In: Lymphatic tissue and germinal centers in immune response. Advances in Exp. Med. and Biology, FIORE-DONATI, L., HAMA, M.G. (eds.), Vol. V, pp. 83–92. New York: Plenum Press 1969.

THORBECKE, G.J., JACOBSON, E.B., ASOFSKY, R.: γ-Globulin and antibody formation in vitro. IV. The effect on the secondary response of X-irradiation given at varying intervals after a primary injection of bovine-γ-globulin. J. Immunol. 92, 734–746 (1964).

TINBERGEN, W.J.: Rat kidney transplantation. An evaluation of immunosuppression. Thesis, Leiden, The Netherlands 1971.

TISON, V., BARUZZI, G.: Anatomical aspects of transplanted lung. Lancet 1, 266–267 (1969).

TOLEDO-PEREYRA, L.H., CONDIE, R.H., MALMBERG, R., SIMMONS, R.L., NAJARIAN, J.S.: A fibrinogen-free plasma perfusate for preservation of kidneys for one hundred and twenty hours. Surg. Gynecol. Obstet. 138, 901–905 (1974a).

TOLEDO-PEREYRA, L.H., SIMMONS, R.L., NAJARIAN, J.S.: Two-to-three day intestinal preservation utilizing hypothermic pulsatile perfusion. Ann. Surg. 179, 454–459 (1974b).

TOLEDO-PEREYRA, L.H., SIMMONS, R.L., NAJARIAN, J.S.: Prolonged survival of canine orthotopic small intestinal allografts preserved for 24 hours by hypothermic bloodless perfusion. Surgery 75, 368–376 (1974c).

TRAEGER, J., CARRAZ, M., RIES, D., PERRIN, J., SAUBIER, E., BERNHARDT, J., BONNET, P., ARCHIMBAUD, J.: Studies of anti-lymphocyte globulins made from thoracic duct lymphocytes. Transplant. Proc. 1, 455–459 (1969).

TRENTIN, J.J.: The arterial obliterative lesions of human renal homografts. Ann. N.Y. Acad. Sci. 129, 654–656 (1966).

TRUMP, B.F., BULGER, R.E.: Experimental modification of lateral and basilar plasma membranes and extracellular compartments in the flounder nephron. Fed. Proc. **30**, 22–41 (1971).

TUBERGEN, D.G., FELDMAN, J.D.: The role of thymus and bone marrow cells in delayed hypersensitivity. J. Exp. Med. **134**, 1144–1153 (1971).

TURK, J.L.: Action of lymphocytes in transplantation. J. Clin. Pathol. Suppl. **20**, 423–429 (1967).

TURK, J.L., POULTER, L.W.: Selective depletion of lymphoid tissue by cyclophosphamide. Clin. Exp. Immunol. **10**, 285–296 (1972).

TURK, J.L., STONE, S.H.: Implications of the cellular changes in lymph nodes during development and inhibition of delayed type hypersensitivity. In: Cell bound antibodies, AMOS, B., KOPROWSKI, H. (eds.), pp. 51–60. Philadelphia: Wistar Institute Press 1963.

TURNER, M.D.: Organ storage. In: Human organ support and replacement, HARDY, J.D. (ed.). Springfield: C.C. Thomas 1971.

TYAN, M.L., NESS, D.B.: Modification of the mixed leukocyte reaction with various antisera. Transplantation **13**, 198–201 (1972).

TYSON, R.R., LAUTSCH, E.V., DI PIETRANTONIO, S., REICHLE, F.A.: Endothelialization of arterial prothetics. In: Current topics in surgical research, SKINNER, D.B., EBERT, P.A. (eds.), Vol. III, pp. 1–19. New York: Academic Press 1971.

UHR, J.W., BAUMANN, J.B.: Antibody formation. I. The suppression of antibody formation by passively administrated antibody. J. Exp. Med. **113**, 935–957 (1961).

UNANUE, E.R., DIXON, F.J.: Experimental glomerulonephritis. V. Studies on the interaction of nephrotoxic antibodies with tissues of the rat. J. Exp. Med. **121**, 697–714 (1965).

UPHOFF, D.E.: Immunological tolerance: The modified self-recognition hypothesis. J. Natl. Cancer Inst. **42**, 255–268 (1969).

VALENTINE, F.T., LAWRENCE, H.S.: Lymphocyte stimulation: transfer of cellular hypersensitivity to antigens in vitro. Science **165**, 1014–1016 (1969).

VANWIJCK, R., SIMAR, L.J., LEJEUNE, G.: Infiltrats mononuclées en transplantation rénale allogénique expérimentale. Société Belge de Biologie **162**, 2324–2327 (1968).

VEITH, F.J., BLUMENSTOCK, D.A.: Lung transplantation. J. Surg. Res. **1**, 33–55 (1971).

VEITH, F.J., LUCKS, R.J., MURRAY, J.E.: The effects of splenectomy on immunosuppressive regimens in dog and man. Surg. Gynecol. Obstet. **121**, 299–308 (1965).

VEITH, F.J., SIEGELMAN, S.S., HAGSTROM, J.W.C., RICHARDS, K., SINHA, S.B.P.: Advances in lung transplantation. Transplant. Proc. **3**, 519–523 (1971).

VEITH, F.J., HAGSTROM, J.W.C., ANDERSON, W.R., KOERNER, S.K., HARDY, J.D., MAGOVERN, G.J., WHITE, J.J., MCLEAN, L.D., BUCHERL, E.S., NASSERI, M., HAJATA, Y., TSUJI, Y., GAGO, O., LOGAN, A., BEALL, A.C., COOLEY, D.A., HALLMAN, G., DEROM, F., ROSS, D.N., JOHNSON, H.R.M., STEVENS, A., VAN DER HOEFF, P., KAHN, D., LILLEHEI, C.W., HAGLIN, J.J.: Alveolar manifestation of rejection: An important cause of the poor results with human lung transplantation. Ann. Surg. **175**, 336–348 (1972a).

VEITH, F.J., SINHA, S.B.P., DOUGHERTY, J.C., BECKER, N.H., SIEGELMAN, S.S., HAGSTROM, J.W.C.: Nature and evolution of lung allograft rejection with and without immunosuppression. J. Thorac. Cardiovasc. Surg. **63**, 509–520 (1972b).

VEITH, F.J., SINHA, S., SIEGELMAN, S.S., GLIEDMAN, M.L., HAGSTROM, J.W.C.: Canine lung allograft rejection with and without immunosuppression. In: Morphology in lung transplantation, WILDEVUUR, CH.R.H., JERUSALEM, C.R., LAUWERIJNS, J.M., WILDEVUUR-VAN HAMERSVELD, C. (eds.), pp. 85–95. Basel: Karger 1973.

VELDMAN, J.E.: Histophysiology and electron microscopy of the immune response. Thesis, Groningen, The Netherlands 1970.

VOGT, W., HAUSSMANN, P., BOHLE, A.: Über die lympho-epithelialen Beziehungen in menschlichen Nierentransplantaten. Klin. Wochenschr. **48**, 1327–1330 (1970).

VOLKMAN, A., GOWANS, J.L.: The production of macrophages in the rat. Br. J. Exp. Pathol. **46**, 50–61 (1965a).

VOLKMAN, A., GOWANS, J.L.: The origin of macrophages from bone marrow in the rat. Br. J. Exp. Pathol. **46**, 62 70 (1965b).

VRIESENDORP, H.M.: Major histocompatibility of the dog. Thesis, Rotterdam, The Netherlands 1973.

WAGENVOORT, C.A., WAGENVOORT, N., WILDEVUUR, CH.R.H.: Morphological changes in long-term denervated and reimplanted lungs. In: Morphology in lung transplantation, WILDEVUUR, CH.R.H., JERUSALEM, C.R., LAUWERIJNS, J.M., WILDEVUUR-VAN HAMERSVELD, C. (eds.), pp. 223–235. Basel: Karger 1973.

WAGNER, H.: Synergy during in vitro cytotoxic allograft responses. I. Evidence for cell interaction between thymocytes and peripheral T-cells. J. Exp. Med. **138**, 1379–1397 (1973 a).

WAGNER, H.: Cell-mediated immune responses in vitro: Interaction of thymus derived cells during cytotoxic allograft responses in vitro. Science **181**, 1170–1172 (1973 b).

WAGNER, H., WYSS, C.: Cell-mediated immune responses in vitro. V. A comparative study of in vitro immunogenicity of splenic lymphocytes, neoplastic lymphoid cells and fibroblasts. Eur. J. Immunol. **3**, 549–555 (1973).

WAKEFIELD, J.D., THORBECKE, G.J.: Relationship of germinal centers in lymphoid tissue to immunological memory. I. Evidence for the formation of small lymphocytes upon transfer of primed splenic white pulp to syngeneic mice. J. Exp. Med. **128**, 153–169 (1968 a).

WAKEFIELD, J.D., THORBECKE, G.J.: Relationship of germinal centers in lymphoid tissue to immunological memory. II. The detection of primed cells and their proliferation upon cell transfer to lethally irradiated syngeneic mice. J. Exp. Med. **128**, 171–187 (1968 b).

WALKER, S.M., LUCAS, Z.J.: Cytotoxic activity of lymphocytes. II. Studies on mechanism of lymphotoxin mediated cytotoxicity. J. Immunol. **109**, 1233–1244 (1972).

WANG, N.S., HUANG, S.N., SHELDON, H., THURLBECK, W.M.: Ultrastructural changes of Clara and type II alveolar cells in adrenalin-induced pulmonary edema in mice. Am. J. Pathol. **62**, 237–252 (1971).

WARD, P.A., REMOLD, H.G., DAVID, J.R.: Leukotactic factor produced by sensitized lymphocytes. Science **163**, 1079–1081 (1969).

WARNER, N.L., SZENBERG, A.: Immunologic studies on hormonally bursectomized and surgically thymectomized chickens: Dissociation of immunologic responsiveness. In: The thymus in immunobiology, GOOD, R.A., GABRIELSEN, A.E. (eds.), pp. 395–411. New York: Harper (Hoeber) 1964.

WARNIER, B., JERUSALEM, C., JAP, P., HESS, F., HEYDE VAN DE, M.N.: The ultrastructural and histochemical aspect of auxiliary heterotopic rat liver homografts up to 22 months. In: Liver transplantation, LIE, T.S., GÜTGEMAN, A. (eds.), pp. 135–141. Baden-Baden: Witzstrock 1974.

WARREN, B.A., DE BONO, A.H.B.: The ultrastructure at early rejection phenomena in lung homografts in dogs. Br. J. Exp. Pathol. **50**, 593–599 (1969).

WATKINS, G.M., PRENTIS, N.A., COUGH, N.P.: Successful 24-hour preservation with simplified hyperosmolar hyper-kalemic perfusate. Transplant. Proc. **3**, 612–615 (1971).

WATSON, J.: The role of humoral factors in the initiation of in vitro immune responses. III. Characterization of thymus cell replacing factors. J. Immunol. **111**, 1301–1313 (1973).

WEBB, W.R.: Discussion remarks. Ann. Surg. **169**, 904–905 (1969).

WEBBER, M.M.: Allograft survival following antibody suppression with radioiodine-labelled antigen. Transplantation **5**, 1198–1203 (1967).

WEGMANN, R., LÉGER, L., MONSALLIER, F., CHAPUIS, Y., LENRIOT, J.P., LEMAIGRE, G., CHARBONNIER, A.: Etude métabolique cellulaire d'un foie humain d'hépatite fulminante et d'un foie de babuin transplanté en hétérotopie sur les vaisseaux fémoreauz de la patiente. C.R. Acad. Sci. (Serie D) **269**, 2113–2116 (1969).

WEIL, R., REEMTSMA, K.: The mechanism of xenograft rejection. In: Liver transplantation, LIE, T.S., GÜTGEMANN, A. (eds.), pp. 273–276. Baden-Baden: Witzstrock 1974.

WEISS, L.: Interaction of sensitized lymphoid cells and homologous target cells in tissue culture and in grafts: An electron microscopic and immunofluorescent study. J. Immunol. **101**, 1346–1362 (1968).

WEISS, M.L., DIGIUSTI, D.L.: Active immunization against Plasmodium berghei malaria in mice. Am. J. Trop. Med. Hyg. **15**, 472–482 (1966).

WEISSMANN, G., ZURIER, R.B., HOFFSTEIN, S.: Leukocytic proteases and the immunologic release of lysosomal enzymes. Am. J. Pathol. **68**, 539–563 (1972).

WEISSMANN, G., DINGLE, T.: Release of lysosomal protease by ultraviolet irradiation and inhibition by hydrocortisone. Exp. Cell Res. **25**, 207–210 (1961).

WELCH, L.T., FLANIGAN, W.J.: Kidney preservation. Lancet **2**, 1444–1445 (1973).

VAN DER WERF, A.J.M.: Immunologisch enhancement en bescherming van zwangerschap. Thesis, Nijmegen, The Netherlands 1972.

WESSLEN, T.: Passive transfer of tuberculin hypersensitivity by mobile lymphocytes from thoracic duct. Acta Tubercol. Scand. **26**, 38–53 (1952).

WEYMOUTH, R.J., SEIBEL, H.R., LEE, H.M., HUME, D.M., WILLIAMS, G.M.: The glomerulus in man one hour after transplantation. An electron microscopic study. Am. J. Pathol. **58**, 85–104 (1970).

WHITTINGHAM, S., MACKAY, I.R., IRWIN, J.: Autoimmune hepatitis: Immunofluorescence reactions with cytoplasm of smooth muscle and renal glomerular cells. Lancet **1**, 1333–1335 (1966).

WIDDICOMBE, J.G.: Respiratory reflexes. In: Handbook of physiology. Respiration, Sect. 3. FENN, W.O., RAHN, H. (eds.), pp. 585–630. Washington: Am. Physiol. Soc. 1964.

WILDEVUUR, CH.H.R., VAN DEN BROEK, A.A., JERUSALEM, C.R.: Prolonged lung allograft survival in T-cell deprived (T.D.) dogs. Eur. Surg. Res. **5**, 50 (1973a).

WILDEVUUR, CH.H.R., JERUSALEM, C.R., LAUWERIJNS, J.: Morphological alterations after simultaneous bilateral lung homotransplantation under various conditions. In: Morphology in lung transplantation, WILDEVUUR, CH.R.H., JERUSALEM, C.R., LAUWERIJNS, J.M., WILDEVUUR-VAN HAMERSVELD, C. (eds.), pp. 96–111. Basel: Karger 1973b.

WILLIAMS, R., CALNE, R.Y., ANSELL, I.D., ASHBY, R.S., CULLUM, P.A., DAWSON, J.L., EDDLESTON, A.L.W.F., EVANS, O.B., FLUTE, P.T., HERBERTSON, P.M., JOYSEY, V., MCGREGOR, A.M.C., MILLARD, P.R., MURRAY-LYON, I.R., RAKE, M.O., SELLS, R.A.: Liver transplantation in man — III. Studies of liver function, histology and immunosuppressive therapy. Br. Med. J. **3**, 12–19 (1969).

WILLIAMS, G.M., ALVAREZ, C.A.K.: Host repopulation of the endothelium in allografts of kidney and aorta. Surg. Forum **20**, 293–294 (1969).

WILLIAMS, G.M., LEE, H.M., WEYMOUTH, R.F., HARLAN, W.R., HOLDEN, K.R., STANLEY, C.M., MILLINGTON, G.A., HUME, D.M.: Studies in hyperacute and chronic renal homograft rejection in man. Surgery **62**, 204–212 (1967).

WILLIAMS, G.M., HUME, D.M., HUDSON, R.P., MORRIS, P.J., KANO, K., MILGROM, F.: "Hyperacute" renal homograft rejection in man. N. Engl. J. Med. **279**, 611–618 (1968).

WILSON, C.B., DIXON, F.J., FORTNER, J.G., CERILLI, G.J.: Glomerular basement membrane-reactivite antibody in anti-lymphocyte globulin. J. Clin. Invest. **50**, 1525–1535 (1971).

WILSON, D.B.: The reaction of immunologically activated lymphoid cells against homologous lymphoid cells against homologous target tissue cells in vitro. J. Cell. Comp. Physiol. **62**, 273–286 (1963).

WILSON, D.B.: Quantitative studies on the behavior of sensitized lymphocytes in vitro. I. Relationship of the degree of destruction of homologous target cells to the number of lymphocytes and the tissue of contact in culture and consideration of the effects of isoimmune serum. J. Exp. Med. **122**, 143- 166 (1965).

WILSON, D.B., BILLINGHAM, R.E.: Lymphocytes and transplantation immunity. Adv. Immunol. **7**, 189–273 (1967).

WISLÖFF, F., FRÖLAND, S.S.: Antibody-dependent lymphocyte-mediated cytotoxicity in man: No requirement for lymphocytes with membrane-bound immunoglobulin. Scand. J. Immunol. **2**, 151–157 (1973).

WOLF, J.S., FAWLEY, J.C., HUME, D.M.: In vitro quantitation of lymphocyte and serum cytotoxic activity following renal homograft rejection in man. Transplant. Proc. **3**, 449–452 (1971).

WOGLOM, W.H.: Immunity to transplantable tumor. Cancer review **4**, 129–314 (1929).

WOLBERG, G., HIEMSTRA, K., BURGE, J.J., SINGLER, R.C.: Reversible inhibition of lymphocyte-mediated cytolysis by dimethyl sulfoxide (DMSO). J. Immunol. **111**, 1435–1443 (1973).

WOODROW, J.C.: Rh immunisation and its prevention. Ser. Haematol. **3**, 1–151 (1970).

WOODRUFF, M.F.A., FORMAN, B.: Evidence for production of circulating antibodies by homografts of lymphoid tissue and skin. Br. J. Exp. Pathol. **31**, 306–315 (1950).

WOODRUFF, M.F.A., ANDERSON, N.A.: Effect of lymphocyte depletion by thoracic duct fistula and administration of antilymphocytic serum on the survival of skin homografts in rats. Nature **200**, 702 (1963).

WRIGHT, P.W.: Studies on the mechanism of immunological enhancement of tumor homografts: Demonstration of specific tolerance to homograft H-2 isoantigens. In: Advance in Transplantation, DAUSSET, J., HAMBURGER, J., MATHÉ (eds.), pp. 41–45. Oslo: Munksgaard 1968.

WRIGHT, P.W., HARGREAVES, R.E., BANSAL, S.C., BERNSTEIN, I.D., HELLSTRÖM, K.E.: Allograft tolerance: Presumptive evidence that serum factors from tolerant animals that block lymphocyte mediated immunity in vitro are soluble antigen-antibody complexes. Proc. Natl. Acad. Sci. **70**, 2539–2543 (1973).

YU, D.T.Y., CLEMENTS, P.J., PAULUS, H.E.: Human lymphocyte subpopulations: effect of corticosteroids. J. Clin. Invest. **53**, 240–246 (1974).

ZANDER, E.: Changes in blood vessels (capillary fragility) with inflammation. J. Exp. Med. **66**, 637–651 (1937).

ZELDER, O., HESS, F., JERUSALEM, C.R.: The influence of environmental factors on the fate of the rat auxiliary liver homograft. Eur. Surg. Res. **5**, 132 (1973).

ZEMBALA, M., PLAK, W., HANCZAKOWSKA, M.: Macrophage and lymphocyte cooperation in target cell destruction in vitro. Clin. Exp. Immunol. **15**, 461–466 (1973).

ZIMMERMANN, G., HELL, E.: Transplantation und Gefrierkonservierung des Pankreas am Hund. Langenbecks Arch. Chir. **328**, 328–348 (1971).

ZIMMERMANN, W.E., REHFELD, K.H.: Function and importance of the RES-system during perfusion with different solutions for the preservation and transplantation of the liver. In: The reticuloendothelial system and immune phenomena, DI LUZIO, N.R. (ed.), pp. 119–127. New York: Plenum Press 1971.

ZMIJEWSKI, C.M., ZMIJEWSKI, H.E., HUNEYCUTT, H.C.: The relationship of the frequences of white cell antibodies and red cell antibodies in the sera of multiparous women. Int. Arch. Allergy **32**, 574–582 (1967).

ZOLLINGER, R.M., LINDEN, M.C., FILLER, R.M., CORSON, J.M., WILSON, R.E.: Effect of thymectomy on skin-homograft survival in children. N. Engl. J. Med. **270**, 707–709 (1964).

ZÜHLKE, V.: Das Verhalten der Serum-Lipoproteine und Serum-Immunglobuline nach homologen Nierentransplantationen beim Menschen. Langenbecks Arch. Chir. **322**, 542–547 (1968).

Bone Transplantation in Animals and in Man

Leonhard Schweiberer and Florian Eitel

With 11 Figures

A. Introduction and Historical Review

Theories concerning the various types of bone transplant — autograft, homograft, or heterograft; fresh or deep-frozen, chemically preserved, or macerated — have been subject to fluctuation ever since Ollier (1867) laid the scientific groundwork for free bone transplants. The literature that has grown up around the many problems of free bone transplantation is so vast as to be almost unassimilable. This is why we mention here only the most significant papers that have contributed to its historical development.

Ollier in his writings emphasized the supreme importance of the periosteum in the regeneration of bone transplants. He further believed that, when the periosteum was transplanted along with the bone, it sustained life in the hard bone substance to which it was attached. He was also the first to make a distinction between transplanting one part of the body tissue to another part of the same body (autografting), transplanting tissue from one individual to another of the same species (homografting), or from one individual to another of a different species (heterografting). Because he observed regeneration induced by the transplanted periosteum only in auto- and homografts, but never in heterografts, he did not advise the use of animal bone for surgical purposes. Ollier's teaching was to determine the course of events for many years.

Barth (1893, 1894, 1895) demonstrated that even on auto- and homografts with a covering of periosteum, the hard bone substance always dies off, to be replaced by hard bone substance produced by local tissue capable of ossification. However, Barth's research was all done on the replantation of trepanized portions of skull and did not take particular account of the behavior of the periosteum. He assumed that the transplanted bone tissue was always reconstructed from the layer of bony tissue. In his opinion the periosteum played no particular role in the reconstruction process, but simply died off.

In the end it was G. Axhausen (1908a, b, 1909) who cleared up the contradiction between the still current theories based on the views of Ollier and Barth and surgical practice. He did this on the basis of histologic studies of surgical specimens and a large series of experimental transplants. He showed that in fresh periosteum-covered transplants from the same species, the hard bone substance always degenerated whereas the periosteum, or most of it, survived; both the deposition of new bone on the necrotic transplanted bone tissue and the early stage of regeneration of the dead bone started from the periosteum. G. Axhausen's work indicated that the difference between auto- and homografting was less a matter of quality than of quantity: in autografts more of the soft bone tissue survived, thus generally permitting more vigorous bone production and more rapid turnover. In heterografts, on the other hand, he noted a complete absence of osteogenic activity.

In all the early research, scientific interest was focused on the periosteum and the adherent cortical bone. It was not until 1932 that Matti, following extensive animal experiments and excellent clinical results in the treatment of pseudarthrosis, pointed out that the vital factor was the transplantation of autologous cancellous bone.

In modern clinical applications preference is given to the use of the cancellous bone autograft. The change from the use of cortical bone to cancellous bone — quite apart from the high osteogenic value of the latter, which is discussed in detail below — can be ascribed in no small measure to the fact that in the past the cortical transplant also served the purpose of stabilization, whereas in modern surgery sophisticated internal fixation techniques take care of stabilization, so that the graft has only to trigger the process of osteogenesis, bridge the gap, and fill bone defects.

B. Anatomy and Physiology of Intact Bone

A basic knowledge of the structural elements of bone and their physiologic behavior is essential for an understanding of the biological reactions that occur after bone transplantation.

1. Structural Elements of Bone

Bone has three basic components: cells, the organic stroma, and calcium phosphate crystals. During the development of the embryo, bone is laid down on the pattern of the cartilage by the mesenchymal cells. These mesenchymal cells are predetermined for osteogenesis and seem to be osteogenic stem cells; they are the origin of all the cellular elements of bone and appear later as periosteum, endosteum, contents of the Haversian canals, and osteocytes.

1.1. Osteoblasts

Recent research with tritiated thymidine has shown that only the stem cells take up this building block of DNA synthesis and pass it on through numerous mitoses to their daughter cells, the osteoblasts. Mitoses are rare in osteoblasts and have little influence on their total number (Kember, 1960; Tonna, 1961; Young, 1962). The generation cycle of stem cells from mitosis to mitosis averages

36 hours in the tibial metaphysis of rats (YOUNG, 1962). The cells then undergo transformation to preosteoblasts or osteoblasts, or remain in the developmental stage of stem cells. An osteoblast remains active for only about 3 days, after which it is incorporated into the bone tissue as an osteocyte; during this period the osteoblast produces two to three times its own volume of intercellular substance (OWEN, 1963). However, not all osteoblasts are incorporated as osteocytes; the fate of the majority has still to be elucidated. It is probable that most of them return to the reservoir of stem cells (YOUNG, 1962). This assumption rests on the observation that necrotic or degenerating cells are very seldom seen. Alternatively, they may be degraded with the release of hyaluronidase and disappear into the bone matrix (KNESE and KNOOP, 1958).

1.2. Osteoclasts

Osteoclasts probably have the same origin as osteoblasts. There is some difficulty in determining where they originate, mainly because in normal, undisturbed development they appear only at certain times of life and only in particular parts of the skeleton (HANCOX, 1956; KNESE and KNOOP, 1961; KNESE, 1963; YOUNG, 1963). Osteoclasts labeled with ^{3}H do not undergo mitosis and usually contain one labeled nucleus and never more than two (TONNA, 1961). Osteoclasts are therefore thought to be formed by the union of several cells. As with osteoblasts, degenerating or necrotic cells are seldom observed. It seems likely that, in this case too, when the osteoclasts have ceased their function, they are reincorporated into the mesenchymal reservoir from which they came (YOUNG, 1962). Polynuclear osteoclasts are extremely rare under physiologic conditions. Nevertheless, it is clear that if bone is being continuously regenerated, it must also be resorbed. Certainly, morphologists consider the polynuclear osteoclast to be the usual type of bone-resorbing cell, but it is possible that resorption may also be effected by mononuclear osteoclasts (KÖLLIKER, 1873; EGER, 1960, 1963; KNESE, 1963).

It follows that osteoblasts and osteoclasts are simply transitional forms of the osteogenic mesenchymal cells, in other words, they represent different functional states of the same cell. It is the tissue medium that determines cell specialization with regard to function (YOUNG, 1963; PUTSCHAR, 1963).

Whether the pluripotent mesenchymal cells can be considered universal stem cells is controversial. It is more likely that the mesenchyme itself is derived from several sources (presumptive germinal areas) and that the presumptive skeletal areas are laid down very early (KNESE, 1966). The cells of the supporting tissue series thus cannot be traced back to one mesenchymal cell; theirs is a polyphyletic rather than a monophyletic pedigree. The cells of the primordial skeleton are not undifferentiated but are destined from the start for specific tasks.

1.3. Osteocytes

When osteoblasts are transformed into osteocytes by incorporation into the ground substance, they retain the mitochondria and enzymes proper to osteoblasts (Putschar, 1963). They form some ground substance and the boundary sheath, while the lacunae become smaller and the osteocyte is inactivated (Lipp, 1954; Dudley and Spiro, 1961). Under pathologic conditions osteocytes can be reactivated and the lacunae enlarged by resorption. In these circumstances, alkaline phosphatase is again shown to be present (Rutishauser and Majno, 1951). The normal fate of the osteocyte is cell death, after which the lacunae fill up with mineral substance. Frost (1960) called this micropetrosis. We do not know whether osteocytes liberated by osteoclastic resorption return to the mesenchymal reservoir.

1.4. Collagen

The organic components of osseous stroma are collagenous fibers and the amorphous intercellular substance, a semifluid colloid system of proteins and proteoglycans. The collagenous fibers are produced by the osteoblasts and are laid down in a definite order. They make up a fabric with several levels of organization (Rollet, 1871; Petersen, 1927, 1930; Knese et al., 1954; Fleisch, 1961). Each fiber is made up of protofibrils. The elasticity of bone is due to the spiral arrangement of the three polypeptide chains that make up the collagen molecule and the way in which the fibers are laid down.

1.5. Amorphous Intercellular Substance

The amorphous intercellular substance is an unstructured material consisting mainly of proteoglycans, and it is also derived from osteoblasts and osteocytes. Its formation commences with the appearance around the osteoblasts and osteocytes of an intercellular substance that is metachromotropic and reacts to periodate. It is noted that there is a close topographic association between reactivity to periodate and phosphatase activity (Moog and Wenger, 1952). Neutral and acid mucopolysaccharides also occur in the form of chondroitin sulfate. As in cartilage, this substance binds to protein to give proteoglycan (Eger, 1960). The proteoglycans are initially bound to the fibrous structure but rapidly disperse throughout the osteoid tissue and form an integrating component of the juvenile trabeculae. During the phases of ossification and resorption, the intercellular substance shows enhanced reactivity to periodate, particularly in the vicinity of cells (Heller and Steinberg, 1951).

During the formation of osteons, even in the adult organism, the proteoglycans are neutral when liberated and are only secondarily esterified prior to mineralization. Autoradiographic studies (Duthie and Barker, 1955a) have shown that appositional bone growth is accompanied by increased synthesis of chondroitin sulfate.

Even in mature bone, proteoglycans are continously synthesized by the osteocytes. Periodate-reactive proteoglycans are found in osteocytes; these granular substances are, to a degree, indicators of bone-tissue activity (Heller, 1950; Heller and Steinberg, 1951).

The following information was obtained from a very thorough study of fracture healing in the rat (Duthie and Barker, 1955b): 48 hours after fracture, hyperplasia of the periosteal cells is seen in the inner cambium layer, with simultaneous intra- and intercellular metachromotropia and ^{35}S activity: The cambium cells form a sulfomucopolysaccharide containing matrix into which nearly all the sulfur is incorporated. These very interesting observations of mucopolysaccharide metabolism were obtained by means of autoradiography with the radioisotope in inorganic form (DZIEWIATKOWSKI, 1952, 1954; BELANGER, 1954; DAVIES and YOUNG, 1954; FRIBERG and RINGERTZ, 1954, 1956; AMPRINO, 1955). The periosteal blastema that has formed after 7 days is characterized by its high ^{35}S activity. After 10 days an amorphous metachromotropic substance is observed between chondrocytes; on day 14 metachromotropia and radioactivity are further intensified in the matrix. After 21 days the start of enchondral ossification is apparent in the metachromotropic and radioactive areas.

Within 2 hours of death—and this observation has important implications for transplantation—a slight increase in periodate reactivity occurs in the bone tissue. Clearly, this is not due to a decalcification effect but is an expression of the depolymerization caused by fermentation (GRAUMANN, 1964).

It can be deduced from the above findings that the highly polymerized mucopolysaccharideprotein complex is an essential building block for bone ground substance. The bone matrix can display considerable biochemical reactivity under certain physiologic and pathophysiologic conditions.

1.6. Hydroxyapatite

The hard substances of bone consist, for the most part, of the crystalline calcium phosphate known as hydroxyapatite. The crystals are deposited on the collagenous fibers in a special order. The apatite crystals in bone have been shown to be present in the form of thin plates of about $400 \times 200 \times 50$ Å (ROBINSON and WATSON, 1953), having a surface area of more than $200 \ \mathrm{m^2/g}$ of the salt. Only about one-quarter of the crystal surface is in contact with the intercellular fluid because of the way the crystals lie on top of one another (FLEISCH, 1961). The large surface area ensures constant ion exchange with the intercellular fluid which, in turn, is in exchange with the blood.

2. Transformation of Bone Tissue

2.1. Physiologic Transformation

Throughout life, bone is subject to continuous transformation (BURKHARDT and PETERSEN, 1928; DEMETER and MATYAS, 1928; HEULER, 1928; AMPRINO and BAIRATI, 1939; LIPP, 1954; PONLOT, 1960; ENLOW, 1963; WAGNER, 1965); the process is most active in youth, declining in intensity with age. During the growth period ossification predominates; between the ages of 20 and 50 years ossification and resorption are in balance, with the mass of bone substance remaining constant; in old age ossification declines, resulting in slow depletion of the bone tissue (WAGNER, 1965). The turnover rate varies tremendously in different parts of the skeleton and is about three times faster in cancellous bone than in compact bone (Frost, 1964).

Bone transformation is effected by means of cellular activity. The fact that the osteocytes retain their extraordinary capacity right into old age is due in no small measure to the continuous, very slow regeneration undergone by the skeleton (Uehlinger and Puls, 1967). Some very careful research has been done on this by means of modern methods and great progress has been made as a result: autoradiography (Ponlot, 1960), as well as microradiography (Sissons et al., 1959), and fluorescence microscopy of juvenile bone tissue labeled with tetracycline (Milch et al., 1957). Radioisotope studies in particular have revealed that bone tissue, or its components, is subject to continuous transformation, characterized by constant ion exchange and the reforming of complicated protein compounds. The process goes on, not only on the surface of bone tissue, but also in the interior, and is kept in equilibrium by intra- and extraosseous regulatory mechanisms. The interior surface areas include not only the surfaces of capillaries and cells but also all interfaces between the microcrystals and the organic intermediate substance (Eger, 1962).

This constant ossification and resorption occurs at small foci which, under physiologic conditions, are generally some 100–1000 μ in length, measured along the longitudinal axis of the osteon. There appears to be a "field effect" involved, causing stimulation of the resting osteogenic stem cells, expressed in either bone-forming or bone-resorbing activity (Cohen and Harris, 1958). Resorption by osteoclasts proceeds much faster than ossification, the activity of 100 osteoblasts being required to fill the defect caused by one osteoclast.

In the case of transformation in the interior of bone, the newly formed bone substance is deposited in thin seams of osteoid. The osteoblasts lie side by side in single-row cell position and deposit the matrix on the old bone as it is secreted. Along with the organic matrix, the osteoblasts secrete alkaline phosphatase. This enzyme plays an important part in the mineralization of the uncalcified matrix, which contains a great deal of tissue water (Robison, 1932; Gomori, 1941; Majno and Rouiller, 1951; Dulce, 1960; Fleisch and Neuman, 1960; Fleisch, 1961, 1967). At 10 days after activation of the osteoblasts, calcium salts appear in the osteoid and within 4 days they make up 70% of the total mineral content (Frost, 1963). Subsequent mineralization proceeds with increasing slowness, extending over many years. Mineral uptake in maturing and mature bone tissue is due less to the "calcium-capturing property" of the acid mucopolysaccharides than to the ability of the neutral mucopolysaccharides to absorb phosphatase (Eger, 1960), which then combines with the calcium ions to form bone salt. Calcification can occur in a great variety of tissues, given the right conditions. Ossification, however, cannot take place unless a bone matrix is present to provide the necessary basic shape.

2.2. Adaptation of Bone to Mechanical Forces

The continuous regeneration of bone that occurs under physiologic conditions receives a tremendous stimulus from any change in physiologic stress. Mechanical forces induce the maintenance, reinforcement, destruction, or redistribution of bone structure. Heavy stressing has been shown to cause elastic dislocation of the collagen fibrils in lamellar bone; an impulse is then sent via the canal system to activate the osteocytes. The bone tissue reacts to such external stimuli with transformation processes that continue for weeks and even months (TISCHEN-DORF, 1951). Piezoelectric forces have recently been invoked as intermediaries between mechanical stress and cell activity (JOHNSON, 1951; ALLGÖWER, 1967).

Acute stress situations evoke a physiologic response within seconds (FUKADA and YASUDA, 1957; BASSETT and BECKER, 1962; BASSETT, 1964; PERREN and STRAUMANN, 1967). Acute bending stress instantly induces the formation of a negative potential on the concave surface. The bone acts as a semiconductor, with the apatite-crystal-collagen unit operating like the positive-negative contact of a diode system (BASSETT and BECKER, 1962). Negative potentials have been measured on the regions under compression and positive potentials on the regions under tension. It has been demonstrated experimentally that, by passing a constant 1 mA current, a bone callus can be induced between the poles and appear as vigorous bone formation at the cathode. This fact fits in with the observation that bending evokes a negative potential on the concave surface of bone. Bone adapts to stress by appositional growth (ALLGÖWER, 1967). Currents in excess of 1000 mA induce resorption (JASUDA *et al.*, 1955).

2.3. Pathologic Bone Transformation

The bone transformation processes that occur in patients with systemic disease are particularly impressive; they are ultimately due to a change in the activity of the osteogenic cells and loss of equilibrium between osteoblasts and osteoclasts. In the rare condition of osteogenesis imperfecta, the activity of the osteoblasts is inhibited, which reduces both the quality and the quantity of new bone formed. In osteopetrosis, or marble bone disease, it is the osteoclasts that are affected, with partial inhibition of both primary and secondary transformation (PUTSCHAR, 1963). In osteoporosis the relationships are less clearcut and morphologically hard to account for. Until recently the cause of osteoporosis was thought to be depression of bone formation due to an imbalance between anabolic and catabolic steroids (ALBRIGHT and REIFENSTEIN, 1948). Today we know that osteoporosis is due not so much to reduced bone formation as to accelerated resorption (HEANEY, 1962; FROST, 1963; LANDRY and FLEISCH, 1964; JOWSEY, 1965). The resorbing cells include, in addition to polynuclear osteoclasts or mononuclear osteolyocytes, osteocytes (BELANGER, 1965). The demineralization process is followed by degradation of the organic matrix by proteolytic enzymes. The overriding control mechanism is now known to be the parathyroid hormone and calcitonin. With increasing calcium loss, or hypocalcemia, the bone mineral is liberated by hormonal action. If the cause of the hypocalcemia is not remedied, there is accelerated deossification, leading to osteoporosis. This is an example of the adaptation of bone to unphysiologic stress (FLEISCH, 1967).

C. Bone Transplantation

The previous chapter dealt with the anatomy of bone and its transformation under both physiologic and pathologic conditions. This topic is important because we may assume that bone transformation in grafts follows the same course and is subject to the same natural laws. It is scarcely likely that biological laws that apply to tissular, cellular, and humoral reactions do not apply in the same way to transplantation, so long as certain, quite specific preconditions are satisfied. Two of the most important of these are (1) that the graft has an adequate blood supply and (2) that the transplant is autologous tissue.

1. Blood Supply to Transplanted Bone Tissue

Research on fresh, nondecalcified microsections from fracture zones has shown that osteocytes in the walls of the Haversian system, when cut off from their blood supply, survived for 1 to 2 weeks before nuclear pyknosis and cytoplasmic disintegration set in (Schenk and Willenegger, 1964).

A bone graft is completely cut off from its blood vessels; the survival of its cellular elements depends on the graft bed from which it is supplied by diffusion or revascularization. Diffusion and revascularization in turn, depend upon the shape and structure of the graft, since the wider the mesh of its supporting structure, the more readily it is penetrated by the vessels from the bed. Cancellous bone is much more rapidly vascularized than cortical bone and hence forms new bone much faster (Matti, 1932; Abbott, 1947).

It is still not definitely established whether the vascular network of the graft survives and forms anastomoses with the invading capillaries. Recent studies failed to reveal any clear "kissing contact" or direct connection between the new and preexisting vascular network (Holmstrand, 1957). Numerous publications are devoted to the question of revascularization, or rather taking over of the function of blood supply by the vessels of the graft (Hancox, 1947; Kiehn et al., 1948; Maatz et al., 1952a, b; Peer, 1954, 1955; Stringa, 1957). A functioning vessel was observed after 5 hours in grafts of embryonal bone on to the allantois of hen's egg (Hancox, 1947). In the cancellous bone test (Maatz et al., 1954), which involves a defect of predetermined size in cancellous bone, on day 1 hyperemia is seen around the chip, on day 2 the capillaries of the bed begin to sprout in the vicinity of the chip, on day 3 the capillaries bridge the gap between bed and chip, and on day 4 one-quarter to one-third of the capillaries in the center of the autologous chip fill with dye (Graf, 1959). It really does not matter in this situation whether these are newly formed capillaries or whether they arose by anastomoses between the new and the transplanted vascular system. What does matter is that the vascularization of a cancellous bone graft proceeds very fast, thus ensuring both the supply of blood to the transplanted cells and the vital reaction of resorption of bone ground substance.

During the first few hours a graft can only be supplied by means of diffusion.

Transplantation experiments have been carried out on dogs in order to study the survival capacity of osteocytes (MAATZ *et al.*, 1952a, b; LENTZ, 1955). Autologous bone chips stored for various periods in preserved blood or "tyrode solution" with 10% serum were implanted into the dorsal muscles of dogs. With preservation for up to 8 days, there was new bone formation rapidly commencing in the heterotopic bed. With a preservation period of 10 days or more, there was a marked decline in bone formation, which ceased altogether when preservation in a suitable nutrient solution exceeded a period of 16 days. It is thus clear that bone tissue can survive in an appropriate medium for 8 days without deterioration, and for up to 16 days to some extent. In vivo experiments indicated that osteocytes in the marginal areas of a graft could survive for up to 250 days (HELSOP *et al.*, 1960).

It has now been proved that nutrients can be supplied to bone grafts by diffusion. The cells of bone grafts transplanted intraperitoneally in millipore diffusion chambers with 0.45 μ-diameter pores survive and form new bone (ALGIRE *et al.*, 1954; ROSIN and ZAJICEK, 1959; ROSIN *et al.*, 1963; SEGMÜLLER, 1967; ECKE, 1967a, b). Cells cannot pass pores of this size but body fluids can. *These experiments prove that autologous bone cells are able to survive, provided they are transplanted into a suitable milieu or into a bed that is capable of vascularization.*

2. Osteogenesis in Autografts

The first requirement is that the graft is tolerated by the host and heals without infection. However, bone grafting is not usually undertaken just for temporary closure of a defect in bone. The transplanted bone is also required to initiate osteogenesis from its own resources, or to stimulate osteogenesis in the host bed. Finally, it is necessary for the graft to be integrated into the host organism, and this involves restructuring of the graft. *The ground substance of a bone graft cannot be assimilated by the host organism until it has been restructured to match the host substance. The entire process of restructuring is effected by means of accelerated osteogenesis. The process is triggered by the cells of the graft or the bony bed that are programmed for osteogenesis, but it has to be completed by the differentiation of unspecific mesenchymal cells into osteblasts.*

For over a century there has been unceasing scientific debate concerning the merit of transplanted osteoblasts. There was, for a long time, confrontation between the two seemingly diametrically opposed theories of causal osteogenesis—osteoblast theory and induction theory. W. AXHAUSEN was able, in 1952, to clear up this dual approach to osteogenesis by demonstrating experimentally that osteogenesis could occur in both ways (AXHAUSEN, W., 1952, 1956). New research techniques have been applied to osteogenesis—electron microscopy, fluorescence microscopy, autoradiography, tissue culture, etc.—and they appear to confirm that the transplanted soft tissue plays an active part in the formation of new bone. They also show that induced osteogenesis does occur; it is the humorally regulated transformation of mesenchymal cells into osteoblasts. Both routes to osteogenesis involve the degradation of bone ground substance, because during this process substances are liberated that can either very quickly stimulate the osteoblasts, or cause nonspecific cells to change gradually into osteoblasts.

It is important to distinguish according to the structure of the graft between grafts with a covering of periosteum and grafts of cortical or cancellous bone. Every graft, whether of cortical or cancellous origin, has to undergo complete restructuring; it has to be integrated into the load-bearing architecture and be able to withstand both compressive and bending stress. It cannot become part of the functional microarchitecture until the graft has been completely restructured (Schweiberer, 1971, 1976).

2.1. Osteogenesis in Transplanted Periosteum

The osteogenic contribution of transplanted periosteum has long been the object of scientific curiosity. The periosteum was always looked upon as the typical osteogenic tissue and hence used for comparative tests. However, to clarify the contribution made by the cellular part of the graft, it was necessary to use soft tissue for the transplantation site. In the growing organism the deeper levels of the periosteum contain large numbers of preosteoblasts and osteoblasts, which make up the cambium layer; in the adult, the periosteum has to receive a proliferative stimulus before its specific activity is triggered. This stimulus is provided by the degradation of the periosteum-bound ground substance (Axhausen, G., 1908, 1909, 1920). The fate of the transplanted ground substance has been known since the end of the 19th century: it is resorbed and replaced by newly formed bone ground substance (Barth, 1893, 1894, 1895). The stimulus provided by the degradation of the ground substance causes the systematically proliferating osteoblasts of the cambium layer to deposit new bone on the necrobiotic transplanted hard substance. This fact can readily be demonstrated by heterotopic grafting of the chips of cortical bone with and without a covering of periosteum. With the periosteum removed, there is no vigorous, rapid subperiosteal new bone formation, and resorption and restructuring of the cortical graft proceed much more slowly. In the periosteum-covered graft new bone begins to form a network subperiosteally on day 3 to 4 (Fig. 1) (Axhausen, G., 1909; de Jong and v.d. Kemp, 1928; Axhausen, W., 1962). On chips of bone without periosteum new bone starts to form later and notably begins on the medullary side or at the ends of the chip where the open Haversian canals and their osteoblasts have made contact with the vascular system. If the periosteum is activated by scraping out the medullary cavity, vigorous new bone formation proceeds very fast after transplantation (Danis, 1958). With transplanted periosteum, the functional imprint, i.e., whether the graft was taken from a zone where osteoblasts or osteoclasts were active, or from a resting zone, is retained for some time in the new environment (Krompecher, 1958, 1959). The boneforming capability of the periosteum, however, is still dependent on vascularization, as demonstrated by transplants in the anterior lens of the eye. Here, there is very little new bone formation, if any, because the lens is supplied by diffusion alone (Cohen and Lacroix, 1955).

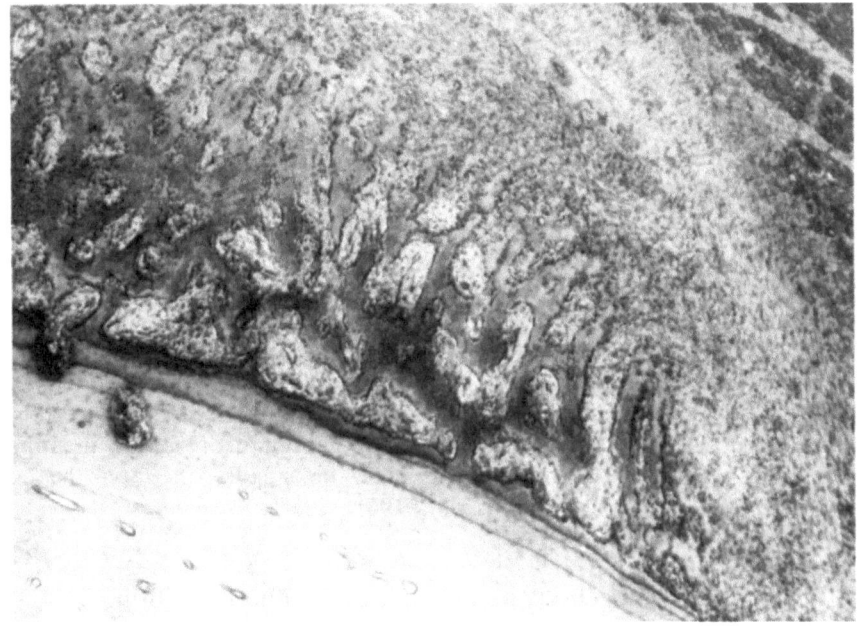

Fig. 1a. Periosteal-covered autologous cortical chip, 8 days after transplantation in muscle tissue. Marked subperiosteal new bone formation

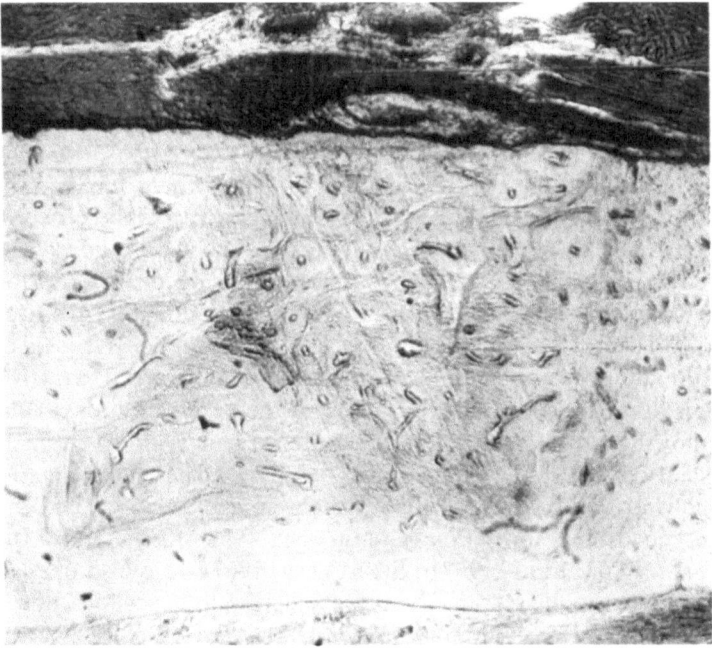

Fig. 1b. Autologous cortical chip without periosteal, 8 days after transplantation in muscle tissue. In contrast to periosteal-covered chip, still no new bone formation evident. (Specimens made available by W. AXHAUSEN)

2.2. Osteogenesis in Transplanted Compact Bone

Compact bone consists mainly of hard bone substance. The Haversian canals alone contain cell elements capable of osteogenesis, apart from the activable osteocytes. Compact cortical bone is not very suitable for grafting as it contains fewer osteogenic cells than cancellous bone, and vascular access to the Haversian system is much more difficult. However, it is not true that compact bone lacks all osteogenic potency, as is sometimes claimed (GEISER, 1963). When chips of compact bone without periosteum are grafted into the muscle bed, new bone is always seen to be formed, although to a lesser extent and with more delay than with periosteum-covered chips (AXHAUSEN, W., 1962). Compact bone is perfectly capable of osteogenesis, as shown by experiments designed to exclude the influence of periosteum and endosteum on the healing of a defect in compact bone. If the defect is separated by means of millipore or silastic membranes from both periosteum and endosteum, new bone still penetrates the defect via the Haversian canals (BASSETT et al., 1961).

2.3. Osteogenesis in Transplanted Cancellous Bone

The principal restructuring processes of bone continues throughout life in the cancellous bone of the metaphyseal regions, the medullary cavity, and the flat bones. Turnover in cancellous bone is three times that in compact bone (FROST, 1963). It has always been recognized that cancellous bone has certain osteogenic capabilities, but it was long believed to be inferior to periosteum. Finally, conclusive clinical and experimental evidence revealed the importance of cancellous bone (Fig. 2) (MATTI, 1932; ABBOTT et al., 1947; SCHWEIBERER, 1971, 1976).

After implantation of particles of cancellous bone in the anterior lens of rat eye, de novo bone formation was always observed so long as there were cells adhering to the graft. When the cells were removed, there was no osteogenesis (RAY et al., 1952; URIST and MCLEAN, 1952; DANIS, 1958; ANDERSON, 1961). The lens of the eye was chosen for heterotopic implantation because it is supplied by diffusion, so that osteogenesis can only proceed from the implant itself. The demonstrative value of this choice is, however, somewhat impaired by the fact that secondary, metaplastic de novo bone formation in the eye is not particularly rare after trauma or inflammatory diseases (BÖRNER, 1956; HAGER and EBEL, 1964). More credence can be given to experiments with millipore diffusion chambers which allow undisturbed growth of isolated tissues. A pore size of 0.45 microns prevents the penetration of cellular elements while allowing quite large protein molecules to pass (ALGIRE et al., 1954; SHELTON and RICE, 1958; GABOUREL and FOX, 1959). The transplantation of fresh autologous or homologous cancellous bone in a diffusion chamber always induces de novo bone formation (GOLDHABER, 1958; ROSIN and ZAJICEK, 1959; ROSIN et al., 1963; ECKE, 1967b; SEGMÜLLER, 1967). Radioisotope labeling fully confirms that osteoblasts survive and proliferate in cancellous bone autografts in rats and mice (RAY and SABET, 1963; URIST et al., 1965).

All experiments set up to study the osteogenic potency of autografts of periosteum, compact, and cancellous bone indicate that specific osteogenic cells

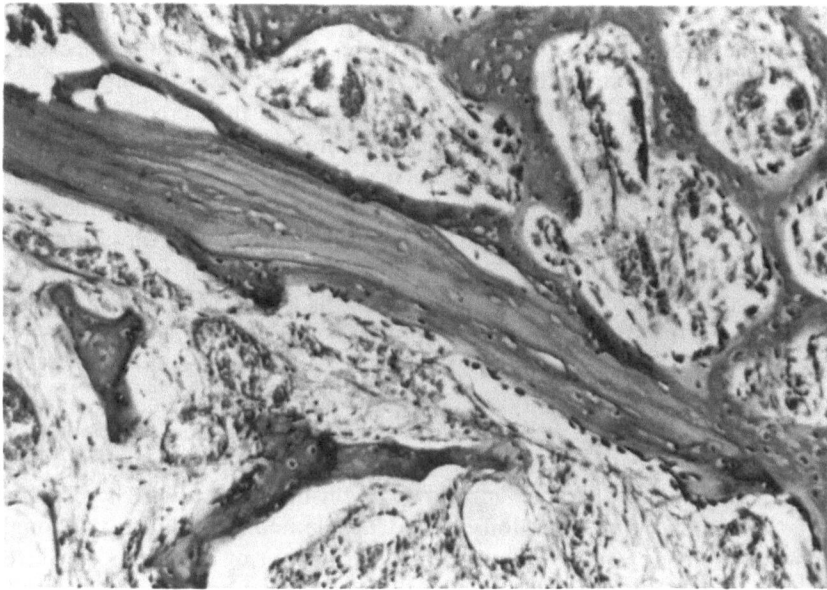

Fig. 2. Autologous cancellous bone, 8 days after transplantation in muscle tissue: very intensive new bone formation on surface of transplanted cancellous bone trabeculae and in surrounding area

will survive so long as the blood supply is adequate. They thus support the so-called osteoblast theory (AXHAUSEN, G., 1908a, b, 1909; LEXER, 1924; AXHAUSEN, W., 1945), which states that the major part of the osteogenesis in a graft derives from the osteoblasts transplanted with it. At the same time, all these experiments do not exclude the other route to osteogenesis: induction, i.e., the differentiation of nonspecific mesenchymal cells under the influence of transplanted bone ground substance in course of degradation.

2.4. Osteogenesis by Induction

For many years it was believed that the two theories of causal osteogenesis, osteoblast theory and induction theory, were diametrically opposed. But, from the start, both theories were based on the knowledge that transplanted bone ground substance is degraded and replaced by new bone. Bone ground substance, in the course of both formation and degradation, exerts a specific stimulus which, in osteoblast theory, acts on nonspecific osteoblasts and, in induction theory, acts on the pluripotent mesenchymal cells growing in from the transplantation site.

After injection of cell-free alcoholic extract of bone into rabbit muscle, de novo formation of bone, or cartilage was observed in a large proportion of the experiments (LEVANDER, 1938, 1941; ANNERSTEN, 1940, 1941; OBERDAHLHOFF, 1947; LACROIX, 1947; ROTH, 1950, 1951). Attempts to define the chemistry of a substance called K-factor or osteogenin were unsuccessful (WILLERSTAEDT *et al.,* 1950). Comparative tests with extracts of autologous, homologous, or heterologous bone tissue established that this hypothetical substance was not specific either to the individual or the species (Annersten, 1940).

These tests were all performed on the rabbit, and their credibility was much shaken when it was discovered that injections of pure alcohol into rabbit muscle also induced metaplastic bone formation in a certain percentage of cases (Heinen *et al.,* 1949). Rabbit muscle often reacts to the trauma induced by the injection of a nonspecific tissue-damaging substance with de novo bone formation (v. Seemen, 1929). Injection of bone extracts into the muscles of white mice, guinea pigs (Lindahl and Orell, 1951), rats (Danis, 1956), dogs (Axhausen, W., 1950), and man (Lindahl and Orell, 1951) failed to induce de novo bone formation. Nevertheless, induced osteogenesis is demonstrable and has subsequently been demonstrated.

When the adherent soft tissues are washed out of cancellous bone without causing any chemical change in the ground substance, its osteogenic potency, though much reduced, is not entirely extinguished. New bone is also formed by the red marrow of cancellous bone transplanted in isolation, although its osteogenic potency is very slight compared with that of autografts of untreated cancellous bone containing bone ground substance. Impregnating the cell-free ground substance with red marrow greatly enhances the osteogenic potency, which then almost equals that of the untreated autograft. It is clearly immaterial whether the bone ground substance used in such tests is autologous or homologous (Burwell, 1963, 1964, 1965). These tests appear to show that the degrading bone ground substance has an inductive effect upon the transplanted soft tissue. However, the inductive substances have, as their target, specific osteoblasts in the marrow, even though it may be the case that reticulum cells or endothelial cells (both present in abundance in the marrow) have first to be transformed into osteoblasts. The evidence obtained is more convincing when cell-free material is transplanted into a bone-free bed, if the study is directed to the pure effect on undifferentiated pluripotent cells.

Even when all cells adhering to a cortical or cancellous bone graft are killed by slow freezing to $-35°$ C before transplanting to a soft-tissue bed, de novo bone formation still occurs in man and dog (Engström and Orell, 1943; Axhausen, W., 1962). There is, however, a fundamental difference between this type of osteogenesis and that observed with fresh autografts. Osteogenesis does not start for at least 30 days after transplantation, whereas with fresh autografts the period is 3–4 days, and its intensity is much less. The late form of osteogenesis is seen mainly in cases where the bone ground substance is resorbed by the tissue of the bed, e.g., at the slightly splintered ends of cortical chips. Both mono- and polynuclear osteoclasts are found in locations of this type. Resorption is followed by osteoplasia, an interesting pointer to the causal genesis of bone formation. It is not enough that young, proliferating mesenchymal tissue should be in juxtaposition with decomposing bone ground substance; there must also be cellular bone degradation, which is a sign of graft viability (Axhausen, W., 1951, 1952, 1956, 1962).

Detailed information concerning the first (osteoblastic) phase and the second (induced osteogenic) phase was first obtained in 1951/52 but was not confirmed until 1959 for homografts of cancellous bone chips (CHALMERS, 1959). When fresh, homologous chips of cancellous bone are transplanted into the muscle bed, new bone forms from day 4, as with autologous material. The osteoblastic phase lasts until day 8, after which regressive changes set in, terminating in the death of all the cells in the newly formed bone tissue. This marks the onset of an antigen-antibody reaction to the homograft and to its cells in particular. If the chips are allowed to remain in the bed, new lamellar bone growth begins on the surface of the graft after 4 weeks. This second phase that begins 4 weeks later must be regarded as induced osteogenesis. The untreated species-specific bone ground substance, in undergoing resorption, exerts an inductive effect on the immature tissue of the bed, thus causing the mesenchymal cells to differentiate into osteoblasts.

Further confirmation that new bone formation can be both osteoblastic and inductive was again obtained from experiments in millipore chambers. Cancellous bone was placed in a diffusion chamber and transplanted into the subcutaneous tissue of mice. New bone formation, although not seen in every case, was found both inside and outside the chamber (GOLDHABER, 1961). After transplantation of homologous chips of epiphyseal plate under the described conditions, new bone formation also occured outside the chamber (ECKE, 1967a).

The stages in the differentiation of each individual cell have still not been fully elucidated. It is, however, reasonable to assume that chemical compounds from the proteoglycans (SCHWEIBERER, 1970) in the dying or decomposing bone ground substance "act upon the regulator genes in the cells of the bed tissue with the result that operator genes assemble the appropriate structure genes into operons. These operons constitute a matrix for protein synthesis" (JAKOB and MONOD, 1961).

It can be regarded as definitely proved today that osteogenesis can be effected by induction as well as by the predetermined osteoblastic cells. Thus, osteogenesis in the graft takes places in two phases: phase 1 starts after 3–4 days with the transplanted osteoblasts at the edge of the graft forming new bone, while in phase 2 the transplanted bone ground substance, namely the proteoglycans, induces nonspecific cells in the bed to differentiate into osteoblasts (SCHWEIBER-ER, 1970).

3. Immunology of Homologous and Heterologous Bone Transplantation

The problem of homo- and heterografting is that it evokes immunopathologic reactions. This is equally true of both organ and tissue grafts, although the antigenic potency of bone, cartilage, and connective tissue is low in comparison with that of the cell-rich, well-differentiated epithelial organs. Let us deal first with homografting. The immune response depends on the degree of histocompatibility and is determined by the specific protein structure in the nuclear fractions, but not in the plasma fractions, of an individual (BILLINGHAM et al., 1956). The antigens localized in the cell nucleus—the ribonucleoproteins—are protein structures unique to the individual and they evoke an immune response, even in an individual of the same species. When a graft is transplanted from one individual to another, rejection is inevitable. The first phase is vascularization of the lymph and blood vessels at the site of the graft (Medawar, 1954), which allows the graft antigens to reach the antibody-producing cells of the host's lymph nodes. There is a certain latency period before antibodies are produced, but rejection begins after a period of 7–30 days with an invasion of lymphocytes, plasma cells, and histiocytes. So far as is known to date, this process invariably ends in total necrosis of the transplanted cells.

3.1. Bone Homografts

Applied to bone homografts, the above statement means that not only does the ground substance perish, as indeed it always does in bone grafting, but the osteoblastic cells of the graft, which are so essential for osteogenesis, are also destroyed. Today we distinguish two types of antigen, H- and T-antigens. The H-antigens are formed by the mucopolysaccharides and have the physical property of thermostability. At first, however, the H-antigen plays a subordinate role in immunologically induced rejection of homografts. It has seldom been possible to demonstrate that humoral antibodies are produced in response to the H-antigens of a homograft; only very low concentrations have been found, which makes it clear that this route to sensitization in homografting is not the main one. The decisive immunologic factor is the T-antigen produced by the cells (Billingham et al., 1956). T-antigen is thermolabile. The antigenic substances are bound to the host's lymphatic system (Burwell, 1961). Fresh homografts of cancellous bone fragments implanted subcutaneously in rabbit ear always cause enlargement of the regional lymph nodes, measurable by the increase in weight, and in certain sections of the cortex and medulla there is proliferation of large and medium-sized pyroninophilic cells (Scothorne and McGregor, 1955; Chalmers, 1959). These lymphoid cells are generally believed to be the source of the tissue antigens.

The events in the graft itself, however, are the main focus of interest. Fresh autografts show no round-cell infiltration, and they quickly heal and start to form bone. Homografts also form a network of new bone after 3–4 days, but as soon as the round-cell infiltrates appear, from day 8 onward, the proliferating osteoblasts and vascular sprouts perish and the newly formed bone is destroyed again (Axhausen, W., 1953; Burwell, 1961; Deleu and Trueta, 1965; Gilman and Enneking, 1965). After homografting of deep-frozen chips, the early osteogenic phase does not occur, and there is no visible or measurable immune reaction. This clearly shows that the host response is directed against the cellular elements of the graft.

Thus, the fate of a chip of homologous bone is determined by the reactions of the immune response. The data were obtained for a soft-tissue bed and they are equally applicable to a bony bed; but, it is not so easy to demonstrate the process histologically because of the activity of the host bone itself. These processes account for the universal clinical experience that, while homografts usually do heal, the proportion of failures is much larger and healing takes much longer than in autografts.

Chemically preserved or deep-frozen homologous bone chips are superior to fresh ones, because the antigen-antibody reaction to the cellular components is eliminated, or at any rate reduced. Healing of homografts can be accelerated by presensitization (HUTZSCHENREUTER, 1972). In sheep and rats firmly attached homografts after sensitization healed much faster than fresh homografts. This is thought to be due, not to "enhancement" but to accelerated degradation in the second graft. With presensitization, the immune response is immediate, so that the cells of the homograft are destroyed at once and inductive new bone formation in the graft is hardly delayed at all (HUTZSCHENREUTER, 1972).

3.2. Bone Heterografts

The healing processes in a heterograft follow an entirely different course. There is a violent tissue reaction with round-cell infiltration and hemorrhage extending deep into the bed tissue; the host immune response is much stronger than with a fresh homograft. Deep freezing to destroy the cells fails to suppress the antigen–antibody reaction (AXHAUSEN, W., 1954). The date obtained from histologic preparations were confirmed by antigen research. Whereas humoral antibodies are rarely found after homografting, after heterografting there is always an increase in humoral antibodies formed in reaction to H-antigens (ALLGÖWER et al., 1952; BURWELL, 1963, 1964). There is no second osteogenic phase like that seen in homografts, and no induced new bone formation, for the osteoinductive substance is specific for the species.

In any body bed with good bone-forming capability, both fresh and deep-frozen heterografts are enclosed in new bone tissue formed from the bed. The abundance of cells in the vicinity of the graft, always indicates a reaction to tissue from a different species. Tissue buds that are capable of ossification then grow from the bone wound surface of the bed into the Haversian canals of the now dead graft and begin its resorption, but the graft cannot play an active part. Resorption proceeds slowly and is restricted to the parts near the surface of the graft; the rest of the dead graft remains in the bed as a foreign body.

4. Transplantation of Pretreated Bone Ground Substance

It remains to be discussed whether a cell-free bone graft, including chemically and physically pretreated bone, can make any contribution to osteogenesis. BARTH's opinion (1893, 1894, 1895) was that the entire bone graft died, then formed a guide structure, and was ultimately replaced over many years. This view influenced clinical practice for a long time, with the result that it was not considered necessary to distinguish between auto-, homo-, and heterografts. Failures were thus common with fresh and deep-frozen homografts, and almost inevitable with heterografts. Homografting, however, is beset with difficulties as regards obtaining material. Once the immune response was explained, it was realized that if heterologous material was to be used in clinical applications, it was not sufficient to remove the cells; the proteins in the bone matrix must also be extracted, or at least denatured, in order to suppress the H-antigens that produced the immune reaction. It had long been known that boiled or heat-treated bone tissue could be replaced by newly formed bone after implantation to fill a bone defect, but it was not known whether, if at all, the treated bone ground substance had an active role in the process of osteogenesis, because the respective contributions of bed and graft tend to overlap. As early as 1912 boiled bone was experimentally implanted in a soft-tissue bed; as no new bone formation occurred, whereas freshly taken bone autografts always formed new bone in soft tissue, the difference in the outcome was attributed to differences in the physicochemical behavior of treated and untreated grafts (ORELL, 1934). Later experiments with heat-treated bone also failed to show osteogenesis. In an alternative approach, it was established that suitable metering of the calcium salt concentration led to bone formation in connective tissue (v. DITTRICH, 1926). The calcium phosphate concentration was believed to effect a change in the behavior of the connective tissue.

Some very important comparative tests were carried out with autografts of fresh bone fragments and bone grafts treated by prolonged boiling in potash lye, or by extraction with acetone, etc. It was found that fresh, untreated grafts always showed new bone formation after 15 days, while the pretreated bone fragments showed none for at least 3 months, and even then it was very restricted (ORELL, 1934). The conclusion drawn was that "the connective-tissue cells outside the skeleton must be made to change by prolonged physicochemical treatment of the implant, which would then not only form collagen but also take on bone-forming and calcium-depositing functions." As a whole, however, preservative measures involving boiling, heat-treating, and macerating were never very satisfactory.

In the last 20 years some publicity has been given to heterografts subjected to a special process of maceration in hydrogen peroxide, known in clinical practice as Kiel bone chips (MAATZ, 1957; BAUERMEISTER, 1958). Objective proof of the efficacy of the denaturation of bone chips prepared in this way was furnished by immunologic investigational methods (KIENHOLZ and KEMKES, 1956). Freeze-dried and thus protein-containing cattle bone was implanted in rabbit with subsequent injection of cattle serum. Symptoms of shock ensued with fatal outcome. Simultaneous implantation and injection produced extensive necrosis at the site of implantation in two out of five cases. Clearly, the antigenic, sensitizing properties of cattle bone were not removed by freeze-drying. However, when cattle bone was macerated with H_2O_2 and implanted under the same experimental conditions, there were no symptoms of immunologic rejection and healing proceeded normally (KIENHOLZ and KEMKES, 1956). Nothing was said about whether the macerated bone retained its osteogenic potency or not.

The bone matrix, as stated in the section on anatomy, is made up of collagenous fibrils on which thin plates of apatite are deposited in a definite order and surrounded by a semifluid colloid system of protein molecules consisting mainly of proteoglycans. Now, if bone matrix is capable of osteogenic induction, the question to be answered is: Is osteogenic induction due to the bone ground substance as a whole, or is it only certain components that are responsible? The answer is provided by some animal experiments.

If an auto-, homo-, or heterograft is subjected to a process of maceration with H_2O_2, this leads to the breakdown not only of the cells, but also of the amorphous intercellular substance or proteoglycan complex. This does not

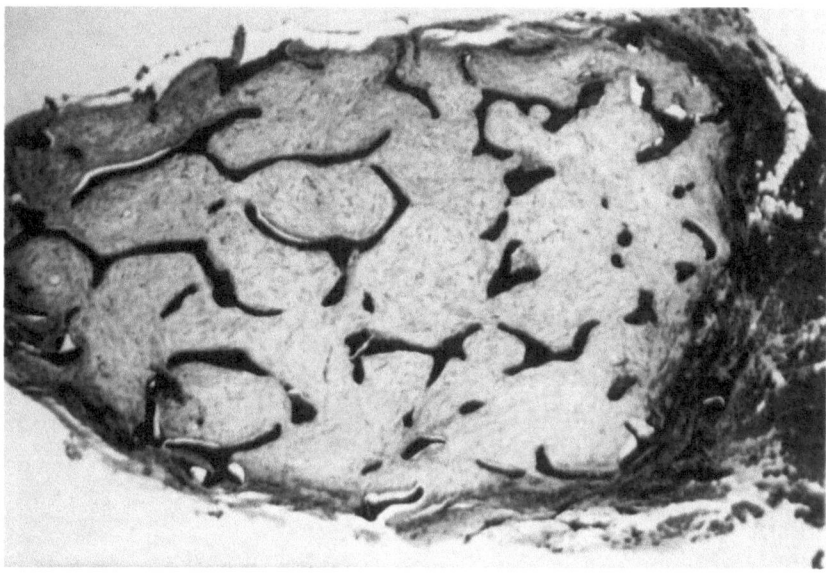

Fig. 3. H_2O_2-denatured heterologous bone chip transplanted into abdominal musculature of man; 93 days after implantation. Fibrous, cell deficient connective tissue infiltrates implant. No osteoclasis, no new bone formation visible. Implant is incorporated as a foreign body

reduce the protein content of the bone ground substance to any great extent, for the amorphous intercellular substance accounts for a mere 1.25% of the ground substance. The macerated bone contains about 25–30% of protein in the form of collagenous fibrils, which is about the same amount of protein as there is in nonmacerated bone. However, the removal of the amorphous intercellular substance makes a tremendous difference: There is no immune response, resorption and restructuring of the bone ground substance are delayed, and the graft is incorporated into the organism as a foreign body. This result has been obtained by implanting in both extraskeletal and bony beds (SCHWEIBERER, 1965, 1967, 1970) (Figs. 3, 4).

When only the calcium phosphate supporting structure of bone is transplanted, that is, when the collagenous fibrils have been burned out in a quartz oven (SCHWEIBERER, 1970), there is still a vigorous connective-tissue reaction, but no acceleration of osteogenesis. These observations are in agreement with the data obtained with labeled calcium (^{45}Ca) and show that, even when regeneration is localized, the inorganic compounds of bone matrix are always obtained from the circulating blood (COHEN et al., 1957) (Fig. 5).

When the collagenous supporting structure is transplanted after the amorphous intercellular substance and the apatite crystals have been removed, there is again a complete absence of osteogenic induction (SCHWEIBERER, 1970). Both the apatite crystals and the collagen fibrils succumb to phagocytosis without participating in osteogenic induction (Fig. 6).

In extensive transplantation and implantation experiments, URIST et al. (1972) showed that the matrix of devitalized and demineralized bone transplants

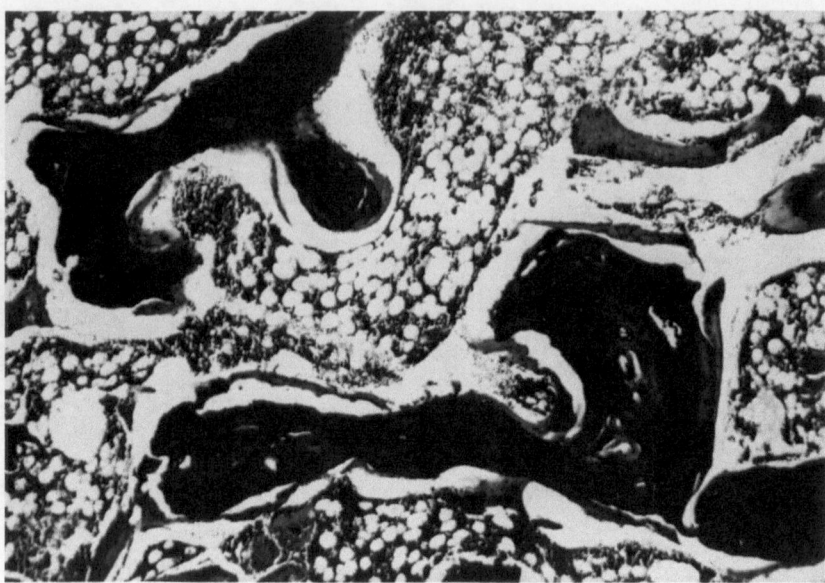

Fig. 4. H$_2$O$_2$-denatured autologous cancellous bone implanted in cancellous tibia; 62 days after implantation. Denatured osseous trabeculae are surrounded by newly formed bone, originating in osseous transplantation site. Resorption of the denatured bone transplant does not occur. Denatured bone is incorporated into organism as a foreign body

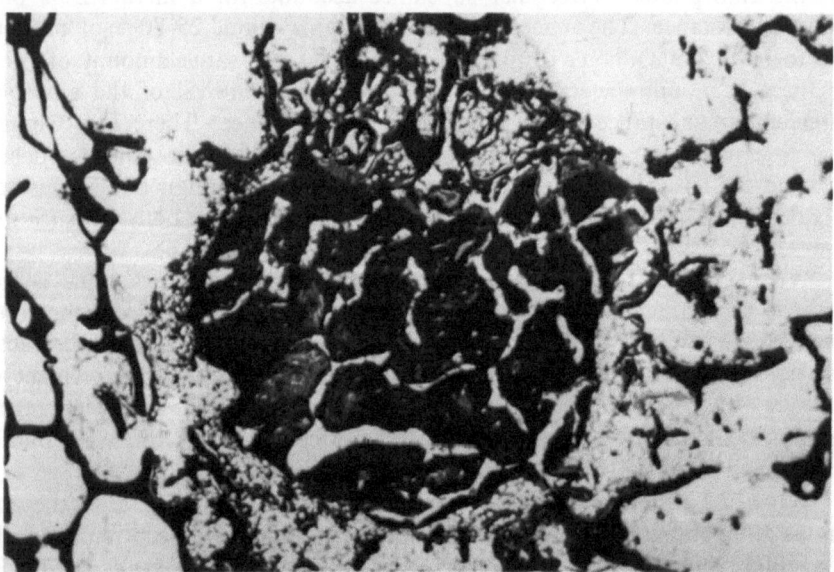

Fig. 5. Calcium salt framework of cancellous bone, following incineration of organic substances in a quartz oven, implanted in a cancellous area of long bone; 35 days after implantation. Marked connective tissue reaction in vicinity of calcium salt structure; no osteogenesis originating from implant

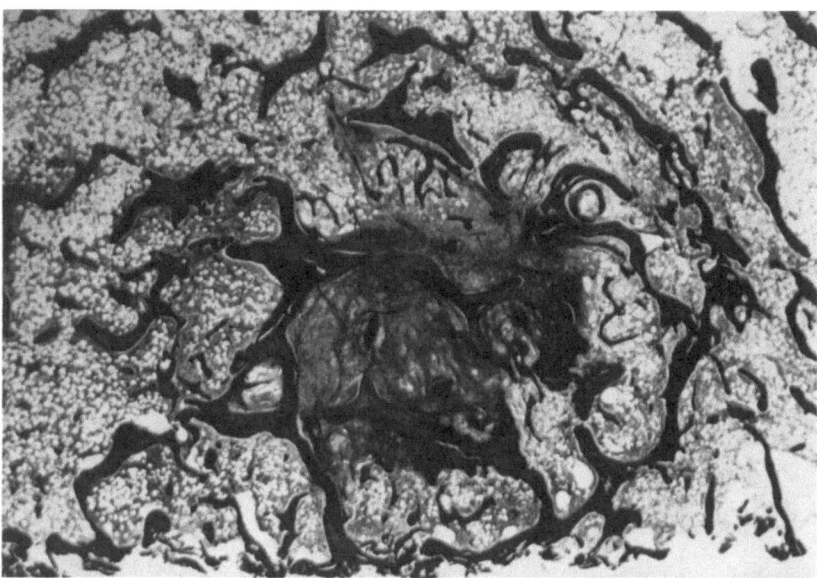

Fig. 6. Collagen structure of cancellous bone following removal of amorphous intercellular substance and the apatite crystals; implanted in cancellous transplantation site; 35 days after implantation. Marked connective tissue reaction in vicinity of the collagen structure. No osteogenesis originating from implant

induced new bone formation. Also URIST *et al.* claimed an extracellular control mechanism which, through differentiation, induces a specific behavior (osteogenesis) in mesenchymal tissue. Using histochemical and biochemical methods, this study group succeeded in more closely describing such a "bone inducting principle" (BIP): it involves a protein complex which is bound to collagen but is not a component of the same. The efficacy of this so-called bone morphogenetic protein (BMP) seems to be influenced by a specific proteolytic enzyme (BMP-ase) (URIST *et al.*, 1974).

The function of the BMP-BMPase-complex is apparently dependent on non-collagen proteins and proteoglycans, which are released from the organic bone matrix by the BMPase activity and may inhibit the BMPase. These proteins and proteoglycans possibly shift the equilibrium of the reaction in favor of BMP, so that a secondary inductive effect would be attributed to them in the model of URIST *et al.* (1972).

Among other things, these metabolic reactions are dependent on pH, which in turn is changed by biolectric potentials. Consequently, BASSETT *et al.* (1972) indicated, in this connection, that stress-induced electric potentials have an osteogenic effect. This opens the way to a modern interpretation of WOLFF's law, which claims the influence of mechanical stress on cell function and so provides a model for morphogenesis of bone.

It is thus clear that the amorphous intercellular substance, or proteoglycan complex, is a vital factor in the induced form of causal osteogenesis (SCHWEIBERER, 1970). *The incorporation of the transplant resembles the physiologic transformation*

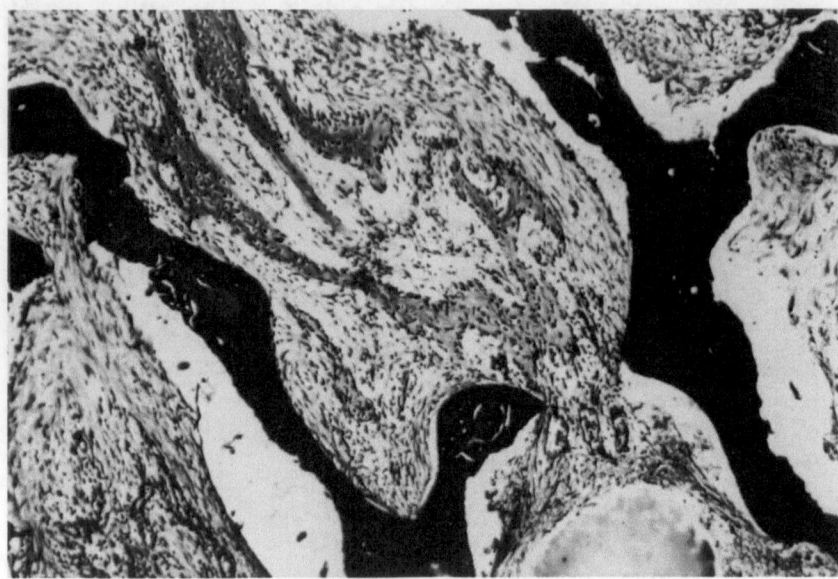

Fig. 7a. Osseous regeneration in a cancellous bone defect, which was packed with H_2O_2-denatured cancellous bone: New bone formation does not occur next to implanted trabeculae but to budding vessels. Implanted cancellous bone does not function as a guiding structure for new bone formation, rather it is incorporated as a foreign body by connective tissue

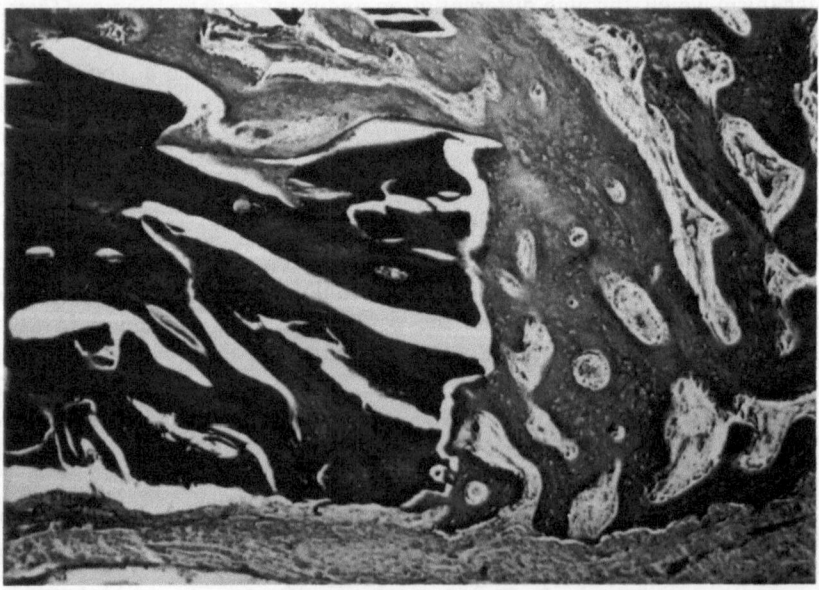

Fig. 7b. Osseous regeneration in a cortical defect which was packed with H_2O_2-denatured cortical bone: Denatured implant hinders osseous regeneration of transplantation site. All support for an organic incorporation of the transplant is missing

of bone with osteon formation, in that neutral mucopolysaccharides are produced initially, then esterified in preparation for mineralization. It is impossible for the graft to be regenerated in the absence of the amorphous intercellular substance, which exerts a strong influence on the cellular metabolism.

The substraction experiments, however, failed to make clear whether it was merely the guide structure of the chemically pretreated bone matrix that accelerated the spread of the newly formed bone from the bony bed. A critical study of implants in cancellous and cortical beds established that the fibrous bone that forms first from the bed does not grow along any existing guide when bridging over or filling in a defect; on the contrary, it grows along the lines of vascular penetration (SCHWEIBERER, 1970, 1971). Comparative planimetric studies of empty cavities and of cavities packed with macerated chips indicated that growth into the implanted cavities was impeded, the rate being some 32% slower than in the empty cavities (SCHWEIBERER, 1970, 1971) (Fig. 7).

5. Conclusions Drawn From the Results of Experimental Bone Transplantation

As noted in the introduction, ideas concerning the various types of bone graft have been subject to theoretical fluctuations ever since OLLIER's pioneering studies (1867). The outstanding merit of autografts has even been challenged on occasion. The most recent data, however, indicate that the essential features of bone transplantation are as follows:

1. Bone grafting involves complete restructuring of the graft. This is the only way to obtain a functional, completely satisfactory repair of the microarchitecture of the bone appropriate to the site.

2. Restructuring is completed first on the surface of the graft and, only if revitalization is successful, does it finally reach the interior of the graft.

3. Bone regeneration is an expression of enhanced osteoblastic activity, extending to:

(a) predetermined osteoblastic germinal tissue in the graft;

(b) predetermined osteoblastic germinal tissue in the bed;

(c) differentiation into osteoblasts of nonspecific, immature mesenchymal cells from the budding transplantation site tissue.

4. The multicentric osteoblastic activity is of differing origins and cannot perform its task without the influence of certain organic chemical compounds belonging to the proteoglycan complex of the bone ground substance. The substances in question have yet to be characterized but are known to be formed during the degradation of bone ground substance.

5. Bone homografts possess osteoinductive potency due to their species-specific bone matrix, but healing is delayed and sometimes placed in jeopardy by the course run by the immune response.

6. Heterologous bone tissue cannot be used for grafting, because both the plasma fractions and the cell nuclear fractions trigger a very violent host reaction.

7. Osteogenic induction cannot take place when the intercellular substances, or proteoglycan complex, have been removed from the bone ground substance by maceration.

8. The hydroxyapatite crystals have no effect on osteogenesis in a graft. During degradation of the bone ground substance they either go into solution or are engulfed by phagocytes. The mineral in the newly formed bone is obtained from the circulating blood, not from the graft.

9. Bone regeneration is not accelerated by the presence of a guide structure consisting of macerated trabeculae. The newly forming trabeculae follow the line of the vessels growing out of the bed, not an artificial framework.

D. Clinical Aspects of Bone Transplantation

Both experimental findings and clinical experience indicate that the autograft is the only reliable solution when the purpose is to initiate new bone formation, provide an adequate supporting structure, or bridge over bone defects. It is usually possible to follow the acceptance and restructuring of the graft by means of clinical and radiologic examinations. There arise, first around the graft and later within it, cloudy callus formations, proliferating unsystematically and displaying no particular order. These callus masses consist of fibrous bone and they form a connection with the local bone. They become cemented and fixed in position. Once a firm union has been created, muscle activity and stress induce compressive and bending loads on the newly formed bone. Another prolonged process of restructuring then begins, in which the fibrous bone is resorbed and restructured into trajectorially aligned lamellar bone (Schweiberer, 1971). Finally, we see the reappearance of longitudinally aligned osteons appropriate to the functional architecture (Fig. 8).

Fig. 8. Transplanting of cancellous bone next to a pseudarthrosis: in the beginning, production of fibrous bone similar to a fixation callus. After a firm connection to transplantation site exists, fibrous bone is remodeled to trajectorially aligned lamellar bone

1. Cancellous Bone Autografts

There are significant differences between the various types of autograft as regards osteogenic merit, speed of healing, and restructuring, and these are very important in clinical applications. For decades clinical interest did not go beyond the periosteum and the cortical chip. It was not until 1932 that MATTI, on the basis of numerous animal experiments and excellent clinical results, drew attention to the outstanding merit of cancellous bone autografts. Today cancellous bone autografts are almost the only type of graft used in clinical applications.

The honeycomb structure of cancellous bone does not place an obstacle in the way of the ingrowing blood vessels. Capillaries from the surrounding soft tissues or from the local bone penetrate in a matter of days into cancellous bone packed into a cavity or next to a bone. In the first few days only the marginal parts are supplied with blood but, if healing proceeds normally, the whole graft is gradually vascularized. As mentioned in the experimental section, it should be borne in mind that the chief regeneration of bone throughout life occurs in the cancellous parts of the flat bones, in the metaphyseal areas, and in the medullary cavities of the long bones. Here the rate of turnover is three times faster than in compact bone (FROST, 1963). *Its cellular "reactibility," combined with the loose, easily vascularizing structure of cancellous bone, makes it the best graft material.*

This is not to say that compact bone grafts do not possess osteogenic properties, too. However, the thicker the chip of compact bone, the slower its vascularization—and hence its restructuring—is completed. When compact bone is transplanted in small chips, restructuring proceeds more quickly, as with the Phemister chip. Its cortical fracture plane usually splinters along the lamellae and is therefore readily vascularized and restructured.

2. Clinical Scale of Merit of Autografts

A clinical scale of merit for bone autografts can be obtained from experimental and clinical results. The order is as follows:

1. Pure cancellous bone from the trochanter major or iliac bone.

2. Cortical-cancellous bone from the os ilium or the proximal metaphysis of the tibia.

3. Thin, splintered Phemister chips with a covering of periosteum, or fine chips of cortical bone.

4. Thick chips of cortical bone.

Now that techniques have been developed for the internal fixation of fractures, allowing complete relief of instability in a fracture, pseudarthrosis, or continuity defect, it is no longer necessary for a graft to contribute to stability. When LEXER (1924) started to treat pseudarthroses and even continuity defects by means of bone autografts, he had to use strong chips of cortical bone with the aim of achieving some stability by fitting the graft into the continuity of the unstable long bone. Cancellous bone taken in thin flakes or small chips from the anterior face of the os ilium or trochanter major is first bedded into a bone defect in small, separate grafts, or laid alongside the bone. Within a period ranging from a few days to 3 weeks a callus block is produced; this callus is so solid it can only be broken up by force. The callus block becomes stabilized, forms a bridge, and provides the foundation for the regeneration of a load-bearing long bone (Schweiberer, 1971).

3. Graft Bed

Even when the very best material is chosen for the graft, a bone transplant cannot give the desired therapeutic success unless the tissue of the bed is capable of revitalizing and integrating the implanted bone. Here it is important to distinguish between grafting into:

   1. a stable, well-vascularized bed;
   2. a secondarily stable bed with impaired vascularization (fractures and pseudarthroses);
   3. continuity defects of the long bones;
   4. a septic milieu.

3.1. Stable, Well-Vascularized Bed

Transplantation into aseptic osseous cavities presents the fewest problems. Juvenile osseous cysts, in particular, are so free from complications and local bone regeneration is so excellent that the quality of the graft itself hardly matters. Traumatic defects in cancellous bone are equally free from complications; when packed with autologous cancellous bone, they achieve complete healing, regeneration, and assimilation of the graft within a few weeks (Fig. 9).

3.2. Secondarily Stable Bed With Impaired Vascularization (Pseudarthroses and Fresh Fractures)

Nonunion does not necessarily present problems regarding vascularization; in such cases biomechanical difficulties tend to be more important. Without going into detail on the relationships involved in the vascularization of long bones, we must note that the shaft of long bones is supplied mainly from the medullary cavity and not from the periosteum. Only the outer layers of the cortex are supplied by the periosteal vessels. If the soft-tissue covering is badly damaged and the periosteal vascularization disrupted by fibrosis and sclerosis of the soft-tissue covering, as can happen in so-called atrophic pseudarthroses, the outer layers of bone will also become sclerotic and ischemic. In cases like this it is essential that the graft should be in direct contact with the medullary vascular system and with the muscular covering, from which the scar tissue must have been removed. The sclerotic outer cortical layers must be chiseled away (decortication) to enable the graft to be in contact with the vascular system of the medullary cavity of the host bone. When the cortical bone has been debrided, connection is quickly made between the host bone and the

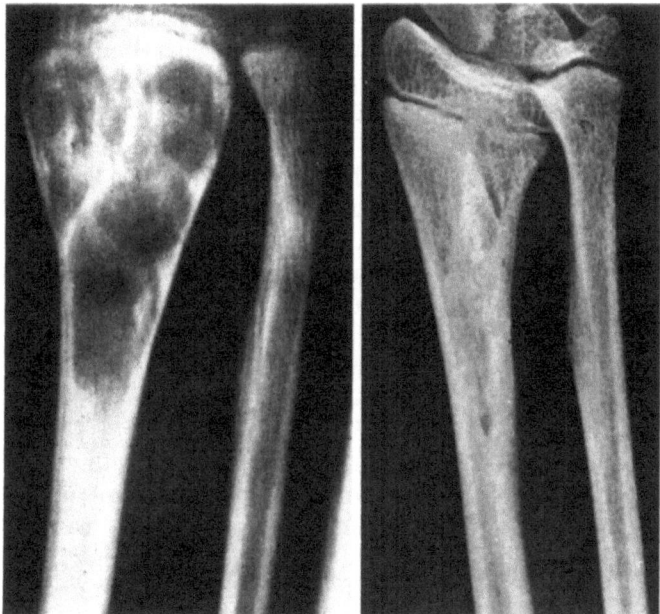

Fig. 9a and b. Transplantation of autologous cancellous bone in well vascularized osseous transplantation site. (a) Juvenile osseous cyst in radius. Packing with cancellous bone. After 2 years, normal bone structure

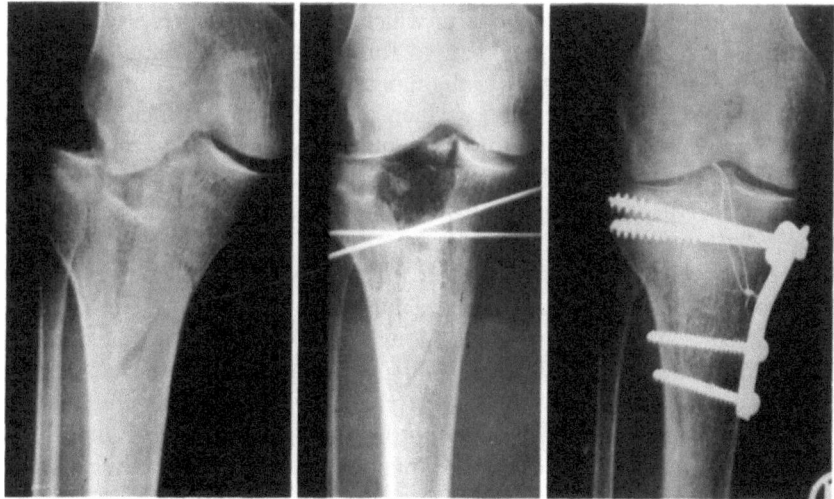

Fig. 9b. Impression of tibia head by femorocondyle with a large cancellous bone defect, in a 65-year-old woman. Reduction and fixation of fracture by osteosynthesis. Packing of defect with autologous cancellous bone. After 1 year, normal bone structure

cancellous bone graft. First, a bridge forms, consisting of a callus of fibrous bone, which is secondarily converted into lamellar bone. Vascularization of a so-called hypertrophic pseudarthrosis is usually very good, and internal fixation under compression generally suffices to ensure osseous consolidation. A supplementary bone graft will encourage the process of bone union.

Fresh, fragmented fractures of the diaphysis, and open fractures in particular, are more likely to be ischemic than are hypertrophic pseudarthroses. The primary injuries to the vessels supplying the bones and soft tissue often create very difficult conditions. The best course here seems to be to remove any devitalized fragments of cortical bone and replace them with cancellous bone, after which vascularization and osseous consolidation will proceed much faster.

3.3. Continuity Defects of the Long Bones

Resections of invasive tumors fall into the category of continuity defects. Autologous cortical bone able to withstand compression is not usually available in sufficient quantity, so that in certain circumstances it may be justifiable to have recourse to a homograft. As already explained in the theoretical and experimental discussion, a homograft must be deep-frozen or presensitized before it is used. However, with modern internal fixation procedures, it is very seldom necessary to resort to homografting. Cancellous bone autografts have given good, indeed, excellent results even when used to bridge quite large defects (Figs. 10, 11).

3.4. Grafting into a Septic Milieu

When bone grafting is used in treating an infection of the bone, a distinction has to be made between cases where stability is impaired and cases where it is not. A stable cylindrical bone in which continuity is preserved, containing a defect with sclerotic margins, caused for example by osteomyelitis, presents grave problems, quite apart from the danger of further infection. The sclerotic margins of the bone are ischemic, which makes it more difficult for the graft to form a connection with the transplantation site. The correct treatment in such cases is to debride the sclerotic margins of an osteomyelitic cavity in the course of the operation to expose well-vascularized bone tissue able to connect with the graft.

In cases where both infection and instability are present, the problem is even more severe. Clinical experience has shown that only cancellous bone is revitalized and restructured fast enough to offer any hope of curing both the infection and the instability. Homografts should never be considered for high-risk cases of this kind. The homograft may indeed react initially like an autograft, forming new bone in the first few days, but the subsequent rejection reactions will inflict further damage on the milieu, so that reinfection is the norm rather than the exception.

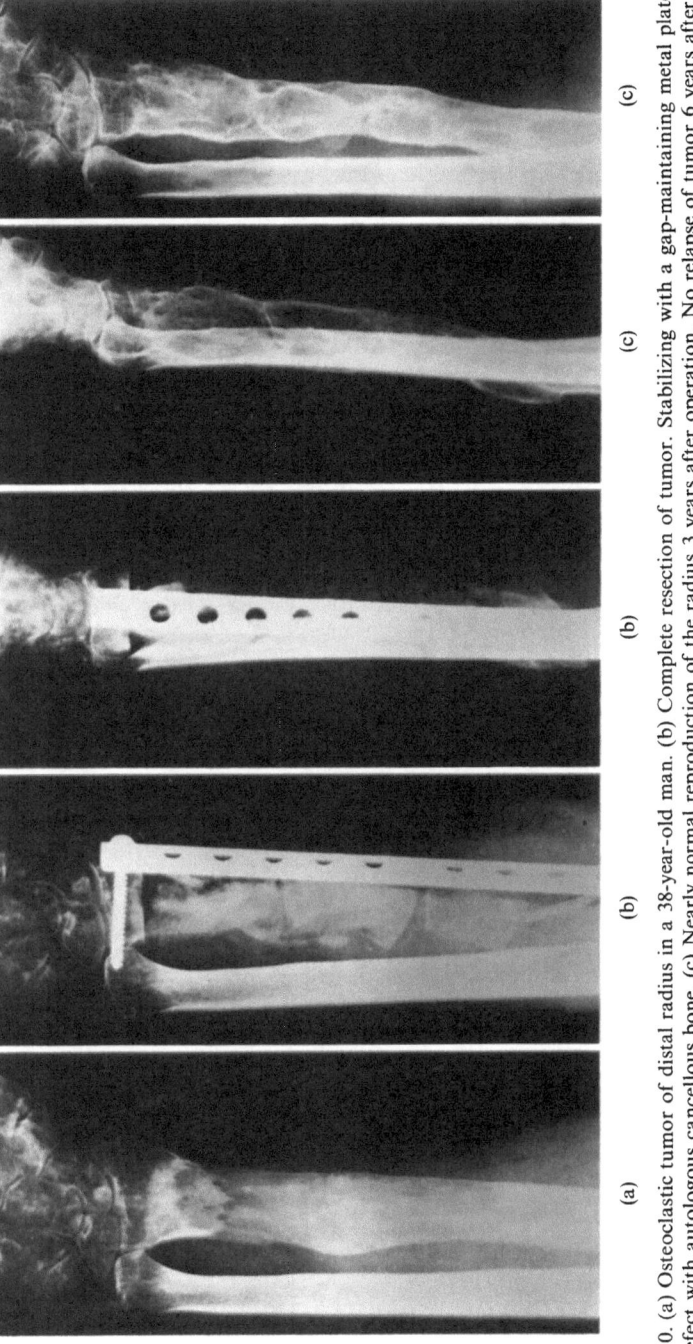

Fig. 10. (a) Osteoclastic tumor of distal radius in a 38-year-old man. (b) Complete resection of tumor. Stabilizing with a gap-maintaining metal plate. Packing of defect with autologous cancellous bone. (c) Nearly normal reproduction of the radius 3 years after operation. No relapse of tumor 6 years after resection

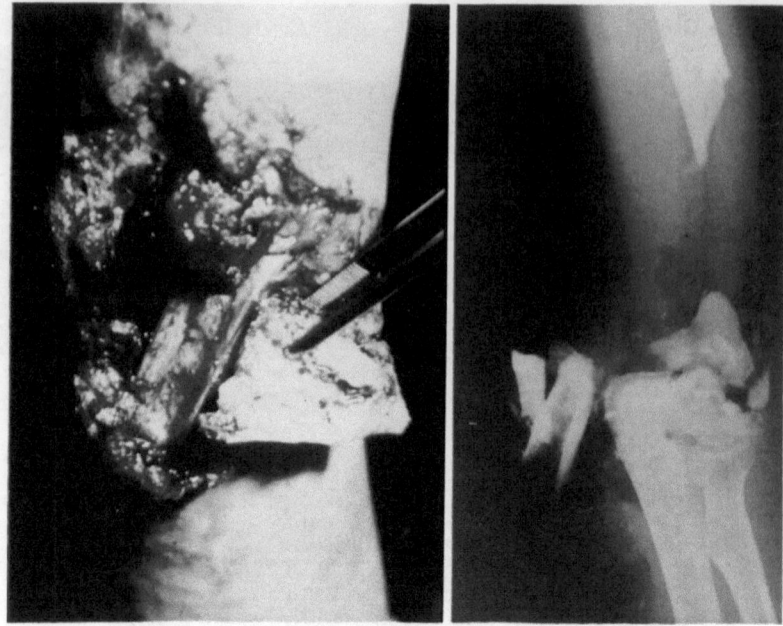

Fig. 11a. Open fracture with bone defect of distal humerus and parts of elbow joint in 20-year-old woman. Stabilizing with gap-maintaining metal plate. Packing of defect with autologous cancellous bone

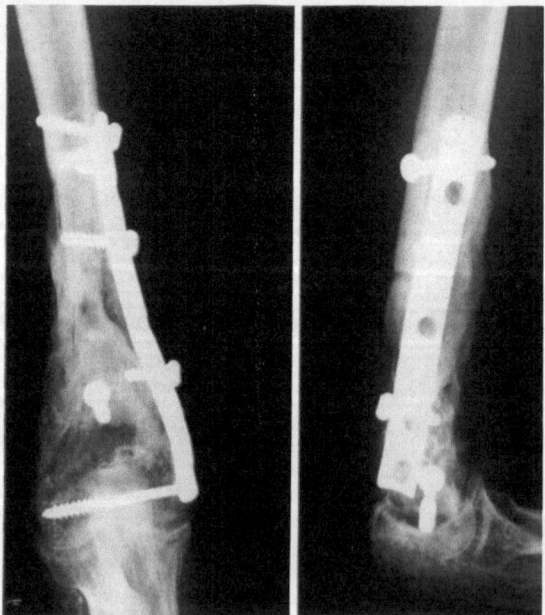

Fig. 11b. Completed trajactorial remodeling of transplanted cancellous bone 8 months after the accident

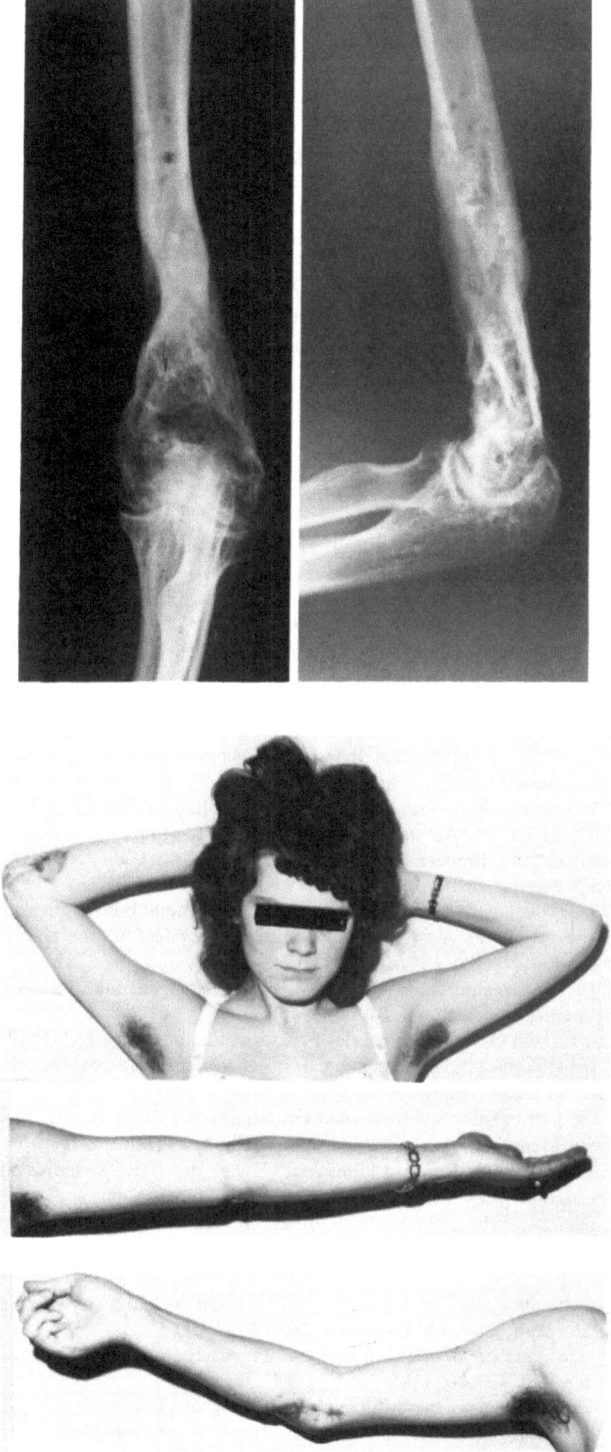

Fig. 11c. Completely restored bone 1 year and 8 months after the accident. Good function of elbow joint

E. Conclusion

Summarizing our knowledge of bone transplantation obtained from experimental surgery and clinical experience, we may say in conclusion that the cancellous bone graft is the best type of autograft because its open structure allows rapid vascularization, physiologic resorption, and ossification are enhanced in cancellous bone, and there is consequently rapid restructuring of the graft. When a transplant is connected with the bone of the host, it is governed by the law listed by WOLFF in his 1892 work, *Das Gesetz der Transformation der Knochen.* WOLFF's law states that a bone of given shape adapts its internal architecture by means of regeneration and resorption in orientation to the mechanical load.

References

ABBOTT, L.C., SCHOTTSTAEDT, E.R., SAUNDERS, J.B., BOST, F.C.: The evaluation of cortical and cancellous bone grafting material. J. Bone Jt Surg. **A29**, 381 (1947)

ALBRIGHT, F., REIFENSTEIN, E.C.: The parathyreoid glands and metabolic bone disease. Selected studies. Baltimore: Williams & Wilkins Co. 1948

ALGIRE, G.H., WEAVER, G.M., PREHN, R.T.: Growth of cells "in vivo" in diffusion chambers. T. Survival of homografts in immunized mice. J. nat. Cancer Inst. **15**, 493 (1954)

ALLGÖWER, M.: Funktionelle Anpassung des Knochens auf physiologische und unphysiologische Beanspruchung. Langenbecks Arch. klin. Chir. **319**, 383 (1967)

ALLGÖWER, M., BLOCKER, T.G., ENGLEY, B.W.D.: Some immunological aspects of auto- and homografts in rabbits, tested by in vivo and in vitro techniques. Plast. reconstr. Surg. **9**, 1–21 (1952)

AMPRINO, R.: Autoradiographic research on the S^{35} sulphate metabolism in cartilage and bone differentiation and growth. Acta anat. (Basel) **24**, 121–163 (1955)

AMPRINO, R., BAIRATI, A.: Processi di riconstruzioni e di riassorbimento della sostanza compatta delle ossa del' uomo. Z. Zellforsch. **24**, 439 (1939)

ANDERSON, K.J.: The behaviour of autogenous and homogenous bone transplants in the anterior chamber of the rat's eye: A histological study of the effect of the size of the implant. J. Bone Jt Surg. **A43**, 980 (1961)

ANNERSTEN, S.: Experimentelle Untersuchungen über die Osteogenese und die Biochemie des Frakturcallus. Acta chir. scand., Suppl. **84**, 60 (1940)

ANNERSTEN, S.: Über die Osteogenese bei der Frakturheilung. Chirurg **13**, 76 (1941)

AXHAUSEN, G.: Histologische Untersuchungen über Knochentransplantationen am Menschen. Dtsch. Z. Chir. **91**, 388 (1908a)

AXHAUSEN, G.: Die pathologisch-anatomischen Grundlagen der Lehre von der freien Knochentransplantation beim Menschen und Tier. Med. Klin. Beih. **2**, 23 (1908b)

AXHAUSEN, G.: Die histologischen und klinischen Gesetze der freien Osteoplastik auf Grund von Tierversuchen. Langenbecks Arch. klin. Chir. **88**, 23 (1909)

AXHAUSEN, G.: Diskussionsbemerkung. Verh. dtsch. Ges. Chir. **44**, 192 (1920)

AXHAUSEN, W.: Die histologischen Gesetze der freien Knochenüberpflanzung. Inaug.-Diss. Berlin 1945

AXHAUSEN, W.: Experimentelle Untersuchungen zur Theorie der „induzierten" Knochenneubildung (LEVANDER). Langenbecks Arch. klin. Chir. **266**, 381 (1950)

AXHAUSEN, W.: Die Quellen der Knochenneubildung nach freier Transplantation. Langenbecks Arch. klin. Chir. **270**, 439–442 (1951)

AXHAUSEN, W.: Die Knochenregeneration, ein zweiphasisches Geschehen. Zbl. Chir. **77**, 435 (1952)

AXHAUSEN, W.: Der biologische Wert kältekonservierter Knochentransplantate. Langenbecks Arch. klin. Chir. **273**, 856 (1953)

AXHAUSEN, W.: Der biologische Wert heteroplastischer Knochentransplantate. Langenbecks Arch. klin. Chir. **279**, 48 (1954)

AXHAUSEN, W.: The Osteogenetic Phases of Regeneration of Bone. J. Bone Jt. Surg. A 38, 593 (1956)

AXHAUSEN, W.: Die Bedeutung der Individual- und Artspezifität der Gewerbe für die freie Knochen-überpflanzung. Hefte Unfallheilk. 72, 1962

BARGMANN, W.: Histologie und mikroskopische Anatomie des Menschen. Stuttgart: G. Thieme 1967

BARTH, A.: Über histologische Befunde nach Knochenimplantationen. Langenbecks Arch. klin. Chir. 46, 409 (1893)

BARTH, A.: Über Osteoplastik in chirurgischer Beziehung. Langenbecks Arch. klin. Chir. 48, 466 (1894)

BARTH, A.: Histologische Untersuchungen über Knochenimplantationen. Beitr. path. Anat. 17, 65 (1895)

BASSETT, C.A.L.: Environmental and cellular factors regulating osteogenesis. In: Bone biodynamics. New York: Little, Brown & Co. 1964

BASSETT, C.A.L.: Biologic significance of piezoelectricity. Calc. Tiss. Res. I, 252 (1968)

BASSETT, C.A.L., BECKER, R.O.: Generation of electric potentials in response to mechanical stress. Science 137, No. 3535, 1063 (1962)

BASSETT, C.A.L., CREIGHTON, D.K., STINCHFILD, F.E.: Contribution of endosteum, cortex and soft tissues to osteogenesis. Surg. Gynec. Obstet. 112, 145 (1961)

BASSETT, C.A.L.: Clinical Implications of Cell Function in Bone Grafting. Clin. Orthop. 87, 49 (1972)

BAUERMEISTER, A.: Experimentelle Grundlagen für den Aufbau einer Knochenbank. H. Unfallheilk. 58. Berlin-Göttingen-Heidelberg: Springer 1958

BÉLANGER, L.F.: Autoradiographic visualization of the entry and transit of S^{35} in cartilage, bone and dentine of young rats and the effect in hyaluronidase in vitro. Canad. J. Biochem. 32, 161 (1954)

BÉLANGER, L.F.: Osteolysis: An outlook on its mechanism and causation. In: P.H. GAILLARD, R.V. TALMAGE, A.M. BUDY (eds.). The parathyreoid glands: Ultrastructure, secretion and function. P. 137. Chicago: Chicago University Press 1965

BILLINGHAM, R.E., BRENT, L., MEDAWAR, P.B.: The antigenic stimulus in transplantation immunity. Nature (Lond.) 178, 514 (1956)

BOSWORTH, D., WRIGHT, H., FIELDING, J.: A study in the use of bank bone for spine fusion in tuberculosis. J. Bone Jt. Surg. A 35, 329 (1953)

BURKHARDT, L., PETERSEN, H.: Über den Umbau im wachsenden Knochen. Z. Zellforsch. 7, 55 (1928)

BURWELL, R.G.: Studies in the transplantation of bone. J. Bone Jt. Surg. B 45, 386 (1963)

BURWELL, R.G.: Studies in the transplantation of bone. J. Bone Jt. Surg. B 46, 110 (1964)

BURWELL, R.G.: Osteogenesis in cancellous bone grafts: Considered in terms of cellular changes, basic-mechanism and the perspective of growth-control and its possible aberrations. Clin. Orthop. 40, 35 (1965)

BURWELL, R.G., GOWLAND, G.: Studies in the transplantation of bone. II. The changes occurring in the lymphoid tissue after homografts and autografts of fresh cancellous bone. J. Bone Jt. Surg. B 43, 820 (1961)

CHALMERS, J.: Transplantation immunity in bone homografting. J. Bone Jt. Surg. B 41, 160 (1959)

COHEN, J., HARRIS, W.H.: The three-dimensional anatomy of Haversian systems. J. Bone Jt. Surg. A 40, 419 (1958)

COHEN, J., MALETSKOS, C.J., MARSHALL, J.H., WILLIAMS, J.B.: Radioactive calcium tracer studies in bone grafts. J. Bone Jt. Surg. A 39, 561 (1957)

COHEN, J., LACROIX, P.: Bone and cartilage formation by periosteum. Essay of experimental autogenous grafts. J. Bone Jt. Surg. A 37, 717 (1955)

DANIS, A.: L' ostogénine existe-t-elle? Acta orthop. belg. 22, 501 (1956)

DANIS, A.: L' os néoformé dans une greffe de perioste homologue presente une evolution histologiquement differente de celle d'une greffe autologue. Acta orthop. belg. 24, 160 (1958)

DAVIES, D.V., YOUNG, L.: The distribution of radioactive sulphur (S^{35}) in the fibrous tissues, cartilages and bones of the rat following its administration in the form or inorganic sulphate. J. Anat. (Lond.) 88, 174 (1954)

Deleu, J., Trueta, J.: Vascularisation of bone grafts in the anterior chamber of the eye. J. Bone Jt. Surg. **B47**, 319 (1965)

Demeter, G., Matyas, J.: Mikroskopisch-vergleichend anatomische Studien am Röhrenknochen mit besonderer Berücksichtigung auf die Unterschiede menschlicher und tierischer Knochen. Z. Anat. Entwickl.-Gesch. **87**, 45 (1928)

Dudley, R.H., Spiro, D.: The fine structure of bone cells. J. biophys. biochem. Cytol. **11**, 627 (1961)

Dulce, H.J.: Der Stoffwechsel des Knochens im Lichte neuer physiologisch-chemischer Erkenntnisse. Verh. dtsch. orthop. Ges. **48**, 151 (1960)

Duthie, R.B., Barker, A.N.: An autoradiographic study of mucopolysaccharide and phosphate complexes in bone growth and repair. J. Bone Jt. Surg. **B37**, 304 (1955a)

Duthie, R.B., Barker, A.N.: The histochemistry of the preosseous stage of bone repair studied by autoradiography. – The effect of cortisone. J. Bone Jt. Surg. **B37**, 619 (1955b)

Dziewiatkowski, D.D.: Autoradiographic studies of sulfat-sulfur (S^{35}) metabolism in the articular cartilage and bone of suckling rats. J. exp. Med. **95**, 489 (1952)

Dziewiatkowski, D.D.: Effect of age on some aspects of sulfate metabolism in the rat. J. exp. Med. **99**, 283 (1954)

Ecke, H.: Die Transplantation der Epiphysenfuge. Stuttgart: Ferdinand Enke 1967a

Ecke, H.: Neue Wege der quantitativen Bestimmung der ossären Regeneration an Knochentransplantaten. Langenbecks Arch. klin. Chir. **319**, 448 (1967b)

Eger, W.: Der Mineralisationsvorgang des Knochengewebes und seine Störungen. Verh. dtsch. orthop. Ges. **48**, 129 (1960)

Eger, W.: Allgemeine morphologische Physiologie und Pathologie des Knochengewebes. Internist (Berl.) **3**, 267 (1962)

Eger, W.: Calciumnachweis und Mineralisation des Knochengewebes. Verh. dtsch. Ges. Path. **47**, 54 (1963)

Engström, H., Orell, S.: Über Regeneration rings um subcutane Knochenimplantate. Mikrosk. anat. Forsch. **53**, 283 (1943)

Enlow, D.H.: Principles of bone remodeling. Springfield, Ill., USA: Charles C. Thomas 1963

Fleisch, H.: Neue Gesichtspunkte der Kalkablagerung. Schweiz. med. Wschr. **29**, 858 (1961)

Fleisch, H.: Funktionelle Anpassung des Knochens auf physiologische und unphysiologische Beanspruchung. Pathophysiologie und Behandlung der Osteoporose. Langenbecks Arch. klin. Chir. **319**, 374 (1967)

Fleisch, H., Neuman, W.F.: On the role of phosphatase in the nucleation of calcium phosphatase by collagen. J. Amer. chem. Soc. **82**, 3783 (1960)

Friberg, U., Ringertz, N.R.: Autoradiographic studies with S^{35} on the development of the rat embryo. Experientia (Basel) **10**, 67 (1954)

Friberg, U.: An autoradiographic study on the uptake of radiosulphate in the rat embryo. J. Embryol. exp. Morph. **4**, 313 (1956)

Friedebold, G., Witt, A.N., Hanslik, L., Jendryschik, A.: Kritische Untersuchungen über den klinischen Wert homo- und heteroplastischer Knochentransplantation. Arch. orthop. Unfall-Chir. **55**, 627 (1963)

Frost, H.M.: Micropetrosis. J. Bone Jt. Surg. **A42**, 144 (1960)

Frost, H.M.: Bone remodelling dynamics. Springfield, Ill., USA: Charles C. Thomas 1963

Fukuda, E., Yasuda, J.: Zit. nach Allgöwer, M., Langenbecks Arch. klin. Chir. **319**, 383 (1967)

Gabourel, J.D., Fox, K.E.: Cell cultures in vivo. I. Growth of L-fibroblast and sarcoma 180 cell lines in diffusion-chambers in vivo. Cancer Res. **19**, 1210 (1959)

Gattow, G., Münzenberg, K.J.: Die organische und anorganische Fraktion des Kieler Knochenspanes im röntgenographischen Bild. Arch. orthop. Unfall-Chir. **55**, 453 (1963)

Geiser, M.: Diskussionsbeitrag. Kongreßber. Orthop. **50**, 329 (1963)

Gilman, S.H., Enneking, W.F.: Prehistologic changes in the rejection mechanism of bone transplants. J. Surg. Res. **5**, 31 (1965)

Goldberg, V.M., Lance, E.M.: Revascularisation and accretion in transplantation. J. Bone Jt. Surg. **54A**, 807 (1972)

Goldhaber, P.: Preliminary observation on bone isografts within diffusion chambers. Proc. Soc. exp. Biol. (N.Y.) **98**, 53 (1958)

Goldhaber, P.: Osteogenic induction across millipore filters in vivo. Science **133**, 2065 (1961)

GOMORI, C.: The distribution of phosphatase in normal organs and tissues. J. cell. comp. Physiol. **17**, 71 (1941)

GRAF, R.: Gefäßversorgung autoplastischer Spongiosatransplantate und ihre Bedeutung. Bruns' Beitr. klin. Chir. **198**, 390 (1959)

GRAUMANN, W.: Handbuch der Histochemie. Bd. II: Polysaccharide (zweiter Teil). Stuttgart: G. Fischer 1964

HAGER, G., EBEL, K.: Beitrag zur intraokularen Knochenbildung. Klin. Mbl. Augenheilk. **144**, 513 (1964)

HANCOX, N.M.: The survival of transplanted embryonal bone graffed to chorioallantoic-membran and subsequent osteogenesis. J. Physiol. (Lond.) **106**, 269 (1947)

HANCOX, N.M.: The osteoclast. The biochemistry and physiology of bone, ed. by G.H. BOURNE, p. 213. New York: Academic Press 1956

HEANEY, R.P.: Radiocalcium metabolism in disuse osteoporosis in man. Amer. J. Med. **33**, 188 (1962)

HEINEN, J.H., DABBS, G.H., MASSON, H.A.: The experimental production of ectopic cartilage and bone in the muscle of rabbits. J. Bone Jt. Surg. **A31**, 765 (1949)

HELLER, M.: Occurrence of possibly secretory granules in osteogenic cells. Anat. Rec. **106**, 204 (1950)

HELLER-STEINBERG, M.: Ground substance; bone salts and cellular activity in bone formation and destruction. Amer. J. Anat. **89**, 347 (1951)

HELSOP, B.F., ZEISS, J.M., NISBET, N.W.: Studies on transference of bone. I. A comparison of autologous and homologous bone implants with reference to osteocyte survival, osteogenesis and host reaction. Brit. J. exp. Path. **41**, 269 (1960)

HEULER, K.M.: Besteht eine Korrelation zwischen Alter und Knochenstruktur? Z. Zellforsch. **7**, 41 (1928)

HOLMSTRAND, K.: Biophysical investigations of bone transplants. Plast. reconstr. Surg. **19**, 265 (1957)

HUTZSCHENREUTER, P.: Beschleunigte Einheilung von allogenen Knochentransplantaten durch Präsensibilisierung des Empfängers und stabile Osteosynthese. Langenbecks Arch. klin. Chir. **331**, 321 (1972)

JAKOB, F., MONOD, J.: Genetic regulatory mechanism in the synthesis of proteins. J. molec. Biol. **3**, 318 (1961). Cited in: ECKE, H., 1967a: Die Transplantation der Epiphysenfuge

JASUDA, J.K., NOGUCHI, K., SATA, T.: Dynamic callus and electric callus. J. Bone Jt. Surg. **A37**, 1929 (1955)

JOHNSON, L.C.: Cited by PUTSCHAR, W.G.J., Verh. dtsch. Ges. Path. **47**, 113 (1963)

JONG, J. DE, KEMP, P.H. v.d.: Experimentelle Untersuchungen über die Autotransplantation von Knochengewebe. Beitr. pathol. Anat. **79**, 268 (1928)

JOWSEY, J., KELLY, P.J., RIGGS, B.L., BIANCO, A.J., SCHOLZ, D.A., GERSHON-COHEN, J.: Quantitative microradiographic studies of normal and osteoporotic bone. J. Bone Jt. Surg. **A47**, 785 (1965)

KEMBER, N.F.: Cell division in enchondral ossification. A study of cell proliferation in rat bones by the method of tritiated thymidine autoradiography. J. Bone Jt. Surg. **B42**, 824 (1960)

KIENHOLZ, M., KEMKES, B.: Untersuchungen über den immunologischen Wert heteroplastischer konservierter Knochenspäne. Arch. orthop. Unfall-Chir. **48**, 623 (1956)

KNESE, K.H.: Knochenbildung und Entwicklung der Knochenstruktur. Verh. dtsch. Ges. Path. **47**, 35 (1963)

KNESE, K.H.: Cytologische Aspekte der Knochenbildung. Internist (Berl.) **7**, 581 (1966)

KNESE, K.H., KNOOP, A.M.: Elektronenoptische Untersuchungen über die periostale Osteogenese. Z. Zellforsch. **48**, 455 (1958)

KNESE, K.H., VOGES, D., RITSCHL, J.: Untersuchungen über die Osteon- und Lamellenformen im Extremitätenskelett des Erwachsenen. Z. Zellforsch. **40**, 323 (1954)

KÖLLIKER, A.: Die normale Resorption des Knochengewebes und ihre Bedeutung für die Entstehung der typ. Knochenformen. Leipzig: F.C.W. Vogel 1873

KROMPECHER, S.: Die Beeinflußbarkeit der Gewebsdifferenzierung im Periost mit besonderer Rücksicht auf die Ergebnisse der Transplantation. Verh. anat. Ges., Erg.-Heft zu Bd. 105 (1958). Anat. Anz. 1959, 174

LANDRY, M., FLEISCH, H.: The influence of immobilisation on bone formation as evaluated by osseous incorporation of tetracyclines. J. Bone Jt. Surg. **B46**, 764 (1964)

Lentz, W.: Die Grundlagen der Transplantation von fremdem Knochengewebe. Stuttgart: G. Thieme 1955

Levander, G.: A study of bone regeneration surgery. Surg. Gynec. Obstet. **67**, 705 (1938)

Levander, G.: Über Knochenregeneration. Formulierung einer Fragestellung vom kausal-osteogenetischen Gesichtspunkt aus. Klin. Wschr. **20**, 40 (1941)

Lexer, E.: Die freien Transplantationen. Neue Dtsch. Chir. **26**, 15 (1924)

Lindahl, O., Orell, S.: Experiments with bone extracts. Acta chir. scand. **101**, 136 (1951)

Lipp, W.: Neuuntersuchungen des Knochengewebes. II: Histologisch erfaßbare Lebensäußerungen der Knochenzellen. Acta anat. (Basel) **22**, 151 (1954)

Maatz, R.: Die Knochentransplantation. Verh. dtsch. Orthop. Ges. (1955) Beilageheft Z. Orthop. **87**, 44 (1956)

Maatz, R.: Der Tierspan in der Knochenbank. Dtsch. med. J. **8**, 190 (1957)

Maatz, R.: Klinische Erfahrungen mit einem eiweißarmen Tierspan. Langenbecks Arch. klin. Chir. **292**, 831 (1959)

Maatz, R., Lentz, W., Graf, R.: Die Knochenbildungsfähigkeit konservierter Späne. Ein Beitrag zur Knochenbank. Zbl. Chir. **77**, 1376 (1952a)

Maatz, R., Lentz, W., Graf, R.: Experimentelle Grundlagen der Transplantation konservierter Knochen. Langenbecks Arch. klin. Chir. **275**, 850 (1952b)

Maatz, R., Lentz, W., Graf, R.: Spongiosa test of bone grafts. J. Bone Jt. Surg. **A 36**, 721 (1954)

Majno, G., Rouiller, Ch.: Die alkalische Phosphatase in der Biologie des Knochengewebes (Histologische Untersuchungen). Virchows Arch. path. Anat. **321**, 1 (1951)

Matti, H.: Über freie Transplantationen von Knochenspongiosa. Langenbecks Arch. klin. Chir. **168**, 236 (1932)

Medawar, P.B.: Preservation and Transplantation of normal tissues. Ciba Found. Symp., London 1954

Milch, R.A., Rall, D.P., Tobie, J.E.: Bone localisation of tetracyclines. J. nat. Cancer Inst. **19**, 87 (1957)

Moog, F., Wenger, E.L.: The occurrence of a neutral mucopolysaccharide at sites of high alkaline phosphatase activity. Amer. J. Anat. **90**, 339 (1952)

Oberdalhoff, H.: Zur Frage der Knochenneubildung. Chirurg **17/18**, 123 (1947)

Ollier, L.: Traité experimentale et clinique de la régénération des os et de la production artificielle du tissu osseux. Paris: Masson & Cie. 1867

Orell, S.: Studien über Knochentransplantation und Knochenneubildung. Acta chir. scand. **74**, Suppl., 31 (1934)

Owen, M.: Cell population kinetics of an osteogenic tissue. J. Cell Biol. **19**, 19 (1963)

Peer, L.A.: Autogenous bone transplants in humans. Plast. reconstr. Surg. **19**, 56 (1954)

Perren, S., Straumann, F.: Zit. nach Allgöwer, M., Langenbecks Arch. klin. Chir. **319**, 383 (1967)

Petersen, H.: Über den Feinbau der menschlichen Skeletteile. Wilhelm Roux' Arch. Entwickl.-Mech. Org. **112**, 112 (1927)

Petersen, H.: Die Organe des Skelettsystems. In: Handbuch der mikroskopischen Anatomie des Menschen, Bd. II/3, S. 521. Berlin: Springer 1930

Ponlot, R.: Le radiocalcium dans l'étude des os. Paris: Masson & Cie 1960

Putschar, W.G.J.: Allgemeine Morphologie und Dynamik des Knochenumbaus unter normalen und pathologischen Bedingungen. Verh. dtsch. Ges. Path. **47**, 113 (1963)

Ray, R.D., Degge, J., Gloyd, P., Mooney, G.: Bone regeneration—an experimental study of bone grafting materials. J. Bone Jt. Surg. **A 34**, 638 (1952)

Ray, R.D., Sabet, T.Y.: Bone grafts; cellular survival versus induction: an experimental study. J. Bone Jt. Surg. **A 45**, 337 (1963)

Recklinghausen, F.v.: Die fibröse oder deformierende Ostitis, die Osteomalazie und die osteoplastische Karzinose in ihren gegenseitigen Beziehungen. Festschrift für R. Virchow. Berlin: G. Reimer, 1891

Robinson, R.A., Watson, M.L.: In: Metabolic interrelations. V.: J. Macy Found. 1953

Robison, R.: Bone phosphatase. Ergebn. Encymforsch. **1**, 280 (1932)

Rohde, C.: Beitrag zur Frage der Metaplasie des Bindegewebes im Knochen. Langenbecks Arch. klin. Chir. **128**, 302 (1924)

ROLLET, A.: Von den Bindesubstanzen. Leipzig: Strickers Handbuch der Lehre von den Geweben. 1871

ROSIN, A., FREIBERG, H., ZAJICEK, G.: The fate of rat bone marrow, spleen and periosteum cultivated in vivo in the diffusion chamber with special reference to bone formation. Exp. Cell. Res. **29**, 176 (1963)

ROSIN, A., ZAJICEK, G.: Bone formation in diffusion chamber cultures of rat bone marrow in vivo. Haematol. lat. (Milano) **2**, 69 (1959)

RUTISHAUSER, E., MAJNO, G.: Physiopathology of bone tissue: The osteocytes and fundamental substance. Bull. Hosp. Jt. Dis. (N.Y.) **12**, 468 (1951)

SCHENK, R., WILLENEGGER, H.: Zur Histologie der primären Knochenheilung. Langenbecks Arch. klin. Chir. **308**, 440 (1964)

SCHRAMM, W.: Klinische und tierexperimentelle Untersuchungen über die Transplantation autoplastischer Spongiosa. H. Unfallheilk. 104. Berlin-Heidelberg-New York: Springer 1970

SCHWEIBERER, L.: Experimentelle Untersuchungen von Knochentransplantaten mit unveränderter und mit denaturierter Knochengrundsubstanz. H. Unfallheilk. 103. Berlin-Heidelberg-New York: Springer 1970

SCHWEIBERER, L.: Neue Ergebnisse zur Knochenregeneration und ihre klinische Bedeutung. Langenbecks Arch. klin. Chir. **329**, 986 (1971a)

SCHWEIBERER, L.: Der heutige Stand der Knochentransplantation. Chirurg **42**, 252 (1971b)

SCHWEIBERER, L.: In: BURRI, C.: Posttraumatische Osteitis. Bern, Stuttgart, Wien: Hans Huber 1974

SCHWEIBERER, L.: Theoretisch-experimentelle Grundlagen der autologen Spongiosatransplantation im Infekt. Unfallheilk.-Traumatology **79**, 151 (1976)

SCHWEIBERER, L., AXHAUSEN, W.: Zur Frage der osteogenetischen Potenz des „Kieler Knochenspans". Langenbecks Arch. klin. Chir. **313**, 959 (1965)

SCHWEIBERER, L., LINDEMANN, M.: Infektionen nach Marknagelung. Chirurg **44**, 542 (1973)

SCHWEIBERER, L., HOFMEIER, G., MÜLLER, I.: Ist der macerierte heterologe Knochenspan (Kieler Knochenspan) ein Calluslocker? Langenbecks Arch. klin. Chir. **319**, 450 (1967)

SCHWEIBERER, L., DAMBE, L.T., EITEL, F., KLAPP, F.: Revaskularisation der Tibia nach konservativer und operativer Frakturbehandlung. H. Unfallheilk. 119, 18. Berlin-Heidelberg-New York: Springer (1974)

SCOTHORNE, R.J., McGREGOR, J.A.: Cellular changes in lymph nodes and spleen following skin homografting in the rabbits. J. Anat. (Lond.) **89**, 233 (1955)

SEEMEN, H.v.: Über die Entstehungsbedingungen metaplastischer Knochenbildungen. Dtsch. Z. Chir. **217**, 60 (1929)

SEGMÜLLER, G.: Spongiosaregeneration in der Milliporekammer. Helv. chir. Acta **34**, 5 (1967)

SHELTON, E., RICE, M.E.: Studies on mouse lymphomas II. Behaviour of three lymphomas in diffusion chambers in relation to their invasive capacity in the host. J. nat. Cancer Inst. **21**, 137 (1958)

SISSONS, H.A., JOWSEY, J., STEWART, L.: Microradiographic appearance of normal bone tissue at various ages. Proc. 2. Intern. Sympos. on x-ray microsc. and x-ray microanalysis. Stockholm, 206 (1959)

STRINGA, G.: Studies of the vascularisation of bone grafts. J. Bone Jt. Surg. **B39**, 395 (1957)

STROEHMANN, J., VORLAENDER, K.O.: Immunologie der Organtransplantation. Wiederbel. u. Organersatz, Erg.-H. z. Z. Kreisl.-Forsch. **4**, 2, 43 (1967)

TISCHENDORF, F.: Das Verhalten der Haversschen Systeme bei Belastung. Wilhelm Roux' Arch. Entwickl.-Mech. Org. **145**, 318 (1951)

TONNA, E.A.: The cellular complement of the skeletal system studied autoradiographically with tritiated thymidine during growth and aging. J. biophys. biochem. Cytol. **9**, 813 (1961)

UEHLINGER, E., PULS, P.: Funktionelle Anpassung des Knochens auf physiologische und unphysiologische Beanspruchung (Die Frakturnagelung und -verschraubung in morphologischer Sicht). Langenbecks Arch. klin. Chir. **319**, 362 (1967)

URIST, M.R.: Osteoinduction in undemineralized bone implants modified by chemical inhibitors of endogenous matrix enzymes. Clin. Orthop. **87**, 132 (1972)

URIST, M.R., McLEAN, F.C.: Osteogenic potency and new bone formation by induction in transplants to the anterior chamber of the eye. J. Bone Jt. Surg. **A34**, 443 (1952)

Urist, M.R., Wallace, T.H., Adams, T.: The functions of fibrocartilaginous fracture callus: observations on transplants labelled with tritiated thymidine. J. Bone Jt. Surg. **B47**, 304 (1965)
Urist, M.R., Silverman, B.F., Buring, K., Dubuc, F.L., Rosenberg, J.M.: The bone induction principle. Clin. Orthop. **53**, 243 (1967)
Urist, M.R., Iwata, H., Boyd, S.D., Cecotti, P.L.: Observations implicating and extracellular enzymic mechanism of control of bone morphogenesis. J. Histochem. Cytochem. **22**, 88 (1974)
Wagner, H.: Präsenile Osteoporose. Stuttgart: G. Thieme 1965
Willerstaedt, H., Levander, G., Hult, L.: Studies in osteogenesis. Acta orthop. scand. **19**, 419 (1950)
Young, R.W.: Cell proliferation and specialization during enchondral osteogenesis in young rats. J. Cell Biol. **14**, 357 (1962)

Radiation-Induced Tolerance

RAINER STORB and C.C. CONGDON

With 5 Figures and 2 Tables

A. Introduction and History

Radiation-induced tolerance in the immunological response is fundamentally a result of cell death and necrosis of lymphatic and hematopoietic tissues. The energy of ionizing radiation is absorbed in a physical sense in tissue, primarily by ionizing water, yielding extremely reactive chemical products of water, which in turn alter macromolecules in cells. During the chemical stages of the interaction with living matter, the initial injury is amplified, leading to cell death according to the intrinsic radiosensitivity of the exposed cells (SMITH and CONGDON, 1968).

Lymphatic tissues and lymphocytes are usually radiosensitive, as is bone marrow in mammals (BLOOM, 1948). Therefore, destruction of lymphatic tissues and cooperating cells from bone marrow might be expected to have a major impact on the immunologic function of the lymphatic tissues, particularly because the immune response is basically a phenomenon of proliferation of cells within tissues. A primary path of injury and cell death in tissues exposed to ionizing radiation is the block to cell division and cell death during mitosis.

The immunologist usually divides the immune response into two types of consequences, one that can be expressed or measured without the presence of cells, humoral immunity, and one that depends on living cells for its expression, cellular immunity. This separation into humoral and cellular immunity has been maintained in the present chapter on radiation effects.

BENJAMIN and SLUKA (1908) were first to report the depressive effects of x-irradiation on the humoral immune response, and HEINEKE (1903) had earlier shown the morphologic injury to bone marrow and lymphatic tissue. These

---

Abbreviations: ALL = acute lymphoid leukemia; ALS = antilymphocyte serum; AML = acute myeloblastic leukemia; ATS = antithymocyte serum; CI = cell inhibition; CML-BC = chronic myelogenous leukemia in blast crisis; CMV = cytomegalovirus; CNS = central nervous system; CRBC = chicken red blood cells; CY = cyclophosphamide; DNCB = dinitrochlorobenzene; GVHD = graft-versus-host disease; HL-A = human leukocyte antigen; LD = lymphocyte defined; LET = linear energy transfer; MHC = major histocompatibility complex; MLC = mixed leukocyte culture; MLD = midlethal dose; MTX = methotrexate; PHA = phytohemagglutinin; RBC = red blood cell; SD = serologically defined; SRBC = sheep red blood cell; TBI = total body irradiation; WBC = white blood cell.

historical discoveries were followed in subsequent years by a continued series of investigations that were expanded by research in many countries in the 1940's and subsequently as the atomic energy era unfolded.

Major reviews by MAKINODAN and GENGOZIAN (1960), TALIAFERRO *et al.* (1964), SIMIC *et al.* (1965), and by MAKINODAN (1966) of radiation effects on the immunological response have been published. COTTIER (1961) gives a systematic review of morphologic changes in lymphatic and hematopoietic tissues exposed to ionizing radiation.

In this chapter major emphasis has been placed on the effect of ionizing radiation on the cellular immune response because it is the mode of immune reaction whose injury by ionizing radiation facilities a tolerance-like state in which foreign grafts can persist in man and animals. The greatest amount of investigation concerns bone marrow transplantation after irradiation, and we have focused our report on grafting of this organ system.

Following the historical development of the research, humoral immunity and irradiation are summarized first. Unless otherwise mentioned, all radiation exposure is penetrating total body and acute, i.e., administered over a short span of time—minutes or hours.

B. Humoral Immunity

I. Primary and Secondary Immune Response

Most investigators have used the classical blood serum antibody production curve to measure radiation effect on humoral immunity. The four indices from this curve are (1) induction period between antigen injection and first appearance of antibody, (2) the rate of appearance of serum antibody, (3) the mean peak titer, and (4) the mean total titer. Acute exposure of an animal to 500 R ionizing total body irradiation (TBI) within a few hours after antigen injection can drastically lengthen the induction or latent period, decrease the rate of antibody production, lower the mean peak titer, and reduce the total antibody produced (TALIAFERRO *et al.*, 1964).

One method of summarizing the four indices of the antibody production curve is to construct a "relative immune status" as MAKINODAN *et al.* (1959) has done to show that the antibody production curve during the secondary immune response is affected by ionizing TBI in a manner that is qualitatively the same as the production curve of the primary response. The secondary response, however, is more resistant to irradiation than the primary, and for equal exposures the relative immune status of the primary responder is more depressed (MAKINODAN, 1966); see Figure 1.

The resistance of the secondary response to radiation injury is attributed by MAKINODAN to the greater number of immunocompetent cells present at the time of second antigen injection in comparison with the first injection. From the point of view of general pathology suppression of humoral immunity

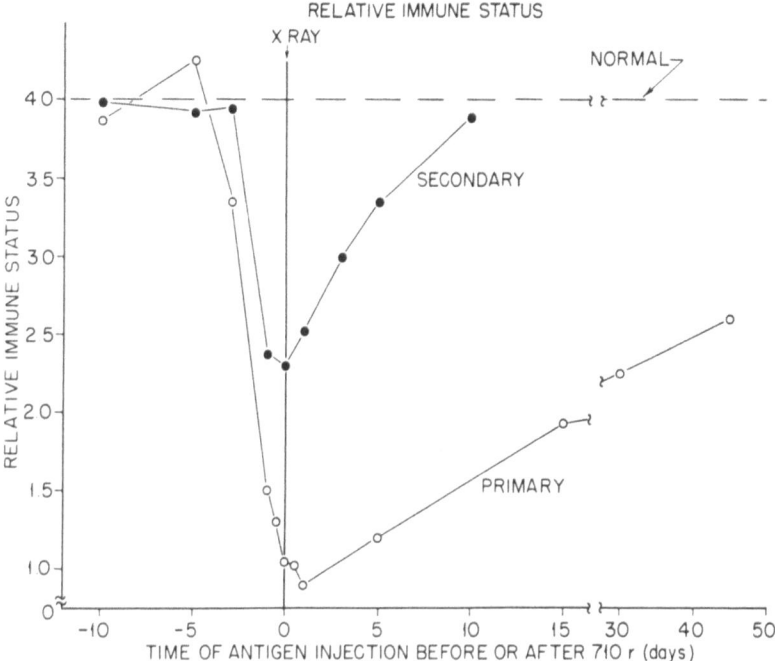

Fig. 1. Relative immune status of primary and secondary immune response after x-irradiation at different times of antigen injection (MAKINODAN *et al.*, 1959; reproduced by permission of Williams and Wilkins Company)

can be further attributed to the radiation cell death and necrosis in lymphatic and hematopoietic tissues and hence loss of cellular compartments from which expansion of lymphatic tissues occurs during an immune response.

II. Time of Irradiation and Antigen Injection

This relationship has been emphasized in all major reviews on radiation immunology (MAKINODAN and GENGOZIAN, 1960; TALIAFERRO *et al.*, 1964; SIMIC *et al.*, 1965; MAKINODAN, 1966). Although there are some species variations, the essential features of the temporal effect are like those shown in Figure 1. The closer the irradiation exposure to the time of antigen injection, the greater is the immune suppression for most species. Increased serum antibody titer when the antigen was injected at certain unique intervals prior to radiation exposure has been noted but not explained.

Studies by CARLSON and GENGOZIAN (1971) demonstrate another variable in the time effect relationship; that of radiation exposure rate. With a common integral exposure of 700 R to mice, the exposure rates of 40 and 72 R/minute were markedly immunosuppressive to sheep red blood cell (SRBC) antigens given 12 hours before or 0–5 days after exposure. At 8 R/minute, the same integral exposure of 700 R was most immunosuppressive when the antigen was

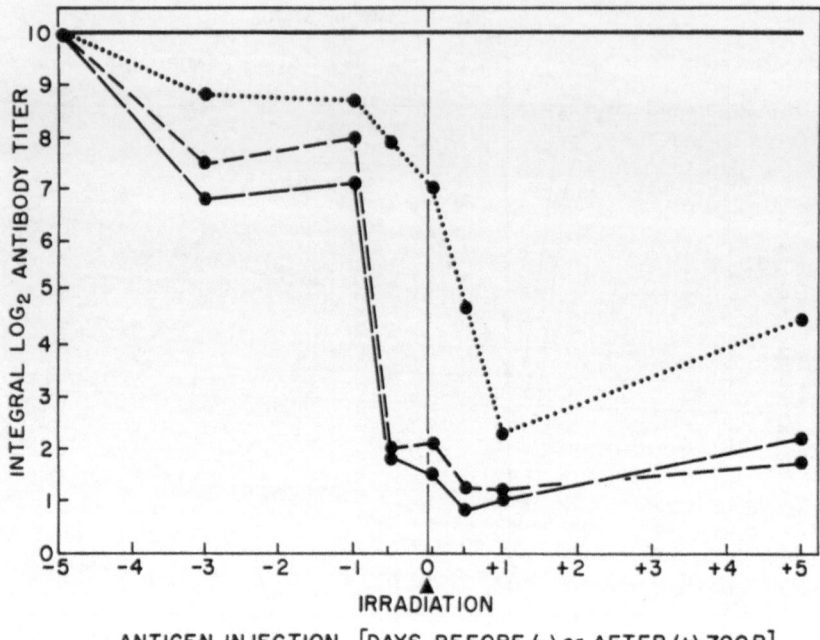

Fig. 2. Primary antibody response to SRBC in mice exposed to 700 R at 8 (dotted line), 40 (dashed line), and 72 R/min (long dashes) (CARLSON and GENGOZIAN, 1971; reproduced by permission of Williams and Wilkins Company)

administered 24 hours after irradiation (Fig. 2, also see GENGOZIAN *et al.*, 1968). This supports the general concept that greatest immunosuppression occurs with antigen injection the day after exposure.

To the general pathologist these temporal relations of exposure and antigen administration are extensions of the relative radiosensitivity and radioresistance of various and changing populations of cells that make up an immune response. Both the preexisting stem cells of the lymphatic tissues and the rapidly proliferating cellular system during the latent or induction phase of a primary humoral immune response are radiosensitive compared with the cellular compartments during serum antibody production. The regeneration of lymphatic tissues is the pathologic process being measured when the antigen is administered days or weeks after exposure.

III. Radiation Type and Amount

Suppression of humoral immunity by TBI is dependent on the amount of radiation exposure. The type of ionizing radiation and its quality, i.e., its penetrance, are also properties of the radiation circumstances. Most studies have been made with x or gamma rays and very few with neutrons or other particulate types of ionizing radiation.

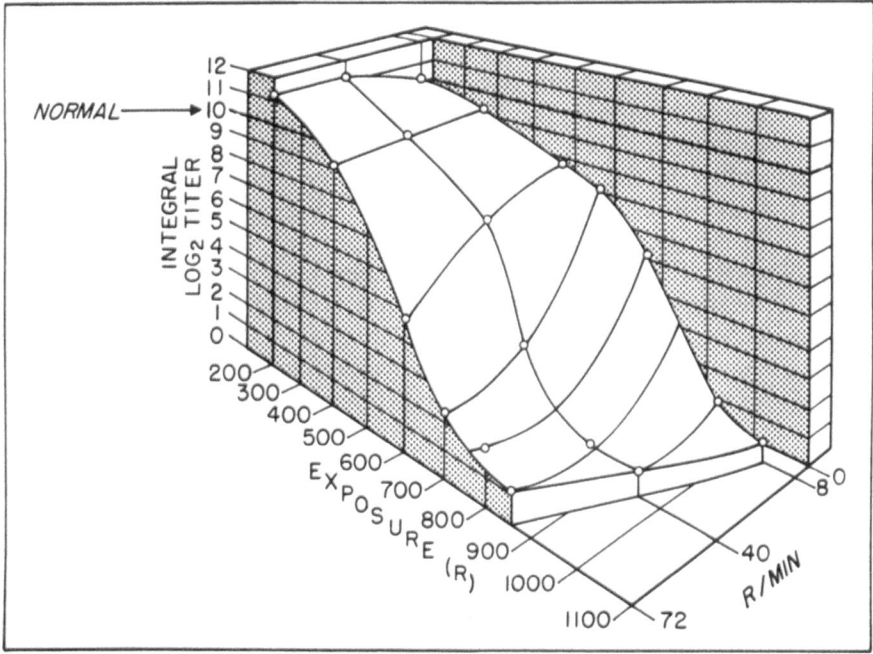

Fig. 3. Antibody formation as a function of radiation exposure and exposure rate (GENGOZIAN *et al.*, 1968)

The radiation effects also can be influenced by partial body versus total body exposure and the exposure rate at which the ionizing radiation is given. Most investigators worked with acute exposure but even here an exposure rate effect can be shown (GOTTLIEB and GENGOZIAN, 1972a, b). Fractionated or intermittent exposure refers to separating exposures by hours, days, or weeks, and chronic irradiation usually implies a relatively low continuous administration of the radiation or small daily exposures.

Between 200 and 104 R of acute gamma rays, immune suppression varied from a just measurable effect to essentially total suppression of humoral immunity (Fig. 3) (GENGOZIAN *et al.*, 1968). At certain integral exposure levels (600–700 R), an exposure rate of 8 R/minute was substantially less immunosuppressive than 72 R/minute. In other studies immunosuppression at 125 R was reported (TALIAFERRO *et al.*, 1964).

For results of fractionated and chronic exposure the reader is referred to the monograph by TALIAFERRO *et al.* (1964).

X and gamma rays have the radiation physics property of low LET or linear energy transfer. When particulate neutron irradiation of high LET was studied, GOTTLIEB and GENGOZIAN (1972a, b) found it to be about four times more efficient than x-rays on an equal rad exposure basis. The acute neutron exposure did not show the exposure rate differences seen with x-rays, which confirms the more general observation that high LET exposure is less exposure rate dependent than low LET for most radiobiological effects.

IV. Type of Antigen

Under this heading attention is called to the existence of a variety of other factors that might influence "radiation induced tolerance" measured by humoral antibody production. The particulate or soluble nature of the antigen, its viable or non-viable state, the dose of antigen, the route of injection, and the genetic relation of the antigen to the irradiated animal could be variables for consideration.

In general, however, the kinds of variables just mentioned have not been noted to be significant in the sense that time of antigen injection and amount of radiation exposure are. MAKINODAN (1966) reviewed the idea of a recognition factor in immunology in which a greater radiation effect is seen with closely related rat red blood cell antigens in exposed mice compared to SRBC antigens.

C. Cellular Immunity

Studies on the influence of irradiation on cellular immunity have predominantly been concerned with the use of TBI. These studies mainly involved attempts at inducing tolerance to marrow allografts and to a lesser degree to grafts of solid organs.

I. Bone Marrow Grafting

Shortly after the discovery of x-rays by Roentgen, several groups of investigators carried out studies on the effect of this new physical agent on living organisms. The investigations of HEINEKE (1903, 1905) and BENJAMIN and SLUKA (1908) were the first to notice the exquisite radiosensitivity of lymphoid and hematopoietic tissues and also of the immune response. The most prominent features of irradiation injury in experimental animals were susceptibility to infection and hemorrhagic complications. Probably the first observations at modifying radiation injury were made by FABRICIOUS-MOELLER (1922). He found that shielding the legs of guinea pigs against irradiation prevented the usual depression of platelet counts and the hemorrhagic problems following TBI. His studies went largely unnoticed, and it was only during the development of the atomic bomb during World War II that further extensive studies on the effects of irradiation on the hematopoietic system were carried out. An important landmark was the finding of JACOBSEN et al. in 1949 that mice could be protected from an otherwise lethal exposure to TBI by exteriorizing and shielding the spleen (JACOBSEN et al., 1949). Soon thereafter LORENZ et al. (1951) observed that mice and guinea pigs could be protected against TBI by the infusion of syngeneic marrow immediately after irradiation. It is interesting to note that these early studies lead to the concept that "humoral factors" were present in the shielded spleen or in the infused hematopoietic tissues, which then induced rapid restoration of the irradiated hematopoietic tissues in the body. The "humoral" hypothesis was considerably strengthened by observations from COLE *et al.* (1952), who showed that cell "extracts" of the hematopoietic tissues were also therapeutically effective. Other investigators, however, were unable to confirm these results, and it seems now to be certain that COLE's positive findings were due entirely to the presence of intact living cells in the "extract". By 1955 an increasing number of investigators expressed their doubts as to the correctness of the "humoral factor" hypothesis. Three independent groups of investigators in different countries using different experimental designs produced cogent evidence that the life-saving effect of hematopoietic cell infusions was due to a cellular mechanism (MAIN and PREHN, 1955; FORD *et al.,* 1956; NOWELL *et al.,* 1956). Subsequently, a number of other investigators confirmed this evidence, and it can now be stated with certainty that the irradiation-induced marrow aplasia can be reversed by infusion of syngeneic, allogeneic, or even xenogeneic hematopoietic cells.

The implications of these findings reach far beyond the problem of modifying irradiation injury. These initial studies were the baseline for further fundamental investigations of the kinetics of hematopoietic cells and of the immunologic principles that govern the fate of the transplanted hematopoietic tissues and of the recipient of the transplant (TRENTIN, 1972). The fact that the transplanted hematopoietic cells persist in the irradiated host offered a variety of theoretical possibilities not only for the treatment of the patient with marrow failure but also for the replacement of malignant hematopoietic cells by normal ones. In addition, because, as a consequence of the marrow transplant, the host's immunologic system was replaced by donor cells, the host was then conditioned to accept grafts of other organs from the marrow donor.

Encouraged by the studies in the inbred rodent models, clinical application of marrow grafting in a variety of malignant and nonmalignant hematopoietic diseases began in 1957 and lasted approximately six years (THOMAS *et al.,* 1957; MATHE *et al.,* 1965a; BORTIN, 1970). Of the 207 reported cases of human marrow grafts, 11 were successful, and only one patient survived beyond one year with sustained engraftment. It appeared that most of these initial cases were destined to fail from the onset because many of the conditions known from the rodent experiments to be necessary for graft acceptance and survival could not be applied to man. Results showed that extrapolation from inbred rodents to man can be a very difficult undertaking.

Because of these failures, the initial enthusiasm was chilled, and human marrow grafting, except for a few patients with identical twin donors, was almost abandoned over the subsequent years. Advances in several areas of research have lead to renewed interest in clinical marrow grafting. One of these advances was the realization that the reactions of two randombred animal species, dogs and monkeys, to both irradiation and hematopoietic grafting resembled in many respects those of humans. In addition, new knowledge has been gathered in the areas of histocompatibility typing, immunosuppressive drug therapy, and supportive measures for patients with decreased immune mechanisms. Patients with marrow failure due to nonmalignant causes who have an identical twin or patients with certain immune deficiency diseases have benefited from marrow grafts without conditioning by an immunosuppressive agent.

The use of a powerful immunosuppressive agent preceding marrow infusion is imperative, however, for the individual who has achieved immunologic maturity whether he suffers from aplastic anemia or acute leukemia. More recently cyclophosphamide (CY), a chemotherapeutic agent, has received investigative attention and has been used as a conditioning agent in experimental and clinical grafting. Other chemical and biological agents such as antilymphocyte serum (ALS) are currently under investigation. The most widely used conditioning agent, however, has been ionizing TBI. The subsequent paragraphs will discuss studies of irradiation and marrow grafting in animal species and the current status of clinical marrow grafting for marrow failure and hematopoietic malignancy.

1. Irradiation Dose

a) Injury

Extensive investigations in rodents, dogs, and primates as well as isolated observations in man have shown that three different irradiation syndromes can be distinguished: hematopoietic, gastrointestinal, and cerebral (Cronkite, 1960).

α) Hematopoietic

Hematopoietic death has been observed after total body exposures lower than 1,500 rad. The underlying process is an inhibition of hematopoietic cell division with a resulting depletion of the hematopoietic tissues as cells mature and are released into the circulation. The first cell line to disappear from the peripheral blood is the lymphocyte. This has been reported to occur within three days of irradiation even after exposure to as little as 200 rad. After irradiation exposures in the "supralethal" range (more than 800 rad), granulocyte and platelet levels fall after exhaustion of the marrow reserve. Profound granulocytopenia occurs after 5–6 days and profound thrombocytopenia after 7–8 days. After exposures near the LD_{50} level, the decline in granulocyte counts is slower, occurring over an interval of 2–4 weeks. Due to the long life span of the red blood cells (RBC), anemia becomes apparent only at a later time after irradiation. As a consequence of the granulocytopenia, the animals' resistance to bacterial infections decreases, setting the stage for life-threatening bacterial sepsis. Thrombocytopenia is accompanied by life-threatening hemorrhage. The exposure after which hematopoietic death is observed varies from species to species. For instance, in the dog, the LD_{50}^{30} is between 300 and 400 R. In man, the exposure is approximately 400 R, in the monkey 550 R, in the mouse 550 R, in the rat 600 R, and in the rabbit and hamster 800 R. It should be emphasized that most of these data pertain to animals that were not treated with cellular blood elements nor antibiotics nor subject to isolation techniques.

β) Gastrointestinal

The gastrointestinal syndrome, irreversible damage to the intestinal tract, has been observed between 1,500 and 12,000 rad. This syndrome is characterized by anorexia, nausea, vomiting, and excessive watery diarrhea with ultimate sloughing of the gastrointestinal mucosa leading to protein loss and water and electrolyte imbalance resembling in its clinical picture the infection with *Vibrio cholerae*. Animals die between the fourth and sixth day following irradiation. Autopsy findings show severe inflammation of the bowel wall with denudation of the mucosal layer.

γ) Central Nervous System (CNS)

The cerebral syndrome in animals has been observed following exposures exceeding 12,000 rad. Death occurs within 48 hours of irradiation and is probably due to pyknosis of the granular cell layer of the cerebellum accompanied by wide-spread vasculitis, encephalitis, and brain edema.

b) Conditioning of Recipients for Hematopoietic Grafting

α) The Midlethal Dose (MLD) Effect

It is of interest to note that marrow grafting started as a means for protecting against a lethal marrow syndrome following TBI. Investigations in inbred rodents as well as in randombred animal systems — dogs, pigs and monkeys — have shown that this protection could be obtained by infusing syngeneic or autologous marrow obtained before and returned after exposure to irradiation. When allogeneic marrow was infused after irradiation exposure in the near lethal range, a heretofore unknown phenomenon was encountered, the MLD effect (TRENTIN, 1956). This term refers to the observation that infusion of allogeneic marrow caused an increased mortality when compared with animals given identical irradiation exposures but no marrow. Several groups of investigators concluded after exhaustive investigations that the MLD effect is the result mainly of a host-versus-graft reaction and is seen only in a limited number of rodent donor-recipient strain combinations (UPHOFF, 1963; NOUZA and LENGEROVA, 1965). As a matter of fact, it appeared that the MLD effect after infusion of allogeneic marrow is the exception rather than the rule.

β) Rejection of the Marrow Graft and "Reversal"

Studies conducted in dogs did not show evidence or the presence of an MLD effect in this species and also served to illustrate some other features of TBI (THOMAS *et al.,* 1970). Dogs given 400, 500, or 600 R and allogeneic marrow did not die more quickly than those given irradiation only. Consistent and sustained engraftment of allogeneic marrow in the dog was achieved only when the irradiation exposure was raised to above 1,200–1,800 R midline air exposure, which corresponds to a midline tissue exposure of 950–1,500 rad. In these experiments, TBI was delivered from two opposing ^{60}Co sources at a rate of 9.2 R/min. A phenomenon which has been observed in both rodents and monkeys following successful marrow engraftment has been the "reversal" to host type hematopoiesis after exposures of up to 800 rad delivered from a single x-ray source (VAN BEK-

Kum and de Vries, 1967). In the dog, reversal has not been observed. However, after initial successful engraftment, spontaneous disappearance of the graft and death with marrow aplasia have been described in some animals. Such spontaneous disappearance might be the result of an immune reaction of host cells against the graft, i.e., host cells that have not been eradicated even by the very high exposure to irradiation.

γ) Exposure Rate Effects

The TBI exposure most frequently used in man is 1,000 rad midpoint tissue exposure delivered from dual ^{60}Co sources at a rate of 5.5 R/minute (Thomas et al., 1975). As a rule this irradiation exposure has lead to successful engraftment of marrow cells from HL-A identical siblings and in the one patient given a marrow transplant from a sister different for one HL-A haplotype. It has been proposed that the use of higher exposure rates at a given total exposure might lead to more consistent engraftment (Gengozian et al., 1969). These data have been obtained in mice, and no thorough studies have yet been carried out to determine whether they apply to larger animals or to man.

δ) Conditioning by Irradiation Other Than Total Body (TBI)

Theoretically it should be possible to condition a recipient for marrow grafting using internally administered radioactive isotopes. This approach has the advantage of a rather homogeneous exposure to irradiation or of selective irradiation of certain body tissues. In studies using ^{90}Y to prepare dogs for allografts it was pointed out that the exposure to lymphatic tissue was about $2^1/_2$ times greater than that to the marrow (Winchell et al., 1966). Internally administered isotopes, however, present many problems with irradiation safety procedures. One cannot "turn off" long-lived isotopes at an optimal time for grafting, and short-lived isotopes present problems in logistics and dosimetry. However, it seems worthwhile to further investigate this approach.

ε) Time of Marrow Infusion in Relation to Irradiation

Most data dealing with the question as to what interval after irradiation is the most suitable for the infusion of marrow cells have been obtained using transplants between syngeneic rodents. On the basis of these studies and of data concerning the primary antibody response to various antigens in rodents following lower radiation exposures, it has been suggested that an interval of 24 hours between TBI and marrow grafting is advantageous (van Bekkum and de Vries, 1967). These studies conducted in rodents have not yet been tested in larger animals. In human patients as well as in dogs, marrow infusions have been carried out within 1–4 hours after TBI with consistently successful engraftment (Storb and Thomas, 1972; Thomas et al., 1975). Obviously, the administration of the marrow immediately following TBI has the advantage of shortening the period of post-irradiation pancytopenia, thus decreasing the length of time required for supportive care.

2. Histocompatibility Differences Between the Host and Donor

There is abundant evidence to implicate an immunologic barrier as the key stumbling block to successful organ transplantation. The induction of the immune response to transplantation antigens as well as the intensity of the response depends on the genetic, i.e., the antigenic differences between donor and recipient. We owe much of the present understanding of the role of transplantation or histocompatibility antigens in marrow grafting to work in inbred rodent species. Many mouse histocompatibility (H) loci (H1-H13, H-Y, and H-X, etc.) have been defined. Differences at any one of these loci lead to graft rejection. One of these loci, the H-2 locus, seems to be of greater importance and has been termed the major histocompatibility locus in the mouse. A major immunogenic system of histocompatibility has been described for every mammalian species studied so far including rats, guinea pigs, pigs, dogs, rhesus monkeys, and chimpanzees. Intensive studies of serologic histocompatibility testing in man have culminated in the definition of a major system of human histocompatibility, the HL-A (human leukocyte antigen) system (DAUSSET and COLOMBANI, 1972). It has been found that the HL-A antigens are genetically determined by a region on an autosomal chromosome. In man, extensive population and family studies over the past decade have resulted in the definite identification of at least two HL-A or serologically defined (SD) loci and have raised speculation regarding a third and a fourth sublocus. The first or LA locus determines at least 13 antigens as alternative alleles. The second, or four locus determines at least 15 antigens. A great number of alleles determined by the two SD loci probably are still unknown. Nevertheless, despite the polymorphism of the HL-A system, one can find HL-A identical individuals amongst siblings because there are only four possible combinations of the parental haplotypes.

The serologic histocompatibility typing has been complemented by the in vitro mixed leukocyte culture (MLC) test (BACH and AMOS, 1967). In family studies, the MLC test and serologic typing were correlated. It was found that HL-A disparity caused stimulation in MLC, while HL-A identity resulted in nonreactivity. The MLC is a one-way test in which peripheral blood lymphocytes of one individual enlarge and divide in response to antigens on lymphocytes of a second individual. These antigens are determined by a lymphocyte defined (LD) locus closely associated with the four locus. The stimulating lymphocytes are made incapable of reacting by irradiation or mitomycin C. The response is assayed by measuring the incorporation of radioactive thymidine into the responding cells. In some cases, HL-A identity cannot be established by serologic histocompatibility typing alone if an insufficient number of family members are available for haplotype analysis. In these cases, HL-A identity can be verified by nonreactivity in MLC.

The importance of histocompatibility differences between donor and recipient has been illustrated in rodents by investigating the number of hematopoietic cells required in various strain combinations in order to obtain a 30-day survival following an LD_{100} of TBI. The 30-day survival rate is a good indicator for hematopoietic engraftment and continued proliferation of the hematopoietic graft. It was found that approximately 80 times as many marrow cells were required for optimal recovery when the graft was carried out across an H-2 barrier than in the case of a syngeneic graft (VAN BEKKUM and DE VRIES, 1967). Even more cells were required for grafts among xenogeneic combinations (rat or hamster into mouse). Unfortunately, little quantitative information exists for randombred species. Data suggest, however, that differences on the order of 5–15 times exist between autologous and allogeneic situations.

Antigenic differences between host and donor are not only important with respect to achieving engraftment but also with regard to the incidence of graft rejection, development of lethal GVHD, or eventual survival of the recipient following the marrow graft. In mice, fatal GVHD can generally be produced in a proportion of the animals when grafts are carried out across the major H-2 barrier (UPHOFF and LAW, 1959). Fatal GVHD has rarely been observed when grafts were performed among strains congenic for H-2 but differing for one or more of the "minor" histocompatibility loci (UPHOFF and LAW, 1959; UPHOFF, 1969; ELKINS, 1971; SALAMAN et al., 1973). In such combinations, fatal GVHD can in general only be produced with cells from donors immunized against the host.

The dog has been used as a model for studies of histocompatibility and marrow grafting in a randombred species (STORB and THOMAS, 1972). Typing for serologically detected histocompatibility antigens (DL-A) and MLC are carried out in a manner similar to that in man. MLC reactivity was shown to correlate with serologic histocompatibility typing of littermates, and approximately one-fourth of the littermate pairs were nonreactive in MLC (TEMPLETON et al., 1971). Furthermore, studies by a number of investigators have shown

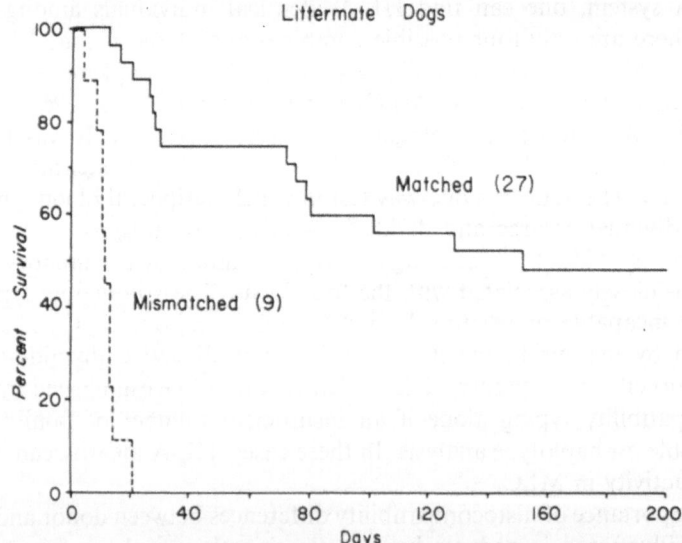

Fig. 4. Survival curves of two groups of dogs given 1,200–1,580 R of TBI followed by infusion of allogeneic hematopoietic cells. No immunosuppressive therapy was given after grafting. The marrow donors were littermates either matched or mismatched at the major canine histocompatibility complex. Numbers of dogs studied are in parenthesis (STORB et al., 1972a; reproduced by permission of LYLE R. HEIM, Ph.D., editor of *Experimental Hematology*)

over 20 preliminary DL-A groups (ALBERT *et al.*, 1973; VRIESENDORP *et al.*, 1973). Segregation analysis yielded information about the allelism of two separate specificities thus confirming earlier suggestions of a two locus histocompatibility system in the dog. Histocompatibility appears to be an important factor governing the fate of a marrow transplant in dogs. When no post-grafting immunosuppression was given, none of the histoincompatible littermates survived beyond day 25, while the survival of histocompatible littermates was significantly prolonged (Fig. 4). A number of the histocompatible dogs have now lived for over eight years. Encouraging as these results are they also indicate that matching for DL-A antigens and MLC negativity alone is not sufficient to guarantee long-term survival. Fatal GVHD was seen in about half of the DL-A matched dogs (STORB *et al.*, 1973a), indicating that some important antigenic differences, probably analogous to the "minor" H-loci in mice, are not detected by the serologic canine histocompatibility testing nor by the MLC test. These data underline the need for post-grafting immunosuppression even in this "compatible" situation. Phenotypic matching for the major dog leukocyte antigen locus not only significantly prolonged the survival of littermate recipients but also that of unrelated dogs when recipients were treated with small doses of an immunosuppressive agent [methotrexate (MTX)] post-grafting (STORB *et al.*, 1970a). It appeared from the studies that not only the development of GVHD but also the acceptance of the transplant by the host was favorably influenced by compatibility for transplantation antigens.

Similar data have been recently described in primates: unrelated monkeys selected for histocompatibility similarities survived better than those that were mismatched (NEEFE *et al.*, 1973).

Two-thirds of histoincompatible canine littermates differ by one DL-A haplotype and one-third differ by two. Most unrelated dogs differ by two DL-A haplotypes on the assumption that the DL-A system is of similar complexity as the HL-A system and that the number of histocompatibility alleles is sufficiently great in the dog population. As expected most recipients in this study died with GVHD despite the use of post-grafting immunosuppression, but littermates survived statistically longer than unrelated recipients (STORB *et al.*, 1972b). This is probably due to the fact that the "amount" of DL-A disparity is important in determining the survival of the marrow graft recipient, i.e., cumulative effects of "major" antigen differences hasten the occurrence and increase the incidence of fatal GVHD in unrelated recipients.

Marrow transplants between human siblings differing by one or two HL-A haplotypes have generally resulted in either failure to show evidence of marrow engraftment or in death with GVHD (THOMAS *et al.*, 1975). One patient with leukemia had a successful marrow graft from a sister differing by one HL-A haplotype post-grafting. The patient showed severe GVHD, which apparently was controlled by treatment with MTX, but he died on day 56 with a cytomegalovirus (CMV) infection.

It appears that HL-A identical siblings offer the optimal donor-recipient combination for marrow grafting in man at the present time. Successful grafts and long-term survival with this donor-recipient combination have already been observed in a number of patients with immunodeficiency diseases (reviewed in VAN BEKKUM, 1972), refractory marrow failure (STORB et al., 1974a), and acute leukemia (THOMAS et al., 1975). The true incidence of fatal GVHD after grafts from HL-A compatible siblings is not known since most patients had been given immunosuppressive therapy post-grafting. It appears from the presently available data that approximately 50–80% of patients with successful grafts will develop GVHD and approximately 25–40% will die of GVHD or complications thereof (STORB et al., 1974a; THOMAS et al., 1975).

The situation in respect to unrelated donor-recipient pairs phenotypically matched for HL-A antigens is unknown. Unfortunately, most such pairs show strong mutual stimulation in MLC, suggesting incompatibility for the locus governing the MLC reaction. Unequivocally successful marrow grafts with such donor-recipient combinations in man have not yet been reported.

3. The Presensitized Recipient

It is known that TBI is most immunosuppressive when administered before exposure of the living organism to antigen. Studies at lower irradiation exposures, carried out predominantly in rodents, have shown that the secondary immune response is more radioresistant than the primary response. This characteristic of TBI is of great importance for marrow grafting in view of the fact that most potential human marrow graft recipients have been exposed to multiple blood transfusions for the treatment of their underlying disease. Since histocompatibility antigens are known to be present on platelets and leukocytes in the transfused blood, recipients may become immunized against a subsequent allogeneic marrow graft. It was hoped that with siblings matched for major histocompatibility antigens immunization would not occur. However, experiments in DL-A matched canine littermates have shown that prior exposure to transfusions with whole blood may jeopardize the success of a subsequent marrow graft even in this "compatible" donor-recipient combination (STORB et al., 1970c). When recipients were given a single transfusion from their intended marrow donor before TBI, marrow graft rejection and early death of the recipient with marrow hypoplasia were seen in many instances. To a lesser degree this phenomenon was also observed after exposure of the recipient to multiple random blood transfusions (STORB et al., 1971). Presumably, rejection was due to immunization of the recipient to histocompatibility antigens other than DL-A. Even very high conditioning doses of TBI, approximately three times the lethal exposure in the dog, were unable to suppress existing immunity sufficiently to prevent graft rejection. In the case of blood transfusions from random donors or from family members other than the marrow donor, immunization of the recipient and rejection of the graft might be expected only when the marrow donor and the transfusion donors share "minor" histocompatibility antigens not present in the recipient. Data similar to those in dogs have been reported in x-irradiated mice and also in mice treated with CY (LOUTIT and MICKLEM, 1961; SANTOS and SENSENBRENNER, 1971). The data obtained in the inbred mouse model and the randombred dog model indicate that a human patient who is a candidate for a marrow graft should be managed without blood transfusions from the intended HL-A identical donor or from other family members. The cumulative experience in human marrow grafting has justified the concern with respect to the harmful effects of preceding blood transfusions. A recent report on the results of allogeneic marrow grafting for the treatment of aplastic anemia has shown that patients who have been given transfusions from family members have a high incidence of failure of marrow engraftment or of marrow graft rejection (STORB et al., 1974a).

Studies in dogs given multiple transfusions from random unrelated donors followed by marrow grafts from histoincompatible littermates have shown that the majority of recipients rejected the graft. This finding, in combination with the observation of a high incidence of fatal GVHD in histoincompatible canine littermates, indicates that successful marrow grafting between histoincompatible humans may be very difficult.

Studies aimed at reducing the incidence of graft rejection by the use of preceding transfusions of buffy coat-poor blood have been disappointing (STORB et al., 1973b). More recently, studies were carried out in the dog model investigating whether immunization by preceding transfusions can be abrogated by a combination of two immunosuppressive agents, procarbazine and rabbit anti-dog antithymocyte serum (ATS) preceding TBI (STORB et al., 1974b). These studies, carried out in DL-A incompatible unrelated dogs of different breeds, have been encouraging and indicate that immunization can be successfully abrogated by a combination of these two agents while either agent alone is not sufficient. It remains to be seen whether this information can be successfully extrapolated to the human marrow graft situation. Initial results have shown that the regimen is well tolerated by human marrow graft candidates and that successful engraftment is possible (Case 19 in STORB et al., 1974a).

4. Successful Hematopoietic Engraftment

a) Evidence of Chimerism

In 1956 three groups of investigators independently succeeded in supplying irrefutable proof that the repopulation of the hematopoietic tissues in allogeneic marrow graft recipients was due to proliferation of cells of donor type (MAIN and PREHN, 1955; FORD et al., 1956; NOWELL et al., 1956). Proof was obtained by cytologic, serologic, and biochemical (hemoglobin electrophoresis) methods. In addition, it was found that grafts of solid organs from the marrow donor, as a rule, survived indefinitely in the marrow recipient. These initial studies were carried out almost uniformly in rodents. Subsequently, the same methods of identification were found to be useful in larger mammals, monkeys and dogs, and also in human patients. Also, additional markers were found such as variants of RBC enzymes, immunoglobulin allotypes, and RBC antigens. Studies in canine radiation chimeras have been carried out for as long as ten years after grafting, and cells in marrow, peripheral blood, and lymph nodes were consistently found to be of donor type (STORB and THOMAS, 1972). In man, such studies have been carried out for more than five years postgrafting with identical results (STORB et al., 1974a; THOMAS et al., 1975).

Thus, dog and human long-term irradiation chimeras show persistent donor type chimerism. Reversal to host type hematopoiesis has been described in some monkeys and also occasionally in mice. Data with xenogeneic rat to mouse transplants and allogeneic mouse transplants have shown that total or partial reversals depended on the amount of irradiation exposure given to the recipient before grafting (GENGOZIAN and MAKINODAN, 1957; SANTOS et al., 1958; WELLING et al., 1959). That is, the incidence of reversal decreased with higher irradiation doses. In addition, it was found that a high degree of incompatibility between host and donor favors the reversion process.

b) GVHD

α) Pathology

In randombred animal species, monkeys, dogs and man, successful hematopoietic engraftment from randomly selected donors is followed by an early, severe, and usually rapidly fatal GVHD. In rodents, depending somewhat on the donor-recipient strain combination, GVHD occurs later, takes a more protracted and milder course, and a variable number of the animals recover. GVHD is presumed to be the result of an immune reaction of the transplanted immunologically active cells against histocompatibility antigens of the host. For unknown reasons, the principal target organs of GVHD in both animals and man are skin, gastrointestinal tract, liver, and lymphoid tissues. Descriptions of these changes have been presented elsewhere (DE VRIES et al., 1961; VAN BEKKUM and DE VRIES, 1967; LERNER et al., 1974; GLUCKSBERG et al., 1974). Briefly, in patients the initial reaction is usually a skin rash that may progress to severe ulcerative skin lesions. Gastrointestinal involvement is reflected by diarrhea, anorexia, nausea, vomiting, and in more severe cases malabsorption, abdominal pain, ileus, and ascites. Liver disease is manifested by moderate hepatomegaly and by rises in serum glutamic oxaloacetic transaminase, alkaline phosphatase, and bilirubin. Fever, wasting, and a decreased clinical performance are also regularly seen with severe involvement. Histologically, skin lesions vary from focal or diffuse vacuolar degeneration of epidermal basal cells and acanthocytes to frank loss of epidermis. The gastrointestinal tract lesions vary from mild to marked mucosal thinning, edema, and ulceration. The changes in the liver involve degeneration and eosinophilic necrosis of parenchymal cells and degeneration necrosis of the epithelium of small bile ducts. Severe lymphoid hypoplasia is usually observed. Lymphoid atrophy may be a consequence of GVHD and may explain the impairment of immunologic defense mechanisms against pathogens seen in animals and patients with allogeneic grafts. Death in dogs and monkeys given marrow from unrelated donors appears between 7 and 25 days (VAN BEKKUM and DE VRIES, 1967; STORB and THOMAS, 1972). The average survival in human patients with GVHD following grafts from histocompatible siblings is longer, perhaps due to the more favorable donor-recipient combinations and due to better supportive care.

β) The Prevention and Treatment of GVHD

Attempts to prevent or delay the complication of GVHD have involved two major approaches. One approach has been the selection of donor and recipient by in vitro methods of histocompatibility testing. In all species studied (mouse, rat, guinea pig, dog, monkey, man) it has been found that the major histocompatibility complex (MHC) is genetically determined by loci on an autosomal chromosome. In each human haplotype at least three loci are involved, two determined serologically and one by MLC. Siblings who have inherited these same two haplotypes are HL-A identical by serologic testing and non-reactive in MLC. The use of these "compatible" sibling pairs has provided the basis for the rapidly increasing number of human marrow transplants. Yet this "compatibility" is imperfect since about two-thirds of such marrow graft recipients develop recognizable GVHD and in more than one-third the GVHD is severe and potentially fatal. This should not be surprising since it was already known that fatal GVHD can occur in littermate dogs despite compatibility for the MHC. Evidently incompatibilities for one or more unknown "minor" histocompatibility loci, undetected by current techniques, are important determinants for the ultimate outcome. Knowledge of these "minor" loci would be useful in selecting the best donor in patients where several HL-A matched siblings are available.

From the animal studies as well as from the clinical marrow grafting experience it has become clear that some forms of immunosuppressive therapy must be used post-grafting to diminish or prevent GVHD. The immunosuppressive regimens usually consist of cytostatic agents with nonspecific immunosuppressive effects. To be effective, treatment with these agents must be begun well before GVHD has become apparent. Of the many agents studied, MTX and CY have been found to be particularly useful. MTX was found effective in mice (UPHOFF, 1958), dogs (THOMAS et al., 1962; STORB et al., 1970a) and monkeys (MULLER-BERAT et al., 1966) when given in the immediate post-grafting period. Studies in dogs have shown that MTX was most effective when continued for a prolonged period of time, and stable long-term chimerism for years was achieved in some DL-A incompatible graft recipients. CY was effective in mice, rats, and monkeys but was ineffective in dogs (STORB et al., 1970b). Controlled studies to compare the effectiveness of MTX and CY have not been carried out in any species other than the dog. Studies using other agents—cytosine arabinoside, procarbazine, 6-mercaptopurine, ATS etc.—in the immediate post-grafting period have been disappointing.

Based on the studies in dogs, the most frequently used post-grafting regimen in human recipients of HL-A matched marrow consists of MTX 15 mg/m² on day 1 and 10 mg/m² on days 3, 6, 11, and weekly thereafter for the first 100 days (STORB et al., 1974a; THOMAS et al., 1975). Other groups have used CY 7.5 mg/kg for five doses on alternate days beginning on the first day after marrow grafting followed by CY at irregular intervals (SANTOS et al., 1971). The incidence of fatal GVHD in patients given a marrow graft from an HL-A matched sibling and no post-grafting immunosuppression is unknown. In dogs given grafts from DL-A compatible littermates, it is approximately 50% when no post-grafting immunosuppression is given and less than 20% with MTX. Despite post-grafting immunosuppression, severe and fatal GVHD has been observed in human marrow graft recipients. An incidence of fatal GVHD on the order of 30–40% is unacceptably high, and better immunosuppressive regimens must be found.

Prevention of GVHD has been attempted using ALS given just before or just after grafting in rodents, dogs, and monkeys with only slight prolongation and survival as recently reviewed (Kolb et al., 1973).

Surprisingly, only a few studies have been reported in which established GVHD was treated either with cytostatic agents or with ALS or ATS. For the most part these studies were negative ones, i.e., the agents used failed to influence the course of events or the authors failed to document sustained chimerism. A detailed review of these studies has been recently presented (Storb et al., 1973c). An exception was the study by Owens and Santos, who inoculated (C57B1/6 × DBA/2) F_1 hybrid mice with BALB/c spleen cells and were able to suppress clinically established GVHD by CY (Owens and Santos, 1971). Almost all surviving mice in their study remained chimeras as determined by immunoglobulin allotype markers (Santos, personal communication). CY was used to treat established GVHD in one patient with aplastic anemia with a marrow graft from an HL-A matched sibling (Storb et al., 1974a). In this patient the treatment proved to be ineffective.

An attempt to influence established GVHD was carried out by treating canine recipients with rabbit anti-dog ATS (Storb et al., 1973c). Unrelated histoincompatible donor-recipient pairs were used, which constitute a severe test model for any immunosuppressive regimen. Even so, the effect of ATS on the GVHD lesions was remarkable. In most instances, skin lesions totally disappeared and diarrhea was reversed. A significant prolongation of survival in the ATS treated group was observed. High doses of prednisone, in the same model, were unable to reverse GVHD or to prolong survival. Recently, application of ATS treatment has been carried out in human marrow graft recipients with GVHD (Storb et al., 1974c). Under ATG therapy, twelve of nineteen patients showed complete resolution of GVHD, five showed improvement of most organ systems involved and two showed no change except for improvement in skin lesions. Six of the nineteen became long-term survivors. Five of the six are alive between 276 and 629 days after grafting, and one died on day 346 with chronic respiratory failure. Of the remaining thirteen patients, eleven died with interstitial pneumonitis of predominantly viral etiology and two died with fungal and bacterial infections. These data demonstrated the relative effectiveness of ATG in reversing human GVHD. Death with interstitial pneumonitis was the single most serious impediment to successful treatment of GVHD with ATG. ATG treatment of established GVHD certainly does not represent the ultimate goal in the solution of the GVHD problem, but it appears to have modified the otherwise grim outlook in a hopeful way. It is obvious from these studies, however, that continued animal and clinical research efforts have to be directed to a better understanding of the nature and control of GVHD.

More recently, albumin gradient and velocity sedimentation techniques have been conducted, aimed at eliminating immunocompetent cells from the marrow inoculum and retaining the hematopoietic stem cell. These techniques have been reported to be useful in preventing the acute GVHD in inbred strain rodents (MILLER and PHILLIPS, 1969; DICKE and VAN BEKKUM, 1971). Proof, however, that this technique is useful in modifying GVHD in grafts between randombred non-rodent animals is as yet missing. Both techniques have been applied in a number of human marrow transplants. The result has been either failure of engraftment or death from GVHD when histoincompatible marrow was employed. This may be due to incomplete separation or loss of stem cells due to prolonged exposure of these cells to room temperature during separation. Aside from the technical problems of the separation, a number of theoretical reasons would argue against the efficacy of "stem cell" separation techniques. Even if it would be possible to perfectly separate lymphoid cells from "stem cells", it is likely that the recipient still might be susceptible to the late form of GVHD, which is presumably caused by a subsequent generation of reactive lymphoid cells derived from the "common" stem cell. If there is not a "common" stem cell giving rise to lymphoid cells, then application of the separation technique would create a recipient who is severely deficient in immune function and thus might succumb easily to infection. At present, therefore, stem cell separation does not appear to be a promising approach.

c) Immunologic Reconstitution of Chimeras

The immunologic system of recipients of marrow grafts is derived from cells of donor origin. In inbred rodent irradiation chimeras, immunologic reactivity was found to be very low in the immediate post-grafting period regardless of whether they were recipients of syngeneic or allogeneic marrow (MAKINODAN et al., 1956; LAVIA et al., 1958; GARVER et al., 1959; HOLLINGSWORTH, 1959; TYAN and COLE, 1963; AGAROSSI and DORIA, 1968; ZARETSKAYA et al., 1968; GREGORY and LAJTHA, 1970). At a later period, syngeneic chimeras showed a more complete recovery of immunologic reactivity than allogeneic chimeras (GENGOZIAN et al., 1958, 1961, 1965, 1971; DORIA et al., 1962; AGAROSSI and DORIA, 1968). These results varied depending on the strain combinations and the antigenic challenges used.

In a recent study, the immune system of randombred canine chimeras was surveyed for periods of up to 8 years after grafting (OCHS et al., 1974). Recovery of granulocytes and return of granulocyte function as determined by iodination tests were complete by day 25 after grafting. Impaired granulocyte function cannot, therefore, explain the frequent infections complicating the early period after grafting. Also, clearance of antigen by the reticuloendothelial system, which presumably represents a first step in the processing of an antigen, did not appear to be impaired in canine chimeras at any stage post-grafting. Chimeras, however, showed lymphocytopenia during the first 200 days post-grafting, and histologically lymphoid hypoplasia was seen with a return to normal after 200 days. Short-term chimeras (less than 200 days post-grafting) showed quantitatively and qualitatively impaired humoral antibody responses to SRBC, chick-

en red blood cells (CRBC), and bacteriophage ØX174 (phage). The cellular
immune reactivity was also generally impaired in short-term chimeras, as indicated by prolonged first- and second-set skin graft survival and by decreased
ability of the dogs' lymphocytes to respond in MLC and to phytohemagglutinin
(PHA). Long-term chimeras showed a delayed rise in antibody titers during
the primary immune response with normal peak titers and a normal quantitative
and qualitative secondary antibody response. Their cellular immune reactivity
was in the normal range. Long-term chimeras were able to live in an unprotected
environment without apparent increased incidence of infection, supporting the
conclusion that after an initial phase of impaired immune function these canine
chimeras regain normal immune reactivity.

One major determinant of the tempo of recovery of the immune reactivity
in chimeras appears to be the speed with which the lymphoid tissues are repopulated by donor cells. This has first been studied in syngeneic mouse chimeras,
and a period of decreased immunologic responsiveness of variable duration
has been observed (Makinodan et al., 1956; LaVia et al., 1958; Garver et al.,
1959; Hollingsworth, 1959; Tyan and Cole, 1963; Agarossi and Doria,
1968; Zaretskaya et al., 1968; Gregory and Lajatha, 1970). Most studies
involved humoral antibody response to SRBC or rat RBC and were limited
to periods of 60–120 days post-grafting. Results showed considerable variation
depending on the mouse strain and the antigenic challenges used. Only one
long-term observation was carried out, and normal antibody responses to SRBC
and rat RBC at 100–300 days post-grafting were reported (Gengozian et al.,
1958). Appearance of cellular immune reactivity was similarly delayed, with
one group of investigators reporting prolonged skin graft survival as late as
350 days post-grafting (Hollingsworth, 1959; Feldman and Yaffe, 1959;
Tyan and Cole, 1963; Riches and Thomas, 1970). Ultimately, syngeneic rodent
chimeras appeared to recover normal immunologic function.

Three patients with advanced hematological malignancies treated by TBI
and infusion of syngeneic marrow were recently studied (Fass et al., 1973).
Results were similar to those seen in rodents with a prolonged period of decreased immunologic reactivity and ultimate immunologic reconstitution. Two
of the three showed normal antibody responses to phage by days 39 and 365
post-grafting and cutaneous reactivity to dinitrochlorobenzene (DNCB) by days
393 and 679.

The recovery of immune reactivity in allogeneic or xenogeneic chimeras
would be expected to be slower than that observed in syngeneic chimeras due
to at least three possible mechanisms: (1) it has been hypothesized that lymphoid
depletion occurs in allogeneic or xenogeneic chimeras as a result of destruction
of donor lymphoid cells during GVHD (Congdon and Urso, 1957; Gorer
and Boyse, 1959). Gengozian et al. have stated that even in animals with
apparent GVHD "an in vivo antigen-antibody reaction persists in these animals
and consequently effects their ability to respond normally to other antigens"
(Gengozian et al., 1971). This concept seems to be supported by recent findings
in canine (Hellstrom et al., 1970) and also in rodent (Hellstrom et al., 1973)
radiation chimeras showing the presence of an immune reaction of chimera
(donor) lymphocytes against host fibroblasts in vitro; (2) allogeneic or xenogen-

eic chimeras have often been treated with immunosuppressive drugs post-grafting, which not only delays or prevents GVHD but also suppresses the response of chimeric lymphocytes to other antigens; and (3) the combination of toxic conditioning regimens, post-grafting immunosuppression, and GVHD causes gut damage leading to a malabsorption syndrome, which, given enough time, can lead to immunodeficiency, as shown in mice placed on a protein deficient diet and in children with protein-calorie malnutrition (SMYTHE *et al.*, 1971; WOODRUFF, 1972). Experimental findings seem to support these theoretical considerations. In general, allogeneic and xenogeneic rodent chimeras were less immunologically active than their syngeneic counterparts even if studied as late as 300 days post-grafting. Most investigations involved SRBC, rat RBC, and *Salmonella typhosa* antigens and, depending upon the strain combination of donor and recipient used, not only quantitative but also qualitative defects were observed. One group of investigators reported that some allogeneic mouse chimeras failed to show normal conversion from 19S to 7S antibody synthesis after repeated immunizations (GENGOZIAN *et al.*, 1965, 1971). Incomplete recovery of some aspects of cellular immunity has also been seen in allogeneic mouse chimeras (HRSAK *et al.*, 1968): pronounced prolongation of skin grafts was found 30 and 65 days after marrow grafting. In contrast, allogeneic mouse chimeras showed positive skin tests to Candida antigen and positive tuberculin conversion after Bacille Calmette-Guerin immunization day 65 (HRSAK *et al.*, 1968).

Recently a number of marrow grafts have been carried out between donor-recipient pairs of beagles that were subject to close breeding for a number of years (RAPAPORT *et al.*, 1972). Chimeras were able to reject skin from unrelated dogs and, after an initial drop, regained significant antidistemper antibody titers.

A number of studies of immune reactivity have been reported in human recipients of allogeneic marrow. Most of these studies were carried out in children with combined immunodeficiency, and improvement and, in some cases, total recovery of cellular and humoral immune reactivity have been reported (reviewed in VAN BEKKUM, 1972). The results obtained in the immunodeficiency patients will not be discussed in the context of the present report since patients did not need to be subjected to an immunosuppressive conditioning regimen and thus are not strictly comparable to TBI chimeras. More recently, a study on ten patients with hematologic malignancy or aplastic anemia given grafts from HL-A compatible sibling donors following 1,000 rad of TBI or high doses of CY was reported (FASS *et al.*, 1973). The patients were observed for 3–30 months after engraftment. In all cases, serum IgG, IgA, and IgM levels declined after grafting and then returned to normal by about day 100. Absolute lymphocyte counts were above $1,000/mm^3$ in all patients within 1–3 months of grafting. Throughout the period of study, patients showed a markedly decreased antibody response to phage, and the antibody, even after repeated immunization, remained predominantly IgM. Several of the patients developed CMV or herpes zoster infections from which they recovered. They developed good antibody titers against these agents. Testing in MLC showed a wide range of responsiveness, but clear stimulation was observed on nearly all occasions even within the first month post-grafting. Similar findings were obtained with PHA. Despite the presence of cellular immune reactivity in vitro, the patients with one exception could not be sensitized to DNCB when tested between days 20 and 365 after marrow grafting. As a clinical corollary to the impaired immune reactivity, pneumonitis, frequently caused by CMV, varicella zoster, *Pneumocystis carinii,* and other infectious agents were the predominant complications in allogeneic human marrow graft recipients (NEIMAN *et al.,* 1973). Viral and parasitic infections are frequent problems in other patients with depressed cellular immunity (RIFKIND, 1965; RIFKIND *et al.,* 1966, 1967; MERIGAN and STEVENS, 1971; GLASGOW, 1970).

The available data on allogeneic rodent chimeras and on human patients with allogeneic marrow grafts thus demonstrate prolonged and apparently indefinite impairment of cellular and humoral immunity while allogeneic canine chimeras show almost complete recovery of both humoral and cellular immunity once they live beyond 200 days post-grafting. The difference in results may be related to species differences or simply due to the fact that dogs were given more marrow (2×10^9 cells/kg) than were patients (3×10^8 cells/kg).

d) Long-term Survivors as Examples of Irradiation Induced Immunological Unresponsiveness: "True Tolerance" or "Enhancement Phenomenon?"

The definition of a stable chimeric state is based upon the persisting presence of a hematopoietic and immunologic system derived from the infused donor cells and the continued absence of GVHD. As discussed in the previous sections,

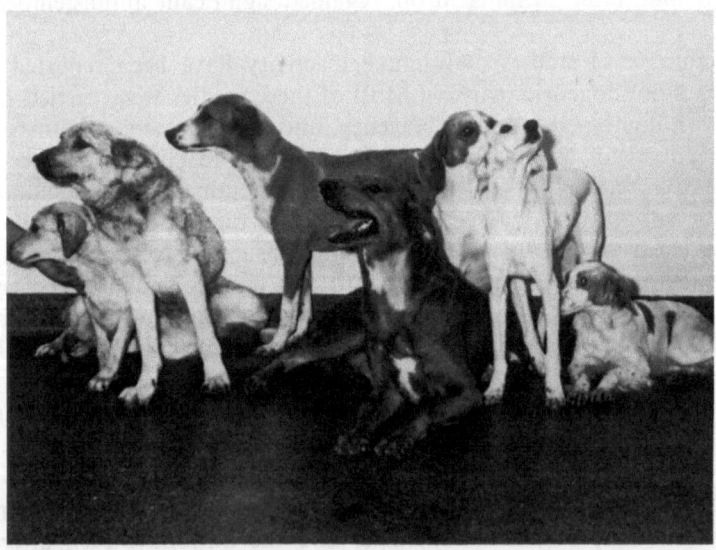

Fig. 5. Seven canine chimeras between $2^1/_2$ and 5 years after marrow transplantation. Six are irradiation chimeras whose hematopoietic and lymphoid systems consist exclusively of cells of donor origin. The large hound in the foreground is a CY chimera with a stable mixed population of donor and host cells

such stable chimerism can be induced by exposure of the recipient to TBI and administration of transient immunosuppressive drug therapy after grafting. Subsequent to the initial induction by immunosuppression, stable chimerism should be self-maintained. Evidence for continued chimerism is provided by appropriate blood genetic markers: sex chromosome markers, RBC antigen markers, white blood cells (WBC) antigen markers, RBC and WBC isoenzymes, immunoglobulin allotypes, or the continued acceptance of a graft of skin or other organs from the marrow donor. Long-term survivors may be defined as those individuals living beyond one year with continued proof of chimerism. The only species in which long-term survival has been observed are rodents, dog, and man. In the dog, more than 50 recipients have survived for more than one year after marrow grafting, and many other animals were killed because of lack of kennel space (STORB and THOMAS, 1972). Figure 5 shows a number of canine chimeras. More than 25 of the dogs have been observed from 3–7 years without evidence of late sequelae and in particular without evidence of malignancies of the reticuloendothelial system as has been described in some rodent strains (SCHWARTZ and BELDOTTI, 1965). The two longest survivors were two male dogs given lethal TBI followed by marrow from unrelated female donors. They continued to show 100% female karyotypes in peripheral blood, marrow, and lymph node cells, which is consistent with findings in other canine TBI chimeras. Table 1 shows an example. One of the two dogs died approximately 10 years after grafting with a metastatic hypernephroma while the other long-term survivor developed a slowly growing carcinoma of the perianal glands with a single metastasis to a cervical lymph node. He was killed approximately 9 years after grafting and was otherwise found to be normal at autopsy. Obviously more long-term survivors following marrow grafting need to be kept for evaluating late irradiation effects in the development of tumors. In man, chimerism seems also to be complete. The longest human TBI chimera, a patient grafted for the treatment of acute lymphoid leukemia (ALL), is now almost 5 years post marrow transplantation and continues to show only cells with the female donor karyotype in marrow and peripheral blood (THOMAS et al., 1975).

Table 1. Karyotype analysis of bone marrow, lymph node, and peripheral blood cells in a male dog 4 years after 1,200 R TBI and transplantation of female hematopoietic cells

Tissue tested	Post-grafting analysis of chromosome counts	
	No. of cells	
	XX	XY
Bone marrow	20	0
Peripheral blood[a]	60	0
Lymph node	20	0
Total	100	0

[a] Cells were stimulated with PHA before analysis

The understanding of the nature of the specific graft-host tolerance in these chimeras is the key to more successful application of clinical marrow grafting. At least two possible broad underlying mechanisms have been proposed: (1) immunologic tolerance in which the lymphocytes of the donor have been rendered specifically unresponsive to host antigen or in which a lymphoid cell clone responding to host antigen has been eliminated (Billingham et al., 1956; Burnet, 1969), and (2) cell-mediated immunity of donor lymphocytes against host antigen that is abrogated by serum blocking factors (Hellstrom et al., 1970, 1971, 1973; Wegmann et al., 1971).

In a previous study in dogs, evidence was presented that stable canine chimeras contained lymphocytes of donor origin responsive to the antigens of the "tolerated" host and that this lymphocyte response was inhibited specifically by serum from the chimera (Hellstrom et al., 1970). These data were obtained using the colony inhibition assay. Subsequently, similar data were obtained in tetraparental mice (Wegmann et al., 1971), mice rendered tolerant neonatally (Hellstrom et al., 1971), and rodent radiation chimeras (Hellstrom et al., 1973). In all of these previous studies consistent colony inhibition or cell inhibition (CI) and blocking have been described, giving rise to the concept of tolerance mediated by a serum blocking factor of some type, possibly an antibody or an antigen-antibody complex (Baldwin et al., 1972; Wright et al., 1974). Similar findings have been reported using the ^{3}H-thymidine release assay in three children with severe combined immunodeficiency grafted with marrow from normal siblings compatible at the MHC (Jose et al., 1971). Chimeric serum inhibited the toxicity of chimeric lymphocytes for chimeric fibroblasts.

In a recent study, the question was reexamined using the microcytotoxicity or CI assay. Nine long-term canine radiation chimeras and their littermate marrow donors matched at the canine MHC were studied between 545 and 1,282 days after 1,200 R TBI and marrow grafting (Tsoi et al., 1975a, b). Before the time of testing, marrow donors were immunized against their chimeras by repeated skin grafts, which they rejected. Skin fibroblasts from chimeras and their donors were tested for CI by exposure to lymphocytes from chimeras, donors, and normal dogs, and the effects of various sera on CI were evaluated. Lymphocytes from sensitized marrow donors consistently inhibited fibroblasts from the chimeras (8 of 9 dogs); CI was abrogated by chimeric serum in only 3 of 8 cases. Only two chimeras showed consistent CI of their own fibroblasts; CI was blocked by chimeric serum in one of the two. The remaining seven chimeras did not show consistent CI.

Sequential studies in 16 additional recipients of littermate marrow matched at the MHC were carried out from 45 to 439 days after marrow grafting. Seven of the 16 did not show CI of chimeric fibroblasts by chimeric lymphocytes at any time. Nine showed CI on one or several occasions. Serum blocking factors were seen on one occasion in each of two chimeras.

It was concluded from these studies that the CI assay is able to detect immunity against "minor" histocompatibility systems in dogs. Both long- and short-term chimeras occasionally demonstrated CI of chimeric fibroblasts, but serum blocking factors did not appear to be necessary for maintaining stable graft-host tolerance in most canine marrow graft recipients matched at the

MHC. The finding of positive CI in some chimeras without serum blocking factors is surprising and remains difficult to explain. It did not correlate with in vivo observations, since none of our chimeras has shown clinical evidence of GVHD. One may be detecting in vitro, due to the enormous lymphocyte: fibroblast ratio used in the CI assay, a population of "sensitized" cells that is too small in numbers to produce any effect detectable in vivo. It may also be that these "sensitized" cells are lymphocytes recently matured from stem cells and in the process of "tolerization" to host antigens.

In a second study, it was attempted to demonstrate in vivo the presence of blocking factors in the serum of canine chimeras using grafts of chimeric skin onto the marrow donor as an indicator system (SCHROEDER et al., 1975). Even very large amounts of chimeric serum (one-fourth of the plasma volume infused daily from day 2 before skin grafting until rejection) failed to modify first- and third-set skin graft rejection patterns. Thus, serum blocking factors could not be demonstrated by this in vivo approach.

A number of other investigators using rodents rendered neonatally tolerant failed to show evidence of serum blocking factors and suggested that tolerance is due rather to a central failure of immune responsiveness (WILSON et al., 1967; SCHWARZ, 1968; WILSON and NOWELL, 1970; ATKINS and FORD, 1972; BRENT et al., 1972; ELKINS, 1973; HERON, 1973; BEVERLEY et al., 1973): (1) spleen cells from tolerant animals failed to produce GVHD when injected into animals of the tolerated strain; (2) GVHD activity of normal spleen cells was not abolished by serum from tolerant animals; (3) attempts to prolong skin graft survival by passive transfer of serum from tolerant animals were negative; (4) it was possible to abrogate tolerance by adoptive transfer of normal spleen cells; (5) the MLC response of tolerant lymphocytes to cells of the tolerated strain was negative while the response to "third party" lymphocytes was positive; and (6) serum from tolerant animals failed to inhibit the MLC response of normal lymphocytes. Others showed that lymphocytes from mouse radiation chimeras were unable to kill tumor cells of host antigenicity in vitro; serum from these animals did not prevent immune cells of donor type being cytotoxic to cells of the host type (GRANT et al., 1972). Evidence against the view that antibody must be involved in serum blocking factors came from studies of ROUSE and WARNER (1972) who were able to induce tolerance to transplantation antigens in agammaglobulinemic chickens.

Evidence for the presence of suppressor cells rather than humoral blocking factors in tolerant animals was reported from studies in tetraparental mice (PHILLIPS and WEGMANN, 1973). It was found that spleen cells from tetraparental mice could block MLC reactivity between the two parental cell types but not between those of unrelated strains. In contrast, WILSON and NOWELL (1970) reported that tolerant cells did not interfere with nontolerant cells in MLC. Similar negative findings have been reported by ELKINS (1973). Others reported that chimeric cells had little, if any, effect on GVH reactions induced by nontolerant cells (ATKINS and FORD, 1972).

The review of the various studies indicates that the stable chimeric state in most rodent chimeras and probably also in the canine irradiation chimeras is not maintained by serum blocking factors. It appears rather that other mechanisms are operational, perhaps suppressor T-cells, perhaps, however, mechanisms operating in the framework of classical tolerance, i.e., elimination or modification of lymphoid clones capable of reacting with host antigens. Currently a number of human irradiation chimeras are being studied with various in vitro tests. These studies might lead to a better understanding of the phenomena of GVHD and graft-host tolerance. They have potentially far reaching clinical implications for the managements of patients with marrow grafts.

e) Clinical Marrow Grafting Studies

As outlined above, marrow grafting started as a means for protecting patients against the lethal marrow syndrome following accidental exposure to TBI. It appears, however, that marrow grafting will not be of practical value for such irradiation accidents. The irradiation exposure would have to be on the order of 800–1,500 rad to the entire body in order to be in the range in which spontaneous recovery would be unlikely to occur, immunosuppression would be adequate to permit engraftment, and gastrointestinal symptoms would be manageable. As pointed out, in the lower but still lethal exposure range, allogeneic marrow grafts would probably not be successful because of inadequate immunosuppression of the host. It is conceivable, however, that progress with additional conditioning regimens may ultimately permit engraftment after such exposures as recently pointed out by GENGOZIAN et al. (1973). They described a patient given horse antihuman ATS for 8 days followed by 500 R and marrow from an HL-A matched sibling. Despite the "low" radiation exposure, engraftment was successful. This regimen could not be applied to an irradiation accident victim since pre-treatment would obviously not be feasible. Much work needs to be done to develop post-irradiation immunosuppressive regimens that might permit successful engraftment of an accident victim, at least for those with an HL-A matched sibling to serve as donor.

The number of patients treated by marrow transplantation after accidental radiation exposure is small. The accident victims at Vinca, Yugoslavia, were given marrow from unrelated donors several weeks after the accident (MATHE et al., 1959). Evidence for engraftment in these patients was weak, and successful engraftment seems unlikely in view of the "midlethal" irradiation exposure and the absence of subsequent GVHD. In addition, a comparison of the clinical course of these patients with the course of the Y-12 accident victims not given marrow led ANDREWS (1962) to conclude that there was no effect of the infused marrow. One radiation accident victim in Pittsburgh, Pennsylvania, had a monozygotic twin to serve as a marrow donor (THOMAS et al., 1971). The patient was exposed to 600 rad TBI and showed prompt hematologic recovery approximately 11–14 days following infusion of the twin marrow. The patient has since been hematologically well for more than 6 years after marrow transfusion.

Encouraged by the advances made in marrow grafting in animal species, in human histocompatibility typing, and in supportive care of patients with decreased defense mechanisms, TBI has now been used as a conditioning agent for marrow grafting in attempts to cure patients with a variety of otherwise fatal diseases. These attempts, described in the following paragraphs, have been characterized by frequent, successful engraftment. A valuable by-product of these studies will be further insight into the basic pathophysiology of diseases such as marrow failure, leukemia, and other diseases of the hematopoietic and lymphoreticular systems. It should be pointed out that these patients were thought to have had the maximum benefit from conventional therapy.

α) Marrow Grafting in Hematologic Malignancy

Antileukemic Effect. The possible use of TBI to eradicate malignant hematopoietic cells has been very attractive. Apparent beneficial effects of TBI and infusion of marrow from syngeneic mice on mouse leukemia were described by BARNES *et al.* (1956). A number of their animals became leukemia-free long-term survivors. This was a rather surprising finding in view of the radiobiologic studies on the radiosensitivity of tumors indicating that complete eradication of mouse leukemia could only be achieved with exposure to several thousand rad (BURCHENAL *et al.*, 1960). The findings by BARNES *et al.* (1956) could only be explained on the basis of further kill of residual leukemic cells by the transplanted cells through a reaction of immunity. MATHE *et al.* (1965b) coined the term "adoptive immunotherapy" to describe the antileukemic effect of the immunologically active foreign marrow. The antileukemic effect of allogeneic hematopoietic cells has been studied by a number of investigators in rodents. BORANIC and TONKOVIC (1971) used inbred AH and RFO mice bearing transplanted lymphoid and myeloid leukemia. Four days after intravenous inoculation of leukemic cells, animals were irradiated with an LD_{10-30} of x-rays followed by injection of spleen and marrow cells from C57Bl/6 mice. Control animals were injected with syngeneic cells after irradiation. Only a transient antileukemic effect was noted with syngeneic cells while a pronounced antileukemic effect was seen in animals injected with allogeneic cells. However, small numbers of leukemic cells still survived during the first 6 days after grafting, and the antileukemic effect of allogeneic cells was complete only after more than 7 days. Other investigators reported that the transplantation of foreign hematopoietic cells following lethal TBI in leukemic rodents could result in prolongation of survival or even in a permanent cure but only in a small proportion of leukemia-bearing animals. The effect of tumor inhibition appears to be most pronounced when, in addition to the marrow inoculum, lymphoid cells were given (reviewed in FEFER, 1973). Based on these findings in rodent models, attempts at treating endstage human leukemias by exposure of the patient to very high doses of TBI and/or chemotherapy followed by transplantation of marrow from either an allogeneic donor or from a normal identical twin have continued. The rationale is that the transplanted lymphoid cells may develop immunity to a residual minimal population of leukemic cells that survives after 1,000 rad TBI. The immunity might be directed against transplantation antigens on the leukemic cells or against leukemia-associated antigens with a resulting effect of "adoptive immunotherapy".

Syngeneic Transplants (THOMAS *et al.*, 1975). Four patients with ALL were given 1,000 rad TBI from opposing ^{60}Co sources followed by intravenous infusion of marrow from a non-leukemic identical twin. All three had remissions and showed recovery of normal hematopoiesis, but leukemia recurred in less than 3 months. These results, in agreement with most studies in rodents, indicated that the TBI exposure that can be tolerated without irreversible gastrointestinal toxicity is not sufficient to eradicate all leukemic cells.

Therefore in 1969, in an attempt to delay or obviate the rapidly recurring leukemia observed, an approach at immunotherapy was tried: immunologically active donor lymphocytes were infused in addition to the marrow. Also, the recipient was given post-grafting subcutaneous injections of previously stored irradiated autochthonous leukemic cells (once weekly) under the assumption of providing a continual stimulus by leukemia-associated antigens to the infused lymphocytes. Accordingly, three such transplants in patients with ALL or acute myeloblastic leukemia (AML) were carried out after 1,000 rads TBI. One patient died on day 51 from an infection without evidence of leukemia. The periods of remission in the other two patients were 97 and 360 days respectively.

Subsequently, therefore, twenty patients were given CY, 120 mg/kg preceding 1,000 rad TBI in an attempt to further decrease the number of leukemic cells. Seven patients did not receive immunotherapy and thirteen were given immunotherapy post-grafting. One patient died of hepatitis too early to be evaluated, and two failed to clear their marrow of leukemic cells. Seventeen experienced complete remissions. Eight of them (3 ALL, 4 AML, 1 lymphosarcoma leukemia) have remained in complete remission at 4–50 months without any maintenance chemotherapy. All normal twin donors remain in excellent health without evidence of hematologic malignancy.

The fact that a number of these patients with endstage hematologic malignancy have now remained in unmaintained remission for up to 50 months is encouraging and suggests that this treatment approach has a definite place for patients who are fortunate enough to have an identical twin.

Allogeneic Transplants (Thomas *et al.*, 1975). The results are summarized in Table 2. Seventy-three patients with ALL, AML, or chronic myelogenous leukemia in blast crisis (CML-BC) were treated between July 1969 and June 1974 by marrow grafts from sibling donors matched for the MHC. All were given 1,000 rad TBI under the assumption that irradiation is effective both against dividing and resting leukemic cells and also effective in suppressing

Table 2. Allogeneic marrow transplantation for the treatment of patients with endstage acute leukemia (Thomas *et al.*, 1975)

Disease[a]	No. of patients	Recurrent leukemia		Survival postgrafting (months) of patients now in remission
		No. of patients	Median no. of months to recurrence (range)	
ALL	34	11[b]	2.5 (0–18)	5, 6, 7, 8, 12, 21, 22, 33, 51
AML	36	4	1.5 (0–6)	5, 5, 5, 6, 7, 9, 14, 18, 25, 31
CML-BC	3	0	–	6

[a] ALL=acute lymphoblastic leukemia; AML=acute myeloblastic leukemia; CML-BC=chronic myeloblastic leukemia in blast crisis
[b] Five of the 11 were prepared for transplantation by 1,000 rads TBI

the host's immune system sufficiently to prevent rejection of the genetically foreign graft. All patients were transplanted at a time when conventional and experimental chemotherapy was failing. The duration of disease from diagnosis averaged 24 months in patients with ALL, spanning an average of three relapses, and in AML an average of 10 months, with fifteen patients not achieving a remission with chemotherapy. Sixty-seven of the seventy-three patients were in relapse. The vast majority had been previously transfused with RBC and/or platelets and twenty-three of the patients were infected at the time of transplantation.

Initially, patients were conditioned with 1,000 rad TBI alone, subsequently with the addition of CY, and recently with additional cytoreduction with other chemotherapeutic agents. Based on the most effective regimen in canine marrow grafting, all patients were given MTX on days 1, 3, 6, 11 post-grafting and weekly thereafter for 100 days to prevent or ameliorate GVHD. In a number of patients, established GVHD was treated by antithymocyte globulin raised in rabbits (STORB et al., 1974c). Nineteen of the thirty-four patients with ALL have remained in unmaintained remission for at least three months. Presently, nine of the thirty-four patients are in remission and well after more than 5–51 months postgrafting. Fourteen of the thirty-six patients with AML have remained in unmaintained remission for more than three months. Ten of the thirty-six are now alive and well in unmaintained remission between 5 and 31 months postgrafting. Only one of the three patients with CML-BC is alive and in remission after more than 6 months. Leukemic relapse was the cause of failure in fifteen patients, four with AML and eleven with ALL. Included are four patients whose leukemic cell populations were so refractory that serial marrow aspirates demonstrated persistence of blast cells immediately following the conditioning regimen. Such refractoriness suggests a spectrum of degrees of reduction of the leukemic cell load. Apparently, after the prolonged period of conventional chemotherapy a substantial fraction of the patients possess a malignant cell population too large or too refractory for the conditioning regimen and the antileukemic effect of the grafted marrow to be effective. Consequently, we have not only observed persistent leukemia but also recurrent leukemia in host type cells appearing after 7–30 weeks following marrow grafting. The relapse rate in our patient population was higher in the early years of our experience where irradiation only was used to condition the patients. With the more aggressive conditioning regimens including cytoreduction chemotherapy and CY preceding TBI, the relapse rate appears to have been modified. Of the first six patients with ALL prepared with TBI alone, five had evidence of recurrence. With the subsequent addition of chemotherapy only six of twenty-nine patients with ALL have shown a recurrence.

Another frequent cause of death in this series of patients was interstitial pneumonia predominantly due to CMV infection. A randomized trial is underway to determine the value of laminar air flow isolation, gut sterilization, and sterile diet in preventing some of the infectious complications. Also, methods for accelerating the recovery of immunologic reactivity are being investigated. Twenty of the seventy-three patients remain in complete remission between 5 and 51 months. Our data indicate that the remission rate is increasing. It is obvious that the overall mortality rate in this series of patients has been high. Considering, however, that the patients had endstage leukemia with a life expectancy of a few weeks the results should not be surprising. We are rather encouraged that marrow grafts between siblings matched at the MHC can be consistently obtained. It appears that long-term control of leukemia is possible by this procedure, and a few patients are living normal lives for up to 51 months.

Leukemic Relapse (THOMAS *et al.,* 1975). Leukemic relapse has been observed in eleven patients with ALL and four patients with AML after engraftment has been established. These recurrent leukemias may have originated either from cells that were resistant to CY and/or TBI and/or not susceptible to the effect of adoptive immunotherapy. These initial speculations had to be revised for at least two patients, both female and both suffering from ALL. They were conditioned by 1,000 rad TBI (no CY) followed by marrow infusion from her brother. In one girl, leukemia recurred after 60 days and in the other after 135 days. Surprisingly, the leukemic blast cells in both cases were of male, donor type as evidenced by cytogenetic analyses associated with autoradiography and with fluorescent Y body staining of cells obtained from the marrow and peripheral blood after recurrence of leukemia. The two donors show no evidence of leukemia $3^1/_2$ and $4^1/_2$ years later. The observation of leukemic transformation of presumably heretofore normal cells is of importance. Theoretical mechanisms explaining the transformation have been discussed in detail elsewhere (THOMAS *et al.,* 1975). The role that viruses play in the etiology of leukemia/lymphoma in other species suggests the possibility of a similar mechanism in man. If one assumes that the observed malignant transformation was due to a virus released from the irradiated leukemic cells, additional therapeutic modalities arise including the delay of marrow infusion until released virus has been cleared, the use of antiviral agents or interferon inducers, the use of lymphoid cells specifically immunized to viral antigens or the use of added chemotherapeutic agents that do not lead to virus release from damaged cells.

β) Marrow Grafting in Aplastic Anemia

Aplastic anemia is a disorder of unknown pathophysiology and high mortality despite the use of androgen therapy and advances in supportive care. The hope of successful treatment of aplastic anemia by marrow grafting is based on the assumption that the etiology of the disease is a hematopoietic stem cell failure rather than a disorder of the marrow microenvironment. Initial attempts at treating aplastic anemia with syngeneic marrow grafts were encouraging (THOMAS *et al.,* 1971). Based on these observations marrow grafting for treatment of this disease using HL-A identical siblings as marrow donors has been continued (STORB *et al.,* 1974a, 1975). Most of the presently evaluable cases have been conditioned for grafting by the immunosuppressive agent CY. In six patients, however, 1,000 rad of TBI were used as conditioning agent in the hope of shortening the period of supportive care before the transplant. The duration of marrow aplasia before transplantation in these patients ranged from 2–15 months, and all had been unsuccessfully treated with conventional therapy. Many of them were infected at the time of admission and some of them were refractory to platelets from random donors. One patient died on day 6 with a pseudomonas septicemia, too early for the graft to be evaluated. One patient who had been given blood transfusions from family members failed to show marrow engraftment and died on day 24 with infection and aplastic marrow. Another patient who had only received random preceding blood transfusions showed initial engraftment followed by rejection of the marrow graft. A second marrow graft attempt following 200 mg of CY/kg failed and the patient died on day 41 with infection and an aplastic marrow. Three patients had successful and sustained marrow engraftment. Two of these died on days 45 and 84 with severe GVHD. One patient is alive more than $3^{1}/_{2}$ years following hematopoietic grafting with sustained engraftment. He has returned to normal activities. This series of cases shows no real difference between patients conditioned by TBI and those conditioned by CY. Although the CY regimen requires a longer period of supportive care, only 2 patients died too early to demonstrate engraftment. The long-term survival rate of 1 of 6 patients after the TBI regimen versus 20 of 37 after CY (STORB et al., 1974a, 1975) is not significantly different in view of the uncontrolled major variables of GVHD and prior sensitization.

These data demonstrate that normal stem cells will repopulate the marrow in aplastic anemia patients and show that long-term stable chimerism is possible in man. They suggest that marrow grafting in patients with complete marrow failure and an HL-A matched sibling should be undertaken before major infections and refractoriness to blood transfusions complicate their course.

γ) Conclusions and Summary of Outstanding Problems in the Field of Irradiation and Clinical Marrow Grafting

After five years of extensive clinical marrow grafting following TBI it can be concluded that marrow transplants from identical twins or from HL-A compatible siblings into patients with otherwise refractory aplastic anemia or endstage acute leukemia have a useful therapeutic effect. A number of transplanted patients have become long-term survivors without recurrence of their initial disease and without maintenance therapy.

In addition to the therapeutic benefit to the patient, important information has been gathered about the pathogenesis of hematologic diseases as shown by the successful repopulation of previously empty marrow spaces in aplastic anemia. This is most consistent with the correction of an underlying stem cell defect and provides a strong argument against other etiologic hypotheses such as the absence of an essential nutrient, persistence of a toxic factor, or a defect in the marrow microenvironment. An unexpected finding was the recurrence of leukemia in cells of donor origin, providing strong circumstantial evidence for transmission of leukemia by a viral agent. This has lead to revisions of the conditioning regimen for transplantation by adding intensive chemotherapy preceding TBI and marrow grafting. Other treatment modalities might involve the use of antiviral agents.

Many problems in the field of marrow transplantation remain to be solved. Sensitization of the marrow recipient against his intended marrow donor by preceding blood transfusions remains a serious problem. Marrow grafting at an earlier stage of the patient's disease might avoid this problem. Recent laboratory studies offer hope of recognizing and eliminating sensitization by blood transfusions. GVHD with fatal outcome is still a major stumbling block despite matching of donor and recipient by currently available histocompatibility typing techniques and the use of postgrafting immunosuppression. Better immunosuppressive agents or the use of combinations of immunosuppressive drugs may offer hope of control of GVHD. Many patients with successful marrow grafts have died of infection. Studies in animal systems as well as in human marrow graft recipients have shown that impaired immune defenses and increased susceptibility to infection exist for prolonged periods after transplantation. Methods for accelerating the immunologic reconstitution of the marrow graft recipient need to be developed perhaps by adding donor lymphocytes or fetal thymus to the marrow inoculum. Such accelerated immunologic reconstitution not only may prevent infectious complications but also may provide the graft with a more profound antileukemic effect. Application of marrow grafting may be expanded to the treatment of other malignant diseases, particularly lymphomas and to non-malignant genetic diseases such as sickle cell disease, thalassemia major, or cyclic neutropenia. In addition, it should be pointed out that a recipient of a successful marrow transplant will subsequently accept the graft of any other organ from the marrow donor without the necessity of continued immunosuppressive therapy. As the safety of marrow transplantation improves, it may become possible to employ this principle for grafting of paired organs.

Finally, the particular attraction of the field of marrow grafting is that increase of our knowledge of normal and abnormal immunology and physiology of disease and of beneficial and adverse effects of TBI can take place in the setting of an endeavor of therapy for the patient with otherwise fatal illness.

II. Other Organ Grafts

As outlined above, marrow transplantation following TBI has been used in rodents and dogs as a means of conditioning a recipient for accepting a renal or skin allograft from the marrow donor without need for further immunosuppressive therapy. Attempts have been described in man to achieve kidney graft survival using this approach (reviewed in HUME and WOLF, 1967). These attempts have all met with failure due to the death of the recipient, and the technique has been largely abandoned in clinical renal allografting (MURRAY et al., 1960). Failures for the most part appeared to be due to lack of knowledge on the amount of immunosuppression needed to establish a successful marrow graft, on the need for histocompatibility matching, etc. In view of the recent progress in clinical marrow transplantation, however, it is conceivable that the approach of marrow transplantation followed by renal grafting from the same donor may one day become reality.

A number of studies in rats and mice have shown moderate prolongation of histoincompatible skin allografts following sublethal TBI (ODELL and CALDWELL, 1958; PIOMELLI et al., 1961). Sublethal TBI was used in the early phase of human renal grafting in preparation for transplantation (HAMBURGER *et al.*, 1959; MERRILL *et al.*, 1960; MURRAY *et al.*, 1962; SHACKMAN *et al.*, 1962). Most extensive studies were carried out in Paris by HAMBURGER *et al.* (1962), who used 400–600 rad in split doses 2–5 days apart. Similar total exposures together with additional splenic irradiation were reported by other groups. Most patients were then given immunosuppression with prednisone and azathioprine. In view of the many different regimens applied and the variable survival times of the kidney grafts, it is difficult to become enthusiastic about the use of sublethal TBI prior to renal grafting. At the present time, most major renal transplant groups have abandoned this technique. It appears, however, that it is worthwhile to carry out further laboratory studies before definitely discarding this approach.

Acknowledgments

We wish to thank N. GENGOZIAN of Oak Ridge Associated Universities for helpful discussions about radiation immunology, and JANIS LEE and SUZETTE MOULIN for secretarial help.

References

AGAROSSI, G., DORIA, G.: Recovery of the hemolysin response in mouse radiation chimeras. Transplantation **6**, 419–426 (1968).

ALBERT, E.D., ERICKSON, V.M., GRAHAM, T.C., PARR, M., TEMPLETON, J.W., MICKEY, M.R., THOMAS, E.D., STORB, R.: Serology and genetics of the DL-A system. I. Establishment of specificities. Tissue Antigens **3**, 417–430 (1973).

ANDREWS, G.A.: Criticality accidents in Vinca, Yugoslavia, and Oak Ridge, Tennessee. J. Amer. Med. Assoc. **179**, 191–197 (1962).

ATKINS, R.C., FORD, W.L.: The effect of lymphocytes and serum from tolerant rats on the graft-versus-host activity of normal lymphocytes. Transplantation **13**, 442–444 (1972).

BACH, F.H., AMOS, D.B.: Hu-1: Major histocompatibility locus in man. Science **156**, 1506–1508 (1967).

BALDWIN, R.W., PRICE, M.R., ROBINS, R.A.: Blocking of lymphocyte-mediated cytotoxicity for rat hepatoma cells by tumour-specific antigen-antibody complexes. Nature (London) **238**, 185–186 (1972).

BARNES, D.W.H., CORP, M.J., LOUTIT, J.F., NEAL, F.E.: Treatment of murine leukaemia with x rays and homologous bone marrow. Preliminary Communication. Brit. Med. J. **2**, 626-627 (1956).

BENJAMIN, E., SLUKA, E.: Antikörperbildung nach experimenteller Schädigung des hematopoetischen Systems durch Röntgenstrahlen. Wien. Klin. Wschr. **21**, 311–314 (1908).

BEVERLEY, P.C.L., BRENT, L., BROOKS, C., MEDAWAR, P.B., SIMPSON, E.: In vitro reactivity of lymphoid cells from tolerant mice. Transpl. Proc. **5**, 679–684 (1973).

BILLINGHAM, R.E., BRENT, L., MEDAWAR, P.B.: Quantitative studies on tissue transplantation immunity. III. Actively acquired tolerance. Philos. Trans. Royal Soc. Lond. Biol. **239**, 357–414 (1956).

BLOOM, W.: Histopathology of Irradiation from External and Internal Sources. New York: McGraw-Hill 1948.

BORANIC, M., TONKOVIC, I.: Time pattern of the antileukemic effect of graft-*versus*-host reaction in mice. Cancer Res. **31**, 1140–1147 (1971).

BORTIN, M.M.: A compendium of reported human bone marrow transplants. Transplantation **9**, 571–587 (1970).

BRENT, L., BROOKS, C., LUBLING, N., THOMAS, A.V.: Attempts to demonstrate an in vivo role for serum blocking factors in tolerant mice. Transplantation **14**, 382–387 (1972).

BURCHENAL, J.H., OETTGEN, H.F., HOLMBERG, E.A.D., HEMPHILL, S.C., REPPERT, J.A.: Effect of total-body irradiation on the transplantability of mouse leukemias. Cancer Res. 20, 425–430 (1960).

BURNET, F.M.: Cellular Immunology. Cambridge, London: University Press 1969.

CARLSON, D.E., GENGOZIAN, N.: The effect of acute radiation exposure rates on formation of hemagglutinating antibody in mice. J. Immunol. 106, 1353–1362 (1971).

COLE, L.J., FISHLER, M.C., ELLIS, M.E., BOND, V.P.: Protection of mice against x-irradiation by spleen homogenates administered after exposure. Proc. Soc. Exp. Biol. (N.Y.) 80, 112–117 (1952).

CONGDON, C.C., URSO, I.S.: Homologous bone marrow in the treatment of radiation injury in mice. Amer. J. Pathol. 33, 749–767 (1957).

COTTIER, H.: Strahlenbedingte Lebensverkürzung. Berlin: Springer-Verlag 1961.

CRONKITE, E.P., BOND, V.P.: Radiation Injury in Man. Springfield, Illinois: C.C. Thomas (ed.) 1960.

DAUSSET, J., COLOMBANI, J.: Histocompatibility Testing 1972. Baltimore, Maryland: The Williams & Wilkins Company 1972.

DE VRIES, M.J., CROUCH, B.G., VAN PUTTEN, L.M., VAN BEKKUM, D.W.: Pathologic changes in irradiated monkeys treated with bone marrow. J. Nat. Cancer Inst. 27, 67–97 (1961).

DICKE, K.A., VAN BEKKUM, D.W.: Allogeneic bone marrow transplantation after elimination of immunocompetent cells by means of density gradient centrifugation. Transpl. Proc. 3, 666–668 (1971).

DORIA, G., GOODMAN, J.W., GENGOZIAN, N., CONGDON, C.C.: Immunologic study of antibody-forming cells in mouse radiation chimeras. J. Immunol. 88, 20–30 (1962).

ELKINS, W.L.: Cellular immunology and the pathogenesis of graft versus host reactions. Progr. Allergy 15, 78-187 (1971).

ELKINS, W.L.: The cellular basis of transplantation tolerance. Transpl. Proc. 5, 685-689 (1973).

FABRICIOUS-MOELLER, J.: Experimental Studies of the Hemorrhagic Diathesis from X-ray Sickness. Copenhagen: Levin & Munksgaards Forlag 1922.

FASS, L., OCHS, H.D., THOMAS, E.D., MICKELSON, E., STORB, R., FEFER, A.: Studies of immunological reactivity following syngeneic or allogeneic marrow grafts in man. Transplantation 16, 630–640 (1973).

FEFER, A.: Adoptive tumor immunotherapy in mice as an adjunct to whole-body X-irradiation and chemotherapy. A review. Israel J. Med. Sci. 9, 350–365 (1973).

FELDMAN, M., YAFFE, D.: Immunogenetic studies on x-irradiated mice treated with hematopoietic cells and grafted with tumor tissues. J. Nat. Cancer Inst. 23, 109–131 (1959).

FORD, C.E., HAMERTON, J.L., BARNES, D.W.H., LOUTIT, J.F.: Cytological identification of radiation-chimaeras. Nature (London) 177, 452–454 (1956).

GARVER, R.M., SANTOS, G.W., COLE, L.J.: Specific hemagglutinins in x-irradiated, bone-marrow treated mice following differential immunization of host and donor. J. Immunol. 83, 57–65 (1959).

GENGOZIAN, N., MAKINODAN, T.: Mortality of mice as affected by variation of the x-ray dose and number of nucleated rat bone marrow cells injected. Cancer Res. 17, 970–975 (1957).

GENGOZIAN, N., MAKINODAN, T., CONGDON, C.C., OWEN, R.D.: The immune status of long-term survivors of lethally x-irradiated mice protected with isologous, homologous, or heterologous bone marrow. Proc. Nat. Acad. Sci. (Wash.) 44, 560–565 (1958).

GENGOZIAN, N., URSO, I.S., CARTER, R.R., MAKINODAN, T.: Immune status of irradiated mice treated with adult bone marrow and fetal hematopoietic tissue. Transpl. Bull. 27, 87–90 (1961).

GENGOZIAN, N., RABETTE, B., CONGDON, C.C.: Abnormal immune mechanisms in allogeneic radiation chimeras. Science 149, 645–647 (1965).

GENGOZIAN, N., CARLSON, D.E., ALLEN, E.M.: Transplantation of allogeneic and xenogeneic (rat) marrow in irradiated mice as affected by radiation exposure rates. Transplantation 7, 259–273 (1969).

GENGOZIAN, N., CARLSON, D.E., GOTTLIEB, C.F.: Radiation exposure rates: Effects on the immune system. In: Dose Rate in Mammalian Radiation Biology, a Symposium, pp. 16.1–16.22. Conf-680410, UT-AEC Agri. Res. Lab. and U.S. A.E.C. 1968.

GENGOZIAN, N., CONGDON, C.C., ALLEN, E.A., TOYA, R.E.: Immune status of allogeneic radiation chimeras. Transpl. Proc. 3, 434–436 (1971).

GENGOZIAN, N., EDWARDS, C.L., VODOPICK, H.A., HUBNER, K.F.: Bone marrow transplantation in a leukemic patient following immunosuppression with antithymocyte globulin and total body irradiation. Transplantation 15, 446–454 (1973).

GLASGOW, L.A.: Cellular immunity in host resistance to viral infections. Arch. Intern. Med. 126, 125-134 (1970).

GLUCKSBERG, H., STORB, R., FEFER, A., BUCKNER, C.D., NEIMAN, P.E., CLIFT, R.A., LERNER, K.G., THOMAS, E.D.: Clinical manifestations of graft-versus-host disease in human recipients of marrow from HL-A-matched sibling donors. Transplantation 18, 295–304 (1974).

GORER, P.A., BOYSE, E.A.: Pathological changes in F_1 hybrid mice following transplantation of spleen cells from donors of the parental strains. Immunology 2, 182–193 (1959).

GOTTLIEB, C.F., GENGOZIAN, N.: The humoral immune response in mice after neutron or x-irradiation at different dose rates. J. Immunol. 109, 711–718 (1972a).

GOTTLIEB, C.F., GENGOZIAN, N.: Radiation dose, dose rate, and quality in suppression of the humoral immune response. J. Immunol. 109, 719-727 (1972b).

GRANT, C.K., LEUCHARS, E., ALEXANDER, P.: Failure to detect cytotoxic lymphoid cells or humoral blocking factors in mouse radiation chimaeras. Transplantation 14, 722–727 (1972).

GREGORY, C.J., LAJTHA, L.G.: Recovery of immune responsiveness in lethally-irradiated mice protected with syngeneic marrow cells. Int. J. Radiat. Biol. 17, 117–226 (1970).

HAMBURGER, J., VAYSSE, J., CROSNIER, J., TUBIANA, M., LALANNE, C.M., ANTOINE, B., AUVERT, J., SOULIER, J.P., DORMONT, J., SALMON, C., MAISONNET, M., AMIEL, J.L.: Transplantation of a kidney between nonmonozygotic twins after irradiation of the receiver. Good function at the fourth month. Presse Med. 67, 1771–1775 (1959).

HAMBURGER, J., VAYSSE, J., CROSNIER, J., AUVERT, J., LALANNE, C.M., HOPPER, J., JR.: Renal homotransplantation in man after radiation of the recipient. Experience with six patients since 1959. Amer. J. Med. 32, 854–871 (1962).

HEINEKE, H.: Über die Einwirkung der Röntgenstrahlen auf Tiere. Münch. Med. Wschr. 50, 2090–2092 (1903).

HEINEKE, H.: Experimentelle Untersuchungen über die Einwirkung der Röntgenstrahlen auf innere Organe. Mitt. Grenzg. Med. Chir. 14, 21–94 (1905).

HELLSTROM, I., HELLSTROM, K.E., STORB, R., THOMAS, E.D.: Colony inhibition of fibroblasts from chimeric dogs mediated by the dogs' own lymphocytes and specifically abrogated by their serum. Proc. Nat. Acad. Sci. (Wash.) 66, 65–71 (1970).

HELLSTROM, I., HELLSTROM, K.E., ALLISON, A.C.: Neonatally induced allograft tolerance may be mediated by serum-borne factors. Nature (London) 230, 49–50 (1971).

HELLSTROM, I., HELLSTROM, K.E., TRENTIN, J.J.: Cellular immunity and blocking serum activity in chimeric mice. Cell. Immunol. 7, 73–84 (1973).

HERON, I.: Is transplantation tolerance in the rat serum-mediated? Transplantation 15, 534–539 (1973).

HOLLINGSWORTH, J.W.: Immunologic mechanisms in heavily irradiated mice treated with bone marrow. Blood 14, 548-557 (1959).

HRSAK, I., NOUZA, K., KOLAR, V., MATHE, G.: Essai de restauration immunitaire de radiochimeres hematopoietiques allogeniques. Rev. Franc. Etudes Clin. Biol. 13, 887–893 (1968).

HUME, D.M., WOLF, J.S.: Modification of renal homograft rejection by irradiation. Transplantation 5, 1174-1191 (1967).

JACOBSON, L.O., MARKS, E.K., ROBSON, M.J., GASTON, E.O., ZIRKLE, R.E.: The effect of spleen protection on mortality following x-irradiation. J. Lab. Clin. Med. 34, 1538–1543 (1949).

JOSE, D.G., KERSEY, J.H., CHOI, Y.S., BIGGAR, W.D., GATTI, R.A., GOOD, R.A.: Humoral antagonism of cellular immunity in children with immune-deficiency disease reconstituted by bone-marrow transplantation. Lancet 2, 841–843 (1971).

KOLB, H.J., STORB, R., GRAHAM, T.C., KOLB, H., THOMAS, E.D.: Antithymocyte serum and methotrexate for control of graft-versus-host disease in dogs. Transplantation 16, 17–23 (1973).

LAVIA, M.F., SIMMONS, E.L., DONKO, J.D.: Antibody formation in x-irradiated rats protected with rat or rabbit hematopoietic cells. Proc. Soc. Exp. Biol. (N.Y.) 98, 215–218 (1958).

LERNER, K.G., KAO, G.F., STORB, R., BUCKNER, C.D., CLIFT, R.A., THOMAS, E.D.: Histopathology of graft-vs.-host reaction (GvHR) in human recipients of marrow from HL-A-matched sibling donors. Transpl. Proc. 6, 367-371 (1974).

LORENZ, E., UPHOFF, D., REID, T.R., SHELTON, E.: Modification of irradiation injury in mice and guinea pigs by bone marrow injections. J. Nat. Cancer Inst. 12, 197–201 (1951).

Loutit, J.F., Micklem, H.S.: Active and passive immunity to transplantation of foreign bone marrow in lethally irradiated mice. Brit. J. Exp. Path. **42**, 577–586 (1961).

Main, J.M., Prehn, R.T.: Successful skin homografts after the administration of high dosage X radiation and homologous bone marrow. J. Nat. Cancer Inst. **15**, 1023–1029 (1955).

Makinodan, T., Gengozian, N., Congdon, C.C.: Agglutinin production in normal, sublethally irradiated, and lethally irradiated mice treated with mouse bone marrow. J. Immunol. **77**, 250–256 (1956).

Makinodan, T., Friedberg, B.H., Tolbert, M.G., Gengozian, N.: Relation of *secondary* antigen injection to time of irradiation on antibody production in mice. J. Immunol. **83**, 184–188 (1959).

Makinodan, T., Gengozian, N.: Effect of radiation on antibody formation. In: Radiation Protection and Recovery, pp. 316–351. New York: Pergamon Press 1960.

Makinodan, T.: Changes in immunobiological processes caused by radiation. In: Encyclopedia of Medical Radiology, Part 2 Radiation Biology, pp. 303–333. Berlin: Springer-Verlag 1966.

Mathe, G., Jammet, H., Pendic, B., Schwarzenberg, L., Duplan, J.F., Maupin, B., Latarjet, R., Larrieu, M.J., Kalic, D., Djukic, Z.: Transfusions et greffes de moelle osseuse homologue chez des humains irradies a haute dose accidentellement. Rev. Franc. Etudes Clin. Biol. **4**, 226–238 (1959).

Mathe, G., Amiel, J.L., Schwarzenberg, L., Cattan, A., Schneider, M., de Vries, M.J., Tubiana, M., Lalanne, C., Binet, J.L., Papiernik, M., Seman, G., Matsukura, M., Mery, A.M., Schwarzmann, V., Flaisler, A.: Successful allogeneic bone marrow transplantation in man: Chimerism, induced specific tolerance and possible anti-leukemic effects. Blood **25**, 179–196 (1965a).

Mathe, G., Amiel, J.L., Schwarzenberg, L., Cattan, A., Schneider, M.: Adoptive immunotherapy of acute leukemia: Experimental and clinical results. Cancer Res. **25**, 1525–1531 (1965b).

Merigan, T.C., Stevens, D.A.: Viral infections in man associated with acquired immunological deficiency states. Fed. Proc. **30**, 1858–1864 (1971).

Merrill, J.P., Murray, J.E., Harrison, J.H., Friedman, E.A., Dealy, J.B., Jr., Dammin, G.J.: Successful homotransplantation of the kidney between nonidentical twins. N. Engl. J. Med. **262**, 1251–1260 (1960).

Miller, R.G., Phillips, R.A.: Separation of cells by velocity sedimentation. J. Cell. Physiol. **73**, 191–201 (1969).

Muller-Berat, C.N., van Putten, L.M., van Bekkum, D.W.: Cytostatic drugs in the treatment of secondary disease following homologous bone marrow transplantation: Extrapolation from the mouse to the primate. Ann. N.Y. Acad. Sci. **129**, 340–354 (1966).

Murray, J.E., Merrill, J.P., Dammin, G.J., Dealy, J.B., Jr., Walter, C.W., Brooke, M.S., Wilson, R.E.: Study on transplantation immunity after total body irradiation: Clinical and experimental investigation. Surgery **48**, 272–284 (1960).

Murray, J.E., Merrill, J.P., Dammin, G.J., Dealy, J.B., Jr., Alexandre, G.W., Harrison, J.H.: Kidney transplantation in modified recipients. Ann. Surg. **156**, 337–355 (1962).

Neefe, J.R., Jr., Merritt, C.B., Vaal, L., Darrow, C.C., II, Rogentine, G.N., Jr.: Histocompatibility and bone marrow transplantation between unrelated rhesus monkeys. Transplantation **16**, 365–370 (1973).

Neiman, P., Wasserman, P.B., Wentworth, B.B., Kao, G.F., Lerner, K.G., Storb, R., Buckner, C.D., Clift, R.A., Fefer, A., Fass, L., Glucksberg, H., Thomas, E.D.: Interstitial pneumonia and cytomegalovirus infection as complications of human marrow transplantation. Transplantation **15**, 478–485 (1973).

Nouza, K., Lengerova, A.: Specific features of the outcome of transplantation of foreign haematopoietic and lymphoid cells in the midlethal irradiation range. Folia Biol. (Praha) **11**, 17–32 (1965).

Nowell, P.C., Cole, L.J., Habermeyer, J.G., Roan, P.L.: Growth and continued function of rat marrow cells in X-radiated mice. Cancer Res. **16**, 258–261 (1956).

Ochs, H.D., Storb, R., Thomas, E.D., Kolb, H.J., Graham, T.C., Mickelson, E., Parr, M., Rudolph, R.H.: Immunologic reactivity in canine marrow graft recipients. J. Immunol. **113**, 1039–1057 (1974).

Odell, T.T., Jr., Caldwell, B.C.: Transplantation of homologous erythropoietic elements in rats after sublethal doses of x radiation. J. Nat. Cancer Inst. **20**, 851–858 (1958).

OWENS, A.H., JR., SANTOS, G.W.: The effect of cytotoxic drugs on graft-versus-host disease in mice. Transplantation **11**, 378–382 (1971).

PHILLIPS, S.M., WEGMANN, T.G.: Active suppression as a possible mechanism of tolerance in tetraparental mice. J. Exp. Med. **137**, 291–300 (1973).

PIOMELLI, S., BEHRENDT, D.M., O'CONNOR, J.F., MURRAY, J.E.: Survival of skin homografts in radiation chimeras. Transpl. Bull. **27**, 431–436 (1961).

RAPAPORT, F.T., WATANABE, K., CANNON, F.D., MOLLEN, N., BLUMENSTOCK, D., FERREBEE, J.W.: Histocompatibility studies in a closely bred colony of dogs. IV. Tolerance to bone marrow, kidney, and skin allografts in DL-A-identical radiation chimeras. J. Exp. Med. **136**, 1080–1097 (1972).

RICHES, A.C., THOMAS, D.B.: Growth of an allogeneic tumor in lethally irradiated mice treated with sensitized and unsensitized spleen cells. Radiat. Res. **44**, 87–96 (1970).

RIFKIND, D.: Cytomegalovirus infection after renal transplantation. Arch. Intern. Med. **116**, 554–558 (1965).

RIFKIND, D., FARIS, T.D., HILL, R.B., JR.: Pneumocystis carinii pneumonia. Studies on the diagnosis and treatment. Ann. Intern. Med. **65**, 943–956 (1966).

RIFKIND, D., MARCHIORO, T.L., SCHNECK, S.A., HILL, R.B.: Systemic fungal infections complicating renal transplantation and immunosuppressive therapy. Clinical, microbiologic, neurologic and pathologic features. Amer. J. Med. **43**, 28–38 (1967).

ROUSE, B.T., WARNER, N.L.: Induction of T-cell tolerance in agammaglobulinemic chickens. Europ. J. Immunol. **2**, 102–104 (1972).

SALAMAN, M.H., WEDDERBURN, N., FESTENSTEIN, H., HUBER, B.: Detection of a graft-versus-host reaction between mice compatible at the *H-2* locus. Transplantation **16**, 29–31 (1973).

SANTOS, G.W., COLE, L.J., ROAN, P.L.: Effect of x-ray dose on the protective action and persistence of rat bone marrow in irradiated, penicillin-treated mice. Amer. J. Physiol. **194**, 23–27 (1958).

SANTOS, G.W., SENSENBRENNER, L.L.: A sensitive and quantitative assay for non-H-2 histocompatibility antigens. Exp. Hematol. **21**, 19–20 (1971).

SANTOS, G.W., SENSENBRENNER, L.L., BURKE, P.J., COLVIN, M., OWENS, A.H., JR., BIAS, W.B., SLAVIN, R.E.: Marrow transplantation in man following cyclophosphamide. Transpl. Proc. **3**, 400–404 (1971).

SCHROEDER, M.L., STORB, R., GRAHAM, T.C., WEIDEN, P.L.: Canine radiation chimeras: An attempt to demonstrate serum blocking factors by an in vivo approach. J. Immunol. **114**, 540–541 (1975).

SCHWARTZ, R.S., BELDOTTI, L.: Malignant lymphomas following allogenic disease: Transition from an immunological to a neoplastic disorder. Science **149**, 1511–1514 (1965).

SCHWARZ, M.R.: The mixed lymphocyte reaction: an in vitro test for tolerance. J. Exp. Med. **127**, 879–890 (+3 unnumbered) (1968).

SHACKMAN, R., DEMPSTER, W.J., WRONG, O.M.: Kidney homotransplantation in the human. Brit. J. Urol. **35**, 222–255 (1963).

SIMIC, M.M., SLJIVIC, V.S., PETROVIC, M.Z., CIRKOVIC, D.M.: Antibody formation in irradiated rats. Bull. Boris Vidric Inst. Nucl. Sci. **16** (Suppl. 1), 1–151 (1965).

SMITH, L.H., CONGDON, C.C.: Biological effects of ionizing radiation. In: Human Transplantation, pp. 510–525. New York: Grune & Stratton 1968.

SMYTHE, P.M., SCHONLAND, M., BRERETON-STILES, G.G., COOVADIA, H.M., GRACE, H.J., LEONING, W.E.K., MAFOYANE, A., PARENT, M.A., VOS, G.H.: Thymolymphatic deficiency and depression of cell-mediated immunity in protein-calorie malnutrition. Lancet **2**, 939–944 (1971).

STORB, R., EPSTEIN, R.B., GRAHAM, T.C., THOMAS, E.D.: Methotrexate regimens for control of graft-versus-host disease in dogs with allogeneic marrow grafts. Transplantation **9**, 240–246 (1970a).

STORB, R., GRAHAM, T.C., SHIURBA, R., THOMAS, E.D.: Treatment of canine graft-versus-host disease with methotrexate and cyclophosphamide following bone marrow transplantation from histoincompatible donors. Transplantation **10**, 165–172 (1970b).

STORB, R., EPSTEIN, R.B., RUDOLPH, R.H., THOMAS, E.D.: The effect of prior transfusion on marrow grafts between histocompatible canine siblings. J. Immunol. **105**, 627–633 (1970c).

STORB, R., RUDOLPH, R.H., GRAHAM, T.C., THOMAS, E.D.: The influence of transfusions from unrelated donors upon marrow grafts between histocompatible canine siblings. J. Immunol. **107**, 409 413 (1971).

STORB, R., THOMAS, E.D.: Bone marrow transplantation in randomly bred animal species and in man. In: Proceedings of the Sixth Leucocyte Culture Conference, pp. 805–840. New York: Academic Press, Inc. 1972.

STORB, R., KOLB, H.J., GRAHAM, T.C., OCHS, H.D., THOMAS, E.D.: Principles of marrow grafting derived from canine studies. Exp. Hematol. 22, 126–137 (1972a).

STORB, R., KOLB, H.J., GRAHAM, T.C., LeBLOND, R., KOLB, H., LERNER, K.G., THOMAS, E.D.: Marrow grafts between histoincompatible canine family members. Rev. Europ. Etudes Clin. Biol. 17, 680–685 (1972b).

STORB, R., RUDOLPH, R.H., KOLB, H.J., GRAHAM, T.C., MICKELSON, E., ERICKSON, V., LERNER, K.G., KOLB, H., THOMAS, E.D.: Marrow grafts between DL-A-matched canine littermates. Transplantation 15, 92–100 (1973a).

STORB, R., KOLB, H.J., GRAHAM, T.C., ERICKSON, V., THOMAS, E.D.: The effect of buffy coat-poor blood transfusion on subsequent hemopoietic grafts. Transplantation 15, 129–136 (1973b).

STORB, R., KOLB, H.J., GRAHAM, T.C., KOLB, H., WEIDEN, P.L., THOMAS, E.D.: Treatment of established graft-versus-host disease in dogs by antithymocyte serum or prednisone. Blood 42, 601–609 (1973c).

STORB, R., THOMAS, E.D., BUCKNER, C.D., CLIFT, R.A., JOHNSON, F.L., FEFER, A., GLUCKSBERG, H., GIBLETT, E.R., LERNER, K.G., NEIMAN, P.: Allogeneic marrow grafting for treatment of aplastic anemia. Blood 43, 157–180 (1974a).

STORB, R., FLOERSHEIM, G.L., WEIDEN, P.L., GRAHAM, T.C., KOLB, H.J., LERNER, K.G., SCHROEDER, M.L., THOMAS, E.D.: Effect of prior blood transfusions on marrow grafts: Abrogation of sensitization by procarbazine and antithymocyte serum. J. Immunol. 112, 1508–1516 (1974b).

STORB, R., GLUCKMAN, E., THOMAS, E.D., BUCKNER, C.D., CLIFT, R.A., FEFER, A., GLUCKSBERG, H., GRAHAM, T.C., JOHNSON, F.L., LERNER, K.G., NEIMAN, P.E., OCHS, H.: Treatment of established human graft-versus-host disease by antithymocyte globulin. Blood 44, 57–75 (1974c).

STORB, R., THOMAS, E.D., BUCKNER, C.D., CLIFT, R.A., JOHNSON, F.L., FEFER, A., GLUCKSBERG, H., LERNER, K.G., NEIMAN, P.E., WEIDEN, P.L., WRIGHT, S.E.: Aplastic anemia (AA) treated by allogeneic marrow grafting. Transpl. Proc. 7, 813–816 (1975).

TALIAFERRO, W.H., TALIAFERRO, L.G., JAROSLOW, B.N.: Radiation and Immune Mechanisms. New York: Academic Press 1964.

TEMPLETON, J.W., THOMAS, E.D.: Evidence for a major histocompatibility locus in the dog. Transplantation 11, 429–431 (1971).

THOMAS, E.D., LOCHTE, H.L., JR., LU, W.C., FERREBEE, J.W.: Intravenous infusion of bone marrow in patients receiving radiation and chemotherapy. N. Engl. J. Med. 257, 491–496 (1957).

THOMAS, E.D., COLLINS, J.A., HERMAN, E.C., JR., FERREBEE, J.W.: Marrow transplants in lethally irradiated dogs given methotrexate. Blood 19, 217–228 (1962).

THOMAS, E.D., LeBLOND, R., GRAHAM, T., STORB, R.: Marrow infusions in dogs given midlethal or lethal irradiation. Radiat. Res. 41, 113–124 (1970).

THOMAS, E.D., RUDOLPH, R.H., FEFER, A., STORB, R., SLICHTER, S., BUCKNER, C.D.: Isogeneic marrow grafting in man. Exp. Hematol. 21, 16–18 (1971).

THOMAS, E.D., STORB, R., CLIFT, R.A., FEFER, A., JOHNSON, F.L., NEIMAN, P.E., LERNER, K.G., GLUCKSBERG, H., BUCKNER, C.D.: Marrow transplantation. N. Engl. J. Med. 292, 832–843, 895–902 (1975).

TRENTIN, J.J.: Mortality and skin transplantability in x-irradiated mice receiving isologous, homologous or heterologous bone marrow. Proc. Soc. Exp. Biol. (N.Y.) 92, 688–693 (1956).

TRENTIN, J.J.: Signposts and landmarks. Exp. Hematol. 22, 18–22 (1972).

TSOI, M.S., STORB, R., WEIDEN, P.L., SCHROEDER, M.L., THOMAS, E.D.: Canine marrow transplantation: Do serum blocking factors maintain stable graft-versus-host "tolerance"? Transpl. Proc. 7, 841–843 (1975).

TSOI, M.S., STORB, R., WEIDEN, P.L., GRAHAM, T.C., SCHROEDER, M.L., THOMAS, E.D.: Canine marrow transplantation: Are serum blocking factors necessary to maintain the stable chimeric state. J. Immunol. 114, 531–539 (1975b).

TYAN, M.L., COLE, L.J.: Dissociation of homograft response to allogeneic versus xenogeneic skin grafts in irradiated mice. Science 141, 813–814 (1963).

UPHOFF, D.E.: Alternation of homograft reaction by A-methopterin in lethally irradiated mice treated with homologous marrow. Proc. Soc. Exp. Biol. (N.Y.) 99, 651–653 (1958).

UPHOFF, D.E., LAW, L.W.: An evaluation of some genetic factors influencing irradiation protection by bone marrow. J. Nat. Cancer Inst. 22, 229–241 (1959).

UPHOFF, D.E.: Genetic factors influencing irradiation protection by bone marrow. III. Midlethal irradiation of inbred mice. J. Nat. Cancer Inst. 30, 1115–1141 (1963).

UPHOFF, D.E.: Immunologic competence of bone marrow of different genotypes. J. Nat. Cancer Inst. 43, 1055–1066 (1969).

VAN BEKKUM, D.W., DE VRIES, M.J.: Radiation Chimeras. New York: Academic Press 1967.

VAN BEKKUM, D.W.: Use and abuse of hemopoietic cell grafts in immune deficiency diseases. Transpl. Rev. 9, 3–53 (1972).

VRIESENDORP, H.M., WESTBROEK, D.L., D'AMARO, J., VAN DER DOES, J.A., VAN DER STEEN, G.J., VAN ROOD, J.J., ALBERT, E.D., BERNINI, L., BULL, R.W., CABASSON, J., EPSTEIN, R.B., ERICKSON, V., FELTKAMP, T.E.W., FLAD, H.D., HAMMER, C., LANG, R., LARGIADER, F., VON LORINGHOVEN, K., LOS, W., MEERA KHAN, P., SAISON, R., SERROU, B., SCHNAPPAUF, H., SWISHER, S.N., TEMPLETON, J.W., UHLSCHMIDT, G., ZWEIBAUM, A.: Joint report on 1st International Workshop on Canine Immunogenetics. Tissue Antigens 3, 145–163 (1973).

WEGMANN, T.G., HELLSTROM, I., HELLSTROM, K.E.: Immunological tolerance: "forbidden clones" allowed in tetraparental mice. Proc. Nat. Acad. Sci. (Wash.) 68, 1644–1647 (1971).

WELLING, W., VOS, O., WEYZEN, W.W.H., VAN BEKKUM, D.W.: Identification and follow-up of homologous and heterologous bone marrow transplants in radiation chimeras. Int. J. Radiat. Biol. 1, 145–152 (1959).

WILSON, D.B., SILVERS, W.K., NOWELL, P.C.: Quantitative studies on the mixed lymphocyte interaction in rats. II. Relationship of the proliferative response to the immunologic status of the donors. J. Exp. Med. 126, 655–665 (1967).

WILSON, D.B., NOWELL, P.C.: Quantitative studies on the mixed lymphocyte interaction in rats. IV. Immunologic potentiality of the responding cells. J. Exp. Med. 131, 391–407 (1970).

WINCHELL, H.S., POLYCOVE, M., LOUGHMAN, W.D., RICHARDS, V., KIM, L., LAWRENCE, J.H.: Homotransplantation studies in dogs following selective radioisotopic lymphatic ablation. J. Nucl. Med. 7, 416–423 (1966).

WOODRUFF, J.F.: Thymolymphatic deficiency and depression of cell-mediated immunity in protein-calorie malnutrition. Lancet 1, 92–93 (1972).

WRIGHT, P.W., HARGREAVES, R.E., BERNSTEIN, I.D., HELLSTROM, I.: Fractionation of sera from operationally tolerant rats by DEAE cellulose chromatography; Evidence that serum blocking factors are associated with IgG. J. Immunol. 112, 1267–1270 (1974).

ZARETSKAYA, Y.M., PANTELEYEV, E.I., KOVALCHUK, L.V.: Antibody formation in radiation chimaeras. Folia Biol. (Praha) 14, 386–389 (1968).

Immunosuppression by Antibodies

K. WONIGEIT and R. PICHLMAYR

With 4 Figures

A. Introduction

The prevention or reversal of the immunological processes leading to allograft rejection is the most difficult task in present day organ transplantation. The ideal solution to this problem would be the selective suppression of the rejection process without impairing other functions of the immune apparatus or causing damage to other organs of the graft recipient. To achieve this, a method of treatment is required which either modifies the antigenicity of the graft or which selectively interacts with those cellular components of the immune system which cause allograft rejection. Because of the high specificity of their effects, *antibodies* appear to be useful tools for these purposes. A great variety of antisera containing antibodies directed against the different components of the immune reaction have therefore been tested as immunosuppressants both experimentally and clinically. In the first section of this paper the *various types of antisera are classified according to origin and specificity* and a *general view of the concepts underlying their use for the purpose of immunosuppression* is given. In the following sections two particularly well studied approaches are discussed in greater detail namely *xenogeneic antilymphocyte sera* and *passive enhancement*.

B. Concepts of Immunosuppression by Antibodies

The development of an immune response is a complex sequence of events, the initial step of which is the interaction between antigen and antigen-reactive cells. Other important steps in this sequence are the proliferation and differentiation of the antigen-reactive cells and their cooperation with accessory and regulatory cells. Antibodies of different types can interfere with these events and thereby induce suppression of the immune response. The way in which this suppression is brought about by a particular type of antibody primarily depends on its specificity, that is, on the type of target structure at which it is directed

and with which it will react when injected into the allograft recipient. According
to this criterion the types of antibodies used so far for the purpose of immunosuppression can be classified into three major groups as follows:

1. Antibodies directed against the cell type specific antigens of lymphocytes
   and macrophages
2. Antibodies directed against the specific recognition structures of the antigen-
   reactive cells
3. Antibodies directed against the sensitizing antigen itself; in the case of organ
   transplantation, against the histocompatibility antigens of the graft

It is obvious that the concepts lying behind the use of these types of antibodies
are as different as the antibodies themselves. The above classification therefore
also represents a very general classification of the underlying concepts and
mechanisms which will now be discussed for each of the three groups of antisera.

1. *Immunosuppression by antibodies directed against lymphocytes and macro-*
phages. Lymphocytes and macrophages possess cell type specific differentiation
antigens against which cell type specific antibodies can be raised. The use of
this type of antibody for the purpose of immunosuppression is based on the
premise that they may be able to remove or inhibit the cells carrying the respective antigens without impairing other organ systems. Although such sera had
been known for a long time, their use as immunosuppressants dates back less
than two decades. It was the rapidly increasing knowledge about the immunological functions of lymphocytes during this period that opened the door for their
use as immunosuppressants.

Antibodies with serological activity against *lymphocytes* can be raised in
both allogeneic and xenogeneic systems. Most of the allogeneic and some of
the xenogeneic antisera posses antibodies specific for single lymphocyte subpopulations. These sera have become useful tools in the investigation of lymphocyte
physiology, in particular for the examination of specific functions of the respective subpopulations in in vitro experiments, but they have only a very limited
immunosuppressive potency. More effective are xenogeneic antilymphocyte sera
which contain antibodies directed against antigenic determinants common to
all lymphocyte subpopulations and which usually possess these antibodies in
much higher concentrations than allogeneic sera. The excellent experimental results obtained with xenogeneic antilymphocyte sera have already led to their
clinical application. A detailed discussion of this type of antiserum will be
given in Section C ("Xenogeneic Antilymphocyte Sera").

Antisera against *macrophages* have not been examined to the same extent
as antilymphocyte sera. It is nevertheless well established that highly specific
xenogeneic antisera can be produced which are able to reduce selectively the
number of macrophages in vivo and to inhibit their phagocytic capacity (UN-
ANUE, 1968; PANIJEL and CAYEUX, 1968). A marked effect on allo- and xenograft
survival has also been reported (THIEDE et al., 1974; CHAUSSY et al., 1975).

2. *Immunosuppression by antibodies directed against the specific recognition*
structures of lymphocytes. The specific receptor molecules of B lymphocytes
are generally believed to be of immunoglobulin nature and to share specificity
with the antibody secreted subsequent to antigenic stimulation (WIGZELL, 1973).
The structure of the T-cell receptor is still a matter of dispute but there is

increasing evidence for a close relationship to immunoglobulin as well (MARCHA-
LONIS *et al.*, 1972; BINZ and WIGZELL, 1975a–c). Antibodies against these receptors can be directed either against allotypic or idiotypic determinants. Allotypic
determinants are localized on the constant part of the polypeptide chains and
antisera directed against them are usually raised in individuals of the same
species lacking that particular allotype. Allotypic determinants are always shared
by a great number of antibody clones with specificity for different antigens.
Idiotypic determinants on the other hand are located on the variable regions
of the polypeptide chains and are characteristic for single antibody clones.
Their number is extremely high, most likely in the order of millions. Antisera
against idiotypic determinants can be raised in xenogeneic, allogeneic and autologous systems.

Findings relevant for the purpose of immunosuppression have been obtained
by passive immunization with both antiallotype and antiidiotype antisera.
Complete and long-lasting suppression of the corresponding allotypes has been
achieved in rabbits (DRAY, 1962; MAGE, 1967) and mice (HERZENBERG and
HERZENBERG, 1974) by neonatal exposure to antiallotype sera. Since there
is no indication that T cell receptors share allotypic determinants with immunoglobulin, this allotype suppression is probably directed exclusively against B
cells (HERZENBERG *et al.*, 1975). All antibody clones expressing the corresponding
allotype are suppressed. This does not mean however that antibody production
against the respective antigen is totally abolished. Most antigens elicit immune
responses comprising more than one allotype.

By passive administration of antiidiotype antibody suppression of single
clones of antibody producing cells has been achieved. This means that idiotype
suppression is much more specific than allotype suppression. Thus a selective
inhibition of antibody formation directed against antigens such as p-azophenyl-
arsonate-KLH (HART *et al.*, 1972; PAWLAK *et al.*, 1973, 1974), streptococcal
A carbohydrate (EICHMANN, 1974), or phosphorylcholine (COSENZA and KÖHLER,
1972a, b) has been possible. Similar to allotype suppression only a partial inhibition of the antibody response to the particular antigen is achieved since most
antigens elicit the production of more than one idiotype. The only exception
so far has been the response to phosphorylcholine which is of oligoclonal origin
and therefore can be suppressed almost completely by means of antiidiotype
antibody (COSENZA and KÖHLER, 1972a, b).

With regard to organ transplantation it is of particular importance to determine whether idiotype suppression is restricted to B-cells like allotype suppression or whether it can also act on T-cells and thereby suppress the immune
response leading to allograft rejection. Sera directed against the lymphocyte
receptors which recognize histocompatibility antigens have recently been prepared by RAMSEIER and LINDENMANN (1972). Their data, as well as the results
of BINZ and WIGZELL with the same type of antiserum, provide convincing
evidence that this antireceptor antibody reacts specifically with receptors on
T- as well as B-cells and is antiidiotype antibody (BINZ and WIGZELL,
1975a, b, c). With antibody of this type the GvH and MLC reactivity of rat
lymphocytes could be abrogated specifically (JOLLER, 1972; BINZ *et al.*, 1973;
MCKEARN *et al.*, 1973; MCKEARN, 1974). Furthermore it was possible to demon-

strate the production of autologous antiidiotype antibodies in rats immunized either by induction of a GvH reaction (Fitch et al., 1974) or by repeated injections with allogeneic tumor or lymphoid cells (McKearn et al., 1974a, b, c). These antibodies appeared later in the course of immunization than the corresponding alloantibodies directed against the sensitizing antigen. Moreover the respective idiotypes of the alloantibody usually disappeared when the anti-idiotype antibody became demonstrable. The conditions under which anti-idiotype antibodies were produced were strikingly similar to those under which enhancement of allografts could be induced (Stuart et al., 1974).

3. *Immunosuppression by antibodies directed against the histocompatibility antigens of the graft.* This type of antibody is different from antilymphocyte and antireceptor antibody in that it is not directed against a component of the immune system but against the *sensitizing antigen itself.* It is thought to bind with the antigen and to modify thereby the interaction between the antigen and the immune system in such a way that suppression of the immune response will occur. Since the early finding that the immunogenicity of diphtheria toxoid was reduced when antitoxoid was given simultaneously, numerous examples have proved the validity of this approach for suppression of antibody formation against soluble antigens and also for allograft rejection (for review see Uhr and Möller, 1968). Prolongation of allograft survival by this type of immunosuppression has been termed "passive enhancement" (Kaliss, 1956), "facilitation reaction" (Voisin, 1971) and "immunological blockade" (Feldman, 1972). The immunosuppression achieved by passive immunization is specific. Despite this great advantage compared with antilymphocyte serum or immunosuppressive drugs its clinical application has been very limited so far. The enormous potential of this type of specific immunosuppression, however, can be seen from the results obtained with passive immunization in the prophylaxis of anti-Rh sensitization in humans.

The findings of McKearn et al. (1974c) mentioned above have related idiotype suppression to enhancement. In many experimental systems in which prolongation of allograft survival has been ascribed to the action of antigen-specific antibody alone, it may be difficult to exclude additional or even preponderant effects of contaminating anti-idiotype antibody. In Section D ("Passive Enhancement") both types of antibody will be dealt with.

C. Xenogeneic Antilymphocyte Sera

I. General Aspects

Xenogeneic antilymphocyte serum (ALS) is an immune serum raised in one species against the lymphocytes of another species. Its essential feature is the presence of antibodies which react specifically with lymphocytes of the sensitizing species. The prerequisite for the formation of such antibodies is the presence of antigens preferentially or exclusively expressed on lymphocytes. Metchnikoff is credited with the first demonstration of such antigens on lymphocytes and the production of the first antilymphocyte sera as early as 1899. During the first half of this century such antisera were repeatedly examined for their various in vivo and in vitro properties but their immunosuppressive potency was not detected until 1956 when INDERBITZIN reported the inhibition of delayed hypersensitivity by xenogeneic antilymphocyte serum in guinea pigs. WAKSMAN et al. (1961) and WOODRUFF and ANDERSON (1963, 1964) achieved prolongation of allograft survival and suppression of autoimmune phenomena in rats. The work of WOODRUFF and ANDERSON in particular prompted many other researchers to investigate the production, specificity, and biological activity of such sera. LEVEY and MEDAWAR (1966a, b) demonstrated that ALS is the most potent immunosuppressant in mice. Subsequent work with canine renal allotransplantation (MONACO et al., 1966b; PICHLMAYR, 1966, 1967; STARZL et al., 1967) quickly led to the clinical application of ALS in human renal allograft recipients (STARZL et al., 1966, 1967, 1968) and in patients with autoimmune diseases (TREPEL et al., 1968; BRENDEL, 1971; PIROFSKI et al., 1969, 1971). Since the work of WOODRUFF and ANDERSON the literature about ALS has gone through a period of exponential growth. Previous reviews have already discussed many aspects in detail (JAMES, 1969; LANCE et al., 1973; MONACO, 1972).

II. Types of Xenogeneic Antilymphocyte Sera

A great number of effective xenogeneic antisera against lymphocytes of various species, including man, have been described. The methods used for their preparation have differed widely. Hence it is not surprising that the in vivo and in vitro properties of the resulting sera show remarkable variation. Since standardization of procedures is still lacking, sera are best characterised by a description of their preparation. Therefore current methods and their various advantages will be summarized here. (For a more detailed review together with references see LANCE et al., 1973). Points of relevance are the source and the purity of antigenic material, the animal species used for immunization, the immunization protocol, and finally the purification of the active antibodies.

The *antigenic material* most commonly used for immunization consists of suspensions of living lymphocytes. Blood and thoracic duct lymph as well as the various lymphatic tissues can be used as the lymphocyte source. All these cell populations contain the relevant antigenic structures although they differ in purity. Spleen cell suspensions in particular are difficult to obtain without contamination by other tissue components which may give rise to a broad spectrum of toxic antibodies. Lymphoblastoid cell lines are an exceptionally pure antigen which is even superior to thoracic duct cells (NAJARIAN et al., 1969, 1970). There is, however, the danger of dedifferentiation of cells in culture and subsequent loss of antigenic determinants. Furthermore human lymphoblast cell lines available so far are B-cell lines and therefore lack T-cell specific antigens. Studies with subcellular fractions have shown that the lymphocyte membrane is the main source of antigen (LEVEY and MEDAWAR, 1966b). Crude membrane fractions as well as solubilized lipoproteins are active although their immunogenicity is low when compared to that of intact cells (LANCE *et al.*, 1968, 1970a; ZOLA *et al.*, 1970; GRABAR, 1970).

Many different animal species have been used in the production of antisera. These include rabbit, horse, sheep, goat, cow, pig, and even various avian species. Avian antibodies however have been shown to have only little or no immunosuppressive potency. Most data has been collected on rabbit and horse sera directed against mouse, rat, dog, and human lymphocytes. Several immunization schedules have been employed. In general one has to distinguish between antisera produced by a short course of antigen administration (two or three pulse sera) (LEVEY and MEDAWAR, 1966a; LANCE, 1968a, b; SHORTER *et al.*, 1967; GOZZO *et al.*, 1971) and antisera produced by hyperimmunization with many repeated antigen injections (WOODRUFF *et al.*, 1967a, b; IWASAKI *et al.*, 1967; PICHLMAYR, 1967; TRAEGER *et al.*, 1967). A third group of antisera has been obtained with schedules using adjuvants (LANCE *et al.*, 1973). The question of which immunization schedule is the most appropriate depends largely on the species used for immunization and the purity of the antigen. Certainly the risk of eliciting the formation of toxic antibodies is lowest with short-course immunization schedules which therefore are favored by most workers in this field. Nevertheless highly purified preparations such as thoracic duct lymphocytes (PICHLMAYR, 1967; PICHLMAYR *et al.*, 1967a, c; 1970; TRAEGER *et al.*, 1970) or cultured lymphoblasts (NAJARIAN *et al.*, 1969, 1970) have also proved to be suitable for the production of strong antisera by hyperimmunization. Adjuvants have been extremely effective in raising potent sera against subcellular membrane fractions which otherwise exhibit only low antigenicity (LANCE *et al.*, 1968, 1970a).

Antilymphocyte sera prepared according to the described procedures usually contain antibodies reactive not only against lymphocytes but also against serum proteins, platelets, erythrocytes, granulocytes, monocytes, and other cell types (PICHLMAYR *et al.*, 1967b). Since antibodies directed against most of the latter can lead to serious complications upon injection, they have to be removed. This is usually achieved by absorption of the antiserum with erythrocytes and serum proteins, resulting in only a slight reduction in antilymphocytic activity (IWASAKI *et al.*, 1967; PICHLMAYR *et al.*, 1967a).

The specificity of the antilymphocyte antibodies has been analyzed in detail in several rabbit-anti-mouse and rabbit-anti-rat lymphocyte sera (CHEN *et al.*, 1974; COLLEY *et al.*, 1970; GRABAR, 1970; SHIGENO *et al.*, 1968; RABINOWITZ *et al.*, 1974). These studies revealed the complexity of the lymphocyte-specific antigens in these species. Several separate antigenic entities were demonstrated and were characterized by physicochemical methods. It was found, however, that antisera directed against complex mixtures of several antigens had a stronger immunosuppressive effect than T-cell–specific antisera (GRABAR, 1970). Since SMITH and WOODY in a more recent study were able to demonstrate in several antihuman antisera a good correlation between T-cell–specific antibodies and immunosuppressive potency, this question should be reevaluated (SMITH and WOODY, 1974).

Numerous studies have shown that most of the antilymphocyte and all or nearly all of the immunosuppressive activity of ALS lies in the IgG fraction

(WOODRUFF et al., 1967b; JAMES and MEDAWAR, 1967; RIETHMÜLLER, 1967; RIETHMÜLLER et al., 1968; IWASAKI et al., 1967; MONACO et al., 1967a, b). The use of isolated IgG for in vivo experiments means that the administration of large amounts of serum protein other than IgG can be avoided. This reduces the load of immunogenic and potentially toxic foreign protein (JAMES and ANDERSON, 1967). Furthermore, the number of hemagglutinins and hemolysins which are predominantly IgM can be reduced by the fractionation procedure making absorption easier (JAMES and ANDERSON, 1967; WOODRUFF et al., 1967a). Fractionation can be done according to standard procedures (JAMES, 1969). For the clinical use of ALS, isolation of the IgG fraction is generally regarded as indispensible (JAMES 1969).

A further step in purification is the separation of specific antibodies from the residual immunoglobulins. WOODRUFF (1968) achieved this by absorption of ALS with lymphoid cells and subsequent elution of the membrane-bound antibodies. Specific antibodies isolated in this way have proved to be extremely valuable for various experimental purposes (LANCE, 1969). The procedures for this purification step, however, are not yet suitable for large-scale performance.

III. Effects on Lymphoid Cells in Vitro

The specific antilymphoid antibodies of ALS primarily react with antigens localized in the outer cell membrane. The presence of these antibodies, therefore, can most easily be demonstrated by classical serological procedures such as agglutination tests (GRAY et al., 1966; ABAZA et al., 1966; PICHLMAYR, 1967) and complement-mediated cytolysis (ABAZA and WOODRUFF, 1966; GRAY et al., 1966; PICHLMAYR, 1967). The localization of the bound antibody on the membrane can be visualized by autoradiography (LANCE, 1969) and indirect fluoresence (LEVEY and MEDAWAR, 1966a; RUSSELL and MONACO, 1967). Other very sensitive methods for the measurement of antilymphocyte antibody are the uptake of radioactively labeled antibodies (WOODRUFF et al., 1967c) and passive agglutination (MONACO et al., 1973). Furthermore, the coating of lymphocytes with antibodies alters their interaction with other cells types. This effect is used in assays measuring the opsonizing capacity of ALS and the inhibition of spontaneous rosetting of lymphocytes with xenogeneic erythrocytes. In the opsonization assay (GREAVES et al., 1969; MARTIN, W.J., 1969a) antibody-coated lymphocytes are mixed with macrophages which then bind the lymphocytes via the Fc part of the attached antibody and ingest them. An inhibitory effect of ALS on the spontaneous rosette formation of lymphocytes with erythrocytes from various species was detected by BACH and ANTOINE (1968). Rosette forming cells are regarded as antigen binding T-cells (BACH, 1970; BACH et al., 1970). Inhibition of rosette formation would thus indicate interference with the antigen-binding process. This interpretation, however, is only valid in rodents. In humans and primates, spontaneous rosette formation with sheep red blood cells is a property of all T-cells and is not related to antigen recognition (JONDAL et al., 1972).

Another in vitro effect of ALS on lymphoid cells is its ability to activate blast transformation when added to lymphocyte cultures in the absence of complement (GRÄSBECK et al., 1963, 1964; SELL et al., 1965; HOLT et al., 1966; BACH and BACH, 1970). This phenomenon is called sterile activation as no antigen is involved (LEVEY and MEDAWAR, 1967). The detection of this effect has very much influenced speculation about the mode of action of ALS. When cultured lymphocytes are stimulated specifically by allogenic cells (mixed lymphocyte culture) or nonspecifically by mitogens, the addition of ALS either enhances or suppresses the reaction depending on the concentration and the type of ALS used. Enhancement probably reflects a combination of specific stimulation by the antigen and sterile activation by ALS, suppression an interaction of ALS with antigen recognition or even a direct toxic effect on the cultured cells (BROCHIER and REVILLARD, 1971; REVILLARD, 1972).

IV. Effects on the Lymphatic System

The effects of ALS on blood lymphocytes can best be observed after intravenous injection. It is usually followed by a pronounced but transient lymphopenia (DENMAN et al., 1968a, b; GRAY et al., 1964, 1966; IWASAKI et al., 1967; PICHL-MAYR, 1967; PICHLMAYR et al., 1967a, b; TAUB and LANCE, 1968). This is due to the destruction of antibody-coated cells via complement-mediated lysis or phagocytosis in the RES (LANCE, 1969; BARTH et al., 1974). Repeated injections often cause a longer lasting lymphopenia, the degree and duration of which depend on the relationship between lymphocyte destruction by ALS and the

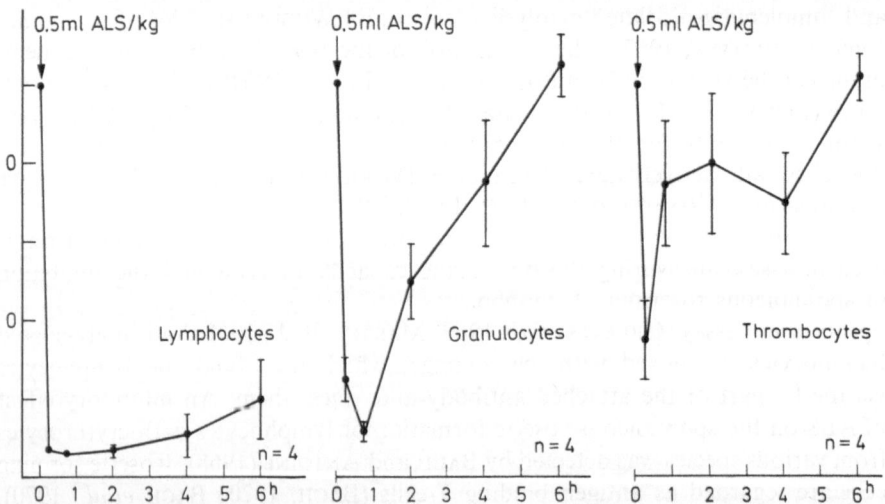

Fig. 1. Lymphopenic effect of horse-anti-dog ALS. Changes in the peripheral lymphocyte, granulo-cyte, and platelet counts of 4 dogs over a 6-h period subsequent to a single i.v. injection are depicted. The dosage was 0.5 ml/kg body weight. Results are expressed as percentage decrease from the absolute count immediately before injection. Mean values ±1 SD are given. All cell types showed a marked reduction in number. Whereas the granulocyte and platelet counts recovered within a few hours, the lymphocyte count remained depressed over the whole time of observation

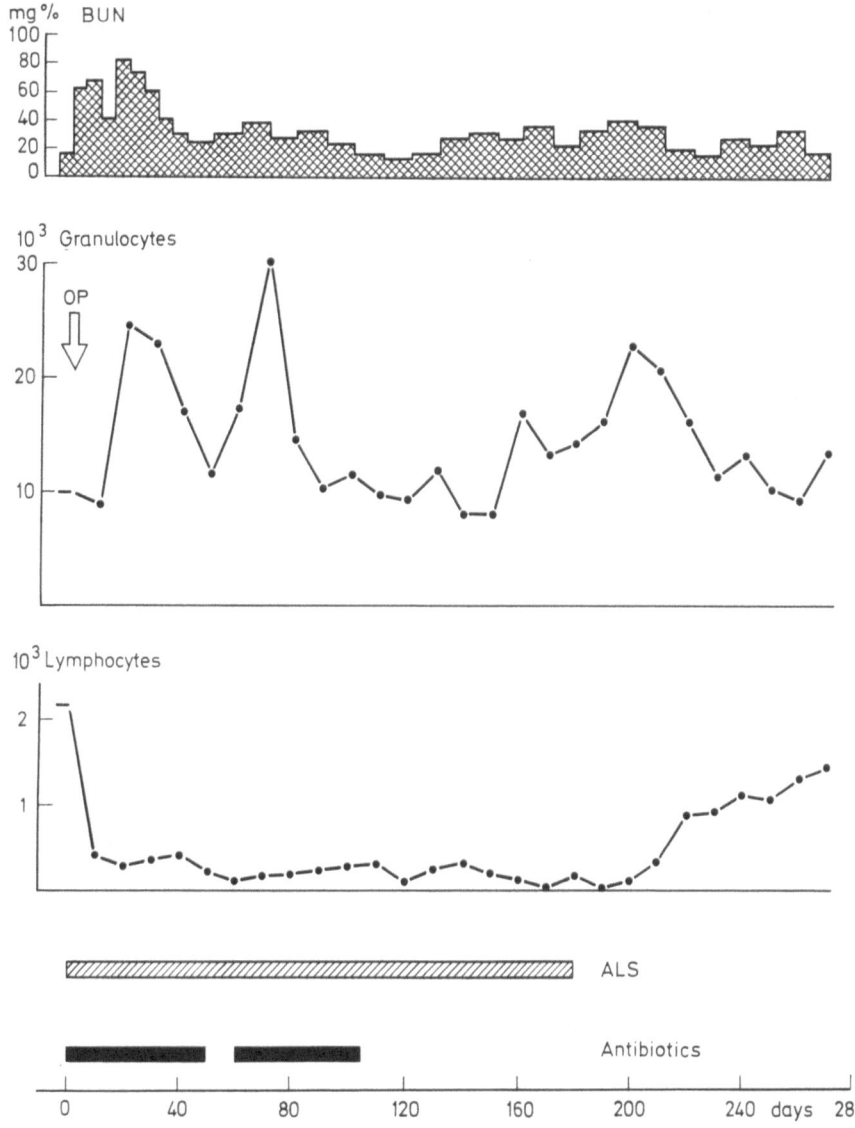

Fig. 2. Effect of long-term treatment with horse-anti-dog ALS on the peripheral lymphocyte count. BUN, granulocyte, and lymphocyte counts of a single dog subsequent to renal allotransplantation and treatment with ALS are depicted. 0.5 ml/kg body weight were injected i.v. twice a day, the lymphocyte count was depressed immediately upon beginning treatment and remained reduced over the whole period of ALS administration. It recovered slowly after ALS treatment had been interrupted. The allograft was permanently accepted

kinetics of lymphocyte release from the lymphatic tissues (PICHLMAYR, 1967; PICHLMAYR *et al.*, 1967a, b). Even when no lymphopenic effect occurs, an accelerated turnover of the lymphoid cells in circulation is detected, indicating that ALS enhances the elimination of lymphocytes from blood. Long-lived recircula-

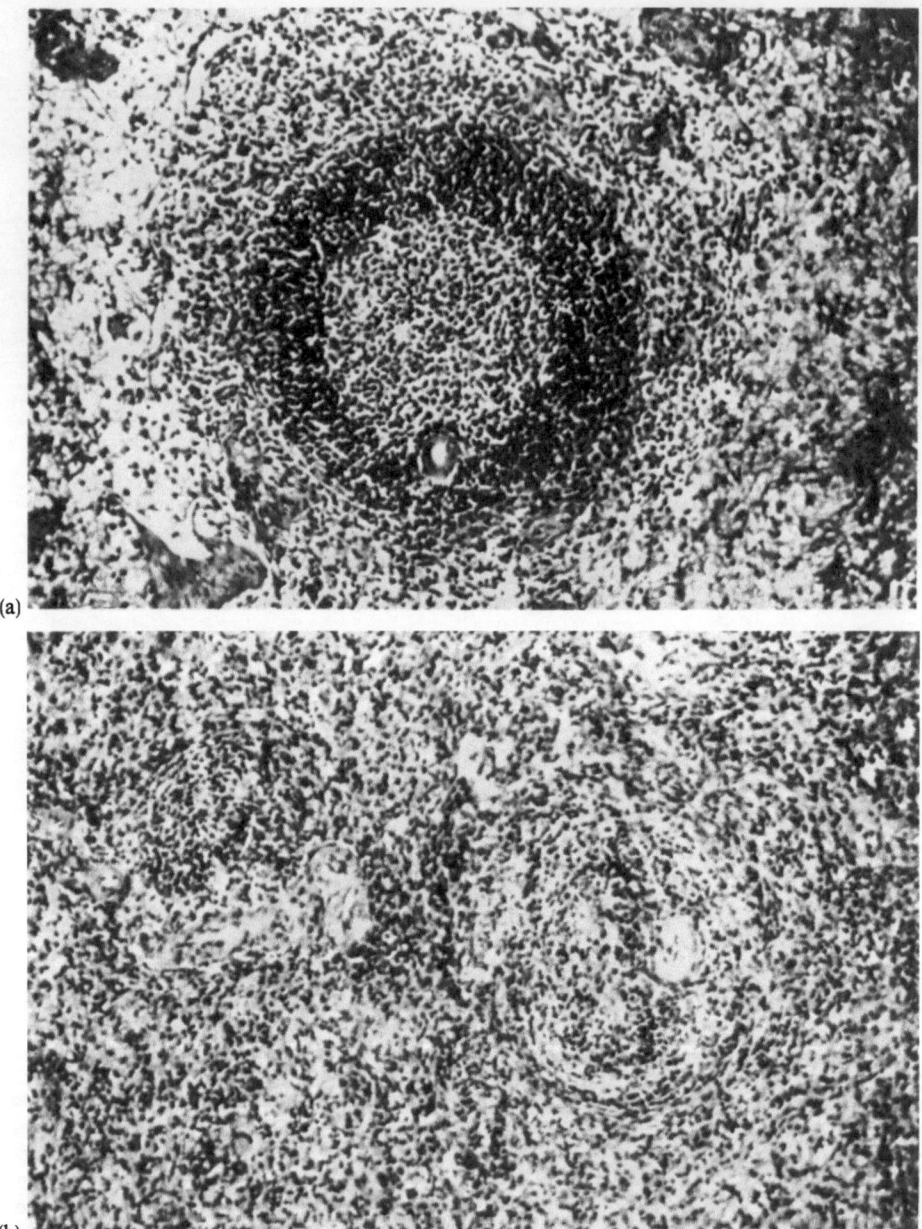

Fig. 3a and b. Normal spleen (a) and spleen of a dog after 1 week of treatment with horse-anti-dog ALS (b). The treatment has led to complete depletion of mature lymphocytes in the periarteriolar sheaths. (Stain: H & E, magnification × 125)

ting lymphocytes are replaced by short-lived populations (DENMAN and FRENKEL, 1968a, b; DENMAN et al., 1968a, b; RAFF and WORTIS, 1970; TAUB and LANCE, 1968). An illustration of the strong lymphopenic effect which can be achieved with some sera is given in Figures 1 and 2.

During the early period following moderate doses of ALS, signs of hyperplasia have frequently been observed in the lymphatic tissue (CHEW and LAWRENCE, 1937; LEVEY and MEDAWAR, 1966a). This has been attributed to the stimulation of cells in tissue by sublytic concentrations of ALS (LEVEY and MEDAWAR, 1966a; TAUB and LANCE, 1968) or to the antigenic stimulation exerted by the xenogeneic serum proteins (IWASAKI et al., 1967; GUTTMAN et al., 1967b, c). Continuous treatment with potent ALS results in a marked depletion of small lymphocytes from the thymus-dependent areas of lymph nodes and spleen. These are the deep paracortical areas in lymph nodes and the periarteriolar sheeths in the white pulp of the spleen (LANCE, 1968a; PARROT, 1967; PICHLMAYR, 1967; TAUB and LANCE, 1968; TURK and WILLOUGHBY, 1967). The B-cell areas are not altered to the same extent (TAUB and LANCE, 1968). The characteristic lesions of spleen and lymph node structure are demonstrated in Figures 3 and 4. Indiscriminate destruction of lymph node architecture has also been reported with some sera when given in high dosage (DENMAN and FRENKEL, 1967; MONACO et al., 1965a, b; NAGAYA and SIEKER, 1965). The morphologic alterations in the peripheral lymphatic tissues are reversible subsequent to the interruption of ALS treatment. Complete restoration, however, requires many weeks or months. The thymus is usually only slightly altered or completely unaffected by ALS treatment, but exceptions have been reported (DENMAN and FRENKEL, 1967; MONACO et al., 1965a, b; NAGAYA and SIEKER, 1965). The latter were probably due to the high toxicity of the sera employed which caused severe shock reactions. It is well known that stress can result in severe damage to the thymus (TAUB and LANCE, 1968).

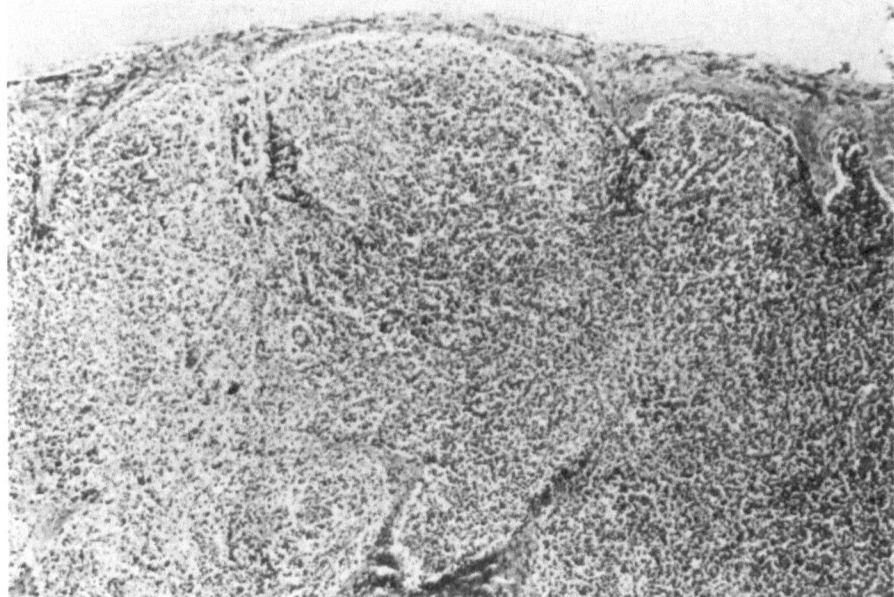

Fig. 4. Lymph node of a dog after 3 weeks treatment with horse-anti-dog ALS. Thymus-dependent areas are depleted of mature lymphocytes; germinal centers have disappeared. (Stain: H & E, magnification × 40)

V. Immunosuppressive Activity of ALS

1. Humoral Immunity

ALS suppresses most humoral immune reactions to thymus-dependent antigens when given in sufficient dosage prior to or simultaneous with the primary antigenic stimulus. This has been demonstrated in many experimental systems with a wide variety of antigens including xenogeneic erythrocytes (ANDERSON et al., 1972; JEEJEEBHOY, 1965a, b; MONACO et al., 1966c; KERBEL and EIDINGER, 1971) and serum proteins (JAMES, 1970; KERBEL and EIDINGER, 1971; LANCE, 1970b), bacterial antigens (LANCE, 1970b; PICHLMAYR, 1967) and synthetic haptens coupled to various carrier proteins (MITCHISON, 1970). The cause of this effect is the inactivation of cooperating T-cells (MARTIN and MILLER, 1968; MITCHISON, 1970). In contrast, primary responses to thymus-independent antigens are much less sensitive to ALS (KERBEL and EIDINGER, 1971; BARTH et al., 1973) and secondary humoral responses in normally primed animals only slightly affected if at all (JAMES, 1970; MARTIN and MILLER, 1968).

One very unexpected finding was that when ALS treatment was started several days after antigen administration, there was an occasional enhancement of antibody responses (ANDERSON et al., 1972). This phenomenon has now been confirmed by several investigators and has been attributed to T suppressor cells being particularly sensitive to ALS (for review with references see KATZ and BENACERRAF, 1972).

2. Delayed Hypersensitivity

The original finding of WAKSMAN et al. (1961) that cutaneous delayed hypersensitivity in guinea pigs was suppressed by doses of ALS which had no effect on antibody mediated immune reactions has been confirmed and extended to other species and antigens by numerous workers (for review see LANCE et al., 1973). IWASAKI et al. (1967) and MONACO et al. (1967a) have established the validity of this observation for man as well.

3. Transplantation Immunity

ALS has proved to be the most potent reagent in the suppression of allo- and xenograft rejection in rodents (LEVEY and MEDAWAR, 1966a, b). Most of the antilymphocyte sera produced in rabbits or horses can prolong the survival time of skin allografts in rats and mice for long periods (ANDERSON et al., 1967; GRAY et al., 1964; MONACO et al., 1965a, b, 1966c; WOODRUFF and ANDERSON, 1963, 1964). Even with skin grafts across strong histocompatibility barriers, significant prolongation has been achieved by short courses of treatment (LEVEY and MEDAWAR, 1966a). In rats the rejection of cardiac and renal allografts is already suppressed by remarkably small doses (GUTTMAN et al., 1967a–d; VAN BEKKUM et al., 1969). In higher species such as dogs and monkeys the effects are less dramatic but marked improvement of allograft survival has also been achieved (ABAZA et al., 1966; MONACO et al., 1966b; PICHLMAYR

et al., 1967a, c; Starzl *et al.*, 1967; Iwahashi *et al.*, 1970; Balner *et al.*, 1968b).
The results obtained in humans will be dealt with in Section X.

In contrast to humoral immune reactivity, transplantation immunity is also markedly influenced by ALS when this reagent is administered several days after transplantation or to presensitized animals (Levey and Medawar, 1966a). Its ability to affect already established transplantation immunity is one of the outstanding characteristics of ALS. Erasure of immunologic memory has been achieved by no other immunosuppressive drug so far. Established humoral immunity is not impaired by subsequent ALS treatment. This proves that the effect of ALS on cellular immune reactions is stronger than on antibody formation. This property renders ALS particularly suitable for use as an immunosuppressant in organ transplantation. In comparison with other immunosuppressants, another advantage of ALS is its effect on the rejection of xenografts in rodents. Monaco *et al.* (1966c) demonstrated that rat skin will be accepted by mice when they are injected with rabbit antiserum. This finding was confirmed by several workers and extended to various other xenogeneic combinations (Lance and Medawar, 1968; Phillips and Gazet, 1967, 1969; Monaco, 1970). The effect of ALS on xenotransplantation, however, is restricted to species in which xenograft rejection is not mediated by preformed antibodies, since ALS does not affect the latter.

4. Autoimmune Phenomena

Autoimmune phenomena represent a great variety of very different types of immune reactions, both cellular and humoral. Under experimental conditions the efficiency of ALS in suppressing autoimmune processes very much depends on the time of application (e. g., simultaneously with antigen administration, subsequent to immunization but before manifestation of symptoms or after the onset of disease with full-blown symptoms) and the type of immune reactions. A detailed discussion of this wide area of research would be beyond the scope of this article. The relevant information and references can be obtained in the reviews by Denman (1969) and Monaco (1972).

5. Graft-versus-Host Immunity

Three different types of approach to abolish graft-versus-host immunity have been used: (1) pretreatment of the donor, (2) in vitro exposure of cells to ALS before inoculation, (3) treatment of the recipient. Pretreatment of the donor has been a very effective method of preventing GvH in rodents (Levey and Medawar, 1967; Brent *et al.*, 1967, 1968; Boak *et al.*, 1968) but was found ineffective in monkeys (Balner *et al.*, 1968b; Balner, 1969). Treatment of donor cells in vitro has also only been effective in rodents (van der Werf *et al.*, 1967; Ledney and van Bekkum, 1968; Brent *et al.*, 1968; Field and Gibbs, 1968). In other species, however, the production of antisera with a sufficient degree of specificity has been a great problem since most sera exhibit some cross reactivity with bone marrow stem cells which is extremely difficult to remove.

The third approach, that of preventing or curing GvH disease by treatment with ALS, has been shown by Balner to be effective in his monkey system (Balner, 1969) and is now in clinical use (Storb et al., 1974).

VI. Cooperative Effects with Other Immunosuppressive Regimens

The effect of ALS is strongly enhanced by procedures which deplete recirculating T-lymphocytes or prevent their regeneration. Thoracic duct drainage was shown by Woodruff and Anderson (1963, 1964) to augment the effect of ALS on skin allograft survival in rats. This finding has been repeatedly confirmed and extended to other species (Jeejeebhoy, 1965a, b; Monaco et al., 1965a, b, 1969; Davis and Lewis, 1968). Adult thymectomy is even more effective (Jee-jeebhoy, 1965a; Monaco et al., 1965a, b). It prevents the regeneration of depleted recirculating T-cells and so gives rise to a long-lasting state of nonspecific immunosuppression which allows prolonged survival of skin allografts even when transferred up to 100 days after ALS treatment has ceased. Corticosteroids strongly enhance the effect of ALS in mice and rats (Levey and Medawar, 1966b), no prolongation of renal allograft survival, however, has been found in dogs when a preoperative regimen of ALS was combined with postoperative corticosteroids (Weil and Simmons, 1968). The cooperative effect of corticosteroids with ALS in mice and rats has been ascribed to the lympholysis brought about by corticosteroids in these species which leads to a type of functional thymectomy (Lance et al., 1970b). In other species such as dogs and guinea pigs, corticosteroids, although immunosuppressive as well, have no comparable lympholytic activity (Claman, 1972). It remains to be clarified whether this relative "cortisone resistance" of lymphocytes has been responsible for the results obtained by Weil and Simmons (1968) in dogs. Since humans are also considered to have a cortisone-resistant population of lymphocytes (Claman, 1972) this question has to be re-evaluated. Irradiation prior to ALS treatment (Levey and Medawar, 1966a) and the administration of various cytotoxic drugs with or subsequent to ALS both enhance its immunosuppressive effect (Hoehn and Simmons, 1966, 1967; Levey and Medawar, 1966a; Perper et al., 1970a, b; Simmons et al., 1968).

The combination of ALS with chemical immunosuppressants such as antiproliferative drugs and corticosteroids is advantageous in that it augments their immunosuppressive effect without increasing the occurrence of most of their nonimmunologic side-effects. Independent of the drug used, however, the resulting immunosuppression is not the only effect and its potentiation may lead to serious complications such as viral, bacterial, and fungal infections. The solution to this problem might be provided by the combination of ALS treatment with tolerance induction. Monaco et al. (1966a) first showed that ALS can facilitate the induction of tolerance to histocompatibility antigen in adult thymectomized mice. Subsequent studies in rodents as well as in dogs and monkeys clearly demonstrated that ALS alone can also be used for this purpose (Lance and Medawar, 1969a, b; Monaco et al., 1971; Brent and Kilshaw, 1970; Brent et al., 1971). Wood et al. (1973) reported the occurrence of blocking antibodies in mice carrying skin allografts for prolonged periods subsequent to treatment with donor marrow cells and ALS. This indicates that ALS may also facilitate the induction of active enhancement of allografts. Potentiation of passive enhancement by ALS was achieved in renal allotransplantation in rats (BATCHELOR et al., 1972). If ALS were able to facilitate the induction of specific nonreactivity by tolerance or enhancement in humans as well, this could solve most of the problems organ transplantation is facing today.

VII. Assays for Immunosuppressive Potency

Comparisons between different antilymphocyte sera, are very much complicated by the lack of generally accepted standards for this type of reagent. The only fully reliable and objective method of determining their immunosuppressive potency is to measure their capacity to prolong allograft survival in well-defined donor recipient combinations. The induction of lymphopenia, which was originally thought to be a good parameter of immunosuppressive capacity (JEE-BEEBHOY, 1965a; DENMAN and FRENKEL, 1968a; PICHLMAYR et al., 1967a, b), is only of limited predictive value. Sera causing pronounced lymphopenia usually do suppress allograft rejection, but not all sera with high immunosuppressive potency evoke a long-lasting reduction of the peripheral lymphocyte count (BAL-NER et al., 1968a, b; STARZL et al., 1967). The correlation might be better if T- and B-cells were examined separately, a procedure that has recently become possible in most species (GREAVES et al., 1974). Assays that have been found to be of some value are the rosette inhibition assay (BACH, 1970; BACH et al., 1970), indirect immunofluorescence (EDWARDS et al., 1972; GILKERSON et al., 1970; ROLAND et al., 1971; THOMAS et al., 1971), indirect passive hemagglutination (GOZZO et al., 1972; MONACO et al., 1973), and the examination of the opsonizing capacity of the immune serum by in vivo (MARTIN, 1969b, c; MARTIN and MILLER, 1969) or in vitro (GREAVES et al., 1969; ROITT et al., 1970) procedures. Cytotoxicity and agglutination tests are usually not very useful for the assessment of immunosuppressive activity. Not all sera with high titers are effective in immunosuppression, whereas others with low activity in these assays are effective (JOOSTE et al., 1968; SKAMENE, 1970). A major factor in the failure of cytoxicity and agglutination tests to detect the lack of immunosuppressive activity has probably been the use of unpurified material. It is well known that IgM antibodies, which have little or no immunosuppressive potency, have strong agglutinating and cytoxic effects in vitro. Unabsorbed sera furthermore contain antibodies with broad specificity which also do not contribute to immunosuppression (SKAMENE and RUSSELL, 1971). As was recently pointed out by LANCE, the use of highly purified IgG fractions which have undergone absorption, could most likely improve the correlation between in vitro results and immunosuppressive activity (LANCE, 1972). The most conclusive results are probably obtained when several different in vitro tests are performed in parallel. It may well be that immunosuppressive activity depends on the presence of different types of antibodies, not all of which are detected in one single assay (MONACO et al., 1973).

Evaluation of the potency of antihuman ALS prior to its clinical application represents a particularly difficult problem. For this purpose Balner et al. (1968 a, b) have introduced the surrogate host assay. This method uses monkeys and apes for the pretesting of antihuman ALS in vivo because of their phylogenetic closeness to man. Antisera prolonging skin allograft survival in these animals are regarded as being immunosuppressive in humans as well. Untreated controls usually reject allogeneic skin within 12 days, whereas with maximal doses of antihuman ALS survival times up to 30 days have been obtained in speciosa monkeys and chimpanzees (Balner, 1972). This assay is at present the most important method for monitoring both immunosuppressive potency and toxicity of antihuman antilymphocyte sera.

VIII. Mode of Action

The multiplicity of in vitro and in vivo effects of ALS has given rise to numerous suggestions regarding its mode of action. Levey and Medawar (1966a) originally proposed that antigen recognition was blocked by specific antilymphoid antibody ("blindfolding"). Later they suggested an inactivation of antigen reactive cells by sterile activation (Levey and Medawar, 1966b). Other hypotheses have been antigenic competition (Guttman et al., 1967c), blocking of antigenic determinants by ALS (induction of passive enhancement) (Guttman et al., 1967b, c; Raju et al., 1969) or an anti-inflammatory effect of ALS (Turk et al., 1968; Turk and Polak, 1969). It is not possible to rule out the existence of these mechanisms completely but there is now widespread agreement that none of these has a significant role in ALS-mediated immunosuppression (for a detailed discussion see Lance, 1970a). The relevant effect of ALS in immunosuppression is its selective depletion of the recirculating lymphocyte pool. Only the evidence for this mechanism will be given here.

The selectivity for recirculating lymphocytes is not an inherent property of ALS which is able to react with and to destroy lymphocytes belonging to all subpopulations. It is due to the fact that lymphocyte destruction by ALS is confined to the periphery. This was first suggested by Levey and Medawar (1967) and later substantiated by Denman et al. (1968a, b), Lance (1969, 1970a), and Martin and Miller (1968).

By studying the distribution of ^{125}I-labeled antibodies Lance (1969) was able to demonstrate convincingly that only small amounts penetrate to lymphoid tissue. The bulk of the antibody was absorbed by the lymphocytes in the periphery and then together with the lymphocytes rapidly cleared from circulation and degraded by the reticuloendothelial system. Since sessile cells within the lymphatic tissue will be spared, the consequence of repeated ALS treatment will be a selective depletion of recirculating cells. This hypothesis is supported by the hematologic and histologic findings in ALS-treated animals. The selective removal of recirculating T-cells usually found in the diffuse cortex (paracortex) of lymph nodes and the periarteriolar sheathes of the Malpighian bodies is the predominant finding after prolonged ALS treatment (Taub and Lance, 1968). Quantitative changes in the different lymphocyte subpopulations under

ALS treatment have been shown by several independent methods. SCHLESINGER and YRON (1969) demonstrated that in lymph nodes of ALS-treated mice, theta positive cells (theta being a marker for thymus-dependent lymphocytes) were reduced to very low numbers. Studies on the output of lymphocytes from the thoracic duct have revealed that this is still very much reduced even when the blood lymphocyte count has already recovered (AGNEW, 1968; TYLER et al., 1968). This directly demonstrates a selective diminution of recirculating cells. The detailed functional analysis of T-cells remaining in the peripheral lymphatic tissues subsequent to ALS treatment revealed that these cells represent a separate subpopulation with functional capabilities different from those of the recirculating T-cells. The former have been designated T1 cells, the latter T2 cells (for review together with literature see GREAVES et al., 1974).

The theory of selective destruction of recirculating lymphocytes fits well with the type of immunodeficiency induced by ALS treatment. It clearly explains the excellent effect of ALS on delayed hypersensitivity and allograft rejection. The cells giving rise to both types of reactions are exclusively T-cells and belong to the recirculating pool. When ALS is given prior to immunization, it will reduce the number of antigen-reactive cells and this will lead to diminished reactivity of the treated individual. When ALS is given subsequent to effective immunization, the antigen-induced proliferation and differentiation of the antigen-reactive cells within the lymphatic tissue will occur, but the effector cells released into circulation and destined to bring about the specific lesion at the site of the antigen will be destroyed by ALS. In this manner the efferent arc of these immune reactions will be inhibited.

The strong effect of ALS on primary antibody formation against T-dependent antigens can be explained along the same lines. The development of antibody secreting plasma cells from B-cells is dependent on the cooperation of the precursor B-cells with antigen-activated T-cells which are also recruited from recirculating T-cells. When ALS is given prior to immunization, the depletion of recirculating T-cells will therefore lead to strong inhibition of antibody formation. In later stages of the immune response when cooperation with T-cells is no longer required, the effect of ALS is less pronounced. MARTIN and MILLER (1968) were able to demonstrate that the antibody response against sheep red blood cells can be restored in ALS-treated mice by adoptive transfer of normal thymus cells. This provided direct evidence that antigen-reactive B-cells are spared.

IX. Side-Effects and Complications

ALS causes various side-effects in experimental animals. These can result from (1) a direct toxic effect of ALS on nonlymphoid cells and tissue structures; (2) its antigenic properties as a xenogeneic protein which can evoke the full spectrum of known hyperergic reactions; and (3) the suppression of immune responsiveness to infections due to the lack of antigen specificity in its immunosuppressive activity. A further, poorly understood complication is (4) an increase in the frequency of malignant lymphoreticular tumors in ALS-treated rodents.

All these findings are extremely relevant with regard to the use of ALS in man. The discussion here will deal with the general aspects. Clinical experiences will be reviewed in Section X.

1. Toxic Effects

The reaction between ALS and the recipient's lymphocytes is a typical antigen-antibody interaction which causes several characteristic symptoms such as local pain and inflammation at the site of injection as well as systemic reactions such as fever and even a short period of hypotension (Monaco et al., 1967a; Pichlmayr, 1967; Brendel, 1971; Starzl et al., 1967, 1969; Traeger et al., 1971). Hematologically there is often a concomitant decrease in the number of platelets and some fluctuation in the levels of polymorphonuclear neutrophils (PMN) and monocytes (Pichlmayr, 1967; Pichlmayr et al., 1967b; Trepel et al., 1968). These symptoms are inevitable insofar as they are a consequence of the desired therapeutic effect of ALS on the lymphatic system. When the intravenous route is used for administration, the local symptoms can usually be avoided (Pichlmayr, 1967; Traeger et al., 1971). The oral application of ALS has been suggested as another elegant way to circumvent local symptoms (Seifert et al., 1974). It has been shown to allow effective immunosuppression in rodents; its suitability for other species remains to be established.

Every active ALS preparation when administered in effective dosage will provoke general reactions of the abovementioned type. Severe shock reactions, marked thrombocytopenia, and hemolytic reactions, however, should not occur. When they do take place in recipients not previously sensitized to the xenogeneic proteins, this invariably indicates the presence of toxic antibodies directed against cells and tissue components other than lymphocytes. The development of such nonspecific antibodies cannot always be avoided in widely disparate xenogeneic systems. Antibodies directed against red cells, platelets, granulocytes, and serum proteins have to be carefully absorbed. Because of the wide cross reaction between different tissues, absorption with red blood cells alone is sufficient in many instances (James, 1969; Pichlmayr, 1967). The appropriate procedure for absorption has to be worked out for each particular type of serum. Human red cells, for instance, do not possess the HLA antigens common to nearly all human tissues and so will not absorb xenogeneic antibodies directed against these antigens, whereas murine red cells will absorb antibodies against the homologous H-2 antigens.

Difficulties have been reported with the absorption of high antiplatelet titers. Occasionally it has not been possible to remove antibodies without a significant decrease in antilymphocyte and immunosuppressive activity. Such sera frequently have to be discarded. Antibodies against basement membranes also can be removed only with great difficulty. They may occur in antisera against homogenates of lymphoid tissue, spleen in particular. If not removed from the serum they will cause toxic nephritis (Iwasaki et al., 1967; Guttman et al., 1967c; Skamene et al., 1972; Thiel et al., 1971). It is a common finding that pure lymphocyte suspensions such as thoracic duct cells or cultured lymphoblasts do not induce the formation of this type of antibody (Pichlmayr, 1967; Brendel, 1971; Najarian et al., 1969, 1970).

Another possibility to reduce the toxic side-effects would lie in the use of antibody fragments lacking the Fc piece. Extensive studies with different antibody fragments produced by enzymatic treatment of the isolated IgG fraction have shown a loss of immunosuppressive potency. The Fc piece of the antibody molecule which mediates C'fixation and binding of complexed antibody to the phagocytic cells of the reticuloendotheliol system (RES) appears to be essential for the immunosuppressive effect of ALS (WOODRUFF et al., 1967b, RIETHMÜL-LER et al., 1968, JAMES, 1969, LANCE et al., 1973).

2. Hyperergic Reactions

The immunogenicity of xenogeneic sera, both normal and immune, is in itself a cause of serious side-effects such as severe anaphylactic shock, skin reactions, immune complex nephritis, and serum sickness (IWASAKI et al., 1967; LANCE, 1968a; PICHLMAYR, 1967; STARZL et al., 1967). These hyperergic complications can be distinguished from the toxic effects of ALS by their delayed appearance, usually one to several weeks after beginning treatment. The risk of hyperergic reactions is largely reduced by the use of purified IgG fractions instead of whole serum (STARZL et al., 1969). As pointed out earlier the use of ALS-IgG (ALG) is indispensible for clinical application and is now mostly used in animal experiments as well. Nevertheless hyperergic reactions due to antibodies against the xenogeneic ALS-IgG are still a major problem. The severity of these reactions largely depends on the species involved and the time schedule of ALG adminis-tration. Whereas mice and rats rarely develop severe anaphylactoid complica-tions, they are common in guinea pigs, dogs, and humans (for a detailed discus-sion together with references see LANCE et al., 1973 and BRENDEL et al., 1974). If injections are repeated at short intervals the frequency and severity of the reactions appear to be reduced in comparison with injections given after intervals of several days (PICHLMAYR, 1967). This can be explained by the accumulation of antibodies during the intervals between successive ALS injections. Besides hyperergic reactions another side-effect of antibody production against ALS is partial or complete inactivation of the antilymphocytic antibody (BUTLER et al., 1971a, b). Both types of unwanted effects can be avoided by the induction of immunologic tolerance to the xenogeneic immunoglobulin prior to ALS treatment (BRENDEL et al., 1974, DENMAN and FRENKEL, 1967).

3. Infections

The immunosuppressive effect of ALS is not specific. Consequently treatment with this reagent will enhance the risk of microbial infections. The degree of ALS-induced suppression of responsiveness to a particular pathogen depends on the importance of the cell-mediated component of the response. In mice the rate of infectious diseases caused by common bacterial pathogens is not increased by doses strongly affecting transplantation immunity (LANCE et al., 1973). The responsiveness to *Mycobacterium tuberculosis* and *M. leprae*, both of which predominantly elicit cellular reactions was, however, heavily impaired (GAUGAS, 1968; GAUGAS and REES, 1968). Influenza and rabies infections, which evoke mainly humoral responses, are not significantly aggravated by ALS (Hirsch, 1970) whereas the course of most other viral infections is more severe or can even be fatal under ALS treatment. In mice, for instance, morbidity and mortality subsequent to infection with vaccinia virus and herpes simplex is increased by ALS treatment (Hirsch, 1970). The same is true for yellow fever (Hirsch and Murphy, 1967), mousepox (Blanden, 1970), and MHV-1 virus (Allison, 1970). Furthermore the primary responses to most oncogenic viruses are depressed in the mouse (Hirsch, 1970). When viral antigens induce antibody formation as well as cellular immune reactions, the humoral response usually is not markedly changed.

Activation of latent infection by ALS has also been shown. In dogs previously immunized with attenuated virus, canine distemper developed subsequent to ALS treatment (Abaza et al., 1966) and in monkeys a number of deaths from preexisting viral infections occurred (van Bekkum et al., 1967). Little is known about the effect of ALS on resistance to fungal and protozoal infection (for review see Hirsch, 1970, and Lance et al., 1973).

4. Neoplasms

ALS treatment increases the incidence of virus-induced tumors. This has been particularly well documented in rodents with viruses such as SV 40, adenovirus type 12 (Allison et al., 1967; Allison and Law, 1968), murine sarcoma virus (Law et al., 1968), and polyoma virus (Vandeputte, 1969). An increase in spontaneously occurring or chemically induced tumors has not been observed (Nehlsen, 1971; Simpson and Nehlsen, 1971).

A higher frequency of tumors is a complication of all types of therapy that result in nonspecific immunosuppression (for review with references see Gleichmann and Gleichmann, 1973). This has also been described in humans treated with conventional immunosuppression with and without additional ALS. For example, the risk of developing neoplasia for patients who receive a renal allograft and have to be treated by immunosuppression is markedly increased. This is particularly true for all types of lymphoreticular tumors and for skin and cervix cancers (Penn et al., 1969, 1971; Penn and Starzl, 1972; Starzl et al., 1971; Hoover and Fraumeni, 1973; Melief and Schwartz, 1975; Birkeland et al., 1975). The risk of mammary carcinoma, the most common tumor in humans, is not increased indicating that the tumor-promoting effect of immunosuppression is not present in all types of oncogenesis. Little is known about the nature of this effect. For some time it has been thought that a major factor is the suppression of a hypothetical immunologic surveillance mechanism which is supposed to eliminate transformed cells in untreated animals (Burnet, 1970). The very existence of this mechanism has recently been questioned, however (Gleichmann and Gleichmann, 1973; Möller and Möller, 1976; Prehn, 1976). One of the main arguments against it is the fact that the frequency of chemically induced tumors is not increased in immunosuppressed animals. Another explanation for the high tumor incidence in ALS-treated animals has been that ALS itself is carcinogenic. This is very unlikely since mice under ALS treatment and kept free of oncogenic viruses do not show an increased tumor frequency (NEHLSEN, 1971; SIMPSON and NEHLSEN, 1971). A simple, but highly relevant explanation is that the reduced resistance to viral infections brought about by nonspecific immunosuppression leads to an increased rate of infections with oncogenic viruses and thereby to greater exposure to whatever factors are responsible for the induction of tumors by this agent.

X. Immunosuppression with ALS in Humans

During the last decade ALS has been prepared against human lymphoid cells and used therapeutically on a large scale. It is not the purpose of this section to review all the clinical observations and results obtained during this time. The emphasis instead will be on the evidence that ALS does have marked immunosuppressive activity in humans, on the complications reported, and on some general considerations about the value of ALS for therapeutic purposes.

There is only a limited number of studies in which volunteers or patients have been treated with ALS as the sole immunosuppressive agent. Nevertheless these investigations provide the best information about its in vivo effects on the lymphoid system and its immunosuppressive properties in humans. In general its effects very much parallel the respective findings in animals. Humoral antibody formation is only mildly affected. Primary antibody responses to T-dependent antigens are moderately suppressed but secondary responses do not show any significant change (PIROFSKY et al., 1974). Cellular immune reactions on the other hand are markedly influenced even by small doses of ALS. The survival time of skin grafts between randomly selected donor recipient pairs is significantly prolonged (MONACO et al., 1967a, b; SIMMONS et al., 1971; PIROFSKY et al., 1974) and the development of the primary cellular response to DNCB is markedly suppressed (PIROFSKY et al., 1974). Furthermore even established delayed hypersensitivity to a variety of substances including bacterial, fungal, and viral antigens is suppressed or temporarily abrogated (MONACO et al., 1967a, b; PIROFSKY et al., 1974). Thus the type of immune deficiency induced by ALS in man very much resembles that found in the more detailed and refined animal studies and there is no evidence against the assumption that the effects of ALS in humans are basically brought about by the same mechanisms demonstrated in animals.

It was expected that clinical organ transplantation would provide conclusive evidence for the therapeutical value of ALS. This hope has not yet been fulfilled despite the widespread use of ALS in this field. Evaluation of the effectiveness of ALS therapy is complicated by several factors, probably the most important of which is that ALS treatment is combined with other standard immunosuppressants. Thus a clear distinction cannot be drawn between the effects of each of the drugs involved. Furthermore the type of serum used and the methods of preparation are not standardized, nor are the dosage and the time course of injections. It is ironic that the generally held belief in the great therapeutic value of ALS held back controlled studies for several years. Moreover comparisons between consecutive series of patients have not been very conclusive since the improvements in results could also have been caused by other factors such as better donor recipient matching or an increase in experience with immunosuppressive treatment in general. Nevertheless, among those workers who have used ALS, there is widespread agreement that it has a beneficial effect and is a valuable addition to other immunosuppressive regimens. In patients with cadaver kidney allografts Starzl et al. (1967) achieved some improvement in the 1-year survival rates and in addition were able to reduce the dosage of corticosteroids. During the following years these experiences were confirmed by several investigators (Monaco et al., 1970; Simmons et al., 1971; Traeger et al., 1970; Turcotte et al., 1973; Diethelm et al., 1974) but were difficult to verify statistically because of the above-mentioned reasons. Recently the first results from controlled clinical studies in renal allograft recipients have become available (Sheil et al., 1973; Birkeland, 1976). They did not reveal that ALS dramatically improved the overall results but showed that the outcome in ALS-treated patients usually was superior with regard to the 1–2 year survival rate or to the number and/or severity of rejection episodes or both. Similar results were obtained in patients with liver or heart allografts, although their limited number renders critical evaluation even more difficult than in renal allograft recipients (Starzl et al., 1969; Fortner et al., 1971).

Apart from organ transplantation, ALS has been used in the treatment of autoimmune diseases such as dermatomyositis, temporal arthritis, lupus nephritis, and some other disorders of unknown etiology such as myasthenia gravis, sympathetic ophthalmia, and multiple sclerosis (Brendel, 1971; Brendel et al., 1970; Pirofsky et al., 1969, 1971, 1974; Ring et al., 1973, 1974; Trepel et al., 1968). Although all these diseases are somewhat unpredictable in their outcome, several groups of workers have reported results which they believe superior to those to be expected without treatment (Brendel, 1971; Ring et al., 1974). The repetition of these results in a controlled study would have enormous therapeutic implications and furthermore provide strong evidence for the autoimmune character of these diseases.

Encouraging results with ALS immunosuppression in skin allotransplantation have recently been obtained in heavily burned patients (Burke et al., 1974). Coverage of the burned areas with foreign skin prevents infection and reduces the danger of metabolic disorders associated with the extensive, open wounds. In patients with normal immune reactivity, however, the allografts are rejected before their replacement with autologous skin is possible. Burke et al. (1974) have demonstrated that immunosuppression with moderate doses of ALS effectively prolongs allograft survival for up to 50 days without increasing the frequency of infection. This period is usually sufficient for the replacement of the allografts with autologous skin, even when only very restricted donor sites are available.

ALS has been used with some success in clinical bone marrow transplantation by Storb et al. (1974). In a group of patients who were HL-A identical with the bone marrow donor and also nonreactive in the mixed lymphocyte culture test, GvH disease occurred in about 50% after transplantation. ALS treatment of 19 such patients suffering from established GvH disease resulted in 6 becoming long-term survivors. Thus ALS can cure GvH disease even when given after the onset of symptoms. Other immunosuppressive drugs are only effective when administered well before GvH disease has become established.

Side-effects of the types described in Section B IX are the main causes of complications in humans. Severe anemia and thrombocytopenia as well as nephrotoxic nephritis have been reported (STARZL *et al.*, 1967; TRAEGER *et al.*, 1971; THIEL *et al.*, 1971; BUSCH *et al.*, 1971; MICHEL *et al.*, 1975) but usually can be avoided by the proper pretesting of the serum and the discarding of batches with toxic antibodies that cannot be removed by absorption and fractionation. Fever, chills, and local inflammatory reactions with severe pain, however, occur frequently and can only be treated symptomatically (KASHIWAGI *et al.*, 1968; MONACO *et al.*, 1967 a, b). In most patients mild to moderate hyperergic reactions appear after 1–2 weeks. The most common symptoms are shivering, high fever, and urticaria. ALS treatment has to be stopped in 20–30% of patients because of these complications (PICHLMAYR *et al.*, 1976). Severe anaphylactic reactions with shock are rare in humans but have also occurred (STARZL *et al.*, 1969; TRAEGER *et al.*, 1971).

Histologic evidence for serum nephritis has repeatedly been demonstrated in kidney biopsies taken during or after a course of ALS treatment. The granular patterns of IgG deposits characteristic of immune complex nephritis could be shown by electron microscopy as well as immunofluorescence. The histologic alterations were found to be reversible after the cessation of ALS treatment. Clinical symptoms of nephritis have been found very seldom and moreover are difficult to distinguish from rejection (THIEL *et al.*, 1971).

Infections have not been a problem in patients treated with ALS as the sole immunosuppressant. The situation is more difficult to assess when ALS is combined with other immunosuppressive regimens as is usually done in clinical organ transplantation. Under these circumstances bacterial, fungal, and viral infections are frequent and represent the main cause of death (BARNES *et al.*, 1975; MONACO *et al.*, 1970). ALS certainly enhances the chances of infection when it is added to unmodified conventional immunosuppressive regimens. The risk is lower when smaller doses of corticosteroids and azathioprine are used. It is not yet clear if the type and the frequency of infectious complications, the most serious side-effect of nonspecific immunosuppression, has been changed by the use of ALS in clinical organ transplantation. With regard to the other very frightening complication — oncogenesis — there is now some evidence that the rate of spontaneous neoplasms in patients having undergone ALS treatment in combination with chemical immunosuppression is not enhanced when compared with patients under the latter treatment alone (LANCE *et al.*, 1973; BIRKELAND *et al.*, 1975).

From the above-mentioned evidence it is clear that ALS is strongly immunosuppressive in humans but that its usefulness in clinical immunosuppression is still a matter of discussion. The main issue in dispute is whether or not ALS treatment by itself or in combination with other immunosuppressants has any advantages over conventional immunosuppression achieved by corticosteroids and antiproliferative drugs alone. Theoretically such advantages should exist. The profile of effects of ALS on the different types of immune reactions, in particular its preferential effect on cellular immunity, clearly distinguishes it from the other immunosuppressive drugs currently in clinical use. Furthermore since it has none of the various nonimmunologic side-effects of cytotoxic drugs, antimetabolites and corticosteroids, it should be able to complement their immunosuppressive effects without potentiating their multiple nonimmunologic side-effects. One of the reasons why the full potential of ALS for immunosuppression in humans has not yet been realized lies in its largely indiscriminate use. This is a consequence of our still very limited insight into the mechanisms bringing about allograft rejection or autoimmunity. For instance, the recent observation that in humans lymphocyte-dependent antibody may have a crucial role in certain types of renal allograft rejection which have so far been ascribed to the action of effector T-cells (Ting and Terasaki, 1974; Stiller et al., 1975) could explain why these types of rejection are not susceptible to ALS treatment. More detailed knowledge about the mechanisms involved in diseases requiring immunosuppressive therapy would permit a more rational use of those immunosuppressants with relatively selective action such as ALS. In view of the rapid development taking place in immunology, however, it can be anticipated that the therapeutic value of ALS in clinical medicine will soon be more clearly defined.

D. Passive Enhancement

I. General Aspects

Specific antibody is one of the end products of the immune response. When it is passively administered to an unprimed individual who is then exposed to the corresponding antigen, the development of humoral and cellular immune reactions against that particular antigen can be inhibited by some type of feedback regulation. The relevance of this type of specific immunosuppression for tissue transplantation was first demonstrated by Kaliss and associates (1953, 1956, 1958). Through passive immunization of mice with specific alloantiserum these authors were able to achieve the acceptance of tumor allografts which were rejected in untreated controls. Since the early work of Flexner and Jobling (1907) it had been known that pretreatment of recipients with nonviable tumor cells prolonged the survival and growth of subsequently inoculated viable cells. The experiments of Kaliss, however, revealed that this phenomenon, named "tumor enhancement", could be attributed to the induction of specific antibody formation by the first inoculum. This observation provided a link between enhancement and the suppression of antibody formation by passively administered antibody as well as the whole field of homeostasis of immune responses (for review together with references see Uhr and Möller, 1968).

The protective effects of antibodies on allografts are not restricted to neoplastic tissues (Billingham et al., 1956). Therefore the meaning of the term "enhancement" has been expanded to include any inhibition or delay of allograft rejection by antibodies evoked by donor type histocompatibility antigens. In *active enhancement* these antibodies have been induced by active immunization of the graft recipient; in *passive enhancement* they have been transferred from another individual. For a long time it has been assumed that only antibodies directed against the antigens of the graft play a major role, but the recent findings of MCKEARN (1974) and MCKEARN *et al.* (1974a, b) suggest that anti-idiotype antibody may be a regular and important component of effective antisera as well (see Section B and below). In addition to the enhancement of allografts there is also strong evidence for enhancement of syngeneic and autochtonous tumors by antibodies that are directed against tumor-specific antigens and are produced spontaneously by the tumor-bearing individual (HELLSTRÖM and HELLSTRÖM, 1971, 1974). Whereas in transplantation research the ultimate goal is usually the induction of immunologic enhancement, the problem in tumor research is to abolish the protective effects elicited by specific antibodies.

The topic of this section is *immunosuppression* with specific antibody. So the main emphasis will be on the passive enhancement of allografts. The discussion will be restricted to enhancement of normal tissues; enhancement of tumor allografts will only be mentioned where necessary for an understanding of the basic principles and mechanisms of this phenomenon. Additional information can be gathered from several reviews covering the whole field of active and passive enhancement of allografts (FELDMAN, 1972; KALISS, 1972; VOISIN, 1971; WINN, 1974). The enhancement of syngeneic and autochtonous tumors is totally beyond the scope of this section. The reader's attention is directed to the recent review on this subject by HELLSTRÖM and HELLSTRÖM (1974).

II. Types of Antibodies Initiating Enhancement

Antisera which effectively prolong allograft survival have been produced using a variety of methods. Normal and neoplastic tissues, single cell suspensions, and subcellular fractions have been used as the source of antigen. The time course of immunization has also differed, ranging from very short to long-term schedules with many booster injections (KALISS, 1956; ZIMMERMAN and FELDMAN, 1969a). Effective sera so obtained usually contain agglutinating, complement-fixing, and cytotoxic antibodies. There is however no clear correlation between serologic and enhancing activity. Antisera highly reactive in serologic assays may be without effect on allograft survival. This is particularly true for sera obtained after short-term immunization. Other in vitro assays such as the blocking of proliferative (mixed lymphocyte culture) or cytotoxic (cell-mediated lympholysis) T-cell responses have also failed to provide a reliable prediction as to whether a certain serum pool will be able to inhibit rejection or not.

This lack of correlation with serologic results may be caused by the partial dependence of the enhancing capacity of the serum on antireceptor antibody or on antigen-antibody complexes rather than on free antibody. Strong evidence for the importance of antigen-antibody complexes has come from the experiments of SJÖGREN *et al.* (1971). He compared the activity of free antibody with that of antigen-antibody complexes in a tumor allograft model and found that the complexes were clearly superior. Anti-idiotype antibodies were recently demonstrated to be regular components of many immune sera (McKearn *et al.*, 1974a, b; Fitch *et al.*, 1974). Therefore the question arises as to whether this type of antibody has a physiologic role in the normal regulation of the immune response and whether this regulatory role may also be responsible for the specific immunosuppression exerted by these sera (Jerne, 1973; Nisonoff and Bangasser, 1975; Stuart, 1973; Stuart *et al.*, 1974). The first direct evidence for the validity of this hypothesis has recently been reported by Lucas and Enomoto (1973) who achieved significant prolongation of renal allograft survival in rats with anti-idiotype antiserum. Thus it seems that free antibody directed against the alloantigens of the graft, soluble antigen-antibody complexes, and the respective anti-idiotype antibody may all be active in immunologic enhancement and may exert synergistic regulatory effects on different parts of the immune response (see below).

Alloantibodies directed against the H-antigens of the graft have been thoroughly investigated with regard to their enhancing activity. Particular attention has been paid to the effectiveness of different antibody classes. Most workers found that the IgG fraction had high enhancing activity whereas the purified IgM had little or none (Kaliss and Kandutsch, 1956; Takasugi and Hildemann, 1969; Kinsky *et al.*, 1972; Zimmerman and Feldman, 1969a, b, 1970; Jones *et al.*, 1972). As Winn (1974) has pointed out, however, this may have been due to the use of hyperimmune antisera by most workers. Fuller and Winn (1973) were able to demonstrate enhancement of a strongly incompatible sarcoma in mice by antibodies of the IgG_{2a}, IgG_{2b}, and IgM subclasses. Voisin *et al.* (1969) even described a blocking effect of separated IgA in the guinea pig. Nevertheless the majority of investigators who have examined this question assume that the predominant role is played by IgG antibodies (for further references see Feldman, 1972).

Several early studies on the specificity of enhancing antisera suggested that effective enhancement was only achieved when the serum used contained antibodies against all antigenic specificities of the graft (Möller, 1963a, b). In the light of improved knowledge about qualitative differences between the various antigenic determinants coded for by the major histocompatibility complex (MHC) this view probably should be modified. MHC disparity usually includes differences in serologically defined (SD) and lymphocyte-defined (LD) determinants (Yunis and Amos, 1971; Bach, 1973; Eijsvoogel, 1974). In the mouse the loci coding for the latter map in the so-called Ir region of the MHC (Shreffler and David, 1975). It has recently been demonstrated in mice that passive immunization with antibodies directed against Ir region—associated antigens also suppresses immune reactions directed against SD antigens (Davies and Alkins, 1974; Staines *et al.*, 1974; Jansen *et al.*, 1975). Antigenic differences in clinical organ transplantation are usually complex and antibodies directed against all incompatible antigens will frequently not be available. The observation that antibodies against selected determinants are sufficient for the induction of enhancement might therefore greatly facilitate the clinical application of this type of immunosuppression (see below).

III. Prolongation of Allograft Survival by Passive Enhancement

The strongest effects of passive immunization on allograft survival have been observed in tumor transplantation systems. With effective antisera even strong histocompatibility barriers can frequently be overcome and tumors that are normally rejected within 10 days grow indefinitely and kill the recipient. In contrast to neoplastic cells, long-lasting takes of normal tissues are usually difficult to achieve. The degree of prolongation that can be obtained by passive immunization depends on the type of tissue grafted and on the strength of the histocompatibility barrier between donor and recipient, as well as on the species and the immune status of the recipient.

The type of tissue used for transplantation has a strong influence on the effectiveness of passively administered antibody. Particularly resistant are skin grafts which often are rejected in normal fashion despite passive immunization. Even with antisera extremely potent in tumor systems, prolongation of skin graft survival usually does not exceed 2–3 days. Vascularized grafts such as heart and kidney are more susceptible. Prolongations of several weeks or even indefinite survival have been achieved. The model giving the best results and which also is the most thoroughly investigated is renal allotransplantation in rats (STUART *et al.*, 1968; FRENCH and BATCHELOR, 1969; WHITE and HILDE-MANN, 1969; LUCAS *et al.*, 1970). The reason for the remarkable variation in results obtained for different types of tissues is not known. Differences in their antigenic composition (LANCE *et al.*, 1971), in the way they present their antigens to the immune system of the host (LINSCOTT, 1970), and differences in their susceptibility to the immune assault by effector mechanisms of the rejection reaction have been suggested.

The influence of different histocompatibility barriers on normal allograft survival has been studied by HILDEMANN and MULLEN (1973). They found it was clearly dependent on the strength of the barrier. The weaker the barrier was, the easier long-lasting enhancement could be achieved. In strongly incompatible systems there may be a difference between homozygous grafts and heterozygous grafts sharing one haplotype with the recipient. This is particularly evident in rat renal allotransplantation. Whereas takes of MHC-different kidneys from homozygous donors are only prolonged for short periods, heterozygous F 1 grafts in the same strain combination usually survive much longer or even indefinitely (HILDEMANN and MULLEN, 1973).

The ease with which enhancement is induced varies greatly between different species. Excellent results have been obtained in mice and rats. It has been extremely difficult to achieve similar effects in dogs and rabbits. This may be caused by differences in the strength of antibody-dependent rejection mechanisms. In animals susceptible to hyperacute rejection, passive immunization may evoke severe damage to the graft instead of prolongation of survival time (see Section on Complications and Side Effects).

IV. Immune Status of Passively Immunized Allograft Recipients

One of the outstanding characteristics of the immunosuppression induced by passive enhancement is its specificity (Möller, 1963 a, b). Passive antibody selectively inhibits the immunologic rejection of grafts carrying the corresponding antigens without interfering with immune responses directed against unrelated antigens. This property distinguishes passive enhancement from the immunosuppression induced by ALS and by chemical drugs. Consequently the discussion about the immune status of passively immunized allograft recipients can be limited to the status of the lymphocyte clones specifically reactive toward the histocompatibility antigens of the allograft. The results referred to in this article have mainly been obtained in rats which had received either kidney, heart, or skin allografts. There is extensive information available about the immune status of recipients of tumor allografts but this will not be discussed here.

In contrast to animals rendered tolerant by the neonatal injection of donor type hemolymphopoietic cells, in recipients of passively enhanced allografts lymphocyte clones responsive to donor type alloantigens can be found at all times. Thus recipient lymphocytes usually show a normal response in the mixed lymphocyte culture test (Heron and Meyer, 1973) and in GvH assays (French et al., 1971), both of which measure T-cell reactivity. The presence of specifically reactive B-cell clones can often be demonstrated by the formation of small amounts of cytotoxic antibody (Lucas et al., 1970; French and Batchelor, 1972). In rats with "enhanced kidney allografts" which do not produce detectable amounts of specific antibody, the formation of the latter can be induced by the injection of donor-type lymphocytes without any deterioration in the allograft function (French et al., 1971; French and Batchelor, 1972).

The demonstration of specifically responsive T- and B-lymphocytes in rats bearing effectively enhanced kidney allografts raises the question of whether these cells have been sensitized by the allograft or remained in an unprimed state. In such rats a transient deterioration in the allograft function has frequently been observed at the time when kidneys are rejected in untreated controls (French and Batchelor, 1972). Furthermore it has been clearly shown that cell-mediated immunity does exist, indicating that sensitization of the recipient had taken place (Stuart et al., 1971; Biesecker et al., 1973a, b; Mullen et al., 1973). Detailed studies comparing the development of immunologic effector mechanisms in passively enhanced and untreated allograft recipients, however, have revealed that the pattern of cellular and humoral immune responses is modified by the passively administered antibody. Thus in a number of different models the occurrence of effector T-cells with lytic activity for ^{51}Cr-labeled target cells in vitro is both delayed and suppressed (Peter and Feldmann, 1972; Biesecker et al., 1973b, c; Burgos et al., 1974; Wonigeit et al., 1974, 1975). Moreover these fully differentiated effector cells can only be demonstrated during the early postoperative course and disappear later despite the continuous presence of the allograft. During this latter phase "blocking factors" that specifically inhibit cell-mediated immunity in the so-called microcytotoxicity assay can frequently be demonstrated (Hellström and Hellström, 1972; Biesecker *et al.,* 1973 b, c). These data have led to the hypothesis that the immuno-suppressed state of passively enhanced allograft recipients consists of two phases, one of initial suppression of cellular immune reactions and the other character-ized by homeostasis of the immune response at low levels for extended periods (BIESECKER *et al.,* 1973 c). The first phase is dependent on the passively admin-istered antibody, the second on the production of blocking factors by the recip-ient himself or some other type of adaptation of the recipient's immune system to the allograft.

In order to characterize further the nature of this homeostasis in rats with long-surviving allografts, these animals were either challenged with a second graft of the same donor type or injected with effector cells strongly cytotoxic for donor-type target cells. Whereas a second kidney graft of the same antigenic composition is always readily accepted without additional treatment, skin grafts are usually rejected with only a slight delay (STUART *et al.,* 1970). Despite the rejection of the skin, the kidney allograft does survive. Adoptive transfer of effectively sensitized cells does not provoke rejection either (BOWEN *et al.,* 1974; STUART *et al.,* 1974). The maintenance of the homeostatic state is dependent on the continuous presence of the graft. When the enhanced kidney is removed and replaced a month later by a second graft of the same donor strain, rejection does occur (ROWLEY *et al.,* 1973).

The possibility that the graft looses its antigenicity subsequent to long-lasting survival in an allogeneic host has been excluded convincingly for kidney trans-plants. When effectively enhanced kidney allografts are transferred to a second untreated recipient they are rejected in only a slightly delayed fashion (STUART *et al.,* 1970; FRENCH and BATCHELOR, 1972). Another line of evidence comes from experiments in which the clearance of specific alloantibodies injected into recipients of effectively enhanced kidney grafts was examined (FRENCH, 1973). In these animals the injected antibody disappeared much faster from circulation than in controls not possessing an allograft. This could only be explained by the binding of the antibodies with free antigenic sites of the graft. Therefore it can be concluded that antigenic determinants are not only continuously expressed in the graft but that a high proportion of them are also accessible, i.e., they are not masked by antibodies produced by the graft recipient. These data of course do not exclude the possibility that antibody-induced loss of antigenic determinants or some other type of antigenic modulation can occur in other types of grafts. This may in fact be a major factor in the enhancement of tumors (for review see HELLSTRÖM and HELLSTRÖM, 1974).

V. Mechanisms of Enhancement

The broadened definition of enhancement used in this article (see section on Concepts of Immunosuppression by Antibodies) includes states of unresponsive-ness of different kinds which are induced by different mechanisms. It is obvious that antibody directed against the antigens of the graft, antigen-antibody com-plexes, and anti-idiotype antibody all will operate in a different way. The purpose of this section is to review the various hypotheses which have been proposed and to present some of the data advanced in their support. It is most likely that the mechanisms to be described are not mutually exclusive and that effective enhancement may only occur when the immune reactions that otherwise lead to allograft rejection are interfered with by more than one mechanism at more than one stage.

Theories of antibody-mediated immunosuppression are usually classified according to the part of the immune response which is supposed to be affected (BILLINGHAM et al., 1956). This correlates roughly with the type of antibody involved. When inhibition of the *afferent* and *efferent* parts is considered, usually only antibody directed against the antigenic determinants of the graft is thought to be involved; inhibition of the *central* part on the other hand is ascribed either to antigen-antibody complexes or anti-idiotype antibody or both.

Specific antibody when administered passively to an allograft recipient will enter the graft and bind with its antigenic determinants. The basic assumption behind all theories of peripheral blockade is that this process leads to complete masking of the antigenic determinants of the graft, thereby interfering with the interaction of recipient lymphocytes with donor antigens. In the case of afferent blockade it is assumed that the recipient lymphocytes do not become sensitized (SNELL et al., 1960; MÖLLER, 1963a), while in efferent blockade effectively sensitized cells are thought not to recognize the antigenic determinants of the graft and therefore not to induce graft rejection (MÖLLER, 1964). The most convincing evidence for the existence of afferent as well as efferent blocking comes from in vivo experiments using tumor allografts (for review together with references see KALISS, 1972, and FELDMAN, 1972) and from studies with various in vitro models of T-cell responses. An in vitro analogue of the afferent arc of the immune reaction is provided by the mixed lymphocyte reaction. In this model complete inhibition of allo-antigen recognition by specific antibody has been achieved (CEPPELLINI et al., 1971; MILLER et al., 1971). In vitro analogues of the efferent phase are the various assays for cell-mediated immunity, and in those complete inhibition has also been shown (BRUNNER et al., 1967, 1968).

Although the existence of both types of peripheral blocking in a number of experimental models is well established, there is some doubt as to whether masking of antigenic determinants alone is sufficient for the induction of long-term survival of nonneoplastic allografts. Since it is nearly always possible to detect humoral as well as cellular immunity in passively enhanced allograft recipients (see previous section) it has to be concluded that afferent blockade usually is not complete. A strong argument against the relevance of efferent blocking is the general finding that passive enhancement has little or no influence on allograft survival in effectively presensitized recipients and that a high proportion of antigenic sites in effectively enhanced grafts remains unmasked (FRENCH, 1973).

Antigen-antibody complexes, either formed within the graft and subsequently released or already present in the passively administered antiserum, are thought to interfere with the central part of the rejection reaction. The mechanism of their blocking effect has not yet been elucidated but several appealing hypotheses have been advanced. FELDMANN and DIENER (1970) have proposed a detailed model of the molecular changes which could be induced in the cell membranes of the antigen-reactive cells subsequent to their interaction with antigen-antibody complexes and which could be responsible for the alteration in their functional capabilities. These authors were able to show that B-cells could be made specifically nonreactive to salmonella flagellin when they were exposed to it in the presence of a critical amount of antibody. They suggested that the fluid membrane of the lymphocyte will be immobilized by the multipoint binding of antigen-antibody complexes which may either result in the inactivation of that particular cell (FELDMANN and DIENER, 1970; DIENER and FELDMANN, 1972) or a switch in activity leading to its differentiation into a suppressor cell (FELDMANN, 1974; BASTEN et al., 1975). According to this model the specific changes in immune reactivity of passively immunized allograft recipients are a consequence of either a decrease in the number of reactive cells or the active suppression of reactive cells. It remains to be seen whether direct evidence in favor of these mechanisms can be obtained from in vivo models of passive enhancement. Another hypothesis that has been put forward is that antigen-antibody complexes exert central inhibition in a more indirect way by the induction of anti-idiotypic antibody. Experimental induction of anti-idiotype antibodies within the same or in a syngeneic animal is usually not achieved by the inoculation of the purified antibody alone. It either has to be chemically modified (JANEWAY and PAUL, 1973), polymerized (McKEARN et al., 1974b; FRAKER et al., 1974; RODKEY, 1974) or injected in the form of antigen-antibody complexes (EICHMANN, 1972; McKEARN et al., 1974c). Of these three, only the complexes also occur under physiologic conditions and therefore it is tempting to speculate that the induction of anti-idiotype antibody is one of the most important functions of antigen-antibody complexes in the regulation of immune responses.

How does anti-idiotype antibody suppress immune reactions? The initiating event for all its immunoregulatory effects most likely is its direct interaction with the specific receptors of antigen-reactive lymphocytes. Convincing evidence that antigen receptors on T- and B-cells can react with anti-idiotype antibody has recently been reported by BINZ and WIGZELL (1975a, b, c). The serum these authors used was directed against receptors for alloantigens and had been raised by immunization of F 1 rats with parental T-cells. F 1 hybrids possess the whole set of parental antigens but they lack the lymphocyte receptors for these antigens. When injected with T-cells from one parental strain they will therefore mount an immune response against the recognition structures of these cells for the alloantigens of the other parental strain. The resulting antibody is directed against the receptor and is anti-idiotypic antibody (RAMSEIER and LINDEMANN, 1971, 1972). In the studies of BINZ and WIGZELL (1975a, b, c) the binding of this type of antibody to a low number of T- and B-lymphocytes could be visualized by direct immunofluorescence and by autoradiography. The specificity of the antiserum for cells with reactivity against the respective alloantigens was demonstrated convincingly by the finding that cell populations enriched for anti-idiotype sensitive cells displayed increased reactivity against the specific antigen whereas the reactivity of cell populations depleted of anti-idiotype sensitive cells was diminished. In vitro exposure of lymphocyte suspensions to anti-idiotype antibody plus complement wiped out their reactivity against the specific antigen in the mixed lymphocyte culture test as well as in the GvH assay.

Receptor blockage or lysis of the receptor-bearing cell, however, are not the only ways in which anti-idiotype antibody can interfere with immune reactions. Suppression of the immune response against streptococcal carbohydrate A in the mouse by anti-idiotypic antibody from guinea pigs has been shown to involve an idiotype-specific suppressor T-cell (Eichmann, 1975). This suppressor cell is only generated after treatment with anti-idiotype antibody of the IgG_1 subclass; injection with IgG_2 leads to enhancement of the immune response, indicating that some type of idiotype stimulation had taken place. Since the binding of anti-idiotype antibody to the idiotypic determinants of the receptor molecule probably is very similar to the interaction between antigen and the receptor, it is conceivable that not only receptor blockage but also specific stimulation may result from the interaction between antigen-reactive cells and anti-receptor antibody. Depending on the type of antibody and its concentration, this may lead to stimulation either of cells cooperating in the immune response or cells suppressing it (Eichmann, 1975).

A definitive evaluation of the many different mechanisms that contribute to the induction and maintenance of enhancement is not possible. The fact that there are so many ways for antibody to interfere with immune reactions, however, raises the hope that their further investigation can provide us with effective methods for the specific control of immune reactions in humans.

VI. Side-Effects and Complications

Specific antibody can exert protective effects on allografts leading to enhancement but it is also capable of attacking that same tissue. In fact this latter function is probably the more physiologic one. Despite the fact that in most types of allograft rejection sensitized T-lymphocytes play the predominant role, there is no doubt that antibody can induce allograft destruction as well. This has been demonstrated convincingly in rabbits, dogs, and guinea pigs in which hyperacute rejection of primarily vascularized organ grafts can easily be induced by passive immunization with specific antiserum when given in appropriate dosage (Holter et al., 1972, 1973). The initial finding that this humoral type of rejection could not be elicited in mice and rats has now been explained by their low levels of complement. Antibody-mediated rejection can be induced in these species but requires the injection of normal rabbit or guinea pig serum as an additional source of complement. Tolerability of passively administered antibodies therefore is a peculiar property of these rodents. In other species all attempts to induce enhancement by passive immunization are accompanied by the risk of causing antibody-mediated damage or even hyperacute rejection. Information about the toxic effects of specific alloantibodies in humans comes from clinical experience with renal allotransplantation. Kidney grafts are nearly always rejected by the preformed ABO antibodies when transplanted into an ABO-incompatible recipient and in a high proportion when antibodies against the serologically defined MHC antigens of the graft are detectable in the preoperative cross match (KISSMEYER-NIELSEN *et al.*, 1966; PATEL and TERASAKI, 1969).

Whereas sensitized T-cells have a direct cytotoxic effect on donor-type target cells, interaction of humoral antibody with donor-type antigens does not necessarily cause cell death. In order to effect tissue damage the bound antibody has to activate nonspecific effector systems. These can either be the complement system, the K-cell system (antibody-dependent cytotoxic lymphocytes), phagocytic cells such as macrophages and granulocytes, or all of these. The activation of all these effector systems is mediated via the Fc part of the immunoglobulin molecule (for review with references see SPIEGELBERG, 1975). Since removal or inactivation of the Fc part can render antibodies nontoxic without changing their binding capacity for the specific antigen, the question arises as to whether this pretreatment diminishes toxicity without abolishing the enhancing effect. In rats and dogs it has been possible to induce enhancement of kidney allografts with $F(ab')_2$ fragments (SHAIPANICH *et al.*, 1971, 1973; WREN *et al.*, 1974) indicating that the protective effect on allograft survival had been retained. On the other hand there is strong evidence for a marked reduction in the immunosuppressive potency of specific antibody subsequent to the removal of the Fc part. SINCLAIR (1969, 1970) compared the capacity of $F(ab')_2$ fragments and intact antibody to suppress the antibody response to sheep erythrocytes in mice and rats and found that intact IgG was one hundred to a thousand times more effective. WASON and FITCH (1973) confirmed these results in an in vitro spleen culture system. Because of the high risk of hyperimmune rejection in humans only the use of antibody fragments appears justified at present, despite their reduced enhancing capacity. It has to be stressed, however, that these considerations are only relevant when antibodies against the alloantigens of the graft are used. They do not apply, of course, to antireceptor antibody which does not interact with the graft but with the immune system of the recipient.

VII. Immunologic Enhancement in Humans

The lack of specificity of immunosuppressive therapy is still the main cause of complications other than rejection in clinical organ transplantation. As a consequence patients run a continuous risk of infection. Specific control of the rejection process by means of active or passive enhancement could help to resolve this problem. Little is known, however, about the feasibility of inducing a state of immunologic enhancement in humans. Intentional induction by active immunization of the recipient appears to bear too high a risk of sensitization and subsequent hyperacute rejection. The problems arising with passive immunization are the provision of sufficient quantities of immune serum as well as the lack of in vitro assays which can predict the enhancing capability of a particular serum and exclude toxicity.

The question has been posed as to whether it will be at all possible to induce enhancement in man, a species prone to antibody-mediated hyperacute rejection. Strong support for the assumption that the same mechanisms which lead to immunologic enhancement of allografts in laboratory animals are also effective in humans comes from the statistical analysis of kidney graft survival in patients who had been preimmunized by a previous unsuccessful graft (OPELZ et al., 1972) or by multiple blood transfusions (OPELZ et al., 1973). The prognosis of those patients who received a second graft because the first had been rejected depended largely on how and when rejection took place. If the rejection was hyperacute or occurred during the first 3 months after transplantation, the prognosis for the second kidney transplant was very poor. In contrast patients rejecting the first graft later than 3 months had markedly better prognoses when compared to patients receiving a kidney for the first time (OPELZ et al., 1972). Similarly, patients who were given multiple blood transfusions but did not produce cytotoxic antibodies ran a lower risk of losing a subsequent kidney allograft than patients who received only a few or no transfusions. This data would seem to indicate that there had been induction of immunologic enhancement subsequent to previous active immunization. At present, however, there is no way to prove this hypothesis. These findings could also be explained by the induction of immunologic tolerance or by the selection of patients with genetically determined low responsiveness.

The treatment of kidney allograft recipients with passive immunization could provide the most convincing evidence for the effectiveness of immunologic enhancement in humans. First trials with this method of therapy were reported by BATCHELOR and associates (BATCHELOR et al., 1970; FRENCH and BATCHELOR, 1972). All patients received their graft from a living related donor so that the specific antiserum used for passive immunization could be produced by intrafamilial immunization. Another advantage of this approach may be that antibodies directed against all major histocompatibility complex (MHC) determined antigens were raised irrespective of whether they are known and detectable by present typing techniques or not. In order to avoid hyperacute rejection the antisera so raised were subjected to digestion by pepsin. The antiserum was given immediately after transplantation. In all three cases reported urine production ceased subsequent to injection of antibody but recovered a few days later. The authors admit that the transient anuria might have been caused by the antibody treatment but stress the point that no signs of antibody-induced damage could be demonstrated in the biopsies taken in two of the three patients. During the immediate postoperative course, azathioprine and corticosteroids were given. After restoration of good renal function, however, all three patients could be maintained for long periods with only little or no azathioprine and without corticosteroids. One patient rejected his graft after 18 months; the other two suffered rejection episodes which were reversed under short intermediate courses of prednisone. The question remains open as to whether passive enhancement had been induced in these patients. What was demonstrated very clearly, however, is that passive immunization could be carried out without causing permanent damage to the allograft.

Passive immunization of recipients of cadaver kidneys has not yet been reported. One of the problems which remains to be solved is the provision of adequate amounts of antibody of the required specificity. Possible donors are postpartum women who very frequently produce antibodies against the paternal antigens of their child or patients who have received blood transfusions. Even the planned immunization of volunteers has been taken into consideration. Since man is disposed to hyperacute rejection, it is generally assumed that the Fc part of the antibodies used should be digested or inactivated despite the reduction of enhancing activity observed in animal studies subsequent to this pretreatment of the antiserum.

Another crucial question is whether the antibody has to be directed against all antigenic determinants in which the graft differs from the recipient or whether antibodies against certain groups of antigens would be sufficient for the induction of enhancement. The latter hypothesis is strongly supported by the already mentioned results of JANSEN et al. (1975) which indicated that antibodies directed against Ir region–associated antigens of the MHC play a predominant role in the mediation of immunologic enhancement in the mouse. Prolonged survival of skin allografts incompatible in both classical serologically defined antigens and Ir region–associated (Ia) antigens of the MHC was achieved by passive immunization with an antiserum from which antibodies directed against SD antigens had been removed. This was done by absorption with red cells which do not express Ia antigens. Furthermore the absorbed serum had lost its capability to induce rejection. In contrast, the unabsorbed material induced hyperacute rejection provided the mice received a simultaneous injection of rabbit complement. It therefore can be concluded that in the mouse the capability to reject a skin graft is a function of anti-SD antibodies only.

If human MHC antigens exhibit the same functional differentiation, the identification of the human homologue of the murine Ia antigens would have far-reaching implications for passive enhancement in clinical transplantation. At present there are two possible candidates for this role: alloantigens defined by the mixed lymphocyte culture test and coded for by the D locus of the MHC (EIJSVOOGEL, 1974), and a group of B-cell antigens detectable by serologic methods and also determined by a locus closely linked to the MHC (VAN ROOD et al., 1975; WERNET et al., 1975; MANN et al., 1975; WINCHESTER et al., 1975). It is not yet clear whether these antigens are in fact separate entities or rather the same antigens detected by different methods. They exhibit a number of similarities to the murine Ia antigens, in particular a very restricted tissue distribution. One could speculate that the lack of toxicity of anti-Ia antibody for murine allografts is caused by the weak phenotypic expression of the respective antigens in the graft. If the same rules apply for the human homologues of the murine Ia antigens, separation of antibodies directed against the former and mediating enhancement from toxic antibodies directed against serologically defined MHC antigens coded for by the A and B locus might be possible. Purified enhancing antibody could then be administered in an undigested form thus retaining its full activity.

Once passive enhancement can be used without risk in humans most of the immunologic problems of organ transplantation will be solved. It cannot be decided yet if the use of antibodies corresponding to the murine anti-Ia antibodies will really provide this solution. Another field the importance of which for clinical purposes cannot be evaluated as yet is antireceptor or anti-idiotype antibody. It may well have the potential to change the whole field of clinical immunosuppression. In any case further improvement of the knowledge about the antigens determining histocompatibility and the antibodies elicited by these antigens will open up the way to new approaches to the problem of specific immunoregulation in clinical medicine.

References

ABAZA, H.M., WOODRUFF, M.F.A.: "In vitro" assay of antilymphocytic serum. Rev. franç. Et. clin. biol. 11, 821 (1966).

ABAZA, H.M., NOLAN, B., WATT, J.G., WOODRUFF, M.F.A.: Effect of antilymphocytic serum on the survival of renal homotransplants in dogs. Transplantation 4, 618 (1966).

AGNEW, H.D.: The effect of heterologous antilymphocyte serum on the small lymphocyte population of rats. J. exp. Med. 128, 111 (1968).

ALLISON, A.C.: Effects of antilymphocytic serum on bacterial and viral infections and viral oncogenesis. Fed. Proc. 29, 1677 (1970).

ALLISON, A.C., LAW, L.W.: Effects of antilymphocyte serum on virus oncogenesis. Proc. Soc. exp. Biol. (N.Y.) 127, 207 (1968).

ALLISON, A.C., BERMAN, L.D., LEVEY, R.H.: Increased tumour induction by adenovirus type 12 in thymectomized mice and mice treated with antilymphocyte serum. Nature (Lond.) 215, 185 (1967).

ANDERSON, N.F., JAMES, K., WOODRUFF, M.F.A.: Effects of antilymphocytic antibody and antibody fragments on skin-homograft survival and the blood-lymphocyte count in rats. Lancet 1, 1126 (1967).

ANDERSON, H.R., DRESSER, D.W., IVERSON, G.M., LANCE, E.M., WORTIS, H.H., ZEBRA, J.: The effects of ALG on the murine immune response to sheep erythrocytes. Immunology 22, 277 (1972).

BACH, F.H.: The major histocompatibility complex in transplantation immunology. Transplant. Proc. 5, 23 (1973).

BACH, F.H., BACH, M.L.: In vitro actions of antilymphocyte sera. Fed. Proc. (Fed. Amer. Soc. exp. Biol.) 29, 130 (1970).

BACH, J.F.: In vitro assay for antilymphocyte serum. Fed. Proc. 29, 120 (1970).

BACH, J.F., ANTOINE, B.: In vitro detection of immunosuppressive activity of anti-lymphocyte sera. Nature (Lond.) 217, 658 (1968).

BACH, J.F., DORMONT, J., DARDENNE, M., BALNER, H.: Correlation of in vitro rosette inhibition and skin allograft prolongation in sub-human primates by anti-human antilymphocyte sera. In: BERTELLI, A. and MONACO, A.P. (eds.): Pharmacological Treatment in Organ and Tissue Transplantation. Amsterdam: Excerpta Medica Foundation, p. 251 (1970).

BALNER, H.: Immunology of experimental transplantation in primate animals. Ann. N.Y. Acad. Sci. 162, 437 (1969).

BALNER, H.: Standardization of anti-human lymphocyte sera by in vivo testing. Behring Inst. Mitt. 51, 1 (1972).

BALNER, H., EIJSVOOGEL, V.P., CLETON, F.J.: Testing of anti-human lymphocyte sera in chimpanzees and lower primates. Lancet 1, 19 (1968a).

BALNER, H., VAN BEKKUM, D.W., DE VRIES, M.J., DERSJANT, H., VAN PUTTEN, L.M.: Effect of anti-lymphocyte sera on homograft reactivity and graft versus host reactions in rhesus monkeys. In: "Advance in Transplantation" (J. DAUSSET, J. HAMBURGER, G. MATHÉ eds.), p. 449 Munksgard, Copenhagen Proceedings of the 1st Int. Congr. Transplantation Society, Paris, Munksgaard Copenhagen, 1968b.

BARNES, B.A., BERGAN, J.J., BRAUN, W.E., FRAUMENI, J.F., KOUNTZ, S.L., MICKEY, M.R., RUBIN, A.L., SIMMONS, R.L., STEVENS, L.E., WILSON, R.E.: The 12th report of the human renal transplant registry. JAMA 233, 787 (1975).

BARTH, R.F., SINGLAR, O., AHLERS, P.: Effects of antilymphocyte serum on thymic independent immunity. I. Lack of immunosuppressive action on the antibody response to E. coli lipopolysaccharide. Cell. Immunol. 7, 380 (1973).

BARTH, R.F., SINGLAR, O., WARD, P.A.: Immunosuppressive effects of anti-lymphocyte serum in complement deficient mice. II. Evidence that activity is mediated by C 3 independent antibodies. J. Immunol. **112**, 858 (1974).

BASTEN R.F., SINGLAR, O., WARD, P.A.: Immunosuppressive effects of anti-lymphocyte serum in complement deficient mice. II. Evidence that activity is mediated by C 3 independent antibodies. J. Immunol. **112**, 858 (1974).

BASTEN, A., MILLER, J.F.A.P., JOHNSON, P.: T-cell dependent suppression of an Anti-Hapten Antibody response. Transplant. Rev. **26**, 130 (1975).

BATCHELOR, J.R., FRENCH, M.E., CAMERON, J.S., ELLIS, F., BEWICK, M., OGG, C.S.: Immunological enhancement of a human kidney graft. Lancet **2**, 1007 (1970).

BATCHELOR, J.R., FABRE, J., MORRIS, P.J.: Passive enhancement of kidney allografts, potentation with antilymphocyte serum. Transplantation **13**, 610 (1972).

BIESECKER, J.L., FITCH, F.W., ROWLEY, D.A., SCOLLARD, D., STUART, F.P.: Cellular and humoral immunity after allogeneic transplantation in the rat. II. Comparison of a 51 Cr-Release assay and a modified microcytotoxicity assay for detection of cellular immunity and blocking serum factors. Transplantation **16**, 421 (1973a).

BIESECKER, J.L., FITCH, F.W., ROWLEY, D.A., STUART, F.P.: Cellular and humoral immunity after allogeneic transplantation in the rat. III. The effect of passive antibody on cellular and humoral immunity after allogeneic renal transplantation. Transplantation **16**, 432 (1973b).

BIESECKER, J.L., FITCH, F.W., ROWLEY, D.A., STUART, F.P.: Passive antibody delays development of cell-mediated immunity in rats receiving renal allografts. Transplant. Proc. **5**, 667 (1973c).

BILLINGHAM, R.E., BRENT, L., MEDAWAR, P.B.: "Enhancement" in normal homografts, with a note on its possible mechanism. Transplant. Bull. **3**, 84 (1956).

BINZ, H., WIGZELL, H.: Shared idiotypic determinants on B and T lymphocytes reactive against the same antigen determinants. I. Demonstration of similar or identical idiotypes on IgG molecules and T-cell receptors with specificity for the same alloantigens. J. exp. Med. **142**, 197 (1975a).

BINZ, H., WIGZELL, H.: Shared idiotypic determinants on B and T lymphocytes reactive against the same antigenic determinants. II. Determination of frequency and characteristics of idiotypic T and B lymphocytes in normal rats using direct visualization. J. exp. Med. **142**, 1218 (1975b).

BINZ, H., WIGZELL, H.: Shared idiotypic determinants on B and T lymphocytes reactive against the same antigenic determinants. III. Physical fractionation of specific immunocompetent T lymphocytes by affinity chromatography using antiidiotypic antibodies. J. exp. Med. **142**, 1231 (1975c)

BINZ, H., LINDEMANN, J., WIGZELL, H.: Inhibition of local graft-versus-host reaction by anti-alloantibodies. Nature (Lond.) **246**, 146 (1973).

BIRKELAND, S.A.: The use of ALG in renal allograft rejection. A controlled study. Postgrad. med. J., in press (1976).

BIRKELAND, S.A., KEMP, E., HAUGE, M.: Renal Transplantation and Cancer. The Scandia Transplant Material. Tissue Antigens **6**, 28 (1975).

BLANDEN, R.V.: Mechanisms of recovery from a generalized viral infection: mousepox. J. exp. Med. **132**, 1035 (1970).

BOAK, J.L., DAGHER, R.K., CORSON, J.M., WILSON, R.E.: Modification of the graft-versus-host syndrome by antilymphocyte serum treatment of the host. Chir. exp. Immunol. **3**, 801 (1968).

BOWEN, J.E., BATCHELOR, J.R., FRENCH, M.E., BURGOS, H., FABRE, J.W.: Failure of adoptive immunization or parabiosis with hyperimmune syngeneic partners to abrogate long-term enhancement of rat kidney allografts. Transplantation **18**, 322 (1974).

BOYSE, E.A., MIYAZAMA, M., AOKI, J., OLD, L.J.: Ly-A and Ly-B: two systems of lymphocyte isoantigens in the mouse. Proc. roy. Soc. B **170**, 175 (1968).

BRENDEL, W.: The clinical use of ALG. Transplant. Proc. **3**, 280 (1971).

BRENDEL, W., LAND, W., PICHLMAYR, R.: Intravenous treatment with horse anti-human lymphocyte globulin (ALG) in organ transplantation and autoimmune dieseases. In: Bertelli, A., Monaco, A.P. (eds.): Pharmacological Treatment in Organ and Tissue Transplantation, Amsterdam: Excerpta Medica Foundation, p. 208 (1970).

BRENDEL, W., RING, J., SEIFERT, J.: Experimental and clinical aspects of ALG. Progr. Immunol. II, **5**, 245 (1974).

BRENDEL, W., SEIFERT, J., RING, J.: Die klinische Anwendung von Antilymphocytenglobulin (ALG). Münch. med. Wschr. **117**, 1361 (1975).

Brent, L., Kilshaw, P.J.: Prolongation of skin allograft survival with spleen extracts and antilymphocyte serum. Nature (Lond.) **227**, 898 (1970).

Brent, L., Courtenay, T., Gowland, G.: Immunological reactivity of lymphoid cells after treatment with antilymphocytic serum. Nature (Lond.) **215**, 1461 (215) (1967).

Brent, L., Courtenay, T., Gowland, G.: Anti-lymphocytic serum: Its effect on the reactivity of lymphocytes. In: "Advance in Transplantation" (J. Dausset, J. Hamburger, G. Mathé eds.) p. 1117 Munksgaard, Copenhagen 1968.

Brent, L., Hansen, J.A., Kilshaw, P.J.: Unresponsiveness to skin allografts induced by tissue extracts and antilymphocyte serum. Transplant. Proc. **3**, 684 (1971).

Brochier, J., Revillard, J.P.: In vitro stimulation or inhibition of lymphocyte activation by antilymphocyte serum. Transplant. Proc. **3**, 788 (1971).

Brunner, K.T., Mauel, J., Schindler, R.: Inhibitory effect of isoantibody on the in vivo sensitization and on the in vitro cytotoxic action of immune lymphocytes. Nature (Lond.) **213**, 1246 (1967).

Brunner, K.T., Mauel, J., Cerottini, J.-C., Chapuis, B.: Quantitative assay of the lytic action of immune lymphoid cells on 51 Cr-labeled allogeneic target cells in vitro; inhibition by isoantibody and by drugs. Immunology **14**, 181 (1968).

Burgos, H., French, M.E., Batchelor, J.R.: Humoral and cell-mediated immunity in rats with enhanced kidney allografts. Transplantation **18**, 328 (1974).

Burke, J.F., May, J.W., Albright, N., Quinby, W.C., Russell, P.S.: Temporary skin transplantation and immunosuppression for extensive burns. New Engl. J. Med. **31**, 269 (1974).

Burnet, F.M.: The concept of immunological surveillance. Progr. exp. Tumor Res. **13**, 1 (1970).

Busch, C.J., Birtch, A.G., Lukl, P., Kobayshi, K., Galvanek, E.G., Carpenter, C.B.: Human renal allografts. Glomerular deposits of horse immunoglobulin G and nephritis following administration of antilymphocyte globulin. Hum. Path. **2**, 299 (1971).

Butler, W.T., Rossen, R.D., Reisberg, M.A., Nazow, F.B., Trentin, J.J., Judd, K.P.: Antibody formation to equine anti-lymphocytic globulin (ALG) in man: Effect on absorption, distribution and effectiveness of the ALG. J. Immunol. **106**, 1 (1971a).

Butler, W.T., Rossen, R.D.: Increasing effectiveness of antilymphocytic globulin by prevention of antibody formation to horse IgG. Transplant. Proc. **3**, 733 (1971b).

Ceppellini, R., Bonnard, G.D., Coppo, F., Miggiano, V.C., Pospisil, M., Curtoni, E.S., Pellegrino, M.: Mixed leukocyte cultures and HL-A antigens. II. Inhibition by Anti-HL-A sera. Transplant. Proc. **3**, 63 (1971).

Chaussy, C., Hammer, C., Pongratz, H., von Scheel, J., Pfeifer, K.J., Land, W., Sollinger, H.-W., Pielsticker, K., Brendel, W.: Prolongation of graft survival in rats and dogs by a specific antimacrophage serum (AMS). Transplant. Proc. **7**, 779 (1975).

Chen, C.H., Sabbadini, E., Sehon, A.H.: Specificity of xenoantisera against mouse cell surface antigens. Transplantation **17**, 22 (1974).

Chew, W.B., Lawrence, J.S.: Antilymphocytic serum. J. Immunol. **33**, 271 (1937).

Clagett, J., Peter, H.H., Feldman, J.P., Weigle, W.O.: Rabbit antiserum to brain associated thymus antigens of mouse and rat. II. Analysis of species-specific and cross-reacting antibodies. J. Immunol. **110**, 1085 (1973).

Claman, H.: Corticosteroids and lymphoid cells. New. Engl. J. Med. **287**, 388 (1972).

Colley, D.G., Malakian, A., Waksman, B.H.: Cellular differentiation in the thymus. II. Thymus-specific antigens in rat thymus and peripheral lymphoid cells. J. Immunol. **104**, 585 (1970).

Cosenza, H., Köhler, H.: Specific inhibition of plaque formation to phosphorylcholine by antibody against antibody. Science **176**, 1027 (1972a).

Cosenza, H., Köhler, H.: Specific suppression of the antibody response by antibodies to receptors. Proc. nat. Acad. Sci. (Wash.) **69**, 2701 (1972b).

Cotton, J.R., Sarles, H.E., Remmers, A.R. jr., Lindley, J.D., Beathard, G.A., Cottom, D.L., Fish, J.C., Townsend, C.M. jr., Ritzmann, S.E.: The appearance of reticulum cell sarcoma at the site of antilymphocyte globulin injection. Transplantation **16**, 154 (1973).

Davis, R.C., Lewis, J.L.: The effect of adult thymectomy on the immunosuppression obtained by treatment with antilymphocyte serum. Transplantation **6**, 879 (1968).

Davies, D.A.L., Alkins, B.J.: What abrogates heart transplant rejection in immunological enhancement. Nature (Lond.) **247**, 294 (1974).

Denman, A.M.: Anti-lymphocytic antibody and autoimmune Disease: A Review. Chir. exp. Immunol. **5**, 217 (1969).

DENMAN, A.M., FRENKEL, E.P.: Studies of the effect of induced immune lymphopenia. I. Enhanced effect of rabbit anti-rat lymphocyte globulin in rats tolerant to rabbit immunoglobulin G.J. Immunol. 99, 498 (1967).

DENMAN, A.M., FRENKEL, E.P.: Mode of action of antilymphocyte globulin. I. distribution of rabbit antilymphocyte globulin injected into rats and mice. Immunology, Lond. 14, 107 (1968a).

DENMAN, A.M., FRENKEL, E.P.: Mode of action of antilymphocyte globulin. II. Changes in the lymphoid cell population in rats treated with anti-lymphocyte globulin. Immunology Lond. 14, 115 (1968b).

DENMAN, A.M., DENMAN, E.J., HOLBORROW, E.J.: Immunosuppressive effects of lymphoid cell proliferation in mice receiving anti-lymphocyte globulin. Nature (Lond.) 217, 177 (1968a).

DENMAN, A.M., DENMAN, E.J., EMBLING, P.H.: Changes in the life-span of circulating small lymphocytes in mice after treatment with antilymphocyte globulin. Lancet 2, 321 (1968b).

DEODHAR, S.D., KUKLINGER, A.G., VIDT, D.G., ROBERTSON, A.L., HAZARD, J.B.: Development of reticulum-cell sarcoma at the site of antilymphocyte-globulin injection in a patient with renal transplant. New Engl. J. Med. 280, 1104 (1969).

DIENER, E., FELDMANN, M.: Relationship between antigen and antibody-induced suppression of immunity. Transplant. Rev. 8, 76 (1972).

DIETHELM, A.G., ALDRETE, J.S., SHAW, J.F., COBBS, C.G., HARTLEY, M.W., STERLING, W.A., MORGAN, J. McN.: Clinical evaluation of equine antithymocyte globuline in recipients of renal allografts: Analysis of survival, renal function, rejection, histocompatibility, and complications. Ann. Surg. 180, 20 (1974).

DRAY, S.: Effect of maternal isoantibodies on the quantitative expression of two allelic genes controlling gamma globulin allotype specificities. Nature (Lond.) 195, 677 (1962).

EICHMANN, K.: Idiotypic identity of antibodies to streptococcal carbohydrate in inbred mice. Europ. J. Immunol. 2, 301 (1972).

EICHMANN, K.: Idiotypic suppression. I. Influence of the dose and of the effector functions of antiidiotypic antibody on the production of an idiotype. Europ. J. Immunol. 4, 296 (1974).

EICHMANN, K.: Idiotypic suppression. II. Amplification of a suppressor T-cell with anti-idiotypic activity. Europ. J. Immunol. 5, 511 (1975).

EIJSVOOGEL, V.P.: Histocompatibility in vivo and/or in vitro. Progr. Immunol. II 5, 107 (1974).

EDWARDS, D.C., THOMAS, D., MOSEDALE, B., WOODROOFE, J.G., ZOLA, H.: The immunosuppressive potency of Antilymphocytic Sera and Globulins predicted by the Use of the Immunofluorescence Test. Behring Inst. Res. Commun. 51, 28 (1972).

FABRE, J.W., MORRIS, P.J.: Experience with passive enhancement of renal allografts in a (DA × Lewis) F$_1$ to Lewis strain combination. Transplantation 13, 604 (1972).

FABRE, J.W., BATCHELOR, J.R.: Passive enhancement of renal allografts. Specificity of the enhancing antisera. Transplantation 20, 269 (1975).

FELDMAN, J.D.: Immunological enhancement: A study of blocking antibodies. Advanc. Immunol. 15, 167 (1972).

FELDMANN, M.: T-cell suppression in vitro. II. Nature of specific suppressive factor. Europ. J. Immunol. 4, 667 (1974).

FELDMANN, M., DIENER, E.: Antibody mediated suppression of the immune response in vitro. I. Evidence for a central effect. J. exp. Med. 131, 247 (1970).

FIELD, E.O., GIBBS, J.E.: Cross-reaction of anti-lymphocyte serum with haemopoetic stem cells. Nature (Lond.) 217, 561 (1968).

FITCH, F.W., HAMADA, Y., McKEARN, T.J., STUART, F.D.: Serum factors associated with resistance to graft-versus-host-disease in adult F$_1$ rats. Fed. Proc. 33, 803 (1974).

FLEXNER, S., JOBLING, J.W.: On the promoting influence of heated tumor emulsions on tumor growth. Proc. Soc. exp. Biol. (N.Y.) 4, 156 (1907).

FORTNER, J., SHIU, M.H., BALNER, H., WILSON, C.B., SICHUK, G., KAWANO, N., HOLMES, J.T., BEATTLE, E.J. JR.: Observation on prolonged immune suppression for human liver homografts. Transplant. Proc. 3, 383 (1971).

FRAKER, P.J., CICUREL, L., NISONOFF, A.: Enhancement of immunogenicity of a BALB/c myeloma protein in BALB/c mice. J. Immunol. 113, 791 (1974).

FRENCH, M.E.: Antibody turnover by enhanced rat kidneys. Transplant. Proc. 5, 621 (1973).

FRENCH, M.E., BATCHELOR, J.R.: Immunological enhancement of rat kidney grafts. Lancet 2, 1103 (1969).

FRENCH, M.E., BATCHELOR, J.R.: Enhancement of renal allografts in rats and man. Transplant. Rev. **13**, 115 (1972).

FRENCH, M.E., BATCHELOR, J.R., WATTS, H.G.: The capacity of lymphocytes from rats bearing enhanced kidney allografts to mount graft-versus-host reactions. Transplantation **12**, 45 (1971).

FULLER, T.C., WINN, H.J.: Immunochemical and biologic characterization of alloantibody active in immunologic enhancement. Transplant. Proc. **5**, 585 (1973).

GAUGAS, J.M.: Enhancing effect of antilymphocytic globulin on human leprosy infection in thymectomized mice. Nature (Lond.) **220**, 1246 (1968).

GAUGAS, J.M., REES, R.J.W.: Enhancing effect of antilymphocytic serum on mycobacterial infections in mice. Nature (Lond.) **219**, 408 (1968).

GILKERSON, S.W., SCOTT, S.M., GADDY, L.: Titres of antilymphocyte serum determined by immunofluorescence. Amer. J. clin. Path. **53**, 928 (1970).

GLEICHMANN, H., GLEICHMANN, E.: Immunosuppression and Neoplasia. I. A critical review of experimental carcinogenesis and the immunesurveillance theory. Klin. Wschr. **51**, 255 (1973a).

GLEICHMANN, E., GLEICHMANN, H.: Immunosuppression and Neoplasia. II. Is deficient immunesurveillance the only mechanism by which immunosuppression promotes neoplasia? A speculative review. Klin. Wschr. **51**, 260 (1973b).

GOZZO, J.J., WOOD, M.L., MONACO, P.A.: Use of minimal doses of lymphoid cells for production of heterologous antilymphocyte serum. Transplant. Proc. **3**, 779 (1971).

GOZZO, J.J., WOOD, M.L., POMPEI, R., MONACO, A.P.: In vitro assay for immunosuppressive potency of antilymphocyte serum by the technique of passive hemagglutination. Behring Inst. Res. Commun. **51**, 40 (1972).

GRABAR, P.: Choix d'antigenes pour la préparation d'immunserums inhibiteurs des rejets de greffes. Symp. Ser. Immunobiol. Stand. **16**, 29 (1970).

GRAY, J.G., MONACO, A.P., RUSSELL, P.S.: Heterologous mouse anti-lymphocyte serum to prolong skin homografts. Surg. Forum **15**, 142 (1964).

GRAY, J.G., MONACO, A.P., WOOD, M.L., RUSSELL, P.S.: Studies on heterologous anti-lymphocytic serum in mice. I. In vitro and in vivo properties. J. Immunol. **96**, 217 (1966).

GRÄSBECK, R., NORDMAN, C., DE LA CHAPELLE, A.: Mitogenic action of antileucocyte immune serum on peripheral leucocytes in vitro. Lancet **2**, 385 (1963).

GRÄSBECK, R., NORDMAN, C.T., DE LA CHAPELLE, A.: The leucocyte-mitogenic effect of serum from rabbits immunized with human leucocytes. Acta med. scand. Suppl. **412**, 39 (1964).

GREAVES, M.F., TURSI, A., PLAYFAIR, J.H.L., TORRIGIANI, G., ZAMIR, R., ROITT, J.M.: Immunosuppressive potency and in vitro activity of antilymphocyte globulin. Lancet **1**, 68 (1969).

GREAVES, M.F., OWEN, J.J.T., RAFF, M.C.: T and B lymphocytes: origins, properties and roles in immune responses. Excerpta Medica Amsterdam, American Elsevier Publishing Co., Inc. New York (1974).

GUTTMAN, R.D., CARPENTER, C.B., LINDQUIST, R.R., MERRILL, J.P.: An immunosuppressive site of action of heterologous antilymphocyte serum. Lancet **1**, 248 (1967a).

GUTTMAN, R.D., CARPENTER, C.B., LINDQUIST, R.R., MERRILL, J.P.: Treatment with heterologous anti-thymus sera: nephritis associated with modification of renal allograft rejection and the immune status of the host to foreign protein. Transplantation **5**, 1115 (1967b).

GUTTMAN, R.D., CARPENTER, C.B., LINDQUIST, R.R., MERRILL, J.P.: Renal transplantation in the inbred rat. III. A study of heterologous anti-thymocyte sera. J. exp. Med. **126**, 1099 (1967c).

GUTTMAN, R.D., CARPENTER, C.B., LINDQUIST, R.R., MERRILL, J.P.: Studies of heterologous anti-thymocyte antibody (AT IgG) and its pepsin digestion product. In Proceedings of the First International Congress of the Transplantation Society, Paris, June 1967 Munksgaard, Copenhagen 1967d.

HART, D.A., WANG, A., PAWLAK, L.L., NISONOFF: Suppression of idiotypic specifities in adult mice by adminstration of antiidiotypic antibody. J. exp. Med. **135**, 1293 (1972).

HATTLER, B.G. JR., DAVIS, M., SOEHNLEN, B., MILLER, J.: Prospective in vitro prediction of enhancement of canine renal allografts. Surgery **74**, 163 (1973).

HELLSTRÖM, I., HELLSTRÖM, K.E.: The role of the immunological enhancement for the growth of autochthonous tumours. Transplant. Proc. **3**, 721 (1971).

HELLSTRÖM, I., HELLSTRÖM, K.E.: Cell-mediated immunity and blocking antibodies to renal allografts. Transplant. Proc. **4**, 369 (1972).

HELLSTRÖM, K.E., HELLSTRÖM, I.: Lymphocyte-mediated cytotoxicity and blocking serum activity to tumor antigens. Advanc. Immunol. **18**, 209 (1974).

HERON, I., MEYER, H.: Cell-mediated immune response in rats during acute allograft rejection and in rats developing allograft acceptance due to passive enhancement. Tissue Antigens 3, 348 (1973).

HERZENBERG, L.A., HERZENBERG, L.A.: Short-term and chronic allotype suppression in mice. In: Contemp. Topics in Immunobiol. 3, eds.: Cooper, M.D., and Warner, N.L. p. 41 Plenum Press New York 1974.

HERZENBERG, A.L., OKUMURA, K., METZLER, CH.M.: Regulation of immunoglobulin and antibody production by allotype suppressor T-cells in mice. Transplant. Rev. 27, 57 (1975).

HILDEMANN, W.H., MULLEN, Y.: The weaker the histoincompatibility, the greater the effectiveness of specific immunoblocking antibodies: A new immunogenetic role of transplantation. Transplant. Proc. 5, 617 (1973).

HIRSCH, M.S.: Effects of antilymphocytic serum on host responses to infectious agents. Fed. Proc. 29, 169 (1970).

HIRSCH, M.S., MURPHY, F.A.: Effects of anti-lymphocyte serum on 17-D yellow fever infection in adult mice. Nature (Lond.) 216, 179 (1967).

HOEHN, R.J., SIMMONS, R.L.: Immunosuppressive drugs combined with heterologous antilymphocyte serum: A clinical regimen for homograft prolongation. Surg. Forum 17, 251 (1966).

HOEHN, R.J., SIMMONS, R.L.: Immunosuppressive drugs combined with heterologous anti-lymphocyte serum for allograft prolongation. Transplantation 5, 1409 (1967).

HOLT, L.J., LING, N.R., STANWORTH, D.R.: The effect of heterologous antisera and rheumatoid factor on the synthesis of DNA and protein by human peripheral lymphocytes. Immunochemistry 3, 359 (1966).

HOLTER, A., McKEARN, T.J., NEU, M.R., FITCH, F.W., STUART, F.P.: Renal transplantation in the rabbit. I. Development of a model for study of hyperacute rejection and immunological enhancement. Transplantation 13, 244 (1972).

HOLTER, A.R., NEU, M.R., McKEARN, T.J., LYNCH, A.F., STUART, F.P.: Abrogation of hyperacute rejection of renal allografts by pepsin digest fragments of antidonor antibody. Transplant. Proc. 5, 593 (1973).

HOOVER, R.N., FRAUMENI, J.F. JR.: Risk of Cancer in renal transplant recipients. Lancet 2, 55 (1973).

INDERBITZIN, T.: The relationship of lymphocytes, delayed cutaneous allergic reactions and histamine. Int. Arch. Allergy 8, 150 (1956).

IWAHASHI, H., NAGAYA, H., SEALY, W.C., SIEKER, H.O.: Immunosuppressive effect of antilymphocyte serum on the canine lung allograft as a single immunosuppressive agent. Transplantation 9, 558 (1970).

IWASAKI, Y., PORTER, K.A., AMEND, J.R., MARCHIORO, T.L., ZÜHLKE, V., STARZL, T.E.: The preparation and testing of horse anti-dog and anti-human anti-lymphoid plasma or serum and its protein fractions. Surg. Gynec. Obstet. 124, 1 (1967).

JAMES, K.: The preparation and properties of antilymphocytic sera. Progr. Surg. 7, 140 (1969).

JAMES, K.: Effect of antilymphocytic antibody on humoral antibody formation. Fed. Proc. 29, 160 (1970).

JAMES, K., ANDERSON, N.F.: Effect of anti-rat lymphocyte antibody on humoral antibody formation. Nature (Lond.) 213, 1195 (1967).

JAMES, K., MEDAWAR, P.B.: Characterization of antilymphocytic antibody. Nature (Lond.) 214, 1052 (1967).

JANEWAY, C.A. JR., PAUL, W.E.: Hapten-specific augmentation of the antiidiotypic response to hapten-myeloma protein conjugates in mice. Europ. J. Immunol. 3, 340 (1973).

JANSEN, J.L.J., KOENE, R.A.P., VAN KAMP, G.J., HAGEMANN, J.F. LT. M., WIJDEVELD, P.G.A.B.: Hyperacute rejection and enhancement of mouse skin grafts by antibodies with a distinct specificity. J. Immunol. 115, 392 (1975).

JEEJEEBHOY, H.E.: Effects of rabbit anti-lymphocyte plasma on immune response of rats thymectomized in adult life. Lancet 2, 106 (1965a).

JEEJEEBHOY, H.F.: Immunological studies on the rat thymectomized in adult life. Immunology 9, 417 (1965b).

JEEKEL, J.J., McKENZIE, I.F.C., WINN, H.J.: Immunological enhancement of skin grafts in the mouse. J. Immunol. 108, 1017 (1972).

JERNE, N.K.: The diffuse organ has the assigment of monitoring the identity of the body. Its basic constituents are lymphocytes and antibody molecules, which recognize both foreign molecules and one another. Sci. Amer. 229, 52 (1973).

JOLLER, P.W.: Graft-versus-host reactivity of lymphoid cells inhibited by antirecognition structure serum. Nature (New Biol.) (Lond.) **240**, 214 (1972).

JONES, J.M., PETER, H.-H., FELDMAN, J.D.: Binding in vivo of enhancing antibodies to skin allografts and specific allogeneic tissues. J. Immunol. **108**, 301 (1972).

JONDAL, M., HOLM, G., WIGZELL, H.: Surface markers on human T and B lymphocytes. I. A large population of lymphocytes forming nonimmune rosettes with sheep red blood cells. J. exp. Med. **136**, 207 (1972).

JOOSTE, S.V., LANCE, E.M., LEYEY, R.H., MEDAWAR, P.B., RUSKIEWICZ, M., SHARMAN, R., TAUB, R.N.: Notes on the preparation and assay of anti-lymphocytic serum for use in mice. Immunology **15**, 697 (1968).

KALISS, N.: Course of production of an isoantiserum affecting tumor homograft survival in mice. Proc. nat. Acad. Sci. (Wash.) **42**, 269 (1956).

KALISS, N.: Immunological enhancement of tumor homografts in mice. A review. Cancer Res. **18**, 992 (1958).

KALISS, N.: Immunological enhancement. In: Najarian, J.S., Simmons, R.L. (eds.) "Transplantation", München-Berlin-Wien 1972 p. 195.

KALISS, N., KANDUTSCH, A.A.: Acceptance of tumor homografts by mice injected with antiserum. I. Activity of serum fractions. Proc. Soc. exp. Biol. (N.Y.) **91**, 118 (1956).

KALISS, N., MOLUMUT, N., HARRISS, J.L., GAULT, S.D.: Effect of previously injected immune serum and tissue on the survival of tumor grafts in mice. J. nat. Cancer Inst. **13**, 847 (1953).

KASHIWAGI, N., BRANTIGAN, C.O., BRETTSCHNEIDER, L., GROTH, C.G., STARZL, T.E.: Clinical reactions and serologic changes after the administration of heterologous antilymphocyte globulin to human recipients of renal homografts. Ann. intern. Med. **68**, 275 (1968).

KATZ, D.H., BENACERRAF: Regulatory influence of activated T-cells on B-cell responses to antigen. Advanc. Immunol. **15**, 1 (1972).

KERBEL, R.S., EIDINGER, D.: Variable effects of antilymphocyte serum on humoral antibody formation: role of thymus dependency of antigen. J. Immunol. **106**, 917 (1971).

KINSKY, R.G., VOISIN, G.A., DUC, H.T.: Biological properties of transplantation immune sera. III. Relationship between transplantation (facilitation or inhibition) and serological (anaphylaxis or cytolysis) activities. Transplantation **13**, 452 (1972).

KISSMEYER-NIELSEN, F., OLSEN, S., PETERSEN, P.V., FJELDBORG, O.: Hyperacute rejection of kidney allografts, associated with preexisting humoral antibodies against donor cells. Lancet **2**, 662 (1966).

LANCE, E.M.: The effects of chronic ALS administration in mice. In: "Advance in Transplantation". (J. Dausset, J. Hamburger, G. Mathé eds.) p. 107. Munksgaard, Copenhagen (1968a).

LANCE, E.M.: Erasure of immunological memory with antilymphocyte serum. Nature (Lond.) **217**, 557 (1968b).

LANCE, E.M.: The mechanism of action of antilymphocyte serum. Studies of antibody eluate. J. exp. Med. **130**, 49 (1969).

LANCE, E.M.: The selective action of antilymphocyte serum on recirculating lymphocytes: A review of the evidence and alternatives. Clin. exp. Immunol. **6**, 789 (1970a).

LANCE, E.M.: The effect of heterologous antilymphocyte serum (ALS) on the humoral antibody response to salmonella typhi "H" antigen and bovine serum albumin. J. Immunol. **105**, 108 (1970b).

LANCE, E.M.: Summary statement for Session (1) on in vivo and in vitro testing of ALG. Behring Inst. Mitt. **51**, 270 (1972).

LANCE, E.M., MEDAWAR, P.B.: Survival of skin heterografts under treatment with antilymphocyte serum. Lancet **1**, 1174 (1968).

LANCE, E.M., MEDAWAR, P.B.: Quantitative studies on tissue transplantation immunity. IX. Induction of tolerance with anti-lymphocytic serum. Proc. roy. Soc. B **173**, 447 (1969a).

LANCE, E.M., MEDAWAR, P.B.: Induction of tolerance with antilymphocytic serum. Transplant. Proc. **1**, 429 (1969b).

LANCE, E.M., FORD, P.J., RUSZKIEWICZ, M.: The use of subcellular fractions to raise antilymphocytic serum. Immunology **15**, 171 (1968).

LANCE, E.M., FORD, P., RUSZKIEWICZ, M.: Use of subcellular lymphocyte fractions to raise antilymphocyte serum. Fed. Proc. (Fed. Amer. Soc. exp. Biol.) **29**, 106 (1970a).

LANCE, E.M., MEDAWAR, P.B., NEHLSEN, S.L., COOPER, S., GUNN, A.: Synergistic effects of antilymphocyte serum and hydrocortisone on lymphoid populations. Symp. Ser. Immunobiol. Stand. **16**, 231 (1970b).

LANCE, E.M., BOYSE, E.A., COOPER, S., CARSWELL, E.A.: Rejection of skin allografts by irradiation chimaeras: evidence for skin-specific transplantation barrier. Transplant. Proc. **3**, 864 (1971).

LANCE, E.M., MEDAWAR, P.B., TAUB, R.N.: Antilymphocyte serum. Advanc. Immunol. **17**, 2 (1973).

LAND, W., FRICK, E., ROSCHER, R., BRENDEL, W., BAETHMANN, A.: Wirkung eines heterologen Antilymphocytenserums auf die experimentelle allergische Encephalomyelitis. Klin. Wschr. **97**, 633 (1969).

LAW, L.W., TING, R.C., ALLISON, A.C.: Effects of antilymphocyte serum on induction of tumours and leukaemia by murine sarcoma virus. Nature (Lond.) **220**, 611 (1968).

LEVEY, R.H., MEDAWAR, P.B.: Some experiments on the action of antilymphoid antisera. Ann. N.Y. Acad. Sci. **129**, 164 (1966a).

LEVEY, R.H., MEDAWAR, P.B.: Nature and mode of action of anti-lymphocytic antiserum. Proc. nat. Acac. Sci. (Wash.) **56**, 1130 (1966b).

LEVEY, R.H., MEDAWAR, P.B.: Further experiments on the action of antilymphocytic antiserum. Proc. nat. Acac. Sci. (Wash.) **58**, 470 (1967).

LEDNEY, G.D., VAN BEKKUM, D.W.: Suppression of acute secondary disease in the mouse with antilymphocyte serum. In: "Advance in Transplantation" (J. Dausset, J. Hamburger, Mathé eds.) p. 441, Munksgaard, Copenhagen 1968.

LINSCOTT, W.D.: Effect of cell surface antigen density on immunological enhancement. Nature (Lond.) **228**, 824 (1970).

LUCAS, Z.J., ENOMOTO, K.: Enhancement of renal grafts by anti-receptor site serum. Fed. Proc. **32**, 971 (1973).

LUCAS, Z.J., MARKLEY, J., TRAVIS, M.: Immunologic enhancement of renal allografts in the rat. I. Dissociation of graft survival and antibody response. Fed. Proc. **29**, 2041 (1970).

MAGE, R.G.: Quantitative studies on the regulation of expressions of genes for immunoglobulin allotypes in heterozygous rabbits. Cold Spr. Harb. Symp. quant. Biol. **32**, 203 (1967).

MANN, D.L., ABELSON, L., HARRIS, S., AMOS, D.B.: Detection of antigens specific for B-lymphoid cultured cell lines with human alloantisera. J. exp. Med. **142**, 84 (1975).

MARCHALONIS, J.J., CONE, R.E., ATWELL, J.L.: Isolation and partial characterization of lymphocyte surface immunoglobulins. J. exp. Med. **135**, 956 (1972).

MARTIN, W.J.: Assay for the immunosuppressive capacity of antilymphocyte serum. I. Evidence for opsonization. J. Immunol. **103**, 979 (1969a).

MARTIN, W.J.: Assay for the immunosuppressive capacity of antilymphocyte serum. II. Nature and specificity of opsonizing antibody. J. Immunol. **103**, 990 (1969b).

MARTIN, W.J.: Assay for the immunosuppressive capacity of antilymphocyte serum. III. Opsonizing activity of anti-human lymphocyte serum. J. Immunol. **103**, 1000 (1969c).

MARTIN, W.J., MILLER, J.F.A.P.: Cell to cell interaction in the immune response. IV. Site of action of antilymphocyte globulin. J. exp. Med. **128**, 855 (1968).

MARTIN, W.J., MILLER, J.F.A.P.: Assay for the immunosuppressive capacity of antilymphocyte serum based on its action on thymus-derived cells. Int. Arch. Allergy **35**, 163 (1969).

McKEARN, T.J.: Antireceptor antiserum causes specific inhibition of reactivity to rat histocompatibility antigens. Science **183**, 94 (1974).

McKEARN, T.J., FITCH, F.W., STUART, F.P.: Inhibition of reactivity to transplantation antigens by antibody against alloantibody. Fed. Proc. **32**, 971 (1973).

McKEARN, T.J., HAMADA, Y., STUART, F.P., FITCH, F.W.: Anti-receptor antibody and resistance to graft-versus-host disease. Nature (Lond.) **251**, 648 (1974a).

McKEARN, T.J., STUART, F.P., FITCH, F.W.: Anti-idiotypic antibody in rat transplantation immunity. I. Production of anti-idiotypic antibody in animals repeatedly immunized with alloantigens. J. Immunol. **113**, 1876 (1974b).

McKEARN, T.J., NEU, M., FITCH, F.W., STUART, F.P.: Presence of antibody and antiantibody in Lewis anti BN sera. Fed. Proc. **33**, 811 (1974c).

MELIEF, C.M., SCHWARTZ, R.S.: Immunocompetence and malignancy. In press (1975).

METCHNIKOFF, E.: Recherches sur l'influence de l'organisme sur lex toxines. Ann. Inst. Pasteur Lille **13**, 737 (1899).

MICHEL, R.P., GUTTMANN, R.D., KNAACK, J., KLASSEN, J., BEAUDOIN, J.-G., MOREHOUSE, D.D.: Antilymphocyte globulin in renal transplantation. Nephrotic syndrome and infection as possible complications. Arch. Surg. (Chicago) **110**, 90 (1975).

Miller, J., Hattler, B., Davis, M., Johnson, M.C.: Cellular and humoral factors governing canine mixed lymphocyte cultures after renal transplantation. I. Antibody. Transplantation **12**, 65 (1971).

Mitchison, N.A.: Mechanism of action of antilymphocyte serum. Fed. Proc. **29**, 222 (1970).

Möller, G.: Studies on the mechanism of immunological enhancement of tumor homografts. I. Specificity of immunological enhancement. J. nat. Cancer Inst. **30**, 1153 (1963a).

Möller, G.: Studies on the mechanism of immunological enhancement of tumor homografts. III. Interaction between humoral isoantibodies and immune lymphoid cells. J. nat. Cancer Inst. **30**, 1205 (1963b).

Möller, G.: Antibody induced depression of the immune response: A study of the mechanism in various immunological systems. Transplantation **2**, 405 (1964).

Möller, G., Möller, E.: The concept of immunological surveillance against neoplasia. Transplant. Rev. **28**, 3 (1976).

Monaco, A.P.: Use of antilymphocyte serum in the induction of immunological tolerance to tissue allografts. Fed. Proc. **29**, 153 (1970).

Monaco, A.P.: Antilymphocyte Serum. In: Najarian, J.S., Simmons, R.L. (eds.) "Transplantation", München-Berlin-Wien 1972, p. 222.

Monaco, A.P., Wood, M.L., Russell, P.S.: Effect of adult thymectomy on the recovery from immunological depression induced by anti-lymphocyte serum. Surg. Forum **16**, 209 (1965a).

Monaco, A.P., Wood, M.L., Russell, P.S.: Adult thymectomy: effect on recovery from immunologic depression in mice. Science **149**, 432 (1965b).

Monaco, A.P., Wood, M.L., Russell, P.S.: Studies on heterologous antilymphocyte serum in mice. III. Immunologic tolerance and chimerism produced across the H-2 locus with adult thymectomy and antilymphocyte serum. Ann. N.Y. Acad. Sci. **129**, 190 (1966a).

Monaco, A.P., Abbott, W.M., Othersen, H.B., Simmons, R.L., Wood, M.L., Flax, M.H., Russell, P.S.: Antiserum to lymphocytes: Prolonged survival of canine allografts. Science **153**, 1264 (1966b).

Monaco, A.P., Wood, M.L., Gray, J.G., Russell, P.S.: Studies on heterologous anti-lymphocyte serum in mice. II. Effect on the immune response. J. Immunol. **96**, 229 (1966c).

Monaco, A.P., Wood, N.L., Russell, P.S.: Some effects of purified heterologous anti-human lymphocyte serum in man. Transplantation **5**, 1106 (1967a).

Monaco, A.P., Wood, M.L., van der Werf, B.A., Russell, P.S.: Effect of antilymphocytic serum in mice, dogs and man. In: Ciba Study Group on Anti-Lymphocytic Serum pp. 111–134 (Churchill, London 1967b).

Monaco, A.P., Franco, D.J., Wood, M.L.: Studies on heterologous antilymphocyte serum in mice: IV. Modification in the effects of antilymphocyte serum produced by prior adult thymectomy. Antibiot. et chemother. (Basel) **15**, 328 (1969).

Monaco, A.P., Lewis, E.J., Latzina, A., Hardy, M.A., Quint, J., Schlesinger, R., McDonough, E., Latham, W.C., Madoff, M., Edsall, G.: Clinical use of equine antihuman lymph node lymphocyte serum: Preliminary results in twenty-one mismatched cadaveric renal transplants. In: International Symposium on Antilymphocyte Serum. Versailles. Basel: p. 355 (1970).

Monaco, A.P., Gozzo, J.J., Wood, M.L., Liegeois, A.: Use of low doses of homozygous allogeneic bone marrow cells to induce tolerance with antilymphocyte serum (ALS): Tolerance by intraorgan injection. Transplant. Proc. **3**, 680 (1971).

Monaco, A.P., Gozzo, J.L., Wood, M.L., Pompei, R.: Further studies on the in vitro assay of immunosuppressive potency of antilymphocyte serum by the mixed agglutination. Transplant. Proc. **5**, 527 (1973).

Mullen, Y., Takasugi, M., Hildemann, W.H.: The immunological status of rats with long surviving (enhanced) kidney allografts. Transplantation **15**, 238 (1973).

Najarian, J.S., Merkel, F.K., Moore, G.E., Good, R.A., Aust, J.C.: Clinical application of antilymphoblast serum. Transplant. Proc. **1**, 460 (1969).

Najarian, J.S., Simmons, R.L., Gewurz, H., Moberg, A., Merkel, F.K., Moore, G.E.: Anti-human lymphoblast globulin. Fed. Proc. **29**, 197 (1970).

Nagaya, H., Sieker, H.O.: Allograft survival: effect of antiserums to thymus glands and lymphocytes. Sience **150**, 1181 (1965).

Nehlsen, S.L.: Prolonged administration of antilymphocyte serum in mice. I. Observation on cellular and humoral immunity. Chir. exp. Immunol. **9**, 63 (1971).

NISONOFF, A., BANGASSER, S.A.: Immunological suppression of idiotypic specifities. Transplant. Rev. **27**, 100 (1975).

OPELZ, G., MICKEY, M.R., TERASAKI, P.I.: Prolonged survival of second human kidney transplants. Science **178**, 617 (1972).

OPELZ, G., SENGAR, D.P.S., MICKEY, M.R., TERASAKI, P.I.: Effect of blood transfusion on subsequent kidney transplants. Transplant. Proc. **5**, 253 (1973).

PANIJEL, J., CAYEUX, P.: Immunosuppressive effects of macrophage antiserum. Immunology **14**, 769 (1968).

PARROTT, D.M.V.: The response of draining lymph nodes to immunological stimulation in intact and thymectomized animals. J. clin. Path. **20**, 456 (1967).

PATEL, R., TERASAKI, P.I.: Significance of the positive cross-match test in kidney transplantation. New Engl. J. Med. **280**, 735 (1969).

PAWLAK, L.L., HART, D.A., NISONOFF, A.: Requirements for prolonged suppression of an idiotypic specificity in adult mice. J. exp. Med. **137**, 1442 (1973).

PAWLAK, L.L., HART, D.A., NISONOFF, A.: Suppression of immunological memory for a cross-reactive idiotype in adult mice. Europ. J. Immunol. **4**, 10 (1974).

PENN, I., STARZL, T.E.: Malignant tumors arising de novo in immunosuppressed organ transplant recipients. Transplantation **14**, 407 (1972).

PENN, I., HALGRIMSON, C.G., STARZL, T.E.: De novo malignant tumors in organ transplant recipients. Transplant. Proc. **3**, 773 (1971).

PENN, I., HAMMOND, W., BRETTSCHNEIDER, L., STARZL, T.E.: Malignant lymphomas in transplantation patients. Transplant. Proc. **1**, 106 (1969).

PERPER, R.J., YU, T.Z., KOOISTRA, J.B.: The in vitro specificity of antilymphocyte sera produced by either cultured or noncultured lymphocytes. Int. Arch. Allergy **37**, 418 (1970a).

PERPER, R.J., MONOVICH, R.E., BOUERSOX, B.E.: Long-term skin allograft survival elicited by a finite treatment with antilymphocyte serum combined with cytarabine. J. Immunol. **104**, 1063 (1970b).

PETER, H.-H., FELDMANN, J.: Cell mediated cytotoxicity during rejection and enhancement of allogeneic skin grafts in rats. J. exp. Med. **135**, 1301 (1972).

PETER, H.-H., CLAGETT, J., FELDMAN, J.D., WEIGLE, W.O.: Rabbit antiserum to brain-associated thymus antigens of mouse and rat. I. Demonstration of antibodies crossreacting to T-cells of both species. J. Immunol. **110**, 1077 (1973).

PHILLIPS, B., GAZET, J.C.: Growth to two human tumour cell lines in mice treated with antilymphocyte serum. Nature (Lond.) **215**, 548 (1967).

PHILLIPS, B., GAZET, J.-C.: Growth of human foetal tissue in mice treated with antilymphocyte serum. Nature (Lond.) **222**, 1292 (1969).

PICHLMAYR, R.: Wirkung eines heterologen Antilymphocytenserums auf die Transplantatabstoßung beim Hund. Klin. Wschr. **44**, 594 (1966).

PICHLMAYR, R.: Herstellung und Wirkung heterologer Antihundelymphocytenseren. Z. ges. exp. Med. **143**, 161 (1967).

PICHLMAYR, R.: Aspects in production of antilymphocyte sera. Fed. Proc. **29**, 111 (1970).

PICHLMAYR, R., BRENDEL, W., ZENKER, R.: Production and effects of heterologous anti-canine lymphocyte serum. Surgery **61**, 774 (1967a).

PICHLMAYR, R., BRENDEL, W., WONIGEIT, K.: Blutbildveränderungen nach Gabe eines heterologen Antihundelymphocytenserums. Z. ges. exp. Med. **143**, 305 (1967b).

PICHLMAYR, R., BRENDEL, W., BECK, G., SCHMITTDIEL, E., TIDOW, G., PICHLMAYR, I.: Herstellung heterologer Immunseren gegen Lymphocyten des Hundes. Klin. Wschr. **45**, 199 (1967c).

PICHLMAYR, R., BRENDEL, W., ZENKER, R.: Erfahrungen mit heterologen Antilymphocytenseren beim Menschen. Münch. med. Wschr. **15**, 893 (1968a).

PICHLMAYR, R., BRENDEL, W., MIKAELOFF, P.H., DESCORTES, J., RASSAT, J.P., BOMEL, J., PICHLMAYR, I., FATEH MOGHADAM, A., THIERFELDER, S.T., MESSMER, K., KNEDEL, M.: Survival of renal and liver homografts in dogs treated with heterologous antilymphocyte serum. In: Advance in Transplantation (J. Dausset, J. Hamburger, G. Mathé, eds.) p. 147, Munksgaard Copenhagen (1968b).

PICHLMAYR, R., WAGNER, E., WONIGEIT, K., TIDOW, G., WESTERWELLE, I.: Some aspects in production of antilymphocyte sera. In: Bertelli, A., Monaco, A.P. "Pharmacological Treatment in Organ and Tissue Transplantation". Amsterdam: Excerpta Medica Foundation 1970, p. 309.

PICHLMAYR, R., WONIGEIT, K., MEYER, H.J.: Aspects of routine application of ALG in human kidney transplantation. Postgrad. med. J., in press (1976).

PIROFSKY, B., BARDANA, E.J., JR., BAYRACKI, C., PORTER, G.A.: Antilymphocyte antisera in immunologically mediated renal disease. J. Amer. med. Ass. 210, 1059 (1969).

PIROFSKY, B., REID, R.H., BARDANA, E.J., JR., BAYRACKI, C.: Antithymocyte antisera therapy in nonsurgical immunologic disease. Transplant. Proc. 3, 769 (1971).

PIROFSKY, B., BEAULIEU, R., BARDANA, J. JR., AUGUST, A.: Antithymocyte antiserum effects in man. Amer. J. Med. 56, 290 (1974).

PREHN, R.T.: Do tumors grow because of the response of the host? Transplant. Rev. 28, 34 (1976).

RABINOWITZ, R., COHEN, A.D.A., LASKOW, L., SCHLESINGER, M.: Antibodies specific for the O- and Ly-alloantigens in various rabbit antisera. J. Immunol. 112, 683 (1974).

RAFF, M.C., WORTIS, H.H.: Thymus dependence of O-bearing cells in the peripheral lymphoid tissues of mice. Immunology 18, 931 (1970).

RAJU, S., GROGAN, J.B., HARDY, J.D.: Prolonged survival of skin allografts exposed to heterologous antilymphocyte serum in vitro. J. surg. Res. 9, 327 (1969).

RAMSEIER, H., LINDEMANN, J.: Cellular receptors. Effect of anti-allo-antiserum on the recognition of transplantation antigens. J. exp. Med. 134, 1083 (1971).

RAMSEIER, H., LINDEMANN, J.: Alliotypic antibodies. Transplant. Rev. 10, 57 (1972).

REVILLARD, J.P.: Inhibition of mixed lymphocyte reaction (MLC) and immunosuppressive activity of ALG. Behring Inst. Res. Commun. 51, 44 (1972).

RIETHMÜLLER, G.: Antilymphocyte serum. Lancet 2, 1210 (1967).

RIETHMÜLLER, G., RIETHMÜLLER, D., STEIN, M., MAUSEN, P.: In vivo and in vitro properties of intact and pepsin digested heterologous anti-mouse thymus antibodies. J. Immunol. 100, 969 (1968).

RING, J., SEIFERT, J., LOB, G., LAND, W., COULIN, K., BRENDEL, W.: Zum Risiko einer ALG-Therapie. Mögliche Nebenwirkungen, Prophylaxe und Behandlung. Klin. Wschr. 51, 487 (1973).

RING, J., LOB, G., ANGSTWURM, H., BRASS, B., BACKMUND, H., SEIFERT, J., COULIN, K., FRICK, E., MERTIN, J., BRENDEL, W.: Intensive immunosuppression in the treatment of multiple sclerosis. Lancet 2, 1093 (1974).

RODKEY, L.S.: Studies of idiotypic antibodies. Production and characterization of autoantiidiotypic sera. J. exp. Med. 139, 712 (1974).

RODT, H.V., THIERFELDER, S., EULITZ, M.: Suppression of acute secondary disease by heterologous anti-brain serum. Blut 25, 385 (1972).

ROITT, I.M., GREAVES, M.F., TEIRSE, A., TORRIGIANI, G., PLAYFAIR, J.H.L., VERKI, W.: Correlation between immunosuppressive potency of anti-lymphocyte globulin and its activity in an opsonic adherence test in vitro. In: Bertelli, A., and Monaco, A.P. (eds.): Pharmacological Treatment in Organ and Tissue Transplantation. Amsterdam: Excerpta Medical Foundation 1970 p. 251.

ROLAND, J.M., NAIRN, R.C., DAVIES, D.J.: Assay of antilymphocyte serum by membrane immunofluorescence. J. immunol. Methods 1, 83 (1971).

ROWLEY, D.A., FITCH, F.W., STUART, F.P., KÖHLER, H., COSENZA, H.: Specific suppression of immune responses. Sience 181, 1133 (1973).

RUSSELL, P.S., MONACO, A.P.: Heterologous anti-lymphocyte sera and some of their effects. Transplantation 5, 1086 (1967).

SCHLESINGER, M., YRON, I.: Antigenic changes in lymphnode cells after administration of antiserum to thymus cells. Science 164, 1412 (1969).

SEIFERT, J., RING, J., BRENDEL, W.: Prolongation of skin allografts after oral application of ALS in rats. Nature (Lond.) 249, 776 (1974).

SELL, S., ROWE, D.S., GELL, P.G.H.: Studies on rabbit lymphocytes in vitro. III. Protein, RNA and DNA synthesis by lymphocyte cultures after stimulation with phytohaemagglutinin, with staphylococcal filtrate, with antiallotype serum, and with heterologous antiserum to rabbit whole serum. J. exp. Med. 122, 823 (1965).

SHAIPANICH, T., VANWIJEK, R.R., KIM, J., LUKL, P., BUSCH, G., WILSON, R.E.: Enhancement of rat renal allografts with F(ab)$_2$ fragment of donor specific antikidney serum. Surgery 70, 113 (1971).

SHAIPANICH, T., WREN, S., VON HAEFEN, U., KOPPENHEFFER, T., BUSCH, G., WILSON, R.E.: Evaluation of organ specificity in renal allograft enhancement with F(ab)$_2$ fragments. Transplant. Proc. 5, 581 (1973).

SHEIL, A.G.R., KELLY, G.E., STOREY, B.G., MAY, J., KALOWSKI, S., MEARS, D., ROGERS, J.H., JOHNSON, J.R., CHARLESWORTH, J., STEWART, J.H.: Antilymphocyte globulin in patients with renal allografts from cadaveric donors. Lancet 2, 227 (1973).

SHIGENO, N., ARPELS, G., HÄMMERLING, U., BOYSE, E.A., OLD, L.J.: Preparation of lymphocyte-specific antibody from antilymphocyte serum. Lancet 2, 320 (1968).

SHORTER, R.G., SPENCER, R.J., HALLENBECK, G.A.: Anti-lymphoid sera in clinical renal homotransplantation. J. Amer. med. Ass. 202, 845 (1967).

SHREFFLER, D.C., DAVID, C.S.: The H-2 major histocompatibility complex and the immune response region: Genetic variation, function and organization. Advanc. Immunol. 20, 125 (1975).

SIMMONS, R.L., OZERKIS, A.J., HOEHN, R.J.: Antiserum to lymphocytes: Interactions with chemical immunosupressants. Science 160, 1127 (1968).

SIMMONS, R.L., MOBERG, A.W., GEWURZ, H., SOLL, R., NAJARIAN, J.S.: Immunosuppression of anti-human lymphocytic globulin: Correlation of human and animal assay systems with clinical results. Transplant. Proc. 3, 745 (1971).

SIMPSON, E., NEHLSEN, S.L.: Prolonged administration of antithymocyte serum in mice. I. Histopathological investigations. Chir. exp. Immunol. 9, 79 (1971).

SINCLAIR, N.R.St.C.: Regulation of the immune response. I. Reduction in ability of specific antibody to inhibit long-lasting IgG immunological priming after removal of the Fc fragment. J. exp. Med. 129, 1183 (1969).

SINCLAIR, N.R.St.C., LEES, R.K., CHAN, P.L., KHAN, R.H.: Regulation of the immune response. II. Further studies on differences in ability of F(ab)$_2$ and 7 S antibodies to inhibit an antibody response. Immunology 19, 105 (1970).

SJÖGREN, H.O., HELLSTRÖM, I., BANSAL, S.C., HELLSTRÖM, K.E.: Suggestive evidence that the 'blocking antibodies' of tumorbearing individuals may be antigen-antibody complexes. Proc. nat. Acad. Sci. (Wash.) 68, 1372 (1971).

SKAMENE, E.: Antilymphocyte serum binding to cell surfaces. Fed. Proc. 29, 126 (1970).

SKAMENE, E., RUSSELL, P.S.: A quantitative study of the binding of ALS to various cell types. Clin. exp. Immunol. 8, 195 (1971).

SKAMENE, E., HAWKINS, D., GOLD, PH., SHUSTER, J., FREEDMANN, S.O., TAYLOR, H.E.: Studies on nephrotoxic antibody in antilymphocyte globulin. Transplantation 13, 9 (1972).

SMITH, R.W., WOODY, J.N.: The immunosuppressive potency of antilymphocyte serum is related to activity against human thymic lymphocyte-specific antigens. Transplantation 17, 503 (1974).

SNELL, G.O., WINN, H.J., STIMPFLING, J.H., PARKER, S.J.: Depression by antibody of the immune response to homografts and its role in immunological enhancement. J. exp. Med. 112, 293 (1960).

SPIEGELBERG, H.L.: Biological activities of Immunoglobulins of different classes and subclasses. Advanc. Immunol. 19, 259 (1975).

STAINES, N.A., GUY, K., DAVIES, L., ALLEN, D.: Passive enhancement of mouse skin allografts. Specificity of the antiserum for major histocompatibility complex antigens. Transplantation 18, 192 (1974).

STARZL, T.E., MARCHIORO, T.L., FARIS, T.D., McCARDLE, R.J., IWASAKI, Y.: Avenues of future research in homotransplantation of the liver with particular reference to hepatic supportive procedures, antilymphocytic serum and tissue typing. Amer. J. Surg. 112, 391 (1966).

STARZL, T.E., MARCHIORO, T.L., PORTER, K.A., IWASAKI, Y., CERILLI, G.J.: The use of heterologous antilymphoid agents in canine renal and liver homotransplantation and in human renal homotransplantation. Surg. Gynec. Obstet. 124, 301 (1967).

STARZL, T.E., GROTH, C.G., TERASAKI, P.I., PUTNAM, C.W., BRETTSCHNEIDER, L., MARCHIORO, T.L.: Heterologous antilymphocyte globulin, histocompatibility matching, and human renal homotransplantation. Surg. Gynec. Obstet. 126, 1032 (1968).

STARZL, T.E., BRETTSCHNEIDER, L., PENN, I., SCHMIDT, R.W., BELL, P., KASHIWAGI, N., TOWNSEND, C.M., PUTNAM, C.W.: A trial with heterologous antilymphocyte globulin in man. Transplant. Proc. 1, 448 (1969).

STARZL, T.E., PENN, I., PUTNAM, C.W., GROTH, C.G., HALGRIMSON, C.G.: Iatrogenic alterations of immunologic surveillance in man and their influence on malignancy. Transplant. Rev. 7, 112 (1971).

STILLER, C.R., SINCLAIR, N.R.St.C., et al.: Lymphocytedependent antibody and renal graft rejection. Lancet 1, 953 (1975).

Storb, R., Gluckmann, E., Thomas, E.D., Buckner, C.D., Clift, R.A., Fefer, A., Glucksberg, H., Graham, T.C., Johnson, F.L., Lerner, K.G., Neiman, P.E., Ochs, H.: Treatment of established human graft-versus-host disease by antithymocyte globulin. Blood **44**, 57 (1974).

Stuart, F.B.: Immunological enhancement of transplanted organs. In "Immunological aspects of transplantation surgery" (Calne, R. ed.) Lancaster 1973, p. 191.

Stuart, F.P., Saitoh, T., Fitch, F.W.: Rejection of renal allografts: Specific immunologic suppression. Science **160**, 1463 (1968).

Stuart, F.P., Fitch, F.W., Rowley, D.A.: Specific suppression of renal allograft rejection by treatment with antigen and antibody. Transplant. Proc. **2**, 483 (1970).

Stuart, F.P., Fitch, F.W., Rowley, D.A., Biesecker, J.L., Hellström, K.E., Hellström, I.: Presence of both cellmediated immunity and serum-blocking factors in rat renal allografts 'enhanced' by passive immunisation. Transplantation **12**, 331 (1971).

Stuart, F.P., McKearn, T.J., Fitch, F.W.: Immunological enhancement of renal allografts. Transplant. Proc. **6**, 53 (1974).

Takasugi, M., Hildemann, W.H.: Lymphocyte-antibody interactions in immunological enhancement. Transplant. Proc. **1**, 530 (1969).

Taub, R.N.: Prolongation of skin homograft survival by mouse-antimouse thymocyte isoantiserum. Transplant. Proc. **1**, 445 (1969).

Taub, R.N., Lance, E.M.: Histopathological effects in mice of heterologous antilymphocyte serum. J. exp. Med. **128**, 1281 (1968).

Thiede, A., Sonntag, H.-G., Müller-Ruchholtz, W.: Vergleich von Blutbild und Phagocytose nach intravenöser Gabe heterologer Antimakrophagen- oder Antithymuslymphocytenseren. Res. exp. Med. **163**, 325 (1974).

Thiel, G., Moppert, J., Mahlich, H., Bühler, F., Vischer, T., Enderlin, F., Weber, H., Zollinger, H.U.: Glomerular damage after intravenous administration of antilymphocyte globulin (ALG) in man and rhesus monkeys. Transplant. Proc. **3**, 741 (1971).

Thomas, D., Mosedale, B., Zola, H.: The use of the indirect fluorescent antibody technique in assessing the activity of antilymphocytic sera and antilymphocytic globulins. Clin. exp. Immunol. **8**, 987 (1971).

Ting, A., Terasaki, P.I.: Influence of lymphocyte-dependent antibodies on human kidney transplants. Transplantation **18**, 371 (1974).

Traeger, J., Fries, D., Carraz, M., Brochier, J., Bernhardt, J.P., Veysseyre, C., Prevost, R., Traeger-Fouillet, Y., Bryon, P.A., Manuel, Y.: Préparation, propriétés et activités d'un sérum de cheval antilymphocyte humain. In: Bacq, L.M., Castermans, A., Lejeune, G. (eds.) "Cell bound immunity". Congrès et colloques de l'Université de Liege, Vol. 43, p. 163 (1967).

Traeger, J., Fries, D., Perrin, J., Saubier, E., Carraz, M., Bernhardt, J.P., Revillard, J.P., Plan, R., Archimbaud, J.P., Brochier, J.: Studies on antilymphocyte globulins made from thoracic duct lymphocytes: Two and a half year's experience in kidney transplantation. In: Bertelli, A., Monaco, A.P. (eds.): Pharmacological Treatment in organ and Tissue Transplantation. Amsterdam: Excerpta Medical Foundation p. 315 (1970).

Traeger, J., Touraine, J.L., Fries, D., Berthoux, F.: Evaluation of intravenous route for administration of antilymphocyte globulins in humans. Transplant. Proc. **3**, 749 (1971).

Trepel, F., Pichlmayr, R., Kimura, J., Brendel, W., Begemann, H.: Therapieversuche mit Antilymphocytenserum bei Autoaggressionskrankheiten des Menschen. Klin. Wschr. **46**, 856 (1968).

Turcotte, J.G., Feduska, N.J., Haines, R.F., Freler, D.T., Gikas, P.W., McDonald, F.D., Johnson, A.G., Morrell, R.M., Thompson, N.W., Arbor, A.: Antithymocyte globulin in renal transplant recipients: a clinical trial. Survival of incompatible related allografts was improved with antithymocyte globulin administration. Arch. Surg. (Chicago) **106**, 484 (1973).

Turk, J.L., Willoughby, D.A.: Central and peripheral effects of antilymphocyte sera. Lancet **1**, 249 (1967).

Turk, J.L., Willoughby, D.A., Stevens, J.E.: An analysis of the effects of some types of antilymphocyte sera on contact hypersensitivity and certain models of inflammation. Immunology **14**, 683 (1968).

Turk, J.L., Polak, L.: Action of antilymphocytic sera on reactions caused by immune-complex formation. Lancet **1**, 130 (1969).

Tyler, R.W., Everett, N.B., Schwartz, M.R.: Effect of antilymphocytic serum on rat lymphocytes. J. Immunol. **102**, 179 (1968).

UHR, J.W., MÖLLER, G.: Regulatory effect of antibody on the immune response. Advanc. Immunol. **8**, 81 (1968).

UNANUE, E.R.: Properties and some uses of anti-macrophage antibodies. Nature (Lond.) **218**, 36 (1968).

VAN BEKKUM, D.W., LEDNEY, G.D., BALNER, H., VAN PUTTEN, L.M., DE VRIES, M.J.: Suppression of secondary disease following foreign bone marrow grafting with antilymphocyte serum. In: "Antilymphocytic Serum" (G.E.W. Wolstenholme and M. O'Connor, eds.) p. 97. Churchill, London (1967).

VAN BEKKUM, D.W., HEYSTEK, G.A., MARQUET, R.L.: Effects of immunosuppressive treatment on rejection of heart allografts in rats. Transplantation **8**, 678 (1969).

VANDEPUTTE, M.: Antilymphocytic serum and polyoma oncogenesis in rats. Transpla. Proc. **1**, 100 (1969).

VAN DER WERF, B.A., MONACO, A.P., WOOD, M.L., RUSSELL, P.S.: Immune competence of mouse lymph node cells after in vivo and in vitro contact with rabbit anti-mouse lymphocyte serum. (RAMLS) In: "Advance in Transplantation" (J. Dausset, J. Hamburger, Mathé eds.) p. 133 Munksgaard, Copenhagen 1967.

VAN ROOD, J.J., VAN LEEUWEN, A., KEUNING, J.J., BLUSSE VAN OUD ALBLAS, A.: The serological recognition of the human MLC determinants using a modified cytotoxicity technique. Tissue Antigens **5**, 73 (1975).

VOISIN, G.A.: Immunological facilitation, a broadening of the concept of the enhancement phenomenon. Progr. Allergy **15**, 328 (1971).

VOISIN, G.A., KINSKY, R., JANSEN, F., BERNARD, C.: Biological properties of antibody classes in transplantation immune sera. Transplantation **8**, 618 (1969).

WAKSMAN, B.H., ARBOUYS, S., ARNASON, B.G.: The use of specific "lymphocyte" antisera to inhibit hypersensitive reactions of the "delayed" type. J. Med. **114**, 997 (1961).

WASON, W.M., FITCH, F.W.: Suppression of the antibody response to SRBC with F(ab)$_2$ and IgG in vitro. J. Immunol. **110**, 1427 (1973).

WEIL, R., SIMMONS, R.L.: Combined immunosuppression for canine renal allograft prolongation: Antilymphocyte serum plus prednisolone and azathioprine. Ann. Surg. **167**, 239 (1968).

WERNET, P., WINCHESTER, R., KUNKEL, H.G., WERNET, D., GIPHART, M., VAN LEEUWEN, A., VAN ROOD, J.J.: Serological detection and partial characterization of human MLC determinants with special reference to B-cell specificity. Transplant. Proc. **7**, 193 (1975).

WHITE, E., HILDEMANN, W.H.: Kidney versus skin allograft reactions in normal adult rats of inbred strains. Transplant. Proc. **1**, 395 (1969).

WIGZELL, H.: On the relationship between cellular and humoral antibodies. Contemp. Top. Immunobiol. **3**, 77 (1973).

WINCHESTER, R.J., FU, S.M., WERNET, P., KUNKEL, H.G., DUPONT, B., JERSILD, C.: Recognition by pregnancy serums of non-H-LA alloantigens selectively expressed on B lymphocytes. J. exp. Med. **141**, 924 (1975).

WINN, H.J.: The mechanisms of immunological enhancement. Progr. Immunol. II **3**, 207 (1974).

WONIGEIT, K., WAGNER, E., HÖLLINGS, K., PICHLMAYR, R.: Effect of specific antiserum on the generation of cytotoxic effector cells in skin and kidney grafted rats. Z. Immun.-Forsch. **147**, 340 (1974).

WONIGEIT, K., WAGNER, E., PICHLMAYR, R.: Modification of lymphocyte reactivity by specific alloantiserum in skin-grafted rats. Transplant. Proc. **7**, 455 (1975).

WOOD, M.L., HEPPNER, G., GOZZO, J.J., MONACO, A.P.: Mechanism of augmented graft survival in mice after ALS and bone marrow infusion. Transplant. Proc. **5**, 691 (1973).

WOODRUFF, M.F.A.: Immunological properties of antilymphocyte serum. J. clin. Path. **20**, 466 (1967).

WOODRUFF, M.F.A.: Purification of antilymphocytic antibody. Nature (Lond.) **217**, 821 (1968).

WOODRUFF, M.F.A., ANDERSON, N.: Effect of lymphocyte depletion by thoracic duct fistula and administration of antilymphocytic serum on the survival of skin homografts in rats. Nature (Lond.) **200**, 702 (1963).

WOODRUFF, M.F.A., ANDERSON, N.F.: The effect of lymphocyte depletion by thoracic duct fistula and administration of antilymphocyte serum on the survival of skin homografts in rats. Ann. N.Y. Acad. Sci. **120**, 119 (1964).

WOODRUFF, M.F.A., JAMES, K., ANDERSON, N.F., REID, B.L.: In vivo and in vitro properties of antilymphocyte serum. In Wolstenholme, G.E.W., O'Connor, M. (eds.): Antilymphocytic Serum (Ciba Foundation Study Group No. 29). Boston: Little, Brown and Co., (1967a) p. 57.

WOODRUFF, M.F.A., REID, B.L., JAMES, K.: The effect of anti-lymphocytic antibody and antibody fragments on human lymphocytes in vitro. Nature (Lond.) **215**, 591 (1967b).

WOODRUFF, M.F.A., REID, B.L., JAMES, K.: Quantitative in vitro studies with anti-lymphocytic antibody. Nature (Lond.) **216**, 758 (1967c).

WREN, S.F.G., MARTINS, A.C.P., ROWLEY, D.A. *et al.*: Passive enhancement of canine renal allografts with polyspecific F(ab')$_2$ fragments. Surgery **76**, 112 (1974).

YUNIS, E.J., AMOS, D.B.: Three closely linked genetic systems relevant to transplantation. Proc. nat. Acad. Sci. (Wash.) **68**, 3031 (1971).

ZIMMERMANN, B., FELDMAN, J.D.: Enhancing Antibody: I. Bioassay for normal skin grafts. J. Immunol. **102**, 507 (1969a).

ZIMMERMANN, B., FELDMAN, J.D.: Enhancing Antibody: II. Specificity and heterogeneity. J. Immunol. **103**, 383 (1969b).

ZIMMERMANN, B., FELDMAN, J.D.: Enhancing antibody. III. Site of activity. J. Immunol. **104**, 626 (1970).

ZOLA, H., MOSEDALE, B., THOMAS, D.: The preparation and properties of antisera to subcellular fractions from lymphocytes. Transplantation **9**, 259 (1970).

Medications and Their Toxicity

EDWARD S. HENDERSON and GERHARD R.F. KRUEGER

With 23 Figures and 2 Tables

A. Introduction

Immunosuppressant activities of drugs have been recognized since the early studies of sulfur mustards (HEKTOEN and CORPER, 1921). Clinically, immunosuppression with adrenocorticosteroids was successfully initiated in the 1940s (HENCH et al., 1949) followed by the introduction of antiproliferative drugs in systemic lupus erythematosus and other collagen diseases in the subsequent decade (DUBOIS, 1954; DIAZ et al., 1951).

It is not by coincidence that most immunosuppressive compounds are also antiproliferative agents, and that the search for immunosuppressants has been remarkably abetted by the cancer drug development programs of the last three decades. Accordingly, studies of the effects of drugs in one setting, e.g., against a variety of tumors and corresponding normal tissues in vivo and in vitro, have proven complementary to similar studies of in vitro and in vivo immunologic function. Although the activities of these compounds are modified by individual cell and tissue characteristics, understanding of the pharmacology and mechanism of action of these drugs is usually comparably predictive for antitumor and antiimmunologic effects. For example, agents active only during the stage of cell replication will have little or no influence on tumor cells with little proliferative activity, nor will they prevent immunologic reactivity when given prior to antigen exposure. Similarly, drugs failing to penetrate certain anatomical and/or physiologic compartments, e.g., the central nervous system, can have, with few exceptions, no influence on either tumors or immunologic reactions within the brain or spinal cord. Concurrent evaluations of antitumor and immunosuppressive therapies thus increase the fund of knowledge in both areas of scientific and clinical endeavor.

As a corollary to this interrelationship, one cannot logically speak of toxicities or side-effects of these drugs. Toxicity for the renal transplantation team may be the myelosuppression leading to granulocytopenia and thrombocytopenia which complicates the induction of relative anergy. However, for the physician treating myeloid metaplasia these definitions of benefit and toxicity are reversed. All drugs used for immunosuppression have a variety of biological effects, at least one of which influences host defenses. With careful consideration of the type of immune alteration desired, and the status of the patient being treated, one must select the agent most likely to achieve the desired effect with the least threatening perturbation of other vital functions.

B. Pharmacology and Immunopathology

A knowledge of the pharmacology and toxicity of drugs is important to their most effective use for at least three reasons. First, the mechanism of action of drugs will often determine their utility as a part of a combination as well as their efficacy in different stages of spontaneous disease (or iatrogenic immunosuppression). The schedule of drug administration must be such as to take advantage of periods of susceptibility, e.g., the DNA synthetic phase in the case of pyrimidine antimetabolites, if the drug is to be effective. Second, one must consider the systemic availability of a drug given by various routes, the volume of distribution, and rate and pathways of excretion and metabolism in order to determine proper dosage and route of administration, and in order to appreciate how beneficial and toxic effects may be altered by alterations in organ system function. Finally, for drugs used in combination, one can through pharmacologic and toxicologic study predict whether and at what dose component drugs can be given with safety.

Immunosuppressive drugs can be grouped on the basis of their mechanisms of action, their derivation, or their chemical structure. In general, all these criteria are used in part as in the classification to be followed in this section (Table 1). The resultant outline groups compounds which with a few notable exceptions exhibit similar or identical mechanisms of action with variations

Table 1. Classification of commonly used chemical immunosuppressants

1. Adrenal Corticosteroids
  Hydrocortisone
  Prednisone
  Dexamethasone
	4. Miscellaneous Synthetics
	  Procarbazine
	  Nitrosoureas

2. Alkylating Agents
  Nitrogen mustard
  Cyclophosphamide
  Chlorambucil
  Melphalan
  Busulfan
	5. Natural Products
	  A. Vinca alkaloids
	    vincristine
	    vinblastine
	  B. Antibiotics
	    actinomycin D
	    daunorubicin
	    adriamycin

3. Antimetabolites
  Antipurines
    6-mercaptopurine
    6-thioguanine
    azathioprine
  Antipyrimidines
    cytosine arabinoside
  Antifolates
    methotrexate
	C. Enzymes
	    L-asparaginase

in individual effects dependent largely upon pharmacologic differences. Although in many cases drugs of one class may theoretically appear interchangeable (e.g., corticosteroids or the alkylating agents) there are too few studies conducted to date to establish parity in clinical use, and indeed some studies exist which suggest that effects are distinctive enough to warrant preferences of one drug over another for reasons other than convenience, convention, or familiarity. Examples of this are the demonstration by PETERS *et al.* (1972) of reduced inhibition of inflammatory exudates exhibited by dexamethasone as compared to other adrenal glucocorticoids, the dramatic difference in myelosuppression exhibited by vincristine and vinblastine, and increased duration of effect when the 6-mercaptopurine molecule is substituted at the S position to form azathioprine. Nonetheless, it is logical and convenient to discuss each of the groups listed in Table 1 together, noting in passing the important differences of individual members thereof.

It exceeds the scope of the chapter to discuss the complete list of cancer chemotherapeutic and immunosuppressive drugs; here, only substances of significant practical importance will be mentioned. For a detailed review of additional substances the reader is referred, to other texts (KRUEGER, 1972; CAMIENER and WECHTER, 1972).

I. Adrenocorticosteroids

Adrenocorticosteroids are those steroidal hormones produced by the adrenal cortex from cholesterol. Of the two major subclasses—the mineral corticoids and glucocorticoids—only the latter have significant antiinflammatory and immunosuppressive properties. The major native glucocorticoid is hydrocortisone or pregn-4-3n3-,3,20-dione, 11,17,21-trihydroxy-, (11B)-. It is produced normally in an amount of 25 mg per day under the primary stimulus of pituitary ACTH, and has normal functions which include stimulation of gluconeogenesis and glycogenolysis in liver, interference with the cellular action of insulin and growth hormone, depletion of protein stores, sensitization of blood vessels to adrenergic stimulation, moderate diminution of sodium excretion by the renal tubules, and release of mature blood granulocytes from marrow and peripheral storage areas. Hydrocortisone in pharmacologic concentrations inhibits chemotaxis and the mobilization of circulating polymorphonuclear leukocytes into areas of inflammation (BOGGS *et al.*, 1964). Hydrocortisone is also directly lympholytic to both mature and progenitor lymphoid cells resulting in a reduction of not only circulating blood lymphocytes, particularly of T-lymphocytes, but also a reduction in the T-lymphocyte regions of lymph nodes, spleen, and thymus (DOUGHERTY *et al.*, 1960; YU *et al.*, 1974). It has been claimed that thymocytes and short-lived small lymphocytes are most sensitive to corticosteroid action while long-lived "memory cells" are less so (ERNSTRÖM and LARSSON, 1967; MILLER and COLE, 1967). Cytologically, the administration of corticosteroids is followed by the disintegration of the nuclear membrane of lymphocytes with subsequent chromatinolysis, cytoplasmic bleb formation, and cytoplasmic shedding. When larger doses are given, lymphoreticular tissues become depleted of small lymphocytes and edematous. Secondary follicles are reduced in number, and nuclear-debris macrophages are observed with increasing frequency (starry sky effect). Cessation of corticosteroid action is followed by rapid recovery within a few days (DUSTMANN and STOLPMANN, 1968; CLAESSON and RÖPKE, 1969).

The effects on lymphoreticular tissues are not only the result of lympholysis, but are also due to the shifting of recirculating T-cell subpopulations out of the circulation into the bone marrow. T-cells responsible for delayed hypersensitivity memory reactions are less affected, and at low and/or intermittent doses, delayed skin test responsitivity is retained. In vitro stimulation of lymphocytes is inhibited by corticosteroids. Finally, corticosteroids interfere with uptake of particulate and substrate antigen by the reticuloendothelial system (NETTESHEIM and HAMMONS, 1970).

Immunologically, both primary and secondary antibody responses are suppressed by corticosteroids; this is, however, especially obvious in rodents while man is less sensitive at dose levels normally used. Since lymphocytopenia is probably responsible for the decreased immunological reactivity, corticosteroids need to be administered before the antigenic stimulus, or should be given continously for a longer time (WHITE, 1963; HARRIS, 1970; MANNICK and EGDAHL, 1968; GERMUTH et al., 1952). Besides the specific "anti-immune" effect of corticosteroids, an unspecific anti-inflammatory effect of these substances accounts for the depressed reactivity of an organism against antigenic stimulation. Unlike most immunosuppressants and antineoplastics, glucocorticoids are effective against cells irrespective of whether or not they are in the replicative cycle. However, their activity depends upon the presence of specific membrane receptors for these hormones. Both the number of sites and binding energies differ from cell to cell, explaining the wide variation of steroid effects even within the same tissue and cell type. The corticosteroids do not directly inhibit DNA synthesis, but indirectly reduce both RNA and protein production in susceptible cells.

Many synthetic analogues of hydrocortisol have been prepared, chiefly with the aim of maximizing the anti-inflammatory activity while minimizing complicating metabolic actions. The most commonly used derivatives, prednisone, prednisolone, dexamethasone, methylprednisolone, and triamcinolone all differ from hydrocortisone by desaturation of the linkage between the first and second carbon. Additional modifications have been the addition of a -methyl (dexamethasone) or -OH (triamcinolone) at position 16. These changes have minimized the sodium-retaining activity of the molecule while preserving or enhancing effects on the inflammatory reactions, and on lymphocyte survival and function. However, as noted earlier, there is some evidence for selective changes in the anti-inflammatory effect of dexamethasone, at least in terms of the blood granulocyte migration into areas of inflammation (PETERS, 1972).

All the commonly used glucocorticoids readily cross plasma lipid membranes and are thus efficiently absorbed following oral ingestion. They are widely distributed throughout all tissues including the central nervous system. This latter property, contrasted to the slow passage into the brain and spinal fluid of most immunosuppressive agents, makes glucocorticoids the anti-inflammatory drugs of choice for the control of intracerebral disease. Unconjugated glucocorticoids are poorly soluble in water, but appropriate conjugates are available for parenteral injection by intravenous, intramuscular, intra-articular, and intrathecal routes. Concentrations and dosage of steroid (as with other agents) must be kept low for intrathecal administration to avoid local irritation and convulsions.

Glucocorticoids are transported in plasma largely through loose association with a specific α-globulin carrier, transcortin. The plasma clearance of prednisolone is quite rapid, with a plasma half-life ($T\frac{1}{2}$) of 1–3 hours after intravenous dosage (TALLEY, 1973). Other analogues have somewhat longer half-lives and thus more prolonged effectiveness. Clearance and excretion of these compounds is through a combination of metabolism in the liver followed by excretion chiefly into the urine. Thus, either hepatic or renal dysfunction will influence the duration and intensity of beneficial and adverse effects (see Section C).

II. Alkylating Agents

Alkylating agents were the first drugs shown to interfere with immunologic reactions (HEKTOEN and CORPER, 1921) and certainly remain among the most effective and widely used chemicals for this purpose. Alkylating agents depend for their activity on their modification in vivo to highly reactive nucleophilic (alkyl) groups capable of binding covalently to the phosphate, amine, sulfhydryl, hydroxyl, carboxyl, and imidazole groups of components of biological systems. The most important of these alkylations involves the nitrogen of guanine. Bifunctional alkylating agents can form cross linkages between the 7N of guanines, between guanine and positions 1 or 3 of adenine, or the 6-position oxygen of a second guanine.

In replicating cells alkylating agents appear most active during mitosis and the $G_{1/2}$ interface and are least active during G_2. However, alkylators, as opposed to antimetabolites and most natural product immunosuppressants, are also active against cells not in the replicative (mitotic) cycle. As a result these drugs are either most active when given before the administration of antigen (e.g., nitrogen mustard) or before, during, and after antigen administration (as with cyclophosphamide).

The morphogenic effects of alkylating agents on antibody-forming tissues are similar to those after X-irradiation (radiomimetic effect). Antigenically unstimulated animals show only a mild to moderate depletion of small lymphocytes from lymph nodes, spleen, and thymus with secondary histiocytic activation (phagocytosis of debris). Prominent germinal center necrosis is observed in lymph nodes and spleen of antigenically stimulated individuals. Transformation of lymphocytes (activation) is inhibited in vivo and vitro (ASTALDI et al., 1969; TURK, 1964). After short-term administration of alkylating drugs such as cyclophosphamide, histologic changes in lymphoreticular tissues completely regress except for the presence of a few atypical large and hyperchromatic lymphoid cells.

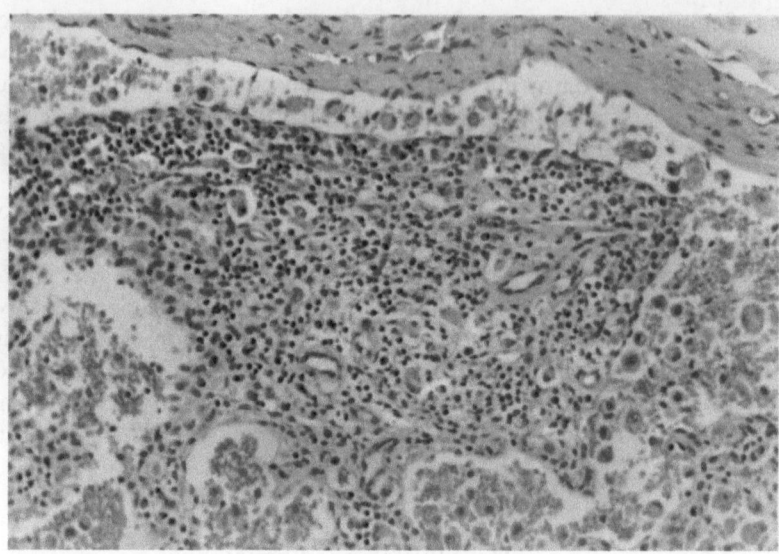

Fig. 1. Lymph node atrophy secondary to sustained cyclophosphamide effects in preparation for bone marrow transplantation: dog. H & E, × 140

Sustained action of alkylating agents lead to severe lymphocytopenia in lymphoreticular tissues with cortical and paracortical atrophy (Fig. 1). Sinus histiocytosis suggests that phagocytosis is not significantly inhibited which was actually demonstrated by a normal carbon-clearance (Zschiesche and Augsten, 1970). Lymphocytopenia comprises both short-lived and long-lived cells, although long-lived cells appear less sensitive to cyclophosphamide effects (Miller and Cole, 1967; Turk and Poulter, 1972). A few persistent lymphoid cells in lymph nodes and spleen show a marked polymorphism and atypia (Fig. 2). Often focal necroses and hemorrhage can be observed following large doses of cyclophosphamide (50–60 mg/kg for a few days). Immunologically, cyclophosphamide was used to induce tolerance toward blood group antigens, to suppress both primary and secondary antibody responses, and to prolong the survival of bone marrow allografts and skin allotransplants (Many and Schwartz, 1970; Karp and Bradley, 1968; Graw et al., 1972). Finally, the local inflammatory response is suppressed by alkylating agents.

Despite their common mechanisms of action, alkylating agents vary considerably in their pharmacology and, as a consequence in their toxicity. Nitrogen mustard is too locally toxic for oral administration. The other compounds are readily absorbed when given by mouth, and cyclophosphamide is frequently given i.m. or i.v.

All alkylating agents are metabolized extensively in vivo. In the case of nitrogen mustard, metabolism is so complete that little or no excretory products other than CO_2 have been identified. Accordingly, this drug can be administered without concern for renal or hepatic function without aggravating its toxic manifestations. Cyclophosphamide (see below), phenylalanine mustard, chlorambucil, and busulfan depend upon the kidneys for excretion of both parent

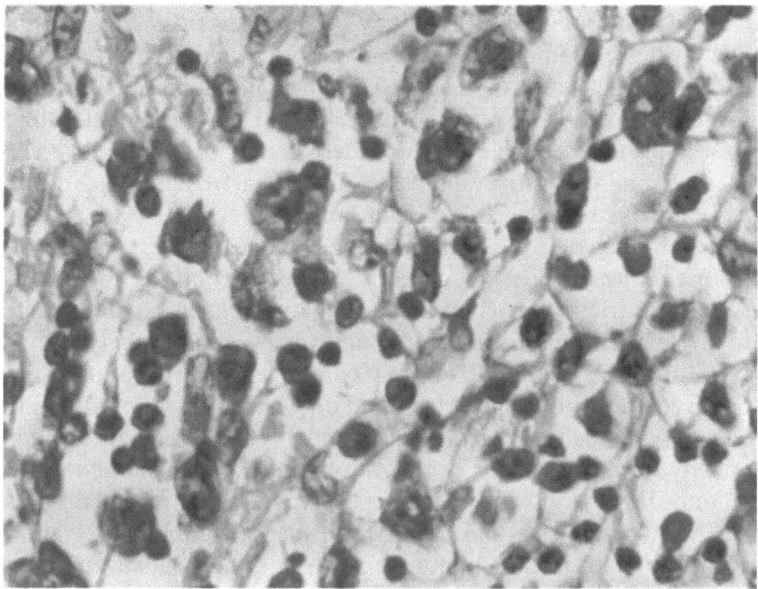

Fig. 2. Lymphoreticular cell polymorphism and atypia secondary to cyclophosphamide treatment:
man. H & E, ×675

compound and metabolites, so caution and, frequently, dose reduction are indicated in patients with renal excretory impairment. With the possible exception
of nitrogen mustard, none of these drugs enters the central nervous system
to any appreciable degree following oral or parenteral administration (see Section C).

Cyclophosphamide (Cytoxan, Endoxan) is unique among alkylating agents
in its requirement to be metabolized to an as yet undefined active derivative,
chiefly by microsomes within the liver. Because of this requirement, the parent
drug has no significant toxicity, is totally safe to handle, and can be given
by any peroral or parenteral route. On the other hand, it is without direct
therapeutic effect when given intrathecally, intraarterially, etc., or when applied
to cells in vitro. Cytoxan is metabolized to a variety of products, many of
which have alkylating activity. These compounds are cleared through the kidney
and retain at least partial activity in the urine.

III. Antimetabolites

The development and clinical introduction of antimetabolites is one of the
most fascinating chapters in medicine. Seeking a substitute for herbs, balms,
elixirs, and other natural toxins, biochemists and physicians joined in an ambi-
tious attempt to "one-up" nature by synthesizing and administering previously
nonexistent chemicals which, by acting as fraudulant substrates, could either
compete for natural enzymes and/or be converted to inappropriate metabolites
which would alter existent cell regulatory and supportive macromolecules. Un-

derstandably, the sought-for specificity of action has rarely been achieved, but in a few instances compounds of great scientific and medical value have been created, including many of the most important antimicrobial, antineoplastic, cardiovascular, renal, and immunosuppressive drugs. Of the latter, methotrexate and azathioprine have achieved the widest clinical use, while mercaptopurine, thioguanine, and cytosine arabinoside have been frequently studied and occasionally employed in specific circumstances. In contrast to adrenal steroids and alkylating agents, the activity of the above antimetabolites is restricted to cells preparing for division, either by killing cells during the period of DNA synthesis or restricting progress through the generative cycle causing reduction in cell division within a tissue or leading to irreversibly imbalanced cell growth (MADOC-JONES and NAURO, 1974). As a consequence the duration of their activity is short-lived following a single dose, and only a small fraction—the proliferating fraction—of a tissue is affected. Understandably then, they are immunosuppressant chiefly during the rapid proliferation phase of the immunologic response which immediately follows antigen exposure. Large or repeated doses will also lead to granulocytopenia and a reduction in both granulocytic and monocyte participation in local inflammatory responses. The relative importance of the latter antigen-processing deficit, and immunocyte proliferation deficit following antimetabolite treatment undoubtedly varies according to dose and individual patient response.

1. Methotrexate

Methotrexate (MTX) is the most widely used folic acid antimetabolite, having utility in acute leukemia, and a variety of solid tumors, psoriasis, transplantation, and certain autoimmune disorders (HARRIS and BAGAS, 1974; WONG and HERSH, 1965; VAN SCOTT et al., 1964). MTX is a weak acid that is relatively insoluble as such, but becomes freely soluble in water as the sodium salt. It is well absorbed by the oral route at low dosage (10 mg or less) though absorption may be erratic and incomplete at higher dosages (HENDERSON et al., 1965b). The drug has only moderate local toxicity and is often administered i.v., i.m., and intrathecally. Once absorbed, it is distributed throughout most of the body water space, with the exception that entry into central nervous tissue, cerebrospinal fluid, and muscle is slow. Following intravenous or oral administration MTX is cleared from the plasma rapidly ($T\frac{1}{2}$ 1.5–2.5 hours) (HENDERSON et al., 1965b; BISCHOFF et al., 1971), the result of tissue distribution and renal clearance. Little of the drug is metabolized in man, and little is excreted in bile (and feces) after a parenteral dose. In rodents, enterohepatic circulation and metabolism by GI bacterial flora is more important (HENDERSON et al., 1965a; BISCHOFF et al., 1971) and as a consequence toxic and therapeutic effects may be altered by the use of gut-sterilizing antibiotics (PREISLER et al., 1971). MTX enters the cell chiefly by a carrier-mediated transport system. At high concentrations passive diffusion may play a major role. Other immunosuppressive agents have been shown in vitro to influence the cellular uptake of the drug, vincristine tending to encourage and corticosteroids to inhibit the transport process (ZAGER et al., 1973).

The intracellular site of action of MTX is dihydrofolate reductase, the enzyme necessary to reduce folic acid to its active coenzyme forms. MTX reversibly but firmly binds to dihydrofolate reductase, decreasing the pool of reduced folates, and thereby inhibiting a variety of chemical reactions. Presumably the most important of these for antiproliferative activity is the methylation of deoxyuridine monophosphate to deoxycytidine monophosphate in the de novo pathway of DNA synthesis. The resultant toxicity can be reversed by thymidine, and more practically for clinical concerns, by the administration of calcium 5-formyl tetrahydrofolate (Calcium Leukovorin).

Immunologically, methotrexate inhibits primarily the 7S antibody response, suppresses cellular immune reactions, and prolongs allograft survival. The immunosuppressive effect of this compound varies markedly with the species investigated: whereas it shows a well-established activity in rats, mice, guinea pigs, and dogs, effects in the rabbit are quite limited (MAKINODAN et al., 1970; SANTOS and OWENS, 1966; RIVAROLA et al., 1967). In man, methotrexate is fairly effectively used to suppress graft-versus-host reaction. In experimental animals, lymphoreticular tissue atrophy is moderate after MTX treatment. Lymphocytes in the lymph node cortex and splenic follicles decrease in number with increasing length of therapy. Also, the thymus becomes moderately to markedly atrophic. When low and intermediate doses of MTX are used over a longer period of time the paracortical tissue of lymph nodes in mice may even become moderately hyperplastic, yet no cellular atypia is observed.

Aminopterin has essentially similar immunosuppressive activities although its therapeutic index is lower than that of MTX. Aminopterin is also immunosuppressive in rabbits.

2. Cytosine Arabinoside

Cytosine arabinoside (ara-C) is an analogue of cytosine which apparently acts to inhibit deoxyribinucleotide polymerase (FURTH and COHEN, 1968). It is poorly incorporated into DNA and retains its effectiveness in cells not dependent upon ribonucleotide reductase for DNA synthesis. Ara-C must be phosphorylated intracellularly to be effective, a step requiring cytidine kinase. It is rapidly deaminated in the presence of cytidine deaminase to uracyl arabinoside, a compound with minimal biological activity. As a consequence the activity of ara-C is markedly influenced by the relative availability of these two enzymes in the various organ systems, and in the plasma and liver.

Ara-C is poorly absorbed from the gastrointestinal tract. However, it can be given with ease and safety by all other conventional routes. It has minimal local toxicity, so that pain and inflammation is rare following i.m., s.c., or i.t. administration. The drug distributes rapidly throughout most aqueous body fluids, and enters the brain and spinal fluid more readily than do methotrexate and the antipurines. However, for optimal effects in CNS tissue, either prolonged intravenous infusion or intrathecal administration are required. Ara-C is rapidly deaminated, the plasma $T_{\frac{1}{2}}$ being about 30 min, and both ara-C and its metabolite ara-U (uracil arabinoside) are promptly excreted by the kidney. Because of the rapidity of its detoxification, ara-C can be given to patients with impaired renal function with greater impunity than is the case with MTX or thiopurines.

For effective immunosuppression, ara-C must be given in multiple doses. It acts apparently on proliferating immunoblastic cells and causes a depressed antibody formation as shown in terms of decreased numbers of plaque-forming cells and in the inhibition of a graft-versus-host reaction (GRAY *et al.*, 1968). Most sensitive to ara-C are cells in DNA synthesis (KESSEL *et al.*, 1969).

3. Antipurines

Of hundreds of synthetic antipurines, only *6-mercaptopurine* (6-MP), *6-thioguanine (6-TG)*, and *azathiopurine* are in wide use. 6-MP and 6-TG find use chiefly in the treatment of acute leukemia. Azathiopurine is most widely employed as an immunosuppressant. Despite extensive study over the last 20 years, the precise mechanism of action of these drugs is still unclear. Both 6-MP and 6-TG must be converted to nucleotides to be active biologically. 6-MP riboside inhibits the conversion of both 5-phosphoribosyl pyrophosphate to 5-phosphoribosylamine and inosinic acid to xanthylic acid and to adenylic acid in the de novo purine synthetic pathway. 6-TG may act in the same way but also competitively inhibits guanine utilization and, unlike 6-MP, is incorporated into RNA and DNA. 6-MP is catabolized by xanthine oxidase to 6-thiouric acid, inorganic sulfate, and a variety of unidentified products. 6-MP is also broken down through methylation and subsequent desulfation. If the vulnerable sulfide is protected by S-substitutions, as in azathiopurine, catabolic deactivation is slowed. Azathiopurine itself acts by being catabolized slowly to 6-MP, and thus serves as a time-release form of 6-MP. 6-TG is catabolized to 6-methylthioguanine and 6-thiouric acid independent of the xanthine oxidase-mediated pathway. Accordingly, while the activity of 6-MP and azathiopurine can be prolonged by the concomitant administration of xanthine oxidase inhibitor (e.g., allopurinol), such inhibitors have no effect on 6-TG metabolism and action.

The metabolism of 6-MP and 6-TG proceeds rapidly in the liver and both the parent compounds and metabolites are excreted chiefly in the urine. The plasma $T\frac{1}{2}$ of the two compounds average 45 and 80 min, respectively (LE PAGE and LOO, 1973; LE PAGE and WHITECAR, 1971). Azathiopurine, following conversion to 6-MP, is handled in an identical fashion. Alterations of hepatic and renal function will influence the toxicity seen with all three compounds.

The three drugs are usually given by mouth, with reasonably consistant and complete absorption. Intravenous forms of 6-MP and 6-TG are available as research drugs, and this formulation is superior when large doses are required or when gastrointestinal dysfunction dictates a parenteral route. 6-MP is too locally toxic to be administered i.m. or i.t. without serious inflammation. These thiopurines do not enter the central nervous system in significant amounts.

The immunosuppressive effect of 6-MP, 6-TG, and azathiopurine is well documented (MAKINODAN *et al.*, 1970). They should be administered during the proliferative phase of the immune reaction, and suppress preferentially the primary antibody response; cellular immune reactions are less effectively influenced, although azathiopurine is used with good results to suppress acute allotransplant rejection (i.e., the cellular phase of allograft rejection) (SCHWARTZ *et al.*, 1958; EPSTEIN and MAYBACH, 1965; SHEHADEH *et al.*, 1970; WINKELSTEIN *et al.*, 1971).

The morphologic changes of lymphoreticular tissues representative of an ongoing immune reaction are not significantly altered by the administration of 6-mercaptopurine: secondary follicles in the lymph node cortex, paracortical pyroninophilic stem cell aggregates ("immunoblastic proliferation"), and plasmacytosis of medullary cords remain uninfluenced. There are species differences in the morphogenic 6-MP effect, however; from dogs to mice to man, there appears a decreasing sensitivity of immunocompetent tissues towards 6-MP.

Sustained azathiopurine (or 6-MP) administration such as in human allotransplant recipients is followed by a moderate to severe lymphocyte depletion of lymph nodes (Fig. 3) and splenic follicles with prominent sinus histiocytosis (the latter representing probably a substitute for the incompetent immune reactivity towards the allograft rather than an immediate reaction to the drug). Discontinuation of short-term therapy with purine antagonists is followed by a masked paracortical proliferation of pyroninophilic blast cells, especially when the individual is immunologically stimulated at the same time.

IV. Vinca Alkaloids

Alkaloids from the periwinkle (*Cantharanthus roseus,* G. Don), first investigated for hypoglycemic properties, were soon known to be myelosuppressive. More recent studies have shown them to be immunosuppressive, and for example, to provide clinical benefit in autoimmune thrombocytopenia (KLENER *et al.,* 1972; AHN *et al.,* 1974). Of the many vinca alkaloids, only two, *vincristine* and *vinblastine* have proved thus far to be of clinical value. These very closely related asymmetrical dimeric indoleindoline compounds have similar pharmacologic properties, and qualitatively similar toxicity. However, in a quantitative

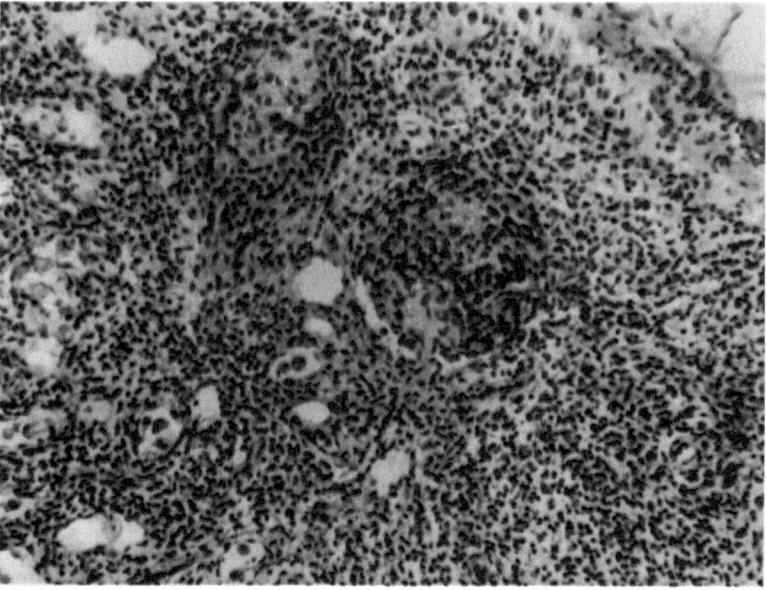

Fig. 3. Lymph node atrophy secondary to sustained azathioprine effects in human renal allotransplant recipient. H & E, × 140

(and practical) sense their side-effects differ markedly, vincristine administration being limited by neurotoxicity and vinblastine by myelotoxicity. Furthermore, the usual weekly dose of vinblastine exceeds that of vincristine by four- to fivefold.

Both vincristine and vinblastine affect cells primarily in the DNA synthesis phase of the cell cycle and cause obvious arrest at the following mitosis. This arrest appears to be the result of disassembly of the microtubular spindle apparatus, a structure which is either missing entirely or appears fragmented or crystallized in vinca alkaloid–treated cells. Although mitotic arrest is the visually striking reflection of vinca alkaloid action, it is not clear that it represents the key antiproliferative effect of these compounds. For example, DNA-dependent synthesis of transfer RNA is increased (Creasey, 1968). There is no known effect of these agents on DNA synthesis, glycolysis, or the synthesis of protein other than microtubular segments.

The vinca alkaloids can be given orally, but since their absorption is erratic and limited by this route, in clinical practice they are given exclusively by the intravenous route. Intravenous injection must be done carefully to avoid painful drug extravasation. Because of technical difficulties, precise pharmacokinetics in humans have never been done adequately and are at best extrapolated from limited animal studies. From these, and from clinical observations, it is clear that the active drug is promptly cleared from the intravascular compartment, and that the major mode of elimination is metabolism and biliary excretion. Hepatic dysfunction apparently aggravates vinca alkaloid toxicity. Enhanced toxicity with concomitant adrenocorticosteroid administration has been reported (Rosner et al., 1975) (see Section C).

Vinca alkaloids inhibit antibody production at toxic doses (Gabrielsen and Good, 1967) and allograft rejection is inhibited as long as an effective serum level of the drug is present. No morphologic changes are known on interphase cells secondary to vincristine and vinblastine administration except for some "roughing" of cell membranes. The effect of these drugs on dividing cells appears to be similar to the effect of radiomimetic agents (i.e., alkylating agents): cytoplasmic and nuclear condensation is observed with disruption of the nuclear membrane and cytoplasmic vacuolization. They have these lesions also in common with other mitotic poisons such as colchicine and podophyllin derivatives. In antigenically stimulated lymph nodes and spleens the formation of secondary follicles may be inhibited.

V. L-Asparaginase

L-Asparaginase is the sole natural enzyme with clinically useful antiproliferative activity. Given intravenously it hydrolyzes exogenous L-asparagine, thus rendering cells incapable of asparagine synthesis deficient in this essential substrate. Certain malignant cells in man and animals, particularly those of lymphoblastic leukemia, are usually deficient in asparagine synthetase, and are thus initially susceptible to the effects of asparaginase. Asparagine synthetase rapidly increases in these cells, so that resistance to the drug rapidly and almost uniformly develops. Although it was hoped, and suggested, from initial clinical trials, that asparaginase might be specific for malignant cells, further trials revealed a multiplicity of side-effects best explained by multiple organ sensitivity to asparagine deprivation.

Most clinical preparations of L-asparaginase are derived from *Escherichia coli,* although enzymes from other sources, notably *Erwinia caratovora,* are also available. These several preparations have virtually identical activity, including toxicity, although they are antigenically distinct. Since the development of humoral antibody to asparaginase is an important cause of both toxicity and lack of effectiveness, these alternate sources of enzyme are of clinical importance when chronic or repeated administration is required.

Asparaginase is completely absorbed intravenously, and slowly absorbed from intramuscular sites. Oral administration is without effect. Once administered the drug remains largely within the plasma, but concentrates to some degree in the liver. Although direct penetration of the central nervous system has not been demonstrated, CNS toxicity and some slight beneficial effect on CNS leukemia has been apparent. At least in part, this CNS action is attributable to depletion of asparagine within nervous tissue (SCHWARTZ *et al.,* 1970). Depending upon the source of asparaginase, its plasma $T\frac{1}{2}$ varies from 8–30 hours. In susceptible cells, which include regenerating liver and PHA-stimulated lymphocytes, asparaginase inhibits mitosis through an as yet undefined mechanism.

Asparaginase has been shown to evoke many forms of immunosuppression, including temporarily decreased antibody production following primary immunization, inhibition of mixed lymphocyte reaction and mitogen stimulation, and suppression of delayed skin hypersensitivity reactions. Clinically and in animals it has been used to reduce graft rejection and to ameliorate the graft-versus-host reaction (GRUNDMANN and OETTGEN, 1970). Secondary humoral immune response appears not to be affected by L-asparaginase. The number of circulating lymphocytes is decreased by the drug. Lymphoreticular tissues contain reduced numbers of small lymphocytes as well, rendering these organs lighter than normal. However, formation of secondary follicles and plasmacytosis post antigenic stimulation are not obviously inhibited by L-asparaginase (ASTALDI *et al.,* 1970).

VI. Miscellaneous Agents

1. Procarbazine

Procarbazine, a methylhydrazine-containing synthetic, has been used for over a decade in cancer therapy, and is also identified as a major immunosuppressive drug (FLOERSHEIM *et al.,* 1975). Procarbazine's mechanism of action remains speculative even after numerous careful studies. Among the suggested bases for activity are alkylation, autooxidation to hydrogen peroxide with resultant peroxidation of DNA and other macromolecules, methylation of tRNA through N-demethylation of procarbazine, and in vivo liberation of formaldehyde. Whatever the mechanism, procarbazine has been shown to inhibit DNA, RNA, and protein synthesis and, in vitro, to degrade DNA.

Procarbazine must be metabolized to be fully active. It is also converted in the liver to both active and inactive metabolites. Procarbazine is readily absorbed following oral administration, and an intravenous preparation is currently under investigation. It distributes rapidly throughout the body, passes freely into the central nervous system, and is rapidly cleared from the plasma ($T\frac{1}{2}$ 8–10 min). The several metabolites are excreted in the urine and, in part, in expired carbon dioxide. This drug has an obvious lymphocytopenic effect, probably secondary to the inhibition of lymphocytopoiesis (Schmähl, 1970). If administered before the antigen, it inhibits humoral and cellular immune responses and prolongs allograft survival (Stock, 1968; Stewart and Cohen, 1969; Stewart and Bell, 1970); its effectiveness, however, varies with the species; whereas immunosuppressive effects were readily demonstrated in rodents, canine allograft rejection was not obviously inhibited (Macdonald et al., 1971).

Histologically, procarbazine administration causes mild to moderate lymphocyte depletion from lymphoreticular tissues accompanied by sinus histiocytosis and some siderosis (hemolysis!).

2. Nitrosoureas

A large number of nitrosourea derivatives have been synthesized as anticancer agents by Montgomery et al. (1970). Many have proved remarkably effective in animal tumor screens and at least three have shown significant activity in clinical trials. These three, the *bis-B-chloroethyl (BCNU)*, *chloroethyl-cyclohexyl* (CCNU), and *methylchloroethylcyclohexyl (MeCCNU) derivatives,* differ slightly in their lipid solubility, pharmacology, and clinical activity, but are in all other respects sufficiently alike to be characterized together.

These compounds are felt to act as alkylating agents (through the formation of vinyl carbonium ions) and/or as inhibitors of de novo purine synthesis. Like most immunosuppressive drugs, their exact mode of action is still unknown. Their toxicity to hematopoietic stem cells is profoundly prolonged, and toxicity is, if anything, more pronounced in nondividing cells (Henderson, 1974; Sensen-brenner, 1972). Nitrosoureas have been shown in experimental systems to lengthen DNA synthesis time (Young and de Vita, 1970), which may contribute to the long duration of observed toxic effects.

Nitrosoureas have rarely been used as immunosuppressives, although they have been used in conjunction with other cytostatics in preparing patients for bone marrow allografts (Herzig et al., 1975). They have been shown in rodents to suppress primary and secondary tumor challenges while not affecting primary antigen recognition (Bonmassar et al., 1969; Einstein et al., 1975). Their chief clinical use remains in the treatment of malignant lymphomas and adenocarcinomas of the gastrointestinal tract.

The substances are highly lipid-soluble, are readily absorbed orally, and distribute rapidly throughout the body including fat, liver, and central nervous system. They are metabolized extensively and the metabolites are excreted largely in urine. Histologically, nitrosoureas cause a generalized atrophy of lymphoreticular tissues which is initiated by loss of lymphocytes from the lymph node cortex and splenic follicles. Severe lymphoreticular atrophy may be accompanied by focal hemorrhage.

3. Cytostatic Antibiotics

Although antineoplastic antibiotics are now rarely used in clinical immunosuppression, they are all immunosuppressive through interference with cell proliferation and protein synthesis. *Dactinomycin* (actinomycin D) is widely used in cancer therapy, and is a fundamental component in the curative treatment of Wilms's tumors. *Daunorubicin* is one of the most active drugs against acute leukemia, and its closely related anthracycline congener, *adriamycin,* is highly effective against a broad spectrum of human carcinomas and sarcomas. All three exert these biological effects through the formation of tenacious complexes with macromolecules, including DNA. Once intercalated to DNA molecules they inhibit both DNA replication and RNA transcription.

All three antibiotics are poorly absorbed when given orally. All must be given by careful intravenous infusion, since extravascular injection results in severe local inflammation and necrosis. Once administered, dactinomycin is cleared from the circulation within minutes. Daunorubicin and adriamycin exit more slowly, with initial plasma $T\frac{1}{2}$ of 45 min and 115 min, respectively, and significant blood levels of active drug are maintained for several days (LENAZ *et al.,* 1971; BENJAMIN *et al.,* 1973) in the case of adriamycin. Dactinomycin is minimally metabolized, whereas the anthracyclines undergo extensive metabolism. Excretion of unchanged dactinomycin and adriamycin is almost entirely through the biliary-gastrointestinal pathway (BENJAMIN *et al.,* 1973), whereas both native and metabolized daunorubicin appear chiefly in the urine and only secondarily in bile.

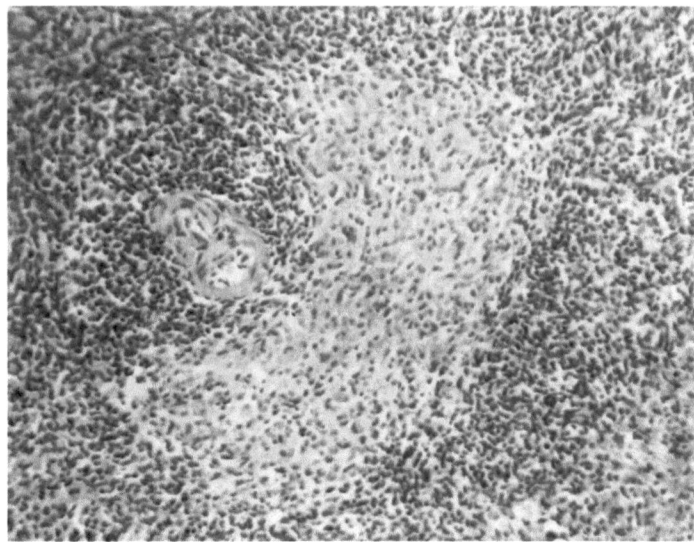

Fig. 4. Actinomycin D effect on spleen of immunologically stimulated mouse: note replacement of secondary follicle by fibroreticular cells. H & E, × 120

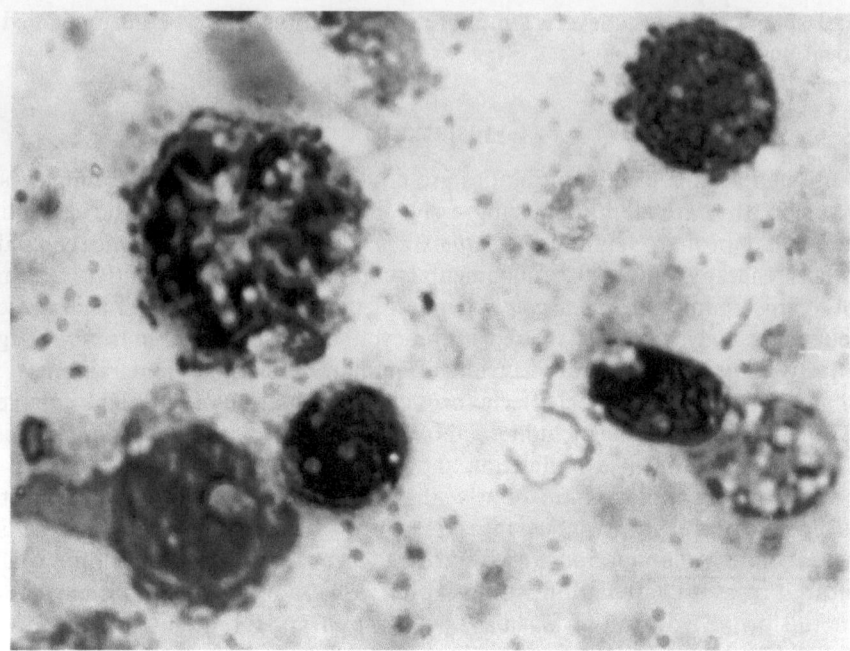

Fig. 5. Daunomycin effect on lymphocytes in culture; note blastic transformation and degeneration of cells with one cell in mitosis. May-Grünwald-Giemsa, × 170

Immunologically, both primary and secondary antibody responses to sheep erythrocytes are suppressed by *dactinomycin;* also, the morphogenesis of a cellular immune reaction is inhibited when the drug is administered shortly after the antigen (Kolin and Landy, 1970; Jennings, 1969). Secondary follicles after antigenic stimulation of immunocompetent tissues are decreased in number by actinomycin probably secondary to a cytotoxic effect on blast cells in the follicle. Already present secondary follicles become depleted of pyroninophilic blast cells rendering this structure a primarily reticulohistiocytic nodule (Fig. 4). Reconstitution of lymphoid follicles occurs within a few days when administration of the drug is discontinued.

Daunomycin, which is readily taken up by lymphoreticular tissues, prolongs skin allograft survival in mice. Even lower doses of the drug cause degeneration of lymphocytes and basophilic stem cells ("immunoblast" type) (Fig. 5) as visualized by cytoplasmic vacuolization, nuclear chromatinolysis, and karyorhexis (Massimo, 1970). Lymphocyte transformation is inhibited (Costa and Astaldi, 1964). Adriamycin, an analogue of daunomycin, has less severe toxic effects.

VII. Antilymphocyte Sera (ALS)

The potential value of ALS for immunosuppression was long anticipated, yet it was only about 10 years ago that it was actually proved. Today it is probably the most specific immunosuppressant with the least toxicity (CAMIENER and WECHTER, 1972).

There are several types of antilymphocyte sera; depending upon the source of antigen, we refer to antilymphocyte serum as such, gained from immunization of animals with mixed (T- and B-) lymphocytes, antithymocyte serum (ATS) obtained from immunization with thymocytes (predominantly T-cells), and specific anti-T-cell serum obtained from immunization with thymocytes or T-cell suspensions from other sources (e.g., from T-cell lymphomas) with subsequent exhaustive absorption of minor antileukocyte and antierythrocyte specificities.

Besides whole cells from thymus, peripheral blood, thoracic duct, lymph nodes or spleen, subcellular fractions served as antigens for the preparation of antilymphocyte sera such as cell membranes and microsomes.

The toxicity of ALS appears especially low when prepared from thoracic duct cells or purified thymic cell suspensions (BACH et al., 1970; STERLIN et al., 1970).

Radiolabeled anti-mouse thymocyte globulin is localized upon i.v. injection in thymus, lymph nodes, spleen, lungs, liver, and kidney (HINTZ and WEBER, 1965; NAVA et al., 1969; LANCE, 1969). This pattern of ATS uptake, however, is probably not representative for the localization of specific ATS since up to 95 percent of the immune globulins in ALS or ATS are nonspecific, and these immune globulins may mask the selective localization of specific ATS or ALS.

When immunocompetent tissues are investigated, antilymphocyte globulin (ATG) is concentrated in the paracortical region of lymph nodes within 2 hours post i.p. injection; at about the same time it is observed in the peripheral follicular area of the spleen. The thymus shows a moderate diffuse retention of ATG (LANCE, 1969). Within the next 4 hours, paracortical ATG increases in lymph nodes, enters the intermediate zone of the splenic follicle, and also increases in concentration in the thymus. After the subsequent 2 days ATG decreases again in the lymphoreticular tissues without changing significantly its pattern of distribution.

The preferential effect of ALS is suggestively mediated by its influence on recirculating lymphocytes and by inhibiting the homing of these cells (LANCE, 1970; TAUB and LANCE, 1972). The immunosuppressive activity of ALS, ATS, and ATG is measured according to several parameters: survival of allografts is prolonged, graft-versus-host reaction is suppressed, cellular immune reactions (i.e., delayed hypersensitivity reactions) are inhibited, growth of induced and transplanted tumors is enhanced, and disseminated infections are facilitated (MONACO et al., 1966; LEVEY and MEDAWAR, 1966; PICHLMAYR, 1966; MATHÉ et al., 1971; KRUEGER et al., 1975; ALLISON and LAW, 1968; VREDEVOE and HAYS, 1969; HIRSCH and MURPHY, 1968). In addition, ALS may show antimacrophage activity, opsonizing potentials, and depression of allogeneic inhibition (MACLAURIN and HUMM, 1970; GILL, 1969; FISHER et al., 1970). There is little effect on humoral immune reactions or on the anamnestic immune response. Histologically, lymphoreticular tissues show lesions after repeated ALS administration which resemble to some extent those after neonatal thymectomy (KRUEGER, 1972). As described above, its overall distribution in these tissues

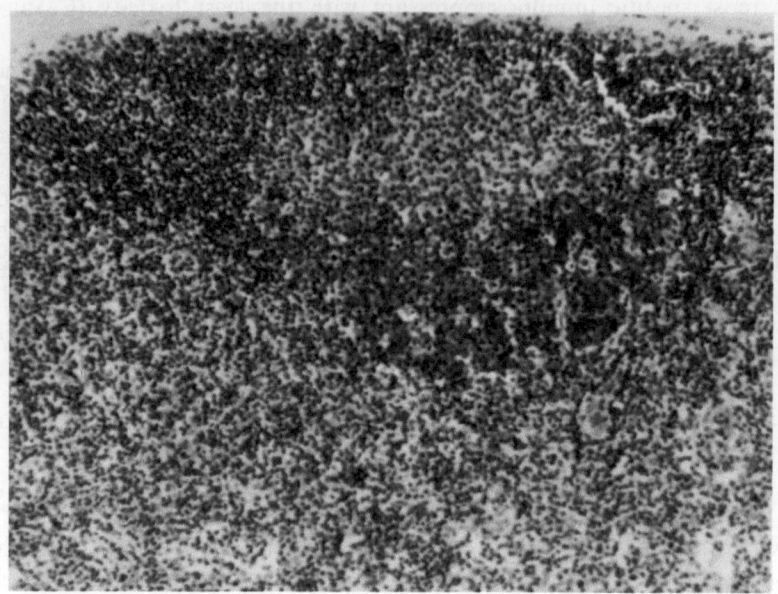

Fig. 6. Lymph node of patient treated with repeated doses of ALS; note combined paracortical atrophy and follicular activation. H & E, ×150

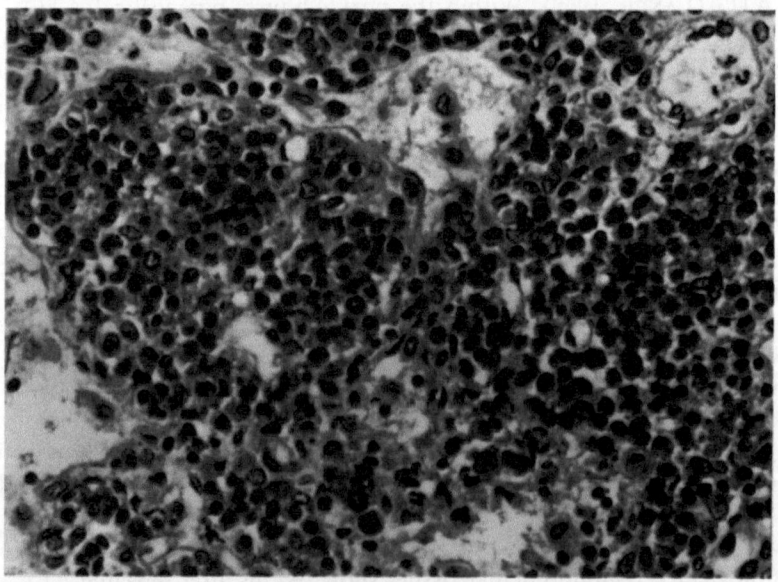

Fig. 7. Severe plasmacytosis of medullary cords of a lymph node in mouse treated with repeated doses of ALS. H & E, ×380

approximates closely that of a proteinaceous antigen (which ALS practically does represent). Morphologic changes usually become apparent 8 hours post ALS administration. Paracortical lymphocytes in the lymph node disintegrate followed by hypertrophy and mild hyperplasia of macrophages with the formation of debris-laden macrophages. If ALS action persists for a longer time, paracortical atrophy results (Fig. 6). This atrophy, however, is accompanied by lymphocytic stimulation with the formation of secondary follicles, basophilic stem cells ("immunoblasts"), and progressive plasmacytosis of medullary cords (Fig. 7). These lesions suggest derivation from stimulation by the antigen ALS (foreign protein!). In the other lymphoreticular tissues, especially in the spleen, corresponding lesions are noted which essentially consist in an atrophy of the T-cell area (centrifollicular region of the spleen) and activation with hyperplasia of the B-cell area (intermediate follicular zone and peritrabecular region of the spleen). Also, the diffuse white pulp of the spleen becomes hyperplastic in rodents, monkeys, and man.

C. Toxicology and Adverse Effects

Few review articles and monographs are available on the general pathology of side-effects of drugs. One such is *Iatrogene Pathologie* by THURNER (1970). A quite extensive coverage of clinical syndromes and diseases induced by drugs is presented by MEYLER (1958–1972) and by MEYLER and PECK (1965, 1968, 1972). For additional information the reader is referred to the *Registry of Tissue Reactions to Drugs,* American Registry of Pathology, Armed Forces Institute of Pathology, Washington, D.C., USA.

In the following sections side-effects of the drugs discussed in this chapter are summarized.

I. Adrenocorticosteroids

The adverse effects of glucocorticoids are legion, and vary depending upon the dosage and chronicity of treatment. Acute large doses of steroids cause hyperglycemia by way of increased gluconeogenesis; and flush, hypertension, and reflex bradycardia by virtue of sodium retention and direct sensitization of vascular smooth muscle to pressor amines. Both gastric hyperchlorhydria and gastrin secretion are stimulated, and as a result gastritis and ulceration is more frequent in patients receiving steroids. Acute and chronic administration cause fluid retention and weight gain in persons with initially normal adrenal function, while at the same time increasing plasma volume, renal plasma flow, globular filtration rate, and clearance of organic acids such as endogenous creatinine and uric acid. Persistent glucocorticoid administration of certain large dose causes lipid depletion from the adrenal cortex with cortical atrophy and storage of birefringent substances (LIEBEGOTT, 1953).

Hematologic changes include an increased hematocrit, granulocytosis, and thrombocytosis associated with an absolute decrement in circulating lymphocytes and eosinophils.

Glucocorticoids lower the brain threshold for neuroexitation, and as a consequence both acute and chronic glucocorticoid administration can result in emotional lability and, rarely, frank psychosis. Sudden withdrawal is regularly attended by some degree of depression whether or not metabolic alterations in mineral balance or energy production can be documented.

Chronic administration regularly reduces protein synthesis and induces protein catabolism resulting in negative nitrogen balance, muscular wasting, and osteoid depletion. Since renal clearance of calcium is enhanced to a greater extent than clearance by the gastrointestinal tract is reduced, significant osteoporosis is a common result of prolonged administration.

Depending on dosage, signs and symptoms of hyperadrenocorticism (Cushing's syndrome) may appear with moon facies, hirsutism, acne, and weakness. Withdrawal of chronic drug administration may leave the patient hypersusceptible to stress for up to a year or more, and he may need adrenocortical supplementation for surgery or severe illness to avoid the consequences of hypoadrenocorticism.

Rare complications of steroid administration include pseudotumor cerebri, syncope and collapse; purpura secondary to vasculitis, posterior cataracts, compulsive hyperphagia, and myocardopathy.

Secondary severe problems associated with chronic steroid administration are tied to the very anti-inflammatory and immunosuppressive actions for which they are prescribed. Both primary infection and exacerbation of latent pathogens, particularly viruses (*Herpes simplex, H. zoster,* etc.), fungi and tubercle bacilli, are not uncommon with long-term steroid administration.

In virtually all cases alternate-day dosing will reduce the incidence and severity of toxicity, while maintaining, at least in the area of anti-inflammatory activity, an efficacy comparable to daily dosing (FAUCI and DALE, 1975; MAC GREGOR et al., 1969).

Steroids freely pass the placental barrier so that during pregnancy the effects cited above will be manifest in the fetus (or newborn) as well. Fetal wastage is high, as is the incidence of specific defects such as cleft palate (CAPIZZI, 1972). Adrenal insufficiency is potentially fatal, but correctable, in newborn offspring of mothers receiving steroids. These infants will exhibit the classic features of Addisonian crisis: hypotension, fever, weakness, eosinophilia, reduced free water clearance by the kidney, and hyperglycemia. Alertness to the diagnosis and prompt replacement therapy may be life saving.

To date, adrenocorticosteroids have not been shown to be carcinogenic per se. Whether their use, or the use of any immunosuppressive agent or procedure, encourages the inception or spread of malignancy remains speculative in man.

II. Alkylating Agents

All alkylating agents in their active form are toxic to rapidly replicating tissues in general, and to blood cell precursors in particular. Bone marrow toxicity is the limiting toxicity in virtually every case requiring reduction of dosage or interruption of drug administration. Although their time of exposure to sensitive cells varies from minutes to a few hours, the results of this exposure may be manifest for days and weeks, and all alkylating agents exert dose-related damage to bone marrow precursors of all types, which, in conventional dosages, causes in reticulocytopenia, granulocytopenia, lymphocytopenia, and, in most cases, thrombocytopenia. High dose and/or chronic administration will prolong these effects and lead to anemia. Anemia and thrombocytopenia can be readily controlled by transfusions of red blood cells and platelets. Granulocytopenia is corrected with greater difficulty and represents the most serious acute and chronic toxic problem. Table 2 lists the usual duration of granulocytopenia following alkylating agent therapy. The increased risk of bacterial and fungal infection ordinarily becomes progressively more significant as granulocyte levels fall below 1,000 per cu mm (Bodey et al., 1966). At lower levels the local inflammatory response becomes impaired (Hersh et al., 1966a; Boggs, 1960) and marrow granulocyte reserves are depleted Vogel (1967). Figures 2, 5, 7, and 9 show the effect of exessive doses of *cyclophosphamide* on bone marrow, spleen, and lymph nodes. Both the degree and duration of granulocytopenia correlate with the incidence of infection, and both are a direct function of the drug dose administered. This predilection to infection is aggravated by the concomitant reduction of immune competence.

Other rapidly replicating organ systems vary in their susceptibility to individual drugs. Thus, *nitrogen mustard* and *cyclophosphamide* cause nausea and vomiting through mucosal irritation within 4–12 hours in almost all patients, and the latter drug in addition causes reversible loss of hair in over 80 percent of patients treated. With the orally administered *phenylalanine mustard, chlorambucil*, and *busulfan* by contrast, alopecia, nausea, and vomiting are rare and generally inconsequential side-effects.

Other, relatively rare, drug-specific toxicities are occasionally observed. High doses of *nitrogen mustard*, particularly when given by the intracarotid route,

Table 2. Duration of granulocytopenia following immunosuppressive drug therapy

	Recovery from Granulopenia (weeks)		Recovery from Granulopenia (weeks)
Alkylating Agents		Antimetabolites	
Nitrogen mustard	2 4	Methotrexate	2–4
Cyclophosphamide	3–5	Mercaptopurine	2–4
Melphalan	3- 5	Thioguanine	2 4
Busulfan	3 -8	Cytarabine	2- 3
Nitrosoureas	5- 12	Antibiotics	
		Actinomycin	2–5
		Daunorubicin/adriamycin	2–4

can cause severe central nervous system toxicities manifested by hyperpyrexia, convulsions, and coma (BETHLENFALVAY and BERGIN, 1972; WEISS et al., 1974). Nitrogen mustard is in addition highly reactive in solution and causes local necrosis if extravasated accidently during intravenous or intrarterial infusion, and severe vesication when it comes in contact with the skin or mucous membranes. Accordingly, great care must be exercised by the therapist to prevent injury to himself and his patient. Should accidental extravascular injection occur, the area should be immediately injected (or washed) in normal saline to dilute the drug, and, if available, sodium thiosulfate should be locally applied as a neutralizing substrate for the alkylating groups.

As indicated before, *cyclophosphamide* is metabolized to a variety of compounds which are excreted through the kidney and retain their alkylating activity in the urine. For this reason, the entire urinary tract epithelium is exposed to these toxic metabolites, and local inflammation is common. Dysuria and hematuria are frequent complaints, and, since the toxicity is directly related to the concentration of metabolites in the urine, are more common and severe when large doses are administered and when urine flow is reduced. Since cyclophosphamide administration reduces the renal clearance of water (DE FRONZO et al., 1973) and thus acts as an antidiuretic, it is important to provide a large fluid load, to encourage frequent voiding during the 24 hours following each dose, and if necessary to administer furosemide to insure a high urine flow and a dilute urine. Exessive cyclophosphamide doses, such as those used for the ablation of lympho- and hematopoiesis in preparation for bone marrow transplantation, cause severe edema and hemorrhage in the bladder mucosa (Fig. 8) progressing to diffuse hemorrhagic urocystitis with mucosal loss. The repetitive acute toxicity associated with long-term cyclophosphamide treatment will occasionally result in bladder fibrosis, apparently from organization of

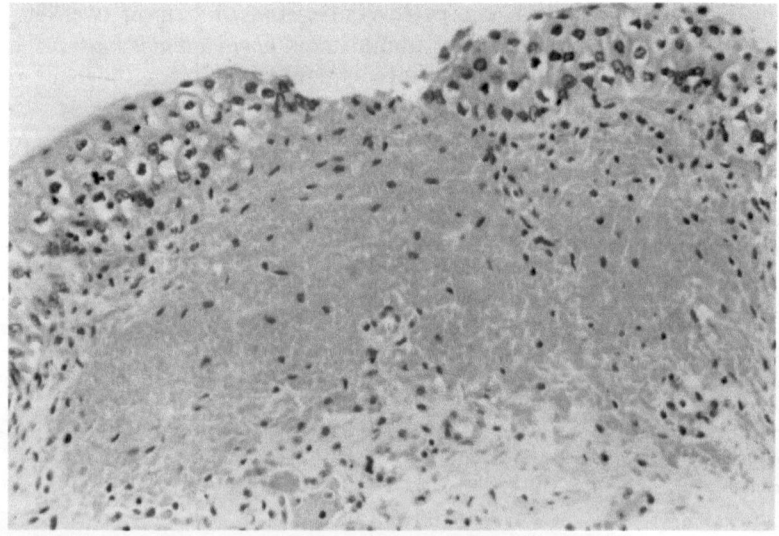

Fig. 8. Hemorrhage and edema of bladder mucosa with focal epithelial loss secondary to cyclophosphamide treatment: dog. H & E, ×150

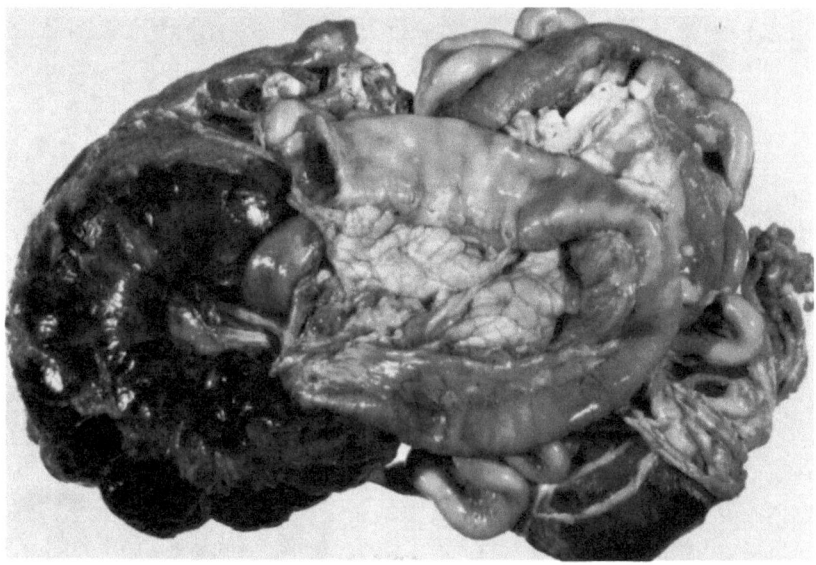

Fig. 9. Intestines of dog with severe hemorrhagic enteritis and intussusception secondary to single dose of cyclophosphamide (100 mg/kg)

chronic edema. Hemorrhagic mucositis is also observed following large-dose cyclophosphamide treatment in the dog (100 mg/kg, one dose); intestinal hemorrhage can be so exessive that blood clots within the intestinal lumen cause intussusception, ileus, and death of the dog (Fig. 9). Microscopically, extensive mucosal and submucosal necroses are accompanied by hemorrhage which may involve all layers of the intestinal wall. The extreme dosages of cyclophosphamide used in preparation for bone marrow transplantation have on occasion led to myocardial necrosis in dogs and in man (BUCKNER *et al.*, 1972; SANTOS, 1974). This becomes especially obvious when the radiomimetic agent cyclophosphamide is combined with therapeutic doses of X-irradiation, or with other cytotoxic agents (BUJA *et al.*, 1973). Histologically one finds necrobiotic muscle cells with multiple contraction bands, diastase-resistant PAS staining, and intracellular fibrin deposits. Vascular microthrombi appear, and the perivascular space contains a hemorrhagic and fibrinous exudate. In addition, nuclear alterations can be seen by electron microscopy: normal chromatin pattern is replaced by a pale fibrous and filamentous material (Fig. 10a–d). The described pathology of combined large-dose cyclophosphamide treatment and therapeutic X-irradiation is at least partially caused by degenerative and necrotic vascular changes. Other organ systems may show severe lesions following this therapy such as hemorrhagic pneumonitis, progressive pulmonary fibrosis (Fig. 11), and centrilobular hepatic necrosis (Fig. 12). We have observed such lesions both in dogs and in man.

Disseminated intravascular coagulation has also been observed post cyclophosphamide treatment (see Fig. 10b, c). The pathophysiology of these toxicities remains obscure.

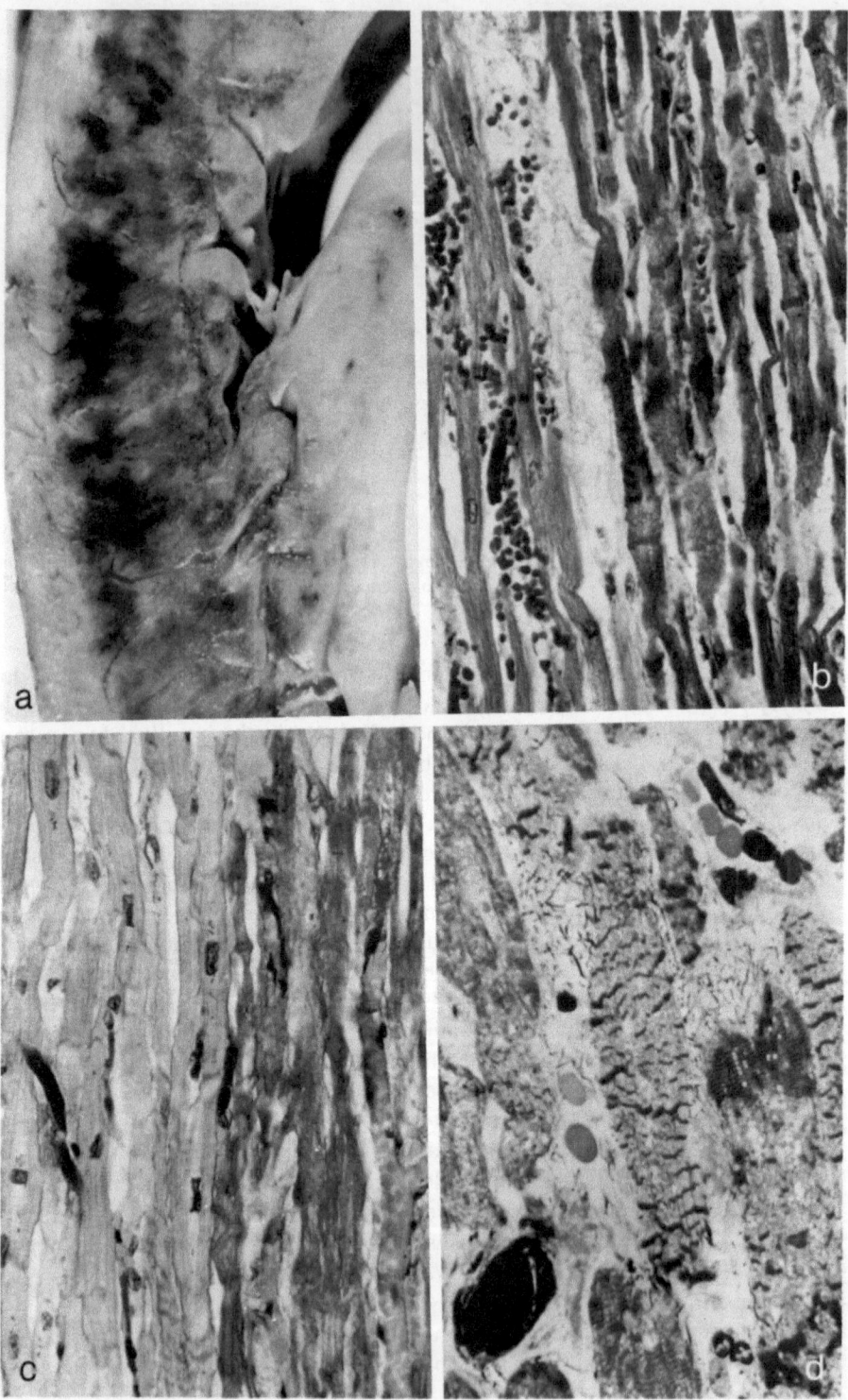

Fig. 10a–d.

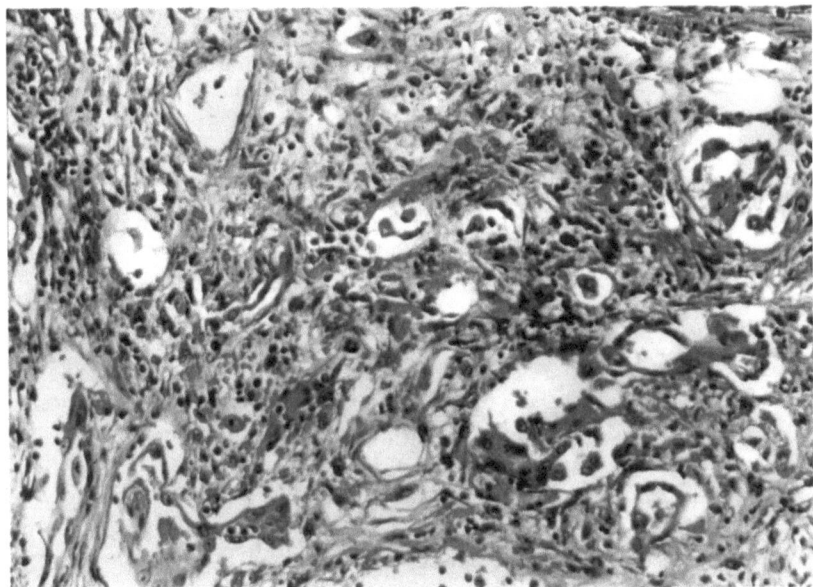

Fig. 11. Severe progressive pulmonary fibrosis in patient with bone marrow allotransplantation and combined cyclophosphamide-radiation therapy. H & E, × 140

Busulfan also causes bizarre side-effects of unclear causation. Weight loss, skin hyperpigmentation, weakness, and diarrhea occasionally form a syndrome mimicking Addison's disease. Adrenocortical function has been shown to be normal in some of these cases (KYLE *et al.*, 1961), whereas in others selective inhibition of ACTH production has been documented (VIVAQUA *et al.*, 1967). Chronic administration has also been associated with gynecomastia, pulmonary fibrosis (SMALLEY and WALL, 1966), and, in one report (WEINBERGER *et al.*, 1975), endocardial fibrosis.

Although alarming, these special side-effects are of much less clinical significance than the risk, apparent in some degree in virtually all alkylating agent-treated patients, of myelosuppression, immunosuppression, chromosomal damage, and gonadal injury. These effects underlie the increased incidence of severe and occasionally mortal infection, the increased incidence of neoplasia, the infertility, fetal wastage, and teratosis which are not infrequent sequelae of these and other forms of chemical immunosuppression.

◁ Fig. 10 a–d. Extensive myocardial necrosis secondary to cyclophosphamide treatment. Patient died unexpectedly of cardiac failure post-bone marrow allotransplantation. a Grossly the inner two-thirds of the myocardium show hemorrhagic necroses. b and c Microthrombi, interstitial edema with mild hemorrhage, necrobiotic muscle cells with multiple contraction bands (H & E, × 300; c diastase-PAS; × 300). d Degenerating muscle fibers with irregular loss of cross striations (semithin section, alkaline toluidine blue n, × 750. (Figs. 10a d were kindly provided by Prof. L.M. BUJA)

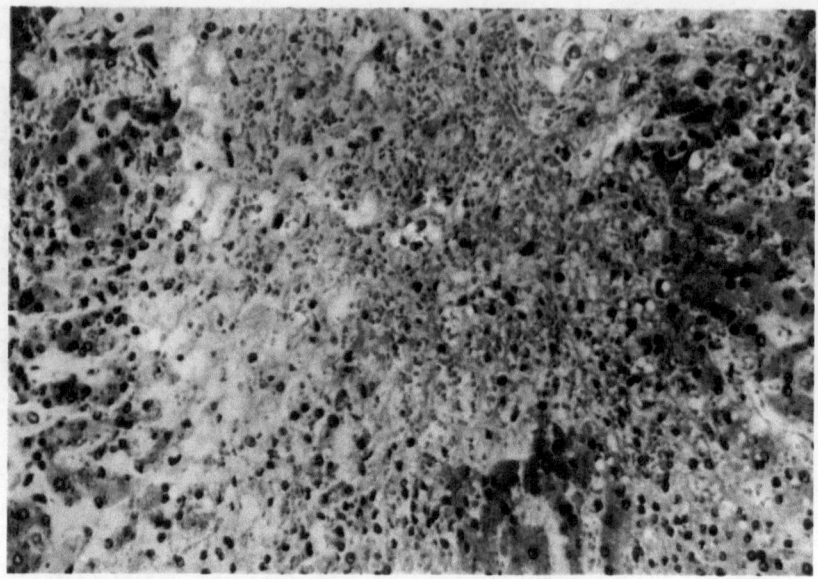

Fig. 12. Severe centrilobular hepatic necrosis in patient with bone marrow allotransplantation and combined cyclophosphamide-radiation therapy. H & E

III. Antimetabolites

1. Methotrexate

The toxicity of *methotrexate* (MTX) is apparent chiefly in the bone marrow, gastrointestinal crypt cells, hair follicles, and—when present—products of conception. Myelosuppression is rapid in onset and rapid in repair, the maximal effect occurring within a week of a single large dose, with complete recovery 1–2 weeks later. MTX affects all marrow cell lines so that some degree of pancytopenia is observed with most dosage schedules. Mild to severe stomatitis is seen in some patients with a degree of unpredictability, which makes careful observations and dose adjustment necessary. Diarrhea is rare except when high prolonged plasma concentrations result from high doses, continuous infusion, and/or impaired renal function.

Less common toxicities include clinically significant hepatic toxicity (liver enzyme elevations are the rule after doses of 10 mg/m² or more, but are usually rapidly reversible), maculopapular skin eruptions, and splenic pain. Hepatic toxicity has usually been clinically reversible following discontinuance of MTX (Hersh *et al.*, 1966; Sharp *et al.*, 1969). Histologic lesions are usually mild and consist of a fine vacuolar fatty degeneration of hepatocytes (primarily centrilobular) and scattered ceroid-laden macrophages suggestive of hepatocellular necrosis (single cell necrosis). Occasionally Councilman's bodies may be seen (Fig. 13). Portal fibrosis is also occasionally seen and an alarming incidence of portal cirrhosis has been observed in patients receiving MTX for psoriasis

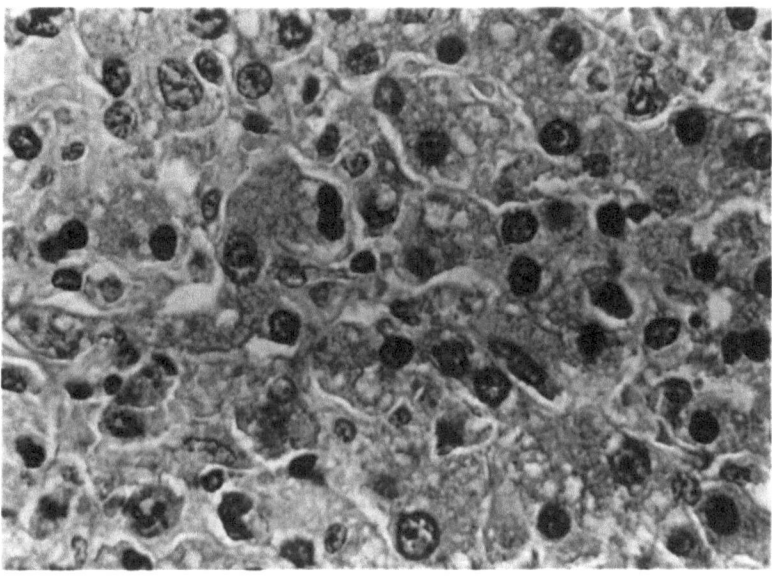

Fig. 13. Mild to moderate fatty degeneration of hepatocytes secondary to methotrexate treatment:
dog. H & E, ×600

(ROENIGK *et al.*, 1972; DAHL *et al.*, 1971). Since excessive alcohol intake and cirrhosis are common in psoriatic populations, the precise role of MTX remains unclear. We can observe portal fibrosis in experimental dogs that received MTX only, yet cirrhosis does not occur in these animals.

Central nervous system toxicity is not uncommon following intrathecal administration. Arachnoiditis with pain, meningismus, and localized neuropathy, and less commonly transverse myelitis, paraplegia, convulsions, and demyelinating encephalopathy has been noted (SAIKI *et al.*, 1972; WEISS, 1974). The latter extreme and usually irreversible complication has also been observed when very high concentrations of MTX are achieved by intravenous or intraarterial infusion (DJERASSI *et al.*, 1967). High-dose MTX has also proved to be directly toxic to renal tubules (CONDIT, 1969). Slight cloudy swelling with focal necrobiosis of epithelial cells in proximal tubules may be observed as well as vacuolar (fatty) degeneration of distal tubules (Fig. 14). Since excretion of the drugs depends on glomerular and tubular function, and since toxicity is inversely related to the rate of renal clearance, MTX-induced nephrotoxicity can initiate a vicious cycle of increasing intoxication. MTX should not be given to patients with creatinine clearances of 30 ml/min (corrected to 1.73 m^2 body surface area) or less and should be given with caution to anyone with a $C_{creat} < 60$ ml/min. If overdosing does occur, with or without renal function impairment, citrovorum factor should be given promptly and repeated at 6–8-hour intervals until methotrexate levels have fallen below the toxic range (as long as 1 week in extreme cases). Chronic methotrexate administration induces both granulopoietic and immunologic function, and thus it is not suprising that a variety of infections

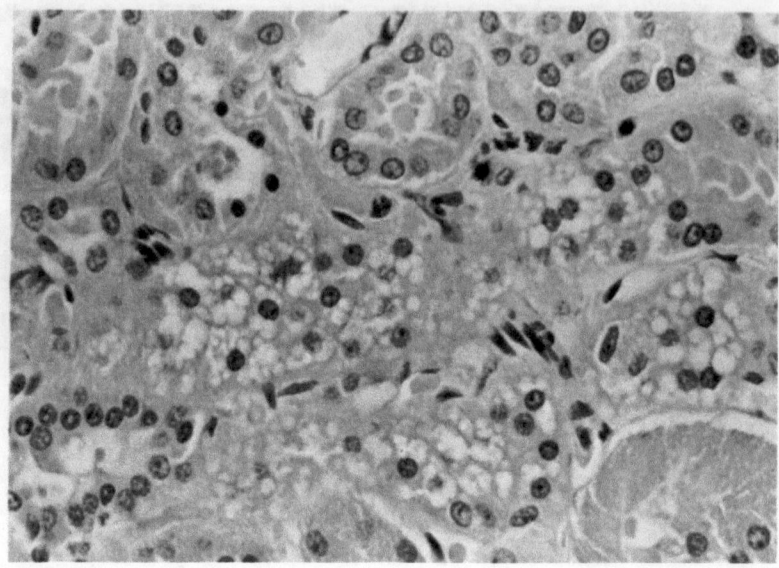

Fig. 14. Focal vacuolar (fatty) degeneration of distal tubules secondary to methotrexate treatment:
dog. H & E, × 380

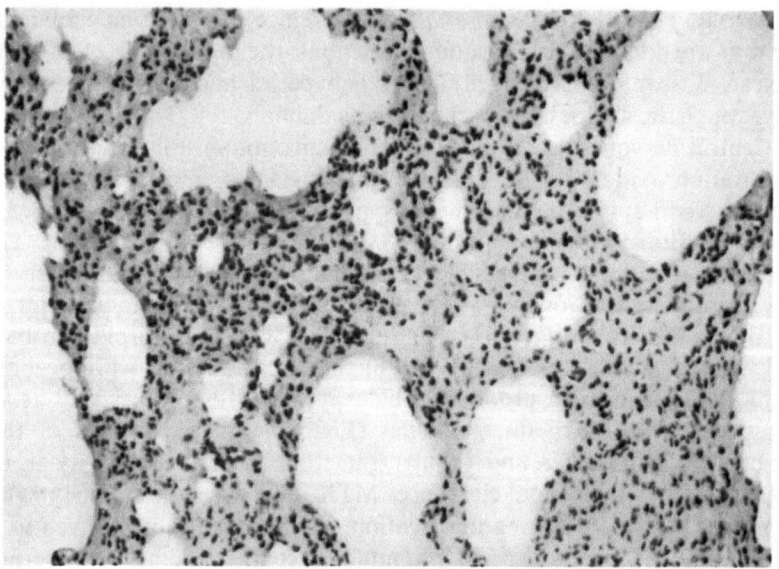

Fig. 15. Pulmonary abacterial inflammation and fibrosis secondary to methotrexate treatment:
dog. H & E, × 150

have been reported. There is evidence that MTX induces bronchial mucosal metaplasia and reduces ciliary function which may account for the relatively high incidence of some pulmonary infections. In addition to fungal, viral, and bacterial etiologies, there have been many cases of *Pneumocystis carinii* pneumonias (see below) in patients receiving MTX, as well as diffuse pulmonary inflammation, for which no microbial etiology could be assigned (CLARYSSE *et al.*, 1969; Acute Leukemia Group B 1969; RAWBONE, 1971) (Fig. 15).

MTX is one of the most powerful abortifacients in existence, and regularly causes fetal wastage or malformations when administered to mothers in the first trimester of pregnancy. Great care must be taken in women of reproductive age to rule out pregnancy before institution of MTX treatment, and to prevent conception during the period of its administration (CAPIZZI, 1972). When early pregnancy is diagnosed in a patient receiving MTX, its termination should be strongly considered and at the very minimum the potential risks of fetal malformation should be discussed with the parents.

2. Cytosine arabinoside

Ara-C toxicity is extremely schedule-dependent. Truly massive doses (3 g/m^2 and more) can be given as a single injection with minimal resultant toxicity. By contrast, prolonged infusion, even with low dosages, is profoundly toxic to the bone marrow. Severe toxicity is virtually restricted to myelosuppression. Reticulocytopenia, granulocytopenia, and thrombocytopenia occur soon after a course of therapy (within 5–7 days) and are rapidly reversible when the drug is discontinued. Mild to moderate anorexia, nausea, occasional vomiting, and reversible alopecia are the only other anticipated side-effects. Ara-C generally causes no overt evidence of liver toxicity. However, a rare patient can be shown to develop toxic hepatitis after even a minimal dose of ara-C (GOODELL, 1971) and liver enzyme elevations with and without hyperbilirubinemia are not uncommon in patients with antecedent liver disease. Intrathecal ara-C may cause headache and meningeal irritation similar to but generally less severe than that seen following the intrathecal administration of MTX (SAIKI *et al.*, 1972).

3. Purine antagonists

The toxicity associated with *6-MP* and *6-TG* is similar. Bone marrow function is regularly reduced, with marrow hypoplasia following large doses. Nausea and anorexia are also common, while vomiting and stomatitis occur less regularly. The drugs are toxic to the liver, and may lead to periportal fibrosis. Acute hepatic toxicity is accompanied histologically by microfocal hepatocellular necroses, cholestasis, and by a mild portal inflammatory reaction.

Rarer complications include alopecia, and generalized skin rash. High doses of 6-MP given intravenously have caused urticaria and pain along the course of the injected vein, and nephrotoxicity with hematuria secondary to the intratubular precipitation of 6-MP crystals (DUTTERA *et al.*, 1972).

IV. Vinca Alkaloids

Vinblastine even at low doses causes myelosuppression with resultant granulocytopenia, thrombocytopenia, and, with repetitive doses, anemia. Alopecia is also frequent. Central and peripheral nervous system side-effects, similar to those described subsequently for vincristine, also occur, but these are usually less severe at therapeutic doses.

Vincristine (VCR) can also cause myelosuppression in patients with antecedent bone marrow injury and/or hepatic dysfunction. Usually, however, neurotoxic side-effects curtail vincristine administration before bone marrow toxicity becomes a clinical concern (Sandler et al., 1969). The neurotoxicity of VCR is both dose- and schedule-related. The drug is rapidly toxic, and is toxic at lower cumulative doses when given daily (Carbone et al., 1963). Weekly doses of $1.5–2.0$ mg/m^2 seem to provide the optimum balance between therapeutic and toxic effects. Virtually all patients receiving such doses may exhibit muscle atrophy, which is apparently secondary to neurotoxicity in man. Initially, fusimotor function is depressed, nerve conduction remaining intact until more drug is given and more profound toxicity is evoked. Cranial nerve palsies, especially III, VI, and VII are not uncommon (Albert et al., 1967). Inadvertently, large doses of VCR have resulted in convulsions, coma, and death. Intrathecal injection of even small doses of VCR are usually fatal, and this route is absolutely contraindicated. The morphology of vincristine-induced neuropathy has been extensively investigated both in man and in experimental animals (Moress et al., 1967; Schochet et al., 1968; Hirano and Zimmermann, 1970). Peripheral nerves show varying degrees of irregular demyelination with numerous deposits of neutral lipids scattered throughout the nerves. Myelin loss is followed by axonal degeneration and, consequently, by severe muscular atrophy. Anterior horn cells of the spinal cord as well as the motor neurons of the medulla are enlarged secondary to irregular clear zones of the cytoplasm alternating with coarsely clumped Nissl bodies. The clear areas contain in some instances argentophilic cords (Bodian stain), are faintly Congo red-positive, and birefringent. By electron microscopy, anterior horn cells exhibit large cytoplasmic areas with interwoven neurofilaments, aggregates of free ribosomes, and short fragments of rough endoplasmic reticulum. There are occasional crystalline inclusions in abnormal neurons. Such crystalline inclusions are also noted in microglial cells; they appear to follow the disappearance of microtubules (and may represent a rearrangement of microtubules or neurofilaments).

A rare but striking side-effect of VCR is its inappropriate stimulation of antidiuretic hormone (ADH) release. The precise mechanism is unclear but certainly the observed increase in plasma ADH (Stuart et al., 1975) and the resultant plasma dilution of electrolytes and proteins is another manifestation of central nervous system toxicity. The syndrome is correctable by fluid restriction and/or furosemide administration. As with most other toxic manifestations of VCR, inappropriate ADH secretion reverses spontaneously even with continued administration of the drug.

Vincristine causes alopecia in most patients. It also causes alarming adynamic ileus, occasionally of such severity that laparotomy has been performed for suspected *gastrointestinal* obstruction or perforation. This GI complaint can be ameliorated by the use of bulk laxatives; it is most severe following the first VCR injection and is rarely a problem thereafter. VCR administration may also be followed by moderate to severe jaw pain, a harmless but occasionally frightening and always distressing side-effect. As with other toxic manifestations, jaw pain becomes less aggravating with time.

V. L-Asparaginase

As mentioned, the side-effects of *asparaginase* are legion. Constitutional symptoms include chills and fever, malaise, anorexia, nausea, weight loss, somnolence, confusion, tremors, and, occasionally, hallucinations and coma. Even more toxicities are documentable chemically. *Asparaginase* inhibits synthesis of many important plasma and tissue constituents, including cholesterol and lipoproteins, insulin, albumin, fibrinogen, and other clotting factors synthesized in the liver. Fatty degeneration of the liver (Fig. 16), toxic pancreatitis, and nonketotic hyperglycemia are almost always present to some degree. In addition, alopecia, ulcerative stomatitis, cardiovascular disorders, and nephrotoxicity are observed after L-asparaginase therapy. Histologically we observed in the kidneys of dogs treated with this drug tubular single cell necroses similar to the formation of Councilman's bodies in the liver (Fig. 17). This may be followed by atrophy of individual distal tubules when the lesion grows more extensive.

Despite these diverse and often frightening abnormalities, the drug rarely needs to be discontinued for such problems, which indeed often are self-limiting and not life-threatening despite continued enzyme administration.

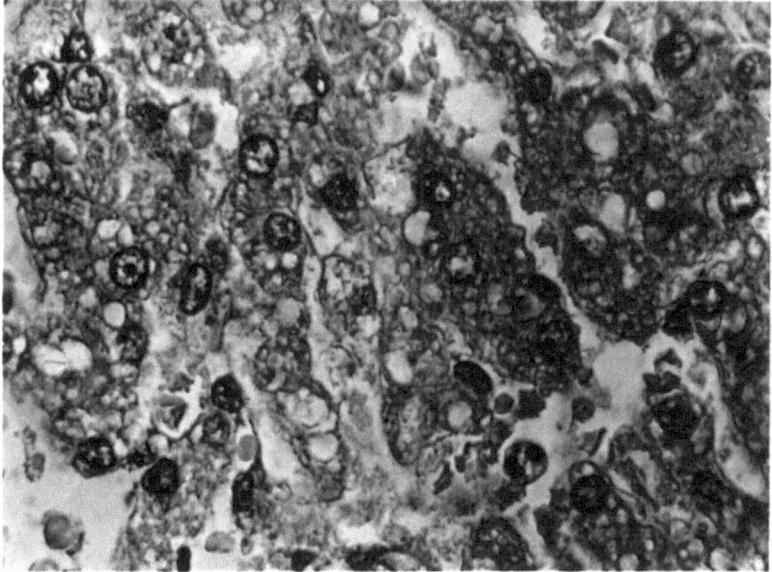

Fig. 16. Fatty hepatocellular degeneration secondary to L-asparaginase treatment: dog. H & E, × 600

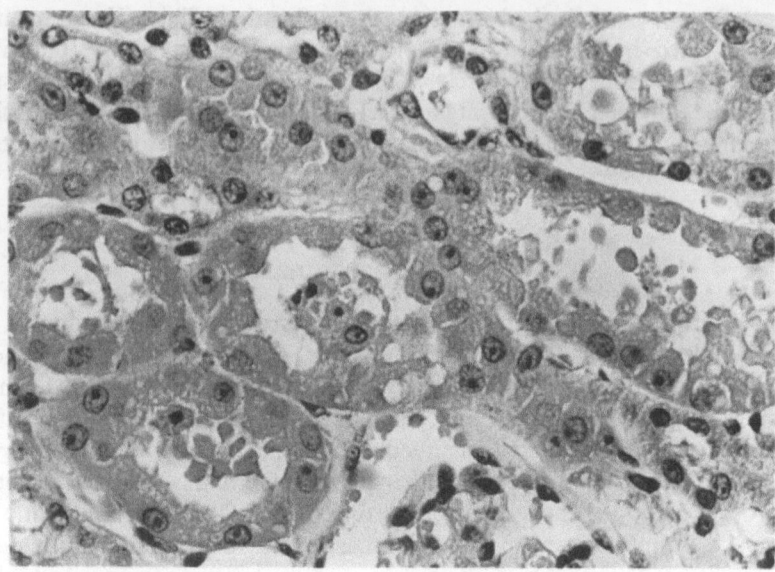

Fig. 17. Renal tubular degeneration secondary to L-asparaginase treatment; note single cell necroses resembling Councilman's bodies. H & E, × 380

Ironically, for an immunosuppressant drug, the major limiting toxicity of all forms of asparaginase comes through the development of antibodies. Repeated injections of asparaginase usually provoke sooner or later moderate to severe allergic reactions, and many instances of anaphylaxis have been observed. As noted earlier, these reactions can temporarily be averted on subsequent dosing by substitution of asparaginase from an alternate source (OHNUMA et al., 1972). Skin testing for sensitivity has not proved to be effective in ruling out severe reactions; the best policy remains slow administration under the watchful eye of the therapist with emergency medication and ventilatory equipment at hand. Daily administration of asparaginase appears to be less allergenic than less frequent application (LEVENTHAL and HENDERSON, 1971). The usual dose is 500 IU/kg daily for 10 days. Higher doses have not been shown to be more effective in eliminating blood asparagine or in achieving biological effects.

Asparaginase is minimally myelosuppressive and is from that standpoint an ideal drug for combination with marrow toxic agents. However, it must be used with caution in combination with drugs such as vincristine, prednisone, 6-mercaptopurine, methotrexate, and cyclophosphamide the activities of which are either dependent or modified by hepatic metabolism or which are themselves hepatic toxins.

The danger of asparaginase to the fetus has not yet been ascertained in man. Since it is a potent inhibitor of protein synthesis, it is likely to be dangerous throughout the period of gestation.

VI. Miscellaneous Agents

1. Procarbazine

The major dose-limiting toxicity of *procarbazine* is myelosuppression, occurring usually within 25 days and reversible in 14 days after discontinuing the drug (HENDERSON, 1974). Nausea, vomiting, stomatitis, myalgia, arthralgia, diarrhea, diplopia, confusion, and somnolence are not uncommon. Severe central nervous system toxicity, including ataxia, coma, psychosis, convulsion, and incapacitating orthostatic hypotension have been observed. These complications are in part a direct result of monoamine oxidase (MAO) inhibition (DE VITA *et al.*, 1965) and pyridoxal phosphate depression (CHABNER *et al.*, 1969), and are seriously aggravated by concomitant use of ethanol, MAO inhibitors, barbiturates, and narcotics, and foods rich in tyramine such as liver, aged cheese, yeast, and caffeine. Generally inconsequential toxicities include xerostomia, hyperpigmentation, and dermatitis.

Finally, procarbazine has the dubious distinction of being the most blatantly carcinogenic compound in active clinical use, inducing pulmonary adenomas, sarcomas, leukemia, and mammary carcinomas in rodents and acute leukemia in Rhesus monkeys (O'GARA *et al.*, 1971; KELLY *et al.*, 1964; SIEBER and ADAMSON, 1975). It is also highly teratogenic in animals, and is contraindicated in pregnancies that are to be carried to term.

2. Nitrosoureas

Given in conventional dosage by an intermittent schedule, the toxicity of the *nitrosoureas* is directed almost entirely at the bone marrow. Pancytopenia may develop within a few days, but the nadir of granulocyte and platelet levels is generally delayed until 4–5 weeks following a single dose, and an additional 2–4 weeks is required until peripheral blood counts return to normal (HENDERSON, 1974). Although liver and kidney toxicity has been observed in animals, it is almost never a problem in man. Nausea and occasional emesis, observed within 24 hours of administration, is similar in duration and severity to that seen with conventional alkylating agents. Despite its rapid entry into the central nervous system, toxicity to this system is rarely encountered.

3. Antibiotics

Cytostatic antibiotics in general are toxic to rapidly dividing cells in the bone marrow, and to gastrointestinal tract and hair follicles, giving rise to nausea, alopecia, and some degree of pancytopenia in most patients. All interact with radiation to cause enhanced dermal and visceral inflammation. In large cumulative doses all can cause cardiac toxicity, although this is of particular severity and clinical concern with *daunorubicin* and *adriamycin*. These latter drugs cause interstitial edema, atrophy, and myofibrillar and nuclear chromatid degeneration of heart muscle (BUJA *et al.*, 1973) leading to congestive heart failure refractory to chemical therapy. Patients in whom the total dose of administered daunorubicin or adriamycin exceeds 500 mg/m^2 are at high risk of this frequently fatal complication (CORTES *et al.*, 1975; DINDOGRU, 1975), and thus these agents are poor candidates for long-term immunosuppression. The histologic findings in life-threatening daunomycin cardiopathy are as follows: myocardial fibers become focally condensed (hypereosinophilia or basophilic degeneration), lose the usual cross striations and show multiple contraction bands instead; other atrophic myocardial fibers exhibit a vacuolar cytoplasm and loss of myofibrils (Figs. 18 and 19). The affected areas show an obvious interstitial edema with activation of mesenchymal cells, in part resembling Anitschkow cells. Adjacent myocardial fibers may show hypertrophy with nuclear hyperchromasia and increased numbers of nuclei. Degenerative atrophic muscle fibers show irregular PAS-positive staining after diastase digestion. The lesions are especially prominent in the subendocardial muscle layers. Ultrastructurally, there are extensive abnormalities of Z-bands with widening of these structures, focal extensions of these bands into adjacent regions of the sarcomere, and replacement of

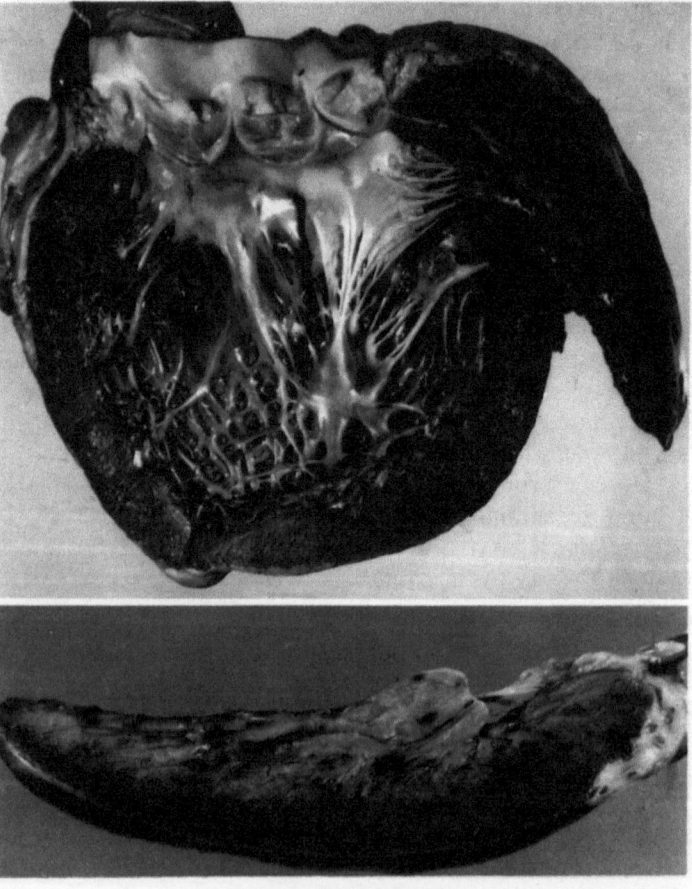

Fig. 18. Heart of a patient with leukemia and daunomycin treatment; acute heart failure 6 weeks post discontinuation of treatment. Note marked hypertrophy and dilatation with mottled appearance of myocardium

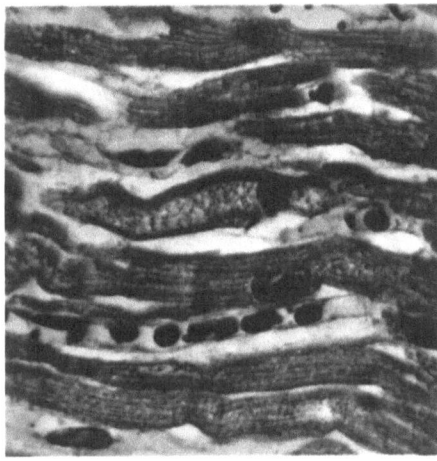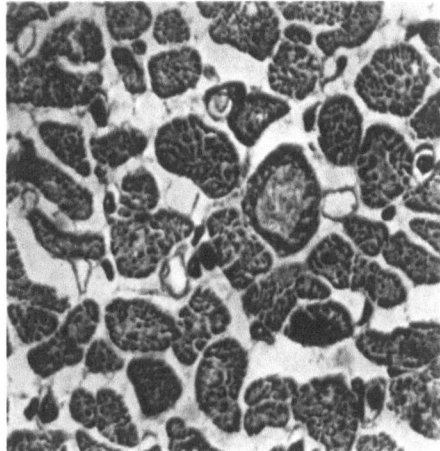

Fig. 19. Histology of heart shown in Fig. 18; note degeneration of myocardial fibers. H & E, × 380

the entire sarcomere by Z-band material (BUJA *et al.*, 1973). In certain cases, clusters of mitochondria exhibit loss of outer membranes and cristae; there is dissolution of myofibrils and formation of multiple myelin figures. In addition, nuclear chromatin disorganization can be noted in a certain number of cases.

VII. Antilymphocyte Sera (ALS)

As indicated above, ALS is probably the least toxic and most specific immuno-suppressant available. Certain side-effects, however, may arise from the restricted specificity of some preparations: besides antilymphocytic antibodies, antibodies against erythrocytes, thrombocytes, granulocytes, serum proteins and glomerular basement membranes were found. Severe anemia and thrombocytopenia are among the most common adverse effects. To avoid adverse effects to such ALS preparations, a careful selection of the antigen used for producing ALS is necessary as well as various absorption methods. Pure thymocytes and thoracic duct cells have proved to be more valuable antigenically than lymph node or spleen cells. Antierythrocyte antibodies, which are found even with the most careful selection of antigen, can be absorbed out fairly easily. Antispleen prepara-tions are probably the most toxic with dangerous antithrombocyte and antiglo-merular basement membrane antibodies. Since the immunosuppressive effective-ness of "anti-spleen-ALS" is usually poor, complete absorption of nonantilym-phocytic antibodies is rarely possible without significant loss of ALS activity. A detailed discussion of the various types of ALS preparations and their contami-nating antibody activities is presented by CAMIENER and WECHTER (1972) as well as by others (TAUB, 1970; MONACO, 1972).

Other adverse effects are caused by the proteinaceous nature of ALS, either by the foreign protein as such or by its antigenicity. Consequently, episodes of allergic and anaphylactoid reactions are described after use of ALS (TRAEGER

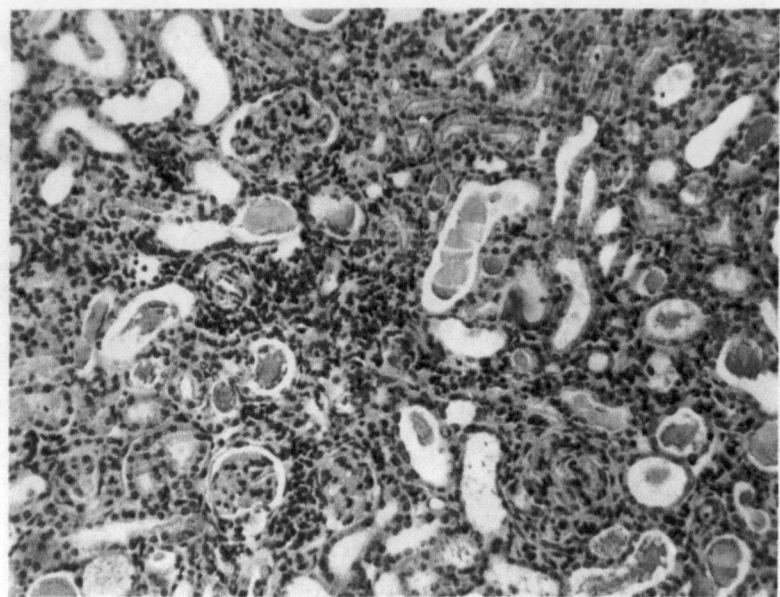

Fig. 20. Severe diffuse glomerulitis with nephrotic syndrome observed in a mouse after sustained ALS treatment. H & E, ×150

et al., 1970). Such reactions include urticaria, serum sickness, glottic edema, and various other minor skin reactions. They can usually be handled by the addition of another immunosuppressant such as steroids or azathioprine. Also, pre-testing is done of ALS recipients with minor doses (skin tests) of the respective preparation to identify presensitized recipients. The significance of such tests with regard to later development of hypersensitivity reactions, however, is limited.

Moreover, the foreign protein as such (effective ALS preparations are xenogeneic sera) can cause nephropathy (neprotic syndrome, "protein nephrosis"). We have observed severe glomerulonephrosis in mice treated for several weeks (once a week) with a quite specific ALS preparation prepared by immunization of a burro against mouse T-cell lymphoma cells (Krueger *et al.*, 1971; Fig. 20).

D. Special Topics

I. Infection

Infection is the single most critical problem with both short-term and long-term immunosuppression. This is the result of three factors; the underlying disease process, the immunosuppressive effects of the drugs, and the almost uniform granulocytopenic toxicity of these same agents (Hersh, 1974; Hersh and Bodey,

1970). Granulocytopenia is related to the incidence of infection in both the absolute and temporal sense, that is, the lower the granulocyte count in the blood and the longer the duration of granulocytopenia, the higher the risk of acquiring a significant infection (BODEY et al., 1966).

The spectrum of infection in immunosuppressed individuals is similar to that seen in patients with acquired granulocytopenia and immune deficiency of other causes. This includes not only common infections caused by aerobic gram-positive pyogenic organisms such as pneumococci and Staphylococcus aureus, but in addition gram-negative and anaerobic bacteria, fungi, viruses, and protozoa (LEVINE et al., 1972, 1974).

Most of the latter organisms are ubiquitous and are included in the endogenous microflora of all patients. Isolation procedures, even when feasible, may therefore fail to reduce the risk of invasive infection although for short-term periods of high risk, that is, during bone marrow transplantation, strict isolation and air filtration may reduce the incidence and severity of gram-negative organism pneumonia (LEVINE et al., 1973; YATES and HOLLAND, 1973; SCHIMPFF et al., 1975). Decontamination with nonadsorbable oral antibiotics increases the degree of protection against bacterial disease and has proved to be valuable in both short- and long-term immune and myeloid deficiency states (LEVINE et al., 1973; YATES and HOLLAND, 1973; SCHIMPFF et al., 1975; DIETRICH and FLIEDNER, 1973).

In chemically immunosuppressed individuals clinical infections caused by the herpes group of viruses, especially cytomegalovirus (CMV), and by the putative protozoa Pneumocystis carinii have been frequent and severe. CMV is the most common infection complicating successful allogeneic bone marrow transplantation (HERZIG et al., 1975; SANTOS, 1974; THOMAS et al., 1975). It usually manifests itself in myalgia, arthralgia, rash, and fever, and occasionally appears as typhoidal disease with fever, chills, malaise, and adenopathy accompanied by atypical lymphocytosis in the peripheral blood. Since antibodies to CMV are common in both adults and children, their presence is of little help in diagnosis. Rising antibody titers are of diagnostic value. Treatment is unsatisfactory, but, fortunately, most patients tolerate and survive this infection with or without antiviral medications.

The pathology is characterized by a mild lymphocyte-infiltrative, and essentially nonproliferative inflammation involving several organ systems such as the exocrine glands, lung, liver, kidney, prostate, and probably also the GI tract. Diagnostic are characteristically enlarged (infected) epithelial and endothelial cells with large purple intranuclear inclusions (Fig. 21).

P. carinii pneumonia is a more dangerous complication being rapidly fatal in 20 percent or more of cases. Its onset is frequently so insidious that the correct diagnosis is delayed until the patient is in critical condition. Pneumocystis causes extensive protein exudates in alveoli, but is associated with little inflammation, and, accordingly, with few of the typical signs and symptoms of acute pneumonitis. Fever is usually present, but rales and rhonchi are frequently absent, and percussion dullness and diminished breath sounds may not be apparent until there is extensive lung involvement. Often the first sign of disease, other than fever, is severe dyspnea and at this juncture pulmonary function is severely compromised and the prognosis is grave. Diagnosis and successful management depend on obtaining early, and where necessary, repeated chest x-rays in febrile patients under chemoimmunosuppression. The diagnosis can be established with certainty only by lung biopsy. Pentamidine sulfate, or, alternatively, pyrimethamine and sulfa should be started as soon as the clinical suspicion of pneumocystis is confirmed by x-ray signs of diffuse infiltration.

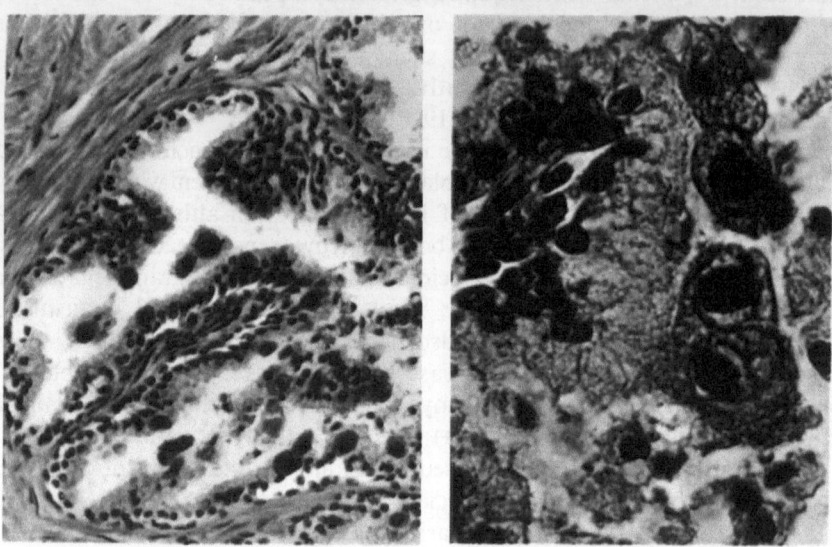

Fig. 21. Inclusion body prostatitis in generalized cytomegalovirus disease in a leukemic patient with combination chemotherapy. H & E, ×150 and ×600

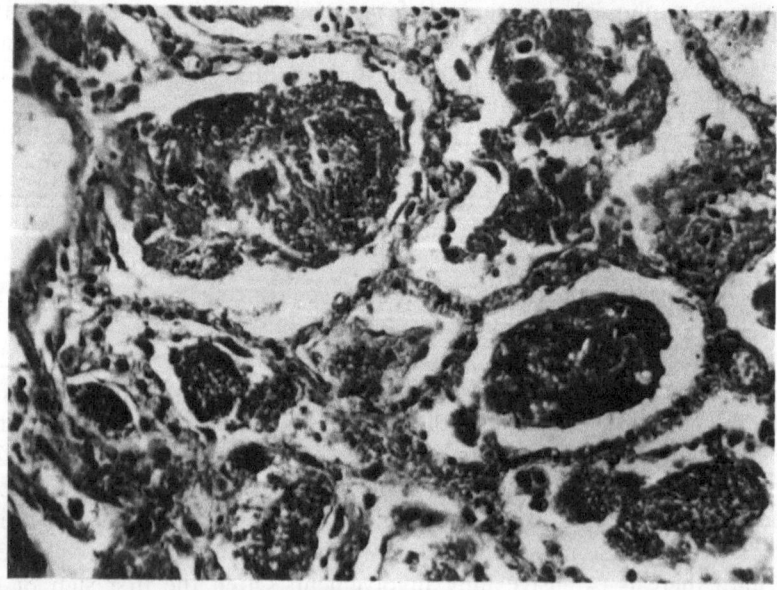

Fig. 22. Pneumocystis pneumonia in a leukemic patient with combination chemotherapy; note proteinaceous foamy exudate. H & E, ×150

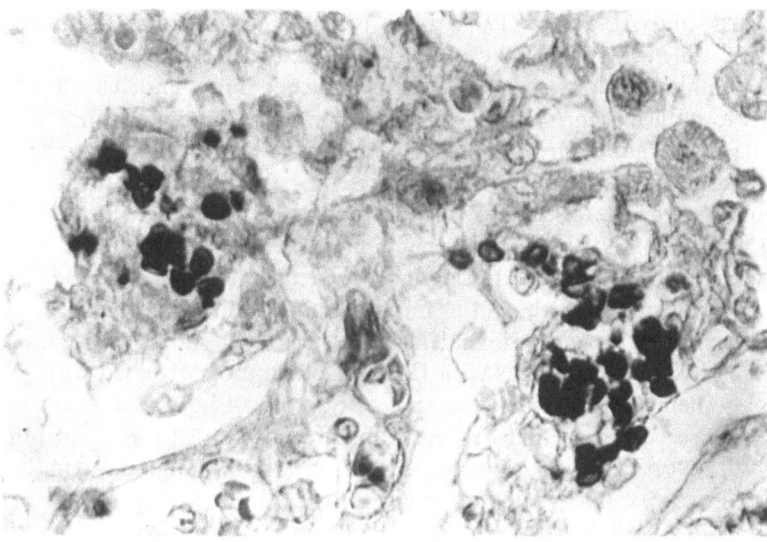

Fig. 23. Pneumocystis pneumonia as shown in Fig. 22; note *P. Carinii* organisms stained with methenamine silver. × 600

Histologically, the pneumonitis is characterized by an eosinophilic foamy alveolar exudate accompanied by interstitial mononuclear cell infiltrates which distend the alveolar septae. The foamy exudate contains few to abundant pneumocystis organisms which stain well with the methenamine silver reaction (Figs. 22 and 23). The interstitial mononuclear cell infiltrate is further complicated by a proliferative response leading to progressing fibrosis, if the initial exudative and infiltrative reaction is not resolved in response to adequate treatment.

Infection complicating acute granulocytopenia, such as may occur during inadvertent overdosage with cytotoxic drugs, may be controlled with antibiotics alone, or may require leukocyte transfusions. Blood granulocytes can be obtained in adequate quantities from normal donors by several techniques (GRAW *et al.*, 1972a; DJERASSI *et al.*, 1972; HIGBY, 1975) and, for best results, should be given daily for at least 4 days in conjunction with appropriate antibiotics.

II. Carcinogenesis

It is perhaps not incongruous that drugs influencing such fundamental processes as immunologic surveillance and cell proliferation should, at the same time, be potent carcinogens. Carcinogenesis was of no material importance when these compounds were used and useful only for short-term palliation of malignant diseases. However, as their indications have broadened to include nonlethal disease, and as their effectiveness in both benign and malignant processes have increased, the specter of the induction of new tumors has become more real and more ominous.

SIEBER and ADAMSON (1975) have recently published an extensive review of this problem, to which the interested reader is referred. In summary, most, if not all immunosuppressive (and antineoplastic) compounds have been demonstrated to induce or promote neoplasia in animals. In man the major offenders have been alkylating agents, especially in patients chronically treated for Hodgkin's disease, multiple myeloma, and, perhaps, carcinoma of the ovary. Great caution must be exercised in reviewing reports of the coincidence of alkylating agent treatment and the appearance of tumors. Second neoplasms in the same patient are not uncommon, and possibly related to host factors which permitted the inception and growth of the initial tumor. Acute leukemia, for example, has a higher than anticipated incidence in patients with multiple myeloma treated with melphalan, and patients with Hodgkin's lymphoma treated with radiotherapy plus chemotherapy. However, the association of both myeloma and Hodgkin's disease with leukemia has been observed in patients who did not receive either drug or radiation therapy. Similarly, while malignant lymphoma has occurred to excess in patients immunosuppressed following renal transplantation (PENN et al., 1969), leukemia incidence has not increased in these patients. Furthermore, malignant lymphomas have been shown to be increased in susceptible mice receiving mismatched allografts in the absence of chemical immunosuppression (SCHWARTZ and BELDOTTI, 1965). Clearly other factors must impinge to cause neoplasms, and one should not forget that the vast majority of patients and animals receiving these drugs survive tumor-free. It has been theorized, therefore, that immunosuppression in coincidence with persistent antigenic stimulation may cause malignant lymphomas (KRUEGER, 1972), or that immunosuppressive mechanisms such as, for instance, chronic graft-versus-host reaction, may activate oncogenic viruses (HIRSCH, 1973).

None theless, the physician using potent immunosuppressants and carcinostatic agents must always weigh the advantages to be gained from immunosuppression with the potential long-term risk that such therapy may enhance the risk of initiation and spread of neoplasia, and, as a logical corollary, must refrain from using such treatment for trivial or frivolous indications.

E. Summary

Diverse chemical compounds exist which can alter immunoreactivity. All of these agents induce untoward effects of considerable consequence in individual patients. The choice of drug, dose, and schedule must be based on the overall status of the patient, taking into due consideration the severity of the illness, the pharmacologic characteristics of the drugs, and the function of critical organs of metabolism and secretion. In this way, the greatest good for the least cost can be realized, which course is, in all circumstances and settings, the goal of rational therapeutics.

References

Acute Leukemia Group B: Acute lymphocytic leukemia in children. Maintenance therapy with methotrexate administered intermittently. J.A.M.A. **207**, 923–933 (1969).

AHN, Y.S., HARRINGTON, W.J., SEELMAN, R.C.: Vincristine Therapy of idiopathic and secondary thrombocytopenias. New Engl. J. Med. **291**, 376–380 (1974).

ALBERT, D.M., WONG, V.G., HENDERSON, E.S.: Ocular complications of vincristine therapy. Arch. Ophthal. **78**, 709–713 (1967).

ALLISON, A.C., LAW, L.W.: Effects of antilymphocyte serum on virus oncogenesis. Proc. Soc. Exp. Biol. Med. **127**, 207–212 (1968).

ASTALDI, G., BURGIO, G.R., KRC, J., GENOVA, R., ASTALDI, A.A., JR.: L-asparaginase and blastogenesis. Lancet **1**, 423 (1969).

ASTALDI, G., BRUCKNER, I., MICU, D., MAXIMILIAN, G., LEAHN, S., BURGIO, G.: 6th Internat. Meeting Reticuloendothel. Soc. Abstr. Freiburg, 1970, p. 4.

BACH, J.F., DARDENNE, M., GALANAUD, P., WATCHI, J.M., ANTOINE, B.: Étude analytique de 69 serums de lapin anti-lymphocytes de souris. I. Activités "in vivo". Path. Biol. **18**, 471–478 (1970).

BENJAMIN, R.S., RIGGS, C.E., JR., BACHUR, N.R.: Pharmacokinetics and metabolism of adriamycin in man. Clin. Pharmacol. Therap. **14**, 592–600 (1973).

BETHLENFALVAY, N.C., BERGIN, J.J.: Severe cerebral toxicity after intravenous nitrogen mustard therapy. Cancer **29**, 366–369 (1972).

BISCHOFF, K.B., DEDRICK, R.L., ZAHARKO, D.S., LONGSTRETH, J.A.: Methotrexate pharmacokinetics. J. Pharm. Sci. **60**, 1128–1133 (1971).

BODEY, G.P., BUCKLEY, M., SATHE, Y.S., FREIREICH, E.J.: Quantitative relationships between circulating leukocytes and infection in patients with acute leukemia. Ann. Int. Med. **64**, 328–340 (1966).

BOGGS, D.R.: The cellular composition of inflammatory exudates in human leukemias. Blood **15**, 466–475 (1960).

BOGGS, D.R., ATHENS, J.W., CARTWRIGHT, G.E., WINTROBE, M.M.: The effect of adrenal glucocorticosteroids upon the cellular composition of inflammatory exudates. Amer. J. Pathol. **44**, 763–773 (1964).

BONMASSAR, E., VADLAMUDI, S., VIEIRA, W., GOLDIN, A.: Influence of Tween 80 on the antileukemic activity of 1,3-bis (2-chloro-etyl)-1-nitrosourea. Arch. Ital. Path. Clin. Tumori **12**, 163–175 (1969).

BUCKNER, C.D., RUDOLPH, R.H., FEFER, A., CLIFT, R.A., EPSTEIN, R.B., FUNK, D.D., NEIMAN, P.E., SLICHTER, S.J., STORB, R., THOMAS, E.D.: High-dose cyclophosphamide therapy for malignant disease: Toxicity, tumor response, and the effects of stored autologous marrow. Cancer **29**, 357–365 (1972).

BUJA, L.M., FERRANS, V.J., MAYER, R.J., ROBERTS, W.C., HENDERSON, E.S.: Cardiac ultrastructural changes induced by daunorubicin therapy. Cancer **32**, 771–788 (1973).

CAMIENER, G.W., WECHTER, W.J.: Immunosuppression—agents, procedures, speculations, and prognosis. Progr. Drug. Res. **16**, 67–217 (1972).

CAPIZZI, R.L.: Hematologic neoplasms during pregnancy. In: Cancer Chemotherapy. New York and London: Grune and Stratton, 1972, Vol. II.

CARBONE, P.P., BONO, V., FREI, E. III, BRINDLEY, C.O.: Clinical studies with vincristine. Blood **21**, 640–647 (1963).

CHABNER, B.A., DE VITA, V.T., CONSIDINE, N., OLIVERIO, V.T.: Plasma pyridoxal phosphate depletion by the carcinostatic procarbazine. Proc. Soc. Exp. Biol. Med. **132**, 1119–1122 (1969).

CLAESSON, M.H., RÖPKE, C.: Quantitative studies on cortisol-induced decay of lymphoid cells in the thymus lymphatic system. Acta path. microbiol. Scand. **76**, 376–382 (1969).

CLARYSSE, A.M., CATHEY, W.J., CARTWRIGHT, G.E., WINTROBE, M.M.: Pulmonary disease complicating intermittent therapy with methotrexate. J.A.M.A. **209**, 1861–1864 (1969).

CONDIT, P.T., CHANES, R.E., JOEL, W.: Renal toxicity of methotrexate. Cancer **23**, 126–131 (1969).

CORTES, E.P., LUTMAN, G., PICKREN, J., WANKA, J., WANG, J.J., WALLACE, J., HOLLAND, J.F.: Adriamycin (ADM) cardiotoxicity (CDTX): A clinicopathological correlation. Proc. AACR/ASCO. **16**, 171 (1975).

COSTA, G., ASTALDI, G.: Effetto della daunomicina sull' attivitá proliferativa di cellule staminale ottenute in coltura da sagne umano normale. Tumori **50**, 471–480 (1964).

CREASEY, W.A.: Modifications in biochemical pathways produced by the vinca alkaloids. Cancer Chemother. Rep. **52**, 501–507 (1968).

DAHL, M.G.C., GREGORY, M.M., SCHEUER, P.J.: Liver damage due to methotrexate in patients with psoriasis. Brit. Med. J. **1**, 625–630 (1971).

DE FRONZO, R.A., BRAINE, H., COLVIN, O.M., DAVIS, P.J.: Water intoxication in man after cyclophosphamide therapy: Time course and relation to drug activation. Ann. Int. Med. **78**, 861–869 (1973).

DE VITA, V.T., HAHN, M.A., OLIVERIO, V.T.: Monoamine oxidase inhibition by a new carcinostatic agent, N-isopropyl-(-2-methyl-hydrazino)-p-toluamide (MIH). Proc. Soc. Exp. Biol. Med. **120**, 561–565 (1965).

DIAZ, C.J., GARCIA, E.L., MERCHANTE, A., PERIANES, J.: Treatment of rheumatoid arthritis with nitrogen mustard: preliminary report. J.A.M.A. **147**, 1418–1419 (1951).

DIETRICH, M., FLIEDNER, T.M.: Gnotobiotic care of patients with immunologic deficiency diseases. Transplant. Proc. **5**, 1271–1277 (1973).

DINDOGRU, A.: EKG changes following adriamycin (ADM) treatment. Proc. AACR/ASCO **16**, 267 (1975).

DJERASSI, I., FARBER, S., ABIR, E., NEIKIRK, W.: Continuous infusion of methotrexate in children with acute leukemia. Cancer **20**, 233–242 (1967).

DJERASSI, I., KIM, J.S., SUVANSRI, U., MITRAKUL, C., CIESIELKA, W.: Continuous flow filtration-leukopheresis. Transfusion **12**, 75–83 (1972).

DOUGHERTY, T.F., BERLINER, M.L., BERLINER, D.L.: Hormonal influence on lymphocyte differentiation from RES cells. Ann. N.Y. Acad. Sci. **88**, 78–82 (1960).

DUBOIS, E.L.: Nitrogen mustard in treatment of systemic lupus erythematosus. Arch. Int. Med. **93**, 667–672 (1954).

DUSTMANN, H.O., STOLPMANN, H.J.: Die Beeinflussung des Lymphknotens durch Glucocorticosteroid. Virchows Archiv Abt. A. Path. Anat. **345**, 121–131 (1968).

DUTTERA, M.J., CAROLLA, R.L., GALLELLI, J.F., GULLION, D.S., KEIM, D.E., HENDERSON, E.S.: Hematuria and crystalluria after high-dose 6-mercaptopurine administration. New Engl. J. Med. **287**, 292–294 (1972).

EINSTEIN, A.B., JR., FASS, L., FEFER, A.: Suppression of secondary cellular immunity to a tumor allograft by cyclophosphamide and 1,3 bis (2-chloroethyl)-1-nitrosourea. Cancer Res. **35**, 492–496 (1975).

EPSTEIN, W.L., MAIBACH, H.I.: Immunologic competence of patients with psoriasis receiving cytotoxic drug therapy. Arch. Dermatol. **91**, 599–606 (1965).

ERNSTRÖM, U., LARSSON, B.: Export and import of lymphocytes in the thymus during steroid-induced involution and regeneration. Acta path. microbiol. Scand. **10**, 371–384 (1967).

FAUCI, A.S., DALE, D.C.: Alternate-day prednisone therapy and human lymphocyte subpopulations. J. Clin. Invest. **55**, 22–32 (1975).

FISCHER, P., GOLOB, E., FRIEDRICH, F., KUNZE-MUHL, E., DOLESCHEL, W., AICHMAIR, H.: Autosomal deletion syndrome 46, XX, 18 p-: a new case report with absence of IgA in serum. J. Med. Genet. **7**, 91–98 (1970).

FLOERSHEIM, G., STORB, R., WEIDEN, P.: Abrogation of sensitization to marrow grafts in dogs. Exper. Hemat. In press (1975).

FURTH, J.J., COHEN, S.S.: Inhibition of mammalian DNA polymerase by the 5 triphosphate of 1-B-D-arabinosfuranosylcytosine and the 5′-triphosphate of 9-B-D-arabinofuranosyladenine. Cancer Res. **28**, 2061–2067 (1968).

GABRIELSEN, A.E., GOOD, R.A.: Chemical Suppression of Adaptive Immunity. Adv. Immunol. **6**, 91–229 (1967).

GERMUTH, F.G., OTTINGER, B., OYAMA, J.: Influence of cortisone on experimental hypersensitivity and circulating antibody in guinea pig. Proc. Soc. Exp. Biol. Med. **80**, 188–191 (1952).

GILL, P.G.: Cytophilic antibody in heterologous antilymphocytic serum: its presence, absorption and possible biologic significance. J. Immunol. **102**, 1329–1331 (1969).

GOODELL, B., LEVENTHAL, B., HENDERSON, E.S.: Cytosine arabinoside in acute granulocytic leukemia. Clin. Pharmacol. Therap. **12**, 599–606 (1971).

GRAW, R.G., JR., HERZIG, G., PERRY, S., HENDERSON, E.S.: Normal granulocyte transfusion therapy: treatment of septicemia due to gram-negative bacteria. New. Engl. J. Med. **287**, 367–371 (1972a).

GRAW, R.G., JR., YANKEE, R.A., LEVENTHAL, B.G., ROGENTINE, G.N., HERZIG, G.P., HALTERMAN,

R.H., MERRITT, C.B., COROLLA, R.L., ALVEGARD, T.A., BULL, J.M., McGINNIS, M.H., KRUEGER, G., GULLION, D.S., LIPPMAN, M.F., BLEYER, W.A., BERARD, C.W., WHANG-PENG, J., TRAPANI, R.J., TERASAKI, P.I., STEINBERG, A.S., GRALNICK, H.R., HENDERSON, E.S.: Bone marrow transplantation in acute leukemia employing cyclophosphamide. Exper. Hematol. **22**, 118–125 (1972b).

GRAY, G.D., MICELSON, M.M., GRIM, J.A.: The immunosupressive activity of ara-cytidine. I. Effects on antibody-forming cells and humoral antibody. Transplant. **6**, 805–817 (1968).

GRUNDMANN, E., OETTGEN, H.E. (eds.): Experimental and clinical effects of L-asparaginase. Recent Res. Cancer Res. **33**, 1–354 (1970).

HARRIS, A.W.: Differentiated functions expressed by cultured mouse lymphoma cells. I. Specificity and kinetics of cell responses to corticosteroids. Exp. Cell Res. **60**, 341–353 (1970).

HARRIS, J.E., BAGAI, R.C.: Clinical utility of immunosuppressive agents. In: Antineoplastic and Immunosuppressive Agents. SARTORELLI, A.C. and JOHNS, D.C. (eds.), Part 1. Berlin-Heidelberg-New York: Springer 1974.

HENCH, P.S., KENDALL, E.C., SLOCUMB, C.H., POLLEY, H.F.: The effect of a hormone of the adrenal cortex (17-hydroxy-11-dehydro-corticosterone: Compound E) and of pituitary adrenocorticotropic hormone on rheumatoid arthritis. Proc. Staff Meet. Mayo Clin. **24**, 181–197 (1949).

HEKTOEN, L., CORPER, H.J.: The effect of mustard gas (dichlorethyl-sulphid) on antibody formation. J. Infect. Dis. **28**, 279–285 (1921).

HENDERSON, E.S., ADAMSON, R.H., DENHAM, C., OLIVERIO, V.T.: The metabolic fate of tritiated methotrexate. I. Absorption, excretion and distribution in mice, rats, dogs, and monkeys. Cancer Res. **25**, 1008–1017 (1965a).

HENDERSON, E.S., ADAMSON, R.H., OLIVERIO, V.T.: The metabolic fate of tritiated methotrexate. II. Absorption and excretion in man. Cancer Res. **25**, 1018–1024 (1965b).

HENDERSON, E.S.: Granulocytopenia induced by cancer chemotherapeutic agents. In: Drugs and Hematological Reactions. New York and London: Grune & Stratton 1974.

HERSH, E.M., WONG, V.G., HENDERSON, E.S., FREIREICH, E.J.: Hepatotoxic effects of methotrexate. Cancer **19**, 600–606 (1966).

HERSH, E.M., BODEY, G.P.: Leukocytic mechanisms in inflammation. Ann. Rev. Med. **21**, 105–132 (1970).

HERSH, E.M.: Immunosuppressive agents. In: Antineoplastic and Immunosuppressive Agents. SARTORELLI, A.C. and JOHNS, D.C. (eds.), Part 1. Berlin-Heidelberg-New York: Springer 1974.

HERZIG, G.P., BULL, B.I., DECTER, J., LOHRMANN, H.P., HERZIG, R.H., KRUEGER, G., POMEROY, T., HENDERSON, E.S., GRAW, R.G., JR.: Bone marrow transplantation in leukemia and aplastic anemia: NCI experience with four grafting regimens. Transplant. Proc. Suppl. 1 **7**, 817–821 (1975).

HIGBY, D.J., YATES, J.W., HENDERSON, E.S., HOLLAND, J.F.: Filtration leukapheresis for granulocyte transfusion therapy: Clinical and laboratory studies. New Engl. J. Med. **292**, 761–766 (1975).

HINTZ, B., WEBBER, M.M.: Antithymic antibody localization in the mouse. Nature **208**, 797–798 (1965).

HIRANO, A., ZIMMERMANN, H.M.: Some effects of vinblastine implantation in the cerebral white matter. Lab. Invest. **23**, 358–367 (1970).

HIRSCH, M.S.: Immunological activation of oncogenic viruses. In: Virus Tumorigenesis and Immunogenesis. CEGLOWSKI, W.S. and FRIEDMAN, H. (eds.). New York: Academic Press, 1973, pp. 131–137.

HIRSCH, M.S., MURPHY, F.A.: Effects of anti-thymocyte serum on Rauscher virus infection of mice. Nature **218**, 478–479 (1968).

JENNINGS, B.R.: The immunosuppressive effects of actinomycin D and radiation. J. Reticuloendothel. Soc. **6**, 50–58 (1969).

KELLY, M.G., O'GARA, R.W., GADEKAR, K., YANCEY, S.T., OLIVERIO, V.T.: Carcinogenic activity of a new antitumor agent, N-isopropyl-(2-methylhydrazino)-p-toluamide, hydrochloride (NSC-77213). Cancer Chemother. Rep. **39**, 77–80 (1964).

KLENER, P., DONNER, L., NEUWIRTOVA, R.: Immunosuppressive therapy of idiopathic thrombocytopenia. Vnitr. Lek. **18**, 228–233 (1972).

KOLIN, A., LANDI, S.: Effect of actinomycin D on the tuberculin skin reaction in guinea pigs. Int. Arch. Allergy **38**, 607–617 (1970).

KRUEGER, G.: Chronic immunosuppression and lymphomagenesis in man and mice. Nat. Cancer Inst. Monogr. **35**, 183–190 (1972).

KRUEGER, G.: Morphology of chemical immunosuppression. In: Advances in Pharmacology Chemotherapy (GARATTINI, S., GOLDIN, A., HAWKING, F., KOPIN, I.J. (eds.). New York: Academic
Press, 1972b, Vol. X, pp. 1–90.
KRUEGER, G.R.F., MALMGREN, R.A., BERARD, C.W.: Malignant lymphomas and plasmacytosis
in mice under prolonged immunosuppression and persistent antigenic stimulation. Transpl. 11,
138–144 (1971).
KRUEGER, G., GRAW, R.G., ROGENTINE, G.N., DARROW, C.C., NEEFE, J.C., LUETZELER, J.: Pathology of modified graft-versus-host disease in bone marrow allografted monkeys treated with antilymphocyte serum. Blut 30, 19–30 (1975).
KYLE, R.A., SCHWARTZ, R.S., OLINER, H.L., DAMESHEK, W.: A syndrome resembling adrenal
cortical insufficiency associated with long term busulfan (Myleran) therapy. Blood 18, 497–510
(1961).
LANCE, E.M.: The mechanism of action of anti-lymphocyte serum. Studies of antibody eluate.
J. Exp. Med. 130, 49–76 (1969).
LANCE, E.M.: The selective action of antilymphocyte serum on recirculating lymphocytes: a review
of the evidence and alternatives. Clin. Exp. Immunol. 6, 789–802 (1970).
LENAZ, L., DI FRONZO, G., MOLINARI, R.: Distribution of daunorubicin and adriamycin in man.
In: Adriamycin Review, Part II. Europ. Press Medikon (1975) 89–98, Ghent, Belgium STAGUET,
M., TAGNON, H., KEHIS, Y., eds.
LE PAGE, G.A., WHITECAR, J.P., JR.: Pharmacology of 6-thioguanine in man. Cancer Res. 31,
1627–1631 (1971).
LE PAGE, G.A., LOO, T.L.: Purine antagonists. In: Cancer Medicine. Philadelphia: Lea & Febiger,
1973.
LEVENTHAL, B.G., HENDERSON, E.S.: Therapy of acute leukemia with drug combinations which
include asparaginase. Cancer 28, 825–829 (1971).
LEVEY, R.H., MEDAWAR, P.B.: Some experiments on the action of antilymphoid antisera. Ann.
N.Y. Acad. Sci. 129, 164–177 (1966).
LEVINE, A.S., GRAW, R.G., JR., YOUNG, R.C.: Management of infections in patients with leukemia
and lymphoma: current concepts and experimental approaches. Sem. Hemat. 9, 141–179
(1972).
LEVINE, A.S., SIEGEL, S.E., SCHREIBER, A.D., HAUSER, J., PREISLER, H., GOLDSTEIN, I.M., SEIDLER,
F., SIMON, R., PERRY, S., BENNETT, J.E., HENDERSON, E.S.: Protected invironments and prophy-
lactic antibiotics: A prospective controlled study of their utility in the therapy of acute leukemia.
New Engl. J. Med. 288, 477–483 (1973).
LEVINE, A.S., SCHIMPFF, S.C., GRAW, R.G., JR., YOUNG, R.C.: Hematologic malignancies and
other marrow failure states: Progress in the management of complicating infections. Sem. Hemat.
11, 141–202 (1974).
LIEBEGOTT, G.: Die Pathologie der Nebennieren. Verh. dtsch. Ges. Path. 36, 21 (1953).
MACDONALD, A.S., CHAN, C.C., FALVEY, C.F.: Use of procarbazine hydrochloride (Natulan) and
procarbazine hydrochloride and azathioprine in canine renal allografts. Transplant. II, 103–104
(1971).
MACGREGOR, R.R., SHEAGREN, J.N., LIPSETT, M.B., WOLFF, S.M.: Alternate-day prednisone thera-
py: Evaluation of delayed hypersensitivity responses, control of disease and steroid side effects.
New Engl. J. Med. 280, 1427–1431 (1969).
MACLAURIN, B.P., HUMM, J.A.: Macrophage specificity of antiserum against thymus lymphocytes.
Clin. Exp. Immunol. 6, 125–136 (1970).
MADOC-JONES, H., NAURO, F.: Site of action of cytotoxic agents in the cell life cycle. In: Antineoplas-
tic and Immunosuppressive Agents. SARTORELLI, A.C., and JOINS, D.C. (eds.), Part 1. Berlin-
Heidelberg-New York: Springer 1974.
MAKINODAN, T., SANTOS, G.W., QUINN, R.P.: Immunosuppressive drugs. Pharmacol. Rev. 22,
189–248 (1970).
MANNICK, J.A., EGDAHL, R.H.: Endocrinologic Agents. In: Human Transplantation. RAPAPORT,
F., and DAUSSET, J. (eds.), pp. 472–481. New York and London: Grune and Stratton, 1968.
MASSIMO, L.: Toxische Nebenwirkungen des Daunomycins bei Kindern. Blut 20, 44–56 (1970).
MATHÉ, G., AMIEL, J.L., SCHWARZENBERG, L., CHOAY, J., TROLAND, P., SCHNEIDER, M., HAYAT,
M., SCHLUMBERGER, J.R., JASMIN, C.: Bone marrow graft in man after conditioning by antilym-
phocytic serum. Transplant. Proc. 3, 325–332 (1971).

MEYLER, L. (ed.): Side Effects of Drugs. Amsterdam: Exerpta Medica-Elsevier, 1958–1972, Vols. I–VII.

MEYLER and PECK (1965, 1968, 1972) — see p. 22.

MILLER, J.J, COLE, L.J.: Resistance of long-lived lymphocytes and plasma cells in rat lymph nodes to treatment with prednisone, cyclophosphamide, 6-mercaptopurine, and actinomycin D. J. Exp. Med. 126, 109–125 (1967).

MONACO, A.P.: Antilymphocyte serum. In: Transplantation. NAJARIAN, J.S., and SIMMONS, R.L. (eds.). Philadelphia: Lea & Febiger, 1972, pp. 222–251.

MONACO, A.P., WOOD, M.L., GRAY, J.G., RUSSELL, P.S.: Studies on heterologous antilymphocyte serum in mice. II. Effect of the immune response. J. Immunol. 96, 229–238 (1966).

MONTGOMERY, J.A., JOHNSTON, T.P., SHEALY, Y.F.: Drugs for neoplastic diseases. In: Medicinal Chemistry, iii4d ed. New York: Wiley-Interscience, 1970.

MORESS, G.R., D'AGOSTINO, A.N., JARCHO, L.W.: Neuropathy in lymphoblastic leukemia treated with vincristine. Arch. Neurol. 16, 377–384 (1967).

NAVA, C., O'KANE, H.O., SHORTER, R.G.: The distribution of rabbit anti-mouse thymus globulin after injection into mice. Proc. Soc. Exp. Biol. Med. 131, 990–994 (1969).

NETTESHEIM, P., HAMMONS, A.S.: Effect of immunosuppressive agents on retention of antigen in the mouse spleen. Proc. Soc. Exp. Biol. Med. 133, 696–701 (1970).

O'GARA, R.W., ADAMSON, R.H., KELLY, M.G., DALGARD, D.W.: Neoplasms of the hematopoietic system in non-human primates: Report of one spontaneous tumor and two leukemias induced by procarbazine. J. Nat. Cancer Inst. 46, 1121–1130 (1971).

OHNUMA, T., HOLLAND, J.F., MEYER, P.: Erwinia carotovora asparaginase in patients with prior anaphylaxis to asparaginase from E. coli. Cancer 30, 376–381 (1972).

PENN, I., HAMMOND, W., BRETTSCHNEIDER, L., STARZL, T.E.: Malignant lymphomas in transplantation patients. Transplant. Proc. 1, 106–112 (1969).

PETERS, W.P., HOLLAND, J.F., SENN, H., RHOMBERG, W., BANERJEE, T.: Corticosteroid administration and localized leukocyte mobilization in man. New Engl. J. Med. 286, 342–345 (1972).

PICHLMAYR, R.: Wirkung eines heterologen Antilymphozytenserums auf die Transplantatabstoßung beim Hund. Klin. Wschr. 44, 594–595 (1966).

PREISLER, H.D., BRUCKNER, H., HENDERSON, E.S.: Reduced production of spleen colonies and granulocytes in antibiotic-treated irradiated mice transplanted with syngeneic bone marrow. Radiation Res. 48, 20–31 (1971).

RAWBONE, R.G., SHAW, M.T., JACKSON, J.G., BAGSHAWE, K.D.: Complication of methotrexate-maintained remission in lymphoblastic leukemia. Brit. Med. J. 4, 467–468 (1971).

RIVAROLA, A., FRIEDMAN, M., LAWRENCE, W., JR.: Methotrexate and the immune response. Transplant. 5, 1223–1230 (1967).

ROENIGK, H.H., JR., MAIBACH, H.I., WEINSTEIN, G.D.: Use of methotrexate in psoriasis. Arch. Dermatol. 105, 363–365 (1972).

ROSNER, F., HIRSHAUT, Y., GRUNWALD, H.W., DIETRICH, M.: In vitro combination chemotherapy demonstrating potentiation of vincristine cytotoxicity by prednisolone. Cancer Res. 35, 700–705 (1975).

SAIKI, J.H., THOMPSON, S., SMITH, F., ATKINSON, R.: Paraplegia following intrathecal chemotherapy. Cancer 29, 370–374 (1972).

SANDLER, S.G., TOBIN, W., HENDERSON, E.S.: Vincristine-induced neuropathy: A clinical study of fifty leukemic patients. Neurology 19, 367–374 (1969).

SANTOS, G.W.: Immunosuppression for clinical marrow transplantation. Sem. Hemat. 11, 341–351 (1974).

SANTOS, G.W., OWENS, A.H., JR.: 19S and 17S antibody production in the cyclophosphamide- or methotrexate-treated rat. Nature 209, 622–624 (1966).

SCHIMPFF, S.C., GREENE, W.H., YOUNG, V.M., FORTNER, C.L., JEPSEN, L., CUSACK, N., BLOCK, J.B., WIERNIK, P.H.: Infection prevention in acute nonlymphocytic leukemia: Laminar air flow room reverse isolation with oral, nonabsorbable antibiotic prophylaxis. Ann. Int. Med. 82, 351–358 (1975).

SCHMÄHL, D.: Entstehung, Wachstum und Chemotherapie maligner Tumoren. Aulendorf: Cantor, 1970.

SCHOCHET, S.S., JR., LAMPERT, P.W., EARLE, K.M.: Neuronal changes induced by intrathecal vincristine sulfate. J. Neuropath. Exp. Neurol. 27, 645 658 (1968).

Schwartz, M.K., Lash, E.D., Oettgen, H.F., Tomao, F.A.: L-Asparaginase activity in plasma and other biological fluids. Cancer 25, 244–252 (1970).

Schwartz, R., Stack, J., Damashek, W.: Effect of 6-mercaptopurine on antibody production. Proc. Soc. Exp. Biol. Med. 99, 164–167 (1958).

Schwartz, R.S., Beldotti, L.: Malignant lymphomas following allogenic disease: transition from an immunological to a neoplastic disorder. Science 149, 1511–1514 (1965).

Sensenbrenner, L.L., Owens, A.H., Jr., Zawatzsky, L.S., Elfenbein, G.J.: The comparative effects of selected cytotoxic agents on transplanted hematopoietic cells. Transplantation 14, 347–351 (1972).

Sharp, H., Nesbit, M., White, J., Krivit, W.: Methotrexate liver toxicity. J. Pediat. 74, 818–819 (1969).

Shehadeh, I.H., Guttman, R.D., Lindquist, R.R.: Renal transplantation in the inbred rat. XV. An assay study of three immunosuppressive drugs. Transplant. 10, 66–74 (1970).

Sieber, S.M., Adamson, R.H.: Toxicity of antineoplastic agents in man: Chromosomal aberrations, antifertility effects, congenital abnormalities, and carcinogenic potential. Advances Cancer Res. In Press (1975).

Smalley, R.V., Wall, R.L.: Two cases of busulfan toxicity. Ann. Int. Med. 64, 154–164 (1966).

Sterlin, W.A., Elveback, L.R., Shorter, R.G.: The immunosuppressive effect of antilymphocyte sera produced by sensitization with different lymphoid tissues. Transplant. 10, 297–301 (1970).

Stewart, P.B., Cohen, V.: Antiserum to lymphocytes and procarbazine compared as immunosuppressants in mice. Science 164, 1082–1083 (1969).

Stewart, P.B., Bell, R.: Procarbazine as an immunosuppressant in animals. J. Immunol. 105, 1271–1277 (1970).

Stock, J.A.: Antimetabolites. In: Experimental Chemotherapy. Schnitzer, R.J. and Hawking, F. (eds.). New York: Academic Press, 1968, Vol. IV, pp. 79–237.

Stuart, M.J., Cuaso, C., Miller, M., Oski, F.A.: Syndrome of recurrent increased secreation of antidiuretic hormone following multiple doses of vincristine. Blood 45, 315–320 (1975).

Talley, R.W.: Corticosteroids. In: Cancer Medicine. Philadelphia: Lea & Febiger, 1973. Holland, J.F. and Frei, E. III, eds.

Taub, R.N.: Biological effects of heterologous antilymphocyte serum. Progr. Allergy 14, 308–258 (1970).

Taub, R.N., Lance, E.M.: Cited by Camiener and Wechter (1972).

Thomas, E.D., Storb, R., Clift, R.A., Fefer, A., Johnson, F.L., Neiman, P.E., Lerner, K.G., Glucksberg, H., Buckner, C.D.: Bone Marrow Transplantation (part 2). N. Engl. J. Med. 292, 895–902 (1975).

Thurner, J.: Iatrogene Pathologie. Munich-Berlin-Vienna, Urban & Schwarzenberg 1970.

Traeger, J., Fries, D., Revillard, J.P., Durix, A., Carraz, M., Plan, M.: Production of human antilymphocytic serum in horse with thoracic duct lymphocytes and peripheral blood lymphocytes. Fed. Proc. 29, 108–110 (1970).

Turk, J.L.: Studies on the mechanism of action of methotrexate and cyclophosphamide on contact sensitivity in the guinea pig. Int. Arch. Allergy 24, 191–200 (1964).

Turk, J.L., Poulter, L.W.: Selective depletion of lymphoid tissue by cyclophosphamide. Clin. Exp. Immunol. 10, 285–296 (1972).

Van Scott, E.J., Auerbach, R., Weinstein, G.D.: Parenteral methotrexate in psoriasis. Arch. Dermat. 89, 550–556 (1964).

Vivaqua, R.J., Haurani, F.I., Erslev, A.J.: "Selective" pituitary insufficiency secondary to busulfan. Ann. Int. Med. 67, 380–387 (1967).

Vogel, J.M., Yankee, R.A., Kimball, H.R., Wolff, S.M., Perry, S.: The effect of etiocholanolone on granulocyte kinetics. Blood 30, 474–484 (1967).

Vredevoe, D.L., Hays, E.F.: Effect of antilymphocytic and antithymocytic sera on the development of mouse lymphoma. Cancer Res. 29, 1685–1690 (1969).

Weinberger, A., Pinkhas, J., Sandbank, U., Shaklai, M., de Vries, A.: Endocardial fibrosis following busulfan treatment. J.A.M.A. 231, 495 (1975).

Weiss, H.D., Walker, M.D., Wiernik, P.H.: Neurotoxicity of commonly used antineoplastic agents. New Engl. J. Med. 291, 75–81; 127–133 (1974).

White, A.: Hormonal influences on immune mechanisms. Ann. Allergy 21, 417–423 (1963).

Winkelstein, A., Craddock, C.G., Lawrence, J.S.: Cell replication in the primary hemolysin response: The effect of six mercaptopurine. J. Reticuloendothel. Soc. 9, 307–322 (1971).

WONG, V.G., HERSH, E.M.: Methotrexate in the therapy of cyclitis. Trans. Amer. Acad. Ophthal. Otolaryng. **69**, 279–293 (1965).

YATES, J.W., HOLLAND, J.F.: A controlled study of isolation and endogenous microbial suppression in acute myelocytic leukemia patients. Cancer **32**, 1490–1498 (1973).

YOUNG, R.C., DE VITA, V.T.: The effect of chemotherapy on the growth characteristics and cellular kinetics of leukemia L1210. Cancer Res. **30**, 1789–1794 (1970).

YU, D.T.Y., CLEMENTS, P.J., PAULUS, H.E., PETER, J.B., LEVY, J., BARNETT, E.V.: Human lymphocyte subpopulations: effect of corticosteroids. J. Clin. Invest. **53**, 565–571 (1974).

ZAGER, R.F., FRISBY, S.A., OLIVERIO, V.T.: The effects of antibiotics and cancer chemotherapeutic agents on the cellular transport and antitumor activity of methotrexate in L1210 murine leukemia. Cancer Res. **33**, 1670–1676 (1973).

ZSCHIESCHE, W., AUGSTEN, K., OZEGOWSKI, W., KREBS, D.: Alkylating anticancer agents and phago-cytosis. I. Effects of a homologous series of 1,2-substituted 5-bis(beta-chloroethyl)-amino-benzim-idazole derivatives on carbon clearance. J. Reticuloendothel. Soc. **8**, 538–549 (1970)

References

Graft-Versus-Host-Reactions*

H.P. Hobik

With 26 Figures

1. Introduction

Transplant rejection is the result of an immune attack of the host against the implanted foreign cells. The graft-versus-host-reaction (GVHR) is the reverse process: the transplant reacts against the host, damages it and may even kill it. GVHR has gained increased attention in the past 20 years since it was first correctly described by BILLINGHAM et al. (1955), TRENTIN (1956), and SIMONSEN (1957).

Four reasons are responsible for this: 1) GVHR is a suitable in-vivo model for the examination of immunocompetent cells. 2) In the experiment, GVHR can lead to "runt disease" (wasting disease), which is largely typical of it. 3) In humans GVHR can lead to graft-vs.-host-disease (GVHD). 4) GVHR can induce or trigger malignant tumors.

A prerequisite for the development of GVHR is the capability of the implanted cells or tissue to give an immune response to an antigen stimulus of the host. This means that the transplant must contain immunocompetent cells and also lymphocytes. Furthermore the host organism must be incapable of rejecting the implanted cells or tissue with a normal transplant rejection. GVHR therefore requires a unilateral immunity reaction, that is, from the transplant against the host. The host must be insufficiently immune. This can be the case, for instance, if the donor's cells are immunocompetent against the host's histocompatibility antigens while this is not he case vice versa. This, for example, is the case with F_1 hybrids of inbred animals. Within certain limits it also applies to embryos which have not yet developed a full immune system. Adult humans or animals can suffer GVHD as hosts if they have inherited or acquired an immune deficiency. Whole-body irradiation is a good example of this: it causes aplasia of the bone marrow in humans and animals. After transplantation of isogenous bone marrow cells these can settle in the bone marrow of the host and so-called radiation chimeras occur. When allogeneic bone marrow is transplanted, GVHR develops regularly, in these cases formerly called "secondary disease" (e.g. COHEN et al., 1957). Today it is certain that this is a typical GVHR (TRENTIN, 1956).

---

* Supported by Ministerium für Wissenschaft und Forschung des Landes Nordrhein-Westfalen.

A similar condition was described as early as 1916 as "embryo disease" in chickens (Murphy, 1916). Murphy observed that inoculation of the chorioallantoic membrane of young chicken embryos with spleen fragments of grown chickens caused a marked enlargement of the spleen of the host animal, and that small whitish nodules appeared on it. These turned out to be necroses surrounded by leukocytes. Enlargement of the spleen was for a long time considered a manifestation of an "organ-specific stimulation of growth" (Ebert, 1954). Only Dempster (1953) and Simonsen (1953) suspected that under certain circumstances implanted cells or tissues could harm the host. Both authors found an early infiltration of plasma cells in kidney transplants on dogs which they took to be host cells.

In 1955 Billingham et al. met with this same phenomenon of "embryo disease" when they injected allogeneic blood cells into 10–11-day-old chicken embryos to obtain tolerance against skin transplants. Ninety-five percent of these animals died just before hatching. The researchers first believed an infection to have been the cause of death. However, since Billingham and Brent (1957) observed typical "runt disease" during experiments to obtain tolerance to skin transplants by injecting spleen cells, the uniformity of this reaction as GVHR has become apparent. The causative type of cells are a form of T-lymphocytes.

In the meantime several good reviews on GVHR have become available to us (e.g., Simonsen, 1962; van Bekkum and de Vries, 1967; Billingham, 1968; Elkins, 1971; Grebe and Streilein, 1976). This report deals especially with the pathology of GVHR in animal experiments and in humans and also with the current information on its causal and formal pathogenesis.

2. Experimental Models

Experimental observations at first took only systemic observations into consideration, i.e. pathological changes which affected the entire organism of the animal and which ended in "runt disease." Closer studies of the phenomena, however, revealed, that local reactions can also be caused which correspond entirely to the conditions of GVHR. These local reactions have made some phenomena of GVHR particularly well interpretable.

Comparable to in-vivo phenomena are in-vitro methods, which grant generally valid insights into cellular immune mechanisms.

In the following the most important methods and findings of systemic, local and in-vitro GVH reactions are presented.

2.1. Systemic GVHR

Prerequisite is an immune insufficiency or immune tolerance of the receiver against the cells of the donor. This can be controlled for instance through genetic selection (p. 796). Embryos and newborns, at least of many species, do not yet have a fully developed immune system.

Thus, experimental studies can be divided into two groups: 1) Experiments with embryonic or newborn receiver animals; that is, the "juvenile form" of GVHR. 2) Experiments with adult animals, which either possess an intact immune system, but for genetic reasons do not recognize the foreign cells as antigen, or else animals which are primarily or secondarily immunoinsufficient. These are the "adult forms" of GVHR. The reaction parameters are identical in both experimental forms so that we can present them together in the some chapter.

2.1.1. Juvenile Forms

These experiments resulted in the most serious general symptoms within the shortest period of time. Birds and small rodents (mice and rats) yielded the best results.

2.1.1.1. Chorioallantoic Membrane Test

This test yielded some of the most important results about the nature of GVHR (BOYER, 1960; BURNET and BURNET, 1960; BURNET and BOYER, 1960, 1961; SZENBERG and WARNER, 1962; WARNER and SZENBERG, 1964; KILLBY et al., 1972; LONGENECKER et al., 1973; WALKER et al., 1973, and others). If one grafts immunologically competent cells onto the chorioallantoic membrane of a chicken, two things happen: individual cells migrate into the embryo and there induce systemic GVHR. Other cells remain on the membrane and cause local GVHR.: Nodules develop with a membrane of lymphocytes and plasma cells (BURNET and BOYER, 1961).

In these experiments it is important that the lymphatic cells which are inoculated come from adult chickens. The importance of genetic differences has not yet been thoroughly analyzed in this model; there is a lack of strictly inbred chickens. It is certain, however, that cells from isogenous or specially immunotolerant donors do not produce this reaction (HILGARD et al., 1962; BURNET, 1969).

These observations led to the conclusion that every single nodule on the chorioallantoic membrane was produced by an individual donor cell which is immunocompetent against the histocompatibility antigens of the host. This was indicated by the fact that there was a direct relationship between the number of inoculated cells and the number of nodules. This was further confirmed by more detailed quantitative studies (COPPLESON and MITCHI, 1965). By using sex chromosomes or other chromosome markers it has been demonstrated that the cells in these nodules which divide by mitosis, are cells from the donor animal.

As early as 1916 MURPHY observed an enlargement of the spleen after injecting spleen cells from adult chickens into chicken embryos, (Fig. 1) a phenomenon, which, later in this test, gained increasing recognition as a prominent characteristic (SIMONSEN, 1962; BILLINGHAM, 1968; ELKINS, 1971). The individual foci ("pocks") on the chorioallantoic membrane originated from antigen-reactive cells which propagated clonally. Serial dilution of the inoculated lympho-

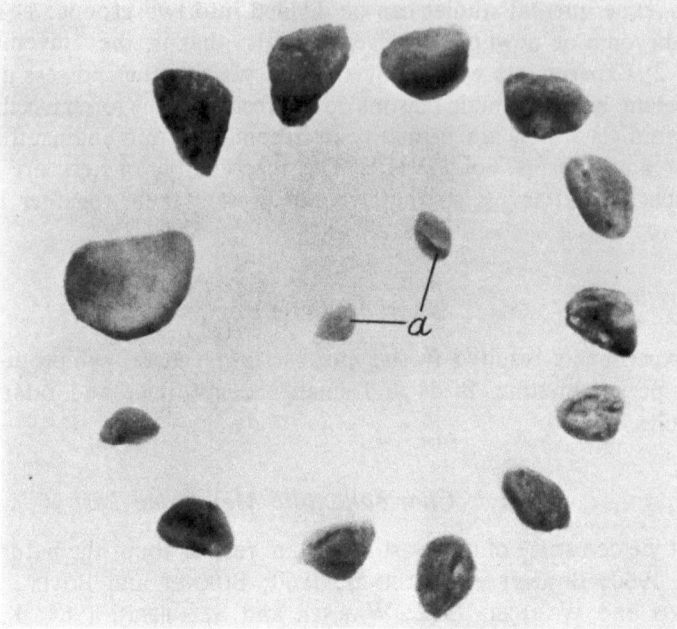

Fig. 1. Splenomegaly in 18-day-old chicken embryos, grafted on the 7th day with small fragments of adult chicken spleen onto the chorioallantoic membrane. a=controls. (Reproduced from Murphy, 1916)

cytes showed that inoculation of the chorioallantoic membrane with 5×10^5 cells causes 10–100 foci to develop. If each focus is the result of *one* immunocompetent cell (Burnet and Burnet, 1960), then only a limited number of lymphocytes can be thus immunocompetent. We shall discuss this further below (p. 808).

2.1.1.2. $A \rightarrow A + B$ Type

The incapability of the host —resulting from immunogenetic conditions—to reject the implanted cells can only be tested on pure strains of inbred animals. For this reason research on mice has yielded the most exact results.

Moreover it is necessary to test the purity of the inbred strain through brother-sister inbreeding or rather, to create pure strains through repeated brother-sister-inbred mating. With two such strains one can obtain F_1 hybrids which, genetically, are clearly defined, after the following principle: AA+ BB→AB. If these AB hybrids are given intraperitoneal, intravenous or intracutaneous injections of spleen cells (or other lymphocytes) from a parent animal, these cells attack the host animal since they recognize the respective other component as a foreign antigen (if A cells are injected the B-component, and vice versa). In mice splenomegaly occurs as a typical first symptom (Simonsen, 1957). If cells of the F_1 hybrids are injected into the parents, no GVHR occurs.

Generally, strict inbreeding is a prerequisite to successfully producing GVHR in this model. The usual purchased inbred strains yield mostly unsatisfactory results. The lack of homozygotes can often be discerned by slight color variations in the fur of the F_1 hybrid mice. However, histocompatibility genes are not strictly linked to color genes.

In practice the production of inbred strains is achieved not only by pairing brothers and sisters but also half-brothers and half-sisters. Mutations are therefore unavoidable (KRAMER and VAN DER VELDEN, 1975). One can, however, gain separate strains for experimental GVHR in this manner.

The spleen index as a measure for the intensity of GVHR makes it possible to test the histocompatibility of the crossbred animal strains by means of their F_1 hybrids.

We have had experience with the following crossbreeds:

A/Jax	× Balb/c	Balb/c	× A/Jax
C_{57}/Bl/6	× Balb/c	Balb/c	× C_{57}/Bl/6
C_{57}/Bl/6	× CPB/N	CPB/N	× C_{57}/Bl/6
Balb/c	× CPB/N	CPB/N	× Balb/c
Balb/c	× Heston	Balb/c	× DBA
CBP/N	× CPB/R	CPB/N	× Str
CPB/N	× C3H	C_{57}/Bl/6	× DBA
C_{57}/Bl/6	× C_{57}/L	Str	× DBA
Heston	× C_{57}/L	AKR	× DBA

The following combinations produced the most pronounced GVHR:

C_{57}/Bl/6	× Balb/c	Balb/c	× C_{57}/Bl/6
C_{57}/Bl/6	× CPB/N	CPB/N	× C_{57}/Bl/6
Balb/c	× CPB/N	CPB/N	× Balb/c

The spleen index of these six combinations was approximately within the same range. On occasion the spleen index is higher after transplantation of spleen cells from male C_{57}/Bl/6 mice than after transplantation of spleen cells from female parent animals, presumably because of the weak H_2 locus in C_{57}/Bl/6 mice which is linked to the male sex chromosome.

With rats good brother-sister-inbred strains have been obtained from the BD III strain (now in its 240th generation) and from Wistar I rats with strong GVHR after the 20th generation (HOBIK, 1969).

With chickens analogous genetic studies have not been carried out yet. GVHR according to type A→A+B is also successful (COCK and SIMONSEN, 1958; ISACSON, 1959). In this case the age of the host animal plays a decisive role: maximal splenomegaly can be obtained after intravenous injection of parental spleen cells from adult chickens into 13–15-day-old hybrid embryos. Chicken embryos between 13 and 17 days of age are also particularly susceptible to the induction of tolerance. (HIRATA and SCHECHTMAN, 1960; SOLOMON and TUCKER, 1962).

The age of the host animal also plays a very important role: in mice-splenomegaly can be produced most easily within the first 24 h after birth, after the second or third day it becomes gradually less marked (SIMONSEN, 1957). According to BILLINGHAM and BRENT (1959) a 100% mortality rate from acute "runt disease" can be obtained if the recipients are no older than 20 h. Here, too, there exists an immediate relationship to immune tolerance: if lymphatic

cells are used which, for genetic reasons, do not cause "runt disease," the
receiver animals can be made immune against this type of cell (BILLINGHAM
and SILVERS, 1962). Accordingly, allogenous skin transplants from the strains
from which the injected cells are derived, are not rejected. If these tolerant
adult animals are later injected with specific antigen-reactive cells of the same
genetic type as the first spleen cells, a serious GVHR can result (STASNY et al.,
1963, 1965).

Under genetically pure conditions, type $A \rightarrow A + B$ has proved a particularly
useful model for experiments as well as for the study of therapy of GVHR
(p. 846).

2.1.1.3. $DA \rightarrow Fischer + DA$-Type

If, 27 to 34 days before delivery, DA skin transplants are grafted onto female
Fischer rats which have been mated with male DA rats, 94% of the young
die of GVHR approximately 4 weeks after birth (cited by GREBE and STREILEIN,
1976). The two strains of rats differ in their locus of histocompatibility, the
AgB-locus, which is the determining factor in rats. The same type of GVHR
can be induced in F_1 hybrids (FISCHER + DA) through transference of 100×10^6
lymphatic cells derived from Fischer rats which have been specially sensitized
against DA alloantigenes (BEER and BILLINGHAM, 1973).

GVHR mortality among F_1 newborns whose mothers had received Fischer
anti-Lewis lymphocytes, amounted to 100%. This demonstrates that the immune
competent cells can pass through the placenta and damage the fetus (p. 811).

2.1.2. Adult Forms

The injection of immunocompetent parental spleen cells into adult F_1 hybrids
does not immediately result in a serious GVHR. This corresponds to the above-
mentioned dependency on age. On the other hand these experiments grant
a better view of the defense mechanisms of the host, since adult animals possess
a fully developed immune system.

If adult F_1 hybrid Syrian hamsters are injected intracutaneously with
200×10^6 sensitized parental lymph node cells, the "epidermolytic syndrome"
sets in (STREILEIN and BILLINGHAM, 1970a, 1970b), which is also fatal: consequent to the destruction of the lymphatic and hemopoietic systems toxic necrosis
of the skin ensues (toxic epidermal necrolysis=TEN) which is fatal within
21 days (STREILEIN, 1971b, 1972c). If the same cells are injected not intracutaneously but intravenously or intraperitoneally, the animals show no reaction
(STREILEIN and BILLINGHAM, 1970b). With rats this reaction is considerably
less reliable, but, interestingly enough, can also be induced intraperitoneally
(cited by GREBE and STREILEIN, 1976). This TEN, however, is probably not
a purely immunologic reaction but a mixed reaction between specific and unspecific factors (SINGH et al., 1972, 1973).

The adult, just as the juvenile form of GVHR, can be noticeably intensified
by sensitizing the donor animals against the antigen of the receiver (DAVIES,

1963; DAVID *et al.,* 1966; UPHOFF, 1969). Lethal irradiation of adult F_1 hybrid mice also encourages the development of GVHR. Experiments in this field have also been conducted with hemopoietic colony-forming units (CFU): lethally irradiated, adult F_1 mice received parental lymphatic cells as well as 2×10^6 syngeneic bone marrow cells, the precursor cells for CFU (BLOMGREN and AN-DERSSON, 1972, 1974; BOGGS *et al.,* 1973). This system largely eliminates the influence of the host lymphocytes which have been killed by the irradiation. Here, GVHR can be induced with only 6×10^4 normal lymph node cells.

2.1.3. Reaction Parameter

Systemic GVHR or rather "runt disease" which it induces, has a characteristic clinical picture (GVHD) with retarded growth, wasting symptoms, splenomegaly, hepatomegaly, lymphatic atrophy, diarrhea and anemia. Outwardly, the animals soon develop a rough fur, a sign of atrophic dermatitis (Fig. 2). These phenomena occur in varying intensity and especially in varying sequence. It is necessary for all of these studies to obtain uniform reaction parameters which can be evaluated quantitatively.

2.1.3.1. Weight of the Spleen

SIMONSEN (1957) found splenomegaly to be a particularly reliable symptom: Six days after intravenous injection of immunocompetent spleen cells into 18-day-old chicken embryos the weight of the spleen had increased fourfold. In principle the same applies to mice (SIMONSEN *et al.,* 1958), in which the weight of the spleen generally reaches its peak 8 to 10 days after injection of spleen cells (SIMONSEN and JENSEN, 1959).

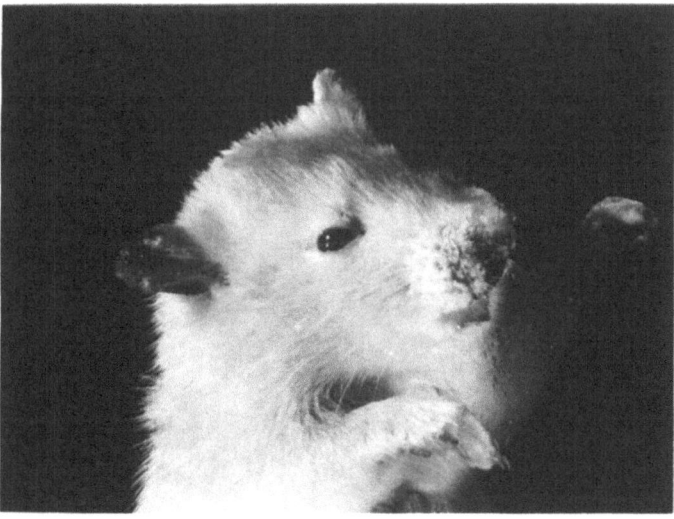

Fig. 2. GVH dermatitis in a 31-day-old (Wistar I × BD III) F_1 rat after i.p. transplantation of 9×10^6 spleen cells from BD III rats at day 16 after birth

Simonsen et al. (1958) have developed a spleen test which is probably the most widely used. It can be applied not only to chickens and mice but also to rats.

Simonsen originally compared the absolute weight of the spleen of test animals with the weight of the spleens of controls of the same age (cf. Isacson, 1959; Terasaki, 1959; Mun et al., 1959; van Alten and Fennell, 1959). Better results, however, were obtained after introduction of the so-called spleen index, i.e., the quotient of the experimental weight of the spleen divided by the body weight of the host. This makes it possible to take into consideration the reduction of body weight which usually accompanies "runt disease." According to Simonsen (1957) and Michie et al. (1961) a spleen index over 1.3 is indicative of GVHR; upon injection of isogeneic cells a maximal spleen index of 1.23 is obtained (Fig. 3).

The discriminant spleen assay (Simonsen and Jensen, 1959) takes into consideration the host-vs.-graft reaction which also occurs, by including a group which had obtained foreign but not parental spleen cells. A prerequisite is that in this case too, the locus of histocompatibility of the cells differs from that of the host cells. These so-called negative controls correct the end result by lowering it and thus yield more accurate data (Simonsen, 1962; see his Table 4).

It must be pointed out, however, that different inbred strains have different spleen indices. Enlargement of the spleen occurs also with local GVHR (Elkins, 1971). It is now certain that splenomegaly is a reaction to GVHR and not a measure of GVHR itself. Thus it is self-evident that other, more specific parameters have been looked for and are still being looked for.

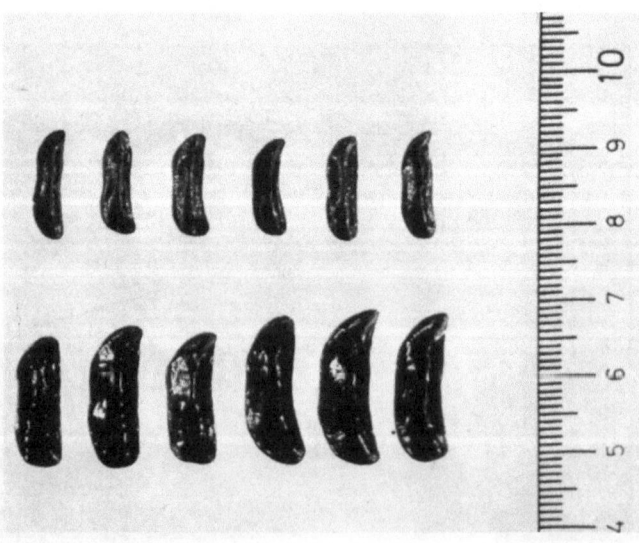

Fig. 3. Splenomegaly in 4-month-old $(C_{57}/Bl/6 \times CPB/N)$ F_1 mice on day 13 after i.p. transplantation of 12×10^6 spleen cells from CPB/N mice. Mean spleen weight: Control = 0.075 g. GVHR = 0.240 g

2.1.3.2. Number of Lymphocytes

Especially in mice lymphopenia was pointed out early (OLINER *et al.*, 1961). According to experimental findings of my own this lymphopenia depends on the number of transplanted cells. BILLINGHAM *et al.* (1962) observed a striking leukocytosis in newborn BN rats after receiving a transplant of lymphatic cells from Lewis rats, which was mainly caused by an increase of granulocytes. The combination of strains we used, however (Wistar I × BD III), showed distinct lymphopenia but no leukocytosis. These leuko- and lymphopenias are correlated to changes in the bone marrow and lymphatic organs.

Lymphopenia in mice, which also occurs with GVHR through parabiosis (CORNELIUS, 1968), has been analyzed in greater detail by WITTING and DETLEF-SEN (1975). Adult F_1 hybrids of strains A/Jax and Balb/c received intraperitoneally up to 200×10^6 parental spleen cells and thus reached a spleen index of over 1.4. The peak was reached after 10 to 12 days and simultaneously the peripheral number of lymphocytes dropped from $2,300/mm^3$ to less than $400/mm^3$. Simultaneously with the subsequent reduction of the spleen index the number of lymphocytes recovered too, and 20 days after injection both spleen index and the peripheral number of lymphocytes were back to normal. According to this, lymphopenia in mice, when high doses of spleen cells are given, is as good a criterion for the degree of intensity of GVHR as the spleen index. However humoral antibodies (ONO *et al.*, 1969) and unspecific reactions, for example, the effects of corticoids, are also assumed to cause lymphopenia with GVHR (HILDEMANN *et al.*, 1964).

2.1.3.3. Body Weight

According to RUSSEL (1960) retarded increase of weight can be considered a criterion for the juvenile form of GVHR. The test animals with the combination of strains DBA/1 × C_{57}/Bl/6 continued to gain weight normally till the 8th day. Then their body weight stagnated and after another 10 days the animals died. This relatively simple test is certainly valid as a rough orientation. Compared to other parameters, however, this test is not specific enough, especially since no strict correlation exists with the number of spleen cells applied (SIMONSEN, 1962).

During our studies, the F_1 combination Balb/c × C_{57}/Bl/6 proved particularly sensitive; it was therefore used to test the change of body weight in greater detail. During the first 7 days there was no difference in 18–32-day-old animals between the untreated F_1 hybrids and the animals which had been treated intraperitoneally with 5×10^6 spleen cells of C_{57}/Bl/6 mice. After the 9th day the animals treated with spleen cells gained no further weight, whereas the untreated control F_1 hybrids showed a normal increase in weight. After the 16th day the animals treated with spleen cells tended to lose weight and the first casualties occurred. With adult animals, i.e., over 2 months of age, there is only a slight, hardly significant difference of 1 to 2 g between the control hybrids and those treated with spleen cells.

If (Wistar I × BD III) F_1 rats were used, 3–7-day-old animals, upon intraperitoneal transplantation of 5 to 7×10^6 spleen cells from male BD III rats, gained

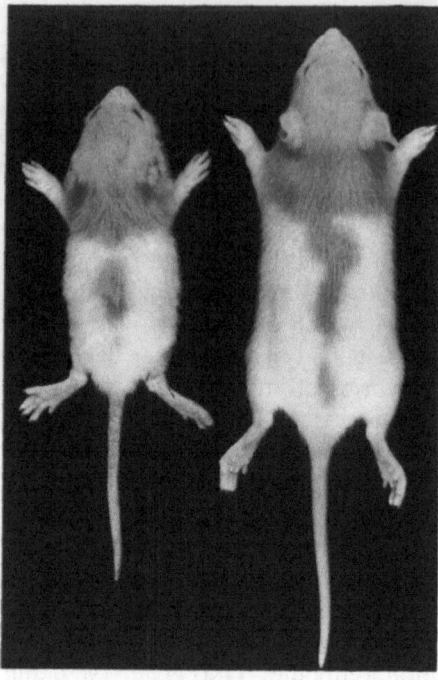

Fig. 4. "Runt disease" of a 25-day-old (BD III × Wistar I) F₁ rat after i.p. transplantation of
5.2×10^6 spleen cells from the Wistar I father on day 5 after birth, and a control animal from
the same litter. Body weight: Control = 34 g. GVHR = 18 g

less weight from the 7th day onward, and on the 13th day their body weight
was 10–15% below that of the untreated control animals (Fig. 4). Thereafter
the animals became increasingly feeble and, upon reduction to approximately
50% of the weight of the control animals, they died of "runt disease." This
difference in body weight, too, depends on the age of the host animals.

2.1.3.4. Survival Time

"Runt disease" is not always lethal. However, if very serious it is 100% lethal,
so that survival rate and survival time can definitely be used as a parameter.
Siskind and Thomas (1959) and Siskind et al. (1960) have thoroughly investigated in various inbred strains the mortality rate between the 5th and the
30th day after the injection of spleen cells. They discovered an accurate dose
dependence and also a dependence on the strength of histocompatibility differences. If the mortality rate is to be used as a reaction parameter, there exists
in rats (Billingham et al., 1960) a dependence on the strain as well as a distinct
relationship to the dose effect if thoracic duct lymphocytes are used as a graft.

The dependence of the survival period on the age of the host animals,
on the amount of injected spleen cells and on the animal strain can be demonstrated in an example.

If at the time of injection of 12×10^6 spleen cells from CPB/N mice, (C$_{57}$/Bl/6 $\times$ CPB/N) F$_1$ mice were 10–12 days old, approximately 25% of the animals died within the first 20 days; after 33 days 50% of the animals were dead. If the mice were 18–32 days old, 10% of the animals died during the first month and only 50% survived 14 months. If the host animals were 2–3 months old, 50% of the animals survived 23 months. After 32 months all animals were dead; in the age group 18–32 days, however, they were already dead after 27 months (Fig. 5). If the host animals were older than 2 months no further change in the mortality rate occurred.

Depending on the number of injected spleen cells, 12×10^6 spleen cells of CPB/N mice cause a 50% mortality after 23 months in (C$_{57}$/Bl/6 $\times$ CPB/N) F$_1$ hybrids; 24×10^6 spleen cells cause a 50% mortality after 4 months. The mortality rates compiled in Figure 6 are comparatively similar although the age of the host animals differed, since at an age upward of 2–3 months no further difference can be recorded with an equal amount of cells.

The dependence on the animal strain can also be proven by comparing various strains of mice. F$_1$ hybrids of the Balb/c $\times$ C$_{57}$/Bl/6 combination die very quickly. While, with an equal amount of transplanted cells, 50% of the animals of this combination are already dead after 30 days, 90% of the F$_1$ hybrids of the C$_{57}$/Bl/6 $\times$ CPB/N combination are still alive.

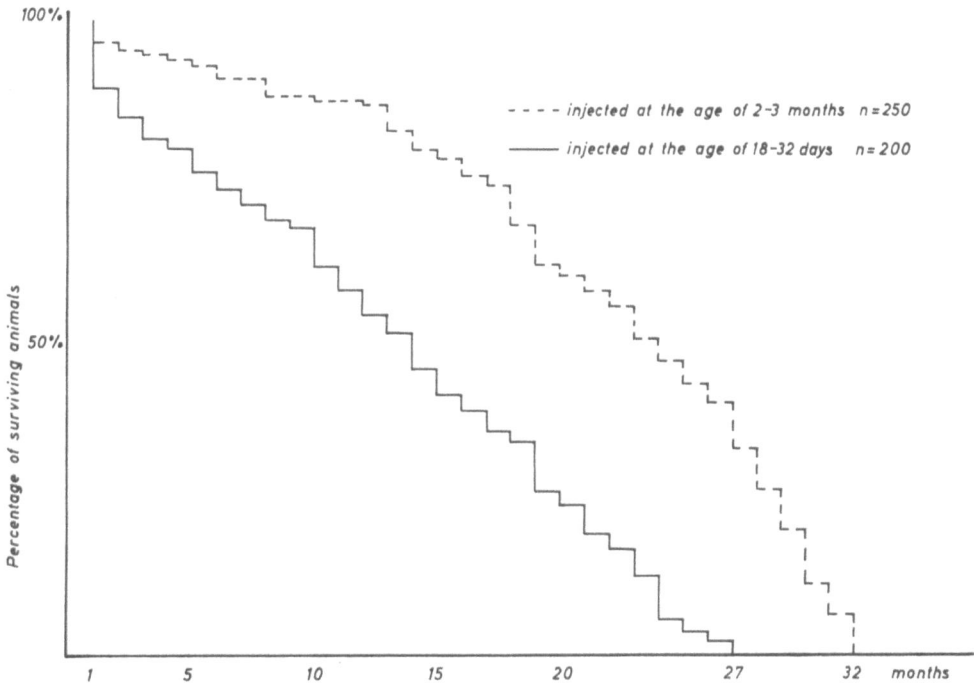

Fig. 5. Mortality in (C$_{57}$/Bl/6 $\times$ CPB/N) F$_1$ mice after i.p. transplantation of 12×10^6 spleen cells from CPB/N mice, at the age of 2–3 months, n=250 (-----) or at the age of 18–32 days, n=200 (———)

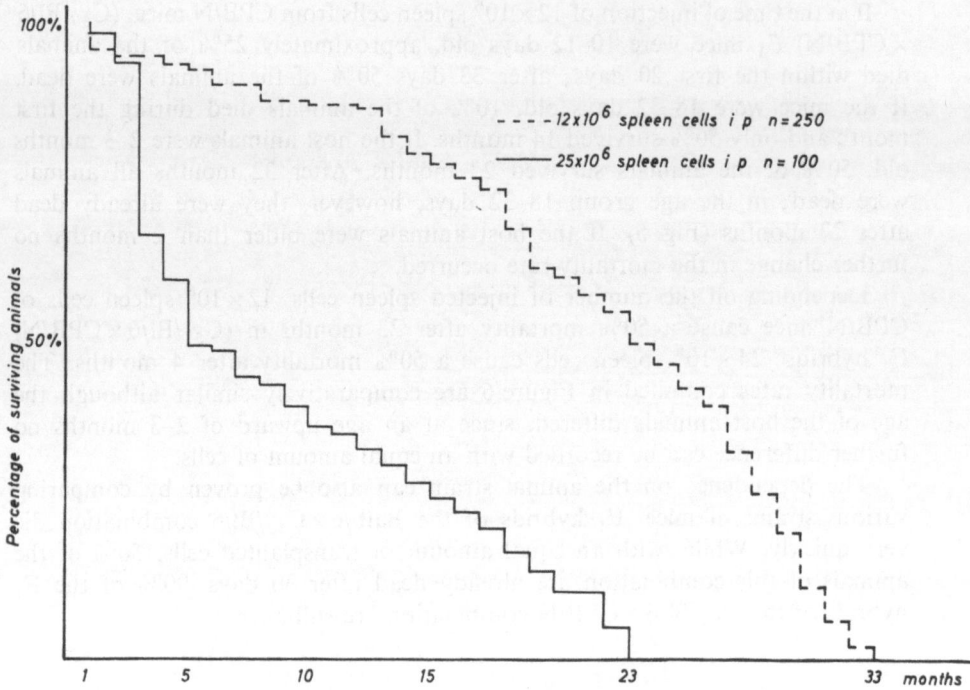

Fig. 6. Mortality in $(C_{57}/Bl/6 \times CPB/N)$ F_1 mice after i.p. transplantation of spleen cells from CPB/N mice: 12×10^6 spleen cells at the age of 2–3 months (------), n = 250, or 25×10^6 spleen cells at the age of 5–6 months (———), n = 100

An analogy can be noted with different strains of rats. Here it is interesting that, upon application of an equal amount of spleen cells of male BD III rats on 3- or 5–7 day-old (Wistar I × BD III) F_1 hybrids, all animals are dead by the 21st or 28th day respectively, whereas, upon application of cells from female Wistar I animals, survival rates ranged up to the 34th day.

Determination of survival time, however, remains an inaccurate parameter since accompanying infections or other unspecific factors influence these data strongly.

2.1.3.5. Phagocytosis Index

Intravenously injected colloidal carbon is *phagocytized* by the reticuloendothelial system. This phagocytosis increases during GVHR (Howard, 1961), up to 10 times its normal rate. This GVHR parameter runs parallel with other signs of GVHR (splenomegaly, loss of weight, etc.), depending on the employed animal strains and on the number of lymphocytes; injections of isologous lymphocytes do not significantly increase the phagocytosis index. The disadvantages of this index are that it is relatively expensive and dependent on unspecific factors.

2.1.3.6. Other Reaction Parameters

Enlargement of the liver has not proved a sufficient parameter. Hepatomegaly does indeed occur regularly but it is not as distinct as the enlargement of the spleen and is much more dependent on unspecific toxic concomitant phenomena.

Based on histologic examinations the periportal infiltration of lymphatic cells in the liver has been recommended as a test (GORER and BOYSE, 1959). MILLER *et al.* (1963) demonstrated that the number of infiltration foci in the liver is directly proportionate to the dose of immunocompetent cells administered. Although in the meantime this test has been used by several authors (e.g., BAIN and ALTON, 1964; LEVINE, 1968a), it, too, depends on numerous unspecific factors. Periportal infiltrates in the livers of rodents occur with virtually all infectious and noninfectious damages.

With chickens, counting the foci on the chorioallantoic membrane (CAM test) has proved a very useful parameter. Details are mentioned by BURNET and BOYER (1961). The number of "pocks" shows a linear dependence on dose. According to SZENBERG and WARNER (1961) an average of 40 lymphocytes is necessary to create a focus.

After comparing the various reaction parameters (cf. SIMONSEN, 1962) the chorioallantoic membrane stands out as the most reliable test for chickens. For rodents the spleen test can be used and—if a large amount of lymphocytes is applied—also the lymphopenia test (WITTING and DETLEFSEN, 1975). Equally significant is the phagocytosis test. Survival period and body weight give approximate clues whereas the weight of the liver and periportal liver cell infiltrates can not be used.

2.2. Local GVHR

Local GVHR is caused by local injection of immunocompetent cells into a host who is immuno-incompetent either for genetic reasons or through immunosuppression. It can be compared more easily than systemic GVHR to local transplant rejection.

2.2.1. The Intrarenal Form

This reaction has been developed in several variations by ELKINS (ELKINS, 1964, 1966, 1970) and has provided us with important general insights into cellular immune reactions (ELKINS, 1971). The experiments were conducted with F_1 hybrid rats which were AgB-incompatible. The immunocompetent parental cells were injected under the renal capsule which led to a rapid enlargement of the kidney tissue with its peak on the 14th day. Histologically, the kidney tissue was largely necrotic but only to the depth to which the immunocompetent cells had penetrated the kidney parenchyma.

In this model the proliferation of the injected immunocompetent cells was particularly easy to observe: it started with the transformation of the injected small lymphocytes into large blasts which soon began mitotic proliferation. This proliferation reached its peak on the 6th day and the necrosis of the kidney parenchyma expanded in a parallel process. During the first week at least, host cells played no part in this. This can be demonstrated by isotopic studies. The rate of incorporation as well as the weight of the kidneys stood in exponential function to the number of injected cells (ELKINS, 1970). The immunologic specificity of this change was confirmed by several investigators (ELKINS and GUTTMANN, 1968; VOLGMANN, 1972; CLANCY et al., 1973, among others).

2.2.2. The Intracutaneous Form

In analogy to the widespread experimental skin transplants the intracutaneous injection of immunocompetent cells was also used to a great extent for production of GVHR. According to BRENT and MEDAWAR (1966a, 1966b) the reaction starts with an inflammation during the first 3 days, followed, after another 3 days, by cell proliferation which greatly enlarges the focus. After 6 days the reaction begins to subside and after 9–10 days it has largely disappeared. In the case of guinea pigs (BRENT and MEDAWAR, 1966a; ZAKARIAN and BILLINGHAM, 1972) the intensity of this reaction is independent of a previous sensitization of the injected cells. This reaction was called "normal lymphocyte transfer reaction" (BRENT and MEDAWAR, 1966a). This test can be easily quantified for counting the newly developed blood vessels within the area of the GVHR. It is then called "lymphocyte-induced angiogenesis" (LIA) and the number of the newly developed blood vessels corresponds—at least within the dose range of 2×10^5 to 4×10^6 cells—to the number of injected immunocompetent cells. This test can also be considered specific depending on the quality of injected cells (SIDKY and AUERBACH, 1975).

In hamsters intracutaneous GVHR can be rendered more sensitive through previous radiation with 1500 r (RAMSEIER and STREILEIN, 1965; RAMSEIER and BILLINGHAM, 1966). The injection of immunocompetent allogeneic and xenogenous lymphocytes produces a skin reaction after 2–4 days which can easily be measured; thereby even weak histocompatibility differences can be detected after previous radiation, even those which can not be attributed to the H_2-locus (CORNELIUS and APONTE, 1974).

In rats, too, the inoculation of 2.5 to 20×10^6 lymphocytes from the thoracic duct of an older animal induces maximal skin reaction after 5 days in AgB-incompatible F_1 hybrids (STREILEIN and BILLINGHAM, 1967; FORD, 1967). The reactive cell proliferation of blasts depends on the strength of the histocompatibility difference (STREILEIN and BILLINGHAM, 1970a, 1970b).

2.2.3. Popliteal Lymph Node Test

The enlargement of the popliteal lymph nodes in Lewis $+$ BN-F_1 hybrid rats upon injection of Lewis spleen cells into the rear foot pad or even directly into the popliteal lymph node has been described as a typical GVHR by LEVINE (1968b). This reaction has several peculiarities: First, the enlargement of the lymph nodes can amount to as much as 50 times their normal size, since the proliferative potency of lymphatic tissue exceeds that of all other organs (GRUNDMANN, 1958). Secondly, there exists a strict relationship between dose and reaction—as with the spleen test (FORD *et al.*, 1970)—with an increase of sensibility by a factor of 10 as opposed to other local GVH reactions. Immunologically incompetent lymphocytes do not react (cf. GREBE and STREILEIN, 1976).

Strictly speaking, however, the popliteal lymph node test (PLN assay) represents not a local but a systemic GVHR. This is confirmed by the reactions of the peripheral blood and of the remaining lymphatic system (GREBE and STREILEIN, 1975a, 1975b, 1976).

With reference to this model the same authors pointed out the differences between a GVHR and a transplant rejection (cf. MEYER and HERON, 1973; TWIST and BARNES, 1973; DORSCH and ROSER, 1974; MONIE and EVERETT, 1974). If, for instance, F_1 lymphoid cells are injected into parental popliteal lymph nodes of rats a hypertrophy occurs as well—the manifestation of a transplant reaction. This reaction, however, reaches its peak on the 4th day, that is 3 days before the maximal reaction of a GVHR. This variation of the popliteal lymph node test is also called the host-versus-graft reaction (HGVR) and is considered a particularly demonstrative model of a transplant-allograft immunity.

The same model was used to investigate problems of immune tolerance and of the enhancement phenomenon (BILDSØE *et al.*, 1971; ATKINS and FORD, 1972; HERON, 1973; COHEN and WEKERLE, 1973; HÁSKOVÁ *et al.*, 1973a, 1973b, among others). Lymphocytes from the spleen and Peyer's patches cause—just as do lymphocytes from the thoracic duct—a typical GVHR upon injection of popliteal lymph nodes from F_1 hybrids (LEVIN *et al.*, 1974). From among the thymus lymphocytes, only the hydrocortison-resistant group shows a reaction (see p. 808). Germ-free rats react just as strongly as ordinary animals (NIELSEN, 1972). The range of variability in this test leads us to expect that popliteal lymph node GVHR will in the future grant us further insights into cellular immunomechanisms.

2.2.4. The Intra-Ocular Form

The injection of parental lymphocytes into the anterior chamber of the eye of F_1 hybrid rats also causes a local GVHR (KAPLAN *et al.*, 1975a, 1975b). The course of the reaction is quicker than under the renal capsule, in the skin or in the popliteal lymph nodes. Speed and duration can also be measured and thus the intensity with allogenous host animals can be compared, so that this test therefore offers advantages as compared to other local reactions of the same type.

2.3. In-Vitro Analogies

All in-vitro experiments are accompanied by numerous reaction factors which
are not at all or else only indirectly of an immunologic nature. There are,
for instance, the influences of the adrenal cortical hormones or of the far
less well known neurovegetative reflexes which occur with every inflammation,
especially, of course, with local GVHR. Such factors of uncertainty are eliminated with in-vitro analogies to GVHR which, in the past 20 years, have not
only greatly improved our understanding of GVHR but which have also enriched
our general knowledge of cellular immune reactions. Several possibilities have
been tested experimentally; two of them proved successful.

2.3.1. The Mixed Lymphocyte Culture

This is an in-vitro confrontation of immunocompetent lymphocytes with other
allogeneic lymphocytic histocompatibility antigens in the presence of macrophages. The mixed lymphocyte culture (MLC) is an important pretest for every
transplant reaction (BAIN and LOWENSTEIN, 1964; BACH and AMOS, 1967; JEAN-
NET et al., 1969; WILSON and NOWELL, 1970, 1971; WILSON and FOX, 1971;
BACH, 1973; EIJSVOOGEL, 1974, among others).

This test is an examination of cell-mediated cytotoxicity (CMC), which is
independent of complement. It only occurs with thymus-dependent cells (WILSON
et al., 1967; KISKEN and SWENSON, 1969) and thus indicates the activity of
those thymus-dependent lymphocytes which is present within the "killer-cell"
population (LONAI et al., 1971). From among the thymus lymphocytes those
that react primarily are the smaller populations (10–20% of the thymus lymphocytes which possess a highly active H_2-locus, are corticoid-resistant, and are
predominantly located in the marrow of the thymus (SHORTMAN et al., 1972)).
Contrary to former belief (cf. GOLDSTEIN and BLOMGREN, 1973) the presence
of B-lymphocytes is also necessary for the MLC, at least for the stimulation
of spleen lymphocytes through thymus cells (BERMAN et al., 1976).

MLC proliferation starts after approximately 2 days, reaches its peak on
the 5th day and lasts altogether about 4 days, that is, until the 6th day after
the beginning of incubation. Lymphocytes from specifically immunized animals
show a stronger proliferation corresponding to the "second set reaction" which
already reaches its peak on the 3rd day. This proliferation is only among parental
cells when parental and F_1 hybrid cells are mixed. As with the in-vivo studies
only 1–3% of the peripheral blood lymphocytes proliferate; this is also the
amount of antigen-reactive cells in allogeneic GVHR. Humoral antibodies obviously play no part in this test. Peripheral blood lymphocytes from germ-free
and from conventional rats show the same MLC.

With this relatively clear in-vitro test, at least three conditions which can
also be transferred to systemic and local in-vivo GVHR, could be determined
most accurately: 1) the exact rate of lymphocytes that are immunocompetent
against the histocompatibility antigens: 1 to 3%; 2) the fact that these immunocompetent cells belong to the minority population of T-lymphocytes; and 3)
the favored primary proliferation of parental cells upon confrontation with
the histocompatibility antigens represented by F_1 hybrid cells (see p. 838).

2.3.2. The Spleen Explant Test

Observations on chickens (MURPHY, 1916; SIMONSEN, 1957; VAN ALTEN and FEN-NELL, 1959) as well as splenomegaly in rodents (see p. 799) kindled interest in an in-vitro test with explanted spleen tissue. GLOBERSON and AUERBACH (1965) have developed such a spleen explant test as a semiquantitative method: they added parental lymphatic cells to a single-cell suspension or to small explants from spleens of F_1 hybrids and measured the growth of the explant. An intensified growth of the explants under the influence of these parental lymphatic cells could indeed be detected. Additions of ^{3}H-labeled leucine (AUERBACH and SHALABY, 1973) proved, as with the MLC, that predominantly the parental lymphocytes incorporated the isotope, which means that they participated in this transformation and proliferation. As compared to the MLC, this test is influenced by a certain number of additional factors of uncertainty since, at least during the implantation into spleen fragments, other cells can be involved apart from the lymphocytes, e.g., sinus endothelia, macrophages and possibly also undifferentiated stem cells.

3. Clinical Observations

In humans GVHR as a disease, that is GVHD, occurs, in analogy to our experiments, when allogeneic immunocompetent cells come into contact with an organism which does possess histocompatibility antigens for these cells but which does not itself react to these alien cells with a specific immune reaction. In principle this can be the case with every transplantation of tissue or organs since immunocompetent cells are practically always implanted along with them. Each time a massive immunosuppression must be carried out in order to curb the transplant rejection, which creates immunologic conditions close to those prerequisite for a GVHR. In most cases, however, these conditions are not quite fulfilled so that GVHR generally plays no part in skin or organ transplantations.

GVHR is, however, the most feared complication in bone marrow transplantations. This operation is always performed in cases of immune insufficiencies, e.g., with congenital immune insufficiency, after iatrogenic or accident-induced whole-body irradiation (i.e., after nuclear explosions or accidents with nuclear reactors) and also after massive drug-induced immune suppression in leukemias, malignant lymphomas, etc. Finally, bone marrow transplantation is also the chosen therapy for true aplastic anemias.

The first—and so far the only one known—nuclear reactor accident with lethal or sublethal irradiation of humans occurred in Vinča near Belgrad. Five men and one woman received a total dose of 95–214 rad each (AUXIER, 1961). At 27 to 32 days after exposure the patients were injected with $8.5–14 \times 10^9$ nucleated bone marrow cells (MATHÉ et al., 1959; JAMMET et al., 1959). This accident occurred at a time during which the possibility of bone marrow transplantation as a clinical therapy was considered and worked on with intense

experimentation (TRENTIN, 1956; MATHÉ and BERNARD, 1958, 1959; MATHÉ
et al., 1958, 1960–1962; DE VRIES and VOS, 1958, 1959; VAN BEKKUM, 1959,
1963, among others). The clinical results, however, remained mostly unsatisfactory (BORTIN, 1970; CONGDON, 1970), for which the frequently lethal GVHR
was not the least important reason. Only the introduction of Hl-A-matching
and of the MLC test (see p. 846) made it possible to obtain, such a far-reaching
isogeneity between donor and host that bone marrow transplants as therapy
was successful. In the meantime identical twins and even isogenous brothers
and/or sisters have successfully undergone bone marrow transplantations in
at least 25 cases (THOMAS et al., 1971; FASS et al., 1973; FEFER et al., 1973;
RUDOLPH et al., 1973; SPECK, 1973, 1975, among others). The maximum survival
rate so far observed is over 12 years (THOMAS, 1974).

Decisive, in this case, are immunogenetics which, however, had a few sur-
prises in store. The Hl-A locus and the MLC locus are very close together
on the same autosome, so that many—about 25%—of the Hl-A-identical
brothers and sisters are MLC-negative (cf., SPECK, 1975). Since the blood group
of the ABO system and other antigens play a part too, the best results are
obtained with Hl-A-identical, MLC-negative brothers and sisters.

Clinical experience, however, shows that even with Hl-A-identity and negative MLC, serious GVH reactions can occur which may even lead to a lethal
GVHD (MEUWISSEN et al., 1971; GRAW et al., 1971; GLUCKSBERG et al., 1974;
SPECK et al., 1971, 1973; among others). This discrepancy gives rise to the
suspicion that differences exist within the Hl-A antigen or that another genetic
factor outside the Hl-A antigen is involved. With mice SALAMANN et al. (1973)
have shown that the M locus of the mouse can cause a GVHR in the same
way as the H-2 locus. KLEIN (1973) described a special GVH locus within
the H-2 locus of the mouse which may be the decisive causative factor for
the GVHR.

Such experimental studies with animals help explain the frequently discourag-
ing clinical experiences with humans. After all the incidence of GVHR with
Hl-A-identical and MLC-negative brothers and sisters is still almost 70% and
the search for histocompatibility antigens which do not belong to the Hl-A-group
is justly given special attention (cf., for example, JEANNET et al., 1969). In over
20% of the cases, the GVHR after bone marrow transplantations is lethal
(GUTTERMANN et al., 1974; THOMAS et al., 1975; SPECK, 1975). Over a period
of over 5 years GLUCKSBERG et al. (1974) observed 43 clear cases of GVHD
in 61 cases of bone marrow transplantation. At the end of the 5-year observation
period about half the patients which had shown no signs of GVHD were still
alive; of those with GVHD only 13% had survived. In many cases it cannot
be determined with certainty what influence the cytostatic therapy had on the
original disease or on the suppression of a GVHD. The same applies when
specific immunosuppressives are used (STREILEIN, 1972b; GENGOZIAN et al.,
1973).

If the donors are Hl-A-incompatible but with negative MLC, it is interesting
to observe that only a slight GVHR sets in (GATTI and MEUWISSEN, 1971;
KOCH et al., 1973; DUPONT, 1974; GALE et al., 1975). Even a positive MLC
test does not necessarily cause a GVHR (GALE et al., 1975). The first bone

marrow transplantations with Hl-A-incompatible brothers or sisters were carried out in 1970 by MATHÉ *et al.* on patients with serious bone marrow aplasias, although under immune suppression and with antilymphocyte-globulin (see p.852). The clinical aspect of GVHD usually begins with a maculopapulous exanthema on the trunk, preferably in the axillae and the flexure of the groin. It can be morbilliform with or without pruritus, but it can also resemble a lichen ruber planus (SAURAT *et al.*, 1975). The skin symptoms can disappear quickly but they can also change into a generalized erythrodermia with rough-leafed flakings. Heavy, watery diarrhea with stomach pain, vomiting and occasionally ileus are the rule, Dehydration follows with general wasting symptoms. The liver-function test has strong positive results and frequently icterus sets in. The hematologic condition shows thrombocytopenia, frequently lymphopenia and hemolytic anemia. The patients mostly die of infections with high fever and in greatly reduced general status. Beside bacterial infections, viruses such as cytomegalovirus with interstitial pneumonia, fungi, and also *Pneumocystis carinii* take part in this.

3.1. "Spontaneous" GVHD in Humans

It is now certain that lymphocytes transfer in utero between mother and child. This exchange has been proven from the 3rd month of pregnancy onward when about 0.3% of the maternal lymphocytes stem from the fetus (SCHRÖDER and DE LA CHAPELLE, 1972). The hypertrophy of the regional lymph nodes of a gravid uterus is considered to be a mild GVHR (BEER and BILLING-HAM, 1973). If the fetus is male, the Y-chromosome in the nucleus of the lymphocytes can be clearly shown by fluorescent microscopy after having been dyed with atebrin, for instance. The mother is normally protected by lymphocyte-blocking antibodies against the alien lymphocytes of the child which, genetically, stem from the male (CEPELLINI *et al.*, 1971). The same applies to the fetus. If this is not the case and father and mother are Hl-A-incompatible, the maternal lymphocytes can cause a GVHD in the embryo in the same way as the A→A+B type of experimental GVHR (see p. 796).

That this can indeed happen is authenticated in at least one case: KADOWAKI *et al.* (1965) have described a lymphatic chimaerism with a congenital immunoinsufficiency syndrome and a typical alymphoplasia. The child was a XX/XY lymphoid cell chimaera.

Meanwhile several further cases have been published (e.g., BERRY, 1970; GROGAN *et al.*, 1975), which presented a similar morphologic aspect of the inner organs but where no lymphocyte chimaerism could be proven. In retrospect it seems likely that the observations of congenital aplastic anemias with histiocytosis and erythrodermia in immunoinsufficient newborns by HATHAWAY *et al.* (1965) and of a child with aplastic anemia, lymphocytosis and hypogammaglobulinemia (HATHAWAY *et al.*, 1966) are to be interpreted in the same way. Similarly, the observations of SHAPIRO (1967) and DOOREN *et al.* (1968), during which either a familiar autohemolytic anemia together with a severe wasting disease or else a sex-specific thymus hypoplasia had appeared, possibly belong to the same category.

It should be investigated—as a hypothesis at least—whether in other cases of congenital immune diseases a uterine exchange of lymphocytes was one of the causative factors.

The first (male) case of Di George syndrome (Di George, 1968) contained 2% female cells as discovered by karyotype analysis. It is unknown why in another case with thymus alymphoplasia and proven XX/XY lymphocyte chimaerism no typical GVHD had ocurred (Githens et al., 1969). Perhaps the child died before the reaction had time to develop. It is also possible, however, that too few male lymphocytes were present since we know from experiments with animals (see p. 803) that the onset and intensity of GVHR depend on the amount of implanted or exchanged lymphocytes.

3.2. GVHD After Bone Marrow Transplantation

3.2.1. In Cases of Primary Immunoinsufficiency or Aplastic Anemia

Today congenital immune deficiency syndromes (IDS), especially the serious combined Swiss-type agammaglobulinemia constitute a domain for bone marrow transplantations. As of 1968 already three apparently successful bone marrow transplantations on children with IDS had been reported (Gatti et al., 1968; Bach et al., 1968; de Koning et al., 1969). So far at least 25 complete bone marrow reconstructions have been reported for such congenital immunopathies (Good, 1973; Hitzig, 1975). Bone marrow transplantation with complete hemopoetic chimaerism is also the chosen therapy for aplastic anemias (Storb et al., 1973a, 1974a, 1974b). The decisive element here is that multipotent stem cells must be implanted together with the bone marrow. In order to reduce the frequency of GVHD as much as possible, very different methods are employed nowadays (see p. 852). Nevertheless, GVHD is the most feared complication especially with this group of patients. Cline et al. (1975) have compiled cases of GVHD after bone marrow transplantations for aplastic anemia. Out of 65 patients 40 were taken ill with GVHD and 11 died from it.

Millers's observations (1967) can be considered characteristic. After bone marrow transplantation for thymus dysplasia with Swiss-type agammaglobulinemia the GVHD set in 6 days after the transplantation with a diffuse edema and a maculous exanthema on the entire body. On the 8th day splenomegaly and on the 10th day hepatomegaly was noted, and on the 12th day the dehydrated child died with symptoms of a respiratory disorder. The autopsy revealed all characteristics of a GVHD (see p. 827) with a considerable alteration of the functions of the reticuloendothelial system (Miller and Hummeler, 1967).

3.2.2. In Leukemias

Especially in cases of acute leukosis a bone marrow transplantation can be life-saving. In order to obtain a complete blood chimaerism, a complete marrow aplasia must be created through high-dosed cytostatic therapy and/or through whole-body irradiation. In so-called sterile tents the patients must be kept free of exogenous infections. By 1967 approximately 60 patients had been treated this way (VAN BEKKUM and DE VRIES, 1967) and, by 1975, 162 patients in three american centers alone (CLINE et al., 1975).

Although this therapy, because of the above-mentioned prerequisites, can only be applied in specially equipped hospitals, bone marrow transplantation is now possible in several centers. Now as then the development of GVHD is the biggest problem (cf. THOMAS and EPSTEIN, 1965, MATHÉ et al., 1969; SPECK, 1973, 1975; THOMAS et al., 1975; CLINE et al., 1975). Among the 162 cases which CLINE et al. (1975) have compiled, 68 were taken ill with GVHD and 26 died of it.

MATHÉ et al. (1965) were able to demonstrate that GVHR can have an immediate antileukemic effect. In the "mouse model" transplantable leukemia in a irradiated mouse was positively influenced by the induction of GVHR (BORANIĆ, 1971, BORTIN et al., 1974). On the other hand it must be remembered that a GVHR can induce malignant tumors, especially of lymphoreticular tissue (see p. 854).

3.2.3. After Blood Transfusions

Less well-known and less taken into consideration in practice, is the fact that a GVHD can set in even after simple blood transfusions. This too, however, applies only to patients with a defective immune system, i.e., with a malignant lymphoma after high-dose cytostatic treatment or in children with a primary immunoinsufficiency. The so-called spontaneous cases of GVHD which are described above, have mostly been treated with blood transfusions only and, according to our present knowledge, it must be assumed that these favored the formation of GVHD. HATHAWAY et al. (1965, 1967), HONG et al. (1968), DOUGLAS and FUDENBERG (1968) and PARK et al. (1974) reported seven cases with serious congenital immune defects who died 2–4 weeks after a blood transfusion from a serious GVHD. In the case of DOUGLAS and FUDENBERG (1968) fresh plasma from the father of the child had been administered; in the other cases whole blood, and in the case of PARK et al. (1974) only 50 ml., had been given. A lethal GVHD can also occur after exchange transfusions with hemolytic disease of the newborn (HATHAWAY et al., 1966). NAIMAN et al. (1969) and PARKMAN et al. (1974) reported on children who died after an intrauterine transfusion and a later exchange transfusion. In all cases a lymphocyte chimaerism existed. RUBINSTEIN et al. (1973) observed GVHD after a plasma infusion in a child with a κ-IGD paraproteinemia. This case is particularly remarkable because here a light – not lethal – GVHD developed without previous injection of lymphocytes. Here the mechanism of the formation of GVHD has not been fully explained.

These experiences show that blood to be transfused into immunoinsufficient patients should previously be irradiated in vitro with 1500 rad in order to inactivate the immunocompetent cells (GROFF et al., 1976).

4. Histopathology

The reaction parameters of the individual species are very similar (see p. 799) and so the histopathologic changes resemble each other correspondingly. In the following, however, the reactions of individual species of animals which times are divergent shall be pointed out. The greatest number of examinations was conducted on the A→A+B type in mice and rats which also yielded the clearest results since with them changes caused by additional factors, as for instance irradiation reactions in radiation chimaeras, can be eliminated (cf. Vos *et al.,* 1959; de Vries and Vos, 1959).

4.1. Mice

4.1.1. Spleen

After 24 h a strong proliferation of large lymphoid cells with basophilic, pyroninophilic cytoplasm can be observed in the center of the splenic corpuscle and perifollicularly, but predominantly subcapsularly, in the red pulp (e.g. Billingham and Brent, 1959; Gowans, 1962; Grundmann and Hobik, 1975). These cells correspond to those which Howard (1961) referred to as plasmoblasts or which Gorer and Boyse (1959) called histiocytes. The same term was adopted by Binet and Mathé (1962) on the basis of electron microscopic studies.

According to follow-up studies by Armstrong *et al.* (1967) over a period of $1^1/_2$ years and our own research on the development of lymphomas (Grundmann and Hobik, 1973a), the propagation of these "blasts," and also of real plasma cells and of reticular cells inside the follicles continues to increase during the first 4 weeks (Fig.7) whereas, in the white pulp, a decrease of the small lymphocytes becomes noticeable already. After this the homogeneity of the reaction discontinues and already the marked differences of extent and nature of the changes in individual animals become apparent: in some of the animals the spleen follicles continue to grow and flow together, a process during which the number of medium-sized and large lymphocytes, of plasma cells and also of reticular cells increases, some of the latter having very pale nuclei.

In contrast to this "pleomorphic" reaction, another group of animals shows a "histiocytic" reaction. In this case a progressive necrosis of the spleen follicles occurs with phagocytosis of the cell fragments and their replacement by histiocytes, ending with complete atrophy and consequent fibrosis. Research by Billingham and Brent (1959) reveals that upon induction of GVHR immediately after birth, the pleomorphic reaction in later stages is barely noticeable while atrophic-fibrous changes predominate. The "secondary disease," namely radiation chimaeras, also results in total atrophy of the follicles (van Bekkum and de Vries, 1967).

The further course often brings localized proliferation of lymphoblasts and reticular cells, similar to the initial symptoms of GVHR ("biphasic reaction"). This can later produce malignant lymphomas, especially since analogous changes

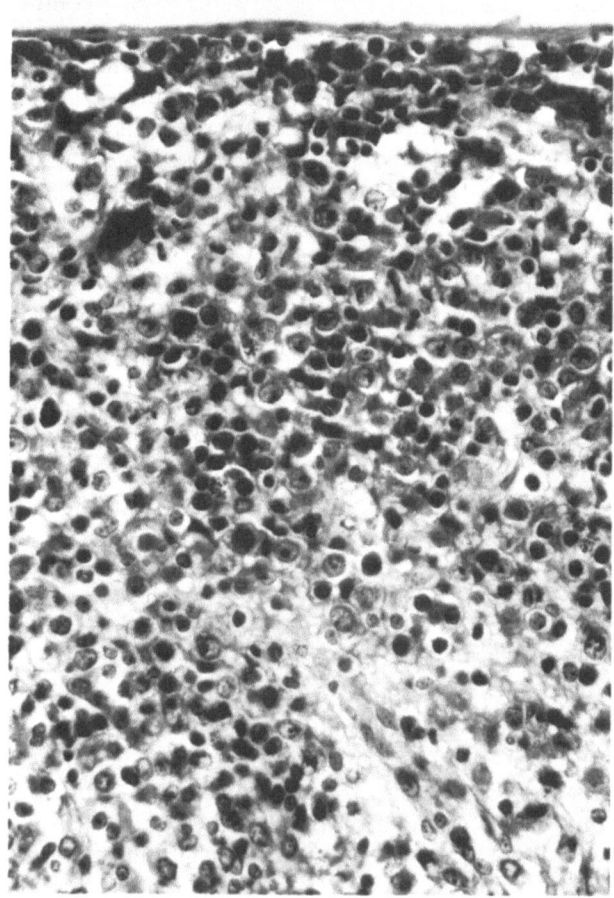

Fig. 7. Spleen of a mouse in acute GVHR on day 15 after transfer of spleen cells. Proliferation
of basophilic "blast cells". H & E × 100

have been observed in immunoinsufficient NZB × NZW mice (HOBIK and SA-
WADA, 1970).

Finally, an extramedullary hematopoiesis of varying intensity, independent
of the kind of above-mentioned changes, is noteworthy. In the A→A+B type
it is to be considered as a consequence of damage to the bone marrow during
the transplantation of spleen cells in irradiated mice, as a manifestation of
a successful repopulation with hematopoietic cells (SILOBRČIĆ and TRENTIN,
1966; GOODMAN et al., 1972).

4.1.2. Lymph Nodes

In the initial phase the changes correspond to those of the spleen. The proliferation of "blasts" is generally less pronounced. A definite multiplication of

histiocytes, however, can be detected in the sinus, which continues to increase with the progress of the disease, with a simultaneous decrease of the small lymphocytes in the follicles. The "pleomorphic" reaction which occurs later, is, according to Armstrong et al. (1967), more unusual in the lymph nodes than in the spleen. The "histiocytic" reaction predominates. In our experience, this depends on the amount of transplanted cells: large numbers of cells (up to 320×10^6 i.p.) produce greater changes which occur earlier, shorten the life span and thus reduce the percentage of animals with "pleomorphic" reactions and biphasic, later premalignant, changes. Comparable changes are observed in experiments with parabiosis (Finerty, 1952), and also in "secondary diseases" from radiation chimaeras (van Bekkum and de Vries, 1967).

The reconstruction of the atrophy of lymph nodes caused by lethal irradiation (Denko, 1956) takes place after transplantation of bone marrow or lymphatic cells by repopulating the lymph nodes from the 6th day on (Congdon and Urso, 1957). If the transplanted bone marrow is isologous, complete restitution can be achieved (van Bekkum and de Vries, 1967), whereas the abovementioned "histiocytic" reaction always sets in—after initial restitution—if homologous cells are used (Kaplan and Rosston, 1959).

4.1.3. Liver

Periportal, perivascular and focal infiltrations of "blasts" are typical as soon as 48 h after the transplantation of cells in, for instance, the $A \rightarrow A + B$ type (Gorer and Boyse, 1959; de Hart et al., 1961; Miller et al., 1963) and also after irradiation (Silobrčić and Trentin, 1966). According to Bain and Fenna (1972) and Bain and Diener (1972), these blast infiltrations, which are also used as reaction parameters for GVHR (cf. 2.1.3.6.), consist predominantly of T-cells. Later on, hypertrophy and an increase of Kupffer cells with increased phagocytosis follow (Howard, 1964; Gotjamanos, 1970). One can also find, in varying degrees, degenerative symptoms and with "secondary disease" even necrotic areas of varying size (van Bekkum and de Vries, 1967) as well as an increase of liver cells with twin nuclei (Siskind and Thomas, 1959; Bain and Alton, 1964; Nowell and Cole, 1959). In some animals Cornelius et al. (1968) found clots in the portal veins and PAS-positive material in the area surrounding them.

In many cases it is difficult to differentiate the consequences of a GVHR from concomitant consequences of infections (Mc Bride, 1966; Keast, 1968b; Keast and Walter, 1968), especially since they may be absent if germ-free animals are used (Pollard, 1969). This applies particularly to reactions which can be detected with the electron microscope (Arakawa et al., 1966) with hypertrophy of Kupffer cells, multiplication of phagosomes and degeneration of hepatocytes. One finds analogous changes in experimental bacterial endotoxinemia (Papadimitriou and Keast, 1969). The typical liver damages resulting from "secondary disease," which are fully comparable to GVHR, are, however, also found in germ-free mice (van Bekkum et al., 1967).

4.1.4. Skin

Changes of the skin are much less frequent in mice than, for instance, in rats and hamsters. Descriptions exist of lesions of varying intensity, from an edema of the subcutaneous tissue via lymphocytic and histiocytic infiltrations to vacuolar degeneration and necrosis of the epithelium, which is permeated by granulocytes (VAN BEKKUM and DE VRIES, 1967; VAN BEKKUM et al., 1967; CORNELIUS et al., 1968; GRUNDMANN and HOBIK, 1975).

4.1.5. Bone Marrow

In the early stage "blast" infiltrations are observed, followed by hyperplasia of the myelopoietic cell group. After 2–3 months aplasia occurs during which the ripe neutrophils remain initially intact. The erythropoiesis is hyperplastic or aplastic. Moreover, histiocyte infiltrations of varying intensity occur. The bone marrow changes are in strict correlation with the changes of the lymphatic tissue (GITHENS et al., 1968; CORNELIUS et al., 1969; SMITANANDA et al., 1972). Our own examinations showed that there exist considerable variations in the changes depending not only on the animal strain, but also on the age of the animals and the amount of implanted cells. Frequently there are differences even between animals of the same experimental group.

4.1.6. Other Tissues

Relatively few histopathologic studies exist regarding changes in other organ systems (kidneys, thymus, heart, pancreas, lungs and intestines). Even these, however, are dependent on the antigen differences of the H_2 locus, the number of transplanted cells and the age of the donors and host animals (KAPLAN and ROSSTON, 1959; SIMONSEN, 1962; LEWIS et al., 1968). During the acute phase of GVHR, "blasts" are often found in the various organs (GORER and BOYSE, 1959), so that the degenerative changes must often be attributed to the consequences of cytotoxic effects from these "blasts" (GRANGER and KOLB, 1968). Some of the changes, however, are probably unspecific consequences of shock.

This certainly does not apply to the atrophy which develops in the thymus. As early as the second day, HILDEMANN et al. (1964) found a narrowing of the thymic cortex together with proliferation of reticular cells and the appearance of large histiocytic cells in the thymus marrow. With the electron microscope (WEISS and AISENBERG, 1965) an edema of the thymus can be detected, and also a swelling of mitochondria and myelin formations in the reticuloepithelial cells. Macrophages, which have developed in increasing numbers, contain fat and other phagocytized material. Necroses, "looking like moth holes," which appear from the 5th day on in the thymic cortex (KAPLAN and ROSSTON, 1959), as well as karyorrhexis of the cortical lymphocytes, which can be observed again and again, eventually dissolve the border between marrow and cortex and lead to a histologic reversal of the thymic structure with a loose cortex and a marrow comparatively rich in cells.

In the *heart* of some animals fibrous necroses occur (Kaplan and Rosston, 1959), in the *lungs* atelectases, hemorrhages and edemas. The *small intestine* shows characteristic necroses with abscesses and localised blast infiltrations (Nowell and Cole, 1959). In newborn mice of the A→A+B type changes are particularly pronounced (Reilly and Kirsner, 1965). An enlargement and flattening of the villi is found with a colonization resembling that found with sprue. The crypts are enlarged and show an increase of mitoses and frequent necroses.

In the *pancreas,* individual foci of necrosis can occur with fat necroses (Gorer and Boyse, 1959; Cornelius *et al.,* 1968), often accompanied by infiltrations of mononuclear cells (Walter, 1966). Strong proliferation of lymphoreticular tissue can cause a granulomatous inflammation.

Amyloid deposits have been described as general reactions in several organs, e.g. in the kidneys and in the walls of the large and small intestine (Cornelius *et al.,* 1968) and also in the spleen (Kaplan and Rosston, 1959). Another general reaction is the increase of the histiocytic macrophage system in all organs. According to Howard *et al.* (1969), at least the pulmonary and alveolar macrophages in mice suffering from GVHR, stem from the donor animal. It is possible that the entire pool of the macrophage-histiocytic system is not only stimulated in a functional and proliferative sense by GVHR but that, temporarily at least, it is formed by lymphocytes from the donor. For radiation chimaera, this has been known for some time (Pinkett *et al.,* 1966; Virolainen, 1968). The multiplication of Kupffer cells in the liver (see above) should probably be interpreted in the same way.

4.2. Rats

4.2.1. Spleen

In our experiments with newborn (Wistar I × BD III) F_1 rats, the reaction after transplantation of 5.4×10^6 spleen cells of adult BD III rats begins on the 4th day with a blast proliferation in the sinusoids, especially subcapsular with a simultaneous decrease of lymphocytes in the spleen follicles. With increasing spleen weight, the blast proliferation becomes even more pronounced from the 7th day onward—now also in the spleen follicles with a marked increase of reticular cells. Intensification of erythropoiesis follows, together, with a strong increase of megakaryocytes. From the 10th day on, the follicles are dissolved through further decrease of lymphocytes with simultaneous increase of reticular cells, and fibrosis sets in which later progresses. On the 13th day the blast proliferation reaches its climax. From the 16th day on, the number of blasts decreases noticeably; a multiplication of reticular cells predominates together with a strong increase of erythro- and myelopoiesis. Degenerative changes of the megakaryocytes take place and localized necroses appear which continue to increase till the 19th day, when the first casualties occur. The changes correspond to those in newborn Lewis rats after transplantation of $18–20 \times 10^6$ lymphatic cells from BN rats (Billingham *et al.,* 1962). In adult rats (Fig. 8),

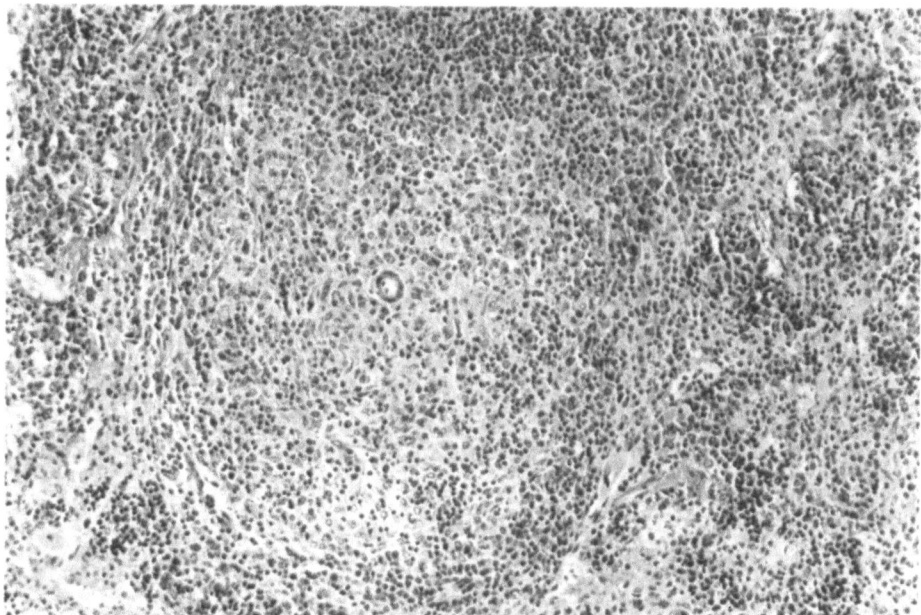

Fig. 8. Depletion of lymphocytes in the lymphatic follicle of the spleen from a 2-month-old (Wistar I × BD III) F_1 rat 15 days after transfer of spleen cells from a parent strain. H & E × 60

the intensity of the above-mentioned changes (STASTNY et al., 1965) depend to a particularly large degree on the number of transplanted cells (BILLINGHAM et al., 1960).

4.2.2. Lymph Nodes

Here, too, a marked blast proliferation can be observed at a very early stage together with an increase of macrophages, particularly in the abdominal lymph nodes. In addition, sinus histiocytosis occurs. The end stage consists of atrophy. Individual animals have small hematopoietic foci in the lymph nodes with megakaryocytes similar to the osteomyelofibrotic animals of BECKER et al. (1968). So far, the "pleomorphic" reaction, which is characteristic for mice, and which sometimes turns into malignant lymphomas, has not been observed in rats in survival periods of as much as 200 days.

4.2.3. Liver

Here, too, periportal cell infiltrations (BILLINGHAM et al., 1962), and an increase of Kupffer cells with individual localized epithelial necroses (STASTNY et al., 1965) are most prominent. According to our observations, all these changes (Fig. 9) depend on the age of the hosts and the number of transplanted spleen cells. In newborn and young rats an increase of hematopoietic foci is occasionally observed, generally in correlation with the osteomyelofibrotic changes of the bone marrow (see p. 821). It is interesting that periportal liver infiltrations

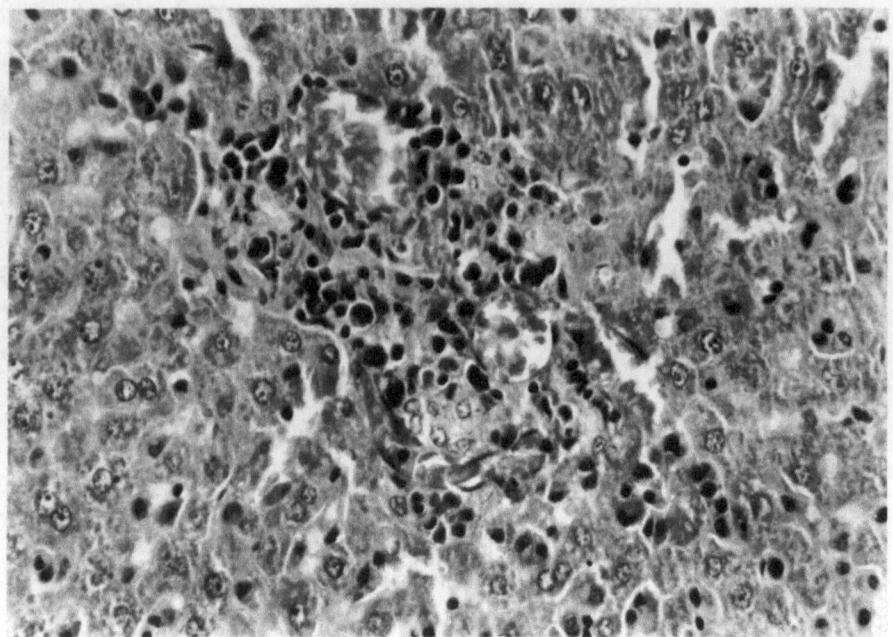

Fig. 9. Liver of rat with acute GVHR. Infiltration of portal spaces with lymphoid "blast cells".
H & E × 100

have also been found after local GVHR of the kidney (ELKINS, 1970). Upon utilization of the A→A+B type, the intensity of these infiltrations was stronger in splenectomized rats than in control animals (LEVINE, 1968a).

4.2.4. Skin

In the acute phase, an infiltration of histiocytes and lymphocytes occurs in the dermis between the 9th and the 11th day (BILLINGHAM et al., 1962; STASTNY et al., 1963). The epidermis above it thickens from normally two to three layers of cells to as many as six or seven. Keratinization increases. After the 12 to 13th day no "stratum granulosum" is visible any more. Vacuoles form between the epithelial cells, localized necroses with granulocytes occur, and also degenerations and necroses of hair, and loss of sebaceous glands with infiltrations of lymphocytes, plasma cells, histiocytes and, in the end stage, also granulocytes.

Homologous transplants, which are not affected by these inflammable changes, have demonstrated that these changes are immediate immunologic reactions (STASTNY et al., 1963).

In the chronic course, the most prominent symptoms are thickening of the skin, formation of scales and alopecia. The dermis is collagenized, a general skin atrophy develops with collagenization of connective tissue. Isolated ulcers appear. According to our experience, these changes, too, depend on the number of implanted cells and the age of the host. Animals which get over GVHR show skin defects. The scaly skin on nose and paws is one of the first exterior signs of GVHR (GRUNDMANN and HOBIK, 1973b, 1975).

4.2.5. Bone Marrow

Depending on the amount of injected cells, the number of cells in the bone marrow decreases with varying rapidity. According to BILLINGHAM et al. (1962) the myelopoiesis/erythropoiesis ratio increases to 4:1 and a strong increase of metamyelocytes, granulocytes and eosinophils sets in. Even with local GVHR, a totally aplastic bone marrow (Fig. 10) with lethal anemia can occur (ELKINS, 1970). After whole-body irradiation and transfusion of $15–70 \times 10^6$ allogenoneic bone marrow cells, BECKER et al. (1968) described myelofibrosis and osteomyelosclerosis in individual animals. The changes start with an increase of reticular cells and of fibroblasts, followed by an osteoid formation and a sclerosation with wide osteoblast seams. We observed such changes during experiments with F_1 (Wistar I × BD III) rats in all animals, their intensity depending on the age of the animals and on the amount of injected cells. The changes start with blast infiltrations, as in spleen and lymph nodes. A few isolated necroses occur (Fig. 11) with interstitial edema and especially with typical fibrin-fiber stars (Fig. 12) which LENNERT et al. (1975) have described for osteomyelofibrosis in humans (cf. BURKHARDT et al., 1964). This is followed by a proliferation of histiocytes which occasionally form nodules (Fig. 13). The megakaryocytes

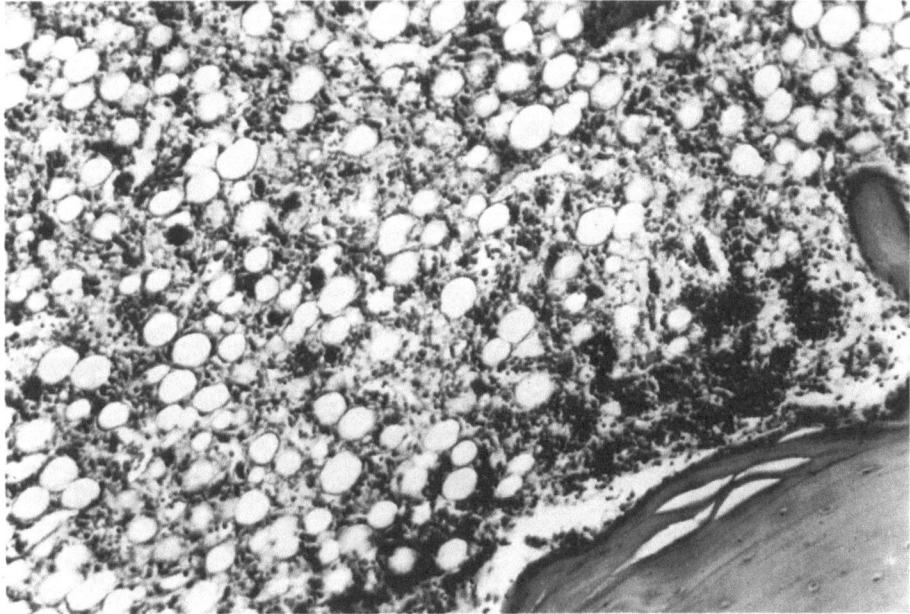

Fig. 10. Aplasia of bone marrow in femur of a 2-year-old (Wistar I × BD III) F_1 rat, 15 days after transfer of 22.5×10^6 spleen cells. H & E × 150

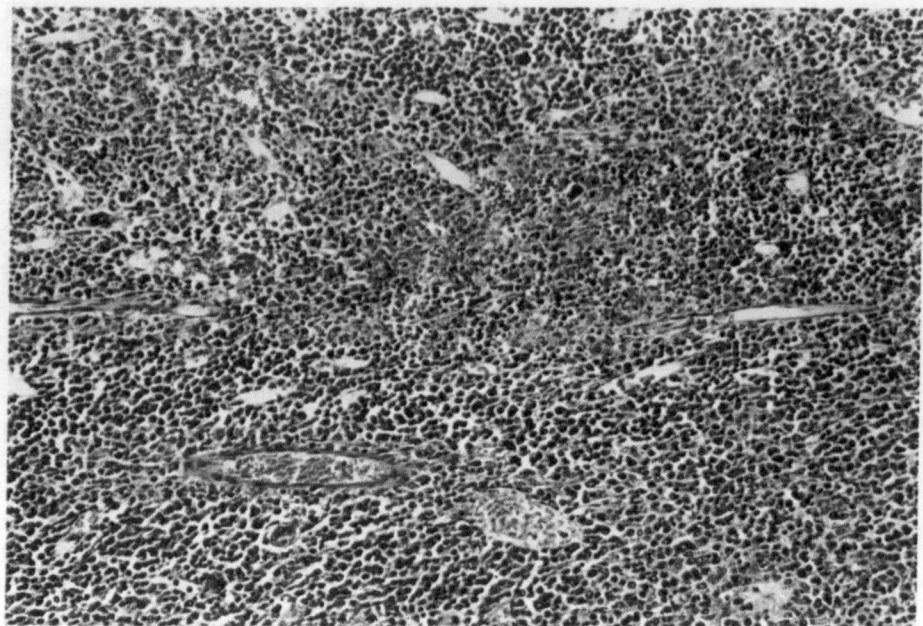

Fig. 11. Necroses in bone marrow surrounded by proliferating "blast cells" in femur of a 2-month-old rat, 15 days after transfer of 8.9×10^6 spleen cells. H & E $\times 150$

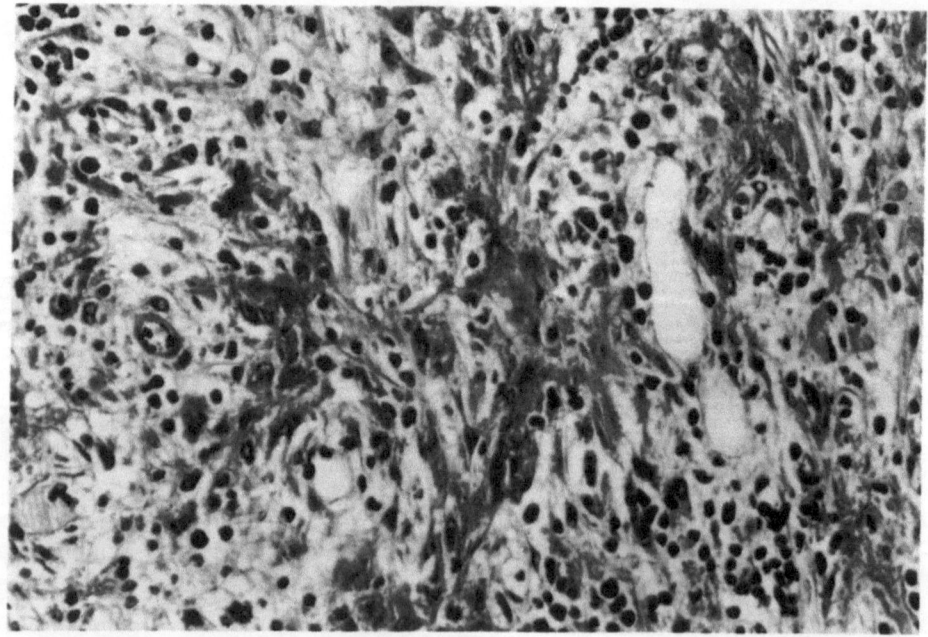

Fig. 12. Myelofibrosis with fibrin deposits (*Fibrinfasersterne*) in femur of a 33-day-old rat, 16 days after transfer of 13×10^6 spleen cells. MSB (Martius scarlet-blue method) $\times 350$

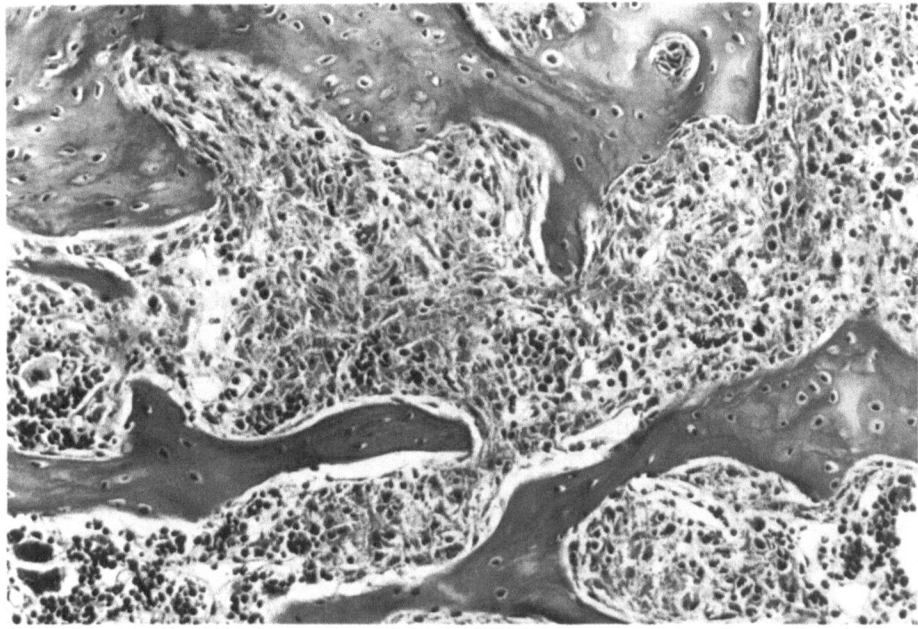

Fig. 13. Myelofibrosis and proliferation of histiocytes in bone marrow of femur from a 36-day-old rat, 20 days after transfer of 13×10^6 spleen cells. H & E $\times 180$

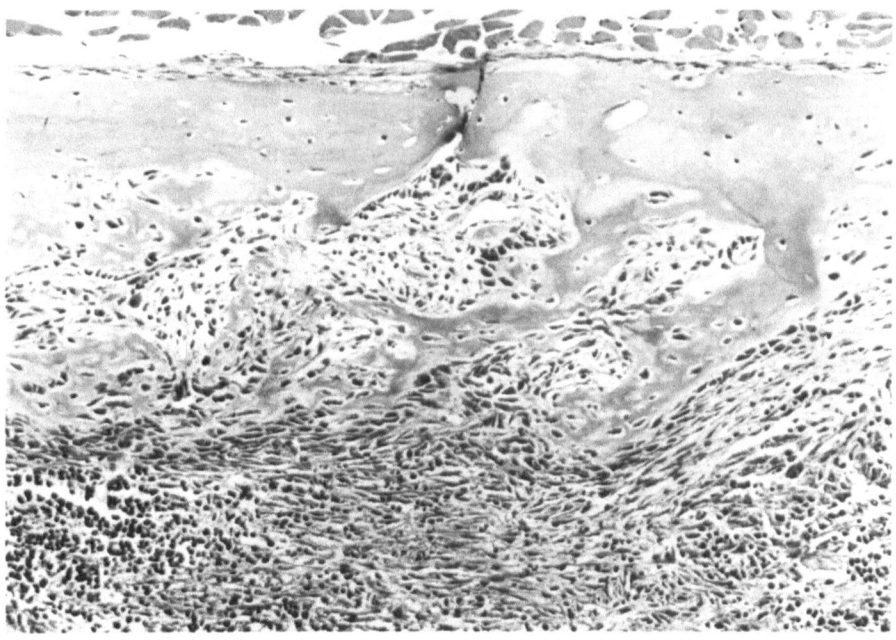

Fig. 14. Osteomyelofibrosis in femur of a 36-day-old rat, 20 days after transfer of 13×10^6 spleen cells. H & E $\times 150$

are increased, gathered in groups, and occasionally pyknotic. Thin collagen fibers multiply parallel to histiocytes and soon lytic trabeculae of bone are to be found in the center of larger fibrotic areas. Erythropoiesis shows a relative increase which proceeds simultaneously with the increase of erythropoiesis in the spleen. In the fibrotic areas, formation of osteoid and widening of the bone trabeculae (Fig. 14) causes atrophy of the medullary zone. In newborn and young animals this process apparently continues unchecked, whereas in adult animals a restitution of the hematopoietic marrow can occur with only slight remnants of fibrosis (Hobik, 1975).

4.2.6. Other Tissue

Here, too, a typical *thymus atrophy* (Billingham *et al.*, 1962) is to be found (Fig. 15) with a narrowing of the cortex and "reversal" of the thymus structure,

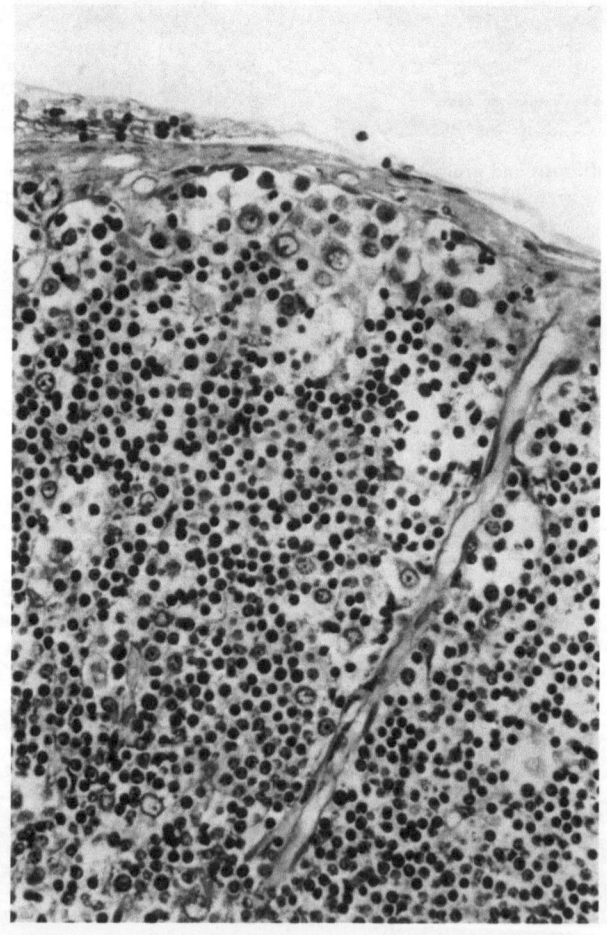

Fig. 15. Depletion of lymphocytes in thymus cortex of a 2-month-old (Wistar I × BD III) F_1 rat, 15 days after transfer of spleen cells from a parent strain. H & E × 350

as well as an increase of mast cells (STASTNY *et al.,* 1965). According to our experience, low numbers of cells cause primarily degenerative changes of the Hassal's bodies with a decrease of PAS-positive matter.

For the *heart* STASTNY *et al.* (1965) have described a focal edema with lymphocyte infiltration, macrophages and plasma cells in the myocardium and endocardium. Later, capillaries and fibroblasts proliferate and the process ends with fibrosis. Individual animals showed a necrotic inflammation with fibrinoid swellings of the coronary arteries. In the *lungs* localized inflammations in various stages of development are found. The reaction in the *intestine* are surprisingly light compared to mice. Only occasionally a slight degeneration of the crypts is found in radiation chimaera (BALNER *et al.,* 1964). For the *kidneys* STASTNY *et al.* (1965) also described perivascular infiltrations of lymphocytes, histiocytes, and plasma cells and, sporadically, a complete glomerulonephritis.

In about 50% of their rats, STASTNY *et al.* (1965) found polyarthritic changes in the *joints* which lasted between 4 and 15 days. The histologic picture showed plethora, edema and effusion into the joint. Massive infiltrations of histiocytes, lymphocytes and plasma cells widened the synovial membrane and the surrounding soft tissue. Occasionally fibrinoid degenerations of the connective tissue occurred, together with proliferation of the layer of synovial surface cells and an increase of capillaries. The diaphysis reacted with periosteal widening. Thus all the changes of polyarthritis had developed.

4.3. Chickens

Seventeen days after transplantation of small pieces of spleen, liver, kidney or bone marrow onto the chorio-allantoic membrane of 7-day-old embryos, gray nodules with central necroses appear in spleen and bone marrow (MURPHY, 1916). On the first day after intravenous injection of spleen cells into 18-day-old chicken embryos, SIMONSEN (1957) found masses of pyroninophilic and basophilic cells in the pulp of the enlarged spleen. These cells proliferated and formed the grey nodules which MURPHY (1916) had described, surrounded by histiocytic cells and syncytial giant cells. In younger embryos (EBERT, 1959), granulopoiesis is accelerated and necrotic and later fibrotic foci appear in several organs (ISACSON, 1959; NISBET and SIMONSEN, 1967).

The changes in other organs are certainly comparable to the initial stages of GVHR in mice and rats. This applies to the periportal foci in the liver (SIMONSEN, 1957), and to nodules with necrotic centers in the "proventriculus," in the bone marrow, in the musculature, subcutis and thymus with relative widening of the thymus marrow and cortical atrophy. The disseminated increased granulopoiesis in chickens (BOYER, 1960), however, differs from GVHR in rodents. According to WALKER *et al.* (1972, 1973a, 1973b), the transplantation of little pieces of spleen or i.v. injection of spleen cells into 4–6-day-old chicken embryos causes massive hemorrhages on the body surface and on the chorio-allantoic membrane. Serious vascular endothelial damages can be shown by electron microscopy.

The degenerative and proliferative changes resulting from GVHR in chicken embryos depend on the development and maturation of the hemopoietic tissue; the cells taken from the vitelline sac are to be considered as stem cells for the proliverative lesions. The earliest date for tracing the first proliferative changes upon cell inoculation in the thymus is between the 6th and 8th day, in the bone marrow from the 10th day and in the bursa of Fabricius from the 14th day on. This timing corresponds to the colonization of the respective organs with hemopoietic stem cells from the vitelline sac.

4.4. Other animals

In *rabbits,* PORTER (1959, 1960) transplanted bone marrow and fetal liver after sublethal irradiation and at the same time he examined young chinchilla rabbits which had received intravenous spleen cell transplants in their embryonic stage on the 20th or 22nd day of pregnancy (gestation period: 31 days). In both experimental groups a typical GVHR set in, which was less pronounced, however, upon transplantation of fetal liver than upon bone marrow transplantations.

The gravity of the histologic changes differed correspondingly. Experiments with embryos resulted in progressive aplasia of the bone marrow with occasional reactive hyperplasia of granulopoiesis and signs of an immunehemolytic anemia. Otherwise, the fibrinoid necroses of spleen follicles, the increased extramedullary hemopoiesis and, in the final stage, the fibrosis in the atrophied spleens, all of which had been described in other rodents, were observed. The lymph nodes and Peyer's patches also showed an initial proliferation of "blasts," and later fibrosis. In addition to this, ulcerating enteritis, necroses of liver cells and, sometimes, bronchial pneumonias occurred.

In F_1-hybrid *guinea pigs,* ANDERSON and NOWELL (1966) described—upon intrathyreoideal implantation of lymphoid cells—primarily hyperplastic and secondarily atrophic changes of the lymphatic tissue and hypoplasia of the bone marrow. A typical "runt disease" with loss of weight and corresponding changes in the skin can also be induced in snapping turtles (*Chelydra serpentina*) through i.p. injection of spleen cells (BORYSENKO and TULIPAN, 1973). The animals, which were treated immediately after hatching, survived for 12–120 days. The spleen, only slightly enlarged, showed a lack of white pulp with massive increase of eosinophilic granulocytes. In irradiated or F_1-hybrid *hamsters* the same changes occur in the lymphatic tissue as in rats and mice (STREILEIN and BILLINGHAM, 1970a, 1970b). Particularly characteristic for hamsters are epidermolyses of the skin which develop within 10 days.

Extensive research on bone marrow transplantations after whole—body irradiation was carried out on *dogs* and *monkeys* (THOMAS *et al.,* 1959, DE VRIES *et al.,* 1961). The aim of these experiments was to develop therapeutic possibilities for humans. It is very difficult to distinguish the purely histologic changes, i.e. those exclusively due to GVHR as a result of bone marrow transplantation, from those resulting from irradiation or cytostatic therapy. Characteristic symptoms, however, are the serious changes in the small intestine with edemas,

blood stases, erosions, disintegration of the crypts, and sometimes ulcers (VAN
BEKKUM and DE VRIES, 1967; WOODRUFF *et al.,* 1969) as well as the changes
of the skin with "satellite cell dyskeratosis" (see p. 830).

4.5. Humans

Only in rare cases does GVHR occur spontaneously in humans, e.g., because
of an XX/XY chimaerism (see p. 811); it sets in more frequently after therapeutic
bone marrow transplantations. This GVHD is lethal in 10–20% of all cases.
In the autopsy reports it is difficult to differentiate the changes caused by
GVHR from the reactions of the organism to the basic disease or to its accompanying infects, or to the cytostatic therapy. Only a target-directed comparison with the results from animal experiments has clarified the autopsy picture
of GVHR.

4.5.1. Spleen

In humans, as in all animals, the spleen, being the largest lymphatic organ,
is particularly affected. In children it is usually enlarged (KADOWAKI *et al.,*
1965; HATHAWAY *et al.,* 1965; MILLER, 1967; GROGAN *et al.,* 1975); in adults,
however, it is atrophic with only narrow remnants of follicles (e.g. KRUEGER
et al., 1971a, 1971b).

Its course can be divided into four stages (SLAVIN and SANTOS, 1973): in
the first, proliferative stage the white pulp especially shows an impoverishment
in lymphocytes (CHOMETTE *et al.,* 1970; KRUEGER *et al.,* 1971b). If the patients
survive this stage, a large number of basophilic, pyroninophilic "blasts," which
are often in mitosis, migrate into the white pulp (CHOMETTE *et al.,* 1970; KRUEGER
et al., 1971b). Among them are also small and medium-sized lymphocytes, lymphoblasts and plasmoblasts. There are, furthermore, always signs of lymphocyte
dissolution with karyorrhexis (ELKINS, 1971; KERSEY *et al.,* 1971). In the second
phase the number of cells in the white pulp is much reduced and now eosinophilic
granulocytes and real plasma cells are found as well (CHOMETTE *et al.,* 1970).
Simultaneously, a proliferation of reticular cells begins in the covering zone
of the follicles and occasionally fibrin clots are found on the border between
white and red pulp. The third phase consists of general lymphatic atrophy
with individual infiltrations of plasma cells and a partial repopulation of the
white pulp with hemopoietic precursors. The infiltrations of plasma cells were
found especially in patients who died from infections (SLAVIN and SANTOS,
1973). If the patient survives this phase, the small lymphocytes in the vicinity
of the follicle-central arteries increase again and lymphocytes settle once more
in the periarterial lymph channels. An interstitial fibrosis, however, remain
(Fig. 16).

Reticulo-histiocytic infiltration is apparently much more marked in children
than in adults (KADOWAKI *et al.,* 1965; MILLER, 1967; GROGAN *et al.,* 1975),
and frequently genuine histiocytic granulomas develop. With children, however,

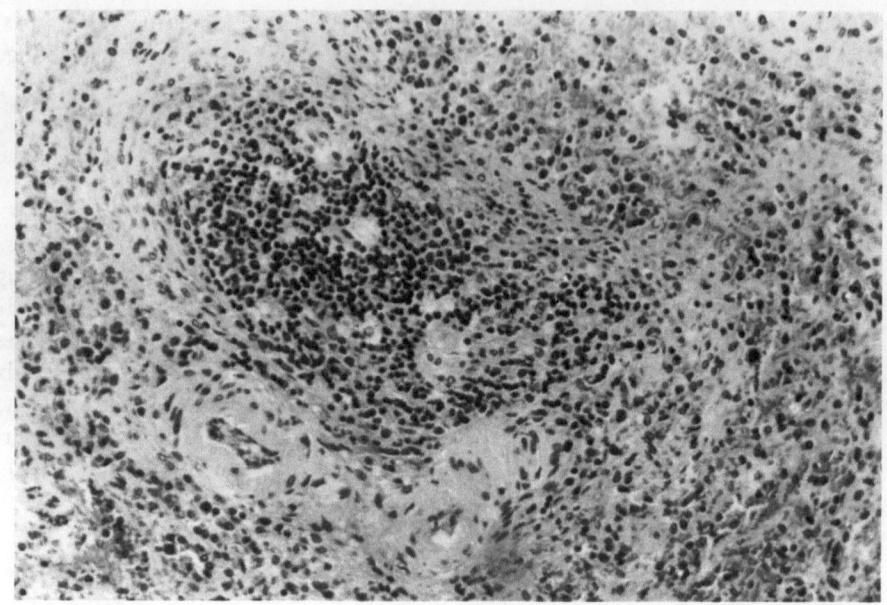

Fig. 16. Depletion of lymphocytes in lymphatic follicle of spleen in an 18-year-old woman, 20 days after transplantation of HL-A-identical and MCL-nonreactive bone marrow. H & E × 187 (Krueger, unpublished)

this is mostly due to congenital immunodefects and it is not possible to determine with certainty the influence of the primary disease on the development of these histiocytic granulomas.

4.5.2. Lymph Nodes

In children with congenital immune defects and with GVHD, the lymph nodes, too, are generally swollen, the germinative centers have largely disappeared, and reticulo-histiocytic cells collect in diffuse or nodular patterns, just as they did in the spleen (Kadowaki et al., 1965; Miller, 1967; Grogan et al., 1975, and others). Kretschmer et al. (1969) described further a remarkable increase of plasma cells, which was not confirmed, however, by Grogan et al. (1975). Histologically, the changes resemble those in the spleen: in the early proliferative phase a primary repopulation of the lymph nodes, which had at first suffered a loss of lymph cells, with small lymphocytes takes place (Woodruff et al., 1969; Chomette et al., 1970), a process during which numerous lymphoblasts appear in the sinusoids of marrow and cortex (Fig. 17). The normal structure of the lymph nodes, however, is not restored. Considerable numbers of lymphocytes and erythrocytes continue to perish, and fibrin clots are found in the sinusoids.

In the second phase, the number of lymphatic cells decreases greatly, followed by a localized proliferation of reticulohistiocytic cells. After about 32 days an extensive lymphatic atrophy sets in with localized cicatrizations. Individual

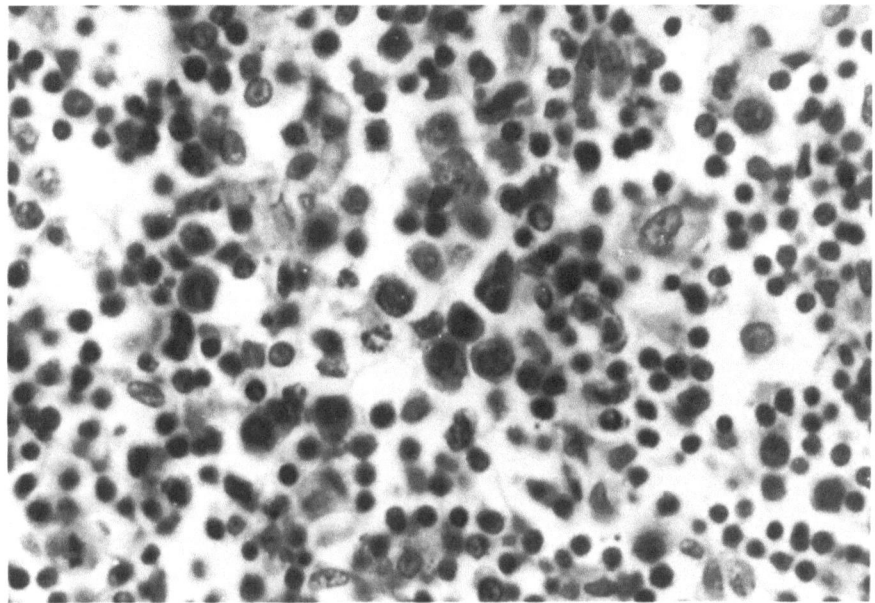

Fig. 17. Proliferation of "blast cells" in lymph node of an 18-year-old woman, 20 days after transplantation of HL-A-identical and MCL-nonreactive bone marrow. H & E × 750 (KRUEGER, unpublished)

follicle remnants, however, can still be detected regularly (KRUEGER *et al.*, 1971a, 1971b).

The state of the lymph nodes is also reversible: if the patients survive this serious lymphatic atrophy without serious infections, lymphocytes can collect once more in marrow and cortex. Normal follicles with germinative centers develop, and finally the lymph node marrow regenerates with lymphocytes and plasma cells (SLAVIN and SANTOS, 1973).

4.5.3. Liver

Here too, differences exist between GVHD in children with immune defects and GVHD, for example, after bone marrow transplantations. The liver of a child reacts with reticulohistiocytic infiltrations in the periportal fields, with bile duct proliferation and necroses of varying extent and fatty degenerations of liver parenchymal cells (e.g. GROGAN *et al.*, 1975). In older children or adults, the liver apparently participates in greatly differing degrees. Some authors (WOOD-RUFF *et al.*, 1969; KRUEGER *et al.*, 1971a, 1971b; GROFF *et al.*, 1976) have described extensive necroses of liver cells and large and small lipid droplets corresponding to the observations made by VAN BEKKUM and DE VRIES (1967) in animal experiments with radiation chimeras. CHOMETTE *et al.* (1970) and KERSEY *et al.* (1971) either failed to mention liver cell necroses or only as isolated phenomena, whereas WOODRUFF *et al.* (1969) reported that hepatocytes as well

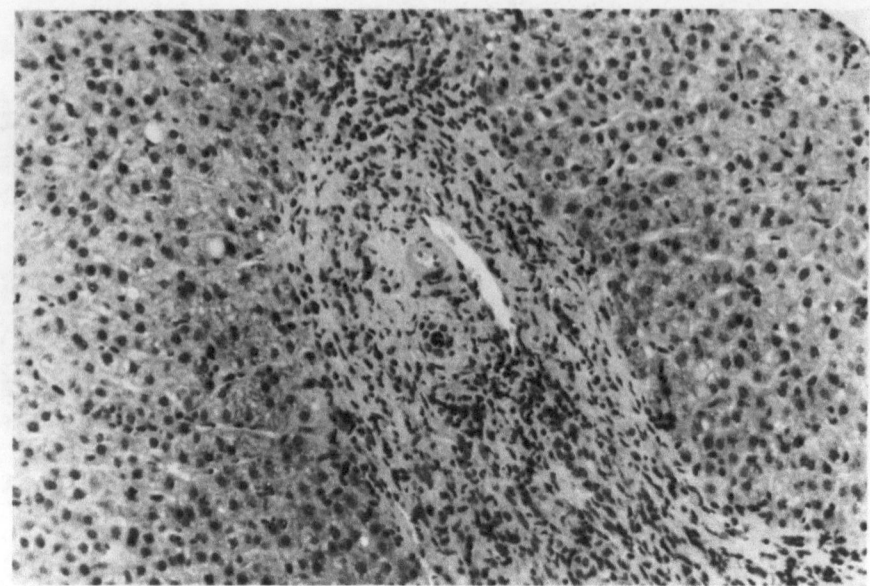

Fig. 18. Infiltration of periportal field with lymphoid cells in the liver of an 8-year-old girl, 16 days after HL-A-identical and MCL-nonreactive bone marrow. H & E × 468 (KRUEGER, unpublished)

as Kupffer cells can become necrotic. A more uniform picture is presented by the reports on lymphatic cell infiltrations in the periportal fields: small and large lymphocytes enter, mixed, in places, with macrophages and eosinophilic granulocytes. The infiltrations can reach the extent of a chronic viral hepatitis, including so-called piecemeal necroses at the edge of the lobules. The bile-duct epithelia, too, become frequently necrotic (WOODRUFF et al., 1969; SLAVIN and SANTOS, 1973; GROFF et al., 1976 etc.). The Kupffer cells generally show a diffuse multiplication, and they can also form nodules (Fig. 18).

In patients who survive GVHD the inflammable infiltrations subside. Remnants of liver cell necroses can still be detected for awhile in the shape of acidophilic corpuscles, and nodules of Kupffer cells are also found (SLAVIN and SANTOS, 1973).

4.5.4. Skin

The first and most impressive phenomena of GVHD in humans are changes in the skin which are specific and occur in a given sequence, as was shown by means of comparative studies in humans and rhesus monkeys (WOODRUFF et al., 1969, 1972; KRUEGER et al., 1971a, 1971b; SLAVIN and SANTOS, 1973; GROFF et al., 1976). In doubtful cases a skin biopsy can verify the diagnosis of GVHD. A specific change is "satellite-cell dyskeratosis" within the epithelium (GROGAN et al., 1975). This signifies the isolated destruction of individual epithelial cells within the epithelial unit during which lymphocytes frequently enter (Fig. 19, 20).

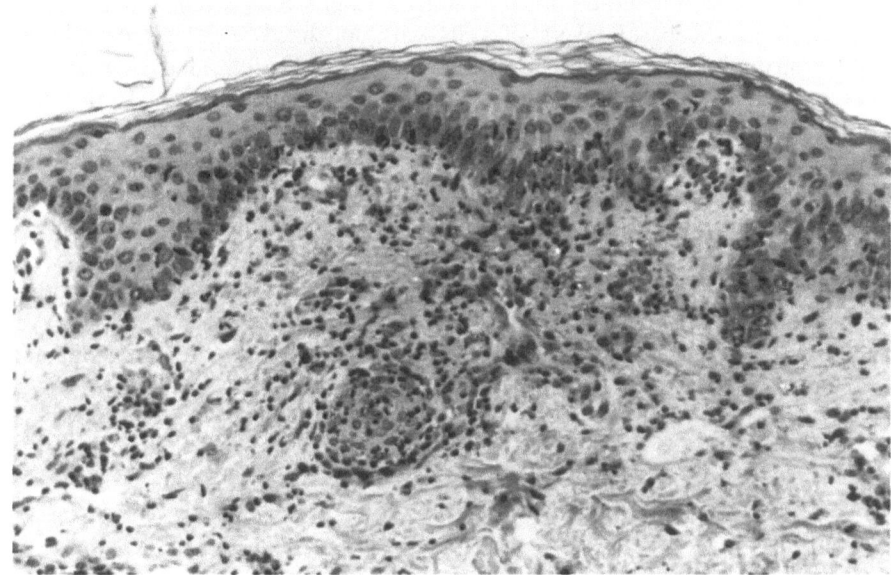

Fig. 19. Infiltration of dermis and epidermis with lymphoid cells in the skin of an 18-year-old woman, 20 days after transplantation of HL-A-identical and MCL-nonreactive bone marrow. H & E × 187 (KRUEGER, unpublished)

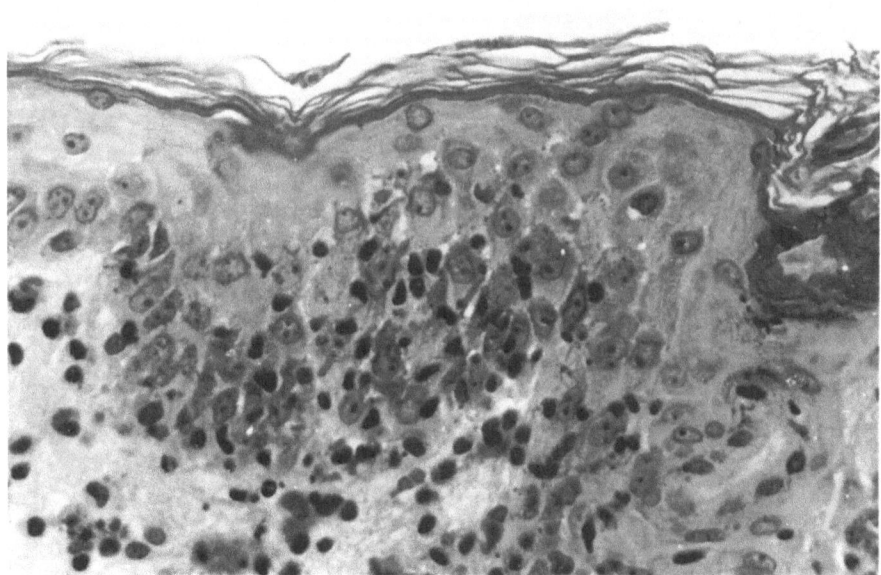

Fig. 20. Necrobiosis of single epidermal cells ("satellite cell dyskeratosis") in the skin of an 18-year-old woman, 20 days after transplantation of HL-A-identical and MCL-nonreactive bone marrow H & E × 468 (KRUEGER, unpublished)

In a more serious grade of skin changes, extensive hydropic swellings occur, especially of the basal layers of cells with localized vesiculation, spongiosis and a strongly marked para- and hyperkeratosis. Localized dyskeratoses and necroses can also comprise larger groups of cells and melanocytes. In the vicinity of the larger necroses, mostly in lacunae, the remnants of the satellite-cell dyskeratoses are found in the shape of "mummified cells" (SLAVIN and SANTOS, 1973). The corium is permeated by lymphocytes of various sizes, but mostly also by macrophages and eosinophilic granulocytes. Dissolved epithelial cells are phagocytized by macrophages. As a result of the melanocyte phagocytosis the macrophages afterwards often contain melanin. The para- and hyperkeratosis cause the typical rough scaling of the epidermis. After the healing of GVHD a skin atrophy generally remains with an extensive loss of the cutaneous accessory glands (CHOMETTE et al., 1970; KRUEGER et al., 1971a, 1971b).

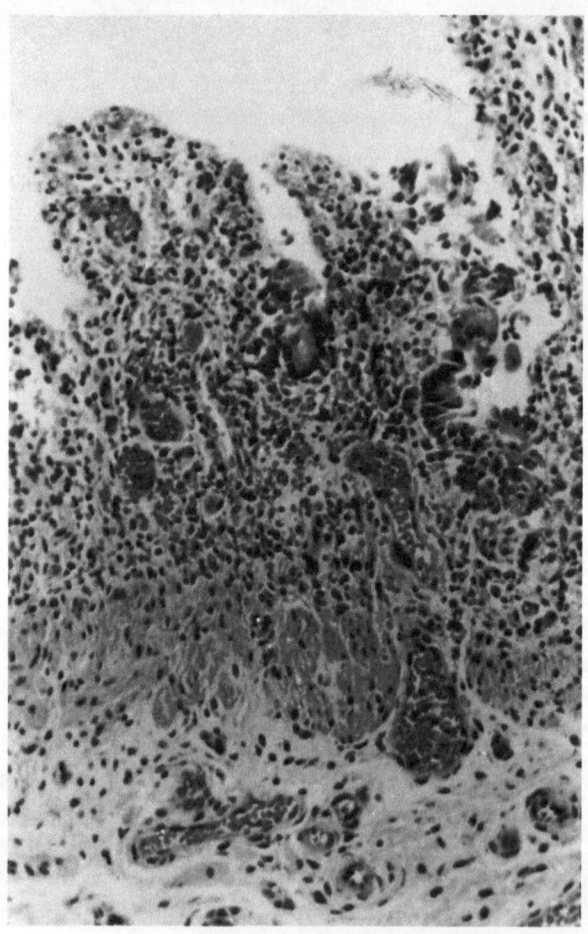

Fig. 21. Focal denudation of intestinal crypts ("acute crypt disintegration") with infiltration of stroma by lymphoid cells in the intestine of a 22-year-old man, 4 weeks after transplantation of HL-A-identical and MCL-nonreactive bone marrow. H & E × 187 (KRUEGER, unpublished)

4.5.5. Gastrointestinal Tract

The same changes as in the epidermis can be detected in the whole gastrointestinal tract, especially in the tongue where the changes manifest themselves particularly early. The esophagus shows a vacuolar degeneration of the epithelium
with an immigration of lymphocytes and histiocytes, a hyperplasia of basal
cells, a kanthosis and necroses of varying extent and even development of ulcers
(KRUEGER et al., 1971 b; GROGAN et al., 1975).

The changes in the stomach vary a great deal. GROFF et al. (1976) found
a total atrophy of the mucous membrane in the antrum which was replaced
by an unspecific granulation tissue. The small and large intestine are regularly
permeated with lymphatic cell infiltrations and histiocytes. Typical symptoms
are necroses of the epithelium and even the development of extensive ulcers
(CHOMETTE et al., 1970; KRUEGER et al., 1971 a, 1971 b). Peyer's plaques have
generally disappeared completely. In the small intestine, further findings are
specific for GVHR: the so-called acute crypt disintegration (GROGAN et al.,
1975), also known as "ghost crypts." It corresponds in principle to the "satellite
cell dyskeratosis" of the epidermis (see p. 830). They are non-collapsed glandular
basal membranes without glandular cells (WOODRUFF et al., 1969), (Fig. 21).

These changes, depending on their extent and state, are either diffuse or
consist of distributed foci, but usually they are particularly pronounced in the
ileum and in the intestine (Fig. 22). The submucous tissue increases, causing
submucous scleroses and atrophy of the musculature. The Brunner's glands
of the duodenum were atrophic and ganglion cells of the autonomic plexus
appeared degenerate (KRUEGER et al., 1971 b).

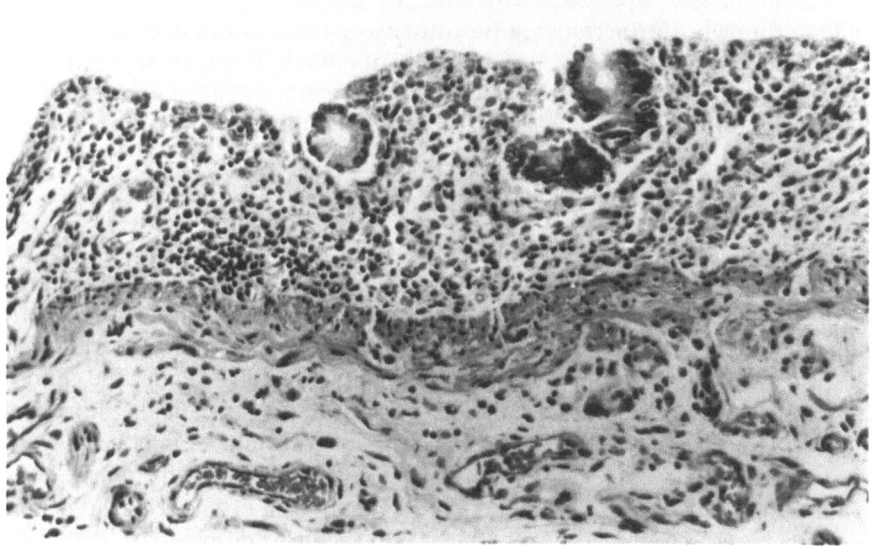

Fig. 22. Advanced atrophy of mucosa with a few remaining crypts and infiltration of lymphoid
cells, in the intestine of a 6-year-old boy, 8 weeks after transplantation of HL-A-identical and
MCL-nonreactive bone marrow. H & E × 187 (KRUEGER, unpublished)

Upon recovery the epithelial cells regenerate. The cystlike enlarged cells are still found with a more or less clearly differentiated epithelium, and frequently numerous macrophages remain in the submucous coating (Slavin and Santos, 1973). The tonsils and the remaining lymphatic tissue of the nose-pharynx area suffer the same degenerative changes as the rest of the lymphatic system. Even in children who suffered from GVHD due to a congenital immune deficiency, the tonsils were usually totally atrophied (Miller, 1967; Grogan et al., 1975). The same applies to the thymus which is reduced in size—the usual differentiation between marrow and cortex is no longer possible. A remarkable phenomenon is the atrophy of "Hassal's corpuscles" (Miller, 1967; Grogan et al., 1975).

4.5.6. Bone Marrow

Here, the changes are frequently determined by the basic disease, e.g., leukemia, or an aplastic anemia. The changes differ correspondingly (cf. Graw et al., 1970; Chomette et al., 1970; Krueger et al., 1971 b; Slavin and Santos, 1973; Groff et al., 1976).

During the first 17 days of a "pure" GVHD, a general aplasia predominates with only discrete foci of erythropoietic and myelopoietic precursors as well as very sporadic megakaryoblasts. Isolated megaloblasts are also found (Slavin and Santos, 1973). Necroses of the hemopoietic cells with subsequent phagocytosis of the erythrocytes stand at the beginning. Sometimes the small lymphoid cells and the plasma cells multiply as well (Groff et al., 1976).

In the 3rd–7th week after a bone marrow transplantation the marrow contains a slightly increased amount of erythropoietic and myelopoietic cells, and also a histiocytic hyperplasia, localized marrow fibroses and, now and then, fibrin clots in the capillaries, especially in the vicinity of fresh necroses of hemopoietic cells. Furthermore, a transitory hyperplasia of eosinophils is noticeable (Slavin and Santos, 1973). From the 3rd month after marrow transplantation, normocellular bone marrow can be found. A continuous osteomyelofibrosis as found in rats (see p. 821) has not been reported for humans so far.

4.5.7. Remaining Tissue

According to recent observations (cf. Buja et al., 1976) changes of the heart musculature after bone marrow transplantations can be a matter of life or death for the patient. In six patients the author detected a diffuse or localized infiltration of histiocytes with typical Anitschkow cells, lymphocytes and plasma cells. These infiltrates could be found in the vessels as well as under the endothelium and between the myocardial fibers. Five of the six patients showed the clinical symptoms of a GVHD. Two patients died from a serious heart failure within the first days after the bone marrow transplantation. A histologic examination revealed necrotic muscle fibers in the heart with extensive fibrin deposits in and between the muscle fibers. But it is difficult to differentiate the cardiac alterations caused by GVHD from direct cardiotoxic effects of immunosuppressive drugs. In this context the observations of Stastny et al. (1973) concerning similar changes in the hearts of rats gain renewed importance (see p. 825).

The most striking changes among the other organs were found in the lungs in the form of either an interstitial or an alveolar pneumonia, caused by bacteria, fungi or viruses (e.g. cytomemegaly). These changes are the consequences of infections and thus secondary diseases of GVHD. Primary consequences, however, are atrophies of the testicles and ovaries (KRUEGER *et al.,* 1971b), as well as a localized medullary fibrosis in the cortex of the suprarenal gland.

As has been mentioned earlier, it is often difficult or even impossible to differentiate between the changes due to the original disease, to GVHD, to therapy or to terminal infections. At least with every bone marrow transplantation a massive immune suppression by means of medicaments must be carried out which can, in its turn, be held responsible for a large portion of the described changes. It is, after all, a defective immune system which is prerequisite for the development of a GVHR.

Therefore the fact that we can nevertheless single out *two histologic changes as being specific for GVHD in humans,* gains increased importance: one is the satellite cell dyskeratosis of the epidermis, the other is the "acute disintegration of the crypts" in the small intestine (WOODRUFF *et al.,* 1969; SLAVIN and SANTOS, 1973; GROGAN *et al.,* 1975). GVHD, therefore, must be considered an independent disease which can be diagnosed reliably by means of an intravital biopsy of the skin or the small intestine.

5. Hematology

Changes in the blood are part of the typical picture of "runt disease." The most prominent changes are those of erythropoiesis: the animals become anemic. Then, the immunologic attack leads to an impairment of the lymphatic system and thus, in most cases, to a lymphopenia. The primary inflammatory reaction can also, in many cases, produce a transitory leukocytosis.

5.1. Mice

In mice the extent and timing of the anemia depend on the strains employed. OLINER *et al.* (1961) found in anemia in one out of four combinations: in C 57 BL/6→DBA + C 57 BL/6. The anemia reached a hematocrit value of only 20–40% of the norm. At the same time the life span of the erythrocytes was greatly reduced and in many cases a positive direct Coombs test was found. HARRISS *et al.* (1961) investigated the anemia in F_1-hybrids more thoroughly and also discovered a dependency on circulating antibodies. Our own investigations confirmed the occurrence of a serious anemia. The result of the histologic examinations of the bone marrow (see p. 817) shows, however, that not only the immunologic component but also an aplasia of the marrow must be taken into consideration as a causative factor. With A/JAX × BALB/c F_1-hybrids and female A/JAX donors, leukopenia together with lymphopenia is a characteristic reaction which reaches its climax between the 9th and 11th day and disappears again after 20 days. Timewise, these observations, made on adult animals

(Witting and Detlefsen, 1975) are correlated with the splenomegaly; there is, however, no causal relation between them since a previous splenectomy has no significant influence on this effect.

5.2. Rats

According to the early observations of Billingham *et al.* (1960), which are still valid today, anemia in newborn rats under the influence of GVHR begins on the 4th day at the latest. A smear reveals symptoms of anisocytosis, poikilocytosis and, occasionally, of spherocytosis. Polychromatic erythroblasts and basophilic cells indicate an increased regeneration of the bone marrow. On the 7th and 8th day, the granulocytes increase rapidly and can attain values of as much as $100,000/mm^3$. This increase in granulocytopoiesis is presumably a result of the unspecific inflammatory irritations caused by the injected cells. The anemia, however, is attributed either to an increased formation of agglutinin, i.e., to humoral antibodies (Simonsen, 1962), or else to an increased phagocytosis in the reticuloendothelial system. This serious anemia is probably one of the causes of death, at least as far as rats are concerned. Together with an increase of the lymphatic atrophy, lymphopenia sets in as well, but it appears to be less constant and less pronounced than in mice.

5.3. Other Species of Animals

Hemolytic anemia is particularly pronounced in rabbits. Reticulocytosis and a multiplication of nucleated erythrocytes in the peripheral blood are always found 2 to 3 weeks after the beginning of the disease (Simonsen, 1962). Whereas terminal leukocytosis occurs in some cases, the lymphocytes gradually decrease from the second week on after induction of GVHR.

A positive, direct Coombs test with serious hemolytic anemia occurs also in chickens (Simonsen, 1957). It is, however, no early symptom. If spleen cells are injected on the 18th day of the embryonic stage, the concentration values of hemoglobin are still normal on the 3rd day after hatching. After that they drop very rapidly to as little as 15% of the norm. Lymphopenia also sets in later and does not reach the same extent as it does in rodents.

In dogs, too, GVHR subsequent to bone marrow transplantations is accompanied by serious anemias of the hemolytic type and by terminal lymphopenias (van Bekkum and de Vries, 1967).

5.4. Humans

The hematologic changes during GVHD in humans correspond to those in rodents in nearly every detail; the extent of the leukocytosis, however, depends on unspecific concomitant infections which are favored by the immune suppression. Here, too, serious anemias of hemolytic character are found together with a positive Coombs test, with temporary reticulocytosis, terminal aplastic anemia and serious lymphopenia, as a manifestation of the general immune suppression.

6. Causal Pathogenesis

Initially, "runt disease" had been considered a consequence of an infection; today, the immunologic character of all forms of GVHR and GVHD is undisputed. Nevertheless, unspecific concomitant factors certainly play a considerable role.

6.1. Immunologic Factors

Anemia is accompanied by a positive Coombs test, which means it is caused by humoral antibodies. These presumably stem from the multiplied plasma cells in the bone marrow, in the spleen, in the liver and in other organs. Thus GVHR is by no means a reaction that is restricted to the cellular immunity.

The latter does, however, play a prominent role. This is proved by the observation of local GVHR as well as by in-vitro tests of MLC and the spleen explant test (see p. 808). To put it more simply: it is an attack of immunocompetent T-lymphocytes on the host cells which, in their turn, respond with an initially unspecific but later specific reaction. We will return later to the details of this immunologic reaction (see p. 844).

6.2. Unspecific Factors

The progressive wasting with the characteristic changes in skin and organs is also very likely influenced by unspecific components. Thus the adreno-cortical hormones are usually reduced and the functioning of the digestive glands is impaired as a consequence of serious changes in stomach and intestines (see p. 833). This serious anemia with hematocrit values of as much as 15% leads, in turn, to serious damages to all parenchymatous organs, especially the heart, liver and brain.

The participation of unspecific factors, produced by T-lymphocytes, has been investigated more thoroughly (PICK and TURK, 1972). The liberation of the macrophage migration inhibition factor (MIF) is delayed and reduced (FALK et al., 1969). A "blastogenic factor" (BF), too, must be considered to constitute an unspecific factor; it is increased and is presumably the reason for the multiplication of blasts in the areas of local GVHR as well as in spleen, bone marrow and kidneys during systemic GVHD. Finally, various lymphotoxins are considered to cause the destruction of the lymphocytes in the germinative centers of the spleen and also in the lymph nodes. Other cytotoxic factors emanating from the lymphocytes or the blasts destroy the organs, e.g., kidney tissue during renal GVHR (see p. 841). Since simultaneously an inflammatory stimulus is given, a cooperation of unspecific cytotoxins is conceivable; for this, however, no verified data are available as yet.

A GVHR animal or a human with serious GVHD is an "immunologic cripple" (Elkins, 1971). This leads to the above-mentioned bacterial, viral and protozoon-induced infections which, in turn, produce unspecific concomitant reactions. Thus a summary picture shows GVHD as the product of many unspecific factors, the beginning of which is formed by an aggression of the immunocompetent cells.

7. Formal Pathogenesis

Since an immunologic reaction stands at the beginning, the question as to the causative antigens arises. Since GVHR appears to be predominantly a reaction of the T-lymphocytes, a second question arises as to the nature of these lymphocytes. Initially at least, the central question concerns the behavior of the lymphocytes which during local or systemic GVHR settle in the tissue where they proliferate and react with each other especially with the host cells. The behavior of the host cells determines the fate of the host animal, which responds with a reactive hyperplasia and eventually ends with the immune suppression.

7.1. Trigger Antigens

All immunogenetic investigations have taught us that the main histocompatibility antigens constitute the decisive triggering factors. With only a slight histocompatibility difference, only a slight GVHR sets in. The importance of these histocompatibility antigens (in humans the HL-A locus or a part of it; in mice the H-2 locus or a special GVH locus (see p. 810); in rats the AG-B locus; in chickens the B-locus, etc.) has been determined in numerous investigations of humans as well as of animals (Uphoff and Law, 1958; Gittes and Russell, 1961; Miller et al., 1963; Ordal and Grumet, 1972; Cantrell and Hildemann, 1972; Klein and Park, 1973; Klein and Egorov, 1973; Huber et al., 1973; Elkins et al., 1973; Salaman et al., 1973; Oppltová and Démant, 1973; Rolstad and Ford, 1974). The effect of these trigger antigens is influenced to a noticeable degree by a leukopenia caused by radiation. Thus there exist indications (cf. Grebe and Streilein, 1976) that the source of the immunogenic stimulus in mice can come from eosinophilic granulocytes, which have on their surface a particularly high concentration of H-2 alloantigens. The same may apply to reticular cells of the thymus, the spleen or the lymph nodes which have a particularly intensive and active H-2 antigen covering (Aoki et al., 1969).

7.2. Immunocompetent Lymphocytes

Prerequisite for the triggering of a GVHR is the presence of alien, immunocompetent lymphocytes. Lymphocytes of the thoracic duct, which contain no or only few so-called large lymphocytes, trigger a particularly serious GVHR (GOWANS, 1962). Since that discovery, a small lymphocyte is generally considered to be an immunocompetent cell (MEDAWAR, 1963). Earlier experiments showed that lymphocytes of the thoracic duct, of the peripheral blood, of the lymph nodes and of the spleen can trigger a GVHR, whereas bone marrow cells and thymus lymphocytes show little or no activity (BILLINGHAM et al., 1962; CANTOR and ASOFSKI, 1970; STREILEIN and BILLINGHAM, 1970a; CANTOR and MOSIER, 1972; DYMINSKI and ARGYRIS, 1973). Since lymphocytes of thymectomized mice or rats were supposed not to produce GVHR (GOOD et al., 1962; RIECKE, 1966; MILLER and MITCHELL, 1967), it was deduced that the thymus plays a role as an activator or carrier of immunocompetent cells. "Immature" and "mature" thymus lymphocytes were accordingly differentiated, the latter of which appear to quickly leave the thymus gland and form approximately 4–5% of the T-lymphocytes in the peripheral blood (TIGELAAR and ASOFSKI, 1973a).

The original idea, that the thymocytes themselves cannot cause a GVHR, is now obsolete (cf. SPRENT and MILLER, 1972a; PIROFSKY et al., 1973): the "minority population" of thymus lymphocytes, i.e., 10–20% of the thymus lymphocytes which are predominantly situated in the marrow and which are corticoidresistant, is the decisive initiating lymphocyte group for GVHR (GREBE and STREILEIN, 1976). At least in rats, the bone marrow, too, contains immunocompetent lymphocytes (McGREGOR, 1968), or at least stem cells which can change into immunocompetent T-lymphocytes.

7.3. Behaviour of Donor Lymphocytes

Only 1–3% of the injected lymphocytes of the donor are immunocompetent cells. The remaining cells perish relatively quickly (BOYSE, 1959; GORER and BOYSE, 1959; SIMONSEN and JENSEN, 1959). A minimum number of cells is necessary, however, contrary to the original conception of Burnet, that *one* single cell was enough to trigger a GVHR. Even for the chorioallantoic membrane test in chickens (see p. 795) 40 immunocompetent cells are presumably necessary for each individual focus.

7.3.1. Nidation

During local GVHR nidation occurs at the very spot where the injection was given. With systemic GVHR, the cells distribute themselves over the entire organism. According to the studies of HESLOP and HARDY (1971), ^{51}Cr-labeled lymph node cells decompose primarily in the liver: this is where the strongest radioactivity is found after 24 h. A lesser activity takes place in the spleen and in the lymph nodes; none, however, in the thymus (HALL et al., 1972). With systemic GVHR, the lymphocytes which have been filtered out in the spleen gather there, but also, at the same time, in the T and B areas of the lymph nodes. According to SPRENT (1973), however, only the T-cells can be traced in the lymph nodes within 24 h while, according to the findings of HOW-ARD et al. (1972) T- und B-lymphocytes circulate in rats. An interesting aspect is presented by the fact that the nidation of the immunocompetent cells can be influenced with ferments such as neuraminidase (GESNER and WOODRUFF, 1969) or trypsin (WOODRUFF, 1974).

Another important aspect is the fact that different cells work together in producing GVHR. In the thoracic duct of adult GVHR rats, FORD and ATKINS (1971) discovered donor as well as host cells among the lymphocytes. In a subsequent popliteal lymph node test (see p. 806), by means of which the specificity of the F_1-hybrid cells was examined, it was found that the specific cells, which react against the host, were filtered out, but that other immune competent cells circulate which can also develop a GVHR against the F_1-hybrids in the popliteal lymph node test. The same authors (ATKINS and FORD, 1975; FORD et al., 1975) discovered that in sublethally irradiated F_1-hybrid rats, paren-tal radiolabeled lymphocytes, are predominantly found in the spleen and less so in the thoracic duct. All these experiments indicate that the nidation of the intraperitoneally or intravenously injected immunocompetent lymphocytes takes place predominantly in the spleen. The ensuing interactions with other lymphocytes, however, have not yet been properly investigated.

7.3.2. Proliferation

The early investigations of GVHR by SIMONSEN (1957) revealed pyroninophilic cells in the spleen, lymph nodes and other organs, which were at first taken for donor cells. GOWANS et al. (1961), by injecting ^{3}H-thymidine-labeled lympho-cytes, proved that these small lymphocytes can develop into larger pyroninophilic cells which, in rats, takes about 24 h. After 42 h, however, the radioactivity had disappeared—presumably as a consequence of dilution due to cell division. Under the electron microscope, these pyroninophilic cells do not correspond to the usual plasma cells (BINET and MATHÉ, 1961); nowadays, since we know in principle the transformation of lymphocytes into proliferating "blasts," they are referred to as "blasts." FOX (1962) proved by means of a T-6-chromosome labeling in mice, that these cells stem from the donor. The mitotic wave of the donor cells reaches its climax after 2–3 days. After 12 days it is still detectable. During these investigations, however, other proliferating lymphocytes were also found in the lymph nodes.

The lymphocyte proliferation of the donor has been investigated with various methods in irradiated animals (BENNETT, 1971; SPRENT and MILLER, 1972a, 1972b; CHEERS et al., 1974). The proliferation of host cells is the second step subsequent to the nidation of immunocompetent cells.

7.3.3. Cellular Interactions

We know from general immunology that T- and B-lymphocytes are mutually dependent in their functions. B-lymphocytes by themselves cannot produce a

GVHR. CANTOR *et al.* (1970a, 1970b) have described a subgroup of T-lympho-cytes which produce a synergistic interaction with B-cells, the so-called T_1-lymphocytes which only circulate in small numbers while the T_2-lymphocytes predominate in the peripheral blood and in the lymph nodes. According to CANTOR and ASOFSKY (1972) there is an interaction between the two thymus-dependent cells during GVHR. These processes have not yet been sufficiently clarified. According to TIGELAAR *et al.* (1975), the addition of thymocytes to the peripheral blood intensifies the GVHR. If the thymocytes are previously treated with anti-thymocyte serum and complement, this intensification effect is neutralized. The two cooperating T-lymphocytes also recover with different rapidity if the animals have been treated with anti-thymocyte serum (MORSE and ASOFSKY, 1974). There also exist suppressor activities, however, which are linked with the proliferation of donor lymphocytes (GERSHON *et al.*, 1972). It is likely that the suppressor T-lymphocytes belong also to the group of corticoid-resistant lymphocytes (BLOMGREN and JACOBSSON, 1974). Macrophages by them-selves cannot produce a GVHR; the macrophages, however, also participate in producing the GVHR via cellular interactions (ARGYRIS, 1974).

7.4. Behaviour of Host Cells

During local GVHR—especially with renal GVHR—the host cells become ne-crotic because of the reaction of the injected immunocompetent cells. This is the consequence of the above-mentioned cellular interactions. At the same time the lymphatic cells in the spleen, in the lymph nodes and in other lymphatic organs react with a hyperplasia, and the final outcome is a general lymphatic atrophy. From these macroscopic and histologic observations it is evident that GVHR is a complex reaction.

7.4.1. Damages

Local GVHR—in the skin for instance—starts with a pronounced inflammation (BRENT and MEDAWAR, 1966; WILSON and BILLINGHAM, 1967, etc.). Local renal GVHR is linked with a splenomegaly which cannot derive from donor cells but is considered to be an unspecific defense of the organism (ELKINS, 1971). In a systemic GVHR, the immunologic destruction of host lymphocytes and of hemopoietic cells constitutes a process which is decisive for the GVHD (STREILEIN, 1971a). The host lymphocytes possess the greatest amount of cellular transplantation antigens. The lymphotoxic products which are thereby released can cause destructions of tissue and also leukopenia and anemia. It has not yet been determined which toxic products injure the hemopoietic stem cells and thus cause the changes in the bone marrow (see p. 837) and the aplastic anemia. It is possible that unspecific toxic products of the tissue have a part in this (STREILEIN and BILLINGHAM, 1970b; STREILEIN and STREILEIN, 1972). In a lethal GVHR such toxic factors may very well trigger the terminal protracted shock.

7.4.2. Reactive Hyperplasia and Allogeneic Effect

Splenomegaly, which Simonsen (1957, 1962) considered to be a criterion for the intensity of systemic GVHR, is predominantly due to a proliferation of host cells. First this is substantiated by the parallel splenomegaly during local GVHR (Elkins, 1971), the intensity of which does not correspond to the intensity of the local renal GVHR. Secondly, this has been proved by numerous studies with ^{3}H-thymidine-labeled lymphocytes and by chromosome-labeling studies.

The first clear result, namely that during a systemic GVHR in chickens the donor cells divide, but that, quantitatively, the reaction of the host cells predominates by far, was presented by Biggs and Payne (1959) (cf. also Owen et al., 1965; Nisbet and Simonsen, 1967). Similar investigations were conducted on newborn mice and they yielded the same results (Davies and Doak, 1960; Zeiss and Fox, 1963; Nakić and Kaštelan, 1967a; Nakić et al., 1967): The proliferating cells in the spleen and in the lymph nodes are a reaction of the host to the reaction of the immunocompetent cells of the donor—only a small portion of them stem from the donor. An interesting result was obtained by Nakić and Kaštelan (1967a, 1967b), namely that more donor cells proliferate in the lymph nodes than in the spleen.

Whereas the first investigations by Silobrčić and Trentin (1966) with sublethally irradiated mice suggested that all mitoses in the spleen stem from the donor, more detailed studies with adult mice (Fox, 1962, 1966; Nakić et al., 1966) furnished the proof that the primary wave of mitoses of the donor cells is followed, a few days later, by a marked increase of mitosis of the host cells in the spleen. Upon irradiation, however, the proliferation of donor cells lasts much longer than in unradiated control animals. Donor cells also get into the bone marrow (Fox, 1966) and multiply there too. Parabiosis studies by Nakić et al. (1966) showed that the partner which outwardly appears to be sick, has a larger number of proliferating donor cells than the seemingly more healthy partner. In rats, the predominance of host-cell proliferations is even clearer than in mice. This applies to newborn animals (Nowell and Defendi, 1964) as well as to adults (Elkins, 1970). In many cases this proliferation is immediately preceded by histologically proven damages, i.e., cell necroses, a fact which could be substantiated particularly well by means of electron microscopic studies (Weiss and Aisenberg, 1965).

Parallel to the proliferation of lymphatic and plasma cellular cells in the entire lymphatic system, runs an increase in immunoglobulin production (Streilein and Stone, 1973), a production of mostly IgM rather than IgG globulins. The reason for this is the presence of antigens which get into the organism of the host together with lymphocytes or even in the form of lymphocytes (Britton, 1972; Armerding and Katz, 1974; Trenker, 1974, etc.).

The injected immunocompetent T-lymphocytes stimulate other T-lymphocytes, and also the B-lymphocytes of the host. Because of the allogeneic lymphocytes, the immune status of the host is changed, one of the results of which is that cells which are confronted with only one specific hapten can produce considerable quantities of specific antibodies (Katz, 1972). Katz et al. (1971)

called this phenomenon the "allogeneic effect" and understood by this a "graft-T-cell-versus-host-B-cell" reaction. This reaction does not interfere with the normal interaction between T- and B-cells (KATZ *et al.*, 1974a).

After this "allogeneic effect" was found in guinea pigs, it was also observed in mice (OSBORNE and KATZ, 1973a, 1973b), and in rats (MCCULLAGH, 1972; ORNELLAS *et al.*, 1974; SCOTT and ORNELLAS, 1974). There were also indications that this allogeneic effect exists in humans, too (DAGUILLARD *et al.*, 1973). It is only found in connection with GVHR and not with transplant reactions.

In vitro investigations have shown that the mediator for the allogeneic effect is a soluble factor, or at least that a soluble factor is involved. Mice, which after a thymectomy or irradiation or for genetic reasons (e.g. nude mice) are incapable or producing sufficient amounts of T-lymphocytes, are stimulated by the supernatant fraction of allogeneic lymph cell mixtures to produce a T-reaction (KETTMANN and SKARVALL, 1974). This supernatant fraction, which also neutralizes the anti-theta treatment of spleen-cell cultures, is in vitro also capable of stimulating antibody production in B-lymphocytes. In this context ARMERDING and KATZ (1974) speak of an "allogeneic defect-factor" with a molecular weight between 30,000 and 40,000, which, moreover, seems to be barely strain-specific. It is presumably a case of a new form of lymphokinins, i.e., of the mediators emitted by lymphocytes.

7.4.3. Immune Suppression

The reactive hyperplasia of the lymphatic tissue is followed, depending on the dose of applied lymphocytes and on the nature of the GVHR, by a lymphatic atrophy (see p. 814) affecting the spleen as well as the lymph nodes, the Peyer's patches of the intestine and the ubiquitous lymphatic system of all organs. Parallel to this runs a lymphopenia which differs in strength in the various species (see p. 835). This lymphatic atrophy with lymphopenia is probably decisive for an understanding of the formal and causal pathogenesis of "runt disease." It is, after all, possible to create, by means of other experimental interventions which also lead to an atrophy of the lymphatic tissue and to a serious lymphopenia, a syndrome which is nearly identical with "runt disease" (for literature, see KEAST, 1968a). Whole-body irradiations with the typical "secondary disease" (BARNES *et al.*, 1962) may be mentioned in this context, or postnatal thymectomy (MILLER and HOWARD, 1964). Furthermore, the phenomena of GVHR are reinforced by immune suppressors (SCHWARTZ and BELDOTTI, 1965a) or through thymectomy plus irradiation (FIELD and GIBBS, 1965). Infusions of syngeneic lymphocytes are capable, at least in the case of allogeneic radiation-chimaera, of improving the clinical picture temporarily (BARNES *et al.*, 1962; THOMPSON *et al.*, 1962).

Thus it is understandable that a marked immune suppression is observed during GVHR (for literature, see ELKINS, 1971). The earliest studies on mice were presented by HOWARD and WOODRUFF (1961): during a serious GVHR the F_1-hybrids showed a delayed transplant rejection as well as a reduced antibody titer against Salmonella typhi. VRUBEL (1961) demonstrated a prolonged autotransplant-rejection reaction during GVHR (cf. LAPP and MÖLLER, 1969).

The reduction in humoral antibody production was described by Koltay et al. (1965) and by Claman et al. (1969) by means of various models. The antibody response to infection with T-2 bacteriophages is also reduced during GVHR (Blaese et al., 1964). Active immunity against sheep erythrocytes can disappear almost entirely if the histocompatibility difference in the H-2 locus of the mice is unequivocal (Lawrence and Simonsen, 1967).

Thus, this GVHR immunosuppression affects the formation of the humoral as well as the cellular immunity (Streilein, 1972a; Treiber and Lapp, 1973). It also occurs if the donor lymphocytes have been presensitized (Möller, 1971), and Zaleski and Milgrom (1973) even consider the suppression of the antitheta response to an F_1-hybrid as a reaction parameter for GVHR. This immune suppression can be ascertained at a very early stage through the lymphopenia in the peripheral blood. The latter is apparently only a rough indicator for the immune competence of an organism.

At times a temporary increase in the formation of antibodies is observed at the beginning of a GVHR (cf., e.g., Blanden, 1969). The resistance of animals against infections with *Listeria monocytogenes* for instance, or with *Salmonella typhimurium,* however, is not contradictory to the above-mentioned immunosuppression but rather a consequence of the increased macrophage activity in the liver, in the spleen and in the peritoneal cavity. This increase in macrophage activity is characteristic for GVHR (see p.804), and Biozzi et al. (1965) have achieved an inhibition of GVHR by previously treating host mice with bacteria which can stimulate the reticuloendothelial system.

The course of immunologic reactions of GVHR goes through two phases: there is first a hyperplasia of the lymphatic organs with a corresponding stimulation also of the B-lymphocytes in the sense of the "allogeneic effect." This is, however, a transitory phenomenon which finally changes into an immune suppression. Grebe and Streilein (1976) presume that in the end both phenomena are caused by the same factor.

7.5. Mechanisms of Immune Regulations

Some special intercellular reactions remain to be pointed out. They are partly interesting from a general immunologic point of view, and are in part necessary especially for the sake of understanding GVHR.

In the mixed lymphocyte culture (MLC) it was found that thymus lymphocytes and lymphocytes from peripheral lymph nodes produce a supra-additive effect if, in the culture, they act together with allogeneic lymphocytes which have been pre-treated with mitomycin-C (Tittor and Walford, 1974; Tittor et al., 1974). Normal spleen or lymph node cells do not react in this way; they do react, however, if they are spleen or lymph node cells of lethally irradiated mice which, 20 h previously, had received compensatory treatment with syngeneic spleen cells.

A study of cell-mediated cytotoxicity reveals a cooperation of T_1- and T_2-lymphocytes. Wagner et al. (1974) presume that the T_2-lymphocytes are precursors of the killer lymphocytes and that the activity of the latter is intensified by a presumably soluble mediator which is produced by the T_1-lymphocytes. The fact that subpopulations of T-lymphocytes exist which act as "suppressor-T cells," has already been mentioned (see p. 841). It is possible that several kinds of suppressor T-lymphocytes exist, and the suppression can also be of an unspecific nature (RICH and RICH, 1974). So far neither the exact functioning of these cells nor the chemical nature of the mediators has been determined. According to OKUMURA and TADA (1974), the "antigen specific T-cell factor" which influence the formation of antibodies in the dinitrophenol-ascaris system is an alpha- or beta-globulin with a molecular weight between 35,000 and 60,000. This factor can be blocked with an anti-thymocyte serum; it is presumably a determinant of the T-lymphocyte membrane.

When the parental immunocompetent cells proliferate in the F_1-hybrids, they react with other T-lymphocytes as well as with B-lymphocytes of the host (see p. 842). A large portion of these histocompatibility antigen-reactive cells (H-ARC) perish. Others may become tolerant towards the host. This is supported by the fact that allogen-antigen-reactive cells which work against other histocompatibility-alloantigens can be found in the host animal (ATKINS and FORD, 1972). Insofar as they retain their antigen reactivity, they can be suppressed by suppressor T-lymphocytes; they can also form anti-host antigens and thus have the local or overall harmful effect of GVHR. Besides this, there are indications than an "enhancing" antibody exists, an antibody which intensifies the reaction (FIELD and GIBBS, 1966). We are still a long way from understanding all the interactions between donor and host cells during GVHR. Altogether, the interest shifts more and more from the donor lymphocytes to the host lymphocytes. The FcR cells too, which multiply very early in the spleen, and which have recently been given increasing attention by CLANCY et al. (1976), are considered to be host cells. Most likely the reaction of these FcR cells has to do with the development of humoral autoantibodies (see p. 842).

There are, furthermore, numerous soluble factors which have no antibody character but which nevertheless influence the immune response. Such an "immune regulatory protein" (IRP), for example, seems to have a suppressive effect on GVHR of the popliteal lymph node-hypertrophic type in F_1-hybrid rats (GREBE and STREILEIN, 1975b). Immune regulatory proteins of the donor can direct themselves against the donor cells, can also attack the host cells; and immune regulatory proteins of the host can have a decisive influence on GVHR. GREBE and STREILEIN (1976) have discussed in detail the possibilities and consequences resulting from this.

More or less specific immunologic regulations, however, are certainly responsible for the fact that GVHR can heal spontaneously, that serial transmissions of GVHR are only possible on a very limited scale (BILLINGHAM et al., 1962; STREILEIN and BILLINGHAM, 1970b; GREBE and STREILEIN, 1975a, 1976) and that in many cases it is impossible, after a GVHR has abated, to induce a new GVHR in the same way (FOX and HOWARD, 1963; FIELD et al., 1967; STREILEIN, 1972a; GREBE and STREILEIN, 1975b).

8. Therapeutic Influence

The best possibility of preventing a GVHR or GVHD lies in an exact examination of the HL-A and ABO differences as well as in an examination of the histocompatibility in the mixed lymphocyte culture (MLC). Even if all these reactions seem to guarantee an optimal effect, a GVHD, which can be lethal, nevertheless occurs in about 10% of the cases. Genetically identical, i.e., monocular twins, are the best guarantee for a successful bone marrow transplantation. For this indication, the American Medical Society has calculated that a patient who is to undergo a bone marrow transplantation has approximately a 40% chance of finding an HLA-compatible donor within his family (Fahey et al., 1969). This percentage is reduced to 1–4% if one takes into consideration the ABO system, the geographic situation and the state of health of the donor (Cline et al., 1975). Since the therapy of an already manifest GVHD is successful in very few cases only, prophylaxis, i.e., a preliminary treatment of the donor or the host, takes a prominent position.

8.1. Results of Experiments with Animals

Closest to the clinical experience comes experimental GVHR after irradiation of the host animals and subsequent transplantation of bone marrow, followed by treatment with immunosuppressive agents. Larger species of animals, e.g., dogs and monkeys, are better suited for this than rodents. This, however, limits to experiments on a larger scale. Among the smaller rodents, the A→A+B type (see p. 796) is most suitable. Larger groups of animals can be subjected to this test which is relatively simple to carry out. The results can easily be reproduced and artificial factors which interfere with the assessment of the mechanism of action of immunosuppressive agents (irradiation etc.), are eliminated.

Today, two methods for treating the donor cells stand in the foreground: one group are the physical methods, based upon the density or the different sizes of the cells. It has been shown that the immunocompetent cells can be largely eliminated by means of density gradient cell centrifugation or deviation cell electrophoresis (Gelfand et al., 1974). These physical methods can be combined with the second method which is based on the immunologic recognition mechanism of the cells which cause GVHR: the basic idea is that the pluripotent stem cells, which determine, for example, the success of a bone marrow transplantation, do not possess histocompatibility antigens. Both the transplant rejection and the GVHR can be influenced in a positive way by means of various methods, e.g., the selective adherence method (Bonavida and Kedar, 1974) or the application of soluble antigen-antibody complexes (Hellström and Hellström, 1974) or even the application of soluble antigens which produce blocking serum antibodies (Rao et al., 1974). Unspecific methods are also suited for reducing the functioning or number of the immunocompetent cells.

Immunosuppressive agents and antisera (ALS, ATS), and also alkylating agents, folic acid antagonists, purine and pyrimidine analogues, antibiotics, enzymes, RES blockers and highly polymeric substances play a prominent role in the treatment of the host animals. Next to monotherapy, combination treatments with various modifications stand in the foreground (c.f. VAN BEKKUM and DE VRIES, 1967; BILLINGHAM, 1968; BRUNE, 1970; BILLINGHAM and SILVERS, 1971; GATTI *et al.*, 1973).

8.1.1. Treatment of Donor Animals

In the A→A+B type of GVHR (see p. 796) in mice, the preliminary treatment of the A donors with soluble antigens of the B-strain or of AB-hybrids has proved favorable (VOISIN *et al.*, 1968). The application of soluble H_2-antigens produced the same effect (HALLE-PANNENKO *et al.*, 1971). In lethally irradiated mice a markedly higher survival rate could be obtained through a pre-treatment of the donor animals with various antigens of viral, bacterial and animal origin such as proteins and lipopolysaccharides. The latter produce a better effect than the former (LIACOPOULOS *et al.* 1967a, 1967b). By means of pre-treatment of the donors with antilymphocyte serum the antigen-specific cell proliferation in the spleen of mice of the A→A+B type could be lowered from 60–90% to as little as 10%, as measured by the T 6-chromosome labeling technique (BAUMANN and THIERFELDER, 1974). If the donor monkeys for bone marrow transplantations receive a pre-treatment with ALS, the GVHR is noticeably reduced (VAN BEKKUM *et al.*, 1972). In irradiated mice, better survival rates could be obtained by immunizing the donor animals with an anti-H2A serum (SAFFORD and TOKUDA, 1970). GVHR of the A→A+B type can also be positively influenced by a treatment with *Bordetella pertussis* vaccine, which is supposed to cause a mobilization of the lymphocytes from the donor organs into the bloodstream (EIKMAN and BOWSER, 1972; LEVINE and IWAHARA, 1969).

MEUWISSEN (1967) achieved a dose-dependent inhibition of the spleen index of A→A+B type mice, after treating the donor animals with mitomycin C. Treatment with cortisone or nitrogen mustard reduces the lymphocytes in the bone marrow of the donor mice, which led to a reduction of the mortality after transplantation into irradiated mice (AMBRUS *et al.*, 1966). Pre-treatment with cyclophosphamide and thalidomide also inhibits GVHR (FIELD *et al.*, 1966; FINK and CLOUD, 1974). According to our experience, 5–13 pre-treatments with L-asparaginase of the donor mice of the CPB/N strain or of the donor rats of the BD III strain, can considerably reduce the GVHR in $(C_{57}$ BL/6 × CPB/N) F_1 mice or in (Wistar I × BD III) F_1 rats respectively, as measured by the spleen index. Pre-treatment with the anti-silicosis agent polyvinylpyridine-N-oxide (PVNO) (SCHLIPKÖTER and BROCKHAUS, 1961) is also, according to our experience, suited for a successful pre-treatment of BD III-donor rats (50 mg/kg, s.c. on 25 consecutive days). The effect shows in a significant reduction of the spleen index, a diminished decrease of body weight (-10% instead of -25%), and a less pronounced lymphopenia. A remarkable phenomenon was the fact that after a pre-treatment with PVNO, no animal showed the skin changes which are otherwise typical for GVHR. Since the PVNO is stored in almost all cells of the reticulo-endothelial system (GRUNDMANN, 1967), the helper function of the macrophages is presumably suppressed in these experiments.

8.1.2. Treatment of Donor Cells

Incubation of the donor cells before injection into the host animals, with various antigens of viral, bacterial and animal origin like proteins, polysaccharides, etc. can, through their immediate cytotoxic effects, reduce the number of immunocompetent cells. Mixing and incubating the parental cells to be injected with neonatal liver cells of the same parental strain (C 57 BL/6 J) reduces the GVHR (BORTIN *et al.,* 1969). Incubation of a mixture of spleen cells and bone marrow cells before transplantation with Fab fragments from horse anti-mouse-thymocyte globulin (HAMTG) also forms part of these not immediately cytotoxic preparations. This can prevent mortality of lethally irradiated mice while the hemopoietic reconstitution is not influenced (RICHIE *et al.,* 1973a, 1973b). In the A→A + B type mice, the spleen index is also inhibited by pre-treatment of the donor cells with Fab fragments (GALLAGHER *et al.,* 1972). ^{51}Cr-labeled spleen cells, which have been incubated with Fab-fragments, settle in smaller numbers in the lymphatic tissues than do untreated spleen cells. In this case inhibition is stronger in the lymph nodes than in the spleen (RICHIE *et al.,* 1975). Fab fragments from univalent rabbit anti-mouse-immunoglobulins could also inhibit the development of the spleen index during GVHR (RIETHMÜLLER *et al.,* 1971). TRENTIN and JUDD (1973) obtained a slight reduction of the GVHR mortality after transplantation of a cell suspension of spleen and bone marrow cells, which had been incubated before transplantation with horse antimouse-thymocyte globulin (HAMTG). A better effect was obtained after incubation of the transplanted cells with spleen-absorbed HAMTG, which lacked the cytotoxic component against the stem cells necessary for hemopoietic reconstitution, but which retained the suppressive potency of the thymus-dependent cellular immunity.

The separation of immunocompetent cells by means of density-gradient centrifugation alone (DICKE *et al.,* 1968, 1970), or through a combination with immunologic methods (see p. 849), can also influence the GVHR in a positive sense. Preincubation of the cells destined for transplantation with spleen or thymus extracts has the same positive effect (GARCIA-GIRALT *et al.,* 1972; KIGER *et al.,* 1973), possibly as a consequence of an effect of tissu-specific chalones. The donor cells can also be treated with antithymocyte globulin (LYDYARD and IVANYI, 1974), with thymus-specific antibodies (POTWOROWSKI *et al.,* 1971), with antisera against light chains (ROUSE and WARNER, 1972) as well as with an "anti-recognition structure serum" (JOLLER, 1972), and thus the GVHR can be reduced. A particularly elegant method seemed to be the application of radioisotopes which kill especially the cells with specific histocompatibility antigens. Thus SALMON *et al.* (1970) have administered high doses of ^{3}H-thymidine in proliferating lymphocytes and have thus, in vitro, killed the cells which were capable of a blastogenic transformation with DNA synthesis. The concavalin A-influenced T-lymphocytes (TYAN, 1974, 1975) or the T-cells which have been treated with antitheta antisera (CANTOR, 1972; TYAN, 1973) are only to a much lesser degree capable of inducing as GVHR.

All these methods, however, are only of limited importance. They are capable of killing many or even all immunocompetent cells. The stem cells, however, which are essential, e.g., for the success of a bone marrow transplantation, remain intact as indeed they must. From these stem cells, however, immunocompetent cells develop again later on and thus the GVHR is only retarded. In hosts, in which — merely theoretically — no immunocompetent cells develop out of the stem cells, immunologic cripples are the result, with all the consequences of immune insufficiency.

8.1.3. Treatment of Host Animals

Because of these drawbacks, most results so far have been obtained from host animals, although the toxic concomitant effects of the immunosuppressors prevent a sufficient dosage and duration of the treatment. Since UPHOFF (1958) reported a positive influence on "secondary disease" in mouse chimaeras, numerous investigations with different substances after bone marrow transplantations have been carried out in lethally irradiated hosts and in the A→A+B type. The parameters were again the spleen index, the dermatitis as an outward symptom, or the survival rate (cf. BRUNE, 1970).

Depending on the presumably differentiated effect of some agents in the initial stage, the immunosuppressive substances can not only influence the GVHR positively, but can, in some cases, even accelerate it. This applies at least to cortisone and 6-mercaptopurine (RUSSEL, 1962; SCHWARTZ and BELDOTTI, 1965; BARNES et al., 1966). FLOERSHEIM and SEILER (1967) could also detect differences in the cutaneous GVHR of chickens. Thus amethopterine, ibenzmethizine, and cyclophosphamide act predominantly in the initial stages of GVHR, while amethopterine acts in the endphase, actinomycine, azathioprine and colchicine during the entire course of the disease. SWINGLE et al. (1973) studied the immunosuppressive effect of 13 agents (steroids, alkylating agents, antimetabolites and colchicine) in popliteal lymph node tests with rats (see p. 806).

Generally, the best effect can be achieved through application together with the transplantation or on the first day, and not only from the 5th day on (OWENS and SANTOS, 1971) or even only after onset of the first clinical symptoms. L-asparaginase (1000 IU/kg) influences the mortality only slightly if applied from the 5th day subsequent to a spleen cell transplantation in the A→A+B type of mice and rats as compared to the animals which had received L-asparaginase from the 2nd day on (Fig. 23), (HOBIK, 1970). ALS and ATS, however, act not only during the initial phase, but also in later phases (KREN et al., 1960, 1962). According to experiments with dogs (STORB et al., 1973b; KOLB et al., 1973) and monkeys (VAN BEKKUM et al., 1967; VAN BEKKUM et al., 1972; MERRITT et al., 1972; NEEFE et al., 1974; KRUEGER et al., 1975), these sera are suitable for monotherapy as well as for combined treatment with cytostatics. An already developed GVHD in dogs can be positively influenced with rabbit anti-dog ATS (STORB et al., 1973b). In most cases the skin changes disappear, the diarrhea lessens and the life-span of the animals increases significantly.

On the other hand, GVHR offers an opportunity to test drugs for their immunosuppressive potency, a process which also discloses other side-effects. The A→A+B type is most suitable for this purpose (HOBIK, 1969b). This

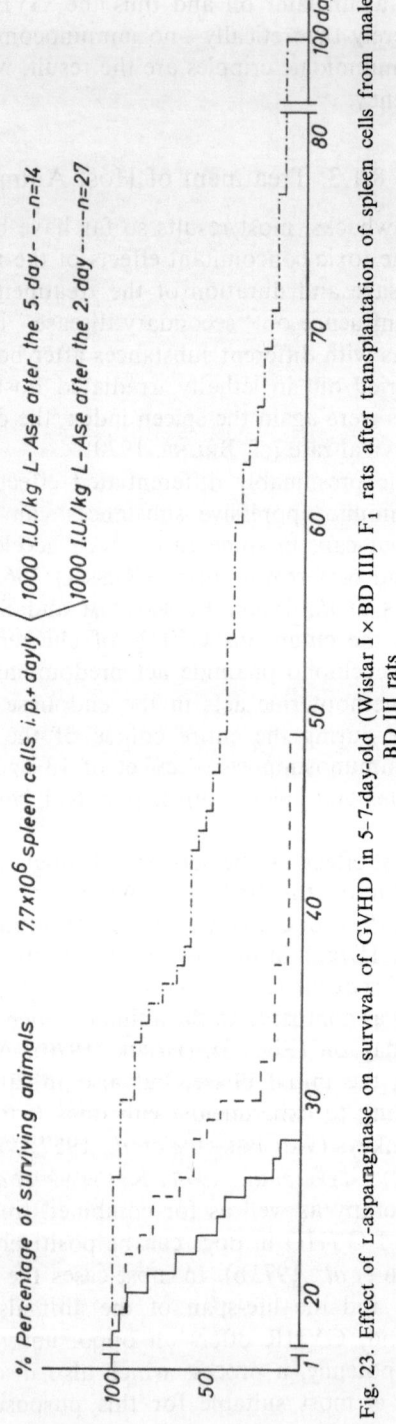

Fig. 23. Effect of L-asparaginase on survival of GVHD in 5-7-day-old (Wistar I × BD III) F_1 rats after transplantation of spleen cells from male BD III rats

makes it also possible to compare the cytolymphotoxic effect with the GVHR, the weight of the thymus and the general damage. According to Table 1, 84 mg/ kg azathioprine have almost the same immunosuppressive effects as do 168 mg/kg, except that the lower dose does not produce the undesirable adverse side-effects. The A→A+B type makes it also possible to determine the doses necessary for the desired effect of various immunosuppressive agents (Fig. 24). For the purpose of long-term testing for instance, GVHR in rats can be prolonged by 10 days by administering 15 times 1000 IU/kg L-asparaginase (HOBIK, 1969a). If the treatment is discontinued, the serious clinical picture of a "runt disease" with development of the typical dermatitis sets in (Fig. 25). Continued treatment with the same doses of L-asparaginase prolongs the average life expectancy by 22 days (Fig. 23). During this time the animals show no exterior signs of changes except for a slower increase of weight. The histopathologic changes of GVHR, however, are less pronounced.

Table 1. Effect of azathioprine on the spleen index in GVHR in 19-day-old $(C_{57}/Bl/6 \times CPB/N)$ F_1 mice, 10 days after transfer of 13.6×10^6 CPB/N spleen cells

mg/kg	GVHR T/C	cyto-lymphotoxic effect		
		spleen index	thymus weight	body weight
5×500	0.11	0.39	-82%	-51.7%
5×168	0.32	0.72	-15.6%	$- 5.9\%$
5×84	0.38	1.2	$+ 0.3\%$	$+ 7.9\%$
5×42	0.68	1.1	$+ 8.1\%$	$+ 3.5\%$

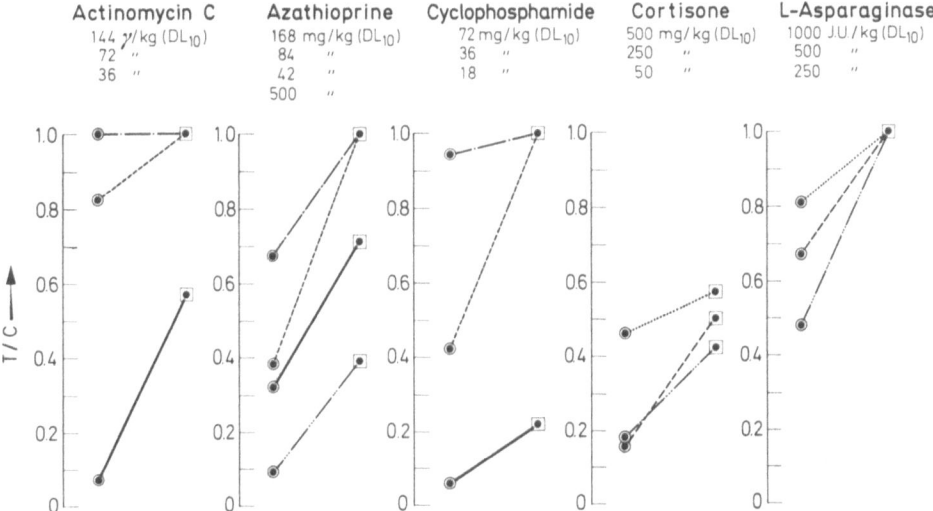

Fig. 24. Comparison of immunosuppressive and cytolymphotoxic effects on GVHR made by actino-mycin C, azathioprine, cyclophosphamide, cortisone and L-asparaginase (see Table 1)

left end of each line = effect on GVHR   (————) = DL_{10}
right end of each line = cytolymphotoxic effect   (- - - - - - - - - -) = $1/2 \, DL_{10}$
                                                                              (-·-·-·-·-·-·-·-·-·-·) = $1.4 \, DL_{10}$

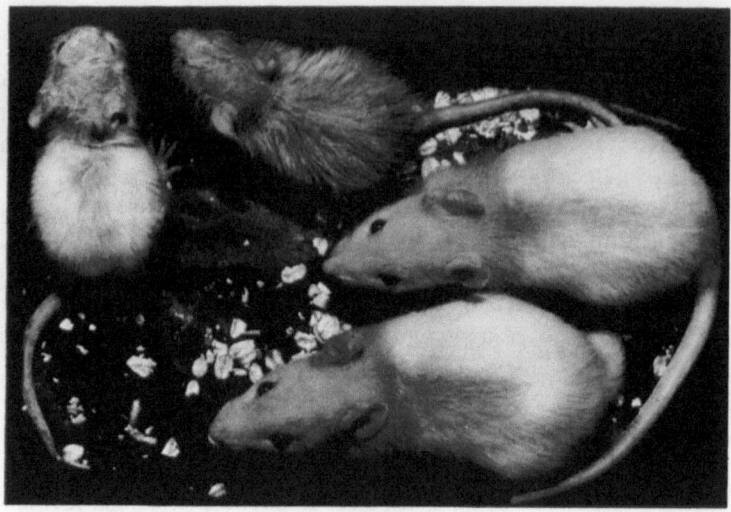

Fig. 25. 43-day-old (Wistar I × BD III) F$_1$ rats from the same litter. *Right:* controls; *left:* after i.p. transplantation of 7.6×10^6 spleen cells from male BD III rats 3 days after birth, followed by daily application of 1000 IU/kg L-asparaginase for 15 days. Development of "runt disease" after cessation of treatment. All untreated animals died until day 21 after cell transfer

8.2. Clinical Results

Compared to the extensive findings in animal experiments, experience with humans is still limited. Nevertheless, several possibilities have presented themselves. Methotrexate treatments with 15 mg/m^2 on the first day and 10 mg/m^2 on days 3, 6 and 11, and then weekly for the first 100 days, are considered to be the standard therapy (Storb et al., 1974a; Thomas et al., 1975). Cyclophosphamide in doses of 7.5 mg/kg in 5 applications on every 2nd day, starting with the 1st day after the bone marrow transplantation, and followed by further administrations of cyclophosphamide at irregular intervals according to the dependency on leukopenia, can also retard a GVHR (Santos et al., 1971). Storb et al. (1974b) treated an already established GVHD with cyclophosphamide but without an effect. Antithymocyte serum (ATS), however, has proved to be an effective treatment for GVHD after bone marrow transplantations in humans (Storb et al., 1974b).

Good prophylactic results have been obtained through pre-treatment of donor cells with the above-mentioned methods (see p. 846). In vitro treatment of lymphocytes stimulated for blastogenic transformation with ^{3}H-thymidine, which kills the immunocompetent cells (see p. 848), has been applied to several children prior to bone marrow transplantations (Sieber et al., 1974). Buckley et al. (1971) discovered a favorable effect of blocking antibodies on the GVHD in humans. In all these investigations, however, the multitude of histocompatibility antigens limits the effect of the antibodies.

9. Late Complications

In addition to the GVHR and to the typical clinical and histopathologic changes of GVHD (see p. 814), reactions have been discussed lately which may only be indirect effects of a GVHR. These late complications give an exemplary significance to the GVHR within the entire immunologic system; the correlations however, are by no means sufficiently known yet.

9.1. Glomerulonephritis

During experimental GVHR of adult animals (see p. 798), in many cases no acute GVHR sets in but rather a chronic clinical picture which is characterized by various symptoms (cf. "allogeneic diseases"; see p. 854). It depends on the nature of the animal strains employed. LEWIS *et al.* (1968) succeeded for the first time in producing a glomerulonephritis by implanting sublethal doses of normal BALB/c spleen cells into adult BALB/c × A/JAX F_1-hybrids. It was accompanied by a serious nephrotic syndrome and histologically and immuno-fluorescence-microscopically, it presented the picture of a membranous glomerulonephritis. These kinds of disease were called "chronic allogeneic diseases." Genetic investigations (GLEICHMANN *et al.*, 1972) could prove that in mice the H_2-locus is again decisive, or at least a locus which is immediately linked with this complex. According to fluorescence microscopic investigations, the immunoglobulins which are detectable on the basement membrane of the glomeruli stem from the donor, the antigens of these glomerular immune complexes, however, from the F_1-hybrids (KANO *et al.*, 1974).

Such immunecomplexes form under the influence of B-lymphocytes. Investigations by GLEICHMANN *et al.* (1974) clearly support the thesis which had already been formulated by ALLISON *et al.* (1971) and BRETSCHER (1973), namely that the immune complexes are formed by B-lymphocytes of the F_1-hybrid host, in the function of autoantibodies, after the autologous F-lymphocytes have been inactivated by the injected parental T-lymphocytes or rendered functionless in some other way. With the same model, KANO *et al.* (1974) also reached the conclusion that the chronic allogeneic glomerulonephritis is triggered and sustained by the activity of B-lymphocytes from the host animal.

9.2. Other Forms of Allogeneic Diseases

It has already been mentioned that other immune diseases occur as well (see p. 835): especially immune hemolytic anemia with a positive Coombs test is typical for GVHD. It is found not only with acute but also with chronic GVHR.

The skin diseases, which often set in only very late, are also chronic reactions (see p. 830). The above-mentioned changes in the heart and in the joints (AISENBERG *et al.*, 1962) belong also among the chronic phenomena. STASTNY *et al.* (1965) succeeded, with high doses of allogeneic lymphocytes, in producing changes not only in the myocardium but also in the cardiac valves and in the epicardium of rats which neonatally had been made tolerant against the donor cells: typical lymphocytic-histiocytic infiltrations developed with fibrinoid swelling of the connective tissue and subsequent fibroblast proliferation, similar to a rheumatic pancarditis (see p. 825). Furthermore, the typical picture of a polyarthritis with lymphocyte and histiocyte infiltrations below the synovial membrane and in the adjoining connective tissue developed in 39 of the 70 animals. This polyarthritis showed very variable localizations and a characteristic feature of human polyarthritis, namely "wandering," i.e. switching from one joint to the other.

The mechanisms on which these reactions are based are not yet known. In analogy to the studies of allogeneic glomerulonephritis (see p. 853), it must be assumed that here too an immune mechanism is at work which is triggered by humoral antibodies, and which probably was made possible by the neutralization of a suppressor function of T-lymphocytes through the injected alien T-lymphocytes.

9.3. Malignant Tumors

GVHR is accompanied by a biphasic reaction pattern of the lymphatic tissue as well as of the immune reactions (see p. 844): first, lymphatic hyperplasia sets in with an increased production of humoral antibodies; it ends with lymphatic atrophy and general immunosuppression. Since the development and growth of malignant tumors are also under the influence of the immune systems, it can be expected that the growth of malignant tumors is also encouraged or inhibited by GVHR, depending on how the test is conducted.

Transplantable tumors are the simplest models for studying the growth of tumors. Data concerning the influence of GVHR vary from an increased resistance (MEDZIHRADSKY, 1966; CARNAUD et al., 1974; BOMFORD et al., 1975) to an extreme growth activation of transplanted lymphomas (ZALESKI, 1975). In the latter experiments, the immune suppression was achieved 6 months after a subliminal GVHR had been induced, at a moment that is, when an immune insufficiency can already be expected. The local renal GVHR also leads to immune suppression with growth stimulus of the transplanted Walker-256 tumors (MEDZIHRADSKY, 1967).

These contradictory results can be explained with the various blocking or activating immunologic mechanisms which play a role in the immune regulation of GVHR (see p.844). In cases in which the tumor growth is inhibited by GVHR, the general increase of phagocytosis, which is regularly observed in GVHR (see p. 804), can be the determining factor.

A more interesting observation is that GVHR by itself produces malignant tumors—invariably of the lymphoreticular tissue (SCHWARTZ and BELDOTTI, 1965; ARMSTRONG et al., 1965 etc.). Here too, the explanation is simple at first, since other experimental conditions of extreme immunosuppression, e.g., neonatal thymectomy, also produce, in mice at least, a high rate of lymphoreticular sarcomas (KEAST, 1968a, 1969; GRUNDMANN and HOBIK, 1973a, etc.).

SCHWARTZ *et al.* (1966) could continue the passage of tumors produced by the GVHR only in special F_1-hybrids. This suggested that the tumors had developed from host cells and not from those of the donor. ARMSTRONG *et al.* (1967) found in the combination BALB/c × A/JAX, through injections of BALB/c cells, also lymphomas of the host type, but, at the same time, an immune complex glomerulonephritis. This could reflect the same induction mechanism for both diseases.

More detailed investigations of this phenomenon have shown that malignant tumors can be of the host type (HAYS, 1972b) as well as of the donor type (ARMSTRONG *et al.*, 1970). GLEICHMANN *et al.* (1975) proved in extensive investigations that in one system both possibilities can be realized: of 92 lymphomas, 12 were of the donor type, 66 of the host type, 14 of an intermediate type. The animals in which lymphomas of the donor type had developed possessed a higher histocompatibility difference between donor and host than the combinations in which no donor-type lymphomas had developed. This at least suggests the possibility that an allogeneic inhibition can suppress the development of tumors of the donor type.

An interesting hypothesis assumes that the T-cells of the donor react continuously with the histocompatibility antigens, which leads to a chronic irritation of lymphatic tissue comparable to a mixed-lymphocyte reaction (MLC) in vivo (GLEICHMANN and GLEICHMANN, 1976). This can have an effect similar to that of a repeated or chronic immune stimulation and thus cause malignant lymphomas (KRUEGER, 1970; KRUEGER *et al.*, 1971c; KRUEGER, 1975). This would also be the best way to explain why tumors can be of the donor as well as of the host or of the intermediate mixed type, since the GVHR-induced lymphomas are presumably polyclonal tumors (GLEICHMANN *et al.*, 1976).

It is also very likely, however, that the activation of tumor viruses plays a major part, be they viruses which are injected together with the spleen cells (HAYS, 1972a), or viruses already present in the host animal.

10. Prospects

According to the hypothesis of GLEICHMANN and GLEICHMANN (1976), this activation of lymphoma-bearing animals, which is brought about by the GVHR, can be of general significance for the development not only of lymphomas but also of other diseases, without requiring the presence of a lymphocyte chimaerism. The only prerequisite is that the structure of the main histocompatibility complex of the lymphocytes are changed, e.g., by viruses, drugs or other chemicals, to such a degree that autologous T-lymphocytes can react against them as if they were alien structures, and thus produce a GVHR. With reference to the clinical symptoms of systemic GVHR, it is deduced that a large number of diseases can be induced by a GVHR-like mechanism. A similar theory was discussed as early as 1961 for the so-called acquired agammaglobulinemia with autoimmune hemolysis (FUDENBERG and SOLOMON, 1961), but it applies probably to an even larger degree to lymphogranulomatosis-X, for instance, which is certainly based on a hyperimmunization reaction (RADASZKIEWICZ and LENNERT, 1975), and which is often associated with an oversensitivity to various drugs (LUKES and TINDLE, 1975) as well as with a dysproteinemia (FRIZZERA et al., 1974). A connection between GVHR and the wasting disease described by HAFERKAMP et al. (1975), the course of which is very rapid with generalized lymphadenopathy, skin involvement and interstitial lung infiltrates, is rejected by these authors, but nevertheless it appears at least possible if the reflections of GLEICHMANN and GLEICHMANN (1976) are taken into consideration.

Smallpox can be mentioned as an example of a virus-induced change of the main histocompatibility complex. At least in mice, they produce a change of the H-2 locus with a strong subsequent cytotoxic reaction of the syngeneic T-cells (KOSZINOWSKI and ERTL, 1975), and they can also induce a lymphoreticular leukosis in the same species (MAZURENKO, 1960) and in humans a nephrotic syndrome (SCHAEFER, 1963; HERRLICH et al., 1965) or a toxic epidermolytic necrosis of the type of LYELL's disease (MARTIN and BINDER, 1971).

Finally, the large group of paraneoplastic syndromes must be pointed out, in which malignant lymphomas are not unfrequently combined with an immune complex glomerulonephritis or a nephrotic syndrome (see JACKSON and Oo, 1971; LONGMIRE et al., 1973) or with an epidermolytic necrolysis (CALDWELL et al., 1971). Combinations of immunecomplex glomerulonephritis and epidermal necrolysis occur also (KRUMLOVSKY et al., 1974).

These conclusions, which are possibly of far-reaching importance for general pathology, show GVHR as a model which can explain the formal and causal pathogenesis of so far unexplained diseases and syndromes. Recently, even arteriosclerosis has been included in the range of GVHR. SCHABEL (1975) pointed out observations by CARREL in the year 1908: In an artery transplantation experiment with a cat which survived the operation for 36 days, CARREL found a massive generalized arteriosclerosis—with the exception of those parts of the artery which came from the donor. Since, according to his illustration, CARREL had included lymph nodes in the transplant, SCHABEL (1975) concluded, that a GVHR could be the reason of this host animal's arteriosclerosis.

So far, the term "allogeneic diseases" is still too poorly defined (GRUNDMANN and HOBIK, 1973b) and it can easily be overstressed. It is certain that the mechanism of GVHR can lead to acute and chronic diseases which are lethal in many cases, that these are always polysymptomatic diseases, and that the pathogenetic causality must not always be clearly recognizable. Maybe the many varieties of autoimmune diseases can be subdivided in a new way by including GVHR. The notion that a condition for allogenieic diseases can be fulfilled on the intrauterine level by diaplacental exchange of lymphocytes between mother and child (GRUNDMANN, 1973; SCHWARTZ, 1974), must be included in this concept. Of course, more questions still remain open in this field than we can answer today.

References

AISENBERG, A.C., WILKES, B., WAKSMAN, B.H.: The production of runt disease in rats thymectomized at birth. J. exp. Med. **116**, 759–772 (1962).

ALLISON, A.C., DENMAN, A.M., BARNES, R.D.: Cooperating and controlling functions of thymus-derived lymphocytes in relation to autoimmunity. Lancet **1971 II**, 135–140.

VAN ALTEN, P.J., FENNELL, R.A.: The effects of chorioallantoic grafts on the developing chick embryo. I. Studies on weight and histology of homologous and heterologous tissues. J. Embryol. exp. Morph. **7**, 459–475 (1959).

AMBRUS, C.M., AMBRUS, J.L., FELTZ, E.T.: Mitigation of secondary disease in mice receiving bone marrow from donors pretreated with cortisone and alkylating agents. Transplantation **4**, 245–249 (1966).

ANDERSON, N.D., NOWELL, P.C.: Fatal agranulocytosis and thrombocytopenia in F_1 hybrid guinea pigs following local inoculation of parental strain lymphoid cells. Fed. Proc. **25**, 660 (1966).

AOKI, T., HÄMMERLING, U., DE HARVEN, E., BOYSE, E.A., OLD, L.J.: Antigenic structure of cell surfaces. J. exp. Med. **130**, 979–1001 (1969).

ARAKAWA, K., JÉZÉQUEL, A.-M., MACVIE, S.I., JOHNSTON, R., PEREZ, Z.M., STEINER, J.W.: The liver in murine transplantation (runt) disease. Observations of the acute lesions by light and electron microscopy. Amer. J. Path. **49**, 257–299 (1966).

ARGYRIS, B.F.: The role of macrophages. Thymus- and bone marrow-derived cells in the graft-versus-host reaction. Transplantation **17**, 387–391 (1974).

ARMERDING, D., KATZ, D.H.: Activation of T and B lymphocytes in vitro. II. Biological and biochemical properties of an allogeneic effect factor (AEF) active in triggering specific B lymphocytes. J. exp. Med. **140**, 19–37 (1974).

ARMSTRONG, M.Y.K., GLEICHMANN, E., GLEICHMANN, H., BELDOTTI, L., ANDRE-SCHWARTZ, J., SCHWARTZ, R.S.: Chronic allogeneic disease. II. Development of lymphomas. J. exp. Med. **132**, 417–439 (1970).

ARMSTRONG, M.Y.K., SCHWARTZ, R.S., BELDOTTI, L.: Neoplastic sequelae of allogeneic disease. III. Histological events following transplantation of allogeneic spleen cells. Transplantation **5**, 1380–1392 (1967).

ASANTILA, T., SORVARI, T., HIRVONEN, T., TOIVANEN, P.: Xenogenic reactivity of human fetal lymphocytes. J. Immunol. **111**, 984–987 (1973).

ATKINS, R.C., FORD, W.L.: The effect of lymphocytes and serum from tolerant rats on the graft-versus-host activity of normal lymphocytes. Transplantation **13**, 442–445 (1972).

ATKINS, R.C., FORD, W.L.: Early cellular events in a systemic graft-versus-host reaction. I. The migration of responding and non-responding donor lymphocytes. J. exp. Med. **141**, 664–680 (1975).

AUERBACH, R., SHALABY, M.R.: Graft-versus-host reaction in tissue culture. J. exp. Med. **138**, 1506–1520 (1973).

AUXIER, J.A.: Dosimetric considerations in criticality exposures. In: Diagnosis and Treatment of Acute Radiation Injury, p. 141–150. Geneva: World Health Organization 1961.

BACH, F.H.: The major histocompatibility complex in transplantation immunology. Transplant. Proc. **5**, 23–29 (1973).

BACH, F.H., ALBERTINI, R.J., JOO, P., ANDERSON, J.L., BORTIN, M.M.: Bone marrow transplantation in a patient with the Wiskott-Aldrich syndrome. Lancet **1968 II**, 1364–1366.

BACH, F.H., AMOS, D.B.: Hu-1: Major histocompatibility locus in man. Science **156**, 1506–1508 (1967).

BAIN, B., LOWENSTEIN, L.: Genetic studies on the mixed leukocyte reaction. Science **145**, 1315–1316 (1964).

BAIN, G.O., ALTON, J.D.: Hepatomegaly in hybrid mice from parental spleen cells. Arch. Path. **78**, 633–642 (1964).

BAIN, G.O., DIENER, E.: Liver infiltration in graft-versus-host reaction. Effect of anti-θ-serum. Transplantation **13**, 626–627 (1972).

BAIN, G.O., FENNA, D.: Lymphoid infiltration in the F_1 hybrid liver as a thymus cell function. Transplantation **13**, 391–399 (1972).

BALNER, H., DE VRIES, M.J., VAN BEKKUM, D.W.: Secondary disease in rat radiation chimeras. J. nat. Cancer Inst. **32**, 419–459 (1964).

Barnes, B.A., Schad, P.B., Pinn, V.W.: Modification of the graft-versus-host reaction in F_1 mice treated with 6-mercaptopurine. Transplantation **4**, 154–158 (1966).

Barnes, D.W.H., Loutit, J.F., Micklem, H.S.: Secondary disease of radiation chimeras: A syndrome due to lymphoid aplasia. Ann. N.Y. Acad. Sci. **99**, 374–385 (1962).

Baumann, P., Thierfelder, S.: Unterdrückung der primären und sekundären Immunantwort durch Antilymphozytenserum (ALS), gemessen an der antigen-spezifischen Proliferationsaktivität im Graft-versus-Host Modell. Blut **28**, 51–55 (1974).

Becker, H., Cronkite, E.P., Fliedner, T.M., Messner, H., Stodtmeister, R.: Osteomyelofibrose in Ratten nach letaler Ganzkörperbestrahlung und Transfusion allogener Knochenmarkszellen. EURATOM Ges. f. Strahlenforschg. (GFS), Assoziation Nr. 031-64-1 BIAD, 1968.

Beer, A.E., Billingham, R.E.: Procurement of runt disease of maternal origin. Transplant. Proc. **5**, 887–891 (1973).

Van Bekkum, D.W.: Factors influencing the take and the rejection of bone marrow grafts. Proc. 7th Congr. Eur. Soc. Haematol, p. 947–952. London-Basel: Karger 1959.

Van Bekkum, D.W.: Foreign bone marrow transplantation following fractionated whole-body irradiation in mice. In: Radiation Effects in Physics, Chemistry and Biology (Ed. M. Ebert, A. Howard), p. 362–371. Amsterdam: North Holland Publishing Co. 1963.

Van Bekkum, D.W., Balner, H., Dicke, K.A., van den Berg, F.G., Prinsen, G.H., Hollander, C.F.: The effect of pretreatment of allogenic bone marrow graft recipients with antilymphocytic serum on the acute graft-versus-host reaction in monkeys. Transplantation **13**, 400–407 (1972).

Van Bekkum, D.W., Ledney, G.D., Balner, H., van Putten, L.M., de Vries, M.J.: Suppression of secondary disease following foreign bone marrow grafting with antilymphocyte serum. In: CIBA Foundation Symposium "Antilymphocytic Serum" (Ed. G.E.W. Wolstenholme, M.O' Connor), p. 97. London: Churchill 1967.

Van Bekkum, D.W., de Vries, M.J.: Radiation Chimaeras. New York-London: Logos Press, Academic Press 1967.

Van Bekkum, D.W., de Vries, M.J., van der Waay, D.: Lesions characteristic of secondary disease in germfree heterologous radiation chimeras. J. nat. Cancer Inst. **38**, 223–231 (1967).

Bennett, M.: Graft-versus-host reaction in mice. Transplantation **11**, 158–169 (1971).

Berman, M., Puryear, K., Argyris, B.F.: In vitro recognition of alloantigens: nature of responding and stimulating cells. Cell. Immunol. **23**, 126 139 (1976).

Berry, C.L.: Histopathological findings in the combined immunity deficiency syndrome. J. clin. Path. **23**, 193–202 (1970).

Biggs, P.M., Payne, L.N.: Cytological identification of proliferating donor cells in chick embryos injected with adult chicken blood. Nature (London) **184**, 1594 (1959).

Bildsøe, P., Ford, W.L., Pettirossi, O., Simonsen, M.: GVH analysis of organ-grafted rat which defy the normal rules for rejection. Transplantation **12**, 189 193 (1971).

Billingham, R.E.: The biology of graft-versus-host reactions. Harvey Lectures **62**, 21–78. New York-London: Academic Press 1968.

Billingham, R.E., Brent, L.: Acquired tolerance of foreign cells in newborn animals. Proc. roy. Soc. B. **146**, 78–90 (1957).

Billingham, R.E., Brent, L.: Quantitative studies on tissue transplantation immunity. IV. Induction of tolerance in newborn mice and studies on the phenomenon of runt disease. Phil. Trans. B **242**, 439 477 (1959).

Billingham, R.E., Brent, L., Medawar, P.B.: Acquired tolerance of skin homografts. Ann. N.Y. Acad. Sci. **59**, 409–416 (1955).

Billingham, R.E., Brown, J.B., Defendi, V., Silvers, W.K., Steinmüller, D.: Quantitative studies on the induction of tolerance of homologous tissues and on runt disease in the rat. Ann. N.Y. Acad. Sci. **87**, 457–471 (1960).

Billingham, R.E., Defendi, V., Silvers, W.K., Steinmüller, D.: Quantitative studies on the induction of tolerance of skin homografts and on runt disease in neonatal rats. J. nat. Cancer Inst. **28**, 365 435 (1962).

Billingham, R.E., Silvers, W.: The immunobiology of transplantation. In: Foundations of Immunology (Ed. A. Osler, L. Weiss), Englewood Cliffs/N.Y.: Prentice-Hall Inc. 1971.

Billingham, R.E., Silvers, W.K.: Some factors that determine the ability of cellular inocula to induce tolerance of tissue homografts. J. cell. comp. Physiol. **60** (Suppl. 1), 183- 200 (1962).

BINET, J.L., MATHÉ, G.: Etude en microscopie optique et électronique des «cellules immunologique-ment compétentes» au cours des réactions de greffe. C. R. Acad. Sci. (Paris) **253**, 1852–1853 (1961).

BINET, J.L., MATHÉ, G.: Optical and electron microscope studies of the immunologically competent cells during the reaction of graft against the host. Ann. N.Y. Acad. Sci. **99**, 426–431 (1962).

BIOZZI, G., HOWARD, J.G., MOUTON, D., STIFFEL, C.: Modifications of graft-versus-host reaction induced by pretreatment of the host with M. tuberculosis and C. parvum. Transplantation **3**, 170–177 (1965).

BLAESE, R.M., MARTINEZ, C., GOOD, R.A.: Immunologic incompetence of immunologically runted animals. J. exp. Med. **119**, 211–224 (1964).

BLANDEN, R.V.: Increased antibacterial resistance and immunodepression during graft-versus-host reactions in mice. Transplantation **7**, 484–497 (1969).

BLOMGREN, H., ANDERSSON, B.: Inhibition of erythroid cell growth in irradiated mice by allogeneic lymphoid cells: a quantitative method for graft-versus-host reactivity of lymphoid cells. Cell. Immunol. **3**, 318–325 (1972).

BLOMGREN, H., ANDERSSON, B.: Cross-reactivity patterns of mouse lymphocytes sensitized against the major histocompatibility complex using a graft-versus-host assay. Cell. Immunol. **11**, 122–129 (1974).

BLOMGREN, H., JACOBSSON, H.: Inhibition of erythroid cell growth by allogeneic murine lymphocytes. Evidence for a synergism between lymph node cells and thymocytes. Cell. Immunol. **13**, 288–303 (1974).

BOGGS, S.S., BOGGS, D.R., NEIL, G.L., SARTIANO, G.: Cycling characteristics of endogenous spleen colony-forming cells as measured with cytosine arabinoside and methotrexate. J. Lab. clin. Med. **82**, 727–739 (1973).

BOMFORD, R., SHAND, F.L., CHRISTIE, G.H.: Observations on the mechanism of antitumor resistance induced by the graft-versus host reaction. Transplantation **20**, 433–435 (1975).

BONAVIDA, B., KEDAR, B.: Transplantation of allogeneic lymphoid cells specifically depleted of graft-versus-host reactive cells. Nature (London) **249**, 658–659 (1974).

BORANIĆ, M.: Treatment of secondary disease in leukaemic mice with host-type and third-party haemopoietic cells and blood. Rev. europ. Et. clin. Biol. **15**, 309–314 (1970).

BORANIĆ, M.: Time pattern of antileukemic effect of graft-versus-host reaction in mice. Transplant. Proc. **3**, 394–396 (1971).

BORTIN, M.M.: A compendium of reported human bone marrow transplants. Transplantation **9**, 571–587 (1970).

BORTIN, M.M., RIMM, A.A., ROSE, W.C., SALTZSTEIN, E.C.: Graft-versus-host leukemia. V. Absence of antileukemic effect using allogeneic H-2-identical immunocompetent cells. Transplantation **18**, 280–283 (1974).

BORTIN, M.M., SALTZSTEIN, E.C.: Graft-versus-host inhibition: fetal liver and thymus cells to minimize secondary disease. Science **164**, 316–318 (1969).

BORYSENKO, M., TULIPAN, P.: The graft-versus-host reaction in the snapping turtle *Chelydra serpentina*. Transplantation **16**, 496–504 (1973).

BOYER, G.S.: Chorioallantoic membrane lesions produced by inoculation of adult fowl leucocytes. Nature (London) **185**, 327–328 (1960).

BOYSE, E.A.: Fate of mouse spleen cells transplanted into homologous and F_1 hybrid hosts. Immunology **2**, 170–182 (1959).

BRENT, L., MEDAWAR, P.B.: Quantitative studies on tissue transplantation immunity. VII. The normal lymphocyte transfer reaction. Proc. roy. Soc. B **165**, 281–307 (1966a).

BRENT, L., MEDAWAR, P.B.: Quantitative studies on tissue transplantation immunity. VIII. The effect of irradiation. Proc. roy. Soc. B **165**, 413–423 (1966b).

BRETSCHER, P.: Hypothesis: A model for generalised autoimmunity. Cell. Immunol. **6**, 1–11 (1973).

BRITTON, S.: When allogeneic mouse spleen cells are mixed in vitro the T cells secrete a product which guides the maturation of B cells. Scand. J. Immunol. **1**, 89–98 (1972).

BRUNE, K.: Graft-versus-Host Reaktionen: Modelle, Beeinflußbarkeit und klinische Analogien. Schweiz. med. Wschr. **100**, 49–58 (1970).

BUCKLEY, R.H., AMOS, B., KREMER, W.P., STICKEL, D.L.: Incompatible bone marrow transplantation in lymphopenic immunologic deficiency. Circumvention of fatal graft-versus-host disease by immunologic enhancement. New Engl. J. Med. **285**, 1035–1042 (1971).

Buja, L.M., Ferrans, V.J., Graw Jr., R.G.: Cardiac pathologic findings in patients treated with bone marrow transplantation. Hum Path. 7, 17–45 (1976).

Burkhardt, R., Bartl, R., Beil, E., Demmler, K., Hoffmann, E., Kronseder, A., Irrgang, U., Ulrich, M., Wiemann, H., Langenecker, H., Saar, U.: Myelofibrosis-Osteosclerosis Syndrome-Review of literature and histomorphology. Advanc. Biosci. 16, 11–56 (1974).

Burnet, F.M.: Cellular Immunology. Melbourne: Melbourne University Press 1969.

Burnet, F.M., Boyer, G.: Loss of specificity on passage of immunologically competent cells in the chick embryo. Nature (London) 186, 175–176 (1960).

Burnet, F.M., Boyer, G.: The chorioallantoic lesion in the Simonsen phenomenon. J. Path. Bact. 81, 141–150 (1961).

Burnet, M., Burnet, D.: Graft-versus-host reactions on the chorioallantoic membrane of the chick embryo. Nature (London) 188, 376–379 (1960).

Caldwell, I.W., Montgomery, P.R., Peachey, R.D.G.: Toxic epidermal necrolysis and malignant lymphoma. Brit. J. Derm. 79, 287–292 (1967).

Cantor, H.: The effects of the anti-theta antiserum upon graft-versus-host activity of spleen and lymph node cells. Cell. Immunol. 3, 461–469 (1972).

Cantor, H., Asofsky, R.: Synergy among lymphoid cells mediating the graft-versus-host response. II. Synergy in graft-versus-host reactions produced by BALB/c lymphoid cells of differing anatomic origin. J. exp. Med. 131, 235–246 (1970).

Cantor, H., Asofsky, R.: Synergy among lymphoid cells mediating the graft-versus-host response. III. Evidence for interaction between two types of thymus-derived cells. J. exp. Med. 135, 764–779 (1972).

Cantor, H., Asofsky, R., Talal, N.: Synergy among lymphoid cells mediating the graft-versus-host response. I. Synergy in graft-versus-host reactions produced by cells from NZB/Bl mice. J. exp. Med. 131, 223–234 (1970a).

Cantor, H., Mandel, M.A., Asofsky, R.: Studies of thoracic duct lymphocytes of mice. II. A quantitative comparison of the capacity of thoracic duct lymphocytes and other lymphoid cells to induce graft-versus-host reactions. J. Immunol. 104, 409–413 (1970b).

Cantor, H., Mosier, D.E.: Maturation of reactivity to histocompatibility antigens. Transplant. Proc. 4, 159–163 (1972).

Cantrell, J.L., Hildemann, W.H.: Characteristics of histocompatibility barriers in congenic mice. Transplant. Proc. 5, 271–274 (1973).

Carnaud, C., Markowicz, O., Trainin, N.: The influence of a graft-versus-host reaction on the incidence of metastases after tumor transplantation. Cell. Immunol. 14, 87–97 (1974).

Carrel, A. (1908), cit. Schabel (1975).

Cepellini, R., Bonnard, G.D., Coppo, F., Miggiano, B.C., Pospisil, M., Curtoni, E.S., Pellegrino, M.: Mixed leukocyte cultures and HL-A antigens. II. Inhibition by anti-HL-A sera. Transplant. Proc. 3, 63–70 (1971).

Cheers, Ch., Sprent, J., Miller, J.F.A.P.: Interaction of thymus lymphocytes with histoincompatible cells. IV. Mixed lymphocyte reactions of activated thymus lymphocytes. Cell. Immunol. 10, 57–67 (1974).

Chomette, G., Mathé, G., Auriol, M., Brocherious, C., Pinaudeau, Y.: Le syndrome secondaire chez l'homme: Etude anatomique de six cas de leucémie traités par greffe allogénique de moelle osseuse après irradiation totale. Virchows Arch. Path. Anat. A 349, 98–114 (1970).

Claman, H.N., Chaperone, E.A., Hayes, L.L.: Thymus marrow immunocompetence. Transplantation 7, 87–98 (1969).

Clancy, J., Adams, B.J., Elkins, W.L.: Fate of deoxyribonucleic acid-synthesizing cells and their progeny in a local graft-versus-host reaction. Transplantation 15, 52–58 (1973).

Clancy Jr., J., Tønder, O., Boettcher, C.E.: The effect of neonatal rat graft-versus-host disease (GVHD) in Fc receptor lymphocytes. J. Immunol. 116, 210–217 (1976).

Cline, M.J., Gale, R.P., Stiehmer, E.R., Opelz, G., Young, L.S., Feig, S.A., Fahey, J.L.: Bone marrow transplantation in man. Ann. intern. Med. 83, 691–708 (1975).

Cock, A.G., Simonsen, M.: Immunological attack on newborn chickens by injected adult cells. Immunology 2, 103–110 (1958).

Cohen, I.R., Wekerle, H.: Regulation of autosensitization. J. exp. Med. 137, 224–238 (1973).

Cohen, J.A., Vos, O., van Bekkum, D.W.: The present status of radiation protection by chemical and biological agent in mammals. In: Advances in Radiobiology (Ed. G.C. de Hevesy, A.G. Forssberg, J.D. Abbatt), p. 134–144. Edinburgh: Oliver & Boyd 1957.

CONGDON, C.C.: Cooperative group on bone marrow transplantation in man. Transplant. Proc. **2**, 342–360 (1970).

CONGDON, C.C., URSO, I.S.: Homologous bone marrow in the treatment of radiation injury in mice. Amer. J. Path. **33**, 749–767 (1957).

COPPLESON, L.W., MICHIE, D.: Comparison of the chorioallantoic membrane and splenomegaly systems of graft-versus-host assay in the chick embryo. Nature (London) **208**, 53–54 (1965).

CORNELIUS, E.A.: Clinical hematological and pathologic changes following parabiosis of syngeneic tolerant and nontolerant mice. Lab. Invest. **19**, 282–289 (1968).

CORNELIUS, E.A., APONTE, L.J.: Sex-linked abrogation of graft-versus-host reaction. Transplantation **17**, 128-131 (1974).

CORNELIUS, E.A., MARTINEZ, C., YUNIS, E.J., GOOD, R.A.: Hematological and pathological changes induced in tolerant mice by the injection of syngeneic lymphoid cells. Transplantation **6**, 33–44 (1968).

CORNELIUS, E.A., YUNIS, E.J., MARTINEZ, M.: Depression of erythrocyte maturation as a result of the graft-versus-host reaction. Proc. Soc. exp. Biol. (N.Y.) **132**, 564–567 (1969).

DAGUILLARD, F., GARNEAU, R., DESCHENES, L., CHOUINARD, C., FUDENBERG, H.H., SCHANFIELD, M.: Hyperactive production of antibody of a boy with thymic dysplasia undergoing graft-versus-host reaction. Clin. Immunol. Immunopath. **2**, 52-61 (1973).

DAVID, L.A., RUTH, R.F., LAW, G.R.J.: Specific detection of cellular transplantation antigen by fluorescent isoantibody. Ann. N.Y. Acad. Sci. **129**, 46–75 (1966).

DAVIES, A.J.S., DOAK, S.M.A.: Fate of homologous adult spleen cells injected into newborn mice. Nature (London) **187**, 610 611 (1960).

DAVIES, D.A.L.: The presence of non-H-2 histocompatibility specificities in preparations of mouse H-2 antigens. Transplantation **1**, 562–568 (1963).

DE HART, R.L., COSGROVE, G.E., UPTON, A.C.: Modification of the foreign spleen reaction: Amelioration of blood and tissue changes. Lab. Invest. **10**, 872–882 (1961).

DE KONING, J., DOOREN, L.J., VAN BEKKUM, D.W., VAN ROOD, J.J., DICKE, K.A., RADL, J.: Transplantation of bone marrow cells and fetal thymus in an infant with lymphopenic immunological deficiency. Lancet **1969 I**, 223–227.

DEMPSTER, W.J.: Kidney homotransplantation. Brit. J. Surg. **40**, 447–465 (1953).

DENKO, J.D.: The histopathology of the irradiation syndrome after homologous injections in mice. Radiat. Res. **5**, 607+ (1956).

DICKE, K.A., VAN HOOFT, J.I., VAN BEKKUM, D.W.: Selective elimination of immunologically competent cells from bone marrow and lymphatic cell mixtures. II. Mouse spleen cell fractionation on a discontinuous albumin gradient. Transplantation **6**, 562 570 (1968).

DICKE, K.A., LINA, P.H., VAN BEKKUM, D.W.: Adaptation of albumin density gradient centrifugation to human bone marrow fractionation. Rev. europ. Etud. clin. Biol. **15**, 305–309 (1970).

DI GEORGE, A.M.: Congenital absence of the thymus and its immunological consequences, concurrence with congenital hypoparathyreoidism. In: (ed.) R.A. GOOD: Immunologic Deficiency Diseases in Man. Birth Defects (Orig. Art. Series) **4**, 116–121 (1968).

DOOREN, L.J., DE VRIES, M.J., VAN BEKKUM, D.W., CLETON, F., DE KONING, J.: Sex-linked thymic epithelial hypoplasia in two siblings. J. Pediat. **72**, 51–62 (1968).

DORSCH, S.E., ROSER, B.: A quantitative lymph node weight assay for allogeneic interactions in the rat. Aust. J. exp. Biol. med. Sci. **52**, 253 -264 (1974).

DOUGLAS, S.D., FUDENBERG, H.H.: Graft-versus-host reaction in Wiskott-Aldrich syndrome: Antemortem diagnosis of human GvH in an immunological deficiency disease. Vox Sang. (Basel) **16**, 172 178 (1968).

DUPONT, B.: Bone marrow transplantation in severe combined immunodeficiency with an unrelated MLC compatible donor. Int. Soc. exp. Hematology, III. Ann. Meeting, Houston 1974, p. 44.

DYMINSKI, J.W., ARGYRIS, B.F.: In vitro sensitization to transplantation antigens. VII. Enhanced graft-versus-host activity of in vitro allosensitized lymphoid cells. Cell. Immunol. **7**, 205–212 (1973).

EBERT, J.D.: Report on the Department of Embryology. Year Book of the Carnegie Institution (Washington) **58**, 361–362, 402–403, (1959).

EBERT, J.D.: The effects of chorioallantoic transplants of adult chicken tissues on homologous tissues of the host chick embryo. Proc. nat. Acad. Sci. (Wash.) **40**, 337–347 (1954).

Eijsvoogel, V.P.: The cellular recognition in vitro of antigens related to human histocompatibility. Semin. Hematol. **11**, 305–324 (1974).

Eikman, E.A., Bowser, R.T.: Alteration in graft-versus-host reactivity and in hematopoietic stem cells of spleen cell inocula from donor mice pretreated with pertussis antigen. J. Immunol. **108**, 253–260 (1972).

Elkins, W.L.: Invasion and destruction of homologous kidney by locally inoculated lymphoid cells. J. exp. Med. **120**, 329–347 (1964).

Elkins, W.L.: The interaction of donor and host lymphoid cells in the pathogenesis of renal cortical destruction induced by a local graft-versus-host reaction. J. exp. Med. **123**, 103–118 (1966).

Elkins, W.L.: Specific and non-specific lymphoid cell proliferation in the pathogenesis of graft-versus-host reactions. Transplantation **9**, 273–301 (1970).

Elkins, W.L.: Cellular immunology and the pathogenesis of graft-versus host reactions. Progr. Allergy **15**, 78–187 (1971).

Elkins, W.L., Guttmann, R.D.: Pathogenesis of a local graft-versus-host reaction: Immunogenicity of circulating host leukocytes. Science **159**, 1250–1251 (1968).

Elkins, W.L., Kavathas, P., Bach, F.H.: Activation of T cells by H-2-factors in the graft-versus-host reaction. Transplant. Proc. **5**, 1759–1762 (1973).

Elves, M.W.: The impairment of graft-versus-host reaction by immunisation of F_1 hybrids with low doses of parental cells. Transplantation **16**, 403–407 (1973).

Fahey, J.L., Mann, D.L., Asofsky, R., Rogentine, G.N.: Recent progress in human transplantation immunology. Ann. intern. Med. **71**, 1177–1196 (1969).

Falk, R.E., Collste, L., Möller, G.: Release of migration inhibitory factors from immune rat lymphocytes confronted with histocompatibility antigens. Nature (London) **224**, 1206–1207 (1969).

Fass, L., Ochs, H.D., Thomas, E.D., Mickelson, E., Storb, R., Fefer, A.: Studies of immunological reactivity following syngeneic or allogeneic marrow grafts in man. Transplantation **16**, 630–640 (1973).

Fefer, A., Buckner, C.D., Clift, R.A., Fass, L., Lerner, K.G., Mickelson, E.M., Neiman, P., Rudolph, R., Storb, R., Thomas, E.D.: Marrow grafting in identical twins with hematologic malignancies. Transplant. Proc. **5**, 927–931 (1973).

Field, E.O., Cauchi, N.M., Gibbs, J.E.: The transfer of refractoriness to GVH disease in F_1 hybrid rats. Transplantation **5**, 241–247 (1967).

Field, E.O., Gibbs, J.E.: Effects of thymectomy and irradiation on graft-versus-host disease. Transplantation **3**, 634–638 (1965).

Field, E.O., Gibbs, J.E.: Reduced sensitivity of F_1 hybrid rats to re-challenge with parental strain spleen cells. Clin. exp. Immunol. **1**, 195–205 (1966).

Field, E.O., Gibbs, J.E., Tucker, D.F., Hellmann, K.: Effect of thalidomide on the graft-versus-host reaction. Nature (London) **211**, 1308–1310 (1966).

Finerty, J.C.: Parabiosis in physiological studies. Physiol. Rev. **32**, 277–289 (1952).

Fink, M.P., Cloud, C.L.: Graft-versus-host disease in rats after donor treatment with cyclophosphamide and spleen cells of host origin. Transplantation **17**, 508–512 (1974).

Floersheim, G.L., Seiler, K.: Differential effects of immunosuppressive drugs on a cutaneous graft-versus-host reaction in chickens. Transplantation **5**, 1355–1370 (1967).

Ford, W.L.: A local graft-versus-host reaction following intradermal injection of lymphocytes in the rat. Brit. J. exp. Path. **48**, 335–345 (1967).

Ford, W.L., Atkins, R.C.: Specific unresponsiveness of recirculating lymphocytes after exposure to histocompatibility antigen in F_1 hybrid rats. Nature New Biology (London) **234**, 178–180 (1971).

Ford, W.L., Burr, W., Simonsen, M.: A lymph node weight assay for the graft-versus-host activity of rat lymphoid cells. Transplantation **10**, 258–266 (1970).

Ford, W.L., Simmonds, S.J., Atkins, R.C.: Early cellular events in a systemic graft-versus-host reaction. II. Autoradiographic estimates of the frequency of donor lymphocytes which respond to each Ag-B-determined antigenic complex. J. exp. Med. **141**, 681–696 (1975).

Fox, M.: Cytological estimation of proliferating donor cells during graft-versus-host disease in F_1 hybrid mice injected with parental spleen cells. Immunology **5**, 489–495 (1962).

Fox, M.: The significance of lymphoid repopulation in the graft-versus-host reaction. Ann. N.Y. Acad. Sci. **129**, 297–309 (1966).

FOX, M., HOWARD, J.G.: An acquired type of refractoriness to graft-versus-host reaction in adult F_1 hybrid mice. Transplantation **1**, 2-14 (1963).

FRIZZERA, G., MORAN, E.M., RAPPAPORT, H.: Angio-immunoblastic lymphadenopathy with dysproteinaemia. Lancet **1974 I**, 1070–1073.

FUDENBERG, H., SOLOMON, A.: "Acquired Agammaglobulinemia" with autoimmune hemolytic disease: Graft-versus-host reaction? Vox. Sang. (Basel) **6**, 68–79 (1961).

GALLAGHER, M.T., RICHIE, E.R., HEIM, L.R., JUDD, K.P., TRENTIN, J.J.: Inhibition of the graft-versus-host reaction. I. Reduction of the GVH potential of mouse spleen cells (with a sparing of stem cells) by treatment with antilymphocyte globulin-derived Fab fragments. Transplantation **14**, 597–602 (1972).

GALE, R.P., OPELZ, G., SPARKES, R.: Bone marrow transplantation between mixed lymphocyte culture-reactive individuals. Transplantation **20**, 194–198 (1975).

GARCIA-GIRALT, E., MORALES, V.H., LASALVIA, E., MATHÉ, G.: Suppression of graft-versus-host reaction by a spleen extract. J. Immunol. **109**, 878–881 (1972).

GATTI, R.A., GOOD, R.A.: Macrophage function in severe combined immunodeficiency disease. J. Pediat. **80**, 285–298 (1972).

GATTI, R.A., KERSEY, J.H., YUNIS, E.J., GOOD, R.A.: Graft-versus-host disease. Progr. clin. Path. **5**, 1-18 (1973).

GATTI, R.A., MEUWISSEN, H.J., ALLEN, H.D., HONG, R., GOOD, R.A.: Immunological reconstitution of sex-linked lymphopenic immunological deficiency. Lancet **1968 II**, 1366-1369.

GATTI, R.A., MEUWISSEN, H.J., TERASAKI, P.I., GOOD, R.A.: Recombination within the HL-A locus. Tissue Antigens (Copenhagen) **1**, 239–241 (1971).

GELFAND, E.W., PHILLIPS, R.A., MILLER, R.G., McCULLOCH, E.A., ROSEN, F.S.: The use of cell separation techniques and isoantibody to host antigens in the treatment of severe combined immunodeficiency disease with HL-A-incompatible maternal marrow. Exp. Hematol. **2**, 122–130 (1974).

GENGOZIAN, N., EDWARDS, C.L., VODOPICK, H.A., HÜBNER, K.F.: Bone marrow transplantation in a leukemic patient following immunosuppression with antithymocyte globulin and total body irradiation. Transplantation **15**, 446–454 (1973).

GERSHON, R.K., COHEN, P., HENCIN, R., LIEBHABER, S.A.: Suppressor T cells. J. Immunol. **108**, 586–590 (1972).

GESNER, B.M., WOODRUFF, J.J.: Cellular Recognition (Ed. R.I. SMITH, R.A. GOOD). New York: Appleton 1969.

GITHENS, J.H., HATHAWAY, W.E., COX, S.M., SUVATTE, V., METZGAR, A.: Serial study of the bone marrow changes in runt disease. Transplantation **6**, 619-623 (1968).

GITHENS, J.H., MUSCHENHEIM, F., FULGINITI, V.A., ROBINSON, A., KAY, H.E.M.: Thymic alymphoplasia with XX/XY lymphoid chimerism secondary to probable maternal-fetal transfusion. J. Pediat. **75**, 87-94 (1969).

GITTES, R.F., RUSSELL, P.S.: Male histocompatibility antigens in mouse endocrine tissues: Functional and histologic evidence. J. nat. Cancer Inst. **26**, 283–303 (1961).

GLEICHMANN, E., GLEICHMANN, H.: Graft-versus-host reaction: a pathogenetic principle for the development of drug allergy, autoimmunity, and malignant lymphoma in non-chimeric individuals. Hypothesis. Z. Krebsforsch. **85**, 91-109 (1976).

GLEICHMANN, E., GLEICHMANN, H., SCHWARTZ, R.S., WEINBLATT, A., ARMSTRONG, M.Y.K.: Immunologic induction of malignant lymphoma. Identification of donor and host tumors in the graft-versus-host model. J. nat. Cancer Inst. **54**, 107-116 (1975).

GLEICHMANN, E., GLEICHMANN, H. WILKE, W.D.: Autoimmunization and lymphomagenesis in parent $-F_1$ combinations differing at the major histocompatibility complex: Model for spontaneous disease caused by altered selfantigens? Transplant. Rev. **31**, 156-224 (1976).

GLEICHMANN, H., GLEICHMANN, E., ANDRÉ-SCHWARTZ, J., SCHWARTZ, R.S.: Chronic allogeneic disease. III. Genetic requirements for the induction of glomerulonephritis. J. exp. Med. **135**, 516–532 (1972).

GLEICHMANN, H., GLEICHMANN, E., PETERS, K.: Induction of immune complex glomerulonephritis in F_1 hybrid mice: Superiority of cortisone-resistent parental thymocytes over spleen cells. Cell. Immunol. **14**, 123–127 (1974).

GLOBERSON, A., AUERBACH, R.: Primary immune reactions in organ cultures. Science **149**, 991–993 (1965).

GLUCKSBERG, H., STORB, R., FEFER, A., BUCKNER, C.D., NEIMAN, P.E., CLIFT, R.A., LERNER, K.G., THOMAS, E.D.: Clinical manifestations of graft versus-host disease in human recipients of marrow from HL-A-matched sibling donors. Transplantation **18**, 295–304 (1974).

GOLSTEIN, P., BLOMGREN, H.: Further evidence for autonomy of T cells mediating specific in vitro cytotoxicity: Efficiency of very small amounts of highly purified T cells. Cell. Immunol. **9**, 127–141 (1973).

GOOD, R.A.: Communication given at the annual meeting of the Int. Soc. exp. Hematol. (1973), cit. SPECK (1975).

GOOD, R.A., DALMASSO, A.P., MARTINEZ, C., ARCHER, O.K., PIERCE, J.C., PAPERMASTER, B.W.: The role of the thymus in development of immunologic capacity in rabbits and mice. J. exp. Med. **116**, 773–796 (1962).

GOODMAN, J.W., BASFORD, N.L., SHINPOCK, S.G.: Marrow stem cell-thymocyte interaction in hemopoiesis. XIV. Internat. Congr. Hematology, Sao Paulo 1972 Abstract No. 95.

GOTJAMANOS, T.: A comparison of the changes produced in reticuloendothelial organs of mice during host-versus-graft and graft-versus-host reaction. Aust. J. exp. Biol. med. Sci. **48**, 567–581 (1970).

GOWANS, J.L.: The fate of parental strain small lymphocytes in F_1 hybrid rats. Ann. N.Y. Acad. Sci. **99**, 432–455 (1962).

GOWANS, J.L., GESNER, B.M., McGREGOR, D.D.: The immunological activity of lymphocytes. In: Biological Activity of the Leucocyte. CIBA Foundation Study Group No. 10, (Ed. G.E.W. WOLSTENHOLME, M. O'CONNOR). p. 32–40. London: Churchill 1961.

GORER, P.A., BOYSE, E.A.: Pathological changes in F_1 hybrid mice following transplantation of spleen cells from donors of the parental strain. Immunology **2**, 182–193 (1959).

GRANGER, G., KOLB, W.: Lymphocyte in vitro cytotoxicity: Mechanisms of immune and non-immune small lymphocyte-mediated target L cell destruction. J. Immunol. **101**, 111–120 (1968).

GRAW, R.G., BUCKNER, C.D., WHANG-PENG, J., LEVENTHAL, B.G., KRÜGER, G., BERARD, C., HENDERSON, E.S.: Complication of bone marrow transplantation: Graft-versus-host disease resulting from chronic-myelogenous-leukemia leucocyte transfusions. Lancet **1970 II**, 338–341.

GRAW JR., R.G., LEVENTHAL, B.G., YANKEE, R.A., ROGENTINE, G.N., WHANG-PENG, J., GINNIF, M.H., HERZIG, G.P., HALTERMAN, R.H., HENDERSON, E.S.: HL-A and mixed leukocyte culture matched allogeneic bone marrow transplantation in patients with acute leukemia. Transplant. Proc. **3**, 405 408 (1971).

GREBE, S.C., STREILEIN, J.W.: (1975 a) cit. GREBE, S.C., STREILEIN, J.W. (1976)

GREBE, S.C., STREILEIN, J.W.: (1975 b) cit. GREBE, S.C., STREILEIN, J.W. (1976).

GREBE, S.C., STREILEIN, J.W.: Graft-versus-host reactions: A review. Advanc. Immunol. **22**, 119–221 (1976).

GROFF, P., TORHORST, J., SPECK, B., NISSEN, C., WEBER, W., CORNU, P., ROSSIER, J., BILAND, L.: Die Graft-versus-Host Krankheit eine wenig bekannte Komplikation der Bluttransfusion. Schweiz. med. Wschr. **106**, 634–639 (1976).

GROGAN, T.M., BROUGHTON, D.D., DOYLE, W.F.:: Graft-versus-host reaction Arch. Path. **99**, 330–334 (1975).

GRUNDMANN, E.: Die Bildung von Lymphocyten und Plasmazellen im lymphatischen Gewebe der Ratte. Beitr. path. Anat. **119**, 217–262 (1958).

GRUNDMANN, E.: Experimentelle Untersuchungen über die zelluläre Speicherung des Polyvinylpyridin-N-oxids. Fortschr. Staublungenforsch. **2**, 223–228 (1967).

GRUNDMANN, E.: Die Rolle der Lymphocyten bei der Wahrung der individuellen Integrität. Verh. dtsch. Ges. inn. Med. **79**, 118 -129 (1973).

GRUNDMANN, E., HOBIK, H.P.: Lymphoretikuläre Sarkome bei immunologisch geschädigten Mäusen. Z. Krebsforsch. **79**, 298–303 (1973 a).

GRUNDMANN, E., HOBIK, H.P.: Graft-versus-Host Reaktion   Allogenkrankheiten — Lymphome. Beitr. path. Anat. **150**, 323–329 (1973 b).

GRUNDMANN, E., HOBIK, H.P.: Studien zur Graft-versus-Host Reaktion. Nova Acta Leopoldina (Halle) **41**, 449–461 (1975).

GUTTERMANN, J.U., HERSH, E.M., RODRIGUEZ, V., McCREDIE, K.B., MAVLIGIT, G., REED, R., BURGESS, M.A., SMITH, T., GEHAN, E., BODEY, G.P., FREIREICH, E.J.: Chemoimmunotherapy of adult acute leukemia. Prolongation of remission in myeloblastic leukemia with BCG. Lancet **1974 II**, 1405-1409.

HAFERKAMP, O., SCHACHENMAYR, W., KLEEBERG, U.R., WILDFEUER, A., BOROWSKI, K., MEISTER, H., KONIETZKO, N., ENGELS, J., SCHREWE, K.H.: Schnell verlaufende Auszehrungskrankheit mit generalisierter Lymphadenopathie, Hautbeteiligung und interstitieller Lungeninfiltration. Dtsch. med. Wschr. **100**, 335-342 (1975).

HALL, J.G., PARRY, D.M., SMITH, M.E.: The distribution and differentiation of lymph-born immunoblasts after intravenous injection into syngeneic recipients. Cell Tiss. Kinet. **5**, 269-281 (1972).

HALLE-PANNENKO, O., MARTYRE, M.C., MATHÉ, G.: Prevention of graft-versus-host reaction by donor pretreatment with soluble H-2 antigens. Transplantation **11**, 414-417 (1971).

HARRISS, E., CURRIE, C., KRISS, J.P., KAPLAN, H.S.: Studies on anemia in F_1 hybrid mice injected with parental strain lymphoid cells. J. exp. Med. **113**, 1095+1112-1113 (1961).

HAŠKOVÁ, V., GANSOVA, E., HAJNÁ, J.: Immunocompetence in regional graft-versus-host reaction of blood cells from skin allografted or ALS-treated rats. Folia biol. (Praha) **19**, 261-266 (1973a).

HAŠKOVÁ, V., KORČÁKOVÁ, L., BEDNARIK, T.: Dissociation of lymphocyte activation and graft-versus-host competence of blood cells after skin grafting in rats treated with antithymocyte and normal pig serum. Transplantation **16**, 325-330 (1973b).

HATHAWAY, W.E., BRANGLE, R.W., NELSON, T.L., ROCKEL, I.E.: Aplastic anemia and alymphocytosis in an infant with hypogammaglobulinemia: Graft-versus-host reaction? J. Pediat. **68**, 713-722 (1966).

HATHAWAY, W.E., FULGINITI, V.A., PIERCE, C.W., GITHENS, J.H., PEARLMAN, D.S., MUSCHENHEIM, F., KEMPE, H.: Graft-versus-host reaction following a single blood transfusion. J. Amer. med. Ass. **201**, 1015 1020 (1967).

HATHAWAY, W.E., GITHENS, J.H., BLACKBURN, W.R., FULGINITI, V., KEMPE, H.: Aplastic anemia, histiocytosis and erythrodermia in immunologically deficient children: probable human runt disease. New Engl. J. Med. **273**, 953-958 (1965).

HAYS, E.F.: Graft-versus-host reaction and the viral induction of mouse lymphoma. Cancer Res. **32**, 270-275 (1972a).

HAYS, E.F.: Development of neoplasia and karyotype analysis in mice with graft-versus-host reaction. Cancer Res. **32**, 276-279 (1972b).

HELLSTRÖM, I., HELLSTRÖM, K.E.: Lymphocyte-mediated cytotoxic reactions and blocking serum factors in tumor-bearing individuals and in rats tolerant to skin allografts; similarities and possible differences. In: Progress in Immunology II, vol. 5, (Ed. L. BRENT, J. HOLBORROW), p. 147-157. New York: American Elsevier Publ. Co. 1974.

HERON, J.: Is transplantation tolerance in the rat serum-mediated? Transplantation **15**, 534-539 (1973).

HERRLICH, A., EHRENGUT, W., SCHLEUSSING, H.: Der Impfschaden. In: Handbuch der Schutzimpfungen, S. 237 239. Berlin-Heidelberg-New York: Springer 1965.

HESLOP, B.F., HARDY, B.E.: The distribution of 51-Cr-labeled syngeneic and allogeneic lymph node cells in the rat. Transplantation **11**, 128-134 (1971).

HILDEMANN, W.H., GALLAGHER, B.A., WALFORD, R.L.: Pathologic changes in lymphoid tissues in early transplantation (runt) disease in mice. Amer. J. Path. **45**, 481-493 (1964).

HILGARD, H., BURNET, D., BURNET, F.M.: Tolerance as shown by the Simonsen reaction on the chorioallantoic membrane. Aust. J. exp. Biol. med. Sci. **40**, 232-240 (1962).

HIRATA, A.A., SCHECHTMAN, A.M.: Studies on immunological depression in chickens. J. Immunol. **85**, 230-239 (1960).

HITZIG, W.H.: Konnatale Defektzustände des lymphatischen Systems. In: Lymphozyt und klinische Immunologie. Hrsg. H. Theml, H. Begemann. S. 112-123. Berlin-Heidelberg-New York: Springer 1975.

HOBIK, H.P.: Die Hemmung der Graft-versus-Host Reaktion in Maus und Ratte durch L-Asparaginase. Verh. dtsch. Ges. Path. **53**, 525-528 (1969a).

HOBIK, H.P.: Der Einfluß immunosuppressiver Agentien auf die Graft-versus-Host Reaktion in der Maus. In: Organtransplantation, Immunologie und Klinik. (Hrsg. A. HEYMER, D. RICKEN), S. 269-274. Stuttgart-New York: Schattauer 1969b.

HOBIK, H.P.: Effect of L-Asparaginase and other immunosuppressive agents on the course of graft-versus-host disease in rats and mice. Exp. Hematol. **20**, 18-20 (1970).

HOBIK, H.P.: Osteomyelosclerosis in experimental graft-versus-host disease. V. Congr. Europ. Soc. Pathology, Vienna 1975 Abstract no. 110, p. 62.

HOBIK, H.P., SAWADA, S.: Zur Morphologie der Milzfollikel von Mäusen der Stämme NZB/NZW und C 57/Bl/6. Verh. dtsch. Ges. Path. **54**, 235-237 (1970).

Hong, R., Kay, H.E.M., Cooper, M.D., Meuwissen, H., Allan, M.J.G., Good, R.A.: Immunological reconstitution in lymphopenic immunological deficiency syndrome. Lancet **1968** I, 503–506.

Howard, J.C., Hunt, S.V., Gowans, J.L.: Identification of marrow-derived and thymus-derived small lymphocytes in the lymphoid tissue and thoracic duct lymph of normal rats. J. exp. Med. **135**, 200–219 (1972).

Howard, J.G.: Changes in the activity of the reticulo-endothelial system (RES) following the injection of parental spleen cells into F_1 hybrid mice. Brit. J. exp. Path. **42**, 72–82 (1961).

Howard, J.G.: The use of reticuloendothelial function for studying graft-versus-host reaction in the presence of potential host-versus-graft reaction. J. reticuloendoth. Soc. **1**, 29–39 (1964).

Howard, J.G., Christie, G.H., Boak, J.L., Kinsky, R.G.: Peritoneal and alveolar macrophages derived from lymphocyte populations during graft-versus-host reaction. Brit. J. exp. Path. **50**, 448–455 (1969).

Howard, J.G., Woodruff, M.F.A.: Effect of the graft-versus-host reaction on the immunological responsiveness of the mouse. Proc. roy. Soc. B **154**, 532–539 (1961).

Huber, B., Peña-Martinez, J., Festenstein, H.: Spleen cell transplantation in mice: Influence of non-H2M-locus on graft-versus-host and host-versus-graft reactions. Transplant. Proc. **5**, 1373–1375 (1973).

Isacson, P.: Cellular transfer of antibody production from adult to embryo in domestic fowls. Yale J. Biol. Med. **32**, 209–228 (1959).

Jackson, R.H., Oo, M.: Nephrotic syndrome with Hodgkin's disease. Lancet **1971** II, 821–822.

Jammet, H., Mathé, G., Pendic, B., Duplan, J.F., Maupin, B., Latarjet, R., Kalic, D., Schwarzenberg, L., Djukic, Z., Vigne, J.: Etude de six cas d'irradiation totale aiguë accidentelle. Rev. franc. Et. clin. Biol. **4**, 210–225 (1959).

Jeannet, M., Wonham, V.A., Winn, H.J., Russell, P.S.: Donor selection for kidney transplantation, based on leukocyte pheno- and genotyping and mixed lymphocyte culture. Transplant. Proc. **1**, 382–384 (1969).

Joller, P.W.: Graft-versus-host reactivity of lymphoid cells inhibited by anti-recognition structure serum. Nature New Biology (London) **240**, 214–215 (1972).

Kadowaki, J., Zuelzer, W.W., Brough, A.J., Thompson, R.I., Woolley jr., P.V., Gruber, D.: XX/XY lymphoid chimaerism in congenital immunological deficiency syndrome with thymic alymphoplasia. Lancet **1965** II, 1152–1155.

Kano, K., Beldotti, L., Milgrom, F., Schwartz, R.S.: Glomerulonephritis in the graft-versus-host reaction: Serologic demonstration of antihost antibodies. J. Immunol. **112**, 410–412 (1974).

Kaplan, H.J., Stevens, T.R., Streilein, J.W.: Transplantation immunology of the anterior chamber of the eye. I. An intra-ocular graft-versus-host reaction (immunogenic anterior uveitis). J. Immunol. **115**, 800–804 (1975a).

Kaplan, H.J., Streilein, J.W., Stevens, T.R.: Transplantation immunology of the anterior chamber of the eye. II. Immune response to allogeneic cells. J. Immunol. **115**, 805–810 (1975b).

Kaplan, H.S., Rosston, B.H.: Studies on a wasting disease induced in F_1 hybrid mice injected with parental strain lymphoid cells. Stanf. med. Bull. **17**, 77–92 (1959).

Katz, D.H.: The allogeneic effect on immune responses: Model for regulatory influences of T lymphocytes on the immune system. Transplant. Rev. **12**, 141–179 (1972).

Katz, D.H., Hamaoka, T., Dorf, M.E., Benacerraf, B.: Cell interactions between histoincompatible T and B lymphocytes. V. Failure of histoincompatible T cells to interfere with physiologic cooperation between syngeneic T and B lymphocytes. J. Immunol. **112**, 855–857 (1974).

Katz, D.H., Paul, W.E., Benacerraf, B.: Carrier function in antihapten antibody responses. V. Analysis of cellular events in the enhancement of antibody responses by the "allogeneic effect" in DNP-DVA-primed guinea pigs challenged with a heterologous DNP-conjugate. J. Immunol. **107**, 1319–1328 (1971).

Keast, D.: Runting syndromes, autoimmunity, and neoplasia. Advanc. Cancer Res. **11**, 43–71 (1968a).

Keast, D.: A simple index for the measurement of the runting syndrome and its use in the study of the influence of the gut flora in its production. Immunology **15**, 237–245 (1968b).

Keast, D.: The murine runting syndrome and neoplasia. Immunology **16**, 693–697 (1969).

Keast, D., Walters, M.N.J.: The pathology of murine runting and its modification by neomycin sulphate gavages. Immunology **15**, 247–262 (1968).

Kersey, J.H., Meuwissen, H.J., Good, R.A.: Graft-versus-host reactions following transplantation of allogeneic hematopoietic cells. Hum. Path. **2**, 389–402 (1971).

KETTMANN, J., SKARVALL, H.: The allogeneic effect: Bystander effect in the primary immune response in vitro. Europ. J. Immunol. **4**, 641–645 (1974).

KIGER, N., FLORENTIN, I., MATHÉ, G.: Inhibition of graft-versus-host reaction by preincubation of the graft with a thymic extract (lymphocyte chalone). Transplantation **16**, 393–397 (1973).

KILLBY, V.A.A., LAFFERTY, K.J., RYAN, M.: Interaction of embryonic chicken spleen cells and adult allogeneic leucocytes. Aust. J. exp. Biol. med. Sci. **50**, 309–321 (1972).

KISKEN, W.A., SWENSON, N.A.: Unresponsiveness of mixed leucocyte cultures from thymectomized adult dogs. Nature (London) **224**, 76- 77 (1969).

KLEIN, J.: The H-2 system: Past and present. Transplant. Proc. **5**, 11- 21 (1973).

KLEIN, J., EGOROV, I.K.: Graft-versus-host reaction with an H-2 mutant. J. Immunol. **111**, 976–979 (1973).

KLEIN, J., PARK, J.M.: Graft-versus-host reaction across different regions of the H-2 complex of the mouse. J. exp. Med. **137**, 1213–1225 (1973).

KOCH, C., HENRIKSEN, K., JUHL, F., WIIK, A., FABER, V., ANDERSEN, V., DUPONT, B., SØNDERSTRUP-HANSEN, G., SVEJGAARD, A., THOMSEN, M., ERNST, P., KILLMANN, S.-A., GOOD, R.A., JENSEN, K., MULLER-BERAT, N.: Bone-marrow transplantation from an HL-A non-identical but mixed-lymphocyte-culture identical donor. Lancet **1973 I**, 1146–1150.

KOLB, H.J., STORB, R., GRAHAM, T.C., KOLB, H., THOMAS, E.D.: Antithymocyte serum and methotrexate for control of graft-versus-host disease in dogs. Transplantation **16**, 17–23 (1973).

KOLTAY, M., KINSKY, R.G., ARNASON, B.G., SCHAFFNER, J.B.: Immunoglobulins and antibody formation in mice during the graft-versus-host reaction. Immunology **9**, 581–590 (1965).

KOSZINOWSKI, U., ERTL, H.: Lysis mediated by T cells and restricted by H-2 antigen of target cells infected with vaccinia virus. Nature (London) **255**, 552–554 (1975).

KRAMER, A.K., VAN DER VELDEN, N.A.: Vererbungslehre und Zucht. In: Versuchstiere und Versuchstiertechnik Vol. II, S. 193–223. Veröff. Gesellsch. f. Versuchstierkunde, Basel 1975.

KŘEN, V., BRAUN, A., ŠTARK, O., KRAUS, P., FRENZL, B., BRDIČKA, R.: Runting syndrome in rats and its inhibition by homologous sera. Folia biol. (Praha) **8**, 341–350 (1962).

KŘEN, V., VESELY, P., FRENZEL, B., ŠTARK, O.: Inhibition of the runting syndrome in rats. Folia biol. (Praha) **6**, 333–341 (1960).

KRETSCHMER, R., JEANNET, M., MEREU, T.R., KRETSCHMER, K., WINN, H., ROSEN, F.S.: Hereditary thymic dysplasia: A graft-versus-host reaction induced by bone marrow cells with a partial 4a series histoincompatibility. Pediat. Res. **3**, 34–40 (1969).

KRUEGER, G.R.F.: Zur Pathogenese von Tumoren des lymphoretikulären Gewebes bei Transplantationsempfängern. Verh. dtsch. Ges. Path. **54**, 175–181 (1970).

KRUEGER, G.R.F.: The significance of immunosuppression and antigenic stimulation for the development of malignant lymphomas. (With special reference to cancer chemotherapy). Rec. Res. Cancer Res. **52**, 88 95 (1975).

KRUEGER, G.R.F., BERARD, C.W., DELELLIS, R.A., GRAW, R.G., YANKEE, R.A., LEVENTHAL, B.G., ROGENTINE, G.N., HERZIG, G.P., HALTERMAN, R.H., HENDERSON, E.S.: Graft-versus-host diseas: Morphologic variation and differential diagnosis in 8 cases of Hl-A-matched bone marrow transplantation. Amer. J. Path. **63**, 179–196 (1971b).

KRUEGER, G.R.F., BERARD, C.W., ELIAS, P.M., GRAW, R.G.: Morphology of graft-versus-host reaction in Hl-A-matched bone marrow transplantation and its differential diagnosis Exp. Hematol. **21**, 4 6 (1971a).

KRUEGER, G.R.F., GRAW, R.G., ROGENTINE, G.N., DARROW, C.C., NEEFE, J.R., LUETZELER, J.: Pathology of modified graft-versus-host disease in bone marrow allografted monkeys treated with antilymphocyte serum. Blut **30**, 19–30 (1975).

KRUEGER, G.R.F., MALMGREN, R.A., BERARD, C.W.: Malignant lymphomas and plasmocytosis in mice under prolonged immunosuppression and persistent antigenic stimulation. Transplantation **11**, 138 144 (1971c).

KRUMLOVSKY, F.A., DEL GRECO, F., HERDSON, P.B., LAZAR, P.: Renal disease associated with toxic epidermal necrolysis (Lyell's disease). Amer. J. Med. **57**, 817–825 (1974).

LAPP, W.S., MÖLLER, G.: Prolonged survival of H-2 incompatible skin allografts on F_1 animals treated with parental lymphoid cells. Immunology **17**, 339–344 (1969).

LAWRENCE, W.L., SIMONSEN, M.: The property of "strength" of histocompatibility antigens, and their ability to produce antigenic competition. Transplantation **5**, 1304–1322 (1967).

LENNERT, K., NAGAI, K., SCHWARZE, E.W.: Patho-anatomical features of the bone marrow. Clin. Hematol. **4**, 331–351 (1975).

LEVIN, D.M., ROSENSTREICH, D., REYNOLDS, H.Y.: Demonstration of graft-versus-host, mixed leuco-cyte reaction and monocyte chemotactic factor production in guinea pig Peyer's patch cells. Fed. Proc. **33**, 803+ (1974).

LEVINE, S.: Graft-versus-host disease. Liver involvement in splenectomized rats. Transplantation **6**, 294-295 (1968a).

LEVINE, S.: Local and regional forms of graft-versus-host disease in lymph nodes. Transplantation **6**, 799-801 (1968b).

LEVINE, S., IWAHARA, M.: Graft-versus-host disease produced with whole blood. Transplantation **8**, 462-465 (1969).

LEWIS, R.M., ARMSTRONG, M.Y.K., ANDRÈ-SCHWARTZ, J., MUFTUOGLU, A., BELDOTTI, L., SCHWARTZ, R.S.: Chronic allogeneic disease I. Development of glomerulonephritis. J. exp. Med. **128**, 653-667 (1968).

LIACOPOULOS, P., MERCHANT, B., HARRELL, B.E.: Inhibition of the graft-versus-host reaction by pretreatment of donors with various antigens. Transplantation **5**, 1423-1435 (1967a).

LIACOPOULOS, P., MERCHANT, B., HARRELL, B.E.: Effect of donor immunization with somatic polysaccharides on the graft-versus-host reactivity of transferred donor splenocytes. Proc. Soc. exp. Biol. (N.Y.) **125**, 958-962 (1967b).

LONAI, P., CLARK, W.R., FELDMAN, M.: Participation of θ-bearing cell in an in vitro assay of transplantation immunity. Nature (London) **229**, 566-567 (1971).

LONGENECKER, B.M., PAZDERKA, F., LAW, G.R.J., RUTH, R.F.: The graft-versus-host reaction to minor alloantigens. Cell. Immunol. **8**, 1-11 (1973).

LONGMIRE, R.L., MCMILLAN, R., YELENOSKY, R., ARMSTRONG, S., LANG, J.E., CRADDOCK, C.G.: In vitro splenic IgG synthesis in Hodgkin's disease. New Engl. J. Med. **289**, 763-767 (1973).

LUKES, R.J., TINDLE, B.H.: Immunoblastic lymphadenopathy: A hyperimmune entity resembling Hodgkin's disease. New Engl. J. Med. **292**, 1-8 (1975).

LYDYARD, P.M., IVANYI, J.: The role of opsonization in antithymocyte globulin-indiced suppression of graft-versus-host reaction in chick embryos. Transplantation **17**, 400-404 (1974).

MARTIN, J., BINDER, T.: Une complication rare de la vaccination jennerienne: La nécrolyse épider-mique toxique (Lyell). Schweiz. med. Wschr. **101**, 1446-1448 (1971).

MATHÉ, G., AMIEL, J.L., BERNARD, J.: Traitement de souris AkR à l'age de six mois par irradiation totale suivie de transfusion de cellules hématopoïétiques allogéniques. Incidences respectives de la leucémie et du syndrome secondaire. Bull. Cancer **47**, 331-340 (1960).

MATHÉ, G., AMIEL, J.L., NIEMETZ, J.: Recherche d'un test d'histocompatibilité pour les essais de greffes allogéniques. I Etude chez la souris. Rev. franc. Et. clin. Biol. **6**, 684-687 (1961).

MATHÉ, G., AMIEL, J.L., MATSUKURA, M., MÉRY, A.M.: Restauration hématopoïétique de souris irradiées par greffe de moelle osseuse allogénique de plusieurs donneurs de diverses lignées. C.R. Acad. Sci. (Paris) **255**, 3480-3482 (1962).

MATHÉ, G., AMIEL, J.L., SCHWARZENBERG, L., CATTAN, A., SCHNEIDER, M., DE VRIES, M.J., TUBIANA, M., LALANNE, C., BINET, J.L., PAPIERNIK, M., SEMAN, G., MATSUKURA, M., MÈRY, A.M., SCHWARZMAN, V., FLAISLER, A.: Successful allogenic bone marrow transplantation in man: Chi-merism, induced specific tolerance and possible antileukemic effects. Blood **25**, 179-196 (1965).

MATHÉ, G., AMIEL, J.L., SCHWARZENBERG, L., CHOAY, J., TROLARD, P., SCHNEIDER, M., HAYAT, M., SCHLUMBERGER, J.R., JASMIN, C.: Bone marrow graft in man after conditioning by antilym-phocytic serum. Brit. med. J. **1970 II**, 131-136.

MATHÉ, G., AMIEL, J.L., SCHWARZENBERG, L., SCHNEIDER, M., CATTAN, A., SCHLUMBERGER, J.R., NOUZA, K., HRASK, Y.: Bone marrow transplantation in man. Transplant. Proc. **1**, 16-24 (1969).

MATHÉ, G., BERNARD, J.: Essai de traitement, par l'irradiation X suivie de l'administration de cellules myéluïdes homologues, de souris AK atteintes de leucémie spontanée très avancée. Bull. Cancer **45**, 289-300 (1958).

MATHÉ, G., BERNARD, J.: Essais de traitement de la léucémie greffée 1210 par l'irradiation X suivie de transfusion de cellules hématopoïétiques normales (isologues ou homologuesm myé-loïdes ou lymphoïdes, adultes ou embryonnaires). Rev. franc. Et. clin. Biol. **4**, 442-446 (1959).

MATHÉ, G., JAMMET, H., PENDIČ, B., SCHWARZENBERG, L., DUPLAN, J.F., MAUPIN, B., LATARJET, R., LARRIEU, M.J., KALIČ, D., DJUKIČ, Z.: Transfusions et greffes de moelle osseuse homologue chez des humains irradiés á haute dose accidentellement. Rev. franc. Et. clin. Biol. **4**, 226-238 (1959).

MATHÉ, G., HARTMANN, L., LOVERDO, A., BERNARD, J.: Essai de protection par l'injection de cellules médulaires isologues ou homologues contre la mortalité produite par l'or radioactif. Rev. franc. Et. clin. Biol. **3**, 1086–1087 (1958).

MAZURENKO, N.P.: Induction of leucoses in mice with infectious viruses and the significance of the latter in the etiology of disease. Probl. Oncol. (N.Y.) **6**, 873–882 (1960).

MCBRIDE, R.A.: Graft-versus-host reaction in lymphoid proliferation. Cancer Res. **26**, 1135–1151 (1966).

MCCULLAGH, P.J.: The abrogation of immunological tolerance by means of allogeneic confrontation. Transplant. Rev. **12**, 180–197 (1972).

MCGREGOR, D.D.: Bone marrow origin of immunologically competent lymphocytes in the rat. J. exp. Med. **127**, 953–966 (1968).

MEDAWAR, P.B.: In: Ciba Foundation Study Group 16. (1963).

MEDZIHRADSKY, J.: Modification of tumor homograft immunity during the graft-versus-host reaction. Neoplasma (Bratisl.) **13**, 223 226 (1966).

MEDZIHRADSKY, J.: Suppression of the tumor transplannation immunity by the local graft-versus-host reaction. Neoplasma (Bratisl.) **14**, 369–375 (1967).

MERRITT, C.B., DARROW, C.C. II, VAAL, L., ROGENTINE, G.N. JR.: Bone marrow transplantation in rhesus monkeys following irradiation. Transplantation **14**, 9–20 (1972).

MEUWISSEN, H.J., GOOD, R.A.: Suppression of graft-versus-host reaction by mitomycin C. Nature (London) **215**, 634–635 (1967).

MEUWISSEN, H.J., KERSEY, J., PABST, H., GATTI, R., CHILGREN, R., GOOD, R.A.: Graft-versus-host reactions in bone marrow transplantation. Transplant. Proc. **3**, 414 417 (1971).

MEYER, H., HERON, I.: Regional lymph node response in rats to injection of semiallogeneic lymphocytes. Acta path. microbiol. scand. B **81**, 724–730 (1973).

MICHIE, D., WOODRUFF, M.F.A., ZEISS, J.M.: An investigation of immunological tolerance based on chimaera analysis. Immunology **4**, 413–424 (1961).

MILLER, J., PIERCE, J.C., MARTINEZ, C., GOOD, R.A.: An assay of graft-host interactions across strong and weak histocompatibility barriers in mice. J. exp. Med. **117**, 863 877 (1963).

MILLER, J.F.A.P., HOWARD, J.G.: Some dissimilarities between the neonatal thymectomy syndrome and graft-versus-host disease. J. reticuloendoth. Soc. **1**, 369–392 (1964).

MILLER, J.F.A.P., MITCHELL, G.F.: The thymus and the precursors of antigen reactive cells. Nature (London) **216**, 659–663 (1967).

MILLER, M.E.: Thymic dysplasia (Swiss agammaglobulinemia). I. Graft-versus-host reaction following bone marrow transfusion. J. Pediat. **70**, 730–736 (1967).

MILLER, M.E., HUMMELER, K.: Thymic dysplasia (Swiss agammaglobulinemia) II. Morphologic and functional observations. J. Pediat. **70**, 737–744 (1967).

MÖLLER, G.: Suppressive effect of graft-versus-host reaction on the immune response to heterologous red cells. Immunology **20**, 597–609 (1971).

MONIÉ, H.J., EVERETT, N.B.: The popliteal node assay for graft-versus-host interaction in mice. I. Location and proliferation of donor and host cells within the popliteal node. Anat. Rec. **179**, 19–25 (1974).

MORSE, H.C., ASOFSKY, R.: In vivo effects of antithymocyte serum on the homing pattern and graft-versus-host reactivity of murine splenic lymphocytes. Cell. Immunol. **11**, 19 29 (1974).

MUN, A.M., KOSIN, J.L., SATO, J.: Enhancement of growth of chick host spleens following chorioallantoic graft of homologous tissues. J. Embryol. exp. Morph. **7**, 512–521 (1959).

MURPHY, J.B.: The effect of adult chicken organ grafts on the chick embryo. J. exp. Med. **24**, 1–5 (1916).

NAIMAN, J.L., PUNNETT, H.H., LISCHNER, H.W., DESTINÈ, M.L., AREY, J.B.: Possible graft versus-host reaction after intrauterine transfusion for Rh erythroblastosis fetalis. New Engl. J. Med. **281**, 697–701 (1969).

NAKIČ, B., KAŠTELAN, A.: Quantitative analysis of chimaeric state in mice. I. Pattern of distribution of donor cells in lymphoid organs of hosts neonatally inoculated with isologous spleen cells. Immunology **12**, 609–614 (1967).

NAKIČ, B., KAŠTELAN, J., MIKUSKA, J., BUNAREVIČ, A.: Quantitative analysis if the chimaeric state in mice. II. Cytological examination of the proportion of proliferating donor and host cells in runt disease in mice. Immunology **12**, 615 627 (1967).

NAKIČ, B., TEPLITZ, R.L., OHNO, S.: Cytological analysis of parabiotic disease in mice. Transplantation **4**, 22–31 (1966).

Neefe, J.R. Jr., Merrit, C.B., Darrow, C.C, II, Rogentine, G.N. Jr.: Beneficial influence of limites histocompatibility of bone marrow grafted to unrelated rhesus monkeys preconditioned with X ray and ALS. Transplant. Proc. **6**, 125–128 (1974).

Nielsen, H.E.: Reactivity of lymphocytes from germfree rats in mixed leukocyte culture and in graft-versus-host reaction. J. exp. Med. **136**, 417–426 (1972).

Nisbet, N.W., Simonsen, M.: Primary immune response in grafted cells dissociation between proliferation of activity and proliferation of cells. J. exp. Med. **125**, 967–981 (1967).

Nowell, P.C., Cole, L.J.: Pathologic changes in old non-irradiated F_1 hybrid mice injected with parental strain spleen cells. Transplant. Bull. **6**, 435–437 (1959).

Nowell, P.C., Defendi, V.: Distribution of proliferating donor cells in runt disease in rats. Transplantation **2**, 375–382 (1964).

Okumura, K., Tada, T.: Regulation of homocytotropic antibody formation in the rat. IX. Further characterization of the antigen-specific inhibitory T cell factor in hapten-specific homocytotropic antibody response. J. Immunol. **112**, 783–791 (1974).

Oliner, H., Schwartz, R., Dameshek, W.: Studies in experimental autoimmune disorders. I. Clinical and laboratory features of autoimmunization (runt disease) in the mouse. Blood **17**, 20–44 (1961).

Ono, K., de Witt, C.W., Wallace, J.H., Lindsey, E.S.: Immunosuppressive activity of allogeneic antilymphocyte serum in the rat. Transplantation **7**, 122–131 (1969).

Oppltová, L., Démant, P.: Genetic determinants for the graft-versus-host reaction in the H-2 complex. Transplant. Proc. **5**, 1367–1371 (1973).

Ordal, J.C., Grumet, F.C.: Genetic control of the immune response. The effect of graft-versus-host reaction on the antibody response to Poly-L (Tyr, Glu)-Poly-D, L-Ala-Poly-L-Lys in non-responder mice. J. exp. Med. **136**, 1195–1206 (1972).

Ornellas, E.P., Sanfilippo, F., Scott, D.W.: Cellular events in tolerance. IV. The effect of a graft-versus-host reaction and endotoxin on hapten- and carrier-specific tolerance. Europ. J. Immunol. **4**, 587–591 (1974).

Osborne, D.P. Jr., Katz, D.H.: The allogeneic effect in inbred mice. III. Unique antigenic structural requirements in the expression of the phenomenon on unprimed cell populations in vivo. J. exp. Med. **137**, 991–1008 (1973a).

Osborne, D.P. Jr., Katz, D.H.: The allogeneic effect in inbred mice. IV. Regulatory influences of graft-versus-host reactions on host T lymphocyte functions. J. exp. Med. **138**, 825–838 (1973b).

Owen, J.J.T., Moore, M.A.S., Harrison, G.A.: Chromosome marker studies in the graft-versus-host reaction in the chick embryo. Nature (London) **207**, 313–315 (1965).

Owens, A.H. Jr., Santos, G.W.: The effect of cytotoxic drugs on graft-versus-host disease in mice. Transplantation **11**, 378–382 (1971).

Papadimitriou, J.M., Keast, D.: The electron microscopy of livers of mice runted as a result of the graft-versus-host reaction and bacterial endotoxin. Brit. J. exp. Path. **50**, 574–577 (1969).

Park, B.H., Good, R.A., Gate, J., Burke, R.: Fatel graft-versus-host reaction following transfusion of allogeneic blood and plasma in infants with combined immunodeficiency disease. Transplant. Proc. **6**, 385–387 (1974).

Parkman, R., Mosier, D., Umansky, I., Cochran, W., Carpenter, W., Rosen, F.S.: Graft-versus-host disease after intrauterine transfusion and exchange transfusions for hemolysis in newborns. New Engl. J. Med. **290**, 359–362 (1974).

Pick, E., Turk, J.L.: The biological activities of soluble lymphocyte products. Clin. exp. Immunol. **10**, 1–23 (1972).

Pinkett, M.O., Cowdrey, C.R., Nowell, P.C.: Mixed hematopoietic pulmonary origin of "alveolar macrophages" as demonstrated by chromosome markers. Amer. J. Path. **48**, 859–867 (1966).

Pirofsky, B., Davies, G.H., Ramirez-Mateos, J.C., Newton, B.W.: Cellular immune competence in the human fetus. Cell. Immunol. **6**, 324–328 (1973).

Pollard, M.: Spontaneous "secondary" disease in germfree AKR mice. Nature (London) **222**, 92–94 (1969).

Porter, K.A.: Use of foetal haematopoietic tissue to prevent late deaths in rabbit radiation chimaeras. Brit. J. exp. Pathol. **40**, 273–280 (1959).

Porter, K.A.: Graft-versus-host reactions in the rabbit. Brit. J. Cancer **14**, 66–76 (1960).

Potworowski, E.F., Zavallone, J.D., Gilker, J.C., Lamoureux, G.: Inhibition of the graft-versus-host reaction by thymus-specific antibodies. Rev. Eur. Et. clin. Biol. **16**, 155–157 (1971).

RADASZKIEWICZ, T., LENNERT, K.: Lymphogranulomatosis X. Dtsch. med. Wschr. **100**, 1157–1162 (1975).

RAMSEIER, H., BILLINGHAM, R.E.: Studies on delayed cutaneous inflammatory reactions elicited by inoculation of homologous cells into hamsters' skins. J. exp. Med. **123**, 629–656 (1966).

RAMSEIER, H., STREILEIN, J.W.: Homograft sensitivity reactions in irradiated hamsters. Lancet **1965 I**, 622 624.

RAO, V.S., BONAVIDA, B., ZIGHELBOIM, J., FAHEY, J.L.: Preferential induction of serum blocking activity and enhancement of skin allograft by soluble alloantigen. Transplantation **17**, 568–575 (1974).

REILLY, R.W., KIRSNER, J.B.: Runt intestinal disease. Lab. Invest. **14**, 102-107 (1965).

RICH, S.S., RICH, R.R.: Regulatory mechanism in cell-mediated immune responses. I. Regulation of mixed lymphocyte reactions by alloantigen-activated thymus-derived lymphocytes. J. exp. Med. **140**, 1588–1603 (1974).

RICHIE, E.R., GALLAGHER, T.M., TRENTIN, J.J.: Prevention of graft-versus-host disease by Fab fragments derived from ALG. Transplant. Proc. **5**, 873–876 (1973a).

RICHIE, E.R., GALLAGHER, M.T., TRENTIN, J.J.: Inhibition of the graft-versus-host reaction. II. Prevention of acute graft-versus-host mortality by Fab fragments of antilymphocyte globulin. Transplantation **15**, 486–491 (1973b).

RICHIE, E.R., MONIÉ, H.J., TRENTIN, J.J., TAUB, R.N.: Inhibition of the graft-versus-host reaction. III. Altered in vivo distribution of spleen cells pretreated with FAB fragments of antithymocyte globulin. Transplantation **19**, 115–121 (1975).

RIEKE, W.O.: Lymphocytes from thymectomized rats: Immunologic, proliferative, and metabolic properties. Science **152**, 535–538 (1966).

RIETHMÜLLER, G., RIEBER, E.P., SEEGER, I.: Suppression of graft-versus-host reaction by univalent antiimmunoglobulin antibody. Nature New Biology (London) **230**, 248-250 (1971).

ROLSTAD, B., FORD, W.L.: Immune responses of rats deficient in thymus-derived lymphocytes to strong transplantation antigens (Ag-B). Transplantation **17**, 405–415 (1974).

ROUSE, B.T., WARNER, N.L.: Suppression of graft-versus-host reactions in chickens by pretreatment of leukocytes with anti-light chain sera. Cell. Immunol. **3**, 470–477 (1972).

RUBINSTEIN, J.R., COTTIER, H., ROSSI, E., GUGLER, E.: Unusual combined immunodeficiency syndrome exhibiting kappa-IgD paraproteinemia, residual gut immunity and graft-versus-host reaction after plasma infusion. Acta paediat. scand. **62**, 365-372 (1973).

RUDOLPH, R.H., FEFER, A., THOMAS, E.D., BUCKNER, C.D., CLIFT, R.A., STORB, R.: Isogeneic marrow grafts for hematologic malignancy in man. Arch. intern. Med. **132**, 285–297 (1973).

RUSSEL, P.S.: The weight-gain assay for runt disease in mice. Ann. N.Y. Acad. Sci. **87**, 445 456 (1960).

RUSSEL, P.S.: In: Ciba Foundation Symposium on Transplantation. London: Churchill 1962.

SAFFORD, J.W., TOKUDA, S.: Suppression of the graft-versus-host reaction by passive immunization of donor against recipient antigens. Proc. Soc. exp. Biol. Med. **133**, 651–654 (1970).

SALAMAN, M.H., WEDDERBURN, N., FESTENSTEIN, H., HUBER, B.: Detection of a graft-versus-host reaction between mice compatible at the H-2 locus. Transplantation **16**, 29–31 (1973).

SALMON, S.E., SMITH, B.A., LEHRER, R.I., MOGERMAN, S.N., SHINEFIELD, H.R., PERKINS, H.A.: Modification of donor lymphocytes for transplantation in lymphopenic immunological deficiency. Lancet **1970 II**, 149 150.

SANTOS, G.W., SENSENBRENNER, L.L., BURKE, P.J., COLVIN, M., OWENS, A.H. JR., BIAS, W.B., SLAVIN, R.E.: Marrow transplantation in man following cyclophosphamide. Transplant. Proc. **3**, 400–404 (1971).

SAURAT, J.H., DIDIER-JEAN, L., GLUCKMAN, E., BUSSEL, A.: Graft-versus-host reaction and lichen planus-like eruption in man. Brit. J. Derm. **92**, 591–592 (1975).

SCHABEL, S.I.: Graft-versus-host atherosclerosis. Lancet **1975 I**, 396.

SCHÄFER, K.H.: Nierenerkrankungen nach Erstimpfung gegen Pocken. Mschr. Kinderheilk. **111**, 361 368 (1963).

SCHLIPKÖTER, H.W., BROCKHAUS, A.: Die Hemmung der experimentellen Silikose durch subcutane Verabreichung von Polyvinylpyridin-N-Oxyd. Klin. Wschr. **39**, 1182-1189 (1961).

SCHRÖDER, J., DE LA CHAPELLE, A.: Fetal lymphocytes in the maternal blood. Blood **39**, 153–162 (1972).

Schwartz, R.S., André-Schwartz, J., Armstrong, M.Y.K., Beldotti, L.: Neoplastic sequelae of allogenic disease. I. Theoretical considerations and experimental design. Ann. N.Y. Acad. Sci. **129**, 804–821 (1966).

Schwartz, R.S., Beldotti, L.: The treatment of chronic murine homologous disease: A comparative study of four "immunosuppressive agents". Transplantation **3**, 79–97 (1965a).

Schwartz, R.S., Beldotti, L.: Malignant lymphomas following allogenic disease: Transition from am immunological to a neoplastic disorder. Science **149**, 1511–1514 (1965b).

Schwarz, J.A.: Die Entwicklung des Immunsystems. Klin. Wschr. **52**, 857–870 (1974).

Scott, D.W., Ornellas, E.P.: Allogeneic interactions in the immune response and tolerance. II. Mechanism of stimulation of TNP plaque-forming cells in normal rats. Cell. Immunol. **11**, 116–121 (1974).

Shapiro, M.: Familial autohemolytic anemia and runting syndrome with Rh-0-specific autoantibody. Transfusion **7**, 281 296 (1967).

Shortman, K., Brunner, K.T., Cerottini, J.C.: Separation of stages in the development of the "T" cells involved in cell-mediated immunity. J. exp. Med. **135**, 1375–1391 (1972).

Sidky, Y.A., Auerbach, R.: Lymphocyte-induced angiogenesis: A quantitative and sensitive assay of the graft-versus-host reaction. J. exp. Med. **141**, 1084–1100 (1975).

Sieber, O., Fulginiti, V., Durie, B., Salmon, S.: Successful immunological reconstitution in severe combined immunodeficiency disease with transplantation from a non-compatible donor. Clin. Res. **22**, 230 (1974).

Silobrčić, V., Trentin, J.J.: On the mechanism of "homologous disease" in sublethally irradiated mice. Transplantation **4**, 719–731 (1966).

Simonsen, M.: Biological incompatibility in kidney transplantation in dogs. Acta path. microbiol. scand. **32**, 1–35 (1953).

Simonsen, M.: The impact on the developing embryo and animal of adult homologous cells. Acta path. microbiol. scand. **40**, 480–500 (1957).

Simonsen, M.: Graft-versus-host reactions. Their natural history, and applicability as tools of research. Progr. Allergy **6**, 349 467 (1962).

Simonsen, M., Engelbreth-Holm, J., Jensen, E., Poulsen, H.: A study of the graft-versus-host reaction in transplantation to embryos, F_1 hybrids, and irradiated animals. Ann. N.Y. Acad. Sci. **73**, 834–841 (1958).

Simonsen, M., Jensen, E.: The graft-versus-host assay in transplantation chimaeras. In: Biological Problems of Grafting, p. 214–238. Oxford: Blackwell 1959.

Singh, J.N., Sabbadini, E., Sehon, A.H.: Cytotoxicity in graft-versus-host reaction. I. Role of donor and host spleen cells. J. exp. Med. **136**, 39–48 (1972).

Singh, J.N., Sabbadini, E., Sehon, A.H.: Detection of nonspecific cytotoxicity in graft-versus-host reaction as a function of target cell type. Cell. Immunol. **8**, 280–289 (1973).

Siskind, G., Leonard, L., Thomas, L.: The runting syndrome. Ann. N.Y. Acad. Sci. **87**, 452–456 (1960).

Siskind, G.W., Thomas, L.: Studies on the runting syndrome in newborn mice. In: Biological Problems of Grafting, p. 176–192. Oxford: Blackwell 1959.

Slavin, R.E., Santos, G.W.: The graft-versus-host reaction in man after bone marrow transplantation: Pathology, pathogenesis, clinical features, and implication. Clin. Immunol. Immunopath. **1**, 472–498 (1973).

Smitananda, N., Nelson, D.S., McRae, J.: Erythropoiesis in mice with graft-versus-host reactions: Effects of cells from various tissues on erythropoiesis and other measures of graft-versus-host reaction. Pathology (Sydney) **4**, 35–46 (1972).

Solomon, J.B., Tucker, D.F.: Influence of age of the chick embryo host on the splenomegaly syndrome in the graft-versus-host reaction. Exp. Cell. Res. **25**, 460–462 (1962).

Speck, B.: Bone marrow transplantation clinical results and problems. Blut **27**, 297–302 (1973).

Speck, B.: Knochenmarkstransplantation bei Leukämie: Möglichkeiten, Probleme. Schweiz. med. Wschr. **105**, 1286–1289 (1975).

Speck, B., Dooren, L.J., de Koning, J., van Bekkum, D.W., Eernisse, J.G., Elkerbout, F., Vossen, J.M., van Rood, J.J.: Clinical experience with bone marrow transplantation: Failure and success. Transplant. Proc. **3**, 409 413 (1971).

Speck, B., Zwann, F.E., van Rood, J.J., Eernisse, J.G.: Allogeneic bone marrow transplantation in a patient with aplastic anemia using a phenotypically HL-A-identical unrelated donor. Transplantation **16**, 24–28 (1973).

SPRENT, J.: Circulating T and B lymphocytes of the mouse. I. Migratory properties. Cell. Immunol. **7**, 10–39 (1973).

SPRENT, J., BASTEN, A.: Circulating T and B lymphocytes of the mouse. II Lifespan. Cell. Immunol. **7**, 40–59 (1973).

SPRENT, J., MILLER, J.F.A.P.: Interaction of thymus lymphocytes with histoincompatible cell. I. Quantitation of the proliferative response of thymus cells. Cell. Immunol. **3**, 361-384 (1972a).

SPRENT, J., MILLER, J.F.A.P.: Interaction of thymus lymphocytes with histoincompatible cells. II. Recirculating lymphocytes derived from antigen-activated thymus cells. Cell. Immunol. **3**, 385–404 (1972b).

STASTNY, P., STEMBRIDGE, V.A., VISCHER, T., ZIFF, M.: Homologous disease in the adult rat, a model for autoimmune disease. II. Findings in the joints, heart and other tissues. J. exp. Med. **122**, 681-692 (1965).

STASTNY, P., STEMBRIDGE, V.A., ZIFF, M.: Homologous disease in the adult rat, a model for autoimmune disease. I. General features and cutaneous lesions. J. exp. Med. **118**, 635–648 (1963).

STORB, R., EVANS, R.S., THOMAS, E.D., BUCKNER, C.D., CLIFT, R.A., FEFER, A., NEIMAN, P., WRIGHT, S.E.: Paroxysmal nocturnal haemoglobinuria and refractory marrow failure treated by marrow transplantation. Brit. J. Haemat. **24**, 743–750 (1973a).

STORB, R., GLUCKMAN, E., THOMAS, E.D., BUCKNER, C.D., CLIFT, R.A., FEFER, A., GLUCKSBERG, H., GRAHAM, T.C., JOHNSON,,F.L., LERNER, K.G., NEIMAN, P., OCHS, H.: Treatment of established human graft-versus-host disease by antithymocyte globulin. Blood. **44**, 57–76 (1974b).

STORB, R., KOLB, H.J., GRAHAM, T.C., KOLB, H., WEIDEN, P.L., THOMAS, E.D.: Treatment of established graft-versus-host disease in dogs by antithymocyte serum or Prednisone. Blood **42**, 601–609 (1973b).

STORB, R., THOMAS, E.D., BUCKNER, C.D., CLIFT, R.A., JOHNSON, F.L., FEFER, A., GLUCKSBERG, E.R., GIBLETT, E.R., LERNER, K.G., NEIMAN, P.: Allogeneic marrow grafting for treatment of aplastic anemia. Blood **43**, 157–180 (1974a).

STREILEIN, J.W.: A common pathogenesis for the lesions of graft-versus-host disease. Transplant. Proc. **3**, 418–421 (1971a).

STREILEIN, J.W.: In: Immunology and the Skin (Ed. W. MONTAGNA, R.E. BILLINGHAM). New York: Appleton 1971b.

STREILEIN, J.W.: Analysis of graft-versus-host disease in Syrian hamsters. IV. The refractory state and immunologic competence. J. exp. Med. **135**, 567–587 (1972a).

STREILEIN, J.W.: In: Cancer Chemotherapy II, the 22nd Hahnemann Symposium (Eds. I. BRODSKY, S.B. KAHN, J.H. MOYER). New York: Grune & Stratton 1972b.

STREILEIN, J.W.: Pathologic lesions of graft-versus-host disease in hamsters: Antigenic target versus "innocent bystander". Progr. exp. Tumor Res. (Basel) **16**, 396–408 (1972c).

STREILEIN, J.W., BILLINGHAM, R.E.: Cutaneous hypersensitivity reactions to cellular isoantigens in rats. J. exp. Med. **126**, 455–473 (1967).

STREILEIN, J.W., BILLINGHAM, R.E.: An analysis of graft-versus-host disease in syrian hamsters. I. The epidermolytic syndrome: Description and studies on its procurement. J. exp. Med. **132**, 163–180 (1970a).

STREILEIN, J.W., BILLINGHAM, R.E.: An analysis of graft-versus-host disease in syrian hamsters. II. The epidermolytic syndrome: Studies on its pathogenesis. J. exp. Med. **132**, 181–197 (1970b).

STREILEIN, J.W., STREILEIN, J.: An analysis of graft-versus-host disease in Syrian hamsters. III. Hematological manifestations: Description and studies in pathogenesis. Transplantation **13**, 378–390 (1972).

STREILEIN, J.W., STONE, M.J.: Graft-versus-host disease: Unmasking of forbidden clones. Transplant. Proc. **5**, 861 865 (1973).

SWINGLE, K.F., GRANT, T.J., VALLE, P.M.: Effect of immunosuppressive drugs on a localized graft-versus-host reaction in the rat. Proc. Soc. exp. Biol. (N.Y.) **142**, 1329–1331 (1973).

SZENBERG, A., WARNER, N.L.: Large lymphocytes and the Simonsen phenomenon. Nature (London) **191**, 920 (1961).

SZENBERG, A., WARNER, N.L.: Quantitative aspects of the Simonsen phenomenon. I. The role of the large lymphocyte. Brit. J. exp. Path. **43**, 123–128 (1962).

TERASAKI, P.I.: Identification of the type of blood-cell responsible for the graft-versus-host reaction in chicks. J. Embryol. exp. Morph. **7**, 394–408 (1959).

Thomas, E.D.: In: Clinical Immunobiology (Ed. F.H. Bach, R.A. Good), Vol. 2. New York: Academic Press 1974.

Thomas, E.D., Ashley, C.A., Lochte, H.L., Jaretzki, A., Sahler, O.D., Ferrebee, J.W.: Homografts of bone marrow in dogs after lethal total-body irradiation. Blood 14, 720-736 (1959).

Thomas, E.D., Epstein, R.B.: Bone marrow transplantation in acute leukemia. Cancer Res. 25, 1521-1524 (1965).

Thomas, E.D., Rudolph, R.H., Fefer, A., Storb, R., Slichter, S., Buckner, C.D.: Isogeneic marrow grafting in man. Exp. Hematol. 21, 16–18 (1971).

Thomas, E.D., Storb, R., Clift, R.A., Fefer, A., Johnson, L., Neiman, P.E., Lerner, K.G., Gluckberg, H., Buckner, C.D.: Bone marrow transplantation II. New Engl. J. Med. 292, 895-902 (1975).

Thompson, J.S., Simmons, E.L., Hofstra, D.: Studies on the immunologic unresponsiveness during the secondary disease period of lethally irradiated mice protected by homologous bone marrow. J. Immunol. 89, 62–71 (1962).

Tigelaar, R.E., Asofsky, R.: Graft-versus-host reactivity of mouse thymocytes: Effect of cortisone pretreatment of donors. J. Immunol. 110, 567–574 (1973).

Tigelaar, R.E., Gershon, R.K., Asofsky, R.: Graft-versus-host reactivity of mouse thymocytes: Effect of in vitro treatment with anti-TL serum. Cell. Immunol. 19, 58–64 (1975).

Tittor, W., Gerbase-Delima, M., Walford, R.L.: Synergy among responding lymphoid cells in the one-way mixed lymphocyte reaction. J. exp. Med. 139, 1488–1498 (1974).

Tittor, W., Walford, R.L.: Synergistic response between thymus and lymph node cells in the mixed lymphocyte culture. Nature (London) 247, 371-375 (1974).

Treiber, W., Lapp, W.S.: Graft-versus-host-induced immunosuppression. Transplantation 16, 211-216 (1973).

Trenkner, E.: The use of allogeneic T lymphocytes and bacterial lipopolysaccharide to induce immune responses to monovalent haptens in vitro. J. Immunol. 113, 918-924 (1974).

Trentin, J.J.: Mortality and skin transplantability in X-irradiated mice receiving isologous, homologous or heterologous bone marrow. Proc. Soc. exp. Biol. (N.Y.) 92, 688-693 (1956).

Trentin, J.J., Judd, K.P.: Prevention of acute graft-versus-host (GVH) mortality with spleen-absorbed antithymocyte globulin (ATG). Transplant. Proc. 5, 865–869 (1973).

Twist, V.W., Barnes, R.D.: Popliteal lymph node weight gain assay for graft-versus-host reactivity in mice. Transplantation 15, 182–185 (1973).

Tyan, M.: Modification of severe GVH disease with antisera to the θ antigen or to whole serum. Transplantation 15, 601-604 (1973).

Tyan, M.L.: Graft-versus-host disease, modification with concanavalin A. Transplantation 18, 305–312 (1974).

Tyan, M.L.: Modification of graft-versus-host disease with Con A and preimmunization. Proc. Soc. exp. Biol. (N.Y.) 150, 628–629 (1975).

Uphoff, D.E.: Alteration of homograft reaction by A-methopterin in lethally irradiated mice treated with homologous marrow. Proc. Soc. exp. Biol. (N.Y.) 99, 651 653 (1958).

Uphoff, D.E.: Immunologic competence of bone marrow of different genotypes. J. nat. Cancer Inst. 43, 1055-1066 (1969).

Uphoff, D.E., Law, L.W.: Genetic factors influencing irradiation protection by bone marrow. II. The histocompatibility 1 (H-2) locus. J. nat. Cancer Inst. 20, 617-624 (1958).

Virolainen, M.: Hematopoietic origin of macrophages as studied by chromosome markers in mice. J. exp. Med. 127, 943–952 (1968).

Voisin, G.A., Kinsky, R., Maillard, J.: Protection against homologous disease in hybrid mice by passive and active immunological enhancement facilitation. Transplantation 6, 187–202 (1968).

Volkman, A.: The host cell response in the local graft-versus-host reaction induced in the kidneys of F_1 rats by parental thoracic duct lymphocytes. J. exp. Med. 136, 21–38 (1972).

Vos, O., de Vries, M.J., Collenreur, J.C., van Bekkum, D.W.: Transplantation of homologous and heterologous lymphoid cells in X-irradiated and non-irradiated mice. J. nat. Cancer Inst. 23, 59–73 (1959).

De Vries, M.J., Crouch, B.D., van Putten, L.M., van Bekkum, D.W.: Pathologic changes in irradiated monkeys treated with bone marrow. J. nat. Cancer Inst. 27, 67-97 (1961).

De Vries, M.J., Vos, O.: Treatment of mouse lymphosarcoma by total-body X-irradiation and by injection of bone marrow and lymph node cells. J. nat. Cancer Inst. 21, 1117–1129 (1958).

DE VRIES, M.J., VOS, O.: Delayed mortality of radiation chimaeras. A pathological and hematological study. J. nat. Cancer Inst. **23**, 1403 1439 (1959).

VRUBEL, J.: Survival of cutaneous homografts after transplantation of lymph nodes immunized against the host. Nature (London) **189**, 853 854 (1961).

WAGNER, H., ROLLINGHOFF, M., SHORTMAN, K.: In: Proc. IInd Internat. Congr. of Immunology, (Ed. L. BRENT, J. HOBROW). Vol. 3. Amsterdam: North-Holland Publ. 1974.

WALKER, K.Z., SCHOEFL, G.I., LAFFERTY, K.J.: The pathogenesis of the graft-versus-host reaction in chicken embryos. Pathological changes in the yolk sac, thymus, bone marrow and bursa of Fabricius. Aust. J. exp. Biol. med. Sci. **50**, 675 689 (1972).

WALKER, K.Z., LAFFERTY, K.J., SCHOEFL, G.I.: Pathogenesis in the graft-versus-host reaction in chicken embryos. Requirement of yolk sac-derived stem cells for the development of proliferative lesions. Aust. J. exp. Biol. med. Sci. **51**, 347 355 (1973a).

WALKER, K.Z., SCHOEFL, G.I., LAFFERTY, K.J., ADAMS, E.P.: Pathogenesis of the graft-versus-host reaction in chicken embryos. The development of hemorrhagic lesions. Aust. J. exp. Biol. med. Sci. **51**, 93–107 (1973b).

WALTERS, M.N.I.: Pancreatitis induced by the graft-versus-host reaction. J. Path. Bact. **91**, 65–69 (1966).

WARNER, N.L., SZENBERG, A.: Quantitative aspects of the Simonsen phenomenon. IV. Effect of immunisation to minor antigenic determinants. Aust. J. exp. Biol. med. Sci. **42**, 100- 108 (1964).

WEISS, L., AISENBERG, A.C.: An electron microscope study of lymphatic tissue in runt disease. J. Cell Biol. **25**, 149–177 (1965).

WILSON, D.B., BILLINGHAM, R.E.: Lymphocytes and transplantation immunity. Advanc. Immunol. **7**, 189–273 (1967).

WILSON, D.B., FOX, D.H.: Quantitative studies on the mixed lymphocyte interaction in rats. VI. Reactivity of lymphocytes from conventional and germfree rats to allogenetic and xenogenetic cell surface antigens. J. exp. Med. **134**, 857–870 (1971).

WILSON, D.B., NOWELL, P.C.: Quantitative studies on the mixed lymphocyte interaction in rats. IV. Immunologic potentiality of the responding cells. J. exp. Med. **131**, 391–407 (1970).

WILSON, D.B., NOWELL, P.C.: Quantitative studies on the mixed lymphocyte interaction in rats. V. Tempo and specificity of the proliferative response and the number of reactive cells from immunized donors. J. exp. Med. **133**, 442–453 (1971).

WILSON, D.B., SILVERS, W.K., NOWELL, P.C.: Quantitative studies on the mixed lymphocyte interaction in rats. II. Relationship of the proliferative response to the immunologic status of the donors. J. exp. Med. **126**, 655–665 (1967).

WITTING, C., DETLEFSEN, W.: Zur Korrelation von Splenomegalie und Blutbildveränderungen bei der Graft-versus-Host Reaktion der Maus. Blut **31**, 229 238 (1975).

WOODRUFF, J.J.: Role of lymphocyte surface determinants in lymph node homing. Cell. Immunol. **13**, 378–384 (1974).

WOODRUFF, J.M., BUTCHER, W.I., HELLERSTEIN, L.J.: Early secondary disease in the Rhesus monkey. II. Electron microscopy of changes in mucous membranes and external epithelia as demonstrated in the tongue and lip. Lab. Invest. **27**, 85–98 (1972).

WOODRUFF, J.M., ELTRINGHAM, R.J., CASEY, H.W.: Early secondary disease in the Rhesus monkey. I. A comparative histopathologic study. Lab. Invest. **20**, 499–511 (1969).

ZAKARIAN, S., BILLINGHAM, R.E.: Studies on normal and immune lymphocyte transfer reactions in guinea pigs, with special reference to the cellular contribution of the host. J. exp. Med. **136**, 1545–1563 (1972).

ZALESKI, M.: Effect of graft-versus-host reaction on the immune response to alloantigens and growth of a syngeneic tumor. Exp. Hematol. **3**, 12–21 (1975).

ZALESKI, M., MILGROM, F.: Immunosuppressive effect of graft-versus-host reaction. Cell. Immunol. **7**, 268–274 (1973).

ZEISS, J.M., FOX, M.: Donor and host contribution to splenomegaly in homologous mouse chimaeras. Nature (London) **197**, 673–675 (1963).

Author Index

Page numbers in *italics* refer to the bibliography

Subject Index

Notes on use of subject index

Main entries are alphabetized on the sequence of letters regardless of space and hyphens which may occur between them, e.g.

blast cell-derived
blast cells
blast cell transformation
blastogenesis

^{51}-Cr-labeled markers
cross immunization
crossing over
cross-match,

and regardless of diacritical letters for characterization of (bio) chemical compounds, e.g.

ASCHER's tectonic keratoplasty
L-asparaginase
assortment

glioma
α-globulin
glomerulonephritis

An exception are compound entries in which individual elements − prefixes and letters − are essential to characterize the whole term. They are alphabetized in that order

antibodies
antibody
antiglobulin
anti-HL-A

H-2 antigens
hard bone substance
H-2 complex

banking of organs
B-cells, lymphocytes
B-cell-T-cell cooperation
beating-heart donor

HL-A antigens
^{3}H-labeled cell markers
HL-A disparity
H-2 ← β 2 m junction

On principle subentries of first and second orders are alphabetized under the main entries, except for conjunctions and prepositions − after, and, as, by, in, of, on, secondary (sec.) to − which may precede subentries to indicate a more detailed relation with the main entry, e.g.

B-cells
— and allotypic determinants
— antiidiotype AB reaction
— in bone marrow
— as killer cells

cornea allografts
— rejection
— — plasma cells
— — and size of graft
— — of stroma
— — treatment

Generally, one hyphen — represents the preceding main entry, two hyphens   refer to the main entry and the preceding subentry. A hyphen between brackets (—) stands for the first word of the preceding phrase, e.g.

delayed type hypersensitivity reaction
— suppression by ALS
— (—) by L-asparaginase

A large number of terms is cross referenced by interchanging main and subentries, e.g.

GVH disease, reaction
— and imm. tolerance
— lymphocytopenia

immunologic tolerance
— and GVHD/R
lymphocytopenia
  – in GVHD/R

Since numerous phrases and subentries serve as collecting terms, they may occur without reference to page numbers. In these instances only subentries of first or second order refer to page numbers, e.g.

kidney allotransplantation
— acute rejection 528, 529
— — blast cell transformation 522
— chronic glomerulopathy
— — and anomalous glomerular AG 553, 554

The multiplicity of terminology necessitated frequently to refer to synonymic terms, if a phrase is unmistakable, and headed only once, e.g.

antilymphocyte serum, see ALS
humoral antibody, see circulating antibody

In other instances reference is made to synonymic terms which also appear as main entries in the index, e.g.

cytotoxic cells, see also cell-mediated cytotoxicity
cell-mediated lymphocytolysis; cytolytic T-cells
cytotoxic lymphocytes, macrophages; cytotoxic T-cells.

No cross references are given for terms differing only slightly and according to the official terminology, e.g.

lymphocytopenia, lymphopenia.

To avoid the excessive extension of phrases because of prevalent multiplicity of terminology, a number of entries appear under compound terms, e.g.

B-cells, lymphocytes
cell-mediated cytotoxicity, immunity
cell-mediated immune reaction, response
GVH disease, reaction

It appeared disadvantageous, however, to pool certain eponymic and synonymic phrases, e.g.

cytotoxic T-cells
T-cell cytotoxicity

circulating antibodies
humoral factors

because of differences in interpretation and to avoid that the desired term is undiscoverable at the place referred to.

Several main entries appear as abbreviation e.g.

ALS (antilymphocyte serum)
MHC/S (major histocompatibility complex, system)

In the case of a less familiar or less frequently used abbreviation, it is cross-referred to the phrase written in full, e.g.

CMC, see cell-mediated cytotoxicity
CML, see cell-mediated lympholysis

If a desired phrase is not listed under one term, it is advisable to seek under an alternative heading or to look in more than one place. This not only holds true for interchangeable expressions like cardiac — heart, hepatic — liver, or renal — kidney, but also for e.g. activity, reactivity, reaction, and numerous other terms.

Surnames as main entries are capitalized.

Page numbers in *italics* indicate figures or tables.

                                         C. Jerusalem, Nijmegen

1008

Handbuch der allgemeinen Pathologie

Herausgeber / Editors:

H.W. Altmann
F. Büchner
H. Cottier
E. Grundmann
G. Holle
E. Letterer
W. Masshoff
H. Meessen
F. Roulet
G. Seifert
G. Siebert

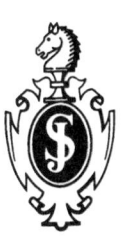

Springer-Verlag
Berlin
Heidelberg
NewYork

1. Band:
Prolegomena einer allgemeinen Pathologie
36 Abbildungen, X, 311 Seiten. 1969
Geb. DM 180,—; US $ 79,20
Subskriptionspreis:
Geb. DM 144,—; US $ 63.40
ISBN 3-540-04515-5

2. Band:
Die Zelle
1. Teil: Das Cytoplasma
246 Abbildungen, XII, 735 Seiten. 1955
Geb. DM 340,—; US $ 149.60
Subskriptionspreis:
Geb. DM 272,—; US $ 119.70
ISBN 3-540-01904-9

2. Teil: Der Zellkern I
335 Abbildungen, XI, 765 Seiten. 1971
Geb. DM 480,—; US $ 211.20
Subskriptionspreis:
Geb. DM 384,—; US $ 169.00
ISBN 3-540-05128-7

3./4. Teil: Der Zellkern II
In Vorbereitung

5. Teil: Stoffwechsel und Feinstruktur der Zelle I
191 Abbildungen, XIV, 799 Seiten. 1968
Geb. DM 530,—; US $ 233.20
Subskriptionspreis:
Geb. DM 424,—; US $ 186.60
ISBN 3-540-04145-1

3. Band:
Zwischensubstanzen, Gewebe, Organe
1. Teil: Gewebe und mesenchymale Substanzen
In Vorbereitung

2.-5. Teil: Die Organe

2. Teil: Blut. Verdauungstrakt und große Drüsen. Musculosceletal System. Genitaltrakt. Haut
220 Abbildungen, zum Teil farbig, XII, 733 Seiten (126 in Englisch). 1960
Geb. DM 400,—; US $ 176.00
Subskriptionspreis:
Geb. DM 320,—; US $ 140.80
ISBN 3-540-02531-6

3. Teil: Allgemeine morphologische Pathologie des Nervengewebes. Die Struktur des zentralen und peripheren Nervensystems als Grundlage seiner Funktion und seiner Erkrankungen. 307 Abbildungen, zum Teil farbig, VIII, 526 Seiten. 1968
Geb. DM 400,—; US $ 176.00
Subskriptionspreis:
Geb. DM 320,—; US $ 140.80
ISBN 3-540-04146-X

4.Teil: Atmungsorgane, Allgemeine Pathologie der Organe des Kreislaufs
327 Abbildungen, zum Teil farbig. VIII, 821 Seiten, 1970
Geb. DM 490,—; US $ 215.60
Subskriptionspreis:
Geb. DM 392,—; US $ 172.50
ISBN 3-540-04844-8

5. Teil: Die Niere
In Vorbereitung

6. Teil: Lymphgefäßsystem/ Lymph Vessel System
272 Abbildungen, XIV, 708 Seiten (216 in englisch). 1972
Geb. DM 460,—; US $ 202.40
Subskriptionspreis:
Geb. DM 368,—; US $ 162.00
ISBN 3-540-05662-9

7. Teil: Mikrozirkulation/Microcirkulation
Etwa 260 Abbildungen. Etwa 1090 Seiten (Etwa 360 Seiten in Englisch). 1977
Geb. DM 560,—; US $ 246.40
Subskriptionspreis:
Geb. DM 448,—; US $ 197.20
ISBN 3-540-07750-2

4. Band:
Der Stoffwechsel
1. Teil: Der Stoffwechsel I
In Vorbereitung

2. Teil: Der Stoffwechsel II
177 Abbildungen, XII, 861 Seiten. 1957
Geb. DM 340,—; US $ 149.60
Subskriptionspreis:
Geb. DM 272,—; US $ 119.70
ISBN 3-540-02155-8

5. Band:
Hilfsmechanismen des Stoffwechsels
1.Teil: Hilfsmechanismen des Stoffwechsels I: Das digestive

System. Verdauung und Resorption. Stofftransport. Atmung. Kreislauffunktion. Blutkreislauf
326 Abbildungen, zum Teil farbig. XVI, 1065 Seiten (65 in Englisch). 1961
Geb. DM 540,—; US $ 237.60
Subskriptionspreis:
Geb. DM 432,—; US $ 190.10
ISBN 3-540-02682-7

2. Teil: Hilfsmechanismen des Stoffwechsels II: Nierenausscheidung, Gallenblase und Gallenwege. Colonresektion. Ausscheidung der Leber. Ausscheidung des Colon. Ausscheidung durch die Lunge. Ausscheidung der Haut
164 Abbildungen, zum Teil farbig. XII, 689 Seiten. 1959
Geb. DM 320,—; US $ 140.80
Subskriptionspreis:
Geb. DM 256,—; US $ 112.70
ISBN 3-540-02400-X

6. Band:
Entwicklung, Wachstum, Geschwülste
1. Teil: Entwicklung, Wachstum I: Embryonale Entwicklung. Teratologie. Biologie und Biochemie des Wachstums. Regeneration
233 Abbildungen, X, 542 Seiten 1955
Geb. DM 230,—; US $ 101.20
Subskriptionspreis:
Geb. DM 184,—; US $ 81.00
ISBN 3-540-01905-7

2. Teil: Entwicklung, Wachstum II: Regernation, Hyperplasie, Cancerisierung
314 Abbildungen, XIV, 833 Seiten. 1969
Geb. DM 490,—; US $ 215.60
Subskriptionspreis:
Geb. DM 392,—; US $ 172.50
ISBN 3-540-04516-3

3. Teil: Geschwülste
98 Abbildungen, VIII, 493 Seiten. 1956
Geb. DM 230,—; US $ 101.20
Subskriptionspreis:
Geb. DM 184,—; US $ 81.00
ISBN 3-540-02020-9

4. Teil: Altern
183 Abbildungen, XIX, 745 Seiten. 1972
Geb. DM 440,—; US $ 193.60
Subskriptionspreis:
Geb. DM 352,—; US $ 154.90
ISBN 3-540-05555-X

5. Teil: Tumors/Geschwülste I: Morphology, Epidemiology, Immunology
Morphologie, Epidemiologie, Immunologie
201 figs., XX, 858 pages (309 in German). 1974
Cloth DM 445,—; US $ 195.80
Subscription price:
Cloth DM 356,—; US $ 156.70
ISBN 3-540-06813-9

6. Teil: Geschwülste/Tumors II: Virale und chemische Carcinogenese
Viral and chemical Carcinogenesis
129 Abbildungen, XVI, 908 Seiten (375 in Englisch). 1975
Geb. DM 460,—; US $ 202.40
Subskriptionspreis:
Geb. DM 368,—; US $ 162.00
ISBN 3-540-06820-1

7. Teil: Geschwülste/Tumors III: Modelle experimenteller Carcinogenese
Models of experimental Carcinogenesis
345 Abbildungen, XVII, 1200 Seiten (256 in Englisch). 1975
Geb. DM 580,—; US $ 255.20
Subskriptionspreis:
Geb. DM 464,—; US $ 204.20
ISBN 3-540-07034-6

7. Band:
Reaktionen
1. Teil: Entzündung und Immunität
164 Abbildungen, X, 742 Seiten 1956
Geb. DM 340,—; US $ 149.60
Subskriptionspreis:
Geb. DM 272,—; US $ 119.70
ISBN 3-540-02021-7

2. Teil: Überempfindlichkeit und Immunität
179 Abbildungen, VIII, 469 Seiten (63 in Englisch). 1967
Geb. DM 380,—; US $ 167.20
Subskriptionspreis:
Geb. DM 304,—; US $ 133.80
ISBN 3-540-03836-1

3. Teil: Immunoreaktionen.
Immune Reactions
129 Abbildungen, XIV, 557 Seiten (219 in Englisch). 1970
Geb. DM 380,—; US $ 167.20
Subskriptionspreis:
Geb. DM 304,—; US $ 133.80
ISBN 3-540-05129-5

8. Band:
Regulationen
1. Teil: Endokrine Regulationsund Korrelationsstörungen
148 Abbildungen, XII, 603 Seiten. 1971
Geb. DM 440,—; US $ 193.60
Subskriptionspreis:
Geb. DM 352,—; US $ 154.90
ISBN 3-540-05379-4

2. Teil: Neurovegetative Regulationen
159 Abbildungen, VIII, 475 Seiten. 1966
Geb. DM 380,—; US $ 167.20
Subskriptionspreis:
Geb. DM 309,—; US $ 136.00
ISBN 3-540-03529-X

9. Band:
Erbgefüge
264 Abbildungen, XIV, 744 Seiten. 1974
Geb. DM 398,—; US $ 175.20
Subskriptionspreis:
Geb. DM 318,40; US $ 140.10
ISBN 3-540-06581-4

10. Band:
Umwelt I
1. Teil: Strahlung und Wetter
283 Abbildungen, X, 434 Seiten. 1960
Geb. DM 290,—; US $ 127.60
Subskriptionspreis:
Geb. DM 232,—; US $ 102.10
ISBN 3-540-02532-4

11. Band:
Umwelt II
1. Teil: Ernährung
173 Abbildungen, XII, 1202 Seiten. 1962
Geb. DM 580,—; US $ 255.20
Subskriptionspreis:
Geb. DM 464,—; US $ 204.20
ISBN 3-540-02829-3

2. Teil: Belebte Umweltfaktoren
173 Abbildungen, XII, 845 Seiten. 1965
Geb. DM 540,—; US $ 237.60
Subskriptionspreis:
Geb. DM 432,—; US $ 190.10
ISBN 3-540-03304-1

Subskriptionspreise gelten bei Verpflichtung zur Abnahme des gesamten Handbuches bis zum Erscheinen des letzten Bandes.

The subscription price is applicable on orders for the complete set of published and unpublished volumes.